The HLA Complex
in Biology and Medicine

The HLA Complex in Biology and Medicine
A Resource Book

Editor
Narinder K Mehra
Professor and Head
Department of Transplant Immunology and Immunogenetics
All India Institute of Medical Sciences, Ansari Nagar
New Delhi, India

Assistant Editor
Gurvinder Kaur
Senior Scientist
Department of Transplant Immunology and Immunogenetics
All India Institute of Medical Sciences, Ansari Nagar
New Delhi, India

Advisory Editors
James McCluskey
Professor, Department of Microbiology and Immunology
Faculty of Medicine Dentistry and Health Sciences
The University of Melbourne, Parkville, Victoria, Australia

Frank T Christiansen
Department of Clinical Immunology and Immunogenetics
PathWest, Royal Perth Hospital and School of Pathology and Laboratory Medicine
University of Western Australia, Australia

Frans HJ Claas
Director, Eurotransplant Reference
Professor, Leiden University Medical Center
Department of Immunohematology and Blood Transfusion
Leiden, The Netherlands

Foreword
Peter C Doherty

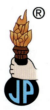

JAYPEE BROTHERS MEDICAL PUBLISHERS (P) LTD

New Delhi • St Louis (USA) • Panama City (Panama) • London (UK) • Ahmedabad
Bengaluru • Chennai • Hyderabad • Kochi • Kolkata • Lucknow • Mumbai • Nagpur

Published by
Jitendar P Vij
Jaypee Brothers Medical Publishers (P) Ltd

Corporate Office
4838/24 Ansari Road, Daryaganj, **New Delhi** - 110002, India, Phone: +91-11-43574357, Fax: +91-11-43574314

Registered Office
B-3 EMCA House, 23/23B Ansari Road, Daryaganj, **New Delhi** - 110 002, India
Phones: +91-11-23272143, +91-11-23272703, +91-11-23282021
+91-11-23245672, Rel: +91-11-32558559, Fax: +91-11-23276490, +91-11-23245683
e-mail: jaypee@jaypeebrothers.com, Website: www.jaypeebrothers.com

Offices in India

- **Ahmedabad,** Phone: Rel: +91-79-32988717, e-mail: ahmedabad@jaypeebrothers.com
- **Bengaluru,** Phone: Rel: +91-80-32714073, e-mail: bangalore@jaypeebrothers.com
- **Chennai,** Phone: Rel: +91-44-32972089, e-mail: chennai@jaypeebrothers.com
- **Hyderabad,** Phone: Rel:+91-40-32940929, e-mail: hyderabad@jaypeebrothers.com
- **Kochi,** Phone: +91-484-2395740, e-mail: kochi@jaypeebrothers.com
- **Kolkata,** Phone: +91-33-22276415, e-mail: kolkata@jaypeebrothers.com
- **Lucknow,** Phone: +91-522-3040554, e-mail: lucknow@jaypeebrothers.com
- **Mumbai,** Phone: Rel: +91-22-32926896, e-mail: mumbai@jaypeebrothers.com
- **Nagpur,** Phone: Rel: +91-712-3245220, e-mail: nagpur@jaypeebrothers.com

Overseas Offices

- **North America Office, USA,** Ph: 001-636-6279734
  e-mail: jaypee@jaypeebrothers.com, anjulav@jaypeebrothers.com
- **Central America Office, Panama City, Panama,** Ph: 001-507-317-0160
  e-mail: cservice@jphmedical.com
  Website: www.jphmedical.com
- **Europe Office, UK,** Ph: +44 (0) 2031708910, e-mail: info@jpmedpub.com

The HLA Complex in Biology and Medicine: A Resource Book

© 2010, Jaypee Brothers Medical Publishers (P) Ltd.

All rights reserved. No part of this publication should be reproduced, stored in a retrieval system, or transmitted in any form or by any means: electronic, mechanical, photocopying, recording, or otherwise, without the prior written permission of the editors and the publisher.

> This book has been published in good faith that the material provided by contributors is original. Every effort is made to ensure accuracy of material, but the publisher, printer and editors will not be held responsible for any inadvertent error (s). In case of any dispute, all legal matters are to be settled under Delhi jurisdiction only.

First Edition: **2010**

ISBN 978-81-8448-870-8

Typeset at JPBMP typesetting unit
Printed at Replika Press Pvt. Ltd.

To
The pioneers who discovered
the Major Histocompatibility complex
and its diverse applications
in Medicine and Biology.

Contributors

Ágnes Szilágyi
Research Fellow
Inflammation Biology and
Immunogenomics
Research Group Hungarian Academy
of Sciences – Semmelweis University
Nagyvárad tér 4
H-1089, Budapest, Hungary
Email: szilagi@kut.sote.hu

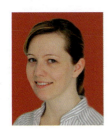

Akinori Kimura
Professor
Department of Molecular Pathogenesis
Medical Research Institute
Tokyo Medical and Dental University
Tokyo, Japan
Email: akitis@mri.tmd.ac.jp

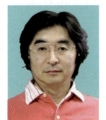

Amit Awasthi
Research Fellow
Center for Neurologic Diseases
Brigham and Womens Hospital
Harvard Medical School
Boston, MA USA
Email: aawasthi@rics.bwh.harvard.edu

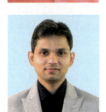

Antonio Arnaiz-Villena
Department of Immunology
University Complutense
The Madrid Regional Blood Center
Madrid, Spain
E-mail: aarnaiz@med.ucm.es;
URL: http://chopo.pntic.mec.es/biolmol

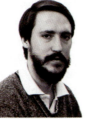

Brian D Tait
Victorian Transplantation and
Immunogenetic Service
Australian Red Cross Blood Service
2nd Floor Rotary Bone Marrow
Research Building
c/o Royal Melbourne Hospital
Parkville, Victoria, Australia
Email: tait@wehi.edu.au

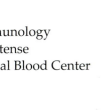

Campbell Stewart Witt
Department of Clinical Immunology
and Immunogenetics
PathWest, Royal Perth Hospital
Perth, Western Australia
Email: campbell.witt@health.wa.gov.au

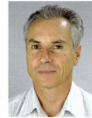

Carlos Parga-Lozano
Department of Immunology
University Complutense
The Madrid Regional Blood Center
Madrid, Spain

D Middleton
Royal Liverpool University Hospital
and School of Infection
and Host Defence
University of Liverpool
Liverpool, L7 8XW
United Kingdom
Email: derek.middleton@rlbuht.nhs.uk

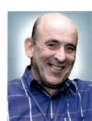

David Charles Sayer
Director
Conexio Genomics
8/31 Pakenham St
Fremantle, Western Australia
Email: david@conexio-genomics.com

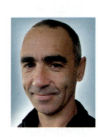

Diego Rey
Department of Immunology
University Complutense
The Madrid Regional Blood Center
Madrid, Spain

Elaine F Reed
Professor of Pathology
Director UCLA Immunogenetics Center
Department of Pathology
David Geffen School of Medicine
at the University of California
Los Angeles, California, USA
Email: ereed@mednet.ucla.edu

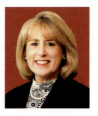

Elham Ashouri
Visiting Research Affiliate
UCLA Immunogenetics Center
Department of Pathology and
Laboratory Medicine
David Geffen School of Medicine
at UCLA
University of California at Los Angeles
Los Angeles, California, USA
Email: eliashouri@hotmail.com

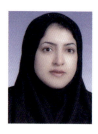

Elizabeth J Phillips
Departments of Clinical Immunology
and Immunogenetics
Royal Perth Hospital
Department of Clinical Immunology
and Infectious Diseases
Sir Charles Gairdner Hospital
Centre for Clinical Pharmacology
and Infectious Diseases
Institute for Immunology and Infectious
Diseases, Murdoch University
Perth, Western Australia
Email: e.phillips@iiid.com.au

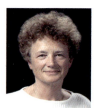

Els Goulmy
Professor
Leiden University Medical Center
Department of Immunohematology
and Blood Transfusion
PO Box 9600, 2300 RC Leiden
The Netherlands
Email: e.a.j.m.goulmy@lumc.nl

Enrique Moreno
Department of Liver Transplant and
Abdominal Surgery
Hospital 12 de Octubre, Madrid
Spain

Eric Spierings
Department of Immunology, F03.821
University Medical Center Utrecht
Postbox 85500
3508 GA, Utrecht, The Netherlands
Email: e.spierings@umcutrecht.nl

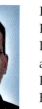

Erik Thorsby
Professor
Institute of Immunology
Rikshospitalet University Hospital
and University of Oslo
0027 Oslo, Norway
Email: erik.thorsby@medisin.uio.no

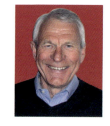

Erwin Schurr
James McGill Professor of Medicine
and Human Genetics
The Research Institute of the
McGIll University
Health Center
Departments of Medicine
Human Genetics and Biochemistry
McGill University, Montreal Quebec
Canada
Email: erwin.schurr@mcgill.ca

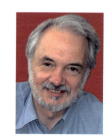

F Gonzalez
Professor
Transplant Immunology
Royal Liverpool University Hospital
and School of Infection
and Host Defence
University of Liverpool
Liverpool, L7 8XW
United Kingdom

Frank T Christiansen
Department of Clinical Immunology
and Immunogenetics, PathWest
Royal Perth Hospital and School of
Pathology and Laboratory Medicine
University of Western Australia
Perth, Australia
Email: frank.christiansen@health.wa.gov.au

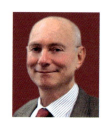

Frans HJ Claas
Professor
Leiden University Medical Center
Department of Immunohematology
and Blood Transfusion
Leiden, The Netherlands
Email: fhjclaas@lumc.nl

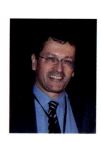

Contributors

George Füst
Research Professor
3rd Department of Internal Medicine
Semmelweis University
BudapestKútvölgyi út 4
H—1125, Budapest, Hungary
Email: fustge@kut.sote.hu

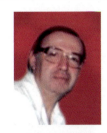

Grant Morahan
Director, Center for Diabetes Research
and Professor of Diabetes Research
The Western Australian Institute
for Medical Research and Center
for Medical Research
University of Western Australia
Email: gem@waimr.uwa.edu.au

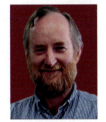

Gurvinder Kaur
Department of Transplant
Immunology and Immunogenetics
All India Institute of Medical Sciences
Ansari Nagar
New Delhi, India
Email: gurvinder@hotmail.com

Indranil Mukhopadhyay
Human Genetics Unit
Indian Statistical Institute
Kolkata, India

JA Madrigal
Director of Research and Professor of
Hematology
The Anthony Nolan Research Institute
Royal Free Hospital, Pond Street
Hampstead, London NW3 2QG
United Kingdom
Email: a.madrigal@medsch.ucl.ac.uk

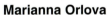

James McCluskey
Professor
Department of Microbiology and
Immunology
Faculty of Medicine Dentistry and
Health Sciences
The University of Melbourne, Parkville
Victoria, Australia
Email: jamesm1@unimelb.edu.au

Jamie Rossjohn
Professor
Australian Research Council
Federation Fellow
Department of Biochemistry and
Molecular Biology
School of Biomedical Sciences
Monash University, Clayton, Victoria, Australia
Email: jamie.rossjohn@med.monash.edu.au

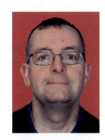

Lars Kjer-Nielsen
Department of Microbiology and
Immunology
Faculty of Medicine Dentistry
and Health Sciences
The University of Melbourne
Australia
Email: lkn@unimelb.edu.au

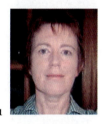

Linda Smith
Department of Clinical Immunology
and Immunogenetics
PathWest Laboratory Medicine
Royal Perth Hospital, Perth
Western Australia
Email: linda.k.smith@health.wa.gov.au

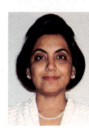

Mandvi Bharadwaj
Department of Microbiology
and Immunology
Faculty of Medicine Dentistry
and Health Sciences
The University of Melbourne
Parkville, Victoria, Australia
Email: mandvi@unimelb.edu.au

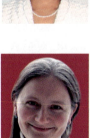

Marianna Orlova
Post-doctoral Fellow
McGill University
Department of Human Genetics
Center for the Study of Host Resistance
Cedar Avenue, Montreal
Quebec, H3G 1A4, Canada
Email: marianna.orlova@mail.mcgill.ca

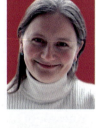

Mary Carrington
Laboratory of Experimental
Immunology
Cancer and Inflammation Program
National Cancer Institute
Frederick, USA

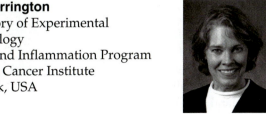

Márton Doleschall
Research Fellow
Inflammation Biology and
Immungenomics Research Group
Hungarian Academy of Sciences –
Semmelweis University
Nagyvárad tér 4., H-1089, Budapest
Hungary
Email: doles@kut.sote.hu

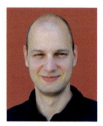

Mary E Atz
Graduate Student Researcher
PhD Candidate
Department of Pathology and
Laboratory Medicine
David Geffen School of Medicine
University of California
Los Angeles, CA USA

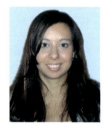

Maureen P Martin
Laboratory of Experimental
Immunology
Cancer and Inflammation Program
National Cancer Institute at Frederick
Frederick, MD USA

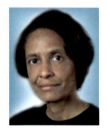

Michael Varney
The Western Australian Institute for
Medical Research and
Centre for Medical Research
University of Western Australia
MRF Building, Level 6, 50 Murray St
Perth, WA, Australia
Victorian Transplantation and
Immunogenetics Service
Australian Red Cross Blood Service
Parkville, Melbourne, Victoria, Australia
Email: mvarney@arcbs.redcross.org.au

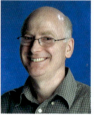

Muhammad Asim Khan
Professor of Medicine
Case Western Reserve University
School of Medicine
Cleveland, OH USA
MetroHealth Medical Center
Division of Rheumatology
2500 MetroHealth Drive
Cleveland OH, USA
Email: mkhan@metrohealth.org

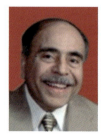

Narinder K Mehra
Professor and Head
Department of Transplant
Immunology
and Immunogenetics
All India Institute of Medical Sciences
Ansari Nagar, New Delhi
India
Email: narin98@hotmail.com

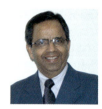

Neeraj Kumar
Department of Transplant
Immunology and Immunogenetics
All India Institute of Medical Sciences
Ansari Nagar
New Delhi, India
Email: neerajkaüms@hotmail.com

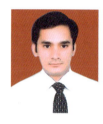

Partha P Majumder
Human Genetics Unit
Indian Statistical Institute
Kolkata, India
Email: ppm@isical.ac.in

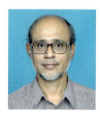

Pablo Gomez-Prieto
Department of Immunology
University Complutense
The Madrid Regional Blood Center
Madrid, Spain

Paras Singh
Department of Transplant
Immunology and Immunogenetics
All India Institute of Medical Sciences
Ansari Nagar
New Delhi, India

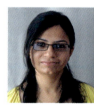

Philippa Saunders
Professor
Department of Microbiology and
Immunology
Faculty of Medicine Dentistry and
Health Sciences
The University of Melbourne, Parkville
Victoria, Australia

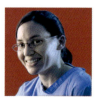

Prashant Sood
Department of Transplant Immunology
and Immunogenetics
All India Institute of Medical Sciences
New Delhi, India
Email: drprashantsood@gmail.com

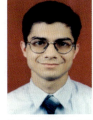

Raja Rajalingam
Assistant Clinical Professor
UCLA Immunogenetics Center
Department of Pathology and
Laboratory Medicine
David Geffen School of Medicine at UCLA
University of California at Los Angeles
Los Angeles California, USA
Email: rrajalingam@mednet.ucla.edu

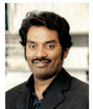

S Kanthi Mathi
Research Associate
Department of Molecular Genetics
Madras Diabetes Research Foundation
No:6B, Conran Smith Road
Gopalapuram
Chennai, India
Email: dr_kanthi@yahoo.co.in

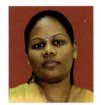

S Tulpule
Medical Officer, Anthony Nolan Trust
The Anthony Nolan Research Institute
Royal Free Hospital, Fleet Road
Hampstead, London NW3 2QG
United Kingdom
Email: satulpule@yahoo.co.uk

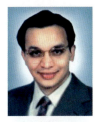

Samantha Fidler
Department of Clinical Immunology
and Immunogenetics, PathWest
Laboratory Medicine
Royal Perth Hospital, Perth
Western Australia
School of Pathology and Laboratory
Medicine
University of Western Australia, Perth
Western Australia
Email: samantha.fidler@health.wa.gov.au

Saurabh Ghosh
Human Genetics Unit
Indian Statistical Institute
Kolkata, India

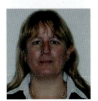

Simon Alexander Mallal
Professor
Royal Perth Hospital, Wellington St
Perth, Western Australia
Institute for Immunology and
Infectious Diseases
Murdoch University, Murdoch
Western Australia
Email: s.mallal@iiid.com.au

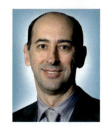

Sophie Caillat-Zucman
Associate Professor
Head of HLA Typing Laboratory
Institut National de la Santé et de la
Recherche Médicale (INSERM) U561
and Hôpital Necker; Université Paris
Descartes
Paris, France
Email: sophie.caillat@inserm.fr

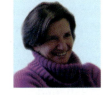

Stephanie Gras
Monash Univeristy
Australia
Email: stephanie.gras@med.monash.edu.au

Steven GE Marsh
Professor of Immunogenetics
Deputy Director of Research
Anthony Nolan Research Institute
and Cancer Institute
University College London
Royal Free Campus, London NW3 2QG
United Kingdom
Email: steven.marsh@ucl.ac.uk

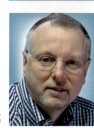

Sudhir Gupta
Division of Basic and Clinical
Immunology
University of California, Irvine
California Medical Sciences I, C-240
University of California, Irvine
CA USA
E-mail: sgupta@uci.edu

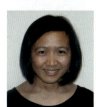

Sue Min Liu
Center for Neurologic Diseases
Brigham and Women's Hospital
Harvard Institutes of Medicine
Boston, MA USA
Email: sliu@rics.bwh.harvard.edu

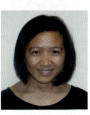

Suraksha Agrawal
Department of Medical Genetics
Sanjay Gandhi Postgraduate
Institute of Medical Sciences
Raebareli Road, Lucknow, UP
India
Email: suraksha@sgpgi.ac.in

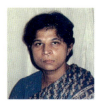

Veena Taneja
Assistant Professor
Department of Immunology
College of Medicine, Mayo
Ist Street SW, Rochester, USA
Email: taneja.veena@mayo.edu

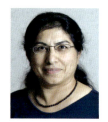

Toshiaki Nakajima
Laboratory of Genome Diversity
School of Biomedical Science, and
Department of Molecular Pathogenesis
Medical Research Institute
Tokyo Medical and Dental University
Tokyo, Japan
Email: tnakajima.tis@mri.tmd.ac.jp

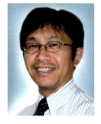

Vijay K Kuchroo
Samuel L Wasserstrom
Professor of Neurology
Harvard Medical School
Brigham and Women's Hospital
Boston, Massachusetts, USA
Email: vkuchroo@rics.bwh.harvard.edu

Uma Kanga
Senior Research Scientist
HLA Laboratory
Department of Transplant and
Immunogenetics
All India Institute of Medical Sciences
Ansari Nagar, New Delhi, India
Email: umakanga@hotmail.com

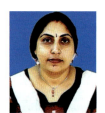

Whitney Macdonald
Department of Biochemistry and
Molecular Biology
School of Biomedical Sciences
Monash University
Clayton, Victoria, Australia
Email: macdonald.whitney@gmail.com

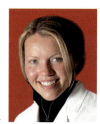

V Mohan
President and Chief of Diabetes
Research
Madras Diabetes Research Foundation
Chairman and Chief Diabetologist
Dr Mohan's Diabetes Specialities Center
No. 6B, Conran Smith Road
Gopalapuram, Chennai, India
Email: drmohans@vsnl.net (or) mvdsc@vsnl.com

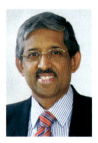

Xiaojiang Gao
Sr Scientist
Laboratory of Experimental
Immunology
Cancer and Inflammation Program
National Cancer Institute at Frederick
Frederick, MD USA
Email: gaoxia@mail.nih.gov

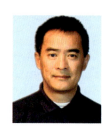

V Radha
Scientist and Head
Department of Molecular Genetics
Madras Diabetes Research Foundation
No 6B, Conran Smith Road
Gopalapuram, Chennai, India
Email: radharv@yahoo.co.in

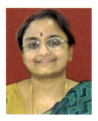

Foreword

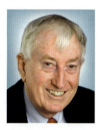

The major histocompatibility complex (MHC), characterized as HLA in humans and H-2 in the mouse, continues to be immensely fascinating in both biology and medicine. The focus of two Nobel prizes (in 1980 and 1996), the MHC specifies a variety of recognition elements and contains genes associated with a spectrum of disease susceptibility profiles. Different MHC-encoded molecules function as receptors for olfactory discrimination, mediate immune protective effects as secreted proteins like TNF and components of the complement cascade, and act as targets for both the "natural killer" immunoglobulin like receptors (KIRs) and the T cell receptors (TCRs) on helper and cytotoxic T lymphocytes.

Discovered more than 50 years back by those grappling with the issue of graft rejection, the MHC provides a classical example of a genetic region named for its first known function. Studies utilizing antibody typing, mixed lymphocyte reactions (MLRs) and genetic back-crossing (in the mouse) allowed identification of the strong transplantation antigens (class I MHC glycoproteins), then the so-called immune response (Ir) genes that were soon found to encode the MHC class II alleles. A further breakthrough came with the discovery that "self" MHCI and MHCII molecules serve primarily to target killer (CD8$^+$) and helper (CD4$^+$) and T lymphocytes to cells modified by an encounter with some "non-self" protein provided, perhaps, by an infecting virus or bacterium.

Then it was recognized that the primary role of the MHCI and MHCII molecules was to carry processed, non-self peptides to cell-surface for lymphocyte recognition via the cognate TCR, the primary event that triggers CD8$^+$ and CD4$^+$ T lymphocyte clonal expansion and differentiation. Some speculate that there may be a further Nobel prize for elucidating the nature of antigen processing and the key role of the antigen-presenting dendritic cell that triggers "adaptive" immunity. If we had the task of naming the MHC now we would, perhaps, choose to call it the "self-surveillance complex!"

When we also consider the more recent discovery of the KIR/MHC interaction, it is apparent that analysis related in some way or other to the MHC is central to at least half of contemporary immunology. While the analysis of the mouse H_2 and the human HLA systems may to some extent run in parallel, the two areas tend to be pursued by separate laboratories that operate in different contexts. The mouse immunologists generally focus on inbred strains that "fix" one or other MHC haplotype. Dealing as they must with a species that outbreeds, those working with HLA continue to be fascinated by questions related to the extraordinary MHC polymorphism and the association with disease susceptibility profiles.

There is thus a very real place for a new book that updates the field and deals specifically with issues related to "The HLA Complex in Biology and Medicine". Covering such a broad spectrum would be extraordinarily daunting for any one individual, so the editors have recruited a group of established investigators to summarize their own areas of expertise in a multi-author format. The result is a text that will be invaluable for introducing graduate students to the full spectrum of HLA-related knowledge while serving also as a conceptual and technical source book for both those focused on or other aspect of HLA-related research and clinical/surgical practice. In addition, it will be a primary point of contact for individuals working in other areas who suddenly find that their research is drawing them into the complexities of HLA genetics.

The focus is essentially on the immunological role of HLA and how that relates to infectious disease resistance, autoimmunity and graft and organ transplantation. The present text deals with more practical matters and does not attempt to cover areas of less immediate clinical relevance that may, nonetheless, have broad implications for understanding both mammalian biology and evolution. The latter would be more adequately addressed in a volume that goes beyond human beings and the other placentals to the non-eutherian mammals, birds, bony fish, the lampreys and so forth. Still, there is sufficient conceptual development here to intrigue those with active intellects and draw at least some into the broader implications of MHC genetics.

This book thus serves those who need to understand how the HLA system impacts on medicine while at the same time providing accounts of practical issues relevant to tissue typing, transplant immunology and clinical immunogenetics. As such, it constitutes an important resource for medical scientists, physicians and surgeons. Given the scope and the undoubted quality of the contributors, it will continue to fulfill those functions in the long-term.

Peter C Doherty
University of Melbourne
Australia

Preface

The postgenomics era has heralded a new beginning in our understanding of the molecular aspects of Clinical Immunology with a considerable impact on developing new perspectives in the field of transplantation and understanding the way disease develops. In this context, the HLA system offers an excellent mini genome model leading to even greater interest in this subject than ever before. The system is a part of the Major Histocompatibility Complex (MHC) that exists in almost all animal species and has been investigated most extensively in the mouse in which it is referred to as the H-2 system. Human MHC research has revealed HLA to be the most polymorphic genetic system in the mammalian genome, with binding of non-self peptides and presenting them for immune inspection as its major function. Its unique gene diversity parallels the need for diverse peptide sites within the MHC to combat a fast evolving range of pathogens.

Although the foundations of genomics and immune recognition were laid in the 20th century, the major focus over the next two decades will be in the area of pharmacogenomics, clinical immunogenetics and personalized molecular medicine. The task of screening for potentially thousands of variations in the global population now appears achievable through advanced chip based and mass spectrometric approaches, with the primary focus on single nucleotide polymorphisms (SNPs) that represent point variations between individuals. The HLA-related knowledge coupled with in-depth understanding of the immune mechanisms is the key for achieving tolerance and long-term success in organ and hematopoietic stem cell transplantation.

The HLA system in man was discovered more than 50 years ago, primarily because of the urge to decipher the mechanism of graft rejection. Soon, it became clear that the set of genes within the complex have far more important functions, associated with the overall survival of the species. We decided to compile and produce a comprehensive resource book on the HLA system with particular reference to its role in medicine and biology. The book is planned on the format of a 'multi-author edited book' carrying detailed and comprehensive information on almost all aspects of the human MHC including its role in immune response, population diversity, organ and bone marrow transplantation and finally as an efficient biomarker for disease. The publication is meant for postgraduate level students and young researchers seeking authentic information on the above aspects. Indeed, a need for such a publication has been felt for a long time and our endeavor has been to provide the reader with updated information on this rapidly growing subject. For this, we recruited a group of established investigators to cover a wide range of topics.

The publication has been aptly entitled *The HLA Complex in Medicine and Biology: A resource Book* with four major sections dealing with immune system in general including the cytokine cascade, general features of the human MHC, including population database and nonclassical HLA molecules, MHC and disease associations and a major section dealing with the transplantation issues. Special chapters deal with the History of HLA and its latest nomenclature as we know of in 2009, as well as the biological significance of minor histocompatibility antigens. Similarly, the book carries a detailed description of the killer immunoglobulin-like receptors (KIRs) in health, disease and transplantation. Special emphasis has been given to the section on HLA and disease associations covering particularly the autoimmune, mycobacterial and rheumatological diseases. Separate chapters deal with host determinants in HIV-1 infection and involvement of HLA in drug sensitivity. Similarly, the section on transplantation deals not only with HLA matching strategies for long-term graft survival, but more importantly for antibody analysis, cross-matching and post-transplant antibody monitoring. The book has been designed to introduce the young doctor and researcher to comprehend the role of HLA in hematopoietic stem cell transplantation and the importance of unrelated donor marrow registries.

Many individuals have made invaluable contributions to this rather daunting task. The list of contributors in extensive but we will like to place in record our special thanks to Erik Thorsby, Brian Tait, Steve Marsh, Derek

Middleton, Antonio Araniz-Villena, Grant Morahan, Mohammed Khan, Veena Taneja, Akinori Kimura, Erwin Schurr, Xiajiang Gao, Sudhir Gupta, Elaine Reed, Els Goulmy, Alejandro Madrigal, Partha Majumdar, Simon and Elizabeth Mallal, Sophie Calliat Zucman, Vijay Kuchroo and Campbell Witt. Our special thanks are due to the excellent team of publishers M/s Jaypee Brothers Medical Publishers (P) Ltd, New Delhi, India who have put in a lot of effort to produce a truly international product.

Lastly, we must state that the inspiration for compiling such a resource book came truly from our numerous students and young researchers grappling with defining the mysteries of human MHC. In the words of Peter C Doherty, who discovered the phenomenon of MHC Restriction together with Rolf Zinkernagel way back in the mid-70s, which won them the Nobel prize in 1996, *"If we had the task of naming the MHC now we would, perhaps, choose to call it the 'Self-surveillance complex !'"*. The editors are ever grateful to Peter for writing the Foreword of the book. We do hope that the publication will provide the transplant physicians, surgeons, internists and biologists with a clear understanding of the biological meaning of the HLA system and encourage them to decipher its translational role in medicine, and discover its hitherto unmet and unknown aspects.

Narinder K Mehra
Gurvinder Kaur
James McCluskey
Frank T Christiansen
Frans HJ Claas

Acknowledgments

The compilation of this resource book has indeed been a milestone in my journey to science, inspired greatly by the remarkable discoveries made by the great pioneers of MHC and HLA biology. Credit for this book rightly goes to my mentors, who introduced me to the legacy of this science, encouraged me at every step as I grew and matured in this field. I feel equally fortunate to have worked with a wonderful bunch of students and associates, whose inquisitive questions and significant contributions expanded my perspectives. I bless them with success and bounty of knowledge, that they may do further good science and contribute towards the welfare of humanity.

It has been a wonderful experience building this book. I thank Gurvinder Kaur, who has been an able and indispensible colleague over the years for shouldering a lot of responsibilities to make this project a success. My sincere gratitude to the team of Advisory Editors comprising of Frank C Christiansen, Frans HJ Claas and James McCluskey with whom I have journeyed wonderful years, exploring and learning MHC science, and whose invaluable advice throughout this project helped us develop this unique compendium of appropriate topics and chapters contributed by the very best in this field. Peter C Doherty who won the Nobel prize together with Rolf Zinkernagel in 1996 for defining the biological meaning of the major histocompatibility complex has been gracious in contributing the Foreword for the book. The Editors are ever grateful to him for the same.

My special thanks are to the large number of contributors who readily agreed to our request, despite short notice. Their contributions reflect knowledge, wisdom and lifetime experience. We truly believe that this book will prove immensely useful to students, researchers, teachers and clinicians from various walks of Medicine and Biology. I express my sincere appreciation to Akinori Kimura, Alejandro Madrigal, Antonio Arnaiz-Villena, Brian Tait, Campbell Witt, David Sayer, Derek Middleton, Elaine Reed, Els Goulmy, Erik Thorsby, Erwin Schurr, Frans HJ Claas, Frank C Christiansen, Grant Morahan, Gurvinder Kaur, Simon Mallal, Elizabeth Phillips, Linda Smith, Michael Varney, Sudhir Gupta, Sophie Caillat-Zucman, James McCluskey, Partha Majumder, Suraksha Agrawal, Steven Marsh, Mohammed Asim Khan, Neeraj Kumar, Raja Rajalingam, George Fust, Uma Kanga, Veena Taneja, Vijay Kuchroo, V Mohan, Xiaojiang Gao and their associates for providing their invaluable inputs and for sticking to the time schedule.

This book and indeed every milestone in my career would not have been possible without the active support of my wife, Raj. She and our two children Nikhil and Neha cheerfully accepted my follies and encouraged me to pursue my research and academic activities with vigor and sincerity. Further, the constant support and academic ambience provided by the All India Institute of Medical Sciences (AIIMS), Ansari Nagar, New Delhi, India has been extremely rewarding.

Finally, our appreciation to Shri Jitendar P Vij (Chairman and Managing Director), Mr Tarun Duneja (Director-Publishing) and members of the publishing team, in particular Mr KK Raman (Production Manager) of M/s Jaypee Brothers Medical Publishers (P) Ltd, New Delhi, India who worked continuously for completing this gigantic task in time for release at the ASEATTA 2009 meeting in New Delhi. We do hope that this unique work brought together by some of the most eminent minds in MHC biology will go a long way in encouraging young minds to this fascinating field of science.

Narinder K Mehra

Contents

Section 1: Introduction to Immune System

1. Immune System—A Primer 3
   Sudhir Gupta

2. Cytokines and T Cell Subsets 19
   Amit Awasthi, Sue Min Liu, Vijay K Kuchroo

3. History of HLA 42
   Erik Thorsby

Section 2: Major Histocompatibility Complex

4. Genetic Structure and Functions of the Major Histocompatibility Complex 61
   Brian D Tait

5. HLA Nomenclature 79
   Steven GE Marsh

6. HLA Molecules of the Major Histocompatibility Complex 86
   James McCluskey, Stephanie Gras, Mandvi Bharadwaj, Lars Kjer-Nielsen,
   Whitney Macdonald, Philippa Saunders, Jamie Rossjohn

7. Immunogenetic Databases 119
   D Middleton, F Gonzalez

8. Complement Genes in the Central Region of the MHC 135
   Ágnes Szilágyi, Márton Doleschall, George Füst

9. HLA-G, -F and -E: Polymorphism, Function and Evolution 159
   Pablo Gomez-Prieto, Carlos Parga-Lozano, Diego Rey, Enrique Moreno, Antonio Arnaiz-Villena

10. HLA Typing Technologies 175
    Linda Smith, Samantha Fidler

11. Computer Programs for the Development of SBT for HLA 188
    David Charles Sayer

Section 3: MHC and Disease

12. The Genetics of Type 1 Diabetes 205
    Grant Morahan, Michael Varney

13. Genetic Determinants of Type 1 Diabetes—Immune Response Genes 219
    Neeraj Kumar, Gurvinder Kaur, Narinder K Mehra

14. Genetics of Type 2 Diabetes 241
    V Radha, S Kanthi Mathi, V Mohan

15. Immunogenetic Mechanisms of Celiac Disease 254
    Sophie Caillat-Zucman

16. HLA and Spondyloarthropathies 259
    Muhammad Asim Khan

17. Immunogenetics of Rheumatoid Arthritis 276
    Veena Taneja

18. HLA Architecture of HIV Disease Pathogenesis 292
    Xiaojiang Gao, Maureen P Martin, Mary Carrington

19. Host Genetics of HIV-1/AIDS Infection 305
    Gurvinder Kaur, Narinder K Mehra

20. HLA and Drug Reactions 332
    Elizabeth J Phillips, Simon Alexander Mallal

21. Comparative Genomics: Insight into Human Health and Disease 350
    Toshiaki Nakajima, Akinori Kimura

22. Genetic Architecture of Mycobacterial Diseases 365
    Marianna Orlova, Erwin Schurr

23. MHC and Non-MHC Genes in Tuberculosis and Leprosy 386
    Narinder K Mehra, Paras Singh, Prashant Sood, Gurvinder Kaur

24. Killer Cell Immunoglobulin-like Receptors in Health and Disease 406
    Raja Rajalingam, Elham Ashouri

25. Role of Non-classical HLA Antigens in Pregnancy 424
    Suraksha Agrawal, Prashant Sood, Narinder K Mehra

Section 4: MHC and Transplantation

26. Donors Selection Strategies for Hematopoietic Stem Cell Transplantation 449
    Uma Kanga, Narinder K Mehra

27. Allorecognition 465
    Frans HJ Claas

28. The Role of HLA Typing in Hematopoietic Stem Cell Transplantation 471
    Frank T Christiansen

29. The Role of HLA Matching and Recipient Sensitization in Organ Allograft Outcome 491
    Brian D Tait

30. Organ Transplantation: Post-transplant Antibody Monitoring and Associated Mechanisms 510
    Mary E Atz, Elaine F Reed

31. The Influence of NK Cell Alloreactivity on Hematopoietic Stem Cell Transplantation 525
    Campbell Stewart Witt

32. Minor Histocompatibility Antigens in Biology and Medicine 544
    Eric Spierings, Els Goulmy

33. Unrelated Marrow Donor Registries 555
    S Tulpule, JA Madrigal

34. An Overview of Statistical Methods for Disease Gene Mapping Using Data on Related
    and Unrelated Individuals 566
    Indranil Mukhopadhyay, Saurabh Ghosh, Partha P Majumder

Index 577

Section 1

Introduction to Immune System

Chapter 1

Immune System—A Primer

Sudhir Gupta

INTRODUCTION

The immune system has evolved primarily to protect the host from microbes, which is achieved by its unique property to discriminate between *self* and *nonself*. This property of the immune system is also critical in transplantation biology, and appears to play a significant role in immune surveillance against tumor cells. Important functional elements of the immune system include central (thymus and bone marrow) and peripheral or secondary lymphoid tissues (lymph nodes, Peyers' patches in the gut, bronchial-associated lymphoid tissue, spleen), several cell types, serum proteins, and small peptides including chemokines, cytokines, and hematopoietic growth factors. Though the components of the immune system interact with each other immunity is broadly categorized into innate immunity and adaptive immunity.

Phylogenetically, the innate immunity is more primitive than adaptive immunity; innate immune response is the earliest immune response to an antigen and sets the stage and is instrumental in the development and shaping of a relatively delayed adaptive immune response. In vertebrates, discrimination between *self* and *nonself* is the property of the adaptive immunity; however, in invertebrates cells of the innate immune system use primitive receptors to distinguish between *self* and *nonself*. What distinguishes between an innate immune response and an adaptive immune response are immunological memory and immunological specificity, which are the characteristics of an adaptive immune response. However, recent evidence has been presented to argue that natural killer cells (a component of innate immunity) may also have a short-term memory but lack a 'true' recall response (rapid and amplified response).

The innate immune responses are mediated by several cell types (professional phagocytes neutrophils, professional antigen presenting cells macrophages and dendritic cells, natural killer [NK] cells), and serum proteins (complement). The adaptive immune responses are mediated by T and B lymphocytes. The majority of cytokines and chemokines are produced by cells of both innate and adaptive immune systems.

INNATE IMMUNITY

One of the major functions of the cells of the innate immune system (macrophages and dendritic cells) is to capture an antigen, process it, and present (antigen processing and presentation) to T cells in context of major histocompatibility complex (MHC), therefore, providing a bridge or link between innate immunity and adaptive immunity. Dendritic cells are critical in the priming of naïve T cells for an immune response, whereas macrophages amplify adaptive immune response of primed naïve T cells. Natural Killer cells play a major role in defense against viruses and certain tumor cells. Other cells of the innate immunity are comprised of professional phagocytes neutrophils, and eosinophils, mast cells, and basophils; however, in this review we will discuss in detail a role of antigen presenting cells (macrophages and dendritic cells) and NK cells in immune responses.

Macrophages

Macrophages are derived by differentiation from circulating monocytes and reside in a variety of tissues (lymph nodes, spleen, liver, lung, brain, peritoneum). Unlike T and B cells they do not have antigen-specific receptors, their important function is to take up antigens, process them by denaturation or partial digestion, and present them on their surface to specific effector T cells. Macrophages express on their surface MHC class I and MHC class II molecules. Macrophages express low levels of MHC class II antigens, which is upregulated by IFN-γ. Macrophages present cytosolic proteins (mostly synthesized inside the cells, and small peptides are generated by cytosolic proteasome), in context of MHC class I antigen and activate cytotoxic CD8+ T cells, whereas endosomal/lysosomal proteins (mostly internalized from extracellular environment, and broken down in slam peptides by lysosomal and endosomal proteases) are presented in context of MHC class II antigen resulting in the activation of CD4+ T cells. Macrophages by virtue of expression of IgGFc receptor, also participate in antibody-dependent cellular cytotoxicity (ADCC). Macrophages are also a factory for the production of a large number of proinflammatory molecules.

Dendritic Cells

Dendritic cells (DCs) were discovered in 1973 by Ralph Steinman and Zanvil Cohen at the Rockefeller University, and were named because of their most striking feature of long cytoplasmic processes. It took several years before their role as "accessory cells" was established. Dendritic cells are derived from hematopoietic stem cells in the bone marrow and following their release from the bone marrow they undergo various stages of differentiation. There are two major subtypes of DCs, the classical DCs (cDCs) and plasmacytoid DCs (pDCs). Monocyte-derived cDCs (mDCs) are long-lived and reside in an immature state in most tissues, where they recognize and uptake various pathogens and other antigens. In addition to peripheral lymphoid tissues cDCs are also present as interdigitating cells of the thymus, and Langerhans cells in the skin. In their immature stage, cDCs are efficient in phagocytosis and induce tolerance. However, upon phagocytosis/uptake of antigens, DCs undergo steps of differentiation and maturation resulting in the induction/upregulation of several cell surface antigens (MHC class II, CD40, CD80, CD86, CCR7) and secretion of a number of cytokines including IL-12, IL-10, and TNF-α. In contrast to immature DCs, mature DCs are poor in phagocytosis; however, they prime naïve antigen-specific T cells to initiate T cell-mediated responses. Immature cDCs in resting tissues, especially at the portal of entry allow them to sample various pathogens and respond to them as well as to danger signals from self antigens via a group of receptors, the toll-like receptors (TLRs). TLRs recognize pathogen-associated molecular patterns (PAMPs), such as viral and bacterial nucleic acids, and repetitive elements within the envelope of viral and bacterial walls. There are 10 human TLR family members (12 in mice) each with distinct ligand and functional properties. TLRs are grouped into extracellular (TLR1, TLR2, TLR4, TLR5, and TLR6), which recognize microbial components of the cell wall from bacteria and fungi, and endosomal TLRs (TLR3, TLR7, TLR8, and TLR9), which recognize bacterial and viral nucleic acid. When DCs encounter microbes or PAMPs, TLR activation initiates the signal transduction pathway that culminates in the activation of NF-κB, interferon regulatory factors (IRFs), and other transcription factors, and production and secretion of cytokines, chemokines, and other biologically active molecules, therefore, contributing to innate immune response.

In addition to innate immune responses, TLRs-activation facilitates cDCs to orchestrate adaptive immune responses via three critical steps: capture of antigen; migration from tissues to T cell areas of lymphoid tissues (primarily lymph nodes and spleen), and presentation of internalized antigen on MHC molecules to naïve T cells. Classical DCs in concert with other cytokines induce differentiation of naïve CD4+ T cells to Th1, Th2, Th17, and Treg (Fig. 1.1). This is important to emphasize that the requirement of cytokines to differentiate naïve CD4+ T cells to Th17 cells in human and mice are significantly different.

Recently, it has been reported that IL-12 secreted by activated human DCs regulate antibody/immunoglobulin production via developing IL-21-producing T follicular helper (Tfh)-like cells and inducing IL-21 secretion by memory CD4+ T cells. Schmitt and colleague demonstrated that activated human DCs induce naïve CD4+ T cells to become IL-21 secreting T Tfh-like cells through IL-12. CD4+ T cells primed with IL-12 induce B cells to produce immunoglobulins, which is dependent upon IL-21 and inducible costimulator (ICOS). IL-12 induces two different IL-21 producing CD4+ T cells: IL-21+IFN-γ+ Tbet+ Th1 cells, and IL-21+IFN-γ-Tbet- non-Th1 cells, which is dependent upon signal induced and activator of transcription 4 (STAT4). IL-12 also regulates IL-21 secretion by memory CD4+ T cells. These observations clearly highlight the differences in the developmental pathways of Tfh cells between mice and humans.

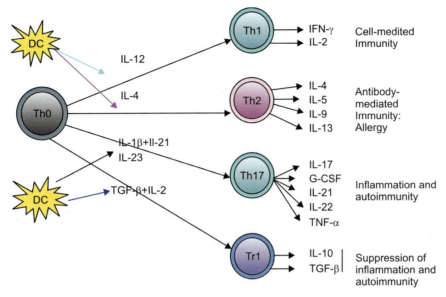

Fig. 1.1: Role of dendritic cells (DC) and different cytokines in the differentiation of naïve CD4+ T cells (Th0) to Th1, Th2, Th17, and Treg (Tr1)

Natural Killer Cells

Natural killer cells are large granular lymphocytes, which lack both classical T and B cell markers, including antigen-specific TCR, kill virus- infected cells, and cells that have lost MHC class I expression. They express CD56, CD57, CD16 (CD2)antigens. The principal physiological role is in defense infection by viruses and other intracellular microbes. NK cells kill various target cells without a need of additional activation (cf CD8+ T cells need to be activated before differentiating into effector CTL). Membrane proteins (CD2, 2B4, CD11a-CD18 and CD69) can induce or modulate NK activity. NK cells develop from hematopoietic cells (HSC) following interaction with Flt3 ligand and in the presence of IL-15 through a series of differentiation steps, express both stimulatory and inhibitory receptors, and perform effector functions, including natural cytotoxicity, antibody-dependent cell-mediated cytotoxicity (ADCC), and cytokine production (Fig. 1.2).

NK cells appear early during gestation and are present in normal numbers by mid to late gestation. Approximately 50 percent are immature (CD56) and have decreased cytotoxicity. Cytotoxicity of mature (CD56+) neonatal NK cells is similar to that of adults, and full function is achieved by one year of age. Neonatal NK cells also respond to IL-2 and IFNs, similar to adults. Cytokines produced by NK cells include IL-12, IL-23, IL-15, and IFNγ. Cytokines regulating functions of NK

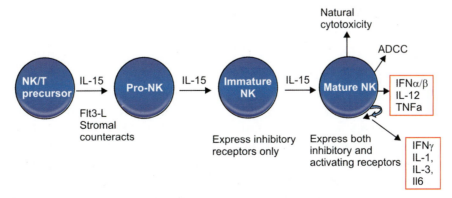

Fig. 1.2: Model of NK cell development. Hematopoietic cells (HSC) following interaction with Flt3 ligand and in the presence of IL-15 undergo a series of differentiation steps to develop into mature NK cells to express both stimulatory and inhibitory receptors, and perform effector functions, including natural cytotoxicity, antibody-dependent cell-mediated cytotoxicity (ADCC), and cytokine production

cells include IL-2, IFN-α, IFN-β, IFN-γ, and IL-12. NK cell activation is regulated by a balance between signals that are generated from two opposite types of receptors, inhibitory receptors and stimulatory receptors. The susceptibility of tumor cells to NK cell killing is inversely related to MHC class I expression ("missing-self" hypothesis). This hypothesis proposes that NK cells survey tissue for MHC class I expression. In the absence of MHC class I, NK cells are released from the negative influence of MHC class I molecules and kill the target. This "missing self" is due to an NK-cell inhibitory receptor specific for MHC class I molecules. These include NKG2-CD94 and human killer cell immunoglobulin receptors (KIRs). KIR will be discussed in detail in another chapter in this book.

More recently NK cells have been assigned a novel function of a critical role in shaping both innate and adaptive immune response via interaction with mDCs. This novel function of NK cells is essentially mediated through the aggression of normal immature mDCs. Only mDCs undergoing optimal maturation become refractory to NK cell cytotoxicity and are able to prime Th1 cells following migration to lymph nodes.

NK Receptors

Most inhibitory and activating NK receptors are encoded by genes in two genomic regions, the NK-gene complex (NKC) and the leukocyte receptor complex (LRC). Molecules encoded in the LRC belong to Ig superfamily, NKC-encodes many molecules that are important for NK-cell activities. NKC-encoded molecules have type II transmembrane protein orientation, share sequence homology with C-type lectins and are expressed as disulphide-linked dimers. Human NKG2-CD94 heterodimers are located in a locus on chromosome 12p13, and most of these genes are conserved across species.

Inhibitory Receptors

In general, the effects of inhibitory receptors dominate over activation receptors. Inhibitory receptors mediate their effects through an immunoreceptor tyrosine-based inhibitory motif (ITIM) in their cytoplasmic tail. Following ligand binding, ITIM becomes tyrosine phosphorylated by an SRC-family tyrosine kinase, which then recruits and activates SH-2 domain-containing tyrosine phosphatase-1 (SHIP-1) and possibly SHIP-2. Activated SHIP-1 inhibits NK functions by dephosphorylation of protein tyrosine kinase (PTK). There are three types of inhibitory receptors on NK cells. Killer Ig-like receptors (KIR), which recognize different alleles of HLA-1,-B, and –C molecules. Binding of HLA molecules to KIR has very fast on- and off- rates, which would be consistent with the ability of NK cells to rapidly "test" for the presence of MHC expression on many cells in a very short-time. Receptors containing Ig-like transcripts (ILTs): ILT2 has broad specificity for many MHC alleles and contain 4 ITIAMs. CMV encodes a molecule UL18, that is homologous to MHC class I, and that can bind to ILT-2 (decoy mechanism to protect it from NK killing. Heterodimer of C-type lectinNKG2A/B covalently bound to CD94. NKG2A/B has two ITIM. This heterodimer binds to HLA-E (non-classsical MHC). Since stable expression of HLA-E depends upon signal peptides derived from HLA-A,-B,-C, or-G, CD94/NKG2A performs surveillance function for the absence of HLA-E, classical MHC class I, and HLA-G molecules.

Activation Receptors

Many NK cell activation receptors have extracellular domains that are similar to those of inhibitory receptors but lack intracellular ITIM. Instead, they generally have charged transmembrane residues that facilitate association with signaling chains that are often required for optimal surface expression. Signaling chains on NK cells include, ITAM containing molecules, DNAX-activating protein of 12 kDa (DAP12), Killer activating receptor associated protein (KARAP), and CD3ξ receptor.

NKG2 Family Receptors

NKG2 Family and CD94: Similar to murine Ly49 and Nkrp1 families, the NKG2 family contains members with activating and inhibitory functions. However, NKG2 molecules must dimerize with the invariant CD94 molecule for the expression of NKG2 on the cell surface and function. CD94 has a short cytoplasmic domain with no apparent functional motifs. The inhibitory NKG2A has two immunoreceptor tyrosine-based inhibitory motifs (ITIMs) in its intracytoplasmic tail and can be alternately spliced to generate NKG2B. When NKG2C, E, or H (E and H are generated by alternate splicing) is disulphide-linked to CD94, the heterodimer can function as an activating receptor by associating with an adaptor molecule DAP12 through its charged membrane residue.

NKG2A-CD94 and NKG2C-CD94 heterodimers recognize the non-classic MHC class I molecule HLA-E. The structure of HLA-E is similar to that of classical MHC class I molecules, but they mainly display peptides that are derived from the signal peptides of classical MHC class I molecules. Therefore, interaction of NKG2-CD94 heterodimers with HLA-E allows NK cells to monitor (indirectly) the expression of MHC class I as well as of HLA-E itself, which requires an intact MHC class I assembly pathway. It appears that NKG2-CD94 inhibitory receptors dominate over NKG2-CD94 activating receptors, which may be due to higher affinity binding of inhibitory receptor NKG2-CD94 to its ligand as compared to activating receptor.

NKG2D

Cloned from human NK cells as a cDNA that was related to NKG2A and NKG2C. However, it is distinct from other NKG2 family members. NKG2D has only limited sequence homology (20% amino acid identity for lectin-like domain) between NKG2D and other NKG2 molecules (70% homology among them). NKG2D is expressed as disulphide-linked homodimer by NKT cells, γδ T cells, CD8+ T cells and macrophages. NKG2D does not have known cytoplasmic motifs and is preferentially associated with a signaling chain, DAP10. DAP10 does not have ITAMs; instead it contains a site for the recruitment for PI-3 kinase and behaves as a co-stimulatory molecule on T cells. Recently two spliced variants of NKG2D have been identified in mice, the long form NKG2D-L (13 amino acid extension at amino terminus) and a short form NKG2D-S. Resting NK cells express NKG2D-L, and after activation NKG2D-S mRNA is upregulated. Neither isoforms are detected on resting CD8+ T cells or macrophages. After TCR activation, expression of both isoforms are upregulated. After activation of macrophages by LPS, the expression of NKG2D-s is preferentially upregulated. NKG2D-L associates only with DAP10, whereas NKG2D-S can associate with both DAP10 and DAP12. Since CD8+ T cells do no express DAP12, the two isoforms that are expressed on activated T cells can associate only with DAP10. Activated NK cells, however, can transmit signals through DAP10 and DAP12. Therefore, NKGD2 can deliver a direct stimulatory signal to NK cells, but only co-stimulatory signal to T cells, because the specificity of T cell signaling would be compromised by direct stimulation of T cells by NKG2D.

NKG2 Ligand

In humans, the NKG2D ligands are: MHC class I-chain-related protein A (MICA), MHC class I-chain-related protein B (MICB), and UL16-binding protein (ULBP) family. *MICA* and *MICB genes* are linked to the HLA region and have limited expression on epithelial and vascular endothelial cells. ULBP molecules are constitutively expressed on a broad array of tissues. Despite marked sequence diversity, the NKG2D ligands have several common features: These include, sequence and structure-related to MHC class I molecules, although they do not associate with β_2 microglobulin or bind peptides, expression of NKG2D ligands is inducible, and MICA and MICB expression by epithelial cells is markedly enhanced in IBD.

Physiological Functions of Activating Receptors

Expression of NKG2D is also upregulated after virus infection, allowing co-stimulation of virus-specific CTLs and efficient killing of infected cells even when virus has downregulated MHC Class I expression. Conversely, CMV contains an ORF, known as UL16, that binds the ULBP family of NKG2D ligands and inhibits their interaction and that of MIC with NKG2D. CMV also has two ORFs that encodes ligands for both structural type of inhibitory receptors, indicating that CMV has evolved mechanisms to specifically evade NK-cell activating receptors.

NKT Cells

NKT cells are a unique subset of lymphocytes that are phenotypically and functionally similar to classical NK cells; however, they are thymus-derived and express TCR α/β, although with restricted repertoire. NKT cells use a rearranged homologous TCR Vα and Jα segments. In contrast to conventional T cells (Fig. 1.3A), the TCR of NKT cells does not interact with peptide antigens presented by MHC class I or II molecules but instead it recognizes glycolipids presented by CD1d, a non-classical antigen-presenting molecule that associates with β2 microglobulin (Fig. 1.3B). The distribution of NK and NKT cells is different; NKT cells are found at locations where T cells are present. NKT cells have been categorized into two subsets: the invariant NKT cells (iNKT or type I NKT) and nonvariant NK cells (type II NKT cells), which is CD1d negative. Type I NKT cells are Vα14+ and contain two subpopulations: a CD4+ and a CD4-CD8- (double negative, DN); they express Vα24-Jα18. Functionally NKT cells are distinct from T cells in that they are autoreactive (recognize self-glycolipids) and produce both Th1 and Th2 cytokines. In addition, NKT cells appear to have an immunoregulatory role. In humans, during early phases of activation NKT cells

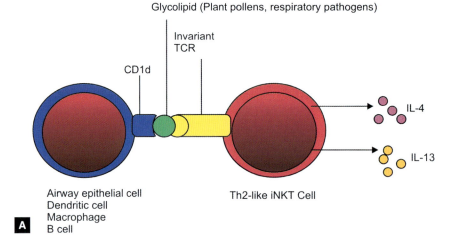

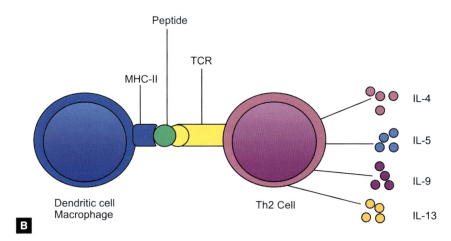

Figs 1.3A and B: Th2-like iNKT cells recognize glycolipids in context of CD1d (A) as compared CD4 Th2 cells, which recognize peptide antigen in context of MHC class II (B)

produce both Th1 and Th2 cytokines, whereas, during late phases of activation predominantly Th1 cytokines are produced. However, there as an evidence to suggest that two types of NKT cells may also differ in their effector functions (cytokine production). CD4+ NKT cells produce exclusively IL-4 and IL-13 (Th2 response), whereas DN NKT cells had restricted Th1 profile. More recently it has been reported that CD4+ and DN NKT cells differentially regulate DC functions by reciprocal NKT-DC interactions resulting in subsequent Th responses. DC stimulated by CD4+ NKT cells preferentially induced Th1 response, whereas DC reacted with DN NKT cells induced shift towards Th2 responses. NKT cells are emerging as an important subset of lymphocytes, with both a protective role in host defense and a pathogenic role in certain immune-mediated disease states, including autoimmune diseases, allergic diseases, inflammatory bowel disease, skin diseases, and atherosclerosis.

Complement

Complement is a system of approximately 30 circulating and membrane-expressed plasma proteins that interacts with pathogens to mark them for destruction. Complement is an important effector of both innate and antibody-mediated acquired immune response. There are three pathways of complement activation, which include. The classical pathway, which is triggered by antibody or by direct binding of C1q to the pathogen surface; [MB lectin pathway], which is triggered by mannan-binding lectin, a normal serum constituent that binds some encapsulated bacteria, and the [Alternative pathway], which is triggered by pathogen surfaces. All these pathways generate a crucial enzymatic activity that, in turn, generates the effector molecules of complement. Three consequences or functions of complement activation are recruitment of inflammatory cells, opsonization of pathogens that enhances phagocytosis of pathogens by neutrophils and macrophages, and direct killing of pathogens (Fig. 1.4A). The early events of all three pathways of complement activation involve a series of cleavage reactions that culminate in the formation of an enzymatic activity (C3 convertase), which cleaves C3 into C3b and C3a (Fig. 1.4B). The production of C3 convertase is the point at which the three pathways converge and the main effector functions of complement are generated. C3b binds covalently to the bacterial cell membrane and opsonizes the bacteria for phagocytosis. C3a is a peptide mediator of local inflammation. C5a and C5b are generated by a C5 covertase formed by C3b bound to the C3 convertase. C5a is also a powerful peptide mediator of inflammation. C5b triggers the late events in which the terminal components of complement

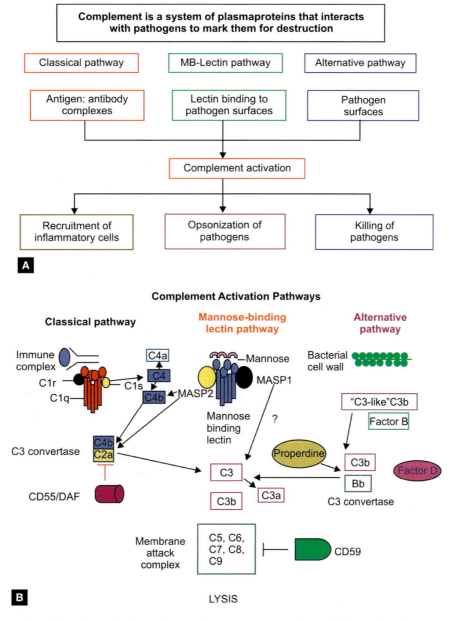

Figs 1.4A and B: Three different pathways of complement activation and their functions (A), and steps of activation of complement proteins by three different pathways (B)

assemble into a membrane attack complex (MAC) that can damage the membrane of pathogens (Fig. 1.6). MHC class III genes encode for serum C2, C4, and factor B.

The majority of complement components are synthesized predominantly by hepatocytes in the liver but are also secreted by monocytes, macrophages, and epithelial cells of the urogenital and gastrointestinal tracts. Proinflammatory cytokines (IL-1α, TNF-β) can induce synthesis and secretion of some complement proteins by other cell types.

Classical Pathway of Complement Activation

It was the first complement pathway that was described and therefore named classical pathway. Antigen-antibody complexes are the predominant activators of classical pathway. Other activators include certain viruses, necrotic cells and subcellular membranes, aggregated immunoglobulins, β-amyloid in Alzheimer's disease, and C-reactive protein (CRP). CRP binds to the polysaccharide phosphocholine expressed on the surface of many bacteria (e.g. *Step. pneumonia*) and activate classical pathway of complement. In the classical pathway the sequence of activation of early component is C1, C4, C2, and C3. C1 complex is made up of subunits, C1q, C1r, and C1s. There are two molecules each of C1r and C1s and one C1q. C1q is produced from six identical subunits, each of which is made up of three similar strands. Each subunit has a collagen-like tail portion (CLR), a flexible arm region that ends in a globular head unit. C1r and C1s are single chain proenzymes that form tetrameric complex. Once the C1q complex has bridged two or more IgG molecules, it undergoes a conformational change that releases C1r and C1s from constraint. Unlike IgG, which requires 2 or more bound antibodies to activate C1, one IgM molecule can bind and activate the C1q rs complex. The C1q binds to the IgM across the joining region of the pentamer. C4b can form co-valent bonds with molecules that are near it when it is formed. This allows it to bind to all kinds of surfaces, including the immune complex or antigen, or another nearby molecule. C4b also participates in the formation of the classical pathway C3 convertase, C4bC2a. C2b is the smaller segment of C2, and it may contain the sequence responsible for the C2-kinin activity associated with hereditary angioedema. C2a is the larger fragment, and it contains a serine esterase active site. In order for C2a to act, it must bound to C4b, and the C4b2a complex is the C3 convertase of the classical pathway.

Alternative Pathway of Complement Activation

The alternative pathway (AP) of complement is triggered by a wide array of factors, including lipopolysaccharide from cell wall of gram-negative bacteria, cell wall of some yeasts, and cobra venom factor. Certain viruses, aggregated Ig, and necrotic cells may also (in addition to classical pathway) activate alternative pathway. The alternative pathway requires three factors analogous to the classical pathway: Factor D is the equivalent of C1s, factor B is equivalent of C2, and C3b takes the place of C4b. Properdine, unique to the alternative pathway, is required for efficient convertase activity. The first step in AP activation occurs when factor B binds to C3b. Factor D cleavesC3b bound factor B. The Ba fragment is released to the fluid phase, and Bb stays bound to the Ce3. C3bBb is the alternative pathway C3 convertase, with the enzymatic activity is in the Bb fragment. Properdine stabilizes the alternative pathway C3-convertase by binding to C3bBb. Factor H binds to C3bBb and displaces the Bb. H acts as a co-factor for I, which cleaves C3b once to produce iC3b, or twice to produce C3c and C3dg. CR1 and MCP can also act as co-factors for I.

The Lectin Pathway of Complement Activation

The lectin pathway is activated by engagement of pathogen oligosaccharides leading to generation of C3 covertase similar to classical pathway. The mannose binding lectin (MBL) recognizes oligosaccharides specific to pathogens (bacteria, yeast, and parasites). The MBL-like proteins have been identified in invertebrates, which may suggest that the lectin pathway may be the most ancient system of complement activation. Following binding to the ligand, MBL undergoes conformational change leading to ac activation of MASP1 and MASP2, two enzymes that are functionally similar to C1r and C1s. MASP2 cleaves C4 into C4b, which binds to cell surface, and C4a. Once C4 is bound to pathogen surface, remaining pathway of activation is similar to classical pathway. MASP1 cleaves C3. Although lectin pathway of complement activation is a component of innate immunity, MLB binds with high affinity to α-galactosyl IgG, which is produced primarily at the time of inflammation. Therefore, this unusual IgG would amplify both classical and lectin pathways at the site of inflammation. Although MLB deficiency is common in general population, it does increase the risk of infection; however, risk of SLE and progression of rheumatoid arthritis is increased. Increased risk of SLE is attributed to the role of MLB in the clearance of apoptotic cells.

The Membrane Attack Complex

Once C3 is cleaved by any of the three pathways it becomes the part of next enzymatic complex, the C5 convertase. C5 covertase is either C4bC2aC3b (in classical and lectin activation pathway) or C3b2Bb (in alternative pathway). The cleavage of C5 results in larger fragment C5b, which become attached to cell surface, and a small fluid phase C5a fragment. C5b binds to C6 and C7 to form a complex. C5b also binds directly to C8, which then becomes incorporated into the complex. This complex of C5b, C6, C7, C8 is sufficient to render the membrane leaky; however, the addition of C9 leads to formation of stable pore. Once stable pore is formed, cell is unable to repair the damage, and cell contents leak from the cell.

ADAPTIVE IMMUNITY

Adaptive immunity is usually exhibited only after an exposure to an antigen either naturally or via immunization. The adaptive immune response is mediated by T lymphocytes and B lymphocytes.

T Lymphocytes

T Cell Development, Differentiation and Maturation

T cell progenitors are derived from common lymphoid progenitors (CLP) in the bone marrow, which enter the thymus, where they interact with thymic stromal cells and dendritic cells to undergo differentiation and maturation prior to their exit into circulation (Fig. 1.5). The process of T cell differentiation and maturation occurs by positive and negative selection, which depends upon the affinity of thymocytes for antigen, and whereby developing T cells that are reactive to self antigens are eliminated. T cells entering the thymus lack TCR complex and CD4 and CD8 antigens. These double negative thymocytes (CD4-CD8-) then induced to express CD1, CD2, CD5, CD7, and CD25. Subsequently these double negative cells undergo TCR α, β, γ, and δ gene rearrangement to generate immature T cells. Cell surface expression of TCR depends upon expression of CD3 complex, which is comprised of δ, γ, ε, and ξ chain. Together, TCR and CD3 complex form the TCR complex. The TCR recognizes antigen presented by APC, whereas CD3 complex, in particular ξ chain is responsible for intracellular signaling. There are primarily two types of T cells that leave the thymus; TCRαβ + CD4+ and TCRαβ + CD8+ T cells. Fewer than 10 percent of T cells emerge from the thymus as TCRγδ + CD4-CD8-. CD4+ T cells recognize antigen presented in context of MHC class II, whereas CD8+ T cells respond to an antigen in context of MHC class I antigen. This is the only unique and single property that distinguishes functionally distinct CD4+ and CD8+ T cells.

T Cell Signaling

T cell activation requires two signals (Fig. 1.6). When TCRαβ binds to a specific antigen in context of MHC molecules it provides first signal, whereas second signal is provided by interaction between co-stimulatory molecules (CD28 on T cells and B7.1/B7.2 [CD80/86] on

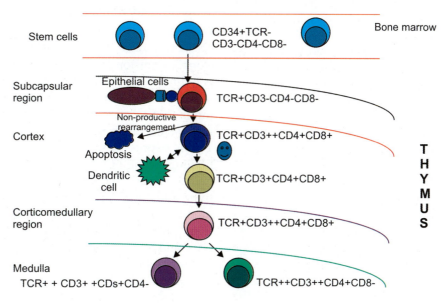

Fig. 1.5: Development of T cells in the thymus

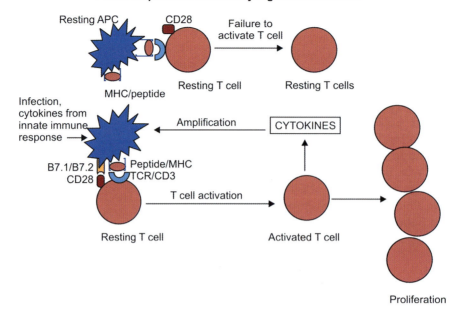

Fig. 1.6: Requirement of two signals in T cells: Recognition of peptide by TCR, and co-stimulation by interaction with CD28-B7

APC). In absence of second signal, T cells are rendered anergic. Binding of antigen to TCR and interaction of co-stimulatory molecules results in downstream sequential intracellular signaling. The earliest detectable event is the activation of Src family tyrosine kinases. The tyrosine kinases associated with CD3 and ξ is *Fyn*, and the tyrosine kinase associated with CD4 is *Lck*. Once activated Fyn and Lck cluster in the region of CD3 and ξ chain and phosphorylate contains immunoreceptor tyrosine-based activation motifs (ITAM). The phosphorylated ITAMs in CD3 and ξ chain then act as docking sites for another tyrosine kinase *Zap70* (belonging to *Syk* family of tyrosine kinases). This step appears to be critical in the activation of T cells, because T cells from patients with Zap70 deficiency do not respond to antigens. Lck activates Zap70, which phosphorylates multiple adapter proteins, two important adapter molecules are LAT and SLP-76. The adapter molecules bind to phospholipase C-γ (PLC-γ), which after being phosphorylated by Zap70 catalyzes the hydrolysis of phospholipid component of lipid membrane PIP2 into IP3 and diacylglycerol (DAG). IP3 increases intracellular calcium due to increased mobilization of calcium from intracellular stores in the endoplasmic reticulum, which in turn activates calcineurin, finally activating the transcription factor NF-AT. DAG activates protein kinase C (PKC), which then activate a cascade of kinases, ultimately leading to the activation of NF-κB. In addition, activated adapter molecules bind to and activate guanosine-nucleotide-binding proteins, Ras and Rac, which in turn activate a cascade of mitogen-activated protein kinases (MAPK), leading to the activation of transcription factor AP-1. These transcription factors enter the nucleus of the T cells and bind selectively to regulatory sequences of several different genes resulting in the secretion of a number of cytokines (Fig. 1.7).

T Cell Effector Functions

Following exposure to an antigen (presented by antigen presenting cells), naïve T cells undergo antigen-specific clonal expansion of effector cells to clear antigen, which is followed by a phase of contraction during which the majority of effector cells undergo apoptosis, and a small number of cells are retained as memory cells, which are responsible for an anamestic immune response. Memory T cells express distinct receptors for chemokines and homing receptors, which allow them to migrate to lymph nodes (central memory) or extralymphoid tissues like liver and lung (effector memory). These subsets of memory T cells are distinct in a variety of functions (Fig. 1.8). Naïve T cells (TN), central memory T (TCM) cells, and effector memory T cells (two types of effector memory cells in CD8+ T cells, CD45RA- TEM and CD45+ TEMRA) are distinct in variety of characteristics (Fig. 1.9). CD8+ cytotoxic effector cells play an important role in killing virus-infected target cells, and some tumor cells.

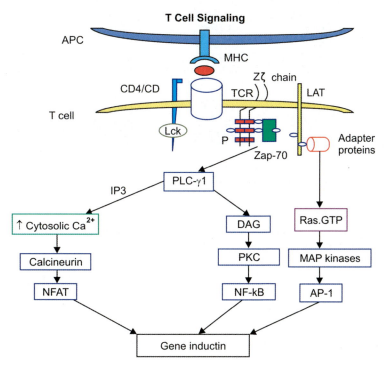

Fig. 1.7: Signaling pathway of T cell activation. DAG= diacylglycerol, PLCγ= phospholipase cγ, IP3=Inositol tris phosphate

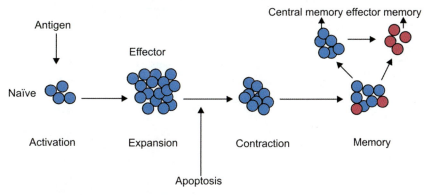

Fig. 1.8: Differences phases of naïve T cell activation into effector and memory subsets

Naïve CD4+ T cells differentiate into Th1 (T-bet-dependent), Th2 (GATA3-dependent), Th17 (RORγt-dependent), and Treg (FoxP3-dependent) cells to mediate effector and immunoregulatory functions (Fig. 1.10). Th1 cells synthesize IL-2, IFN-γ, and TNF-β, and Th2 cells produce IL-4, IL-5, IL-9, IL-10 and IL-13. Th1 cytokines activate CD8+ T cells, NK cells, and macrophages and appear to play major role in cell-mediated immunity. In contrast, cytokines secreted by Th2 cells trigger B cell to class switch to IgE production, and to activate eosinophils, a pattern commonly observed in allergic and parasitic diseases. IFN-γ produced by Th1 cells negatively regulate the development of Th2 cells, whereas cytokines produced by Th2 cells regulate the differentiation of naïve CD4+ T cells to Th1 cells. Th17 synthesize and secrete IL-17, IL-21, IL-22, and TNF-α; appears to play a role in inflammation and autoimmunity. Treg cells appear to mediate (in part) their regulatory effects via IL-10 (and ?TGF-β), and play an important role in immunological tolerance and homeostasis. There are two types of Tregs: natural Treg (nTreg) which are present in the thymus and are FoxP3+ and exported into periphery, and FoxP3- CD4+ T cells in the periphery, which are inducible to become Fox3+CD4+ Treg (iTreg).

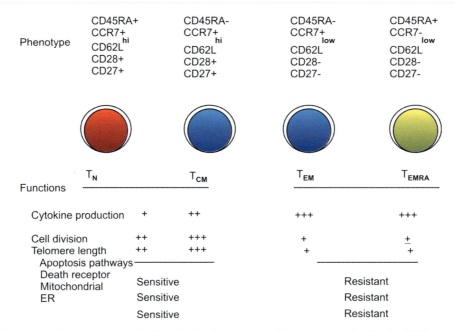

Fig. 1.9: Phenotypic and functional properties of different subsets of memory T cells. Tn = Naïve T cells, TCM = central memort T cells, TEM = CD45RA-effector memory T cells, TEMRA = CD45RA+ effector memory T cells

Functional Responses of T Cells

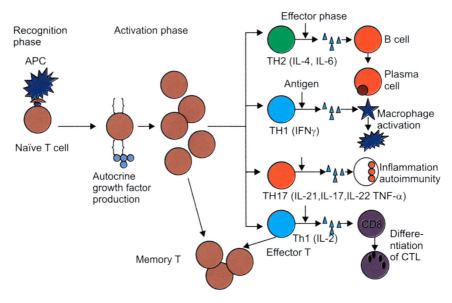

Fig. 1.10: Effector functions of T cell subsets

B Lymphocytes

B Cell Development, Differentiation and Maturation

Similar to T cells, B lymphocyte progenitors are derived from CLPs, interact with bone marrow stroma and factors produced by the stroma, and undergo various differentiation and maturation steps within the environment of bone marrow (Fig. 1.11). During differentiation, B cell precursors undergo a series of DNA rearrangements of immunoglobulin heavy (H) chain and light (L) chain genes by a process of V[D]J recombination, for the expression of membrane bound and secreted immunoglobulin molecules. Recombination-activating gene 1 and 2 (RAG-1 and RAG-2) are two enzymes that are critical in initiating V (variable) D(diversity) J (joining) recombination in precursor cells (at the Pro-B cells and

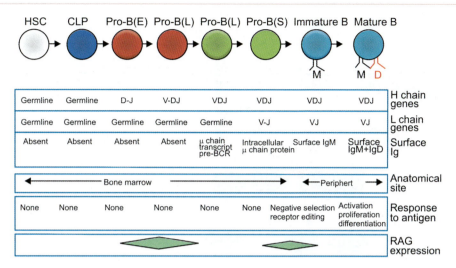

Fig. 1.11: Development of B cells. RAG = recombinase activation gene, L = late, E = early, l = large, s = small, CLP = common lymphoid precursor, HSC = hematopoietic stem cell, V = variable region, J = joining region, D = diversity region

at Pre-B cell level). The pre-B-cell receptor (pre-BCR) is expressed following the productive recombination of the immunoglobulin heavy chain gene. Signals through the pre-BCR are required for initiating diverse processes in pre-B cells, including proliferation and recombination of the light chain gene, which eventually lead to the differentiation of pre-B cells to immature B cells. Recent findings suggest that forkhead box O (FOXO) transcription factors connect pre-BCR signaling to the activation of the recombination machinery that allow the progression of the cell cycle and the recombination of the light chain gene.

As a result of alternative splicing of heavy chain mRNA transcribed from VDJ plus μ and δ genes, mature virgin B cells co-express surface IgM and IgD. The maturation of B cells up to this stage is antigen-independent and occurs within the bone marrow. IgM and IgD expressed on a single B cell have identical antigen specificities. However, subsequent differentiation of IgM+IgD+ B cells in the periphery is antigen-driven. The function of membrane bound IgD is not completely understood; however, IgD bearing B cells do not make antibodies to self antigens, therefore, the expression of IgD may be an inhibitory signal to autoreactive B cells.

B Cell Signaling

B cell activation signaling events are similar to those of T cells. Similar to TCR, Ig H and L chains have very short intracellular domains and do not play a direct role in signal transduction. Igα (CD79a) and Igβ (CD79b) molecules, which are non-covalently associated with IgH and L chain in B cell membrane transmit intracellular signals (Fig. 1.12).

Multivalent antigens with repeating epitopes directly activate B cells. Activation of B cells is initiated by cross-linking of B cell antigen receptor (BCR) with earliest association of tyrosine kinases Lyn, Blk, and Fyn with BCR. Activated kinases phosphorylate ITAM in Igα and Igβ molecules associated with Ig chains. Phosphorylated ITAM recruits Syk to the cluster and then activated Syk recruits and activates adapter molecules, which in turn activates downstream pathways similar to T cells. Transcription factors then enter the nucleus, and promote the transcription of Ig and cytokine receptor genes.

Other molecules that affect signals through BCR include CD19, CD81 (also termed TAPA-1), and CD21, and are associated in the B cell co-receptor complex. Antigens binding to co-receptor enhance the activation signal by BCR by lowering the threshold for stimulating B cell responses.

CD21 is a receptor for C3d, which binds to microbial pathogens. Therefore, CD21 appears to play a major role in increasing antibody responses to pathogens that activate complement pathway. The pathogen can also bind to IgM on the same B cell. This cross-linking of antigen via IgM and C3d on B cells delivers simultaneous stimulating signals to the B cells; CD19 in the coreceptor complex is phosphorylated and activates ITAM in Igα/Igβ. CD21 is also a receptor for Epstein-Barr virus (EBV). CD22 has a negative effect on signaling to the B cells (negatively affects CD19, CD81, CD21 co-receptor.

B Cell Effector Functions

Following antigen stimulation two critical events occur in B cells; isotype or class switching, and somatic

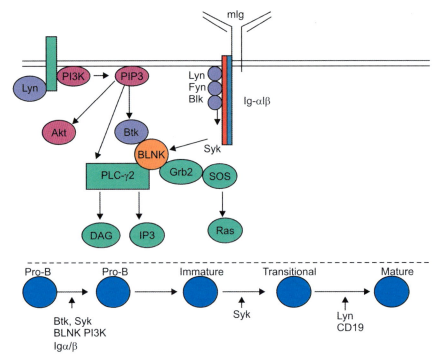

Fig. 1.12: B cell signaling pathway

hypermutation. Individual B cells can switch to make a different class of antibodies such as IgG, IgA, and IgE (Fig. 1.13). This phenomenon is termed class switching or isotype switching. Class switching changes the effector function of the B cells but not the antigenic specificity. Isotype or Ig class switching occurs only in antigen-stimulated IgM+ IgD+B cells and involve further DNA rearrangement, juxtaposing the rearranged VDJ genes with a different heavy chain C (constant) region, and T cell-derived cytokines. In the presence of IFN-γ, cells can rearrange VDJ to the Cγ2 heavy chain, and cell switches of IgG2 synthesis, whereas in the presence of IL-4, B cells can rearrange VDJ to Cε, and cell switches to IgE. There is no class switching in the absence of cytokines. Class switching is a mechanism unique to heavy chains of immunoglobulins. Mutations that occur in V (variable) region of H and/or L chains of B cells also increase the variety of antibodies. In somatic hypermutation, point mutations in the VDJ recombinant unit of antibody V genes results in changes in individual amino acids; it occurs at a rate of at least 10,000 fold higher than the normal rate of mutation. Somatic hypermutation results in observed increased affinity of antibodies (affinity maturation) in the secondary immune response; in primary antibody response antibodies of low affinity are produced. Somatic hypermutation occurs in the germinal center of spleen and lymph nodes. Isotype or class swich is regulated by a number of gene products namely AICD, UNG, and NEMO. Mutations of each of these genes have resulted in defects in class switch and somatic hypermutation resulting in Hyperimmunoglobulinemia M syndromes (HIM).

Effector Functions of Antibodies

Different antibody isotypes can trigger different effector functions. Antibodies perform four major functions: neutralization of antigen, classical complement activation, opsonization, and antibody-dependent cell-mediated cytotoxicity (ADCC). Neutralization of antigen depends exclusively on Fab region of the Ig, and therefore, it is isotype independent. Classical complement activation is isotype dependent because C1q binds to Fc region of certain Ig isotype. In humans, IgM, IgG1, IgG2, and IgG3 are best suited for activating classical complement pathway. Such antibodies are termed as "complement fining antibodies". For opsonization and ADCC, the Fc region of the antibody in the immune complex must interact with Fc receptors on the surface of leukocytes of innate imunity that perform their effector functions. These interactions are isotype-dependent. In opsonization an antigen coated with antibodies enhances recognition of antigen by phagocytic cells like neutrophils and macrophages. IgG1 and IgG3 bound to an antigen are best Igs to mediate opsonization. When a pathogen

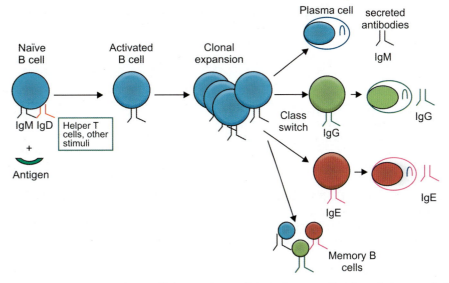

Fig. 1.13: Sequence of B cell activation, proliferation, class switch, and memory B cells and plasma cell differentiation

coated with antibodies is too large to be phagocytosed, ADCC may eliminate a pathogen. ADCC is mediated by several leukocytes that express FcRs and have cytotoxic properties: NK cells, eosinophils, and to a lesser extent neutrophils, monocytes and macrophages. In humans, NK cells express FcγRs, which bind to monomeric IgG1 and IgG3. Eosinophils express FcεR, and FcαR molecules that can bind to IgE-coated or IgA-coated parasitic targets. Such pathogens are resistant to ADCC by NK cells and neutrophils.

CONCLUSION

Immunity against microbes and their products or against other foreign substances is divided into two major components: innate immunity and adaptive immunity. These two types of immunities and their origins, components, and interrelationships are discussed. Innate immune system is evolutionary primitive compared to adaptive immune system, and plays a major role in influencing the nature of adaptive immune responses. In this respect, one of the major players of the innate immune response is DCs. Though adaptive immune system is considered to play a critical role in transplantation biology, NK cells of the innate immune system also play a significant role in transplantation.

BIBLIOGRAPHY

Antigen-presenting Cells

1. Agrawal A, Agrawal S, Gupta S. Dendritic cells in human aging. Exp Gerontol. 2007;42:421-6.
2. Agrawal A, Agrawal S, Tay J, and Gupta S. Biology of dendritic cells in aging. J Clin Immunol 2008;28:14-20.
3. Barton GM, Kagan JC. A cell biological view of Toll-like receptor function: Regulation through compartmentalization. Ann. Rev. Immunol 2009;9:535-42.
4. Barton GM, Kagan JC. A cell biological view of Toll-like receptor function: Regulation through compartmentalization. Nat Rev Immunol 2009;9:535-42.
5. Buckwalter MR, Albert ML. Orchestration of the immune response by dendritic cells. Curr Biol 2009;19(9):R355-61.
6. Buckwalter MR, Albert ML. Orchestration of the immune response by dendritic cells. Current Biol 2009;9: R355-R361.
7. Ferlazzo G, Münz C. Dendritic cell interactions with NK cells from different tissues. J Clin Immunol 2009;29: 265-73.
8. Geijtenbeek TB, Gringhuis SI. Signaling through C-type lectin receptors: Shaping immune responses. Nat Rev Immunol 2009;9:465-79.
9. Gilliet M, Cao W, Liu YJ. Plasmacytoid dendritic cells: Sensing nucleic acids in viral infection and autoimmune disease. Nat Rev Immunol 2008;8: 594-606.
10. Kadowaki N. The divergence and interplay between pDC and mDC in humans. Front Biosci 2009;14:808-17.
11. Onoé K, Yanagawa Y, Minami K, Iijima N, Iwabuchi K. Th1 or Th2 balance regulated by interaction between dendritic cells and NKT cells. Immunol Res. 2007;38(1-3):319-32.
12. Schmitt N, Morita R, Bourdery L, Bentebibel SE, Zurawski SM, Banchereau J, Ueno H. Human dendritic cells induce thee differentiation of interleukin-21-producing follicular helper-like cells through interleukin-12. Immunity 2009;31:158-69.
13. Shortman K, Naik SH. Stead-state and inflammatory dendritic cells development. Nature Rev Immunol 2007;7:19-30.

14. Steinman RM, Cohen ZA. Identification of a novel cell type in peripheral lymphoid organs of mice. I. Morphology, quantitation, tissue distribution. J Exp Med 1973;137:1142-62.

Natural Killer Cells

15. Balato A, Unutmaz D, Gaspari AA. Natural killer T cells: An unconventional T-cell subset with diverse effector and regulatory functions. J Invest. Dermatol 2009;129: 1628-42.
16. Germain RN. An innately interesting decade of research in immunology. Nat Med 2004; 10:1307-20.
17. Hamerman JA, Ogasawara K, Lanier LL. NK cells in innate immunity. Curr Opin Immunol. 2005; 17:29-35.
18. Jonsson AH, Yokoyama WM. Natural killer cell tolerance licensing and other mechanisms. Adv Immunol 2009;101:27-79.
19. Lanier LL, Sun JC. Do the terms innate and adaptive immunity create conceptual barriers? Nat Rev Immunol 2009; 9:302-03.
20. Lanier LL. Evolutionary struggles between NK cells and viruses. Nat Rev Immunol 2008;8:259-68.
21. Malarkannan S. The balancing act: Inhibitory Ly49 regulate NKG2D-mediated NK cell functions. Semin Immunol 2006;18:186-92.
22. Marcenaro E, Ferranti B, Moretta A: NK-DC interaction: On the usefulness of auto-aggression. Autoimmunity Rev 2005;4:520-25.
23. Sun JC, Lanier LL. Natural killer cells remember: An evolutionary bridge between innate and adaptive immunity? Eur J Immunol 2009;39:2059-64.
24. Wu L, Gabriel CL, Parekh VV, Van Kaer L. Invariant natural killer T cells: Innate-like T cells with potent immunomodulatory activities. Tissue antigens 2009; 3: 535-45.

Complement

25. Gál P, Dobó J, Závodszky P, Sim RB. Early complement proteases: C1r, C1s and MASPs. A structural insight into activation and functions. Mol Immunol. 2009; 46:2745-52.
26. Ip WK, Takahashi K, Ezekowitz RA, Stuart LM. Mannose-binding lectin and innate immunity. Immunol Rev 2009;(1) 230:9-21.
27. Pangburn MK, Ferreira VP, Cortes C. Discrimination between host and pathogens by the complement system. Vaccine 2008;30(Suppl 8): 115-21.
28. Ramaglia V, Baas F. Innate immunity in the nervous system. Prog Brain Res. 2009;175:95-123.

B Lymphocytes

29. Brezski RJ, Monroe JG. B-cell receptor. Adv Exp Med Biol 2008;640:12-21.
30. Elgueta R, Benson MJ, de Vries VC, Wasiuk A, Guo Y, Noelle RJ. Molecular mechanism and function of CD40/CD40L engagement in the immune system. Immunol Rev 2009; 229:152-72.
31. Fearon DT, Carroll MC. Regulation of B cell response to foreign and self-antigens by the CD19/CD21 complex. Ann. Rev Immunol 2000;18:393-
32. Herzog S, Reth M, Jumaa H. Regulation of B-cell proliferation and differentiation by pre-B-cell receptor signalling. Nat Rev Immunol 2009;9:195-205.
33. Hodson DJ, Turner M. The role of PI3K signaling in the B cell response to antigen. Adv Exp Med Biol 2009;633: 43-53.
34. Kurosaki T, Hikida M. Tyrosine kinases and their substrates in B lymphocytes. Immunol Rev 2009;228:132-48.
35. Storn U, and Stavnezer J. Immunoglobulin genes: Generating diversity with AID and UNG. Curr Biol 2002; 12: R725-27.

T Lymphocytes

36. Annunziato F, Cosmi L, Liotta F, Maggi E, Romagnani S. The phenotype of human Th17 cells and their precursors, the cytokines that mediate their differentiation and the role of Th17 cells in inflammation. Int Immunol 2008; 20:1361-68.
37. Boros P, Bromberg JS. Human FOXP3+ regulatory T cells in transplantation. Am J Transplant 2009;9:1719-24.
38. Coffman RL. Origins of the T(H)1-T(H)2 model: a personal perspective. Nat Immunol 2006;7:539-41.
39. Gupta S, Gollapudi S. Susceptibility of naïve and subsets of memory T cells to apoptosis via multiple signaling pathways. Autoimmun Rev 2007;6:476-81.
40. Gupta S Bi R, Su K, Yel L, Chiplunkar S, Gollapudi S. Characterization of naïve, memory and effector CD8+ T cells: effect of age. Exp Gerontol 2004;39: 545-50.
41. Lu LF, Rudensky A. Molecular orchestration of differentiation and function of regulatory T cells. Genes Dev 2009;23:1270-82.
42. Oukka M. Th17 cells in immunity and autoimmunity. Ann Rheum Dis 2008; 67 (Suppl 3):iii26-29.
43. Sallusto F, Lanzavecchia A. Heterogeneity of CD4+ memory T cells: Functional modules for tailored immunity. Eur J Immunol 2009;39:2076-82.
44. Samelson SE. Signal transduction mediated by the T cell receptor antigen: The role of adapter proteins. Ann Rev Immunol 2002; 20: 371-94.
45. Sharpe AH, Freeman GJ. The B7-CD28 superfamily. Nat Rev Immunol 2002; 2: 116-26.
46. Shevach EM. Mechanisms of foxp3+ T regulatory cell-mediated suppression. Immunity 2009;30:636-45.
47. Spits H. Development of T cells in the human thymus. Nat Rev Immunol 2002; 2:760-72.
48. Zhou X, Bailey-Bucktrout S, Jeker LT, Bluestone JA. Plasticity of CD4(+) FoxP3(+) T cells. Curr Opin Immunol 2009;21:281-85.

Chapter 2

Cytokines and T Cell Subsets

Amit Awasthi, Sue Min Liu, Vijay K Kuchroo

ABSTRACT

The vertebrate immune system has evolved to protect against a myriad of potentially pathogenic microorganisms. The immune system is comprised of different cell types, which can be broadly divided into innate and adaptive immune systems. *The innate immune system* is composed of macrophages, monocytes, neutrophils and dendritic cells (DC), whereas *the adaptive immune system* is mostly composed of B and T lymphocytes (Fig. 2.1). Powerful non-specific host defense mechanisms prevent invasion of microorganisms via physical barriers, such as epithelial lining, and a variety of secreted antimicrobial factors. Once the physical barriers are breached, pathogens are taken up by phagocytes like macrophages and DCs, which leads to a series of events beginning with the activation of these cells. Pattern recognition receptors (PRRs) expressed by innate cells play an important role in their maturation and activation. Toll-like receptors (TLRs) are the most extensively studied PRRs; e.g. TLR4 recognizes lipopolysaccharides that are components of bacteria, TLR3-mediated activation requires double-stranded RNA molecules and similarly, unmethylated CpG motifs in DNA is recognized by TLR9. Signaling through TLRs not only induces cell activation and microbicidal activity, but also induces accessory functions including the up-regulation of co-stimulatory molecules and cytokine production by macrophages and DCs. Activation of the innate immune system is therefore essential in inducing antigen-specific T and B cell responses. Once activated and loaded with antigen, DCs migrate to the secondary lymphoid organs to activate and initiate T and B cell responses. Activated T cells then migrate to the site of infection and mediate tissue inflammation to control infection. Cytokines are small molecules secreted by different cells of both innate and adaptive immune systems that can initiate immune responses, differentiate T cells, help B cells to class switch and secret antibodies, and mediate tissue inflammation to clear pathogens. In this chapter, we present an overview of T cell activation, differentiation and the specific role of cytokines in this process.

INTRODUCTION

Mosmann and Coffman first classified the T helper (T_H) cells into T_H1 and T_H2 subsets based on their specific cytokine profiles, effector functions, and B cell help and antibody class switching.[1,2] This classification formed the basis for understanding the differential ability of T_H cells to mediate diverse immune reactions and participate in different types of tissue inflammation. T_H1 cells were shown to play a dominant role in mounting immune responses against a variety of intracellular pathogens including *Mycobacteria*, *Trypanosoma* and *Leishmania*. Efficient T_H1 responses not only eliminate intracellular pathogens, by activation of microbicidal functions of macrophages, but also inhibit the functions of T_H2 cells.

Similarly, T_H2 cells are necessary in combating extracellular pathogens, such as helminths, and also cross-regulate the generation of T_H1 cells. T_H1 and T_H2 cells, however, do not efficiently clear fungal infections, which need massive inflammation at the site of tissue infection. Recently, a new subset of T_H cells that predominantly produce IL-17 (T_H17 cells) and induce tissue inflammation has been discovered, and it is believed that this subset may play a major role in orchestrating tissue inflammation to clear fungal infection. In addition to effector T cells (T_H1, T_H2 and T_H17), regulatory T cells occur in the immune system that regulate the functions of effector T cells. In particular, Foxp3+ regulatory T (Treg) cells and IL-10-producing type 1 regulatory T (Tr1) cells are two

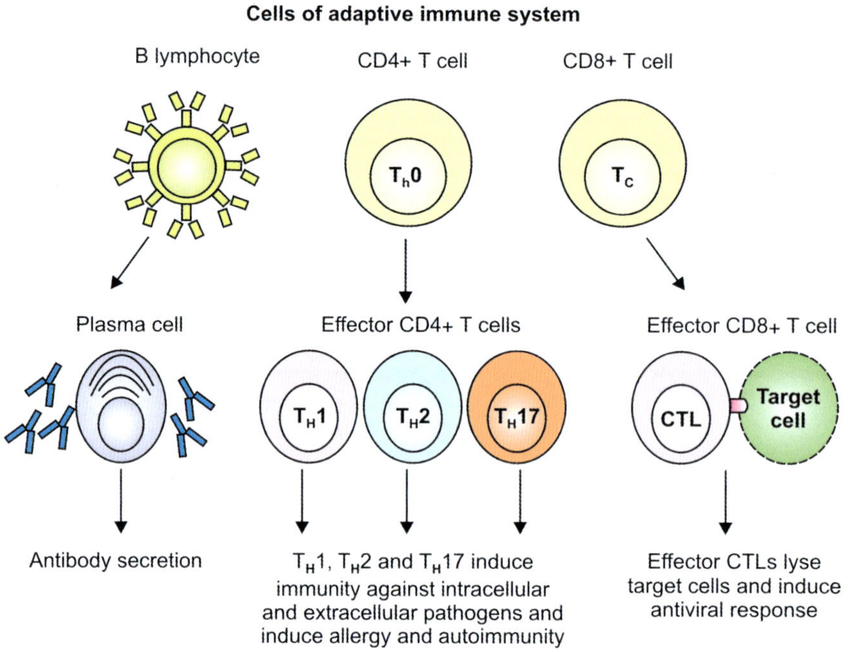

Cells of adaptive immune system

Fig. 2.1: Cells of the adaptive immune system. The adaptive immune system consists of T and B lymphocytes. Upon activation, B cells differentiate into antibody secreting plasma cells. Similarly, CD4+ and CD8+ T cells differentiate into effector helper T cells and CTLs, respectively. Antigen and specific cytokine signals induce differentiation of naïve T cells into various subsets of T helper cells (T_H1, T_H2 and T_H17) and induce specific effector functions. Effector CTLs are essential for antiviral immune responses

types of regulatory T cells that have gained considerable attention and are essential in suppressing tissue inflammation to minimize tissue damage and maintain self-tolerance. Naïve CD4+ T cells ($CD62L^{hi}CD44^{lo}$) have the potential to differentiate into these effectors (T_H1, T_H2 and T_H17) and regulatory (Treg and Tr1) subsets depending on the antigen density and affinity for the TCR, expression of co-stimulatory molecules, and the genetic background of the individual. Cytokines, a group of small proteins secreted by both innate and adaptive immune cells, play the most dominant role in the differentiation of effector and regulatory T cells. How cytokines induce differentiation of naïve T cells into effector and regulatory T cells is the focus of this review.

T_H1 Cells and Immune Responses

T_H1 cells are essential for cell-mediated immunity against intracellular pathogens. Differentiated T_H1 cells secrete interferon (IFN)-γ, interleukin (IL)-2 and TNF-β (or lymphotoxin), which mediate a variety of effector functions including activation of macrophages and DCs. Further, cytokines such as IL-12, IFN-γ and IL-18 play an essential role in T_H1 differentiation (Table 2.1).

IFN-γ

IFN-γ is a type 1 interferon produced by both innate and adaptive immune cells and exerts its effect on both adaptive and innate immune compartments. IFN-γ is produced by different cell types including CD4+ and CD8+ T cells and NK cells. It is believed that NK cells produce the first wave of IFN-γ, which helps in the polarization of naïve CD4+ T cells toward the T_H1 differentiation pathway.[3,4] Recent data demonstrates that in addition to NK cells, both macrophages and DCs can also secret IFN-γ in response to microbial stimuli, which can induce or enhance ability of CD4+ T cells to become T_H1 cells[5,6] (Fig. 2.2). Interestingly, IFN-γ positively regulates its own induction in CD4+ T cells, macrophages and DCs via a receptor complex composed of IFN-γR1 and IFN-γR2 subunits.[7] IFN-γ can further differentiate and amplify T_H1 cells and thus act as a feed-forward loop to enhance the T_H1 response.[7] Upon binding to its receptor, IFN-γ induces the activation of tyrosine kinases, JAK1 and JAK2, which induce phosphorylation and nuclear translocation of the downstream molecule, STAT-1.[8] IFN-γ signaling requires IFN-γR1, IFN-γR2, STAT-1 and downstream transcription factors that induce T_H1

Table 2.1: Features of effector T helper subsets						
Type	Differentiation factors	IL-1 family	Transcription factors	Effector cytokines	Functions	Immuno-pathology
T_H1	IFN-γ, IL-12	IL-18	T-bet, STAT-1 STAT-4	IFN-γ	Clearing intracellular pathogens	Auto-immunity, cell mediated response
T_H2	IL-4	T1/ST2	GATA-3, STAT-6	IL-4, IL-5, IL-13	Clearing extracellular pathogens	Asthma, Allergy, Atopy
T_H17	TGF-β + IL-6 + IL-23	IL-1	ROR-γt, ROR-α, STAT-3	IL-17A, IL-17F, IL-22	Clearing extracellular pathogens (fungal infections)	Auto-immunity and tissue inflammation

responses, and a genetic defect in any of the components in the T_H1 pathway would compromise clearance of intracellular pathogens such as *Leishmania, Mycobacteria,* and others.[9-11]

Although IFN-γ is essential for differentiation of T_H1 cells, the cellular source of IFN-γ during initiation of T_H1 differentiation is elusive. Both NK cells and DCs, which contribute to the early waves of IFN-γ production, have been implicated in initiating T_H1 differentiation. IFN-γ-signaling is indispensable for T_H1 differentiation as IFN-γR- or STAT-1-deficient mice are defective in generating fully mature T_H1 responses *in vivo*. In addition to NK cells and DCs, T cells also induce IFN-γ production upon TCR activation, and therefore likely contribute to initiation of T_H1 differentiation. Recent data suggest that IFN-γ is essential for initiating commitment to the T_H1 pathway by activating the master transcription factor T-bet, a member of the T-box family (also known as Tbx21), in a STAT-1-dependent manner.[12] T-bet further induces IFN-γ induction and also induces expression of the IL-12Rβ2 subunit to maintain functional IL-12R complexes, which make T_H1 cells responsive to IL-12 and stabilize the mature T_H1 phenotype[13] (Fig. 2.2).

A genetic defect in IFN-γ or IFN-γR signaling leads to induction of T_H2 cytokines to that promote T_H2 differentiation by relieving T_H1-mediated T_H2 cross-inhibition. Similarly, developing T_H2 cells extinguish IL-12Rβ2 expression and make them insensitive to the effects of IL-12.[14] The presence of IFN-γ at the time of T_H2 differentiation induces IL-12Rβ2 on T_H2 cells causing these cells to start secreting IFN-γ upon exposure to IL-12.[14] This implies that shutting off IFN-γ responses in the initial phase of T_H2 development is essential for maturation of T_H2 response. Similarly, both IL-12 and IFN-γ also inhibit the differentiation of T_H17 cells and convert them into T_H1 cells.[15] Further, mice deficient in T-bet and STAT-1 show an exaggerated T_H17 response.[16] This plasticity of T_H subsets could be one of the mechanisms by which IFN-γ and IL-12 can convert other effector T cells into IFN-γ-secreting T_H1 cells *in vivo*. IFN-γ and IL-12, therefore, coordinately act to induce mature T_H1 differentiation.

IL-12

IL-12 is a heterodimeric cytokine composed of IL-12p35 and IL-12p40 subunits.[17] Macrophages, monocytes and DCs primarily produce IL-12 upon exposure to microbial stimuli, such as lipopolysaccharides. Stimulation of macrophages and DCs via CD40 can also induce IL-12 production. Initially IL-12 was believed to be a initiation factor for T_H1 differentiation as *Listeria monocytogens* infected macrophages were shown to induce T_H1 differentiation in an IL-12-dependent manner.[18] Interestingly, IL-12 can also act as a growth factor and can further enhance proliferation of NK cells and T cells.[3] Indeed, the IL-12 receptor complex (IL-12Rβ1 and IL-12Rβ2 subunits) is not expressed on naïve CD4+ T cells, which makes these cells unresponsive to IL-12. Upon activation, however, CD4+ T cells begin to express both subunits of IL-12R. The IL-12Rβ2 subunit provides specificity to IL-12-responsive T cells. T_H1 cells express higher levels of the IL-12Rβ2 subunit and therefore are highly sensitive to IL-12 stimulation compared to T_H2 and T_H17 cells.[13] Moreover, T_H2 and T_H17 cells downregulate IL-12Rβ2 expression and provide a mechanism by which IL-12 is not able to convert T_H2

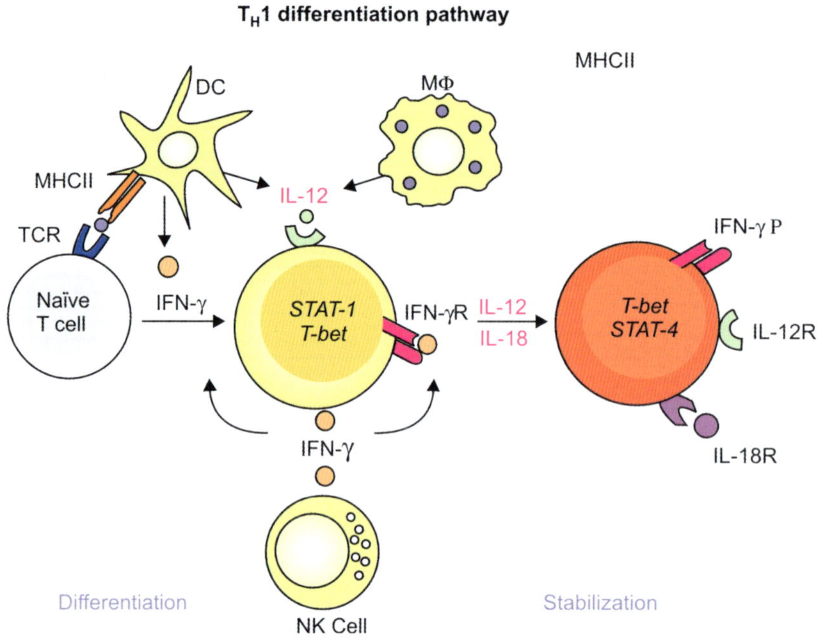

T$_H$1 differentiation pathway

Fig. 2.2: T$_H$1 differentiation pathway. Activated DCs or NK cells produce initial wave of IFN-γ, initiate T$_H$1 differentiation pathway. IFN-γ-STAT-1 signaling induces T-bet expression, which specifically induce expression of IL-12Rβ2, and make T$_H$1 cells responsive to IL-12. Activated macrophages and DCs produce IL-12, which further amplify generation of T$_H$1 cells in a STAT-4-dependent manner. Mature T$_H$1 cells express IFN-γR, IL-12R and IL-18R on their surface

cells into IFN-γ producers. T$_H$17 cells, on the other hand, do not completely extinguish IL-12Rβ2 expression and therefore show a greater plasticity and conversion into T$_H$1 cells.[15] Upon binding to the IL-12 receptor complex, IL-12 initiates a cascade of intracellular signaling events that includes phosphorylation of Jak2 and Tyk2 kinases, which in turn further induces phosphorylation of STAT-1, STAT-3 and STAT-4.[19] Compared to STAT-1 and STAT-3, STAT-4 specifically induces IL-12-mediated activation and plays a dominant role in IL-12 signaling in T$_H$1 differentiation. Mice deficient in STAT-4 show a profound defect in the generation of T$_H$1 responses as T-bet is not able to transactivate the expression of STAT-4-dependent genes in the absence of endogenous STAT-4.[3] Thus T-bet requires STAT-4 for IL-12-dependent T$_H$1 cell differentiation and maturation. Similarly, genetic deficiency of both IL-12Rβ1 and IL-12Rβ2 subunits also results in a defective T$_H$1 response. Altogether, this suggests that in addition to an absolute requirement of IFN-γ, IL-12 is essential for maintaining a mature T$_H$1 phenotype.

IL-18

Interleukin-18, a proinflammatory cytokine from the IL-1 family, primarily produced by activated macrophages and DCs, synergize with IL-12 to enhance IFN-γ production by mature T$_H$1 effector cells.[20] IL-18 signals through a receptor complex consisting of IL-18Rα and β subunits to potentiate T$_H$1 differentiation.[21] The components of IL-18R are widely expressed on a variety of cell types and tissues including spleen, liver, lung, heart, thymus and small intestine. In addition, T$_H$1 clones have been shown to induce highest levels of IL-18Rα expression, however, naïve T cells do not express either of the subunits of the IL-18R. Interestingly, effector T$_H$1 cells maintain both IL-12 and IL-18 receptor expression, even in the resting state. Further, genetic deficiency of IL-18 leads to defective T$_H$1 responses.[22] Interestingly, the failure of T$_H$2 cells to express the IL-18Rα chain led to the discovery that IL-12 signaling is necessary for the induction of IL-18Rα expression.[23] Both IL-12 and IL-18 can enhance T$_H$1 polarization independently, but together, they synergize to induce efficient and enhanced T$_H$1 development.[24] IL-18 utilizes a similar signal transduction pathway as IL-1, involving the receptor-associated kinase IRAK and the adaptor protein MyD88.[25] Activation of IRAK induces activation of TRAF6 and the nuclear translocation of NFκB.[26] IL-18 also induces activation of AP-1 through the JNK pathway. Elevated expression of IL-18 has been observed in patients with rheumatoid arthritis and Crohn's disease, in which T_H1 cells are observed in high numbers at the site of tissue inflammation.[27,28] Interestingly, expression of IL-18 mRNA has been shown to be elevated during the development of experimental autoimmune encephalomyelitis (EAE). Furthermore, neutralization of IL-18 during EAE, reduced the severity of disease.[29] Similarly, IL-18 treatment enhances the development of collagen-induced arthritis.[30] Altogether, these data suggest that the three cytokines IFN-γ, IL-12 and IL-18 act coordinately to induce T_H1 differentiation, whereby IL-12 makes T_H1 cells responsive to the effect of IL-18 by inducing the expression of its receptor, which in turn enhances the development of the T_H1 phenotype.

T_H1 Specific Transcription Factors

In recent years, substantial progress has been made in the identification of transcription factors that induce IFN-γ, a hallmark cytokine of T_H1 responses. Binding sites for a number of other transcription factors such as ATF-2, NFκB, AP-1, YY1, NF-AT, and STAT are found in the promoter or intronic regions of the *Ifnγ* gene.[31] However, none of these factors are directly responsible for the tissue-specific expression of IFN-γ. Glimcher and colleagues found that T-bet specifically induces IFN-γ secretion from naïve CD4+ T cells.[12] T-bet is expressed in lymphoid organs, especially the lymph nodes, spleen and thymus.[12] Furthermore, T-bet expression is restricted to developing T_H1 cells, but not in T_H2 or T_H17 cells.[12-16] IFN-γ-mediated STAT-1 activation is essential for the induction of T-bet during T_H1 development.[32] In addition to IFN-γ, CD3/CD28 stimulation also induces T-bet expression and initiates the first wave of IFN-γ production. IFN-γ further potentiates T-bet expression via STAT-1 and provides a feed-forward loop and amplification of T_H1 differentiation.[32] Interestingly, ectopic expression of T-bet induces its own expression, which further induces IFN-γ production.[13] The induction of endogenous T-bet expression is dependent on STAT-1 activation, as ectopic expression of T-bet in STAT-1-deficient T cells fail to further induce expression of endogenous T-bet.[32] This experiment suggested that the presence of IFN-γ is essential for the initiation of T_H1 differentiation by inducing the expression of this master transcription factor. In addition to CD4+ T cells, NK cells, macrophages and DCs also produce IFN-γ soon after activation, this enhances differentiation of T_H1 cells. Further, T-bet induces the expression of the IL-12Rβ2 subunit in T_H1 cells, which makes them responsive to IL-12, which then promotes differentiation and maintenance of differentiated T_H1 cells.[13] Overexpression of T-bet in developing and fully matured T_H2 cells induces a profound increase in the expression of IFN-γ, with a concurrent dramatic reduction in the production of T_H2 cytokines.[12] Conversely, T-bet knockout mice show a profound reduction in the frequency of IFN-γ-producing T cells with a concomitant increase in production of T_H2 cytokines, such as IL-4.[33] Interestingly, T-bet-deficient mice failed to clear *Leishmania major* infection due to lack of T_H1 cells. Further, higher parasite burden in these mice was accompanied by increased IL-4 production, hence a T_H2 response.[33] Similarly, T-bet-deficient mice also develop spontaneous airway inflammation with increased T_H2 cytokine responses.[34] In addition to T_H2 cells, T-bet also negatively regulates T_H17 responses. However, T-bet-deficient mice were resistant to development of EAE.[16,35] Altogether, these studies suggest that T-bet is the master transcription factor for the generation of T_H1 cells. Molecular mechanisms by which T-bet induces IFN-γ-producing T cells is just beginning to be understood. In addition to T-bet, T_H1 cells also express Hlx, a homeobox gene which genetically interacts with T-bet to synergistically enhance IFN-γ induction.[36] It is now clear that differentiation of T_H1 cells requires the activation of STAT-1, T-bet, Hlx and STAT-4 for the production of mature IFN-γ-producing T_H1 cells (Fig. 2.2).

T_H1 Cells and Infection

T_H1 cells are known to induce protective immune responses against intracellular pathogens such as *Leishmania, Mycobacteria, Toxoplasma,* and others. The protective effects of T_H1 cells has been well documented in *L. major* infection where induction of IFN-γ mediates protection and intracellular killing of the parasite in macrophages by production of nitric oxide.[37] *Leishmania* and *Mycobacteria* both live and survive within macrophages and therefore escape the antiparasitic immune response. Interestingly, parasites subvert protective T_H1 responses by enhancing T_H2 responses, which regulates the protective T_H1 responses and deactivates the effector functions of macrophages and thus helps parasite survival.[38] Mice deficient in T_H1 molecules such as IFN-γ, STAT-1, T-bet, IL-12Rβ2 showed increased parasite burden with non-healing lesions after infection. On the other hand, IL-4-deficient mice are able to clear *Leishmania* infection efficiently with increased T_H1 responses.[39] Similar to defects in expression of T_H1 molecules, IL-12p40-deficient mice also show higher parasite burden.[40] The IL-12p40 subunit is shared by both IL-12 and IL-23. Like IL-12 is required for mature and effective T_H1 responses, IL-23 is essential for the expansion and maturation of T_H17 cells. Higher parasite growth in IL-12p40-deficient mice suggest that, in addition to T_H1 cells, T_H17 cells might play an essential role in eliminating intracellular pathogens. Accumulating data shows that IL-12 is an effective adjuvant for inducing long lasting antiparasitic responses against *Leishmania*, *Mycobacteria* and *Toxoplasma* infection *in vivo*.[41,42] Treatment with recombinant IL-12 at the time of *Leishmania* and *Mycobacteria* infection induces progressive T_H1 responses, which efficiently clears these pathogens. Conversely, both IL-12p35- and IL-12/IL-23p40-deficient mice show a defective anti-*T gondii* immune response, with a substantial decrease in the frequency of T_H1 cells such that the mice die due to uncontrolled replication and increase in parasite burden.[43] However, IL-23p19-deficient mice are able to eliminate infection, implying that T_H1 cells, but not T_H17 cells, are the dominant effector cells in this model of infection.[43] On the other hand, recent data suggest that T_H17 cells play have accessory functions in mediating effective T_H1 responses in mycobacterial infection.[44] In addition to T_H1-inducing cytokines, co-stimulatory molecules that enhance T_H1-response are essential to induce effective antiparasitic responses. Deficiency of co-stimulatory molecules, such as CD40L and CD40, that promote T_H1 responses *in vivo* leads to failure to control *Leishmania* infection.[45] This defect in T_H1 immune responses of CD40/CD40L-deficient mice is attributed to a defect in IL-12 production and generation of nitric oxide.[46] IFN-γ produced primarily by T_H1 cells, not only activates the co-stimulatory functions of both macrophages and DCs, but also induces the microbicidal activity through nitric oxide production.[37] Mice deficient in type 2 nitric oxide synthase (INOS-2), which generates nitric oxide in response to IFN-γ, have been shown to develop a non-healing *Leishmania* infection. Altogether, these studies suggest that T_H1 cells are essential and dominant cell types in generating anti-intracellular parasite responses.

T_H1 Cells and Autoimmunity

T_H1 cells have been associated with many autoimmune diseases including multiple sclerosis, rheumatoid arthritis, type 1 diabetes, systemic lupus erythematosus (SLE), inflammatory bowel disease (IBD) and others.

Recent studies, however, suggest that such autoimmune reactions involve complex interplay between T_H1 and the recently described T_H17 subsets. T_H1 cells have been detected in the target organs in animal models of autoimmunity and patients with various autoimmune diseases. Consistent with the role of T_H1 cells in autoimmunity, T-bet-deficient mice were found to be resistant to the development of EAE and other experimental autoimmune diseases.[35] These observations imply that T_H1 cells play an important role in the development of autoimmunity. Although T_H1 cells are consistently observed at the target tissue of autoimmune inflammation, deficiency of some T_H1-specific molecules (IFN-γ, IFN-γR, STAT-1, IL-12Rβ1, IL-12p35) in mice revealed opposite effects in that these mice developed more severe EAE compared to their wild type counterparts.[47] This suggests that T_H1 cells are dispensable for the development of EAE and that other T_H subset may be required for the development of autoimmunity. The newly described T_H17 cells have been suggested to be the key T cell subset required for the development of organ specific autoimmune inflammation. However, whether these cells alone can induce autoimmunity and tissue inflammation is not fully clear. It has been suggested that T_H17 cells are more plastic and convert into T_H1 cells *in vivo* and that is how they induce autoimmune tissue inflammation.[15] It is therefore possible that the T_H17 cells are required for the initiation of autoimmunity, while IFN-γ and T_H1 cells play a crucial role in propagating tissue inflammation and autoimmunity.[15] These observations highlight the notion that induction of autoimmune tissue inflammation is a complex process that requires interaction of both T_H17 and T_H1 cells. T_H1 cells and IFN-γ also play dominant roles in intestinal inflammation both in mouse and human.[48] For example, transferring of IFN-γ- or IFN-γR-deficient T cells into RAG-deficient hosts failed to induce weight loss or colitis.[49] Similarly, neutralization of IFN-γ or IL-12 by injecting anti-IFN-γ or anti-IL-12 antibody into hosts also inhibited intestinal inflammation.[50] The increased level of IFN-γ, STAT-1 and T-bet expression at the mucosal surface has also been associated with ulcerative colitis in patients. Similarly, T-bet-deficient T cells failed to transfer colitis.[51] On the other hand, IL-10-deficient mice, develop spontaneous colitis with higher expression of IFN-γ and T-bet.[52] Interestingly IL-17 and T_H17 cells have also been detected in different models of autoimmunity (discussed below) emphasizing their role in inducing autoimmune tissue inflammation.[15]

T$_H$2 Cells and Immune Responses

T$_H$1 cells are not the effector T cells in many other inflammatory conditions such as, asthma, atopy and in extracelluar parasitic infections. T$_H$2 cells, which mainly produce IL-4, IL-5, IL-13 and IL-25, play a dominant role in allergic inflammation and in clearing extracellular parasitic infections. GATA-3 and STAT-6 are two key transcription factors involved in the programming of T$_H$2 cell development (Table 2.1). Here we discuss the T$_H$2 differentiation pathway and its implications in various disease conditions.

Differentiation of T$_H$2 Cells

In vitro activation of naïve CD4+ T cells via the TCR with exogenous IL-4 induces differentiation of T$_H$2 cells expressing a distinct cytokine pattern compared to T$_H$1 and T$_H$17 cells (Fig. 2.3). IL-4R, which consists of IL-4Rα and a common cytokine receptor gamma chain, is expressed on naïve T cells.[53] Although, IL-4 has been described as the initiation factor for T$_H$2 differentiation, the initial cellular source of IL-4 at the time of naïve T cell priming is not clear. DCs that take up antigens and present them to naïve T cells do not produce IL-4 upon TLRs activation. Other cell types, such as NKT cells, mast cells, basophils and eosinophils, may be the initial source of IL-4 in inducing T$_H$2 differentiation.[53] While mast cells and basophils require IgE cross-linking for IL-4 production, NKT cells, however, require specialized glycolipids presented via a non-classical MHC molecule (e.g. CD1). The IL-4 locus, which encompasses IL-4, IL-5 and IL-13, has been described as a susceptibility locus for many allergic diseases in humans.[54] The polymorphisms in both the IL-13 promoter and coding sequence have been linked to asthma susceptibility.[55] Other than the initial IL-4 signal, the genetic background of an individual also determines the predominance of the T$_H$2 phenotype. For example, mice on the Balb/c background readily mount a T$_H$2 response as compared to C57BL/6, and in contrast, the B10.D2 strain, which share MHC molecules with Balb/c mice, mount an effective T$_H$1 response. Further analysis of *Leishmania* infection in these inbred mouse strains showed how the genetic background of the species affects T$_H$1 and T$_H$2 responses to the same antigen. *L. major* infection in Balb/c mice effectively initiates T$_H$2 differentiation and mice are susceptible to infection. C57BL/6 mice, on the other hand, mount an effective T$_H$1 response and are resistant to infection. These results suggest that IL-4, along with other factors, polarize naïve T cells to T$_H$2 cells. However,

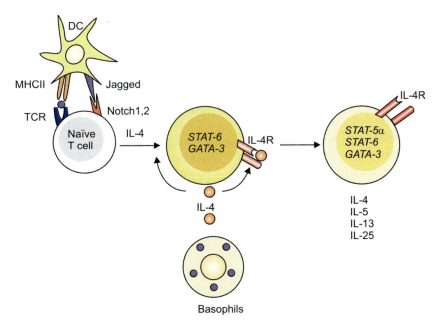

Fig. 2.3: T$_H$2 differentiation pathway. Activated DCs present antigen to naïve T cells and initiates T$_H$2 cells differentiation in the presence of IL-4. Jagged on DCs interacts with Notch1, 2 and helps T$_H$2 differentiation. IL-4 activates STAT-6 phosphorylation, which further induces GATA-3 expression and induces T$_H$2 differentiation. T$_H$2 cells produce a distinct pattern of cytokines (IL-4, IL-5, IL-13, IL-25) and induce specific effector functions in allergic inflammation and helps in clearing extracellular pathogens

the cellular source of IL-4 during the initial T cell priming of the T_H2 response is still elusive. Recent data suggests that the Notch pathway is also essential for the initiation of T_H2 responses. Interestingly, Notch signaling in naïve T cells does not require IL-4 and STAT-6 signaling, indicating that T_H2 differentiation can be initiated without IL-4 initially.

T_H2 Cells and Transcription Factors

Substantial progress has been made in understanding the molecular basis of T_H2 development. STAT-6 is the primary STAT activated in response to IL-4 and required for T_H2 differentiation.[53] Binding of IL-4 to its receptor activates JAK1 and JAK3 as well as phosphorylation of specific tyrosine residues in the cytoplasmic domain of IL-4R, which mediates STAT-6 binding to the SH2 domain and induces STAT-6 phosphorylation.[53] Phosphorylated STAT-6 forms a homodimer and translocates to the nucleus where it binds to genomic DNA to initiate transcription of genes that are required for T cell differentiation. Interestingly, IL-4Rα-deficient T cells revealed essential functions of STAT-6 in the induction of IL-4-responsive genes. Furthermore, mutations in the gene regulation domain (Y575F, Y603F and Y631F) of the IL-4Rα tail was found to be associated with a defect in STAT-6 phosphorylation.[56] These observations suggest that binding of IL-4 to its receptor initiates a signaling cascade, which involves the phosphorylation of a tyrosine motif in the receptor to induce phosphorylation of STAT-6 (Fig. 2.3). The critical role of STAT-6 in the generation of T_H2 responses was shown in STAT-6-deficient mice that failed to develop T_H2 responses and were unable to expel N. brasiliensis after infection.[57] STAT-6-deficient mice have undetectable levels of serum IgE in response to N. brasiliensis infection.[58] Further, CD4+ T cells from STAT-6-deficient mice failed to respond to IL-4 and showed an increase in the production of IFN-γ, thus biased toward a T_H1 profile.[59] These results suggest that IL-4 initiates a T_H2 differentiation pathway through STAT-6, which subsequently upregulates the expression of GATA-3, a master transcription factor required for T_H2 differentiation[60] (Fig. 2.3). Activation of naïve T cells via the TCR also induces the expression of GATA-3 independent of STAT-6. Addition of IL-4, however, further enhances the expression of GATA-3 and potentiates T_H2 differentiation. Similarly, forced expression of GATA-3 in transgenic mice or by retroviral transduction in primary T cells increases the production of T_H2 cytokines, such as IL-4, IL-5 and IL-13.[60-62] Conversely, overexpression of a dominant negative form of GATA-3 inhibits expression of these cytokines and induces production of IFN-γ.[63] GATA-3 enhances its own expression and mediates long-term chromatin changes in the IL-4 locus and also directly transactivates both IL-5 and IL-13 in addition to the IL-4 gene. The essential function of GATA-3 in the development and expansion of T_H2 response was demonstrated using GATA-3 conditional knockout mice (where GATA-3 was specifically deleted in CD4+ T cells) revealed a defect in initiation and maintenance of T_H2 responses.[64] Interestingly, deletion of GATA-3 in CD4+ T cell was sufficient for initiating the T_H1 response even in the absence of T_H1 inducing cytokines, IL-12 and IFN-γ, suggesting that GATA-3 might interact and repress T_H1 transcription factors and therefore inhibit T_H1 responses.[64] In addition to enhancing T_H2 differentiation, GATA-3 represses the expression of STAT-4, thereby inhibiting IL-12 responsiveness in T_H2 cells, and thus further stabilizing the T_H2 phenotype.[65] On the contrary, deletion of GATA-3 in committed T_H2 cells showed a lesser production of IL-4, although the frequency of T cells producing IL-4 was not significantly affected. In addition to STAT-6 and GATA-3, STAT-5 is also essential to stabilize IL-4 production in developing T_H2 cells[54] (Fig. 2.3). IL-2 induces phosphorylation of STAT-5α and, with IL-4, synergistically enhances T_H2 differentiation.[66] Moreover, neutralization of IL-2 or depletion of STAT-5α significantly affects production of IL-4 and T_H2 cell differentiation.[67] Conversely, overexpression of a constitutive active mutant of STAT-5α significantly enhances expression of IL-4 and this effect is independent of both STAT-6 and IL-4Rα.[67] However, STAT-5α is not required for the expression of GATA-3. On the other hand, GATA-3 is essential for STAT-5α-mediated effects on T_H2 differentiation. SOCS-3 is a negative regulator of T_H1 differentiation. Interestingly, STAT-5α enhances the expression of SOCS-3, which inhibits development of T_H1 cells, further enhancing the differentiation of T_H2 cells.[68] Initially, c-Maf was described as a transcription factor for T_H2 development as it binds to the IL-4 promoter and induces IL-4 transcription.[69] However, recent data suggests that c-Maf may be more important for other T cell subsets; expression profiling of various T cell subsets revealed that c-Maf is also expressed by T_H17, Tr1 and T follicular helper (T_{FH}) cells. Moreover, c-Maf expression in these three cell types is much higher than in T_H2 cells.[70] Although, c-Maf is not required for the development of

T_H2 cells, c-Maf-deficient T cells show decrease IL-4 production in T_H2 cells.

In addition to IL-4, Notch signaling also plays critical role in T_H2 differentiation.[71] Since Notch signaling can initiate T_H2 differentiation in the absence of IL-4 and STAT-6, it seems that Notch signaling can initiate T_H2 differentiation pathways, which is further enhanced in an IL-4-STAT-6-dependent manner.[71] Four Notch receptors and five Notch ligands (Delta like (DL)-1, DL-3, DL-4, Jagged-1 and Jagged-2) have been described. Naïve T cells express Notch-1 and Notch-2 and both Jagged-1 and Jagged-2 are expressed on DCs.[72] Ligation of Notch receptors initiates a cascade of intracellular signaling events and releases the intracellular domain (ICD) of the Notch receptors by proteolytic cleavage. The released ICD then translocates into the nucleus and there it acts as a transcription factor. Overexpression of Notch ICD enhances T_H2 differentiation, this effect is dependent on GATA-3. Altogether, these results suggest that initiation of the T_H2 differentiation pathway requires multiple transcription elements. GATA-3 is the dominant and master transcription factor of T_H2 differentiation, but other transcription factors synergize with GATA-3, or act at different stages of T_H2 development to develop a fully mature T_H2 phenotype.

T_H2 Cells and Infections

T_H2 cells have been implicated and are associated with antiparasitic immunity against extracellular pathogens such as *Nippostrongylus brasiliensis*, *Trichinella spiralis*, *Schistosoma mansoni*, and others. Moreover, T_H2 responses inhibit T_H1 anti-intracellular parasitic responses and help intracellular parasite survival within the host. *L. major* is a good example of this phenomena, where T_H1 responses protect mice from *L. major* infection; T_H2 cytokines, such as IL-4, not only inhibit T_H1 responses during infection but also exacerbate infection by deactivating the effector functions of macrophages.[38] Neutralization of IL-4 cytokine using anti-IL-4 antibody at the time of *L. major* infection protects mice from infection and prevents parasite growth by increasing protective T_H1 responses.[73] Moreover, treatment with rIL-12 induces long-lasting protective T_H1 immunity against both *Leishmania* and *Mycobacterium* infection with a significant decrease in IL-4 production.[40,74] Similarly, T_H1 responses are also implicated in exacerbating infection and growth of extracellular pathogens *in vivo*. T_H2 responses are necessary to expel infecting *N brasiliensis* and treatment with rIL-12 did not accelerate worm expulsion. This proparasitic effect of IL-12 is largely due to generation of T_H1 responses, as IFN-γ neutralization or genetic deficiency of IFN-γ have been shown to clear *N brasiliensis* infection.[75] Interestingly, long-lasting IL-4 in the form of IL-4/IL-4 antibody complex (IL-4 and anti-IL-4 antibody mixture) has been shown to have a protective effect in *N brasiliensis* infection in RAG-deficient mice suggesting that IL-4 must activate the innate immune system for clearing these parasites. Similarly, both IL-4Rα- and STAT-6-deficient mice fail to expel the extracellular parasite, whereas IL-4-deficient mice are capable of worm expulsion; this suggests the involvement of T_H2 cytokines other than IL-4 that use both the IL-4Rα and STAT-6 pathway to mediate their effects in this infection model.[76, 77] In addition to IL-4, IL-13 can also induce STAT-6 phosphorylation, and under certain conditions, IL-4Rα helps stabilize IL-13 binding to IL-13 receptor. Hence, it is possible that IL-13 can facilitate expulsion of the parasite and thus provide an alternative mechanism for preventing such infection in the absence of a progressive IL-4 response. Similar observations have been made in other extracellular parasite models where progressive T_H2 responses have been shown to be essential for generating antiparasitic T_H2 immunity.[76]

T_H2 Responses and Allergic Inflammation

Although T_H2 cells are essential components for clearing extracellular pathogens, an exaggerated T_H2 response often leads to atopy and allergic reactions.[78] In asthma, T_H2 cells are the dominant cell type believed to play a role in perpetuating the disease.[78] Although CD4+ T cells represent a small proportion of cells present in the lung, their numbers are increased significantly during disease and a major proportion of these cells produce higher levels of T_H2 cytokines such as IL-4, IL-5 and IL-13. T_H2 cells also express high levels of GATA-3 but not T-bet, the transcription factor required for T_H1 differentiation.[63,79] The mouse model of asthma has further emphasized and demonstrated the role of T_H2 cells in allergic airway inflammation. Interestingly, a detectable number of T_H1 cells have also been reported in some asthmatics raising the possibility of their involvement in allergic inflammation of the airways. Nevertheless, a large body of literature suggest that T_H1 cells are protective for asthma,[80] or may induce a different type of disease in the lungs. In contrast to T_H2 cells, T_H1 cells do not increase mucus secretion and airway hyper responsiveness (AHR). Further, T_H1 cells alone are not able to induce asthma and, in fact, the presence of these cells in the target organ reduces disease severity and

T_H2 mediated inflammation. The reduction in lung inflammation during asthma by T_H1 cells is not due to cross regulation of T_H2 responses by T_H1 cells, rather that IFN-γ directly targets the effector functions of T_H2 cells during asthmatic lung inflammation. It has been shown that rIFN-γ treatment in mild asthmatics reduced the inflammation. Similarly, T-bet-deficient mice, which lack IFN-γ production and have reduced frequency of T_H1 cells and spontaneously develop eosinophilic airway inflammation with increased production of IL-4, IL-5, and IL-13. This further confirms the dominant role of T_H2 responses and a protective role of T_H1 cells in asthmatic inflammation.[63] IL-13, in addition to IL-4, plays a dominant role in inducing allergic inflammation.[81] Similarly, transgenic overexpression of IL-5, IL-13, and IL-9 in mice showed increased AHR and collagen deposition in the airways. Finally, overexpression of the dominant negative form of GATA-3 in mice has been shown to cause a blunted airway inflammation including less eosinophilic infiltration and AHR.[63] Recent data suggests that in addition to T_H2, T_H17 cells may also induce allergic inflammation. Cutaneous sensitization with antigen induces T_H17 cell generation and neutrophilic infiltration in the lung along with bronchial hyperactivity, which can be reversed by neutralizing anti-IL-17 treatment. Accumulating data suggests that T_H17 cells may induce lung inflammation and asthma to environmental pollutants.[82]

T_H17 Cells and Immune Responses

The third subset of effector T_H cells, named T_H17 cells, has recently been discovered and these cells produce a distinct profile of cytokines (IL-17A, IL-17F, IL-21, IL-22) compared to T_H1 and T_H2 subsets. T_H17 cells also express transcription factors (ROR-γt, ROR-α, STAT-3) that are not expressed in T_H1 and T_H2 subsets. Interestingly, T_H17 cells mainly induce autoimmunity and tissue inflammation, although it is now becoming increasing clear that they play a major role in clearing extracellular pathogens especially fungal infections (Table 2.1).

Discovery of T_H17 Cells

The discovery of IL-23 was instrumental in identifying T_H17 cells. In 2000, Kasteline and colleagues discovered a unique cytokine chain called IL-23p19, which associated with the IL-12p40 chain of IL-12 to make a novel cytokine, IL-23.[83] Subsequent experiments using an EAE model showed that whereas IL-12p35-deficient mice were susceptible to EAE, genetic loss of either IL-23p19 or IL-12/IL-23p40 chains made mice highly resistant to EAE.[84] These studies suggested that while IL-12 and T_H1 cells were not critical for the development of EAE, IL-23 was crucial in its pathogenesis. In a subsequent study, Cua and colleagues[84] reported that IL-23 expands a subset of T cells that predominantly produced IL-17 and these cells were named T_H-IL-17 (now T_H17).

Differentiation of T_H17 Cells

Initial studies suggested that IL-23 is required for the differentiation of T_H17 cells, but naïve T cells could not be differentiated into T_H17 cells when activated in the presence of IL-23. Further analysis revealed that IL-23R expression was restricted mainly to the activated effector or memory T cell compartments, hence IL-23 could not act on naïve T cells. This naturally raised the question of what the differentiating factors for T_H17 cells were? In 2006, three seminal papers from different laboratories identified TGF-β and IL-6 as the differentiation factors for the induction of T_H17 cells from naïve CD4+ T cells[85-87] (Fig. 2.4). TGF-β was known as the quintessential immunosuppressive cytokine that induces the generation of Foxp3+ (iTregs) cells from naïve T cells that are able to suppress immune responses *in vitro* and *in vivo*.[85] Interestingly, addition of IL-6 to TGF-β-containing conditions abrogated the induction of Foxp3 expression and resulted in the induction of T cells that predominantly produced IL-17.[85] The *in vivo* role of TGF-β in T_H17 differentiation was further supported using TGF-β transgenic mice in which immunization with myelin antigen in CFA induced severe EAE with an overwhelming generation of T_H17 cells.[85] Conversely, T-cell specific deficiency of TGF-β signaling induced a defective T_H17 response, making mice resistant to the development of EAE.[88] On the other hand, the *in vivo* function of IL-6 in the generation of T_H17 cells was emphasized in both IL-6-deficient and gp130 conditional knockout mice.[89,90] Both of these mice were resistant to EAE induction and, in fact, the peripheral repertoire in these mice contained a higher frequency of Foxp3+ Treg cells.[90] The reciprocal developmental pathways of T_H17 and iTreg cells suggest that these cells share a common precursor of T cells and, depending on the balance of cytokines present at the time of their activation, T cells can differentiate into Treg cells or T_H17 cells depending on the availability of IL-6. This is further supported by a number of other observations. For example,

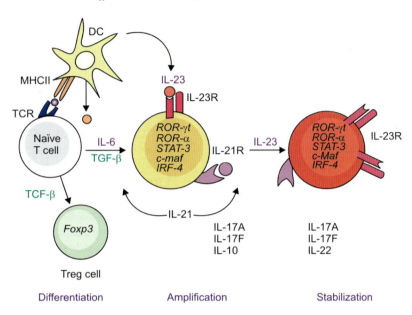

Fig. 2.4: T_H17 differentiation pathway. Activated DCs present antigen to naïve T cells and initiate T cell differentiation. DCs produce IL-6, which in combination with TGF-β initiate T_H17 differentiation pathway. T_H17 cells produce IL-21 that amplifies T_H17 generation in an autocrine manner and induces IL-23R on differentiated T_H17 cells. IL-23 stabilizes the T_H17 cells by inducing IL-17A, IL-17F and IL-22, and helping in acquiring effector functions. STAT-3, ROR-γt, ROR-α, c-Maf, and IRF-4 plays important roles in T_H17 differentiation, amplification and stabilization

(1) IL-2 and retinoic acid, that both promote Treg cell differentiation, suppress the generation of T_H17 cells,[91-93] (2) the transcription factor that induces Treg cells (Foxp3) and T_H17 cells (ROR-γt) physically associate with each other (see below).[94] Thus, depending on the availability of the switch factors (e.g. IL-6), the T cells may differentiate into Treg or T_H17 cells by regulating the expression of key transcription factors involved in the generation of these cells.

Human T_H17 Cells

T_H17 cells and their products are associated with the pathology of many inflammatory and autoimmune diseases. Higher amounts of IL-17 has been reported in the lesions of multiple sclerosis, psoriasis, rheumatoid arthritis and inflammatory bowel disease and others.[95-97] Initial studies on identifying differentiation factors for human T_H17 cells suggested that TGF-β is not required for the generation of T_H17 cells. Instead, a cocktail of IL-1 and IL-6 or IL-1β in combination with IL-23 induces T_H17 differentiation.[98,99] These studies suggested that TGF-β may in fact suppress the generation of human T_H17 cells. It was later found that human serum contains TGF-β and may be responsible for the inhibition.[100] Using serum-free media, subsequent studies demonstrated the need for TGF-β to induce human T_H17 differentiation.[100] Similar to mouse T_H17 cells, a combination of TGF-β plus IL-21 or TGF-β plus IL-6 and IL-23 induced T_H17 differentiation from naïve human T cell.[101] Besides the differentiating factors, human and mouse T_H17 cells express similar cytokines, such as IL-17A, IL-17F, IL-22, and IL-21, and a similar pattern of cell surface receptors, such as IL-23R and CCR6.

IL-21 and Amplification of T_H17 Cells

Differentiating T_H17 cells produce IL-21, which in turn amplifies the expansion of the T_H17 population as a feed-forward loop. Parrish-Novak and colleagues first identified IL-21 in 2000,[102] which is produced by activated T cells and NKT cells, but not by antigen presenting cells.[103] IL-21 plays an important role in the expansion of activated B cells and in the induction of immunoglobulin class switching.[103] Initially, IL-21 was characterized as a T_H2 cytokine,[103] new data suggests that IL-21 is abundantly expressed in certain populations of T cells, including T_{FH}, IL-27-induced IL-10-producing Tr1 cells and T_H17 cells.[70] The inducible co-stimulatory molecule (ICOS)-ICOS ligand (L) pathway is important in inducing IL-21 production in both T_{FH} and Tr1 cells.[70,104] IL-21 production is higher in T_H17, T_{FH} and

Tr1 cells compared to other subsets of T cells.[70, 104,105] STAT-3 is essential for the production of IL-21 in response to IL-6.[105,106] The master T_H17 transcription factor, ROR-γt, is not required for IL-21 production by T_H17 cells.[106] "Self-amplification" is one of the essential features of T_H differentiation. IFN-γ produced by T_H1 cells amplifies further IFN-γ and T_H1 differentiation through STAT-1- and T-bet-dependent pathways. Similarly IL-4 produced by T_H2 subsets amplifies its own differentiation via STAT-6 activation. Unlike IFN-γ and IL-4, which amplify T_H1 and T_H2 differentiation, respectively, IL-17 does not amplify T_H17 cells. IL-21, a member of the IL-2 family of cytokines, which uses a common IL-2Rγ chain expressed on all T and B cells, is essential for amplification of T_H17 cells.[105-107] Cells such as NKT and NK cells that produce IL-21 can support T_H17 differentiation in certain conditions in the absence of IL-6. IL-21 enhances expression of IL-23R on T_H17 cells and makes them responsive to the effects of IL-23, which further expand and stabilize the phenotype of T_H17 cells.[106] IL-21- and IL-21R-deficiency is known to result in a reduction in the expression of IL-23R, resulting in blunted T_H17 generation. Therefore, IL-21 not only amplifies T_H17 differentiation but also helps T_H17 cells to attain a mature phenotype by inducing the expression of IL-23R (Fig. 2.4). Both IL-21R-or IL-21-deficient mice, however, develop EAE at a similar frequency to the wild type control mice,[108] raising the issue of whether IL-21 is indeed essential *in vivo* for the generation and amplification of T_H17 cells. One possible explanation of this unexpected result is that the induction of IL-6 by immunization with CFA might override the need for IL-21 *in vivo* and might thus compensate for the IL-21-deficiency *in vivo* in the development of EAE. Recent reports, however, show that IL-21R-deficient NOD mice are highly resistant to type-1 diabetes, an autoimmune disease that arises spontaneously in NOD mice.[109] Our initial data suggests that the IL-12R-deficient mice on the NOD background have a defect in generating T_H17 cells (Liu SM and Kuchroo VK, unpublished observations) thus supporting the *in vivo* role of IL-21 in T_H17 differentiation and the development of autoimmunity.

IL-23

IL-23, a member of the IL-12 family of cytokines, was described in 2000 with the discovery of the novel IL-23p19 subunit.[83] Initially it was suggested that IL-23p19 dimerizes with the IL-12p40 subunit to promote T_H1 differentiation. The observation that IL-23 induces the generation T_H17 cells began in 2001, when Cua and colleagues showed that IL-23p19- and IL-12/IL-23p40-deficient mice were resistant to EAE.[84] IL-12p35-deficient mice, on the other hand, developed relatively more severe EAE.[110] Interestingly, IL-23p19$^{-/-}$ EAE-resistant mice showed a profound defect in T cells that produce IL-17. Further studies showed that IL-23 expands T_H17 cells from previously activated T cells.[111] These experiments clearly indicated that IL-23 promotes the generation of T_H17 cells rather than T_H1 cells. Further, IL-23 treated T cells, upon adoptive transfer, were able to induce EAE and collagen-induced arthritis (CIA), further emphasizing the role of IL-23-induced T_H17 cells in inducing tissue inflammation. IL-23R is composed of a novel IL-23Rα subunit, which couples with the IL-12Rβ1 subunit of the IL-12 receptor to generate a competent IL-23R complex.[112] Expression analysis of IL-23R demonstrated that it is expressed only on activated effector/memory T cells and not naïve T cells.[113] These data further supported the concept that IL-23, instead of differentiating T_H17 cells, promotes expansion of already existing T_H17 precursors. Discovery of T_H17 differentiation factors (TGF-β and IL-6 or IL-21) revealed that IL-23 is not required for the differentiation of T_H17 cells.[47] IL-23, however, is absolutely required to maintain T_H17 cells in long-term culture. Both IL-23p19- and IL-23R-deficient mice, are resistant to the development of EAE.[84,114,113] Cua and colleagues elegantly showed that IL-23R-deficient T cells are able to differentiate into T_H17 cell *in vivo*, similar to wild type T cells, however, IL-23R-deficient T_H17 cells failed to expand and migrate out of the lymph nodes to the target organs.[114] Our study using IL-23R-GFP reporter mice, on the other hand, revealed that IL-23R is expressed on different cell types including macrophages, DCs, γδ T cells and CD4+ T cells.[113] IL-23R expression on CD4+ T cells, however, was indispensable for the induction and development of EAE.[113] Further analysis of IL-23R-GFP reporter mice revealed that IL-23 enhances the expression of its own receptor on T_H17 cells which further enhances their responsiveness to IL-23.[113] Exposure of T_H17 cells to IL-23 induces phenotypic maturation by inhibiting IL-10 production and enhancing the production of IL-17A, IL-17F and IL-22[115] (Fig. 2.4). ROR-γt has been suggested to be essential for the induction of IL-23R on T_H17 cells as ROR-γt-deficient mice have a defect in IL-23R expression. However, it has not been shown whether ROR-γt directly transactivates the promoter of IL-23R. The importance of the IL-23/T_H17 pathway in human autoimmune diseases have come from genetic studies, showing IL-23R polymorphisms are associated with psoriasis, IBD, and ankylosis spondylitis.[116,117]

T_H17 Responses and Transcription Factors

T_H subsets were mainly recognized by the specific cytokine patterns that they produce, lineage-specific transcription factors, however, are also pivotal in defining specific T_H subsets. A set of defined STAT-signaling proteins work together with the lineage-specific transcription factors to induce T_H differentiation. T_H1 cells require the activation of STAT-4 and STAT-1 together with T-bet to induce differentiation. Similarly, STAT-6 and GATA-3 is essential for T_H2 differentiation. T_H17 cells were identified as a distinct T cell lineage since none of the T_H1 and T_H2 transcription factors were found to be expressed in these cells. TGF-β, IL-6, IL-21 and IL-23, the cytokines that mediate T_H17 differentiation, all induce STAT-3 phosphorylation. T-cell specific deletion of STAT-3 reduced the frequency of T_H17 cells. Mice and patients expressing a dominant negative form of STAT-3 have a defect in generation of T_H17 cells.[118] Moreover, STAT-3 regulates IL-23R and IL-21 expression, both of which are required for amplification and stabilization T_H17 cells. Initial studies showed that T_H17 differentiation conditions (TGF-β plus either IL-6 or IL-21) specifically induce ROR-γt, a member of the retinoic-acid-receptor-related orphan nuclear hormone receptor family, encoded by the *Rorc* gene[119] (Fig. 2.4). Retroviral overexpression of ROR-γt in naïve CD4+ T cells induces both IL-17A and IL-17F production.[119] Analysis of the ROR-γt/GFP reporter mice revealed a correlation of GFP expression and IL-17 induction in lamina propria CD4+ T cells.[119] Furthermore, ROR-γt-deficient mice showed a reduced frequency of T_H17 cell induction and EAE development.[119] In addition to both IL-6 and IL-21, which are the essential components of T_H17 development, recent data, however, revealed that TGF-β alone is sufficient to induce both ROR-γt and Foxp3.[94] The presence of IL-6 or IL-21 with TGF-β, inhibits induction of Foxp3 expression and relieves the ROR-γt to induce T_H17 generation.[94] Runx1 has also been implicated in T_H17 generation by inducing ROR-γt expression. In addition to ROR-γt, Runx1 also interacts physically with Foxp3 and therefore regulates T_H17 differentiation.[120] ROR-α, another member of the retinoic-acid-receptor-related orphan nuclear hormone receptor family, is highly expressed in T_H17 cells and enhances generation of T_H17 cells synergistically with STAT-3.[121] Recent observations demonstrated that ICOS is required for the generation of T_H17 and T_{FH} cells.[122] The generation of T_{FH} cells with the distinct surface phenotype CD4+CCR5+ICOS^{high} is dependent on IL-21, IL-6 and STAT-3.[121,70] Both T_H17 and T_{FH} cells showed a higher expression of c-Maf.[70] c-Maf directly transactivates the IL-21 promoter and IL-21 expression.[104] Deficiency of c-Maf, in turn, resulted in defective IL-21-mediated IL-23R expression. Although the requirement of c-Maf is essential for the expansion of T_{FH} cells, unlike T_H17 cells, the differentiation of T_{FH} cells did not require T_H17-specific transcription factors, ROR-γt and ROR-α.[70,121] Altogether, these observations suggest that ROR-γt, together with STAT-3, ROR-α and c-Maf, induces differentiation of T_H17 cells. It has not been addressed so far, however, whether ROR-γt directly transactivates the expression of IL-17A, IL-17F, IL-22 and IL-21. Recently, IRF-4 has been described as a critical transcription factor for the generation of T_H17 cells. IRF-4-deficient mice failed to develop EAE[123] and T cells from these mice failed to differentiate into T_H17 cells. Interestingly, the effect of IL-21 in the generation/amplification of T_H17 cells is completely dependent on IRF-4.[124] Moreover, IRF-4-deficient T cells showed a defective expression of ROR-γt accompanied by increased Foxp3 expression (Fig. 2.4).

T_H17 Cells and Autoimmunity

Association of T_H1 cells with many organ-specific autoimmune diseases such as EAE, CIA and type 1 diabetes has been well documented. However, the *in vivo* role of T_H1 cells in inducing autoimmunity was questioned when loss of T_H1-specific molecules (IFN-γ, IL-12Rβ2, STAT-1, IL-12p35) did not abrogate induction of autoimmunity, on the contrary, their deficiency enhanced disease severity.[47,125] On the other hand, higher levels of IL-17 expression was detected in many human autoimmune diseases including rheumatoid arthritis, multiple sclerosis, IBD, and psoriasis.[95-97] Patients with rheumatoid arthritis showed increased IL-17 expression in T cells in their arthritic synovium, as well as elevated IL-1, IL-6, IL-8, and TNF-α. Similarly, IL-17 and IL-6 are highly expressed in the active lesions in the brain of multiple sclerosis patients.[126] Other autoimmune diseases such as IBD and psoriasis have also been reported to have T_H17 cells and IL-17 in the tissue lesions. Altogether, these observations imply that T_H17 cells might be required for the induction of tissue inflammation and pathology during autoimmune diseases. The genetic linkage of IL-23R with many of the known autoimmune diseases further supports the role of the IL-23/T_H17 axis in human autoimmune diseases.[116,117] The role of both IL-17A and IL-17F is to activate tissue cells to induce proinflammatory cytokines (IL-6, TNF-α, IL-1β) and chemokines (CXCL1, GCP-2, CXCL8, CINC and MCP-1) to promote tissue inflammation and neutrophil infiltration in the target organ. In addition, IL-17 further potentiates tissue pathology by inducing the production of reactive nitric oxide and matrix-metalloprotinases. Mouse models of autoimmune disease, such as EAE and CIA further provide evidence for a role for T_H17 cells in autoimmune diseases. Mice deficient in T_H17 associated molecules (IL-23p19, IL-12Rβ1, IL-23R, STAT-3, ROR-γt) exhibited a resistance to autoimmunity or reduced disease severity.[47,113,114] In line with elevated expression of IL-17 in the target tissues in animal models of EAE and CIA, mice deficient in IL-17 develop attenuated CIA and EAE.[127,128] Furthermore, in another experimental approach, CD4+ T cells from IL-17-deficient mice failed to transfer EAE to recipient mice, suggesting a CD4+ T-cell intrinsic role of IL-17 in the induction of EAE. Consistently, therapeutic intervention using IL-17-receptor-Fc-protein in acute EAE resulted in reduced disease severity.[129] Increased levels of IL-6 have been shown in autoimmune diseases such as multiple sclerosis and arthritis. IL-6 is one of the dominant factors in T_H17 differentiation, and blockade of IL-6 by humanized IL-6R antibody has shown significant efficacy in a phase II clinical trial in RA and systemic onset juvenile idiopathic arthritis patients.[130] Blocking of IL-6 is expected to decrease the frequency of T_H17 cells in these patients and increase Treg functions. Recent data demonstrated an absolute requirement of IL-23 in the development of mature T_H17 responses. Since IL-23R is expressed on a variety of cell types, including macrophages, DCs, γδ T cells and CD4+ T cells, it is not clear which cells are involved in inducing IL-17 and autoimmunity.[113] In IL-23R-deficient mice, it was clear that CD4+ T cells expressing IL-23R play a dominant role in the induction of EAE; IL-23R deficiency in CD4+ T cells failed to transfer EAE in an adoptive transfer model, but loss of IL-23R on the innate immune system did not alter disease phenotype.[113] Taken together these data suggest that T_H17 cells are the major contributors of autoimmune inflammation in many autoimmune diseases and is a potential therapeutic target for regulating tissue inflammation. However, it should be noted that T_H1 cells specific for autoantigens can also induce tissue inflammation and thus the two cell types (T_H1 and T_H17 cells), collaborate together to induce and amplify tissue inflammation.

T_H17 Responses and Infection

The discovery T_H17 cells came from studies of autoimmune diseases, emerging data emphasize that this newly described subset may also have a very important role in protection from infection and host defense. T_H1 and T_H2 cells have been described as effector subsets that help in clearing intracellular and extracellular pathogens, respectively. However, IL-17A and IL-17F are also induced in several models of infections. IL-17 upregulates expression of specific chemokines, proinflammatory cytokines and colony stimulating factors, and recruits neutrophils and myeloid cells to the site of infection. T_H17 cells have been shown to be most important in clearing fungal infections. A genetic defect in IL-17 production results in an unrelenting *Candida albicans* infection in humans. Furthermore, it has been shown that CD4+ T cells are defective in IL-17 production in patients with hyper IgE syndrome (Job's syndrome). Defective T_H17 responses in these patients were further associated with a dominant negative mutation in the *STAT-3* gene, which is essential for the generation of T_H17 cells, suggesting that T_H17 cells are critical in eliminating fungal and extracellular bacterial infections commonly seen in patients with hyper IgE syndrome.[131] Pathogens such as *Mycobacterium* and *Pneumocystis carinii* induce IL-23 secretion from infected macrophages and DCs that helps in the expansion of T_H17 cells.[132] Consistent with this, IL-23p19-deficient mice were unable to clear *Pneumocystis carinii* infection and similar results were found with IL-17 neutralization in this infection model. Thus indicating that the IL-23-IL-17 axis is essential for generating anti-fungal immune response.[132] In addition to fungal pathogens, IL-17 is also crucial for protecting against gram-negative bacteria, including *Klebsiella pneumoniae*. Mice deficient in IL-17R, IL-23p19 or IL-12/IL-23p40 were susceptible to *Klebsiella pneumoniae* infection associated with a reduced expression of colony stimulating factors and neutrophil recruitment.[133,134] IL-22, a cytokine produced by T_H17 cells, has been shown to increase proliferation of lung epithelial cells and enhance transepithelial resistance to injury in *Klebsiella pneumoniae* infection.[135] In addition to fungal pathogens, IL-17 also appears to play an important role in mediating immune response to intracellular pathogens including *Mycobacterium* infection. Both human and mouse T cells produced higher amounts of IL-17 in response to *Borrellia burgdorferi* infection. New literature convincingly suggests that T_H17 cells might play an important role in inducing/recruiting T_H1 cells to the site of inflammation.[44] This has been shown in *M. tuberculosis* infection, for which an early wave of T_H17 response is essential to attract anti-bacterial T_H1 cells into the infected lung tissue to control the infection.[136] A role for IL-17 has also been described in *T. gondii* infection. IL-17R-deficient mice initially showed a normal adaptive immune response against *T. gondii* infection, however, mice died due to a defect in the migration of neutrophils to the site of infection.[137] These observations suggested an essential role for IL-17 in modulating the migration of neutrophils to the site of infection and helping to clear pathogens that are not effectively handled by T_H1 or T_H2 effector T cells.

Attenuation of T_H17 Responses

T_H17 immunity is essential to protect against certain extracellular and intracellular pathogens. A dysregulated T_H17 response to self-antigens, however, can initiate and induce severe tissue inflammation and autoimmunity. T_H subsets cross-regulate each other's differentiation and effector functions by virtue of the cytokines they produce, thus mediating the amplification of one subset and inhibition of the other. Here we have described the cytokines that negatively regulate the differentiation and effector functions of T_H lineages.

IL-27, IL-10 and T_H17 Responses

IL-27, a member of the IL-12 cytokine family, is composed of two subunits, p28 and EBI3.[138] Initial studies suggested that IL-27 induces T-bet and IFN-γ and thus, induces effector T_H1 responses.[138,139] However, using IL-27R-deficient mice, it became clear that IL-27 is a negative regulator of both T_H1 and T_H2 responses.[140,141] Initial studies have been performed on IL-27R-deficient mice using a *T. gondii*, an intracellular parasite that infect macrophages. IL-12- and IFNγ-deficient mice infected with *T. gondii* died due to uncontrolled parasite growth. *T. gondii* infected IL-27R-deficient mice, however, showed a normal T_H1 immune response and clearance of the parasite but, they ultimately died of severe immunopathology.[142] Similarly, IL-27R-deficient mice are able to clear other intracellular pathogens such as *Leishmania*, *Mycobacterium*, and *Trypanosoma*.[140,143,144] These observations imply that IL-27 is a negative regulator of T_H1 immune responses. The IL-27R complex is composed of the gp130 subunit of the IL-6 receptor with a unique IL-27Rα chain (also called WSX-1 or TCCR);[145] it was difficult to predict whether IL-27 could promote or inhibit T_H17 response. Interestingly, the immunopathology in the IL-27R-deficient mice was associated with an exaggerated T_H17 response, suggesting that IL-27 may also negatively regulate T_H17 cells. Both *T. gondii* infection and MOG peptide-induced EAE in IL-27R-deficient mice revealed an increased frequency of T_H17 cells in the central nervous system in these mice.[146,147] Similarly, addition of IL-27 in T_H17 differentiation conditions (TGF-β plus IL-6) inhibited differentiation of T_H17 cells *in vitro*. IL-27 inhibits the expression of the T_H17 cell master transcription factor ROR-γt, thereby inhibiting the differentiation of T_H17 cells.[148] Similarly, IL-27p28-deficient mice showed severe EAE with an increased frequency of T_H17 cells.[148] Similar to IL-6, IL-27 also inhibits the induction of iTreg cells by inhibiting Foxp3 expression.[149] Altogether, these data suggest that IL-27 is a potent inhibitory cytokine for the T_H1, T_H2 and T_H17 differentiation and raises a possibility that it might induce other factors that inhibit immune responses in general. A series of papers recently showed that IL-27 induces the generation of IL-10-producing Tr1 cells,[149-151] raising the possibility that IL-27 might mediate inhibition of T_H17 differentiation and other effector T cells via IL-10-producing Tr1 cells.

Tr1 Cells and Regulatory Responses

Regulatory T cells are essential cell types that maintain immune homeostasis by induction of peripheral tolerance to self and foreign antigens. A large body of evidence demonstrated an indispensable role for these cells in maintaining immunological tolerance, and loss of these cells may lead to chronic inflammatory and autoimmune diseases. The two most relevant classes of regulatory T cells described so far within the CD4+ subset are CD4+CD25+Foxp3+ Treg and Tr1 cells.[152,153] A major distinction between these regulatory cells is their expression of the transcription factor Foxp3. CD4+CD25+Foxp3+ are generated in the thymus, Tr1 cells, however, differentiate from naïve T cells in the peripheral immune compartment. Tr1 cells induce their effector function in an IL-10-dependent manner.[152] The effector mechanism by which CD4+CD25+Foxp3+ Tregs cells suppress are not clearly defined, but IL-10 produced by these cells may be a part of this mechanism. Here we discuss the generation and functions of IL-10-producing Tr1 cells.

Tr1 Cells and IL-10

Tr1 cells can be distinguished from other known T_H subsets by its cytokine production. Tr1 cells mainly produce IL-10 with variable amounts of IFN-γ.[152] IL-10 was first identified based on its capacity to inhibit effector functions of mouse T_H1 cells.[154] IL-10 has anti-inflammatory and suppressive effects on most hematopoietic cells, and it also inhibits antigen presenting capacity of antigen presenting cells by inhibiting MHC, co-stimulatory molecules and proinflammatory cytokines.[155,156] IL-10 can be produced by a broad range of immune cells such as DCs, macrophages, monocytes, B cells and T cells, which can induce a variety of cellular functions during an immune response. The anti-inflammatory role of IL-10 is well established as IL-10-deficient mice develop spontaneous colitis.[52] The CD4+ T cells that mainly produce IL-10 and TGF-β were designated Tr1 cells.[157] These cells were generated *in vitro* supplemented with IL-10.[157] Further analysis revealed the *in vivo* existence of these cells in a variety of different conditions in both mouse and human.

Differentiation of Tr1 Cells

IL-10-producing CD4+ Tr1 cells are characterized by a profile of cytokines distinct from that of classical T_H1, T_H2 and T_H17 cells. Tr1 cells produce high levels of IL-10, TGF-β and IL-5 with low amounts of IFN-γ and IL-2, and no IL-4.[157] Initially, IL-10 was described as the differentiation factor for Tr1 cells. It has also been proposed that fully differentiated T_H1 and T_H2 cells can also become Tr1 cells upon chronic stimulation, maintaining only their ability to secrete IL-10 but not other cytokines. In addition to IL-10, drugs such as dexomethasone and vitamin D3 have also been described to promote Tr1 differentiation.[158] These cells, however, do not express Foxp3 and inhibit T cell proliferation in an IL-10-dependent manner.[159] Although, IL-10 was described as the differentiation factor for Tr1 cells, the cells cultured in the presence of IL-10 could not be expanded, and therefore, it was difficult to generate these cells in large quantities to characterize their biological properties. Recent data demonstrated that IL-27 and TGF-β, instead of IL-10, are the differentiation factors for Tr1 cells.[149,150] (Fig. 2.5). It was discovered that IL-27, in combination with TGF-β, induces expression of IL-10, but IL-27 alone could also induce IL-10, albeit at a lower level.[149] Interestingly, in addition to IL-10, IL-27 also induces IFN-γ in a STAT-1- and T-bet-dependent manner, which makes these cells different from the previously described Tr1 cells.[139] In contrast to Tr1 cells generated with IL-10, IL-27 and TGF-

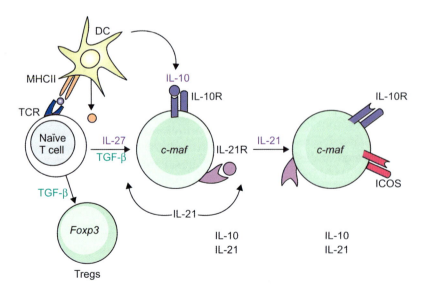

Tr1 differentiation pathway

Fig. 2.5: Tr1 differentiation pathway. Activated DCs produce IL-27 and TGF-β, which initiates differentiation of Tr1 cells from naïve T cells. IL-10 produced by DC further enhance the generation of Tr1 cells. IL-27 also induces the production of IL-21 from Tr1 cells, which further amplify the generation of Tr1 cells. IL-21 induces the expression of c-Maf and ICOS, which maintains generation of Tr1 cells. Tr1 cells produce IL-10 and IL-21, which inhibit effector T cells response

β rapidly induce proliferation of IL-10-producing Tr1 cells, suggesting that IL-27 and TGF-β are the differentiating factors for IL-10-producing Tr1 cells.[149]

Macrophages and DCs are a major source of IL-27. We showed that Foxp3+ Treg cells modify DCs to generate Tr1 cells from naïve T cells.[149] These modified DCs (CD11c^{intermediate}CD45RB^{high}B220^{high}) showed a plasmacytoid-like phenotype and produce both IL-27 and TGF-β necessary to initiate the differentiation of Tr1 cells.[149] Similarly, other DC subsets such as immature DCs and tolerogenic DCs can promote the generation of IL-10-producing Tr1 cells in an IL-10-dependent manner. However, IL-27 production in these DCs was not tested.

Amplification of Tr1 Cells

The autocrine production of IL-10 by Tr1 cells contributes to their low proliferation and expansion. IL-15 has been described as a growth factor for Tr1 cells.[160] Addition of anti-IL10 neutralizing antibody partially restores their proliferation and expansion. It has been demonstrated that IL-15 supports Tr1 cell proliferation, and IL-2 acts synergistically to significantly expand Tr1 cell clones *in vitro*.[160] Interestingly, IL-15 does not alter the phenotype or function of Tr1 cell clones in long-term culture, however, this cytokine might not be a specific amplification factor of Tr1 cells. IL-15 is known to enhance survival of memory T cells. Moreover, the cellular source of IL-15 during Tr1 differentiation is not clear.

We have shown recently that IL-27 induces the expression of IL-21, which in turn expands Tr1 cells.[104] Neutralization of IL-21 *in vitro* or culture of IL-21R-deficient T cells results in reduced IL-10 production in response to IL-27 stimulation.[104,161] Interestingly, IL-27 also increases ICOS expression, and the ICOS-ICOSL pathway further amplifies Tr1 cells via generation of IL-21.[104] ICOS-ICOSL interactions have also been described to enhance IL-10 production in human and murine T cells.[162] IL-27 therefore acts on naïve T cells to produce IL-21, which acts as an autocrine growth factor for developing Tr1 cells.

Tr1 Cells and Transcription Factors

Unlike T_H1, T_H2 and T_H17 cells, a lineage-specific transcription factor has not yet been identified for IL-10-producing Tr1 cells. TGF-β and IL-27 induces the expression of T-bet, which supports IFN-γ induction in IL-10+ T cells.[149] Interestingly, T-bet-deficient mice have increased IL-10 production during *Mycobacterium* infection, thus ruling out the involvement of T-bet as a transcription factor for IL-10 induction in Tr1 cells.[163] A recent study showed that GATA-3 is essential in stabilizing and remodeling of the *Il10* locus.[164] IL-27 alone, or in combination with TGF-β, does not induce GATA-3 expression.[149] In fact, both TGF-β and IL-27 were shown to antagonize GATA-3 expression.[165,166] IL-27 activates STAT-1, STAT-3, STAT-4 and STAT-5. IL-27-mediated STAT-1 is necessary to induce T-bet expression. Notably, the IL-10 promoter has a STAT-binding site, suggesting possible involvement of STAT proteins in the generation of IL-10 via IL-27 and TGF-β. Recent studies revealed that c-Maf, which was initially believed to be a transcription factor for T_H2 cells, is highly expressed in IL-10-producing Tr1 cells. Interestingly, in addition to IL-10, c-Maf transactivates IL-21 transcription, which further amplifies the generation of Tr1 cells.[167] It is interesting to note that both T_H17 and T_{FH} cells produce IL-10 and also express c-Maf, raising the possibility that c-Maf is the transcription factor for IL-10.[70,115,167] Recent data further demonstrated that both the IL-21 and IL-10 promoters have c-Maf binding sites and c-Maf can in turn transactivate their expression.[104,167] We propose that IL-27 induced c-Maf may be the transcription factor involved in induction of both IL-21 and IL-10 in Tr1 cells.[104] (Fig. 2.5).

ACKNOWLEDGMENTS

This work was supported by grants from National Institutes of Health, National Multiple Sclerosis Society and the Juvenile Diabetes Research Foundation Center for Immunological Tolerance at Harvard Medical School. VKK is a recipient of the Javits Neuroscience Investigator Award from the US National Institutes of Health. AA is supported by a post-doctoral fellowship from the National Multiple Sclerosis Society (NMSS), New York.

REFERENCES

1. Mosmann TR, Cherwinski H, Bond MW, Giedlin MA, Coffman RL. Two types of murine helper T cell clone. I. Definition according to profiles of lymphokine activities and secreted proteins. J Immunol 1986;136:2348-57.
2. Mosmann TR, Coffman RL. T_H1 and T_H2 cells: Different patterns of lymphokine secretion lead to different functional properties. Annu Rev Immunol 1989;7:145-73.
3. Kaplan MH, Sun YL, Hoey T, Grusby MJ. Impaired IL-12 responses and enhanced development of T_H2 cells in STAT-4-deficient mice. Nature 1996;382:174-7.

4. Thierfelder WE, van Deursen JM, Yamamoto K, et al. Requirement for STAT-4 in interleukin-12-mediated responses of natural killer and T cells. Nature 1996; 382:171-4.
5. Munder M, Mallo M, Eichmann K, Modolell M. Murine macrophages secrete interferon gamma upon combined stimulation with interleukin (IL)-12 and IL-18: A novel pathway of autocrine macrophage activation. J Exp Med 1998;187:2103-8.
6. Ohteki T, Fukao T, Suzue K, et al. Interleukin-12-dependent interferon gamma production by CD8alpha+ lymphoid dendritic cells. J Exp Med 1999;189:1981-6.
7. Boehm U, Klamp T, Groot M, Howard JC. Cellular responses to interferon-gamma. Annu Rev Immunol 1997;15:749-95.
8. Bach EA, Aguet M, Schreiber RD. The IFN gamma receptor: A paradigm for cytokine receptor signaling. Annu Rev Immunol 1997;15:563-91.
9. Dalton DK, Pitts-Meek S, Keshav S, Figari IS, Bradley A, Stewart TA. Multiple defects of immune cell function in mice with disrupted interferon-gamma genes. Science 1993;259:1739-42.
10. Durbin JE, Hackenmiller R, Simon MC, Levy DE. Targeted disruption of the mouse STAT-1 gene results in compromised innate immunity to viral disease. Cell 1996;84: 443-50.
11. Kamijo R, Le J, Shapiro D, et al. Mice that lack the interferon-gamma receptor have profoundly altered responses to infection with Bacillus Calmette-Guerin and subsequent challenge with lipopolysaccharide. J Exp Med 1993;178:1435-40.
12. Szabo SJ, Kim ST, Costa GL, Zhang X, Fathman CG, Glimcher LH. A novel transcription factor, T-bet, directs T_H1 lineage commitment Cell 2000;100:655-69.
13. Mullen AC, High FA, Hutchins AS, et al. Role of T-bet in commitment of T_H1 cells before IL-12-dependent selection. Science 2001;292:1907-10.
14. Szabo SJ, Dighe AS, Gubler U, Murphy KM. Regulation of the interleukin (IL)-12R beta 2 subunit expression in developing T helper 1 (T_H1) and T_H2 cells. J Exp Med 1997;185:817-24.
15. Lee YK, Turner H, Maynard CL, et al. Late developmental plasticity in the T helper 17 lineage. Immunity 2009;30:92-107.
16. Rangachari M, Mauermann N, Marty RR, et al. T-bet negatively regulates autoimmune myocarditis by suppressing local production of interleukin-17. J Exp Med 2006;203:2009-19.
17. Schulz O, Edwards AD, Schito M, et al. CD40 triggering of heterodimeric IL-12 p70 production by dendritic cells in vivo requires a microbial priming signal. Immunity 2000;13:453-62.
18. Hsieh CS, Macatonia SE, Tripp CS, Wolf SF, O'Garra A, Murphy KM. Development of TH1 CD4+ T cells through IL-12 produced by Listeria-induced macrophages. Science 1993;260:547-9.
19. Gately MK, Renzetti LM, Magram J, et al. The interleukin-12/interleukin-12-receptor system: Role in normal and pathologic immune responses. Annu Rev Immunol 1998;16:495-521.
20. Fantuzzi G, Reed DA, Dinarello CA. IL-12-induced IFN-gamma is dependent on caspase-1 processing of the IL-18 precursor. J Clin Invest 1999;104:761-7.
21. Sims JE. IL-1 and IL-18 receptors, and their extended family. Curr Opin Immunol 2002;14:117-22.
22. Takeda K, Tsutsui H, Yoshimoto T, et al. Defective NK cell activity and Th1 response in IL-18-deficient mice. Immunity 1998;8:383-90.
23. Xu D, Chan WL, Leung BP, et al. Selective expression and functions of interleukin-18 receptor on T helper (Th) type 1 but not Th2 cells. J Exp Med 1998;188:1485-92.
24. Robinson D, Shibuya K, Mui A, et al. IGIF does not drive Th1 development but synergizes with IL-12 for interferon-gamma production and activates IRAK and NFkappaB. Immunity 1997;7:571-81.
25. Adachi O, Kawai T, Takeda K, et al. Targeted disruption of the MyD88 gene results in loss of IL-1- and IL-18-mediated function. Immunity 1998;9:143-50.
26. Cao Z, Xiong J, Takeuchi M, Kurama T, Goeddel DV. TRAF6 is a signal transducer for interleukin-1. Nature 1996;383:443-6.
27. Gracie JA, Forsey RJ, Chan WL, et al. A proinflammatory role for IL-18 in rheumatoid arthritis. J Clin Invest 1999;104:1393-401.
28. Maerten P, Shen C, Colpaert S, et al. Involvement of interleukin-18 in Crohn's disease: Evidence from in vitro analysis of human gut inflammatory cells and from experimental colitis models. Clin Exp Immunol 2004;135:310-7.
29. Wildbaum G, Youssef S, Grabie N, Karin N. Neutralizing antibodies to IFN-gamma-inducing factor prevent experimental autoimmune encephalomyelitis. J Immunol 1998;161:6368-74.
30. Leung BP, McInnes IB, Esfandiari E, Wei XQ, Liew FY. Combined effects of IL-12 and IL-18 on the induction of collagen-induced arthritis. J Immunol 2000;164:6495-502.
31. Szabo SJ, Sullivan BM, Peng SL, Glimcher LH. Molecular mechanisms regulating Th1 immune responses. Annu Rev Immunol 2003;21:713-58.
32. Afkarian M, Sedy JR, Yang J, et al. T-bet is a STAT-1-induced regulator of IL-12R expression in naive CD4+ T cells. Nat Immunol 2002;3:549-57.
33. Szabo SJ, Sullivan BM, Stemmann C, Satoskar AR, Sleckman BP, Glimcher LH. Distinct effects of T-bet in TH1 lineage commitment and IFN-gamma production in CD4 and CD8 T cells. Science 2002;295:338-42.
34. Finotto S, Neurath MF, Glickman JN, et al. Development of spontaneous airway changes consistent with human asthma in mice lacking T-bet. Science 2002;295:336-8.
35. Bettelli E, Sullivan B, Szabo SJ, Sobel RA, Glimcher LH, Kuchroo VK. Loss of T-bet, but not STAT-1, prevents the development of experimental autoimmune encephalomyelitis. J Exp Med 2004;200:79-87.
36. Mullen AC, Hutchins AS, High FA, et al. Hlx is induced by and genetically interacts with T-bet to promote

36. heritable T(H)1 gene induction. Nat Immunol 2002;3: 652-8.
37. Murray HW, Spitalny GL, Nathan CF. Activation of mouse peritoneal macrophages in vitro and in vivo by interferon-gamma. J Immunol 1985;134:1619-22.
38. Awasthi A, Mathur RK, Saha B. Immune response to Leishmania infection. Indian J Med Res 2004;119:238-58.
39. Kopf M, Brombacher F, Kohler G, et al. IL-4-deficient Balb/c mice resist infection with Leishmania major. J Exp Med 1996;184:1127-36.
40. Park AY, Hondowicz BD, Scott P. IL-12 is required to maintain a T_H1 response during Leishmania major infection. J Immunol 2000;165:896-902.
41. Afonso LC, Scharton TM, Vieira LQ, Wysocka M, Trinchieri G, Scott P. The adjuvant effect of interleukin-12 in a vaccine against Leishmania major. Science 1994;263:235-7.
42. Scharton-Kersten T, Contursi C, Masumi A, Sher A, Ozato K. Interferon consensus sequence binding protein-deficient mice display impaired resistance to intracellular infection due to a primary defect in interleukin-12 p40 induction. J Exp Med 1997;186:1523-34.
43. Lieberman LA, Cardillo F, Owyang AM, et al. IL-23 provides a limited mechanism of resistance to acute toxoplasmosis in the absence of IL-12. J Immunol 2004;173:1887-93.
44. Khader SA, Bell GK, Pearl JE, et al. IL-23 and IL-17 in the establishment of protective pulmonary CD4+ T cell responses after vaccination and during Mycobacterium tuberculosis challenge. Nat Immunol 2007;8:369-77.
45. Kamanaka M, Yu P, Yasui T, et al. Protective role of CD40 in Leishmania major infection at two distinct phases of cell-mediated immunity. Immunity 1996;4:275-81.
46. Soong L, Xu JC, Grewal IS, et al. Disruption of CD40-CD40 ligand interactions results in an enhanced susceptibility to Leishmania amazonensis infection. Immunity 1996;4:263-73.
47. Bettelli E, Korn T, Oukka M, Kuchroo VK. Induction and effector functions of T(H)17 cells. Nature 2008;453: 1051-7.
48. Neurath MF, Finotto S, Glimcher LH. The role of Th1/Th2 polarization in mucosal immunity. Nat Med 2002;8:567-73.
49. Ito H, Fathman CG. CD45RBhigh CD4+ T cells from IFN-gamma knockout mice do not induce wasting disease. J Autoimmun 1997;10:455-9.
50. Powrie F, Leach MW, Mauze S, Menon S, Caddle LB, Coffman RL. Inhibition of Th1 responses prevents inflammatory bowel disease in scid mice reconstituted with CD45RBhi CD4+ T cells. Immunity 1994;1:553-62.
51. Neurath MF, Weigmann B, Finotto S, et al. The transcription factor T-bet regulates mucosal T cell activation in experimental colitis and Crohn's disease. J Exp Med 2002;195:1129-43.
52. Kuhn R, Lohler J, Rennick D, Rajewsky K, Muller W. Interleukin-10-deficient mice develop chronic enterocolitis. Cell 1993;75:263-74.
53. Nelms K, Keegan AD, Zamorano J, Ryan JJ, Paul WE. The IL-4 receptor: Signaling mechanisms and biologic functions. Annu Rev Immunol 1999;17:701-38.
54. Ansel KM, Djuretic I, Tanasa B, Rao A. Regulation of Th2 differentiation and Il4 locus accessibility. Annu Rev Immunol 2006;24:607-56.
55. van der Pouw Kraan TC, van Veen A, Boeije LC, et al. An IL-13 promoter polymorphism associated with increased risk of allergic asthma. Genes Immun. 1999;1:61-5.
56. Ryan JJ, McReynolds LJ, Keegan A, et al. Growth and gene expression are predominantly controlled by distinct regions of the human IL-4 receptor. Immunity 1996;4: 123-32.
57. Takeda K, Tanaka T, Shi W, et al. Essential role of STAT-6 in IL-4 signaling. Nature 1996;380:627-30.
58. Urban JF Jr, Noben-Trauth N, Donaldson DD, et al. IL-13, IL-4R alpha, and STAT-6 are required for the expulsion of the gastrointestinal nematode parasite Nippostrongylus brasiliensis. Immunity 1998;8:255-64.
59. Kaplan MH, Schindler U, Smiley ST, Grusby MJ. STAT-6 is required for mediating responses to IL-4 and for development of T_H2 cells. Immunity 1996;4:313-9.
60. Zheng W, Flavell RA. The transcription factor GATA-3 is necessary and sufficient for T_H2 cytokine gene expression in CD4 T cells. Cell 1997;89:587-96.
61. Lee HJ, Takemoto N, Kurata H, et al. GATA-3 induces T helper cell type 2 (T_H2) cytokine expression and chromatin remodeling in committed Th1 cells. J Exp Med 2000;192:105-15.
62. Ouyang W, Ranganath SH, Weindel K, et al. Inhibition of Th1 development mediated by GATA-3 through an IL-4-independent mechanism. Immunity 1998;9:745-55.
63. Zhang DH, Yang L, Cohn L, et al. Inhibition of allergic inflammation in a murine model of asthma by expression of a dominant-negative mutant of GATA-3. Immunity 1999;11:473-82.
64. Zhu J, Min B, Hu-Li J, et al. Conditional deletion of GATA-3 shows its essential function in T(H)1-T(H)2 responses. Nat Immunol 2004;5:1157-65.
65. Usui T, Nishikomori R, Kitani A, Strober W. GATA-3 suppresses T_H1 development by downregulation of STAT-4 and not through effects on IL-12R beta2 chain or T-bet. Immunity 2003;18:415-28.
66. Cote-Sierra J, Foucras G, Guo L, et al. Interleukin-2 plays a central role in T_H2 differentiation. Proc Natl Acad Sci USA 2004;101:3880-5.
67. Zhu J, Cote-Sierra J, Guo L, Paul WE. STAT-5 activation plays a critical role in T_H2 differentiation. Immunity 2003;19:739-48.
68. Takatori H, Nakajima H, Kagami S, et al. STAT-5a inhibits IL-12-induced T_H1 cell differentiation through the induction of suppressor of cytokine signaling 3 expression. J Immunol 2005;174:4105-12.
69. Ho IC, Hodge MR, Rooney JW, Glimcher LH. The proto-oncogene c-Maf is responsible for tissue-specific expression of interleukin-4. Cell 1996;85:973-83.

70. Bauquet AT, Jin H, Paterson AM, et al. The co-stimulatory molecule ICOS regulates the expression of c-Maf and IL-21 in the development of follicular T helper cells and T(H)-17 cells. Nat Immunol 2008.
71. Amsen D, Blander JM, Lee GR, Tanigaki K, Honjo T, Flavell RA. Instruction of distinct CD4 T helper cell fates by different notch ligands on antigen-presenting cells. Cell 2004;117:515-26.
72. Amsen D, Antov A, Flavell RA. The different faces of Notch in T-helper-cell differentiation. Nat Rev Immunol 2009;9:116-24.
73. Nabors GS, Farrell JP. Depletion of interleukin-4 in BALB/c mice with established Leishmania major infections increases the efficacy of antimony therapy and promotes T_H1-like responses. Infect Immun 1994;62:5498-504.
74. Palendira U, Kamath AT, Feng CG, et al. Coexpression of interleukin-12 chains by a self-splicing vector increases the protective cellular immune response of DNA and Mycobacterium bovis BCG vaccines against Mycobacterium tuberculosis. Infect Immun 2002;70:1949-56.
75. Finkelman FD, Madden KB, Cheever AW, et al. Effects of interleukin-12 on immune responses and host protection in mice infected with intestinal nematode parasites. J Exp Med 1994;179:1563-72.
76. Cheever AW, Williams ME, Wynn TA, et al. Anti-IL-4 treatment of Schistosoma mansoni-infected mice inhibits development of T cells and non-B, non-T cells expressing T_H2 cytokines while decreasing egg-induced hepatic fibrosis. J Immunol 1994;153:753-9.
77. Urban JF Jr, Schopf L, Morris SC, et al. STAT-6 signaling promotes protective immunity against Trichinella spiralis through a mast cell- and T cell-dependent mechanism. J Immunol 2000;164:2046-52.
78. Cohn L, Elias JA, Chupp GL. Asthma: Mechanisms of disease persistence and progression. Annu Rev Immunol 2004;22:789-815.
79. Ray A, Cohn L. T_H2 cells and GATA-3 in asthma: New insights into the regulation of airway inflammation. J Clin Invest 1999;104:985-93.
80. Li XM, Chopra RK, Chou TY, Schofield BH, Wills-Karp M, Huang SK. Mucosal IFN-gamma gene transfer inhibits pulmonary allergic responses in mice. J Immunol 1996;157:3216-9.
81. Wynn TA. IL-13 effector functions. Annu Rev Immunol 2003;21:425-56.
82. Wakashin H, Hirose K, Iwamoto I, Nakajima H. Role of IL-23-Th17 cell axis in allergic airway inflammation. Int Arch Allergy Immunol 2009;149 Suppl 1:108-12.
83. Oppmann B, Lesley R, Blom B, et al. Novel p19 protein engages IL-12p40 to form a cytokine, IL-23, with biological activities similar as well as distinct from IL-12. Immunity 2000;13:715-25.
84. Cua DJ, Sherlock J, Chen Y, et al. Interleukin-23 rather than interleukin-12 is the critical cytokine for autoimmune inflammation of the brain. Nature 2003;421:744-8.
85. Bettelli E, Carrier Y, Gao W, et al. Reciprocal developmental pathways for the generation of pathogenic effector T_H17 and regulatory T cells. Nature 2006;441:235-8.
86. Veldhoen M, Hocking RJ, Atkins CJ, Locksley RM, Stockinger B. TGFbeta in the context of an inflammatory cytokine milieu supports de novo differentiation of IL-17-producing T cells. Immunity 2006;24:179-89.
87. Mangan PR, Harrington LE, O'Quinn DB, et al. Transforming growth factor-beta induces development of the T(H)17 lineage. Nature 2006;441:231-4.
88. Veldhoen M, Hocking RJ, Flavell RA, Stockinger B. Signals mediated by transforming growth factor-beta initiate autoimmune encephalomyelitis, but chronic inflammation is needed to sustain disease. Nat Immunol 2006;7:1151-6.
89. Okuda Y, Sakoda S, Bernard CC, et al. IL-6-deficient mice are resistant to the induction of experimental autoimmune encephalomyelitis provoked by myelin oligodendrocyte glycoprotein. Int Immunol 1998;10:703-8.
90. Korn T, Mitsdoerffer M, Croxford AL, et al. IL-6 controls T_H17 immunity in vivo by inhibiting the conversion of conventional T cells into Foxp3+ regulatory T cells. Proc Natl Acad Sci USA 2008;105:18460-5.
91. Laurence A, Tato CM, Davidson TS, et al. Interleukin-2 signaling via STAT-5 constrains T helper 17 cell generation. Immunity 2007;26:371-81.
92. Mucida D, Park Y, Kim G, et al. Reciprocal T_H17 and regulatory T cell differentiation mediated by retinoic acid. Science 2007;317:256-60.
93. Xiao S, Jin H, Korn T, et al. Retinoic acid increases Foxp3+ regulatory T cells and inhibits development of T_H17 cells by enhancing TGF-beta-driven Smad3 signaling and inhibiting IL-6 and IL-23 receptor expression. J Immunol 2008;181:2277-84.
94. Zhou L, Lopes JE, Chong MM, et al. TGF-beta-induced Foxp3 inhibits T(H)17 cell differentiation by antagonizing RORgammat function. Nature 2008;453:236-40.
95. Tzartos JS, Friese MA, Craner MJ, et al. Interleukin-17 production in central nervous system-infiltrating T cells and glial cells is associated with active disease in multiple sclerosis. Am J Pathol 2008;172:146-55.
96. Fujino S, Andoh A, Bamba S, et al. Increased expression of interleukin-17 in inflammatory bowel disease. Gut 2003;52:65-70.
97. Zaba LC, Cardinale I, Gilleaudeau P, et al. Amelioration of epidermal hyperplasia by TNF inhibition is associated with reduced T_H17 responses. J Exp Med 2007;204:3183-94.
98. Acosta-Rodriguez EV, Napolitani G, Lanzavecchia A, Sallusto F. Interleukins 1beta and 6 but not transforming growth factor-beta are essential for the differentiation of interleukin 17-producing human T helper cells. Nat Immunol 2007;8:942-9.
99. Wilson NJ, Boniface K, Chan JR, et al. Development, cytokine profile and function of human interleukin-17-producing helper T cells. Nat Immunol 2007;8:950-7.

100. Manel N, Unutmaz D, Littman DR. The differentiation of human T(H)-17 cells requires transforming growth factor-beta and induction of the nuclear receptor RORgammat. Nat Immunol 2008;9:641-9.
101. Yang L, Anderson DE, Baecher-Allan C, et al. IL-21 and TGF-beta are required for differentiation of human T(H)17 cells. Nature 2008;454:350-2.
102. Parrish-Novak J, Dillon SR, Nelson A, et al. Interleukin-21 and its receptor are involved in NK cell expansion and regulation of lymphocyte function. Nature 2000;408:57-63.
103. Leonard WJ, Zeng R, Spolski R. Interleukin-21: A cytokine/cytokine receptor system that has come of age. J Leukoc Biol 2008;84:348-56.
104. Pot C JH, Awasthi A, Liu SM, Miaw SC, Lai CY, Madan R, Sharpe AH, Karp CL, Ho IC and Kuchroo VK. IL-27 induces the transcription factor c-Maf, cytokine IL-21 and costimulatory receptor ICOS that coordinately act together to promote differentiation of IL-10-producing Tr1 cells. Journal of Immunology. 2009;In press.
105. Korn T, Bettelli E, Gao W, et al. IL-21 initiates an alternative pathway to induce proinflammatory T(H)17 cells. Nature 2007;448:484-7.
106. Zhou L, Ivanov, II, Spolski R, et al. IL-6 programs T(H)-17 cell differentiation by promoting sequential engagement of the IL-21 and IL-23 pathways. Nat Immunol 2007;8:967-74.
107. Nurieva R, Yang XO, Martinez G, et al. Essential autocrine regulation by IL-21 in the generation of inflammatory T cells. Nature 2007;448:480-3.
108. Coquet JM, Chakravarti S, Smyth MJ, Godfrey DI. Cutting edge: IL-21 is not essential for Th17 differentiation or experimental autoimmune encephalomyelitis. J Immunol 2008;180:7097-101.
109. Spolski R, Kashyap M, Robinson C, Yu Z, Leonard WJ. IL-21 signaling is critical for the development of type I diabetes in the NOD mouse. Proc Natl Acad Sci USA 2008;105:14028-33.
110. Gran B, Zhang GX, Yu S, et al. IL-12p35-deficient mice are susceptible to experimental autoimmune encephalomyelitis: Evidence for redundancy in the IL-12 system in the induction of central nervous system autoimmune demyelination. J Immunol 2002;169:7104-10.
111. Langrish CL, Chen Y, Blumenschein WM, et al. IL-23 drives a pathogenic T cell population that induces autoimmune inflammation. J Exp Med 2005;201:233-40.
112. Parham C, Chirica M, Timans J, et al. A receptor for the heterodimeric cytokine IL-23 is composed of IL-12Rbeta1 and a novel cytokine receptor subunit, IL-23R. J Immunol 2002;168:5699-708.
113. Awasthi A, Riol-Blanco L, Jager A, et al. Cutting edge: IL-23 receptor gfp reporter mice reveal distinct populations of IL-17-producing cells. J Immunol 2009;182:5904-8.
114. McGeachy MJ, Chen Y, Tato CM, et al. The interleukin-23 receptor is essential for the terminal differentiation of interleukin 17-producing effector T helper cells in vivo. Nat Immunol 2009;10:314-24.
115. McGeachy MJ, Bak-Jensen KS, Chen Y, et al. TGF-beta and IL-6 drive the production of IL-17 and IL-10 by T cells and restrain T(H)-17 cell-mediated pathology. Nat Immunol 2007;8:1390-7.
116. Duerr RH, Taylor KD, Brant SR, et al. A genome-wide association study identifies IL23R as an inflammatory bowel disease gene. Science 2006;314:1461-3.
117. Rahman P, Inman RD, Maksymowych WP, Reeve JP, Peddle L, Gladman DD. Association of Interleukin-23 Receptor Variants with Psoriatic Arthritis. J Rheumatol, 2008.
118. Harris TJ, Grosso JF, Yen HR, et al. Cutting edge: An in vivo requirement for STAT-3 signaling in T_H17 development and T_H17-dependent autoimmunity. J Immunol 2007;179:4313-7.
119. Ivanov, II, McKenzie BS, Zhou L, et al. The orphan nuclear receptor RORgammat directs the differentiation program of proinflammatory IL-17+ T helper cells. Cell 2006;126:1121-33.
120. Zhang F, Meng G, Strober W. Interactions among the transcription factors Runx1, RORgammat and Foxp3 regulate the differentiation of interleukin-17-producing T cells. Nat Immunol 2008;9:1297-306.
121. Yang XO, Pappu BP, Nurieva R, et al. T helper 17 lineage differentiation is programmed by orphan nuclear receptors ROR alpha and ROR gamma. Immunity 2008;28:29-39.
122. Nurieva RI, Chung Y, Hwang D, et al. Generation of T follicular helper cells is mediated by interleukin-21 but independent of T helper 1, 2, or 17 cell lineages. Immunity 2008;29:138-49.
123. Brustle A, Heink S, Huber M, et al. The development of inflammatory T(H)-17 cells requires interferon-regulatory factor 4. Nat Immunol. 2007;8:958-66.
124. Huber M, Brustle A, Reinhard K, et al. IRF4 is essential for IL-21-mediated induction, amplification, and stabilization of the T_H17 phenotype. Proc Natl Acad Sci USA 2008;105:20846-51.
125. McGeachy MJ, Cua DJ. T_H17 cell differentiation: The long and winding road. Immunity 2008;28:445-53.
126. Lock C, Hermans G, Pedotti R, et al. Gene-microarray analysis of multiple sclerosis lesions yields new targets validated in autoimmune encephalomyelitis. Nat Med 2002;8:500-8.
127. Nakae S, Nambu A, Sudo K, Iwakura Y. Suppression of immune induction of collagen-induced arthritis in IL-17-deficient mice. J Immunol 2003;171:6173-7.
128. Komiyama Y, Nakae S, Matsuki T, et al. IL-17 plays an important role in the development of experimental autoimmune encephalomyelitis. J Immunol 2006;177:566-73.
129. Hofstetter HH, Ibrahim SM, Koczan D, et al. Therapeutic efficacy of IL-17 neutralization in murine experimental autoimmune encephalomyelitis. Cell Immunol 2005;237:123-30.
130. Kishimoto T. Interleukin-6: From basic science to medicine—40 years in immunology. Annu Rev Immunol 2005;23:1-21.

131. Milner JD, Brenchley JM, Laurence A, et al. Impaired T(H)17 cell differentiation in subjects with autosomal dominant hyper-IgE syndrome. Nature 2008;452:773-6.
132. Rudner XL, Happel KI, Young EA, Shellito JE. Interleukin-23 (IL-23)-IL-17 cytokine axis in murine Pneumocystis carinii infection. Infect Immun 2007;75:3055-61.
133. Happel KI, Dubin PJ, Zheng M, et al. Divergent roles of IL-23 and IL-12 in host defense against Klebsiella pneumoniae. J Exp Med 2005;202:761-9.
134. Happel KI, Zheng M, Young E, et al. Cutting edge: Roles of Toll-like receptor 4 and IL-23 in IL-17 expression in response to Klebsiella pneumoniae infection. J Immunol 2003;170:4432-6.
135. Aujla SJ, Chan YR, Zheng M, et al. IL-22 mediates mucosal host defense against gram-negative bacterial pneumonia. Nat Med 2008;14:275-81.
136. Khader SA, Cooper AM. IL-23 and IL-17 in tuberculosis. Cytokine 2008;41:79-83.
137. Kelly MN, Kolls JK, Happel K, et al. Interleukin-17/interleukin-17 receptor-mediated signaling is important for generation of an optimal polymorphonuclear response against Toxoplasma gondii infection. Infect Immun 2005;73:617-21.
138. Pflanz S, Timans JC, Cheung J, et al. IL-27, a heterodimeric cytokine composed of EBI3 and p28 protein, induces proliferation of naïve CD4(+) T cells. Immunity 2002;16:779-90.
139. Takeda A, Hamano S, Yamanaka A, et al. Cutting edge: Role of IL-27/WSX-1 signaling for induction of T-bet through activation of STAT-1 during initial T_H1 commitment. J Immunol 2003;170:4886-90.
140. Holscher C, Holscher A, Ruckerl D, et al. The IL-27 receptor chain WSX-1 differentially regulates antibacterial immunity and survival during experimental tuberculosis. J Immunol 2005;174:3534-44.
141. Artis D, Villarino A, Silverman M, et al. The IL-27 receptor (WSX-1) is an inhibitor of innate and adaptive elements of type 2 immunity. J Immunol 2004;173:5626-34.
142. Villarino A, Hibbert L, Lieberman L, et al. The IL-27R (WSX-1) is required to suppress T cell hyperactivity during infection. Immunity 2003;19:645-55.
143. Rosas LE, Satoskar AA, Roth KM, et al. Interleukin-27R (WSX-1/T-cell cytokine receptor) gene-deficient mice display enhanced resistance to Leishmania donovani infection but develop severe liver immunopathology. Am J Pathol 2006;168:158-69.
144. Hamano S, Himeno K, Miyazaki Y, et al. WSX-1 is required for resistance to Trypanosoma cruzi infection by regulation of proinflammatory cytokine production. Immunity 2003;19:657-67.
145. Pflanz S, Hibbert L, Mattson J, et al. WSX-1 and glycoprotein 130 constitute a signal-transducing receptor for IL-27. J Immunol 2004;172:2225-31.
146. Stumhofer JS, Laurence A, Wilson EH, et al. Interleukin-27 negatively regulates the development of interleukin-17-producing T helper cells during chronic inflammation of the central nervous system. Nat Immunol 2006;7:937-45.
147. Batten M, Li J, Yi S, et al. Interleukin-27 limits autoimmune encephalomyelitis by suppressing the development of interleukin-17-producing T cells. Nat Immunol 2006;7:929-36.
148. Diveu C, McGeachy MJ, Boniface K, et al. IL-27 blocks RORc expression to inhibit lineage commitment of T_H17 cells. J Immunol 2009;182:5748-56.
149. Awasthi A, Carrier Y, Peron JP, et al. A dominant function for interleukin-27 in generating interleukin 10-producing anti-inflammatory T cells. Nat Immunol 2007;8:1380-9.
150. Stumhofer JS, Silver JS, Laurence A, et al. Interleukins-27 and 6 induce STAT-3-mediated T cell production of interleukin-10. Nat Immunol 2007;8:1363-71.
151. Fitzgerald DC, Zhang GX, El-Behi M, et al. Suppression of autoimmune inflammation of the central nervous system by interleukin-10 secreted by interleukin-27-stimulated T cells. Nat Immunol 2007;8:1372-9.
152. Battaglia M, Gregori S, Bacchetta R, Roncarolo MG. Tr1 cells: From discovery to their clinical application. Semin Immunol 2006;18:120-7.
153. Ziegler SF. FOXP3: of mice and men. Annu Rev Immunol 2006;24:209-26.
154. Sher A, Fiorentino D, Caspar P, Pearce E, Mosmann T. Production of IL-10 by CD4+ T lymphocytes correlates with downregulation of T_H1 cytokine synthesis in helminth infection. J Immunol 1991;147:2713-6.
155. Enk AH, Angeloni VL, Udey MC, Katz SI. Inhibition of Langerhans cell antigen-presenting function by IL-10. A role for IL-10 in induction of tolerance. J Immunol 1993;151:2390-8.
156. Ding L, Shevach EM. IL-10 inhibits mitogen-induced T cell proliferation by selectively inhibiting macrophage costimulatory function. J Immunol 1992;148:3133-9.
157. Groux H, O'Garra A, Bigler M, et al. A CD4+ T-cell subset inhibits antigen-specific T-cell responses and prevents colitis. Nature 1997;389:737-42.
158. Barrat FJ, Cua DJ, Boonstra A, et al. In vitro generation of interleukin-10-producing regulatory CD4(+) T cells is induced by immunosuppressive drugs and inhibited by T helper type 1 (T_H1)- and T_H2-inducing cytokines. J Exp Med 2002;195:603-16.
159. Vieira PL, Christensen JR, Minaee S, et al. IL-10-secreting regulatory T cells do not express Foxp3 but have comparable regulatory function to naturally occurring CD4+CD25+ regulatory T cells. J Immunol 2004;172:5986-93.
160. Bacchetta R, Sartirana C, Levings MK, Bordignon C, Narula S, Roncarolo MG. Growth and expansion of human T regulatory type 1 cells are independent from TCR activation but require exogenous cytokines. Eur J Immunol 2002;32:2237-45.
161. Spolski R, Kim HP, Zhu W, Levy DE, Leonard WJ. IL-21 mediates suppressive effects via its induction of IL-10. J Immunol 2009;182:2859-67.
162. Lohning M, Hutloff A, Kallinich T, et al. Expression of ICOS in vivo defines CD4+ effector T cells with high

inflammatory potential and a strong bias for secretion of interleukin-10. J Exp Med 2003;197:181-93.
163. Sullivan BM, Jobe O, Lazarevic V, et al. Increased susceptibility of mice lacking T-bet to infection with Mycobacterium tuberculosis correlates with increased IL-10 and decreased IFN-gamma production. J Immunol 2005;175:4593-602.
164. Shoemaker J, Saraiva M, O'Garra A. GATA-3 directly remodels the IL-10 locus independently of IL-4 in CD4+ T cells. J Immunol 2006;176:3470-9.
165. Gorelik L, Fields PE, Flavell RA. Cutting edge: TGF-beta inhibits Th type 2 development through inhibition of GATA-3 expression. J Immunol 2000;165:4773-7.
166. Yoshimoto T, Yasuda K, Mizuguchi J, Nakanishi K. IL-27 suppresses T_H2 cell development and T_H2 cytokines production from polarized T_H2 cells: A novel therapeutic way for T_H2-mediated allergic inflammation. J Immunol 2007;179:4415-23.
167. Xu J, Yang Y, Qiu G, et al. c-Maf regulates IL-10 expression during T_H17 polarization. J Immunol 2009;182:6226-36.

Chapter 3

History of HLA

Erik Thorsby

INTRODUCTION

The "first" HLA antigen was described by the French immunogeneticist Jean Dausset in 1958, i.e. just over 50 years ago. It was initially detected as an alloantigen on human leukocytes, called MAC,[1] but later became HLA-A2. Since then we have seen a tremendous development in our knowledge of the HLA complex, both concerning the structure and function of its many genes and gene-products. It is impossible to give a full account of this development in a short book chapter. Thus, I will focus on some highlights in the history of HLA class I and II antigens, or molecules as they should be called now, which I consider to be among the most important. Further, it is impossible to mention all who have contributed to this development. I must therefore apologize to those whose important contributions could not be included for lack of space. The chapter is a revised and extended version of a recent short review by the author on the history of HLA.[2] Only some selected key references will be given in the text and are listed at the end of the chapter. References to other work mentioned in the text are found in the review mentioned above.[2] For a more comprehensive treatment of the subject the reader is referred to earlier extensive reviews by others.[3-5]

EARLY EXPERIMENTAL ALLOTRANSPLANTATIONS

Experimental allotransplantations started in the late 1800s, first by surgeons mainly using skin grafts, and later by tumor biologists to study the mechanisms behind tumor growth. It was the latter group of scientists who noted that while transplanted allogeneic tumors usually were rejected, sometimes a tumor would grow in the recipient if it belonged to the same stock as the donor of the tumor. In the early 1900s, two US geneticists, Ernest E Tyzzer and Clarence C Little performed some crucial tumor transplantation experiments in the offspring of crosses between mice who were susceptible or resistant to an allogeneic tumor. Based on the results they arrived at the conclusion that susceptibility to the growth of allogeneic tumors was genetically determined, possibly by as many as 15 genes. The nature of these susceptibility (or rather resistance) genes and their products was, however, unknown. The same was the case of the mechanisms responsible for the rejection.

REJECTION IS CAUSED BY AN IMMUNE RESPONSE

The fact that rejection of allografts was caused by an immune response was first demonstrated by the British biologist, Peter B Medawar in 1944-45. By performing allogeneic skin transplantation in rabbits he observed a massive infiltration of lymphocytes and monocytes in the rejecting grafts. Further, rejection led to *sensitization* which caused a quicker rejection of a second graft from the same donor, but often not of grafts from a third party donor, i.e. the sensitization was *specific* for the donor. In addition, he found that rejection was a *systemic* response and not localized to the site of the graft.[6,7] Based on these observations, Medawar concluded that rejection of an allograft is caused by a specific and systemic immune response against the graft. He received the Nobel prize in 1960 for his seminal observations (shared with another pioneer immunologist, Frank McFarlane Burnet).

IT STARTED IN THE MOUSE: DISCOVERY OF HISTOCOMPATIBILITY ANTIGEN II AND THE H-2 COMPLEX

An antigen responsible for rejection was first discovered by the British physician and pathologist, Peter A Gorer (Fig. 3.1) in 1936, working at that time in the Lister Institute for Preventive Medicine in London. Following a suggestion from the British geneticist JBS Haldane, he studied whether resistance factors to the growth of allogeneic tumors might be associated with some blood group antigens. First he found that his own serum contained "natural" antibodies which could distinguish between erythrocytes of three inbred strains of mice. He next immunized rabbits with erythrocytes from the same three stains of mice and obtained antisera with which he could distinguish three different blood group antigens in mice:[8]

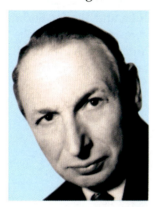

Fig. 3.1: Peter A Gorer (1907-1961)

- *Antigen I:* Shared by strains A and CBA, weakly expressed in C57BL
- *Antigen II:* Expressed strongly in strain A, weakly in CBA, but not in C57BL
- *Antigen III:* Shared by strains A, CBA and C57BL.

The rabbit antiserum recognizing antigen II behaved similar to his own serum.

He then grafted a tumor from a mouse of strain A (carrying antigen II) into mice of strain C57BL (lacking antigen II) and into offspring of crosses between these strains. He found that mice lacking antigen II quickly rejected the tumor, while it grew well in strain A and first and second generation crosses between A and C57BL which expressed antigen II. Further, he made the important observation that sera of mice rejecting the tumor contained antibodies against antigen II.[9] Thus antigen II, shared between malignant and normal cells, apparently was an important resistance factor to the growth of an allogeneic tumor, when present in the donor and absent in the recipient. Note that these findings were made before Peter Medawar first established that rejection of allogeneic transplants was caused by an immune response against the graft.

After World War II, Gorer visited the mammalian geneticist George D Snell (Fig. 3.2) at the Jackson Laboratory, Bar Harbor, Maine, US. Snell was studying tumor resistance genes, which he called *Histocompatibility or H* genes. He had previously found that mice carrying the *Fu* gene, causing mice to develop a deformed tail, were resistant to the growth of tumors from strain A.

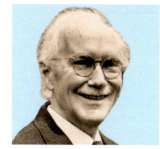

Fig. 3.2: George D Snell (1903-1996)

Thus, he concluded that there was a strong linkage between an *H* gene and the *Fu* gene. During his visit Gorer tested various backcross strains segregating for the *Fu* gene with his antiserum against antigen II, and found that erythrocytes of almost all mice carrying the *Fu* gene tested negative with his antiserum. In contrast, the presence of antigen II on erythrocytes of the host was strongly associated with growth of the tumor from strain A.[10] This was further strong evidence that antigen II was encoded by a gene at an H locus in strain A, and that the mice carrying the *Fu* gene probably carried another allele at the same locus. Their combined results indicated three alleles at this H locus. Since Gorer's antiserum against antigen II was the first to detect an allele at this H locus, it became *Histocompatibility locus 2*, or *H-2*.

The work of Gorer and Snell, extended by Snell and coworkers and others later,[3] established that the H-2 locus encoded strong or *major* histocompatibility antigens, inducing quick rejection, compared to weaker histocompatibility antigens encoded by other loci. The H-2 locus therefore became the *major* histocompatibility locus in mice. Other H loci became *minor* H loci.

Snell received the Nobel prize in 1980 for his contributions. At that time Gorer had passed away (he died in 1961). If not, he would no doubt have shared the prize with Snell.

Later the H-2 locus became more and more complex, seemingly consisting of several different "subdivisions", and where each allele apparently determined many different antigens. In 1970, I first suggested that the hitherto known H-2 genes belonged to two segregant series, encoded by two different loci, *D* and *K* respectively, similar to the at that time two known loci in the HLA complex.[11] Snell and coworkers arrived at a similar conclusion.[12] The two locus model for the H-2 antigens known at that time turned out to be correct. Subsequently, many additional H-2 loci were found, including those encoding the Ia antigens (see later). The H-2 locus became the H-2 *complex*, or the *major histocompatibility complex, MHC,* in the mouse.

DISCOVERY OF THE "FIRST" HLA ANTIGENS

Three papers appeared in 1958, by Jean Dausset, Jon van Rood and Rose Payne and their associates respectively,[1,13,14] which laid the foundation of what was later to become the *HLA complex*. All three papers described antibodies in human sera from multitransfused patients or multiparous women, sera which reacted with leukocytes from many but not all individuals who were tested. Thus, antibodies in these sera detected alloantigens on human leukocytes.

The credit for discovery of the "first" HLA antigen goes to Jean Dausset (Fig. 3.3). Studying sera from patients who had received multiple blood transfusions, he found seven sera which behaved quite similarly in that they agglutinated leukocytes from 11 out of 19 individuals tested.[1] Since leukocytes from the donor of the sera were also not agglutinated, the antisera obviously detected an alloantigen present on human leukocytes. He gave the name "MAC" to this antigen, to honor three individuals who had been important volunteers for his experiments, and whose names began with the initials M, A and C respectively. Antigen MAC (later to become HLA-A2) was present in approx. 60 percent of the French population. At the end of the paper Dausset wrote: "Finally, in a more long-time perspective, the study of leukocyte antigens might become of great importance in tissue transplantation, in particular in bone marrow transplantation" (translated from French). Thus, he was very foresighted! For his discovery, Dausset received the Nobel prize in 1980 (shared with Snell and Baruch Benacerraf).

Jon van Rood and Rose Payne both followed up their initial findings of alloantigens on human leukocytes. Using (at that time) a sophisticated computer analysis of the reaction patterns of 60 sera from multiparous women against leukocytes from a panel 100 donors, van Rood (Fig. 3.4) found some sera which apparently detected a diallelic system of leukocyte antigens, which he called 4a and 4b (later to become HLA-Bw4 and -Bw6, respectively). The results were reported in his PhD thesis in 1962.[15] Two years later Payne (Fig. 3.5), together with Julia and Walter Bodmer (see Fig. 3.9, later), also using sera from multiparous women, detected two leukocyte antigens, LA1 (later HLA-A1) and LA2 (later HLA-A2), apparently controlled by alleles, but also postulated at least one additional antigen, LA3, determined by an additional allele at the same locus.[16]

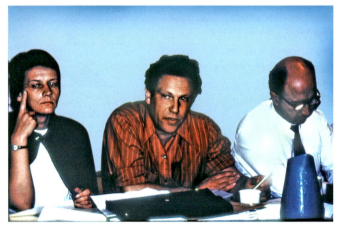

Fig. 3.4: Jon J van Rood (1926-) in the center, with his long-time associate Aad van Leeuwen (1929-2009) to the left, at one of the earlier IHWSs

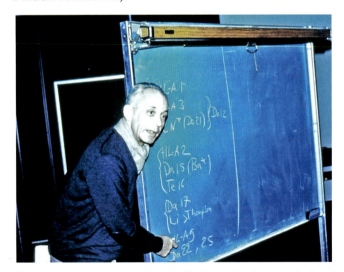

Fig. 3.3: Jean Dausset (1916-2009) discussing the complexity of HLA at one of the earlier International Histocompatibility Workshops (IHWSs)

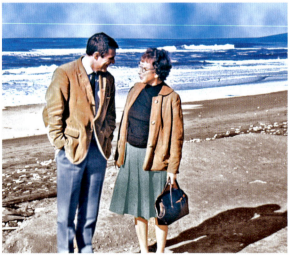

Fig. 3.5: Rose Payne (1909-1999), together with the author (1938-) just after the fourth IHWS in 1970

Several other investigators also made original or "first" identifications of leukocyte antigens in these early days of HLA. They included, among others, Bernard Amos, US; Richard Batchelor, UK; Ruggero Ceppellini, Italy; Paul Engelfriet, The Netherlands; Wolfgang Mayr, Austria; Flemming Kissmeyer-Nielsen, Denmark; Ray Shulman, US; Paul Terasaki, US; Roy Walford, US; and myself.[17]

SOLVING THE COMPLEXITY THROUGH INTERNATIONAL COLLABORATION: THE FIRST THREE INTERNATIONAL HISTOCOMPATIBILITY WORKSHOPS

The relationship between the different leukocyte (later HLA) antigens which had been identified, and their polymorphism and genetics, were difficult subjects to solve. No single laboratory could do this alone. Therefore, very early, *International Histocompatibility Workshops (IHWSs)* were established, where investigators in the field met to compare their reagents, techniques and results, and communicate new findings. The aims and results of all 15 workshops hitherto organized are briefly summarized in Table 3.1 (see later), and comprehensively treated in the proceedings from the workshops.[2]

The first three IHWSs were "wet" workshops where the investigators carried out their experiments together, in the same laboratory, using the same panel of cells. The first IHWS was organized by Bernard Amos (Fig. 3.6) as early as in June 1964, at Duke University, Durham, North Carolina, US. Amos should be considered the "father" of the workshops. He was also able to obtain funds from the National Institutes of Health, NIH, to organize the first workshops. The major aim of the first IHWS was to compare different techniques to detect leukocyte antigens, since a variety were in use by different investigators (leukoagglutination, the indirect antiglobulin consumption test, mixed agglutination, complement fixation, microcytotoxicity, etc.). Twenty-three investigators attended the workshop, testing the same sera and cells with their own techniques. Much to their dismay, most of the results were discordant.

These disappointing results, coupled with the fact that van Rood at the first IHWS had presented evidence also for other clusters of leukocyte antigens in addition to 4a and 4b, prompted van Rood to organize the second IHWS already in August the next year, at the University of Leiden, The Netherlands. Here investigators from 14 different groups tested their own antisera, using their own techniques, on cells from a common panel of 45 individuals. The main aim was to see if "local" specificities defined in one laboratory correlated with those defined in other laboratories. Most encouraging, it was now found that several local specificities were indeed identical or almost identical. These included the specificities MAC (of Dausset), LA2 (of Payne and the Bodmers), 8a (of van Rood), B1 (of Shulman) and Te2 (of Terasaki), later to become HLA-A2. Further, Dausset et al and van Rood et al also presented work suggesting that most of the antigens they could identify were controlled by a single chromosomal complex.

The third IHWS was organized by the well known human geneticist Ruggero Ceppellini (Fig. 3.7) at the University of Turin, Italy, in June 1967. The main aim was to study the genetics of the hitherto identified leukocyte antigens. Thus, the organizers included blood from 11 families, including monozygotic twins, which were tested "blindly" by the different investigators with

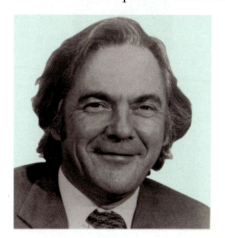

Fig. 3.6: Bernard Amos (1923-2003)

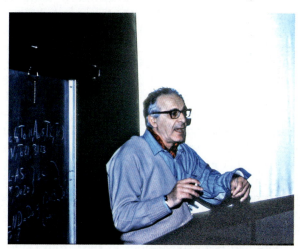

Fig. 3.7: Ruggero Ceppellini (1917-1988), giving a talk at one of the earlier IHWSs

their own typing antisera and techniques. Several investigators were now using the quicker and more reliable microcytotoxicity test, initially developed by Paul Terasaki (Fig. 3.11, later) and McClelland, which later became the standard serological typing technique for HLA antigens. The results demonstrated strong correlations between 13 local specificities. But more importantly, it was now fully established that most of these specificities were encoded by closely linked genes at one chromosomal region. This led to the designation *HL-A* for this chromosomal region, i.e. *human leukocyte; locus A*. This was later changed to *HLA* (without the hyphen), where *A* is now interpreted to mean antigen.

Just after the third IHWS, in 1968, an *HLA Nomenclature Committee* was established (first sponsored by the World Health Organization, WHO), consisting of leading investigators in the field. The Committee, which still exists, is responsible for giving official names to HLA specificities and loci. In the early days, an officially recognized or "accepted" HLA specificity was a specificity which could be recognized by several different investigators, using their own serological reagents. An account of the lively discussions at the first meeting of the Committee in New York in September 1968 is given by Roy Walford in ref. 5. By quickly establishing a common, uniform nomenclature and thus avoiding a long list of various, local specificities, the Committee has played a major role in unravelling the complexity of HLA genes and their products.

SEVERAL LOCI IN THE HLA CHROMOSOMAL REGION

The first to propose two HLA loci were Bodmer and Payne and their associates in 1966. They called the two loci "*LA*" (adapted from the LA antigens of Payne and coworkers) and "*4*" or "*Four*" (adapted from the 4a and 4b antigens of van Rood). At the third workshop in Turin, Ceppellini and coworkers also proposed that there were two different mutational sites within the HLA chromosomal region. It was, however, the work of Flemming Kissmeyer-Nielsen (Fig. 3.13, later) and associates in 1968 which firmly established that there were two HLA loci.[18] In extensive studies of unrelated individuals and families they showed that the two loci, *LA* (later named *HLA-A*) and *4* (later named *HLA-B*), were closely linked and contained at least seven and eight alleles, respectively.

There had been suggestions in 1969 from Dausset, Terasaki and Walford and their associates also of a third locus in the HLA chromosomal region. The strongest evidence came, however, from the studies by a Scandinavian group of an antiserum detecting a "new" leukocyte antigen, AJ, which in population and family studies behaved as if it was encoded by another HLA locus separate from LA and 4.[19] Later, we were able to show in cell-membrane capping experiments that antigen AJ indeed was independent of antigens encoded by the *LA* and *4* loci, which firmly demonstrated the existence of a third HLA locus. This was first called the *AJ* locus (from its "first" antigen), but was later named *HLA-C*.

In 1964, two groups, Bach and Hirschorn, and Bain, Vas and Lowenstein, independently described morphological transformation and cell division if leukocytes from two different individuals were mixed. This was to become the *mixed lymphocyte culture (MLC)* reaction. Fritz H Bach (Fig. 3.8) together with Amos then demonstrated that the MLC reaction was governed by genes in the HLA chromosomal region. Cells from siblings who were genotypically HLA identical generally did not respond to each other in reciprocal MLC tests.[20] Later Amos and Bach also obtained results indicating that the HLA determinants stimulating in the MLC test might not be identical to the serologically defined HLA-A and -B antigens. This was fully confirmed by Yunis and Amos in 1971[21] who demonstrated that there was a separate "*MLC locus*" in the HLA chromosomal region responsible for the determinants inducing the MLC response. From their studies in mice, Bach and co-workers then proposed in 1972 that there were two different types of determinants encoded by genes in the H-2 complex; serologically defined (*SD*) and lymphocyte defined (*LD*)

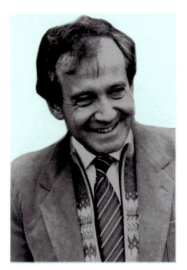

Fig. 3.8: Fritz H Bach (1934-)

determinants, the latter being responsible for stimulation in the MLC test, a concept which was also adapted for man.

This started an extensive hunt for the LD determinants in man. It was Mempel et al[22] who first suggested that MLC stimulating cells which were homozygous at the *LD* locus could be used to type for LD determinants in man, in that non-responsiveness of the responding cells would indicate that the stimulating and responding cells shared the same LD determinant(s). Several investigators showed that this indeed was possible, and multiple LD determinants were identified by what was generally called *MLC typing*. This was also a major topic at the sixth IHWS in 1975, organized by Kissmeyer-Nielsen in Aarhus, Denmark. By exchange of 62 LD homozygous typing cells, eight different LD determinants were clearly defined by MLC typing by the different participating laboratories, of which six LD determinants were accepted by the nomenclature committee and provisionally (by the prefix "w" = workshop) named HLA-Dw1-6. The corresponding "locus" was named *HLA-D*. Sheehy et al reported[23] that LD (or Dw) determinants could also be identified by priming lymphocytes against given LD determinants, which was called *primed LD typing; PLT*. Later studies showed that the provisional HLA-D locus consisted of several different closely linked loci, which encoded three different series of determinants; DR, DQ (previously called DC) and DP (previously called SB).

In the early 1970s, several groups reported that some sera which contained HLA antibodies were able to inhibit the MLC reaction. This was confirmed by van Leeuwen et al in 1973 who also obtained suggestive evidence that the responsible antibodies recognized antigens present on B cells, but not on T cells or platelets.[24] Thus these antisera might serologically detect HLA-D determinants. This was therefore made a major topic at the seventh IHWS in 1977, organized by Julia and Walter Bodmer (Fig. 3.9), in Oxford, UK. Using 177 selected antisera recognizing antigens on B cells, antisera which had been exchanged between the participating laboratories, it was possible to convincingly identify seven different B cell antigens which were closely correlated to the HLA-Dw1-7 determinants, and which therefore were named HLA-DRw1-7 (DR = D Related).

In the early 1980s, the overall picture was that the HLA chromosomal region, found to be present on the short arm of chromosome no. 6, encoded six different very polymorphic series of determinants; A, B and C which were present on most nucleated cells, and DR, DQ

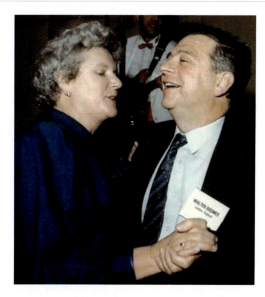

Fig. 3.9: Julia (1934-2001) and Walter Bodmer (1936-). Dancing has been one of the highlights at the farewell dinner of all IHWSs

and DP which were mainly present on B cells, monocytes and dendritic cells. In 1967, Ceppellini had introduced the term HLA *haplotype* for the genetic information carried by each of the two HLA chromosomal regions of an individual. In 1977, Jan Klein introduced the terms *class I* to describe the A, B and C antigens, and *class II* to describe the DR, DQ and DP antigens (and the corresponding antigens in other species), a nomenclature which has since been followed. Further, after the discovery of additional class I antigens, HLA- G, -E and -F, which have a more limited tissue distribution, the latter were named *non-classical* HLA class I antigens, while the HLA-A, -B and -C antigens were named *classical* HLA class I antigens.

Later, many additional loci were detected in the HLA chromosomal region, or the HLA *complex* as it is called now. As a matter of fact, in the extended HLA complex covering a total of 7.6 Mb, as many as 252 genes have been found expressed, of which approx. 28% may have immune functions (Fig. 3.10). This is further treated in other chapters in this book.

THE HLA CLASS I AND II ANTIGENS ARE STRONG HISTOCOMPATIBILITY ANTIGENS

From skin grafting experiments in the early1960s, both Dausset and coworkers and van Rood and coworkers had obtained evidence that the HLA antigens are strong histocompatibility antigens. This was confirmed and extended in studies by Ceppellini et al[25] and Amos et al.[26] They showed that first set skin grafts exchanged

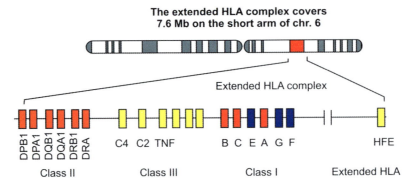

Fig. 3.10: A very simplified picture illustrating just some of the many loci in the extended HLA complex. Red squares: Classical HLA class I and II genes. Blue squares: Non-classical HLA class I genes. Yellow squares: Some other HLA complex genes

between HLA identical siblings (who had inherited the same HLA haplotypes from their parents) had a significantly longer survival time than skin grafts between siblings differing for one or two HLA haplotypes. Since, skin grafting resulted in the production of antibodies against HLA antigens of the donor, this was also evidence that the HLA antigens were important histocompatibility antigens.[27]

The first data suggesting a correlation between HLA matching and kidney allograft survival were presented by Terasaki (Fig. 3.11) and coworkers as early as in 1965.[28] These early results are quite remarkable given the broadly reacting serological typing reagents available at that time, and just typing for a few HLA-A and -B antigens. Other references to early work on the impact of HLA matching on clinical kidney transplantation are found in refs 4 and 27. Taken together, the results from skin and clinical kidney grafting, together with other evidence[27] demonstrated that the HLA complex indeed was the *major histocompatibility complex, MHC,* in man, as it had been previously shown for H-2 in mice.

At the start of the 1970s, it had become accepted that the survival of kidneys transplanted between HLA identical siblings was superior to all other combinations. HLA typing to obtain such or other well matched combinations in kidney transplantations from living related donors became of general use. Following several reports of better survival also of HLA matched compared to mismatched kidneys from cadaveric donors,[27] HLA typing to obtain well matched kidneys in such unrelated combinations was also used in many centers. However, the benefits of the latter application were hit hard by a presentation by Terasaki's group at the Third Congress of the International Transplantation Society in Hague, The Netherlands, in 1970. While HLA matching was found to be of great importance using living related donors, they reported no effects of HLA matching when instead cadaveric donors were used. The results raised such a storm at the Congress that their paper was not included in its proceedings. Instead, it was published separately in an article in *Tissue Antigens* in 1971,[29] accompanied by comments by its editor at that time, Kissmeyer-Nielsen, discussing reasons for the discrepancy between the disappointing results reported by Terasaki's group compared with the beneficial effects of HLA matching in cadaveric donor transplantation as reported by several others. The result was, however, that HLA matching in cadaveric donor transplantation went into a state of limbo. The differences in survival found between grafts from HLA matched and mismatched cadaveric donors were considered by many surgeons to be too small to matter.

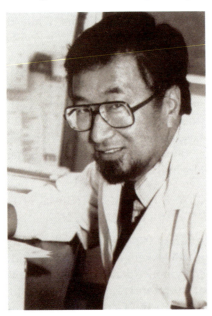

Fig. 3.11: Paul I Terasaki (1929-)

Following the identification of the HLA-DR antigens, the picture changed. Three independent studies published in 1978; one from Oxford, another from Oslo and a third from Leiden, all showed beneficial effects of matching for the HLA-DR antigens in cadaveric kidney transplantation. Our own studies[30] also demonstrated that the HLA-DR matching effect was seen irrespective of matching for the HLA-A and -B antigens (Figs 3.12A and B). The impact of HLA-DR matching was later also confirmed in studies by many others. The further developments in this area and the present use of HLA matching in clinical organ transplantation are treated in other chapters in this book.

While the role of HLA matching in clinical organ transplantation has continued to be a much discussed issue, the role of optimal HLA matching in bone marrow transplantation (BMT) or hematopoietic stem cell transplantation (HSCT) is universally accepted. Graft-versus-host disease (GVHD) is a major barrier to successful HSCT. Early successful HSCTs to children with inborn immunodeficiencies and patients with aplastic anemia were obtained by using HLA identical siblings as donors. It was also shown that it was particularly important that the MLC test between donor and recipient was negative, i.e. their HLA class II antigens had to be matched. Together this has resulted in the formation of large international registries of HLA typed volunteer HSC donors and banks of HLA typed cord blood, which have made it possible to offer HLA matched HSCT to most patients in need of this treatment. The more recent developments in this area are treated in other chapters in this book.

HLA ANTIGENS ARE ASSOCIATED WITH DISEASES

Already at the third IHWS in 1967, Amiel reported that an HLA antigen, 4C (later shown to be a "broad" antigen including several different HLA-B locus antigens), was found significantly more frequently in patients with Hodgkin's disease (51%) than among healthy individuals (27%).[31] The association was not strong, the relative risk, RR, (i.e. how much more frequently the disease occurs among individuals carrying the antigen under study compared to those lacking it) was just 2.8, and the observation has been hard to reproduce by others later. It led, however, to an extensive hunt for other HLA associated diseases.

In 1973 came the "big bang". Brewerton et al[32] and Schlosstein et al[33] independently reported a very strong association between HLA-B27 and ankylosing spondylitis. The studies found that 88-96% of the patients carried HLA-B27, compared to 8-4% of healthy controls, respectively. These data were later confirmed by many other groups, giving an RR of >100 to develop ankylosing spondylitis in individuals being positive for HLA-B27. The reason for this very strong association was unknown, but it was speculated that since the association was so strong, either an immune response (*Ir*) gene in strong linkage (disequilibrium) to the gene encoding HLA-B27 was involved, or there was a cross-reaction between HLA-B27 and the etiologic agent causing the disease. Later the same year Jersild and coworkers[34] first reported a strong disease association to an HLA class II antigen. Multiple sclerosis was found to be more strongly associated to a determinant as established by MLC typing, LD-7a (later to become HLA-Dw2, now -DR2), than HLA-B7.

Since, then many diseases have been found to be associated to given HLA antigens, in particular autoimmune diseases. Autoimmune diseases are the combined result of predisposing genes and precipitating environmental factors, and in almost all autoimmune diseases the strongest genetic predisposition is associated to one or more HLA antigens. Diseases associated to HLA antigens and the possible mechanisms involved are treated in detail in other chapters in this book.

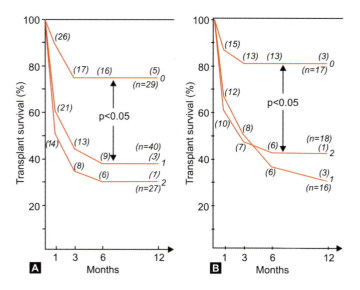

Figs 3.12A and B: Influence of HLA-DR matching in 96 transplants from a cadaveric donor. Left part shows the overall data, the right part shows the data for transplants mismatched for one or two HLA-A or–B antigens. 0, 1 and 2: Transplants mismatched for 0, 1 or 2 HLA-DR antigens respectively. Reprinted from The Lancet 312: 1126-7, copyright 1978, with permission from Elsevier

ROLE OF THE INTERNATIONAL HISTOCOMPATIBILITY WORKSHOPS

Science is of course to a large extent driven by competition between individual investigators. This has also been the case in the HLA field. However, there must be very few other scientific fields where international collaboration has played such a major role for the progress, mainly through the many International Histocompatibility Workshops (IHWSs). They have had an extremely important unifying influence on the studies of HLA. The IHWSs laid the ground for a continuous open and friendly collaboration between involved investigators all over the world, which is an important mark distinguishing this research field from many others. As reported above, the first three IHWSs were "wet" workshops where the investigators carried out their investigations in the laboratory of the workshop chairman. From the fourth IHWS, however, the project studies have been carried out locally in the laboratories of the investigators, to a large extent using exchanged reagents, followed by a joint workshop meeting to discuss the results (Fig. 3.13). More recently, a conference for a broader audience has also been arranged in conjunction with the workshop meetings, where not only the workshop results have been summarized, but also where individual scientists have presented their most recent research on HLA, its applications and related topics.

The important role of the first three "wet" workshops as well as some of the other early IHWSs for identification of the "first" HLA antigens, has been treated above. However, all workshops have been instrumental for the development of the HLA field and its application in research and clinical medicine. To just mention a few additional achievements, the fifth IHWS showed that HLA typing would become an important tool in anthropology; in the eighth IHWS, the role of HLA matching in clinical renal transplantation was an important aim; the ninth IHWS introduced various new techniques for studies of the polymorphism of HLA, as a result of the tenth IHWS a reference panel of well-typed cell lines was established which has been of great help for many investigators, and as a result of the thirteenth IHWS a publicly accessible database was established, which now contains a huge amount of data for future research. And so on, the list of what has been accomplished in the 15 workshops so far organized is long, very long. The work laid down by the workshop chairmen and their associates in organizing these workshops has been extensive, and so has also been the work of the participants. It is, however, impossible in this short review to give a comprehensive account of all projects that has been studied in these workshops, and the results obtained, for which I apologize to all workshop organizers and participants. Table 3.1 just gives a very short and incomplete summary of some important aims and results. For more details, the reader should consult the proceedings from the various workshops,[2] which not only contain the "Joint reports" which summarize the results of the various workshop projects, but also contain a lot of important results of research on HLA and its applications by individual investigators, presented at the workshop conferences. These proceedings are thus a rich source of information, and also demonstrate the extensive development which has taken place during the 45 years since the very first workshop was organized.

If I should try to very briefly summarize some important achievements of the workshops, I would list the following:

1. They have been instrumental for solving the complexity of HLA. This has been the case for all workshops, but in particular the early ones.
2. They have been necessary in order to carry out investigations which need large, international collaboration, involving many different centers. These projects include, among many others, the role of HLA matching in renal transplantation and in BMTs, the role of antibodies in chronic rejection, studies of HLA associated diseases and use of HLA in anthropology.
3. They have been biobanks long before this term was coined, i.e. for collection of reliable typing reagents, important patient sera, reference cell line panels,

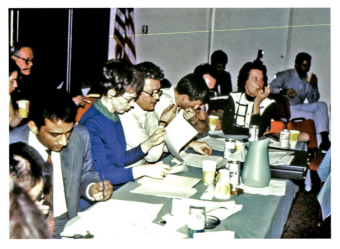

Fig. 3.13: Some members of the Scandinavian group studying their data at the fourth IHWS meeting in 1970. The leader of the group, Flemming Kissmeyer-Nielsen (1921-1991), is seen (with glasses) in the center

Table 3.1: Some major aims and results from the International Histocompatibility Workshops (IHWSs)[1]				
WS nos.	Dates	Places	Chairmen	Some important aims and results
1	June 1964	Durham, NC, US	D Bernard Amos	Comparison of different typing techniques. Results: Very little consistency!
2	August 1965	Leiden, Holland	Jon J van Rood	Comparison of different "local" specificities. Results: Strong correlations between several.
3	June 1967	Turin, Italy	Ruggero Ceppellini	Establish the genetics of leukocyte antigens. Results: Strong correlations between more "local" specificities; most are encoded by genes at one chromosomal region; HL-A.
4	January 1970	Los Angeles, US	Paul I Terasaki	Further definition of HL-A specificities. Eleven HL-A specificities accepted.
5	May 1972	Evian, France	Jean Dausset	Use of HL-A in anthropology. Established HL-A frequencies in different populations.
6	June 1975	Aarhus, Denmark	Flemming Kissmeyer-Nielsen	Focus on HLA LD antigens by exchange of homozygous typing cells. HLA-Dw1-6 accepted. More HLA-A and-B antigens, and five -Cw antigens accepted.
7	September 1977	Oxford, UK	Julia and Walter F Bodmer	Focus on antigens expressed on B cells. HLA-DRw1-7 accepted, strong correlations to corresponding HLA-Dw antigens.
8	February 1980	Los Angeles, US	Paul I Terasaki	Focus on applications. A possible beneficial effect of HLA matching in renal transplantation from unrelated donors. Strong HLA-DR associations to some diseases.
9	May 1984	Munich, Germany	Ekkehard D Albert Wolfgang R Mayr	Further dissection of HLA polymorphism by family studies, also using monoclonal antibodies and biochemistry. More HLA specificities accepted. Beneficial effects of both HLA-A, -B and -DR matching in renal transplantation from unrelated donors.
10	November 1987	Princeton, NY, US	Bo Dupont	Theme: Molecular genetic basis of HLA polymorphism. Comparison of HLA specificities detected by different assays. Established an IHWS reference cell line panel.
11	November 1991	Yokohama, Japan	Kimiyoshi Tsuji Miki Aizawa Takehiko Sasazuki	Establishment of DNA typing of HLA (PCR SSO). New data on the role of HLA in transplantation, disease associations, anthropology, etc.
12	June 1996	Saint-Malo, France	Dominique Charron	Theme: Genetic diversity of HLA. Extensive DNA typing, many new HLA variants detected. More data on applications.
13	May 2002	Victoria, BC, Canada	John A Hansen	Theme: Immunobiology of the human MHC. New data on applications. Establishment of different International Histocompatibility Working Groups (IHWGs). Establishment of a publicly accessible MHC database.
14	November 2005	Melbourne, Australia	Jim McCluskey	New results of work by the different IHWGs and others. New data on KIR-HLA and applications, in particular in BMTs.
15	September 2008	Buzios, Brazil	Maria Elisa Moraes Maria Gerbase-DeLima	Further results of the work by the different IHWGs and others. New data on applications in clinical medicine, anthropology, etc.

[1] The first-three IHWSs were "wet" workshops, were participants carried out their investigations together in the laboratory of the workshop chairman. From the fourth IHWS the participants carried out their investigations locally in their own laboratories, often using exchanged reagents. The investigators then met at the workshop meeting to discuss the results.

oligonucleotides and cDNA probes, and for generation of publicly accessible HLA databases, all of which have been instrumental for workers in the field.
4. They have been platforms for further research and developments in individual laboratories. Many new and original contributions by individual investigators have been based on workshop results or reagents provided by the workshops.
5. They have played an important educational role, making quick technology transfer possible. Many less experienced laboratories have by participation been actively trained and learned new techniques.

The bottom line is that, without these workshops, we would not have been where we are to day with respect to our knowledge of the HLA complex and its applications in research and clinical medicine.

IMMUNOBIOLOGICAL FUNCTION OF THE HLA CLASS I AND II ANTIGENS

But what is the immunobiological function of the HLA class I and II antigens? It was clear very early that they were strong histocompatibility antigens, hence the name *major histocompatibility complex* or *MHC* for the HLA and analogous complexes in other species. But this could not be their real immunobiological function! The first answers mainly came from studies in the mouse.

Baruch Benacerraf and colleagues first reported in 1963, that the antibody response in guinea pigs to a particular synthetic polypeptide antigen (PLL) was controlled by a single gene.[35] Genes controlling specific immune responses were later called *Immune response* or *Ir* genes. Benacerraf received the Nobel prize in 1980 (shared with Snell and Dausset) for his contributions on *Ir* genes. Then, in 1968, came the first data which would lead to an understanding of the immunobiological function of the MHC antigens. Hugh McDevitt (Fig. 3.14) together with Tyan then first showed that the ability of mice to make an antibody response to a series of synthetic polypeptide antigens was a genetic trait which was closely linked to the H-2 complex. The next year McDevitt and Chinitz confirmed and extended these results in further experiments.[36] Using 33 different inbred strains of mice, which were of eight different H-2 types but where strains having the same H-2 type had different genetic backgrounds, they demonstrated that all strains being H-2b responded strongly to the synthetic antigen (T,G)-A--L, while strains of other H-2 types did not respond or responded much more weakly. In contrast,

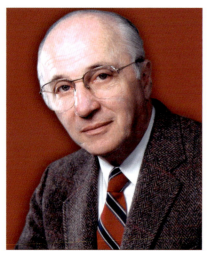

Fig. 3.14: Hugh McDevitt (1930-)

when they instead used another synthetic antigen (H,G)-A--L, different mouse strains being H-2a or H-2k responded strongly, strains being H-2b responded poorly and strains having other H-2 types did not respond or responded variably. Thus genes closely linked to the H-2 complex controlled specific immune responses! The authors concluded that their results were compatible either with multiple *Ir* gene loci, or a single *Ir* gene locus with multiple alleles, but in both cases closely linked to the H-2 complex.

MHC linked *Ir* genes were later identified in several species, and the mechanism of their function became much discussed. It was speculated that they might be identical to the MHC genes themselves, i.e. the genes encoding the MHC class I antigens, and that the MHC antigens on immunocompetent cells in one way or another might modify the antigen receptors on these cells. Alternatively, the *Ir* genes might be different from the genes encoding the MHC class I antigens, and represent a new set of antigen receptors on T cells. Later studies showed that the murine *Ir* genes were separate from and mapped to a position between H-2D and H-2K, and that some antisera recognized the corresponding gene products, called Ia (Immune-response associated) antigens. The Ia antigens were later shown to be encoded by two different loci in the H-2 complex, I-A and I-E, corresponding to HLA-DQ and -DR in man respectively, i.e. class II antigens of mice.

In 1972, it was first shown that cooperation between T and B cells required MHC compatibility between the interacting cells.[37] The next year it was shown that the same was true for the interaction of macrophage-associated antigen with T cells.[38] That the MHC antigens were directly involved in T cell recognition of antigens was, however, first shown in 1974 by Rolf Zinkernagel and Peter Doherty, when they worked together in Canberra, Australia. A very interesting account of how they discovered this is given by Zinkernagel and Doherty.[39] The results of their initial experiments are reported in two short and yet momentous letters in Nature.[40,41]

Very briefly, using mice infected with lymphocyte choriomeningitis virus (LCMV), they observed that T cells from the H-2k strain were only able to kill LCMV infected target cells from the H-2k strain, and not LCMV infected target cells from the H-2d strain. The reverse was true when they instead used T cells from LCMV infected H-2d mice, which were only able to kill LCMV infected target cells from H-2d and not LCMV infected target cells from H-2k mice. Thus, T cell recognition of virus antigens was restricted by the MHC antigens of the T cell donor, which was called *MHC restriction.* They proposed two explanations for their results, either the antigen-specific receptor on T cells, the T cell receptor (TCR), recognizes MHC antigens which have been modified by the virus, or the TCR recognizes a complex formed between virus and MHC antigens (Fig. 3.15). They later proposed a unifying hypothesis that T cell recognition by cytotoxic (CD8) T cells and by helper (CD4) T cells involved similar mechanisms, involving MHC class I and class II antigens respectively, and that this may explain the experiments summarized above on *Ir* gene effects and the need for histocompatibility between interacting immune system cells. Further, they proposed that this may also explain how the MHC antigens are strong histocompatibility antigens and may predispose to diseases.[42] Although the exact mechanism how the MHC antigens were involved in T cell recognition could not be revealed by their experiments, Zinkernagel and Doherty came very close (see later). They received the Nobel prize in 1996 for their seminal observations (Fig. 3.16).

In 1986, it was first shown that MHC restriction, not surprisingly, was also the case for human T cell mediated immune responses. Goulmy et al[43] first demonstrated that human cytotoxic (CD8) T cells were restricted by the HLA class I antigens of the T cell donor, while Bergholtz and myself[44] first showed that human helper (CD4) T cells were restricted by the HLA class II antigens of the T cell donor.

When the natural killer (NK) cells were discovered, it was soon found that the MHC class I antigens also

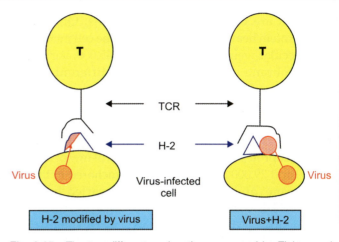

Fig. 3.15: The two different explanations proposed by Zinkernagel and Doherty to explain the results of their experiments, very schematically

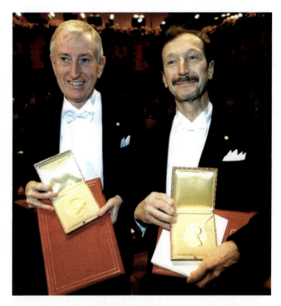

Fig. 3.16: Peter Doherty (left) and Rolf Zinkernagel receiving the Nobel prize in 1996

played an important role in their function. As will be treated in detail in other chapters in this book, some self MHC class I antigens are important inhibitory ligands for activation of NK cells. Thus, MHC or HLA antigens play an important immunobiological function both in adaptive and innate immune responses.

STRUCTURE OF HLA RESOLVED: THE PIECES COME TOGETHER

During 1960s and 1970s a lot of studies on the structure of MHC antigens, both H-2 and HLA, appeared.[3,4] By the early 1980s it had been established that the class I antigens are composed of two chains. One was a glycoprotein heavy chain anchored in the cell membrane of molecular weight (mw) of approx. 45.000, varying in its membrane distal part between different class I molecules. This heavy chain was non-covalently associated with β-2 microglobulin (β2m; mw about 12.000) which was found to be constant in all class I molecules. In contrast, the class II antigens consisted of two glycoprotein heavy chains (α and β) of mw of approx. 34.000 and 29.000 respectively, both anchored in the cell membrane, and where the β chain varied between different HLA-DR antigens.

The studies by Zinkernagel and Doherty summarized above, and studies by many others later, had shown that T cells recognize foreign antigens associated with MHC antigens, or MHC molecules as we should call them from now on. It was shown by Ziegler and Unanue[45] that CD4 T cells recognize fragments of antigens in association with MHC class II molecules in macrophages, and by Townsend et al[46] that CD8 T cells recognize peptide-fragments of antigen in association with MHC class I molecules in target cells. But what is the mechanism?

In 1987, two papers by the Strominger/Wiley group were published back-to-back in *Nature*, which provided the explanation and caused a paradigm shift not only in the HLA field but in immunology in general. In an article to the memory of Don Wiley (1944-2001), Jack Strominger has given a very interesting account on how the group arrived at their results.[47] In the first *Nature* paper, Pam Bjorkman and coworkers,[48] using X-ray crystallography, showed that the part of the HLA-A2 molecule proximal to the cell-membrane contains two domains with immunoglobulin-folds that are paired in a novel manner. However, more importantly, they also demonstrated that the membrane distal domain is a platform of antiparallel β-strands topped by two β helices, which together form a large groove which provides a binding site for processed antigen, probably a peptide. They also showed that an unknown peptide material was found in this site in crystals of HLA-A2 (Figs 3.17 and 3.18, which for many years were the most frequently shown pictures in any talk on HLA or immunology).

In the accompanying paper, Bjorkman and coworkers[49] discussed how some of the polymorphic amino acid residues in the groove of HLA class I molecules, and by inference also in the groove of class II molecules (which was, however, first demonstrated six years later[50]) would interact with a peptide, while other polymorphic residues of HLA molecules would interact

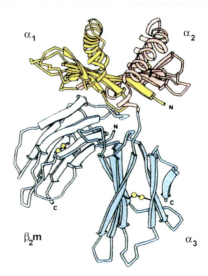

Fig. 3.17: Schematic representation of the four domains of HLA-A2. Reprinted by permission from Macmillan Publishers Ltd: Nature, copyright 1987;329:506-12[48]

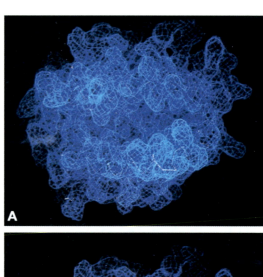

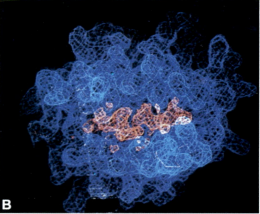

Figs 3.18A and B: Surface representation of the top of the HLA-A2 molecule, showing (A) the deep groove identified as the antigen recognition site and (B) the electron density found in this site, probably a peptide. Reprinted by permission from Macmillan Publishers Ltd: Nature copyright 1987;329:506-12[48]

with the TCR. Thus a given T cell recognizes a particular peptide-HLA complex, where both the peptide and the presenting HLA molecule constitute the ligand. In other words, the HLA molecules present peptide-fragments of antigen to T cells (Fig. 3.19). The pieces had come together.

It is interesting to note that the first HLA molecule whose structure was fully revealed was the same as the very first HLA molecule discovered in man, i.e. MAC or HLA-A2, discovered by Dausset 29 years previously.[1]

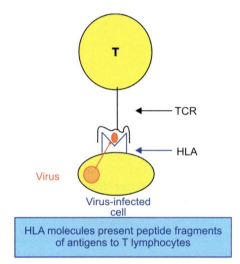

Fig. 3.19: HLA molecules present peptide-fragments of antigen to T cells

THE HLA COMPLEX IS THE HUMAN MAJOR IMMUNE RESPONSE COMPLEX (THE *MIRC*)

The HLA class I and II antigens were first detected because they induced alloantibody formation, and were later shown to be major histocompatibility antigens in man. Less than 30 years, later they were shown to be peptide-presenting molecules for T cells (Fig. 3.19). As will be fully described in later chapters in this book, the HLA class I molecules A, B and C, which are found in almost all nucleated cells, present peptides derived from endogenous proteins to CD8 T cells. In contrast, the HLA class II molecules DR, DQ and DP, which are mainly found in specialized antigen-presenting cells (dendritic cells, monocytes, B cells) present peptides derived from exogenous proteins to CD4 T cells. The HLA molecules do not distinguish between peptides from self proteins or peptides from foreign proteins. Since, however, our T cells by various mechanisms generally are tolerant to our own, self peptide-HLA complexes, i.e. self-tolerance, a T cell immune response will mainly be formed against peptides from *foreign* proteins bound to self HLA molecules.

The studies by Bjorkman et al cited above demonstrated that a given T cell recognizes a particular peptide-HLA complex, where both the peptide and the presenting HLA molecule constitute the ligand. Their studies also suggested that there would be limitations in the ability of a given HLA molecule to bind all types of peptides. This was amply confirmed in later studies by many others of peptide binding to HLA molecules.[51] The polymorphic residues in the peptide-binding groove or cleft of HLA molecules determine which peptides will be bound strongly and which will not be bound or bound more weakly.

This explains the earlier findings of Zinkernagel and Doherty referred to above, namely that T cell recognition of antigen is restricted by the MHC of the T cell donor, i.e. *MHC restriction*. The MHC molecules of the T cell donor will not only determine which peptides may be bound and presented to the T cell, they will also constitute part of the ligand being recognized by the TCR of T cells.

This also explains the earlier findings of McDevitt and coworkers referred to above of *Ir* genes in the MHC. The MHC molecules of an individual will to a large extent determine his or her immune response, i.e. which antigenic peptides will be immunogenic and which will not. Thus, the *Ir* gene effects are not caused by separate genes in the MHC, they are a function of the MHC molecules themselves. It should be noted, however, that both class I and class II molecules have *Ir* effects. The class I and II molecules of an individual will determine the repertoire of peptides which will be presented to CD8 and CD4 T cells respectively, and thus be immunogenic for the individual.

The *Ir* effects of HLA molecules also explain why some HLA molecules are associated with protection against diseases, as will be fully treated later in this book. For example, HLA-B27 is associated with a relative protection against HIV infection, which is most probably caused by preferential binding and presentation by HLA-B27 of some peptides from HIV to T cells. The protective effects of HLA molecules also provide an explanation of their extreme polymorphism. The more HLA molecules to select from in a given population, the more likely it is that some individuals will have optimal HLA molecules for binding and displaying peptides from a foreign intruder to induce an appropriate immune response, and thus survive the infection.

The *Ir* effects of HLA molecules most probably also explain why so many autoimmune diseases are associated to given HLA molecules, as will also be treated in detail in several other chapters later in this book. In celiac disease, it has been shown that the strong association to HLA-DQ2 and -DQ8 is caused by the ability of these two class II molecules to preferentially bind gliadin peptides derived from ingested gluten, the agent causing the disease.[52] It has also been shown, however, that what HLA-DQ2 and -DQ8 preferentially bind are gliadin peptides which have been deamidated by the enzyme tissue transglutaminase, i.e. modified gliadin peptides. The autoantigens inducing an immune response in autoimmune diseases are generally not known. On the basis of the findings in celiac disease, however, one may speculate that the autoimmune response is not initially directed against native autoantigens, but a self-protein which for one reason or another has been post-translationally modified, i.e. a *modified* self-protein. This would also explain the loss of self-tolerance. The HLA associations in autoimmune diseases may then be explained by preferential binding of peptides from some modified self-proteins to the disease-associated HLA molecules.

To complete the picture, it should also be mentioned that some diseases are (also) associated to HLA class I molecules which are inhibitory ligands for NK cells. This is further treated in other chapters in this book.

But how can HLA molecules be major *histocompatibility* antigens? Briefly, since HLA molecules are present in very high concentrations in cells, and thus also in cells of an allogeneic transplant, they will, when foreign to the recipient, constitute a major part of the antigenic challenge of the recipient. After processing, peptides derived from the foreign HLA molecules will be a major source of foreign peptides presented to recipient CD4 T cells by self-HLA class II molecules of recipient dendritic cells (DC). Following activation these T cells will also help B cells to produce antibodies against the foreign HLA molecules. Together this is called *indirect* allorecognition (Fig. 3.20, right part). T cells of the recipient are, however, also able to directly recognize foreign peptide-HLA complexes on the grafted cells, in particular on donor DC. Recipient T cells will be tolerant to self peptide-HLA complexes, but not to allogeneic, foreign peptide-HLA complexes, i.e. complexes of peptides bound to foreign HLA molecules. Even though the T cells of an individual during positive selection in the thymus become biased to recognize peptides presented by *self*-HLA molecules, many of them will because of cross-reactivity also be able to directly recognize complexes of peptides bound to *foreign* HLA molecules. This is called *direct* allorecognition (Fig. 3.20, left part).

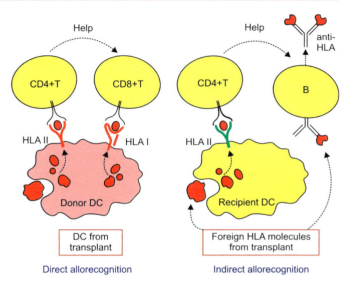

Fig. 3.20: Direct and indirect allorecognition, very schematically (see text)

Indirect and direct allorecognition, leading to alloimmune responses against the graft, play important parts in *acute* rejection. After donor DC in the graft are lost, alloimmune responses as a result of direct allorecognition become less important. In contrast, indirect allorecognition becomes dominant, which may lead to *chronic* rejection where antibodies to foreign antigens in the graft, HLA and others, play a major role. This is treated in other chapters in this book, as is also the role of NK cells in alloimmune responses. For example, after HSCT, NK cells among donor stem cells may be activated by recipient cells lacking donor NK cell inhibitory HLA class I ligands.

It follows that the function of HLA molecules as major histocompatibility antigens may be considered more as a side effect of their function in general immune responses. Thus the term the *major histocompatibility complex*, the *MHC*, for the HLA complex and similar genetic complexes in animals is a misnomer, caused by historical reasons before its true immunobiological functions were known. Given our current knowledge of the instrumental importance of the MHC molecules both in innate and adaptive immune responses, and adding the function of many other products of the MHC in immune responses, a better name for the complex would be the *major immune response complex*, the *MIRC*. But it is too late to change this now!

CONCLUDING REMARKS

It is now just a little more than 50 years since Jean Dausset first discovered a leukocyte antigen in man, which became the "first" HLA antigen; HLA-A2. Since, then the field has moved from histocompatibility to become one of the most central fields in basic and clinical immunology in general.

There are several reasons for the quick and extensive developments of the field. First and foremost are the instrumental contributions by its many pioneers. Some of them have received the Nobel prize (Snell, Dausset, Benacerraf, Zinkernagel and Doherty), but several others would also have been excellent candidates. That such a relatively large number of Nobel prizes has gone to pioneers in this field witnesses its importance. But another factor which must not be underestimated is the extensive international collaboration which has taken place since the early days of HLA, in particular the international histocompatibility workshops. Together the pioneers and the extensive international collaboration are responsible for the giant progress we have seen in this field during the last 50 years.

ACKNOWLEDGMENTS

I am grateful to Walter Bodmer, Jon van Rood and Paul Terasaki for helpful comments to the parts of this review dealing with the early history of HLA, to Hugh McDevitt for helpful comments concerning the part describing the immunobiological function of HLA antigens, and to Torstein Egeland, Ludvig Sollid and Frode Vartdal for careful reading of the manuscript.

REFERENCES

1. Dausset J. Iso-leuko-anticorps. Acta Haemat 1958;20:156-66.
2. Thorsby E. A Short History of HLA. Tissue Antigens 2009;74:101-16.
3. Klein J. Natural History of the Major Histocompatibility Complex. New York etc.: John Wiley & Sons, 1986.
4. Brent L. A History of Transplantation Immunology. San Diego, etc. Academic Press, 1997.
5. Terasaki PI (Ed). History of HLA: Ten Recollections. Los Angeles: UCLA Tissue Typing Laboratory, 1990.
6. Medawar PB. The behaviour and fate of skin autografts and skin homografts in rabbits: A report to the War Wounds Committee of the Medical Research Council. J Anat 1944; 78:176-99.
7. Medawar PB. A second study of the behaviour and fate of skin homografts in rabbits: A report to the War Wounds Committee of the Medical Research Council. J Anat 1945;79:157-76.
8. Gorer P. The detection of antigenic differences in mouse erythrocytes by the employment of immune sera. Br J Exp Pat 1936;17:42-50.
9. Gorer P. The genetic and antigenic basis of tumor transplantation. J Path Bact 1937;44:691-7.
10. Gorer PA, Lyman S, Snell GD. Studies on the genetic and antigenic basis of tumor transplantation. Linkage between a histocompatibility gene and "fused" in mice. Proc Roy Soc B 1948;135:499-505.
11. Thorsby E. A tentative new model for the organization of the mouse H-2 histocompatibility system: Two segregant series of alleles. Eur J Immunol 1971;1:57-9.
12. Snell GD, Cherry M, Demant P. Evidence that the H-2 private specificities can be arranged in two mutually exclusive systems possibly homogenous with the two subsystems of HL-A. Transpl Proc 1971;3:183-6.
13. van Rood JJ, Eernisse JG, van Leeuwen A. Leukocyte antibodies in sera from pregnant women. Nature 1958;181:1735-6.
14. Payne R, Rolfs MR. Fetomaternal leukocyte incompatibility. J Clin Invest 1958;37:1756-62.
15. van Rood JJ. Leukocyte grouping. A method and its application. Den Haag: Pasmans, 1962.
16. Payne R, Tripp M, Weigle J, Bodmer W, Bodmer J. A new leukocyte isoantigen system in man. Cold Spring Harbor Symp Quant Biol 1964;29:285-95.
17. Park I, Terasaki P. Origins of the first HLA specificities. Hum Immunol 1970;61:185-9.
18. Kissmeyer-Nielsen F, Svejgaard A, Hauge M. Genetics of the human HL-A transplantation system. Nature 1968;219:1116-9.
19. Thorsby E, Sandberg L, Lindholm A, Kissmeyer-Nielsen F. The HL-A system: Evidence of a third sub-locus. Scand J Haemat 1970;7:195-200.
20. Bach FH, Amos DB. Hu-1: Major histocompatibility locus in man. Science 1967;156:1506-8.
21. Yunis EG, Amos DB. Three closely linked genetic systems relevant to transplantation. Proc Nat Acad Sci 1971;68:3031-5.
22. Mempel W, Grosse-Wilde H, Albert E. Thierfelder S. Atypical MLC reactions in HL-A typed related and unrelated pairs. Transpl Proc 1973;5:401-8.
23. Sheehy MJ, Sondel PM, Bach ML, Wank R, Bach FH. HL-A LD (lymphocyte defined) typing: A rapid assay with primed lymphocytes. Science 1975; 188:1308-10.
24. van Leeuwen A, Schuit HRE, van Rood JJ. Typing for MLC (LD): II. The selection of nonstimulator cells by MLC inhibition tests using SD-identical stimulator cells (MISIS) and fluorescence antibody studies. Transpl Proc 1973;5:1539-42.
25. Ceppellini R, Mattiuz PL, Scudeller G, Visetti M. Experimental allotransplantation in man. I. The role of the HL-A system in different genetic combinations. Transpl Proc 1969;1:385:9.
26. Amos DB, Seigler HF, Southworth JG, Ward FE. Skin graft rejection between subjects genotyped for HL-A Transp Proc 1969;1:342-6.
27. Kissmeyer-Nielsen F, Thorsby E. Human transplantation antigens. Transplantation Rev. 1970;4:1-176.

28. Vredevoe DL, Terasaki PI, Mickey MR, Glassock R, Merrill JP, Murray JE. Serotyping of human lymphocyte antigens. III. Long-term kidney homograft survivors. In Amos DB, van Rood JJ (Eds): Histocompatibility Testing 1965. Copenhagen: Munksgaard 1965;25-35.
29. Mickey MR, Kreisler M, Albert ED, Tanaka N, Terasaki PI. Analysis of HL-A incompatibility in human renal transplants. Tissue Antigens 1971;1:57-67.
30. Albrechtsen D, Flatmark A, Jervell J, Halvorsen S, Solheim BG, Thorsby E. Significance of HLA-D/DR matching in renal transplantation. Lancet 1978;2:1126-7.
31. Amiel JC. Study of the leukocyte phenotypes in Hodgkin's disease. In Curtoni ES, Mattiuz PL, Tosi RM (Eds): Histocompatibility Testing 1967. Copenhagen: Munksgaard 1967;79-81.
32. Brewerton DA, Caffrey M, Hart FD, James DCO, Nicholls A, Sturrock RD. Ankylosing spondylitis and HL-A 27. Lancet 1973;1:904-7.
33. Schlosstein L, Terasaki PI, Bluestone R, et al. High association of an HL-A antigen, W27, with ankylosing spondylitis. New Engl J Med 1973;288:704-8.
34. Jersild C, Fog T, Hansen GS, Thomsen M, Svejgaard A, Dupont B. Histocompatibility determinants in multiple sclerosis, with special reference to clinical course. Lancet 1973;2:1221-5.
35. Levine BB, Ojeda A, Benacerraf B. Studies on artificial antigens. III. The genetic control of the immune response to hapten poly-L-lysine conjugates in guinea pigs. J Exp Med 1963;118:953-7.
36. McDevitt HO, Chinitz A. Genetic control of the antibody response: Relationship between immune response and histocompatibility (H-2) type. Science 1969; 163:1207-8.
37. Kindred B, Shreffler DC. H-2 dependence of cooperation between T and B cells in vivo. J Immunol 1972;109:940-3.
38. Rosenthal S, Shevach EM. Function of macrophages in antigen recognition by guinea pig T lymphocytes. I. Requirement for histocompatible macrophages and lymphocytes. J Exp Med 1973;138:1194-212.
39. Zinkernagel RM, Doherty PC. The discovery of MHC restriction. Immunology Today 1997;18:14-7.
40. Zinkernagel RM, Doherty PC. Restriction of in vitro T cell-mediated cytotoxicity in lymphocytic choriomeningitis within a syngeneic or semiallogeneic system. Nature 1974;248:701-2.
41. Zinkernagel RM, Doherty PC. Immunological surveillance against altered self components by sensitized T lymphocytes in lymphocytic choriomeningitis. Nature 1974;251:547-8.
42. Doherty PC, Zinkernagel RM. A biological role for the major histocompatibility antigens. Lancet 1975;1:1406-9.
43. Goulmy E, Termijtelen A, Bradley BA, van Rood JJ. Y-antigen killing by T cells of women is restricted by HLA. Nature 1977;266:544-5.
44. Bergholtz BO, Thorsby E. Macrophage-dependent response of immune human T lymphocytes to PPD in vitro. Scand J Immunol 1977;6: 779-86.
45. Ziegler K, Unanue ER. Identification of a macrophage antigen-processing event required for I-region-restricted antigen presentation to T lymphocytes. J Immunol 1981;127:1869-75.
46. Townsend ARM, Rothbard J, Gotch FM, Bahadur G, Wraith D, McMichael AJ. The epitopes of influenza nucleoprotein recognized by cytotoxic T lymphocytes can be defined with short synthetic peptides. Cell 1986;44:959-68.
47. Strominger J. Don Wiley (1944-2001), a reminiscence. Nat Immunol 2002;3:103-4.
48. Bjorkman PJ, Saper MA, Samraoui B, Bennett WS, Strominger JL, Wiley DC. Structure of the human class I histocompatibility antigen, HLA-A2. Nature 1987;329:506-12.
49. Bjorkman PJ, Saper MA, Samraoui B, Bennett WS, Strominger JL, Wiley DC. The foreign antigen binding site and T cell recognition regions of class I histocompatibility antigens. Nature 1987;329:512-8.
50. Brown JH, Jardetzky TS, Gorga JC, et al. Three-dimensional structure of the human class II histocompatibility antigen HLA-DR1. Nature 1993;364:33-9.
51. Engelhard VH. Structure of peptides associated with class I and class II MHC molecules. Ann Rev Immunol 1994;12:181-207.
52. Sollid LM. Coeliac disease: Dissecting a complex inflammatory disorder. Nat Rev Immunol 2002;2:647-55.

Section 2

Major Histocompatibility Complex

Chapter 4
Genetic Structure and Functions of the Major Histocompatibility Complex

Brian D Tait

INTRODUCTION

The genes comprising the human major histocompatibility complex (MHC) are located on the short arm of chromosome 6 in region 6p21.3 (Fig. 4.1) extending over approximately 4 megabases of DNA (see http://www.nature.com/nrg/posters/mchmap/). This map of the MHC is included in a paper by Horton et al listed under Additional Reading). Over the last 40 years the MHC has been the most extensively studied region of the human genome as a result of the discovery of the human leukocyte antigen (HLA) genes contained within this complex, which are critical control elements of immune responsiveness playing a pivotal role in disease susceptibility and clinical transplantation. The impact of the HLA gene products in immune response is mediated via their role as receptors for both self and nonself peptides and initiation of the immune response by presentation of the self HLA molecule/peptide complex to both cytotoxic and helper T cells. As a result of their role in discriminating between self and nonself, the HLA gene products also play a role in clinical transplantation and are central to the graft rejection process.

In addition to the HLA genes the MHC contains over 200 genes some of which play a role in immune response at several levels. For many of these genes however the functions are unknown. In this chapter the organization of the HLA genes and the nature and high degree of polymorphism of their protein products will be discussed. The non-HLA genes within the MHC will also be considered and the role of some of the better characterized genes in immune responsiveness explored.

HLA Gene Organization and Structure

The HLA genes are located in three regions. The class 1 and class 2 regions code for cell membrane receptors differing both in structure and function and between the HLA class 1 and class 2 regions lies the class 3 region which contains genes mainly coding for soluble factors involved in immune responses such as complement factors and cytokines. Figure 4.1 shows the broad structure of the genetic regions containing the HLA genes. The class 1 and class 2 regions are classified based on similarities of sequence and general structure, and similarities of the protein products. However, in both regions some of the gene products have evolved to fulfill differing functions. The numerous genes within the class 1 and class 2 regions with sequence and structural homology have arisen by a process of duplication from an ancestral gene with subsequent mutations and divergence of function. This process has been accompanied by gene deletions and in some cases insertions which has led to heterogeneity in the human population with differences observed in individuals with respect to gene number and overall gene structure. This is particularly evident in the HLA class 2 region. This evolving process has also led to numbers of nonfunctional genes, either non-coding genes or pseudogenes within the MHC. For example, in the class 1 region over 50 percent of the genes do not code for a protein product. The biological purpose, if any, of this large number of nonfunctional genes in the class 1 region is not understood. They may simply be relics of an evolutionary process spanning several millions of years.

HLA Class 1 Region Genes

The class 1 genes are further classified into two groups, classical (1A) and non-classical (1B). The classical class 1 genes comprise HLA-A, HLA-B and HLA-C. These are the most polymorphic of the class 1 genes, their products are expressed on all nucleated cells, and their function with respect to peptide presentation to T cells is

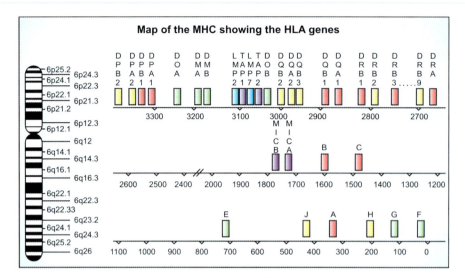

Fig. 4.1: Left hand side shows the broad structure of Chromosome 6. The MHC genes are located on the short arm in region 6p21.3. The right hand side of Figure 1 displays a simplified map of the class 1, 2 and 3 regions of the MHC highlighting some of the genes which are discussed in this Chapter. The classical class 1 and 2 expressed genes are shown in red, the nonexpressed genes in yellow and the non-classical class 1 and 2 genes in green. Also shown are the MIC, LMP and TAP genes. This figure is reproduced from Robinson J, Waller MJ, Parham P, Bodmer JG, Marsh SGE.IMGT/HLA database-a sequence database for the human major histocompatibility complex. Nucleic Acids Research. 2001; 29(1): 210-213

understood in great detail at the molecular level. In contrast the non-classical class 1 genes are less polymorphic, have limited expression and differing functions. The evolution of multiple genes from a single class 1 gene and subsequent divergence of function is evident when we examine the structure and function of both the classical and non-classical class 1 genes.

a. Classical HLA Class 1 Genes

The gene and molecular structure of the class 1 genes is shown in Figure 4.2. The HLA class 1 molecule consists of a glycosylated heavy chain of molecular weight 32K which is non-covalently linked to beta- 2- microglobulin ($\beta 2$ m). $\beta 2$ m coded for by a gene on chromosome 15 is a critical component required for correct folding of the class 1 heavy chain. The importance of $\beta 2$ m for correct folding of the class 1 molecule has been clearly demonstrated in mice who have a deletion of the $\beta 2$ m gene and are unable to express class 1 molecules on the cell surface.

The classical HLA class 1 gene consists of six exons (Fig. 4.2). The first exon comprises the leader sequence which initiates transcription of the gene. The second exon codes for the $\alpha 1$ domain of the class 1 molecule, the third exons the $\alpha 2$ domain and the fourth exons the $\alpha 3$ domain. The remaining two exons code for the transmembrane portion of the molecule and the cytoplasmic tail which anchors the molecule. Finally, there is an untranslated region at the 3′ end of the gene.

The $\alpha 1$ and $\alpha 2$ domains of the class 1 molecule form the cleft responsible for binding both self and nonself peptides and is commonly referred to as the peptide binding cleft. The $\alpha 3$ domain is critical in forming molecular bonds with $\beta 2$ m which ensures correct folding of the molecule on the cell surface.

The class 1 molecules are assembled in the endoplasmic reticulum and bind endogenous peptide which are formed from degradation of intracellular proteins. The peptide/class 1 complex is expressed on the cell membrane for presentation to CD8+ cytotoxic T cells. The process of antigen presentation is discussed fully in the Chapter entitled "Biological and Functional Significance of the Major Histocompatibility Complex".

b. Non-classical Class 1 Genes (HLA-E, F and G)

There are several non-classical class 1 genes consisting of the expressed genes HLA-E, F and G and the non-expressed full length pseudogenes HLA- H, J, K and L. The features that define the non-classical from the classical class 1 genes are their limited polymorphism, and their differing tissue distribution and evolved functions. They have evolved to play specific roles in both innate and adaptive immune systems.

HLA-E

Although HLA-E has a framework structure similar to the HLA 1a molecules and is transcribed in most tissues

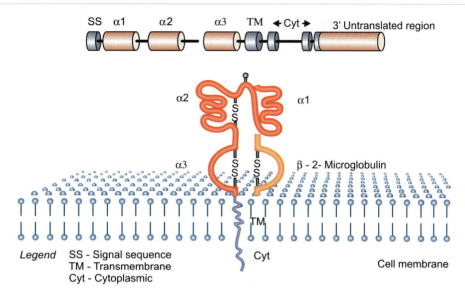

Fig. 4.2: Shows the gene/structure relationship for HLA class 1 (HLA-A,B, C). The gene exons are represented as cylindrical segments and the introns are depicted as black lines. The exons are labeled to indicate the corresponding domain of the class 1 molecule for which they code. The extracellular domains of the class1 molecule are shown in red and β2- m in orange. This figure is from the original figure by Kaufman JF, Auffray C, Korman AJ.The class 2 molecules of the human and murine major histocompatibility complex. Cell.1984, 36(1): 1-13. and reproduced with permission in Tait BD. MHC-from serology to sequence. Today's Life Science 1990;2: page 30

the peptide binding cleft has evolved to bind a nonamer peptide derived from the signal sequence of classical class 1 transcripts and also the leader peptide of HLA-G. Unlike the classical class 1 binding groove, the HLA-E groove has specific binding constraints in several pockets along its length leading to stringent restrictions at positions 2, 3, 6, 7 and 9 of the bound peptide. Due to polymorphism in the classical class 1 leader sequence, some B locus leader peptides bind poorly to HLA-E. The peptide is bound to the HLA-E molecule in the conventional peptide binding pathway involving both TAP and Tapasin (see Chapter "The Biological and Functional Significance of the Major Histocompatibility Complex"). Interestingly there are 9 alleles of HLA-E (Tables 4.1A to C) and some variation in the binding ability of the respective HLA-E molecules. For example, HLA-E*0101 has a lower affinity for the class 1 leader peptide than HLA-E*0103 yet there is only one amino acid difference at position 107 in the α 2 domain, Arginine in *0101 and Glycine in *0103, indicating this is clearly a critical residue in determining the strength of peptide binding.

The HLA-E/signal peptide complex binds to the inhibitory receptor CD94/NKG2 heterodimer found on NK cells and also the NK like αβ CD8 T cells. The HLA-E molecule therefore acts as an indicator of classical class 1 expression. In the presence of normal class1 expression the NK cell will be inhibited from killing and the cell can function normally presenting endogenous peptides via the classical class 1 molecules ensuring the integrity of the cell. However, if a cell loses classical class 1 expression, the NK cell is then released to perform its cell killing function.

Mutations are constantly arising in tumor cells which can alter the function of the cell. One example is the loss of expression of β2 m or mutations in the antigen presentation machinery genes which result in the loss of class 1 expression. Cells which undergo these mutations have a survival advantage due to the loss of recognition of tumor specific endogenous peptides by potentially reactive T cells. However, when class 1 expression is lost HLA-E cannot be expressed due to the lack of the leader peptide. The inhibitory signal to the NK cell is removed and the NK cell is therefore potentially able to kill the tumor cell. The HLA-E molecule is therefore located at the interface between the innate and adaptive immune systems and has evolved to fulfill this role.

HLA-G

HLA-G has limited tissue expression confined mainly, although not exclusively, to immunologically privileged sites. It is expressed in the trophoblast, thymus, cornea and in some erythroid and endothelial precursor cells. HLA-G is unique amongst the class 1 molecules in that it

Table 4.1A: Polymorphism of HLA class 1 genes

Gene	Number of sequenced alleles	Number of protein variants	Number of null alleles
HLA-A	767	600	49
HLA-B	1,178	999	39
HLA-C	440	346	9
HLA-E	9	3	0
HLA-F	21	4	0
HLA-G	43	14	2
MICA	65	55	0
MICB	30	19	2

Figures obtained from the IMGT/HLA database (April 2009)

Table 4.1B: Polymorphism of HLA class 2 genes

Gene	Number of sequenced alleles	Number of protein variants	Number of null alleles
HLA-DRA	3	2	0
HLA-DRB1	618	506	3
HLA-DRB3	50	40	0
HLA-DRB4	13	7	3
HLA-DR5	18	15	2
HLA-DQA1	34	25	1
HLA-DQB1	96	70	1
HLA-DPA1	27	16	0
HLA-DPB1	133	116	3

Figures obtained from the IMGT/HLA database (April 2009)

Table 4.1C: Polymorphism of antigen presentation machinery (APM) genes

Gene	Number of sequenced alleles	Number of protein products	Number of null alleles
HLA-DMA	4	4	0
HLA-DMB	7	7	0
HLA-DOA	12	3	1
HLA-DOB	9	4	0
TAP1	7	5	1
TAP2	4	4	0

Figures obtained from the IMGT/HLA database (April 2009)

exists in a variety of isoforms. Four of the isoforms G1-G4 are expressed on the cell membrane while three exist as soluble forms of HLA-G. The functional significance of these numerous forms is not fully understood. Unlike other class 1 molecules HLA-G is expressed as a dimer on the cell membrane. The expression of HLA-G in the chorionic villi and the amniotic fluid suggests a role in the maintenance of pregnancy. Like other class 1 molecules, the HLA-G molecule has an adapted peptide groove and binds a nonamer peptide derived from several intracellular proteins and the HLA-G/peptide complex interacts with leukocyte Ig-like inhibitory receptors, LIR-1 and LIR-2 and to three KIR receptors. The third domain of the HLA-G molecule has a different structure from other class 1 molecules and this appears to be the putative binding site for LIR-1 and LIR-2.

The mechanism whereby HLA-G protects the allogeneic fetus from immune attack appears to involve the production of soluble forms of the molecule which flood the maternal-fetal interface and have an inhibitory effect on the immune cells of the mother.

It appears that in some human cancers such as melanoma, HLA-G expression is a method utilized by the tumor cells to avoid immunosurveillance. By flooding the local microenvironment with the soluble forms of HLA-G, the tumor cell is able to inhibit immune cells and alter the local cytokine microenvironment.

HLA-F

Less is known about the function of HLA-F. It is not expressed as a mature protein on the cell membrane existing mainly as an intracellular protein in immune system organs such as the spleen, tonsils and thymus but is also found in the villous trophoblast. Its precise function there is not fully appreciated although it may play a supporting role to HLA-G. Like HLA-G it appears to bind to LIR-1 and LIR-2.

Class 1 Pseudogenes

In addition to the expressed class 1 genes there are four pseudogenes HLA-H, K, J and L which by definition are not expressed and serve no obvious function. They are most likely remnants of the duplication, deletion and mutation events of the evolutionary process which has occurred within the MHC. In these cases the mutations have rendered the genes non-functional.

Class 1 Like Molecules

In addition to the classical and non-classical class 1 HLA genes there are a series of genes with class 1 like structure and divergent functions which are widespread throughout the MHC.

MHC Class 1 Chain Related (MIC) Genes and Molecules

There are seven MIC (MHC class 1 chain related gene) genes located within the MHC. Only two of these genes termed MICA and MICB code for functional products. These two genes are located in the class 3 region, MICA being 42.4 Kb centromeric of HLA-B, and MICB 141.2 Kb centromeric of HLA-B. The other five non-functional MIC genes are located in the class 1 region between HLA-F and HLA-E.

The structure of the MIC genes is homologous to the classical class 1 with three extracellular domains but in the case of MIC there is no β2 microglobulin binding nor is there a groove which functions as a peptide binding site. The MIC-A molecule can vary in size from 383 to 389 amino acids long due to variation in the length of the transmembrane region while the MIC-B molecule is 384 amino acids in length.

MIC-A and MIC-B are stress molecules which are upregulated under certain conditions. They have limited cell distribution and are expressed mainly on gastric epithelium, endothelial cells, epithelial cells, monocytes and fibroblasts. Both MICA and MICB are highly polymorphic (Table 4.1A) but the functional significance of this high degree of polymorphism is not understood. The MIC molecules act as a ligand for the NKG2D activating natural killer cell receptor. They therefore bind to γδ T cells and αβ CD8+ T cells which express this receptor. Despite the high degree of polymorphism of these molecules there is only one amino acid substitution which significantly affects the binding to the receptor. Methionine at position 129 results in 10-50 fold greater binding of MICA to NKG2D than valine at that position.

The biological function of the MIC molecules therefore appears to be at the level of the innate immune response in a fashion similar to HLA-G. Tumor cells have been shown to express MICA and MICB molecules and intuitively one would expect this to provide some protection to the host via activation of NK and T cells. However, it appears that tumor cells by virtue of their high turnover rate shed a large amount of soluble MICA and MICB into the microenvironment. This has the effect of blocking the NKG2D receptor and hence inhibiting the interaction of the NK cell or T cell with the tumor target. This would therefore seem to be another mechanism by which tumor cells can evade immune surveillance.

Since, MIC molecules can be upregulated during cellular stress it is not surprising that their expression has been demonstrated on transplanted kidney cells. Due to their high degree of polymorphism donor-recipient matching for MIC alleles is not common in renal transplantation and therefore transplant recipients are exposed to foreign MIC molecules to which they can mount a humoral response. MIC antibodies have been demonstrated in significant proportion of transplanted patients and have been shown to be associated with both acute and chronic rejection.

HFE Gene

Prior to the discovery of the HFE gene by Feder et al in 1996, the association of the disease hemochromatosis with the HLA class 1 allele A3 was well documented in many populations. The discovery of the HFE gene was a landmark event from three major perspectives. Firstly, it identified the gene responsible for hemochromatosis, secondly it was the first example, described of a class 1 like gene with a non-immunological function, and thirdly since, it was mapped 4 Kb telomeric of HLA-A was a clear demonstration that linkage disequilibrium extended telomeric of the class1 loci further than was generally appreciated at the time. The HFE molecule is 343 amino acids in length and has a typical class 1 structure consisting of three extracellular domains, a transmembrane region and a cytoplasmic tail which anchors the molecule into the cell. The molecule requires β2 m for correct folding and presentation on the cell membrane. The α1 and α2 domains form the equivalent of a peptide binding groove which is narrower than that found in the classical class 1 molecule and does not bind peptide but acts as a receptor binding site.

There are two major polymorphisms in the HFE gene. At nucleotide position 845 which is part of the coding triplet for amino acid 282, there is a guanidine to adenine mutation which results in a cysteine to tyrosine substitution. This 282 mutation which is referred to as C282Y interferes with the correct folding of the α3 domain and its correct binding with β2 m resulting in failure of expression. Individuals who are tyrosine homozygous therefore have total failure of expression of the HFE molecule.

The second mutation is at nucleotide position 187 where a cytosine to guanidine substitution results in a histidine to aspartic acid substitution at amino acid position 63 in the α1 domain (H63D). The 282 mutation occurs in approximately 5-10 percent of Caucasian populations studied but is rarely seen in non-Caucasian populations. The homozygous genotype therefore occurs in approximately 1 in 250 to 1 in 100 Caucasian individuals.

Hemochromatosis is a disease of iron overload whose onset usually occurs about the 4th or 5th decade of life. Its features include an increased level of serum iron and biopsy results reveal iron deposits in many organs particularly the liver which eventually results in organ failure. Homozygosity for tyrosine 282 occurs in nearly all patients with the disease and hence has a very strong association with a high relative risk. The 63 mutation on the other hand confers a much lower level of risk but nevertheless is significantly associated with the disease.

The unravelling of the mechanism surrounding the association of the 282 mutation and hemochromatosis represents only one of three instances where an HLA association exists, the responsible gene has been identified, and a likely mechanism of action proposed with supporting experimental evidence.

Proposed Mechanism Explaining the Association of C282Y with Hemochromatosis

Iron is transported in the bloodstream bound to the protein molecule transferrin. This complex is then transported across the cell membrane by binding to the transferring receptor 1 (TfR1). Experiments using human embryonic kidney cells have shown that HFE forms a stable complex with TfR1 and decreases the affinity of TfR1 for the iron-transferrin complex thereby decreasing the amount of iron absorbed. HFE, therefore, acts as a negative regulator of iron transport across the cell membrane. In individuals with the homozygous 282 mutation there is no expression of HFE and hence, there is no negative feedback on iron absorption resulting in high intracellular levels.

Individuals with the H63D mutation have expression of HFE but the mutation is thought to negatively influence the binding of HFE to the transferring receptor and hence decrease its effectiveness as a negative regulator. This explains the weaker clinical expression of this mutation.

HLA Class 2 Region Genes

The HLA class 2 region consists of 3 subregions termed DR, DQ and DP. The HLA genes that comprise these regions while sharing a basic common structure have diverged in terms of sequence and to a lesser extent function. The important feature to note about the class 2 region is that there are different combinations of genes which comprise the varying haplotypes observed. This adds an extra dimension of polymorphism within populations as in addition to the polymorphism seen in individual alleles we have the added degree of variation in terms of the number of genes which comprise the haplotypes. This is most marked within the DR subregion.

DR Subregion

There are 10 HLA genes within the DR subregion named DRA and DRB1-9. Of these DRA1, DRB1, DRB3, DRB4, and DRB5 code for a membrane expressed product. The remaining genes DRB2, DRB6, DRB7, DRB8, and DRB9 are non-expressed. The number and combinations of genes observed on different chromosomes is another striking example of the diversity which has been generated during the evolution of the MHC (Table 4.2). A single ancestral gene by virtue of duplication, deletion and mutation under selective pressure has resulted in the genetic structure we observe today.

The class 2 genes differ in basic structure from the class 1 genes in that they only have five exons. The first codes for the signal sequence, the second and third exons

Table 4.2: HLA-DR region gene structure

DR haplotype	DRA	DRB1	DRB2	DRB3	DRB4	DRB5	DRB6	DRB7	DRB8	DRB9
DR1,10	+	+					+			+
DR 15,16 (DR51)	+	+				+	+			+
DR3,11,12, 13,14 (DR52)	+	+	+	+						+
DR4,7,9 (DR53)	+	+			+			+	+	+
DR8	+	+								+

Table shows the gene arrangements in the class 2 DR subregion. A cross indicates the presence of the gene on the haplotype. Red indicates an expressed gene and blue a non-expressed gene. This complex arrangement is the result of gene duplication, mutation and deletion which is a central characteristic of the human MHC.

DR1, 10, 15, 16, etc. refer to the DRB1 serological subgroups. DR51, DR52 and DR53 refer to serological epitopes on the DRB5, DRB3 and DRB4 coded molecules.

code for two extracellular domains, the fourth exon for the transmembrane portion of the molecule and the fifth exon for the cytoplasmic tail which anchors the molecule into the cell. The most striking difference between the class 1 and class 2 molecules therefore is the number of extracellular domains and the fact that class 2 molecules do not require β2 m for their expression. These features can be explained by the structure of the class 2 molecule which is expressed as a heterodimer consisting of the products of the DRA gene and one of the DRB genes. The class 2 heterodimer therefore consists of four extracellular domains, comprising two from the DRA protein and two from the DRB protein (Fig. 4.3).The first domain of the α and β chains, α 1 and β1 form a peptide binding groove with a basic structure similar to that seen in the class 1 molecule. However in the case of class 2 these molecules have been evolved to present exogenous peptide to CD4 helper cells in contrast to the endogenous peptides presented to CD8 cytotoxic cells in the case of class 1. A fuller description of peptide binding and the mechanism of peptide loading is described fully in the Chapter entitled" Biological and Functional significance of the Major Histocompatibility Complex".

Given the number of expressed DRB genes, four DR different heterodimers can be assembled and expressed on the cell surface: DRA/DRB1, DRA/DRB3, DRA/DRB4, and DRA/DRB5. The combination of these heterodimers found on haplotypes are shown in Table 4.2 with their designated nomenclature. The only heterodimer present on all haplotypes is the DRA/DRB1 molecule which is commonly referred to in the literature as simply DRB1.

DQ Subregion

Five HLA genes are located in the DQ subregion. They are DQA1, DQB1, DQA2, DQB2 and DQB3. As in the DR subregion gene duplication and subsequent mutations have led to the non-expression of DQA2, DQB2 and DQB3. There is therefore only one expressed DQ heterodimer consisting of the non-covalently bound protein products of the DQA1 and DQB1 genes. As with the DR molecules there are four extracellular domains with the α1 and β1 domains forming the peptide binding groove. Like the DR molecule DQ presents peptide to CD4+ helper T cells.

DP Subregion

There is a similarity between the gene structures of the DP and DQ subregions in that there is one expressed DP heterodimer,DPBA1/DPB1 and three non expressed genes DPA2,DPB2 and DPA3. The level of expression of the DP heterodimer however appears to be significantly less than that observed for DR and DQ. As with DR and

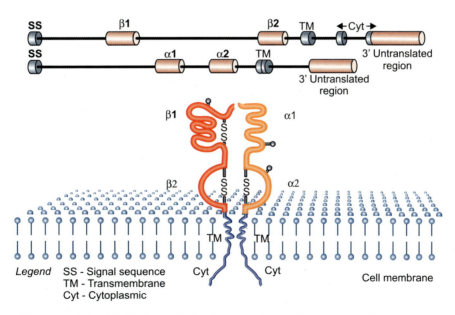

Fig. 4.3: Shows the gene/structure relationship for the HLA class II genes (HLA-DR,DQ,DP).The A and B genes are shown indicating the corresponding domains on the α and β chains respectively for which they code. The α chain is shown in orange and the β chain in red. The two chains are expressed as a dimeric structure on the cell membrane. This figure is from the original figure by Kaufman JF, Auffray C, Korman AJ.The class 2 molecules of the human and murine major histocompatibility complex. Cell.1984, 36(1):1-13. and reproduced with permission in Tait BD. MHC-from serology to sequence. Today's Life Science 1990;2:page 30

DQ the primary role of the DP molecules is to present exogenously derived peptide to T helper cells.

Other HLA Genes within the Class 2 Region

PSMB8 (proteasome subunit beta type 8-also called LMP7) and PSMB9 (proteasome subunit beta type 9 – also called LMP2).

These genes were originally discovered in the early 1980s, when Robert DeMars and his co-workers at the University of Wisconsin-Madison generated cell lines which had been heavily irradiated and undergone chromosomal fracture. One particular cell line generated a great deal of interest as much of the MHC class 2 region had been deleted but the phenotype of the cell included failure to express class 1 molecules on the cell surface. This led to the finding and identification of genes in the class 2 region which influence class 1 molecule expression. There are several genes which are now collectively referred to as antigen processing machinery (APM) genes including PSMB8 and PSMB9 which code for proteasome subunits.

Proteasomes are a family of molecules which exist in most cell types and are involved in the catalytic degradation of short lived proteins within the cell and as such can be considered as an essential part of the normal metabolic turnover of a cell. Amongst the family of proteasomes there are specialized proteasomes which have been designated immunoproteasomes and which are located primarily in the cytoplasm and are involved in the production of peptides for class 1 loading and presentation to T cells. The proteasomes are cylindrical ring shaped molecules whose core is composed of four rings comprised of 28 subunits. Two of the rings are composed of seven α subunits and two of seven β units. Three genes PSMB8, PSMB9 and MECL-1 (which is located on chromosome 16) code for three β subunits which are preferentially incorporated into the ER immunoproteasome after induction with γ interferon (γIFN). These subunits "fine tune" the immunoproteasome so that there is increased efficiency of peptide production and an increase in the number of peptides which include COOH terminal amino acids which preferentially bind to class 1 molecules. Induction by γ IFN ensures that in cases of infection or inflammation the amount of immunoproteasomes is increased and the optimal peptides for class 1 presentation are generated.

TAP1 and TAP2

The TAP1 and TAP 2 genes code for a dimeric ER resident protein called TAP (transport antigen processing) which is responsible for the transport and loading of peptides into the class 1 molecule. TAP is a member of the ATP binding cassette (ABC) subfamily B. The TAP molecule is inserted into the ER membrane via a helical transmembrane domain. There are two binding domains, one of which is located on the cytosol side of the membrane and is the peptide binding domain. There is a second ATP binding domain which is located on a loop of the molecule located in the cytosol (termed the nucleotide binding domain –NBD for TAP1 and NDB2 for TAP2). The transport of peptides from the cytosol into the ER is ATP dependent. When the cytosolic peptide binds to TAP in an ATP independent manner it causes changes in the molecular structure of the transmembrane domain which in turn results in the dimerization of NDB1 and NDB 2, hydrolysis of ATP and release of the peptide into the ER. Transport of the peptide to the ER lumen is therefore an ATP dependent process.

TAPBP (Tapasin)

The TAPBP gene is located within the extended class 2 region approximately 43 Kb centromeric of the DPB1 gene. The TAPBP gene consists of eight exons and codes for an ER transmembrane glycoprotein called tapasin which as a result of alternative splicing can exist in 3 isoforms. Exon 1 codes for the leader sequence, exons 2-5 for a large ER intraluminal domain and exons 6-8 for the transmembrane portion and cytoplasmic tail. The overall structure of tapasin resembles that of class 1 while exon 5 has sequence similarity to the immunoglobulin superfamily suggesting tapasin is a member of that family with a specifically evolved chaperone function.

The tapasin molecule appears to have several functions the most important of which is to bind to the assembled class 1 molecule and bring it in close proximity to the dimeric TAP molecule to facilitate peptide binding into the class 1 groove. In order to achieve this function the tapasin molecule has some interesting structural features. Firstly the intraluminal domain of the molecule expresses a binding site for the assembled class 1 molecule. Residues 334-342 are thought to be the critical residues for interaction with the $\alpha 1$, $\alpha 2$, and $\alpha 3$ domains of the class 1 molecule. The cytoplasmic tail has a KKKAE endoplasmic reticulum retention signal which may assist in the anchoring of the class 1 molecule in the ER prior to interaction with TAP and subsequent peptide binding. The binding site for TAP is located in the C terminal portion of the molecule and the overall binding structure involves four class 1 /tapasin complexes binding to one TAP dimer. In addition to providing a chaperone function for the class 1 molecule and its interaction with TAP, tapasin also appears to have a peptide editing role ensuring only high affinity peptides are bound into the class 1 binding cleft. Interestingly there is variation in the reliance of class 1 molecules for peptide binding. For example, B8 and B*4402 are tapasin dependent while A2 and B*2705 are tapasin independent although peptide binding in the absence of tapasin is not as efficient.

HLA-DM/DO

Class 2 HLA molecules like class 1 are assembled in the endoplasmic reticulum (ER). However, unlike class 1 molecules the peptide binding groove must be prevented from binding endogenous peptides. This is achieved by a molecule called the invariant (I) chain. The I chain acts as a chaperone for the class 2 molecule as it travels through the Golgi apparatus into the late endosome/lysosome vesicles where proteases trim the I chain to produce a short length peptide called CLIP (class 2 associated I chain peptide) which remains bound to the class 2 peptide groove until eventually loaded with exogenously derived peptide. Exogenous proteins are degraded in the endosome and loaded into the class 2 groove in association with DM/DO.

HLA-DM is formed into a heterodimer consisting of DMα and DMβ chains. HLA-DO likewise exists as a DOα/DOβ heterodimer which forms a tetrameric complex with DM in the endoplasmic reticulum. This tetrameric complex is transportd to the late endosome where it plays a critical dual role in stabilizing the class 2 complex and peptide editing orchestrating the replacement of the CLIP peptide with exogenously derived peptides generated in the endosome by protease digestion. While the critical role for DM has been demonstrated by mutant cell lines, the precise role for DO has not been elucidated.

Both DM and DO have class 2 like structure although with functional divergence from classical class 2, there is only weak sequence homology particularly for DM with approximately 30 percent homology compared with 60 percent for DO.

Implications and Relevance of Antigen Processing Machinery (ATM) Molecules in Human Cancers

One of the fundamental functions of the adaptive immune response is to maintain the cellular integrity of the individual. When somatic mutations occur in cells they can produce fundamental molecular changes which can lead to the development of tumors. In normal immune responses the class 1 molecules present tumor associated peptides to the CD8+ T cells which in turn can respond by mounting a cytotoxic response directed at the tumor cell. As previously mentioned in the section dealing with class 1 genes, mutations in β2 m or the heavy chain of the class 1 molecule can result in failure of expression of that gene and hence reduced or complete loss of class 1 expression on the cell surface thereby abolishing the recognition of the mutated peptide/class 1 complex by the cytotoxic CD8+ T cell. Similarly, mutational changes in the genes involved in antigen presentation such as TAP, tapasin and the proteasome genes can also result in failure of expression of class 1 emphasizing the dependence of expression on the efficient functioning of these important accessory molecules.

HLA Class 3 Region Genes

The class 3 region which is an approximately 700 Kb stretch of DNA located between the class1and class 2 regions is the most gene rich segment of the MHC containing a series of 75 genes of which 35 code for protein products. There are basically three types of genes some of which code molecules which operate at several levels of the immune response, some whose gene products have functions unrelated to immune regulation, and non- expressed genes. The precise reason why some genes whose function is clearly non-immunological are located between the class 1 and class 2 genes is not understood. One tandem set of genes the CYP21 and the complement component 4 genes are a classical example of genes who have coevolved, one with an immune function (C4) and one with no apparent role in immune response (CYP21).

The following section describes some of the more interesting class 3 genes and their functions.

Tumor Necrosis Factor (TNF) Superfamily Genes

There are three genes termed LTA, LTB and TNF located within the class 3 region which belong to the tumor necrosis factor superfamily and code for cytokine products that are key mediators of the inflammatory response. The genes each containing four exons are arranged tandemly approximately 220 Kb centromeric of the HLA-B locus.

LTA and LTB

LTA codes for lymphotoxin α (LTα) which is produced by lymphocytes as an inducible cytokine, is secreted and exists in a trimeric form (LTα3). LTA also forms a heterodimer with the product of the LTB gene (lymphotoxin β, LTβ) which stabilizes the membrane form of LTα. This complex is often referred to in the literature as TNFβ. The cell bound heterodimer exists in two forms. The most common is a complex of one α molecule and two β molecules but a less common one consisting of two α and one β also exists. The lymphotoxin complex activates a series of inflammatory responses acting via two receptors, tumor necrosis factor receptors 1 and 2 (TNFR1 and TNFR2). TNFR1 is expressed constitutively on most cell types while TNFR2 is inducible and has a more restricted cell type expression. The signalling processes resulting from this TNFR activation can lead to apoptosis of the cell or NF-κB activation of genes involved in the inflammatory pathway.

TNF

Tumor necrosis factor (originally called Cachectin and referred to in the literature as TNFα) is expressed as a membrane bound trimeric structure which can be enzymatically cleaved by tumor necrosis factor alpha converting enzyme (TACE). TNF is produced by macrophages and both the membrane bound and soluble forms of TNF can also activate the TNFR1 and TNFR2 receptors leading to an apoptopic or inflammatory cascade. It can influence a range of other cell processes including cellular proliferation. It was originally shown to induce death *in vitro* of tumor cell lines which lead to its designation as tumor necrosis factor. However, the name is now somewhat misleading as its properties are more fully understood. It is beyond the scope of this chapter to fully explore the molecular events involving TNF and LT and the reader is referred to other articles under the section Additional Reading.

Clinical Implications of TNF

TNF is a key player in many autoimmune diseases and antiviral responses due to its central role in inflammatory processes. Efforts to produce anti-TNF monoclonal reagents as a therapeutic approach in several diseases have yielded positive results and have proven efficacious in several diseases including rheumatoid arthritis.

There are three antibodies currently used in clinical practice. Adalimubab (Humira, human monoclonal in rheumatoid arthritis, Abbott Laboratories) is a monoclonal of human origin which binds to the TNF molecule reducing its capacity to bind to the TNF receptor and hence reduces the overall inflammatory effect of this molecule. Etanercept (Enbrel, Amgen and Wyeth) is an IgG fusion protein produced by using a DNA construct which combines the TNF receptor with the Fc fragment of human IgG. This molecule acts as a soluble receptor combining with TNF and preventing its binding to cell bound TNF receptor. The third therapeutic reagent is Infliximab (Remicade, Centocor, Schering-Plough) which is a mouse human chimeric antibody that acts in a manner similar to Adalimubab binding to TNF and preventing its interaction with the TNF receptors.

These reagents have been used successfully in recent years in rheumatoid arthritis, psoriatic arthritis, ankylosing spondylitis, Crohn's disease and juvenile idiopathic arthritis.

The use of these therapeutic reagents is an elegant example of how research into the molecular structure and detailed cellular function of an MHC coded gene product and its relevance to disease processes has led to an important breakthrough in the treatment of a cluster of immune related diseases.

The Relevance of Polymorphism in the TNF Gene

Extensive polymorphism has been described in the promoter region of the TNF gene with at least 10 SNPs having been confirmed. Some of these SNPs have clear functional implications. For example, nucleotide position -308 is part of the sequence which binds transcription factors. A substitution of G to A at this position results in a higher level of expression which in turn can have functional effects in inflammatory disease states. One interesting feature of this allele is that it is found on the A1, B8, DR3 haplotype (8.1 haplotype) which is the haplotype showing the strongest association with several autoimmune diseases in Caucasians. Because of this lack of disease specificity with this haplotype it has often been suggested that this haplotype influences autoimmunity in a non disease specific manner perhaps through some alteration in immune regulation. The finding of the -308 SNP and its expression association raises the possibility that this may be a major reason for the strong association of the 8.1 haplotype with autoimmune disease.

Other studies have shown that the presence of the T allele at nucleotide position -857 increases the binding of a specific transcription factor which in turn inhibits the binding of NFκβ at a nearby binding region which has the effect of decreasing TNF production.

For additional information on the effect of polymorphisms on TNF function and disease associations, see the section titled "MHC and Disease" and the Additional Reading section at the end of this Chapter.

CYP21A2 (21-OH gene) and CYP21A1P

CYP21A2 and CYP21A1P are two genes located between the TNF genes and the class 2 region which occur in a tandem gene arrangement with the C4 genes (4th component of complement). The CYP genes like many of the genes within the MHC arose as a gene duplication followed by mutations which rendered the CYP21A1P non-functional. The functional gene CYP21A2 codes for 21-hydroxylase which is a key enzyme involved in steroid synthesis. The CYP21A2 gene consists of 10 exons in which numerous perturbations have been described including point mutations, deletions and base pair insertions which when present in the homozygous state can result in the clinical condition termed congenital adrenal hyperplasia (CAH). CAH can be caused by deficiency in several of the enzymes involved in steroid synthesis but changes in the activity of 21-OH account for the overwhelming majority of CAH cases. The loss of 21-hydroxylase activity which plays a critical role in the aldosterone and cortisol pathways results in shunting of the enzyme substrates progesterone and 17-OH progesterone into the androgen pathway with accumulation of testosterone and reduced cortisol. When this process occurs *in utero* it results in masculinization of a female fetus. Suppression of andrenocorticotrophic hormone (ACTH) normally occurs through a negative feedback loop via the production of cortisol. With the reduced production of cortisol this feedback loop is inhibited resulting in the overproduction of ACTH. The condition is treated by administering the drug Dexamethasone to the mother which crosses the placenta and suppresses ACTH.

In Utero Detection of Fetuses at Risk of Developing CAH

First pregnancies are particularly susceptible to the full clinical implications of CAH since screening for genetic defects in the 21-OH gene is not performed routinely. Once an affected child is recorded in a family, HLA typing of the parents and child are performed to ascertain the HLA haplotypes which contain the relevant 21-OH genetic mutations or deletions. In subsequent pregnancies chorionic villous sampling can be performed early in the pregnancy to obtain tissue for fetal DNA extraction and subsequent molecular typing to ascertain the inherited HLA haplotypes. Since, the 21-OH gene is located in the class 3 region it is important to type for genes both centromeric (HLA-DR/DQ) and telomeric (HLA-A, B) of CYP21A2 to accurately establish the haplotypes.

Dexamethasone is generally given to the mother in the early part of the pregnancy. If the fetus is male or molecular typing indicates that the female fetus is unaffected the treatment is stopped. It is possible to sequence the 21-OH gene and determine the exact defect in the gene and test for this in future pregnancies. However, testing for HLA haplotype segregation and determining haplotypes in most cases is sufficient. The only case where additional testing may be required is where a recombination appears to have occurred between HLA-B and DR on one of the affected haplotypes in which case there is uncertainty as to whether the 21-OH gene has co-segregated with the inherited recombinant haplotype. In this instance sequencing of the 21-OH gene would be recommended.

C4A and C4B

C4 or the fourth component of complement is a glycoprotein consisting of three chains of approximately 200kDa. C4 is involved in both innate and adaptive immunity. It is a central component of the classical complement pathway which is activated in the presence of complement fixing isotypes of immunoglobulin binding to the appropriate antigen. The result of the complement cascade is the membrane-attack complex which has a cytolytic effect on the membrane of the cell on which the antigen is presented. In the case of infection, this can be for example bacteria or in the case of transplanted tissue, the endothelial cells of the transplanted organ. C4d, one of the cleavage products of C4 is measured as an indicator of antibody mediated rejection in biopsies of transplanted organs. The role of C4 in innate immune responses include opsonization and clearance of immune complexes.

Genes of the C4 complex are arranged in a complex pattern with one to four C4 genes present on each haplotype. Each gene can code for either C4A or C4B depending on the sequence located between amino acid positions 1101 to 1106. C4A contains the acidic residue PCPVLD while the basic C4B codes for PCPVIH. The critical difference is the substitution of aspartic acid at 1106 in C4A with histidine in C4B. Further polymorphism in these genes is created by the insertion of the endogenous retrovirus HERV-K in intron 9 which creates two size variations of the gene, 14.2 Kb (short) and 20.6 Kb (long).

The function of C4A and C4B vary in that C4A appears to have more affinity for protein antigens by forming amide bonds while C4B forms ester linkages with carbohydrate antigens. An ability to react with carbohydrate antigens is of importance for example in antibacterial responses.

C4 deficiency characterized as a lower expression of C4A compared with C4B is a central feature of systemic lupus erythematosus (SLE), a disease which has a strong association with the 8.1 haplotype. Examination of the complement gene structure on this haplotype reveals an absence of the C4A gene (C4A null) resulting in reduced levels of circulating C4A. The 8.1 haplotype is increased in frequency in several autoimmune diseases such as type 1 diabetes and glomerulonephritis although the relevance of the C4 gene association to the various disease processes is not clear.

Additional Features of the MHC Genes and Molecules

Polymorphism

The most striking genetic feature of the HLA class 1 and class 2 genes is the degree of polymorphism observed in human populations which is far greater than that seen in any other part of the human genome. Tables 4.1A to C lists the number of alleles currently defined at both the classical and nonclassical class 1 and 2 loci as of April 2009. The greatest degree of polymorphism is observed with the classical class 1 and class 2 genes. This is a direct reflection of their role as presenters of peptide to responding T cells in contrast to the nonclassical genes whose protein products are involved in functions where polymorphism in some cases may be detrimental.

The driving force behind the generation of the classical class 1 and class 2 gene polymorphism is the imperative to provide molecules that are able to bind a host of pathogen derived peptides for the overall benefit of the species. Pathogens are constantly undergoing mutations and are selected based on their ability to thwart the human immune system. One mechanism through which this can be achieved is by alterations in the sequence of the peptide which binds into the HLA class 1 or class 2 groove giving the peptide/MHC interaction a high on/off ratio. In turn the HLA genes within populations mutate and are selected based on their ability to meet the challenges of the changing microenvironment, i.e. their ability to bind relevant pathogenic peptides with high affinity increasing the chances of a successful immune response.

The main evidence for this type of hypothesis is that while the mutations are random, subsequent selection has clearly played a role. Examination of the patterns of polymorphisms reveals that the overwhelming number of polymorphic sites are located in positions that either directly or indirectly affect binding of the peptide in the groove. The patterns of polymorphism vary between class 1 and class 2 molecules and also between the class 2 isotypes. The reader is referred to the IMGT HLA database http://www.ebi.ac.uk/imgt/hla/ which shows the variable regions between both alleles and protein products at the class 1 and class 2 loci. When presented in this form the pattern differences are readily seen. These sequence differences reflect variation in peptide binding to the binding groove and changes to the overall structure of the HLA/peptide complex between class 1 and class 2 and between allelic products at one locus. This theme is explored further in the Chapter, entitled "Biological and Functional aspects of the Major Histocompatibility Complex".

Comparison of the frequency of alleles between different human populations reveals striking differences. These differences are partly due to historical population migration but also to differences in selection patterns due to geographical pathogen variations. The measurement of HLA variation across populations has been an extremely useful tool in human anthropological studies. This aspect is also discussed in detail in the Chapter titled "Major Histocompatibility Complex: Population diversity and significance".

Nomenclature

The early definition of the polymorphism of the HLA genes was described using serological techniques. Sera obtained from multiparous females, transfused patients and transplant rejection patients containing HLA antibodies were used in a microlymphocytotoxicity assay developed by Paul Terasaki and colleagues. This technique involved incubating sera containing HLA antibodies with isolated lymphocytes from the individual being HLA typed. Rabbit serum was added as a source of fresh complement and further incubated with the cells and serum. If antibodies specific for the HLA antigens carried by the cell were present they would bind to the relevant antigen and in the presence of complement cause lysis of the cell. The lysis could be detected by adding the dye eosin which stains dead cells and then fixing the reaction with formaldehyde. This technique became the accepted method for both HLA typing and for screening sera for HLA antibodies to identify potential typing reagents and for screening potential transplant patients for the presence of HLA antibodies.

In the mid to late 1960s; only the HLA- A and B loci had been mapped to the MHC and the serologically defined epitopes were designated numbers as they were discovered. The International HLA community formed a Nomenclature Committee which arose out of the regular international workshops which were held to discuss techniques and share information on the reactivity of sera containing HLA antibodies. When there was general agreement at the workshops on the presence of an antigen specificity detected by several sera with similar patterns of reactivity, the antigen was given a number preceded by the locus to which it belonged, and a 'W' designation which indicated it was a workshop designated antigen, e.g. BW5. After rigorous testing in laboratories worldwide and when there was unambiguous definition of an antigen the W designation was removed, e.g. B5.

There were three major technical phases following this initial definition of the HLA genes which led to our current understanding of their extensive polymorphism. The first was the further refinement of the serological technique, the development of expertise in the use of the assay and the contribution of standardization exercises in order to improve reproducibility of the technique. This led to the realization that some of the antigens hitherto defined consisted of two or more antigens and that what was being defined was a shared epitope. For example B5 was subdivided serologically into B51, B52, B53, and B78. B5 was therefore referred to as a supertypic specificity and B51, etc. as subtypic specificities.

The second technical phase was the introduction of DNA techniques to study HLA polymorphism. The use of techniques such as restriction fragment length polymorphism (RFLP) utilizing restriction enzymes to cut genomic DNA at specified sequences followed by Southern Blotting and then hybridization with full length gene probes enabled further polymorphism of both the class 1 and class 2 genes to be described.

The third and most important technical development in the study of HLA polymorphism was the application of the polymerase chain reaction (PCR) to amplify the gene exons coding for the variation and the use of this amplified product in various molecular typing methods such as the sequence specific hybridization technique (SSO) and more recently nucleotide sequencing. This development led to the realization that the degree of polymorphism was far more extensive than could be defined by serological techniques as many of the sequence variations were not serological epitopes. A new form of nomenclature was required to deal with this next level of polymorphism and hence the basis of the current method of allele naming was devised.

Each sequence based allele is given a prefix designating the gene locus followed by an asterix denoting the fact it is a sequence and not an antigen epitope. The first two digits designate the serological group to which the sequence belongs and the next two digits indicate the number of the sequence which again have been numbered as they have been discovered. Alleles are only given a different sequence number at the third and fourth digit if the difference in sequence is nonsynonymous. For example, HLA-B* 5105 indicates this allele is the fifth allele discovered and sequenced in the serological B51 group and has a different amino acid sequence from other B51 alleles. In order to accommodate differences in synonomous exon nucleotide differences and intron sequence differences two further sets of two numbers are added respectively. Finally the designation N (for null allele) is added if the allele is not expressed for example due to a mis-sense mutation or premature stop codon. Finally alleles which have been demonstrated to be alternatively expressed are given the designations L,S,C,Q or A. Examples of alleles with the above types of designations are shown in Table 4.3. Further descriptions of the polymorphism and Nomenclature can be found at the IMGT database http://www.ebi.ac.uk/imgt/hla/ and also in the Chapter entitled "Nomenclature of the HLA System".

Haplotypes

The term haplotype was originally devised to convey the fact that one or more alleles at neighboring HLA loci occurred on the one chromosome. When the term haplotype is used in the HLA system, it is important to convey the telomeric and centromeric boundaries to

Table 4.3: Basis for naming HLA alleles	
Allele	Explanation
HLA-A*24	Refers to all the alleles in the A24 serologically group
HLA-A*2402	Belongs to the serological group designated A24 and is the second sequenced allele in that group
HLA-A*240201	Identical protein sequence to A*2402 but contains a synonymous substitution.
HLA-A*24020102	Identical sequence to A*240201 but is the second allele containing a substitution in an intron or in the 5' or 3' region.
HLA-A*24020102L	The designation L indicates substitution has Resulted in low expression
HLA-A*2409N	Designation N indicates null allele, i.e. allele is not expressed

which the term is being applied. For example, the most common haplotype observed in Caucasians is A1, Cw7, B8, DR3, DQ2. This is often referred to as the 8.1 haplotype. However, there are two common haplotypes including the above alleles extending to DP and including either DPB1*0101 or DPB1*0401. The term 8.1 is often used in the literature to describe both without indicating the extent of the haplotype boundaries.

The term haplotype which was originally applied to the HLA system is now used to describe cis phase in other areas of the genome. However in this process the term haplotype has been inappropriately used to describe two closely related single nucleotide polymorphisms in cis phase, a departure from it original definition.

The other point to stress is that haplotypes can only be defined by showing segregation in family studies where by definition the presence of the haplotype is proven. The term haplotype applied to describe data from unrelated individuals should be used with caution as the implied presence of a haplotype is based purely on statistical probability using linkage disequilibrium data.

Linkage Disequilibrium

Linkage disequilibrium (LD) occurs when alleles at neighboring loci occur together either more often (positive LD) or less often (negative LD) than is expected given the individual allele frequency. For example, if an allele A occurs at locus X with a frequency of 20 percent and allele B occurs at locus Y with a frequency of 20 percent then with normal recombination rates over a number of generations the frequency of the combination of allele A and allele B occurring together on the one chromosome will approach 5 percent (i.e. 20% × 20%). The two alleles are then said to be in equilibrium. Any statistically significant deviation from this value within a population is reflective of linkage disequilibrium. LD was originally observed between HLA-A and HLA-B but as more data was gathered on other HLA loci it became evident that LD can extend for long distances across the MHC from at least HLA-A to HLA-DP and in some instances both telomeric of HLA-A and centromeric of HLA-DP.

In order to calculate the degree of LD between two alleles, firstly it must be shown that they occur together on one chromosome more often than expected. This is best performed in family studies where segregation studies permit the accurate assessment of how often the two alleles occur on the one chromosome. A Chi-squared test of statistical significance is then performed using the conventional formula:

$$\frac{(ad-bc)^2 n}{(a+d)(b+c)(a+b)(c+d)}$$

where a = the number of cases where allele A and allele B occur together on the one chromosome, b = no of A allele positive B allele negative c = no of A allele negative B allele positive and d = the number of cases where both alleles are absent, i.e. A and B allele negative. n is the total number of observations, i.e. a+b+c+d. Two alleles cannot be said to be in LD unless the value of a is statistically different from the expected value given the frequency of the individual alleles. The degree of LD can then be expressed as a delta (δ) value using the following formula:
δ = Frequency of the two alleles occurring together on the one chromosome (as established by segregation studies) minus the product of the overall frequency of the two alleles, i.e. f (allele A) × f (allele B). The higher the value of δ the greater the degree of positive linkage disequilibrium. In cases where the δ value is negative the two alleles are said to be in negative linkage disequilibrium.

In the absence of family segregation data, an approximation to the δ value can be obtained from population genotype data using the following formula:

$$\Delta \text{ (Delta) value} = \sqrt{\frac{d}{n}} - \sqrt{\frac{(b+d)(c+d)}{n}}$$

(a, b, c and d are defined above)
n = total number of observations.

Haplotype Segregation in Families, Codominant Expression and Recombination

In most families haplotypes extending from HLA-A through to HLA-DPA1/DPB1 are inherited *en bloc* with no evidence of genetic recombination. Table 4.4 shows an example of a family where the HLA genotypes of the first three offspring permit identification of the four haplotypes present in the parents. Sibling 3 in this case has inherited from the mother a meiotic recombination between the B locus and the class 2 DR/DQ loci.

Recombination is not uniform across the MHC but occurs in "hot spots" of recombination. Genetic distances were originally defined as a unit called a centimorgan which was based on the frequency of recombination between genes. With the discovery that recombination is not uniform this measurement ceased to be of practical use. When referring to papers written prior to the 1980s, this important point should be borne in mind.

Recombination in the MHC has been shown to occur between HLA-A and HLA-C, HLA-B and DR/DQ and

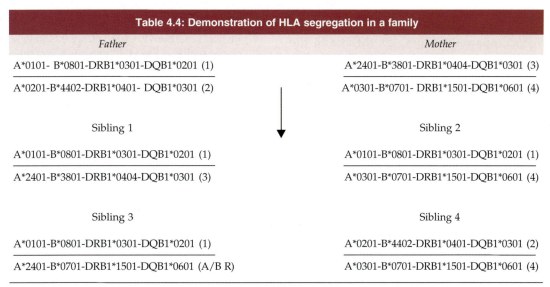

Segregation of HLA haplotypes within a family. For simplicity the C, DRBA, DRB3, DRB4, DRB5 DQA1, DPA1 and DPB1 loci have been omitted. The haplotypes from both parents can be deduced. Note that a new haplotype has been generated in sibling 3 due to a meiotic A/B locus recombination in the mother. This new haplotype has been designated A/B R in the above table

DR/DQ and DPA/DPB. Recombination is rarely observed between HLA-C and HLA-B and has not been convincingly demonstrated between DR and DQ.

The restricted sites of recombination within the MHC has led to the concept that the MHC can be represented as sequences of DNA which are inherited undisturbed as a "block". The MHC therefore can be seen as five blocks consisting of the α block containing HLA-A and surrounding genes, the β block which includes the HLA-B and HLA-C region, the γ region which includes the class 3 genes, the δ block which includes the HLA-DR and HLA-DQ genes and the ε block which includes the DP series of genes. The shuffling of these blocks by meiotic recombination is another mechanism by which the diversity and polymorphism of the MHC is generated within a population.

Since one chromosome 6 from each parent is inherited each individual has two alleles at each of the MHC loci. Both alleles at each locus are fully expressed (with the exception of course of mutations causing non expression). The alleles are therefore said to be codominant which is another feature of the MHC and an additional mechanism whereby the immune repertoire of an individual can be maximized.

The pattern of cell expression however differs between the class 1 and the class 2 genes. Class 1 gene expression is ubiquitous with all nucleated cells having some level of class 1 expression on their cell surface. Since, class 1 molecules present foreign peptide to CD8+ cytotoxic T cells these molecules have evolved a role acting as monitors to maintain the normal integrity of the cell. When foreign proteins in the form of pathogens invade the cell it is the class 1 molecules that convey this information to the relevant T cell which results in the eventual destruction of the cell preventing the pathogen using the cell as a means of continuous proliferation. Since, any cell can potentially become infected it is essential therefore that this monitoring role occurs in every nucleated cell hence the widespread expression of class 1 molecules.

Class 2 molecules on the other hand monitor the protein content of the extracellular environment presenting peptides to the CD4+ helper T cell. They are therefore presented on specialized cells called "antigen presenting cells" which include dendritic cells, macrophages and B lymphocytes. It is essential for optimal immune responsiveness that cells expressing these molecules remain viable and able to continually monitor the external environment. In some instances, however, class 2 molecule expression is induced or upregulated by cytokines produced in response to either infection or inflammation in cell types which are exposed to the external environment such as endothelial cells. Such upregulation has the potential to amplify immune responses.

SUMMARY

The major histocompatibility complex (MHC) in the human is located on the short arm of chromosome 6 (6p21.3) and extends over 4 megabases of DNA. The MHC consists of three regions which have been designated class 1, 2 and 3 based on the structure and function of the gene products. Over 200 genes have been identified in the MHC many of which have a role in regulating immune responsiveness at several levels. However, the function of many of the genes has not been fully elucidated. The best characterized and most polymorphic are the HLA genes. The function of the ubiquitous HLA class 1 gene products (HLA-A,B and C) is to present endogenous peptides to responding cytotoxic CD8+ T cells while the class 2 coded molecules DR,DQ and DP have restricted expression and process exogenous peptide for presentation to CD4+ helper T cells. By functional definition they are present on antigen presenting cells. In addition to these classical class 1 and class 2 genes, there are additional genes in both classes which fulfill other functions described in this Chapter.

The class 3 region contains genes which code for soluble immune regulatory molecules such as tumor necrosis factor and the C4 component of complement. There are also genes which have no immune function such as CYP21 (21-hydroxylase), mutations in which can cause congenital adrenal hyperplasia.

It is beyond the scope of this chapter to describe in detail all the genes comprising the MHC. It is designed rather to convey the basic structure and function of the MHC genes highlighting with specific examples. The reader is referred to the Additional Reading section for more detailed descriptions of specific genes.

ADDITIONAL READING

Map of the MHC and Genomic Structure

1. Shiina T, Inoko H, Kulski JK. An update of the HLA genomic region, locus information and disease associations: 2004. Tissue Antigens 2004;64:631-49.
2. Shiina T, Hosomichi K, Inoko H, Kulski JK. The HLA genomic loci map: Expression, interaction, diversity and disease. Journal of Human Genetics 2009;54:15-39.
3. Horton R, Wilming L, Rand V, Lovering RC, Bruford EA, Khodiyar VK, Lush MJ, Povey S, Talbot CC, Wright MW, Wain HM, Trowsdale J, Ziegler A, Beck S. Gene map of the extended human major histocompatibility complex. Nature Reviews Genetics 2004;5(12):889-99.

Classical Class 1 Region Genes and Molecules

4. Pichon L, Giffon T, Chauvel B, Le Gall JY, David V. The class 1 region of the MHC genes is one of the most complex in the whole human genome. Medicine/Sciences 1996;12(11):1209-18.
5. Le Bouteiller P. HLA class 1 chromosomal region, genes, and products: Facts and questions. Critical Reviews in Immunology 1994;14(2):89-129.
6. Ljunggren HG, Thorpe CJ. Principles of MHC class 1-mediated antigen presentation and T cell selection. Histology and Histopathology 1996;11(1): 267-74.
7. Natarajan K, Li H, Mariuzza RA, Marqulies DH. MHC class 1 molecules, structure and function. Reviews in Immunogenetics 1999;1(1):32-46.
8. Little AM, Parham P. Polymorphism and evolution of HLA class 1 and II genes and molecules. Reviews in Immunogenetics 1999;1(1):105-23.
9. Flutter B, Gao B. MHC class 1 antigen presentation-recently trimmed and well presented. Cellular and Molecular Immunology 2004;1(1):22-30.
10. Yang Y. Generation of major histocompatibility complex class 1 antigens. Microbes and Infection 2003;5(1):39-47.
11. Hammer GE, Kanaseki T, Shastri N. The final touches make perfect the peptide-MHC class 1 repertoire. Immunity 2007;26(4):397-406.

HLA-E, HLA-G, HLA-F

12. Sullivan LC, Clements CS, Rossjohn J, Brooks AG. The major histocompatibility complex class 1b molecule HLA-E at the interface between innate and adaptive immunity. Tissue Antigens 2008;72(5):415-24.
13. Lee N, Goodlett DR, Ishitani A, Marquardt H, Geraghty DE. HLA-E surface expression depends on binding of TAP-dependent peptides derived from certain HLA class 1 signal sequences. J Immunol 1998;160:4951-60.
14. Clements CS, Kjer-Nielson L, Kostenko L, Hoare HL, Dunstone MA, Moses E, Freed K, Brooks AG, Rossjohn J, McCluskey J. Crystal structure of HLA-G: A non-classical MHC class 1 molecule expressed at the fetal-maternal interface. PNAS 2005;102(9):3360-65.
15. Hunt JS, Langat DK, McIntire RH, Morales PJ. The role of HLA-G in human pregnancy. Reproductive Biology and Endocrinology 2006;4 (Suppl 1):S10 (open access journal)
16. Rouas-Freiss N, Moreau P, Menier C, LeMaoult J, Carosella ED. Expression of tolerogenic HLA-G molecules in cancer prevents anti-tumor responses. Seminars in Cancer Biology 2007;17:413-21.

MIC genes

17. Collins RWM. Human MHC class 1 chain related (MIC) genes: Their biological function and relevance to disease and transplantation. European J Immunogenetics 2004;31:105-14.

18. Zwirner NW, Fuertes MB, Girart MV, Domaica CI, Rossi LE. Immunobiology of the human MHC class 1 chain-related gene A (MICA): From transplantation immunology to tumor immune escape. Immunologia 2006;25(1):25-38.
19. Terasaki PI, Ozawa M, Castro R. Four years follow-up of a prospective trial of HLA and MICA antibodies on kidney graft survival. Am J Transplant 2007;7(2):408-15.

HFE

20. Feder JN, Gnirke A, Thomas W, Tsuchihashi Z, Ruddy DA, Basava A, Dormishian F, et al. A novel MHC class 1 like gene is mutated in patients with hereditary Hemochromatosis. Nature Genetics 1996;13(4):399-408.
21. Wheeler CJ, Kowdley KV. Hereditary hemochromatosis: A review of the genetics, mechanism, diagnosis, and treatment of iron overload. Comprehensive Therapy 2006;32(1):10-16.
22. Swinkels DW, Janssen MCH, Bergmans J, Marx JJM. Hereditary hemochromatosis: Genetic complexity and new diagnostic approaches. Clinical Chemistry 2006;52(6):950-68.
23. Jacobs EMG, Verbeek ALM, Kreeftenberg HG, van Deursen CTBM, Marx JJM, Stalenhoef AFH, Swinkels DW, de Vries RA. Changing aspects of HFE –related hereditary hemochromatosis and endeavours to early diagnosis. Netherlands Journal of Medicine 2007;65(11):419-24.
24. Adams PC, Barton JC. Hemochromatosis. Lancet 2007;370 (9602):1855-60.
25. Rosenberg W, Hemochromatosis. Medicine 2007;35(2):89-92.
26. Fix OK, Kowdley KV. Hereditary Hemochromatosis. Minerva Medica. 2008; 99(6);605-17.

Classical Class 2 Genes

27. Creswell P. Assembly, transport, and function of MHC class II molecules. Annual Review of Immunology 1994;12:259-93.
28. Guardiola J, Maffei A, Lauster R, Mitchison NA, Accolla RS, Sartoris S. Functional significance of polymorphism among MHC class II gene promoters. Tissue Antigens 1996;48(6):615-25.
29. Wong FS, Wen L. The study of HLA class II and autoimmune diabetes. Current Molecular Medicine 2003;3(1):1-15.
30. Jones EY, Fugger L, Strominger JL, Siebold C. MHC class II proteins and disease: A structural perspective. Nature Reviews Immunology 2006;6(4):271-82.

DO/DM

31. Brocke P, Garbi N, Momburg F, Hammerling GJ. HLA-DM, HLA-DO and tapasin: Functional similarities and differences. Current Opinion in Immunology 2002;14(1):22-29.
32. Denzin LK, Fallas JL, Prendes M, Woelsung Y. Right place, right time, right peptide: DO keeps DM focused. Immunological Reviews 2005;207:279-92.
33. Chen X, Jensen PE. MHC class II antigen presentation and immunological abnormalities due to deficiency of MHC class II and its associated genes. Experimental and Molecular Pathology 2008;85:40-44.

Proteasomes

34. Brooks P, Murray RZ, Mason GGF, Hendil KB, Rivett AJ. Association of immunoproteasomes with the endoplasmic reticulum. Biochem J 2000;352:611-15.
35. Yewdell JW, Bennink JR. Cut and trim: Generating MHC class 1 peptide ligands. Current Opinion in Immunology 2001;13(1):13-18.
36. Kruger E, Kuckelkorn U, Sijts A, Kloetzel PM. The components of the proteasome system and their role in MHC class 1 antigen processing. Reviews of Physiology, Biochemistry and Pharmacology 2003;148:81-104.
37. Kloetzel PM, Ossendorp F. Proteasome and peptidase function in MHC-class 1 –mediated antigen presentation. Current Opinion in Immunology 2004; 16(1):76-81.
38. Rivett AJ, Hearn AR. Proteasome function in antigen presentation: Immunoproteasome complexes, peptide production, and interactions with viral proteins. Current Protein and Peptide Science 2004;5(3):153-61.
39. Borissenko L, Groll M. Diversity of proteasomal missions: Fine tuning of the immune response. Biological Chemistry 2007;388(9):947-55.

TAP

40. Abele R, Tampe R. The ABC's of Immunology: Structure and function of TAP, the transporter associated with antigen processing. Physiology 2004;19:216-24.
41. McCluskey J, Rossjohn J, Purcell AW. TAP genes and immunity. Current Opinion in Immunology 2004;16(5): 651-59.
42. Paulsson KM. Evolutionary and functional perspectives of the major histocompatibility complex class 1 antigen –processing machinery. Cellular and Molecular Life Sciences 2004;61(19-20):2446-60.
43. Larsen MV, Nielsen M, Weinzierl A, Lund O. TAP-independent MHC class 1 presentation.Current Immunology Reviews 2006;2(3):233-45.

Tapasin

44. Wright CA, Kozik P, Zacharias M, Springer S. Tapasin and other chaperones: Models of the MHC class1 loading complex. Biological Chemistry. 2004;385(9):763-78.
45. Garbi N, Tiwari N, Morrburg F, Hammerling GJ. A major role for tapasin as a stabilizer of the TAP peptide transporter and consequences for MHC class 1 expression. European Journal of Immunology 2003;33(1):264-73.
46. Morrburg F, Tan P, Tapasin –The keystone of the loading complex optimizing peptide binding by MHC class 1

molecules in the endoplasmic reticulum. Molecular Immunology 2002;39(3-4):217-33.
47. Garbi N, Hammerling G, Tanaka S. Interaction of ERp57 and tapasin in the generation of MHC class 1- peptide complexes. Current Opinion in Immunology 2007; 19(1):99-105.
48. Cabrera CM. The double role of the endoplasmic reticulum chaperone tapasin in peptide optimization of HLA class 1 molecules. Scandinavian Journal of Immunology 2007;65(6):487-93.
49. Sadegh-Nasseri S, Chen M, Narayan K, Bouvier M. The convergent roles of tapasin and HLA-DM in antigen presentation. Trends in Immunology 2008; 29(3):141-47.

Class 3

50. Hauptmann G, Bahram S. Genetics of the central MHC. Current Opinion in Immunology 2004;16(5):668-72.

TNF

51. Hehlgans T, Pfeffer K. The intriguing biology of the tumor necrosis factor/tumor necrosis factor receptor superfamily: Players, rules and the game. Immunology 2005;115(1):1-20.
52. Posch PE, Cruz I, Bradshaw D, Medhekar BA. Novel polymorphisms and the definition of promoter "alleles" of the tumor necrosis factor and lymphotoxin α loci: Inclusion in HLA haplotypes. Genes and Immunity 2003; 4:547-58.
53. Fonseca JE, Teles J, Queiroz MV. Tumor necrosis factor α gene promoter and its role in rheumatoid arthritis outcome and pharmacogenetics. Current Pharmacogenomics 2007; 5:275-79.
54. Smith AJP, Humphries SE. Cytokine and cytokine receptor gene polymorphisms and their functionality. Cytokine and Growth Factor Reviews 2009; 20(1):43-59.
55. Tracey D, Klareskog L, Sasso EH, Salfeld JG, Tak PP. Tumor necrosis factor antagonist mechanism of action: A comprehensive review. Pharmacology and Therapeutics 2008;117:244-79.
56. Choo-Kang BSW, Hutchison S, Nickdel MB, Bundick RV, Leishman AJ, Brewer JM, McInnes IB, Garside P. TNF-blocking therapies: An alternative mode of action? Trends in Immunology 2005;26(10):518-22.
57. Borrebaeck CAK, Carlsson R. Human therapeutic antibodies. Current Opinion in Pharmacology 2001;1: 404-08.
58. Bogunia-Kubik K. Polymorphisms within the genes encoding TNF-α and TNF-β associate with the incidence of post-transplant complications in recipients of allogeneic hematopoietic stem cell transplants. Archivum Immunologiae et Therapiae Experimentalis 2004; 52(4):240-49.
59. Tumanov AV, Christiansen PA, Fu YX. The role of lymphotoxin receptor signaling in diseases. Current Molecular Medicine 2007;7(6):567-78.

C4 Genes

60. Crawford K, Alper CA. Genetics of the complement system. Reviews in Immunogenetics 2000;2(3):323-38.
61. Martinez OP, Longman-Jacobsen N, Davies R, Chung EK, Yang Y, Gaudieri S, Dawkins RL, Yu CY. Genetics of the human complement component C4 and evolution of the central MHC. Frontiers in Bioscience 2001; 6:D 904-13.
62. Yu CY, Whitacre CC. Sex, MHC and complement C4 in autoimmune diseases. Trends in Immunology 2004; 25(12):694-99.

CYP

63. Nimkarn S, New MI. Prenatal diagnosis and treatment of congenital adrenal hyperplasia owing to 21-hydroxylase deficiency. Endocrinology and Metabolism 2007; 3(5): 405-13.
64. Riepe FG, Sippell WG. Recent advances in diagnosis, treatment, and outcome of congenital adrenal hyperplasia due to 21-hydroxylase deficiency. Review Endocr Metab.Disord 2007;8:349-63.
65. Demirci C, Witchel SF. Congenital adrenal hyperplasia. Dermatologic Therapy 2008; 21:340-53.

Polymorphism and Nomenclature

66. For information on MHC gene sequences and nomenclature including regular nomenclature reports visit the IMGT/HLA at http://www.ebi.ac.uk/imgt/hla/
67. For detailed information on MHC genes including sequence location and function visit the University of California Santa Cruz site at http:// genome.ucsc.edu/

Chapter 5

HLA Nomenclature

Steven GE Marsh

SUMMARY

Early in their study it was recognized that the genes encoding the HLA molecules were highly polymorphic and that there was a need for a systematic nomenclature. The result was the WHO Nomenclature Committee for Factors of the HLA System that first met in 1968, and laid down the criteria for successive meetings. This committee meets regularly to discuss issues of nomenclature and has published 19 major reports documenting firstly the HLA antigens and more recently the genes and alleles. The standardization of HLA antigenic specificities has been controlled by the exchange of typing reagents and cells in the International Histocompatibility Workshops. Since 1989 when a large number of HLA allele sequences were first analyzed and named, the job of curating and maintaining a database of sequences has been of prime importance. In 1998, the IMGT/HLA database became the official repository for HLA sequences. In addition to the nucleotide and protein sequences the database contains information of the cell from which the sequence was obtained. The database provides tools for sequence analysis and the submission of new data, is updated quarterly and now contains over 4000 HLA allele sequences.

Many of the advances in the HLA field have come about through the collaborative International Histocompatibility Workshops (IHWs). The first of these took place at Duke University, Durham, USA in 1964 organized by Bernard Amos. Following this, workshops have taken place every three to five years with the most recent, the 15th taking place in Buzios, Brazil in 2008. In the early days the numbers of participants was small: only sixteen laboratories took part in the 1st Workshop, where they compared the typing of a panel of eight cells using seven different techniques. The work presented in the most recent workshops has been undertaken by hundreds of laboratories around the world, participating in a variety of different projects, using many different molecular based techniques and typing thousands of samples.[1]

Very early in the study of HLA, the potential complexity of the system was beginning to be recognized and the need for standardized nomenclature understood. This was felt during both the 1st IHW in 1964 and again at the 2nd IHW in 1965 organized by Jon van Rood at the University Hospital, Leiden, in the Netherlands where it became apparent that different groups were each using their own local designations to describe the same serologically defined antigens. During the 2nd IHW a committee was formed to discuss nomenclature. It met only once believing that the time was not ripe to decide on a final nomenclature and suggesting that only provisional terms be used. The report of this meeting signalled to the community that the need for a standard nomenclature had been recognized, and was no more than a single sentence: *"The question of nomenclature of the leukocyte antigens has been raised during the workshop. An advice on this matter will be formulated by a committee on nomenclature, which has been formed during this Workshop."*[2]

During the 3rd IHW organized by Ruggero Ceppellini in Torino, Italy, in June 1967 the issue of nomenclature was discussed again, and following a second meeting in Williamsburg, USA in November that same year, while still awaiting the formation of an official nomenclature committee, the main investigators in the field *"…agreed to use the term HL-A for indicating the major system of leukocyte antigens (previous names: Du-1, Four, Hu-1, LA, etc.)".*[3,4] Contrary to popular belief the name assigned, "HL-A" was not an abbreviation for "Human Leukocyte Antigen" or "Human Locus A" but simply as a contraction of the "H" from "Hu-1" system of Dausset and "LA" from the system named by Payne and Bodmer.[5]

In September 1968 under the auspices of the World Health Organization (WHO) the first meeting of the "WHO Leukocyte Nomenclature Committee" took place in New York, USA. This meeting was recorded and a full verbatim account of the meeting was reported later.[6] The first eight serologically defined HL-A antigens, HL-A1 through HL-A8, were named at this time. These official names together with their previous locally assigned designations, as used in ten different laboratories, were listed in the first full Nomenclature Report.[7] The report also listed guidelines on the use of the new nomenclature and on the criteria used in the assignment of new serologically defined antigens.

After the 4th IHW which took place in Los Angeles in 1970 organized by Paul Terasaki, a further four antigens were deemed worthy of an official designation HL-A10, -A11, -A12, -A13. For some reason HL-A9 was not listed at this time, however, the nomenclature report makes reference to its existence and that it was readily recognisable, suggesting that this antigen had been named in the intervening period between the workshops.[8]

Following the 5th IHW in Evian, France in 1972 organized by Jean Dausset, the Nomenclature Committee announced that the definition of a histocompatibility antigen would pass through four stages. Firstly, a new specificity would be detected by a laboratory and given a local designation. Secondly, if this specificity was confirmed by several of the reference laboratories, it would be given a provisional number preceded by the prefix 'W'. In the third stage, when all the reference laboratories had reached a firm agreement on the definition of the new specificity, an HL-A number would be assigned. In the fourth stage, a chemical or molecular analysis would allow the HL-A specificity to be confirmed.[9] Ten new HL-A specificities were listed in this report, each of which carried the new 'W' prefix, indicating that the antigen had "Workshop" status. It was also recognized by this time that some specificities, for example HL-A9, appeared to represent cross-reactivity between two component antigens. As a consequence the committee introduced the concept of a "Broad" specificity, such as A9 and its components, later to be termed "Splits", which were named AW23 and AW24.

It had been evident for sometime that the relationship between different HL-A antigens was complex, and that the original serologically defined specificities of this system were being assigned to two separate series (first or LA, and second or FOUR) corresponding to two linked genes, each with multiple alleles. As such these two genes would require a separate nomenclature. Following the 6th IHW in Århus, Denmark in 1975 organized by Flemming Kissmeyer-Nielsen, it was decided to remove the hyphen from the name HL-A, and use HLA as a designation of the region or system.[10] This was followed by a hyphen used as a separator, before a gene designation A, B, C, etc. Hence the antigens defined previously were assigned either to the HLA-A (previously LA or first) or HLA-B (previously FOUR or second) gene. The specificities 1, 2, 3, 9, 10, and 11 became HLA-A1, -A2, -A3, -A9, -A10, and –A11; specificities 5, 7, 8, 12, 13, etc. became HLA-B5, -B7, -B8, -B12, -B13. The use of a lower case 'w' to indicate a provisional specificity was retained with the 'w' being inserted between the gene name and antigen number, hence HLA-Aw23. Once antigens had been verified successfully it could be upgraded to full HLA status by omission of the 'w'. In addition at this time two new genes were recognized and named. What had previously been termed AJ or the third locus was named HLA-C. In addition to the serologically defined antigens of the HLA-A, -B and –C loci, the first antigens defined by the cellular technique of Mixed Lymphocyte Culture (MLC), were assigned to the new HLA-D locus, and HLA-Dw1 to –Dw6. A total of 51 different HLA antigens had been recognized and assigned official designations by 1975.

The HLA Nomenclature Report published after the 7th IHW in Oxford, UK organized by Walter Bodmer in 1977, saw the introduction of the HLA-DR locus. The designation DR for 'D' related, indicated that these serological specificities were in some way related to the HLA-D specificities which had previously been defined using MLC.[11] The first seven HLA-DR antigens were named at this time; HLA-DRw1 to DRw7. The notation used to represent antigen splits was revisited at this time with the suggestion that the broad antigen name should follow the split name in parenthesis; for example Aw23,[9] where Aw23 was a split of the A9 antigen. Although the numbers 4 and 6 had been held in reserve since 1968 for the 4a and 4b specificities, it was not until the 1977 report that these were officially named Bw4 and Bw6 and were recognized as public epitopes being present on all of the HLA-B antigens.

The 1980 Nomenclature Report included only a handful of new antigens and saw no major additions or changes to the HLA nomenclature; a total of 92 antigens were listed at this time.[12] The 1984 Nomenclature Report, published after the 9th IHW organized by Ekkehard Albert and Wolfgang Mayr in Munich, Germany, saw the assignment of two new HLA genes, HLA-DQ and HLA-DP.[13] The newly assigned DQ specificities, DQw1, DQw2, and DQw3 were defined by serological techniques; the six new DP antigens, DPw1 to DPw6 were defined using the cellular assay Primed Lymphocyte Typing (PLT). In addition two new DR antigens were named DRw52 and DRw53. At the time it was unclear whether these represented public epitopes on the DR molecule in an analogous way to the Bw4 and Bw6 epitopes of HLA-B. It was later shown that these were the products of secondary HLA-DR genes. By this time an elementary map of the HLA region had been established and the first HLA genes had been cloned, and it was clearly understood that the HLA class II molecules consisted of two polypeptide chains whose genes were both located within the HLA region. The suggestion was made that the genes for the separate chains be called DRA and DRB, etc.

In 1987 following the 10th IHW organized by Bo Dupont in Princeton, USA a molecular nomenclature for both genes and DNA allele sequences was introduced with the recognition that many pseudogenes were also located in the HLA region.[14] Expanding the previously suggested notation, the HLA genes were given official names, the gene encoding the DRα chain was called DRA. Several different genes encoding DRβ chains had been identified and were named HLA-DRB1, -DRB2, -DRB3, and –DRB4. The HLA-DRB2 gene was shown to be a pseudogene. In addition to naming many new genes, it was recognized that many of the antigen specificities previously defined by serology, such as HLA-A2, could be subdivided still further by DNA sequencing. Four different A2 sequences were named at this time, A*0201, A*0202, A*0203, and A*0204. The asterisk was used as a separator between the gene name, and the four-digit code used to distinguish between the alleles. The first two digits indicating the HLA antigen encoded by the allele and the second two digits indicating that number of the allele in that series, where each allele differs from the others by at least one nucleotide substitution that changes the amino acid sequence of the encoded protein. A total of 12 HLA class I alleles and nine class II alleles were named at this time. In addition a further 24 HLA antigens were named at this time.

The meeting of the WHO Nomenclature Committee for Factors of the HLA System in 1989 took place between workshops and recognized the need to assign official names to the many new HLA allele sequences that were being published.[15] A total of 56 HLA class I and 78 class II alleles were named in the report of this meeting. It had become necessary to emphasize the need to deposit the newly discovered sequences in an appropriate database, and that this would need to be continually updated.

It became apparent as early as 1989 that the analysis and assigning of official names to alleles could not wait for periodic histocompatibility workshops or even annual Nomenclature Committee meetings, and so began the process of daily assessing newly defined HLA allele sequences. Julia Bodmer and Steven Marsh at the Imperial Cancer Research Fund (ICRF) in collaboration with Peter Parham at Stanford University carried out this work. It was out of the need to record and manage the HLA sequence data being submitted to the Nomenclature Committee that the first incarnation of an HLA Sequence Databank (HLA-DB) emerged.[16]

Periodically HLA class I[17-20] and class II[21-26] sequence alignments were published in a variety of journals and by 1995 the numbers of new alleles being reported now warranted the publication of monthly nomenclature updates,[27] something which continues to this day. Also by 1995, the expansion of the Internet and the introduction of the World Wide Web (WWW) saw the first distribution of the HLA sequence alignments from the web pages of the Tissue Antigen Laboratory at the ICRF. This work transferred to the Anthony Nolan Research Institute (ANRI) in 1996 where it continues today. In an effort to make the data held in the database available in a more accessible and interactive format the IMGT/HLA Database project was begun in 1997 as part of a European collaboration involving the ICRF, ANRI and the European Bioinformatics Institute (EBI), which maintains the European Molecular Biology Laboratory's nucleotide sequence database (EMBL). The IMGT database project contains a number of distinct databases specializing in sequences of immunological interest. The IMGT/HLA database was first released in 1998,[28, 29] the database combines the sequence data and information previously provided to the WHO Nomenclature Committee for Factors of the HLA System and the additional data found in the original EMBL/GenBank/DDBJ entries. The database can be accessed from www.ebi.ac.uk/imgt/hla. The database is updated every three months and provides a suite of tools for analyzing the nucleotide and protein sequences.

Since 1989, the HLA Nomenclature Committee has continued to meet everyone to two years to establish further guidelines for the naming of HLA genes and alleles and published reports in 1990,[30] 1991 following the 11th IHW,[31] 1994,[32] 1995,[33] 1996 following the 12th IHW,[34] 1998,[35] 2000,[36] 2002 following the 13th IHW[37] and 2004.[38] The HLA allele names were first extended to five digits in 1990 to allow for the discrimination of alleles differing only in non-coding (synonymous) substitutions within the coding sequence.[30] In 1995, they were again extended to seven digits to allow for the naming of alleles which differed only in introns or the 3´ or 5´ regions of the gene.[33]

In addition to the unique allele number there are additional optional suffixes that may be added to an allele to indicate its expression status. Alleles that have been shown not to be expressed, "Null" alleles have been given the suffix 'N'.[32] Those alleles which have been shown to be alternatively expressed which may have the suffix 'L', 'S', 'C', 'A', or 'Q'. The suffix 'L' is used to indicate an allele that has been shown to have "Low" cell surface expression when compared to normal levels.[34] The 'S' suffix is used to denote an allele specifying a protein which is expressed as a soluble "Secreted" molecule but is not present on the cell surface.[37] A 'C' suffix is used to indicate an allele product which is present in the "Cytoplasm" but not on the cell surface. An 'A' suffix to indicate 'Aberrant' expression where there is some doubt as to whether a protein is expressed. A 'Q' suffix when the expression of an allele is "Questionable" given that the mutation seen in the allele has previously been shown to effect normal expression levels.

In 2002, due to the increasing number of alleles being described, an additional digit was inserted between the fourth and fifth digits to allow for more than nine alleles differing only by synonymous substitutions, extending the allele name to eight digits.[37] At this time the idea of roll-over allele names was introduced for the A*02 and B*15 allele families, both of which were rapidly approaching more than one hundred and could not be named within the four-digit system. It was decided that cases where the total number of coding variants exceeded 99, a second-number series would be used to extend the first one. For the B*15 family of alleles, the B*95 series was used to code for additional B*15 alleles, so that B*1599 was followed by B*9501, and for the A*02 family of alleles A*0299 was followed with A*9201. A similar problem existed for HLA-DPB1 where alleles had been named sequentially, and not grouped into families of alleles based on prior serological relationships. With the number of DPB1 alleles approaching one hundred it was decided to assign new alleles within the existing system, hence once DPB1*9901 had been assigned, the next allele was named DPB1*0102, followed by DPB1*0203, DPB1*0302, etc.[37] Neither of these were satisfactory solutions and were destined to be revisited later.

Aside from extending the number of digits used to code for the different alleles, and the adding of optional suffixes to indicate the expression status of an alleles, the nomenclature used for alleles has changed little since it was first introduced in 1987. The first-two digits describe the allele family, which often corresponds to the serological antigen carried by the allotype. The third and fourth digits are assigned in the order in which the sequences have been determined. Alleles whose numbers differ in the first four digits must differ in one or more nucleotide substitutions that change the amino acid sequence of the encoded protein. Alleles that differ only by synonymous nucleotide substitutions within the coding sequence are distinguished by the use of the fifth and sixth digits. Alleles that only differ by sequence polymorphisms in introns or in the 5' and 3' untranslated regions that flank the exons and introns are distinguished by the use of the seventh and eighth digits.

When these conventions were adopted it was anticipated that the nomenclature system would accommodate all the HLA alleles likely to be sequenced. Unfortunately over time this has been shown not to be the case, as the number of alleles for certain genes has exceeded the maximum possible with the current naming convention. At the time of writing, October 2009, a total of 3007 HLA class I alleles and 1154 class II alleles have been named (Fig. 5.1). This issue was discussed at length during the Nomenclature Committee meeting held during the 15th IHW in Buzios, Brazil in 2008, and following this meeting the decision was taken to revise the nomenclature for HLA alleles. This new nomenclature will be implemented in April 2010. It was decided to introduce colons (:) into the allele names to act as delimiters of the separate fields. Hence A*01010101 becomes A*01:01:01:01, the four distinct fields being used as before to indicate firstly, the allele family; the second field to indicate the order in which the allele was described; the third field to distinguish alleles differing only by synonymous nucleotide substitutions; and the forth field to indicate those differing only in their introns, or in the 5' and 3' untranslated regions. The existing leading zeros in the allele names will be maintained, to lessen confusion in the conversion to the new style of nomenclature, but no further leading zeros will be added to allele names. As a result of this change it will become possible to expand each field as

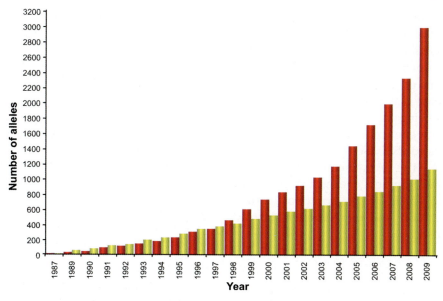

Fig. 5.1: The number of HLA class I and II alleles officially recognized between 1987 and 2009. Class I allele numbers are shown in red and class II allele numbers in yellow

necessary once the number of alleles within an allele family makes this a requirement.

This change will allow the renaming of the rollover alleles A*92 and B*15 in to the A*02 and B*15 families, with A*9201 becoming A*02:101 and B*9501 becoming B*15:101. Likewise it will allow the DPB1 alleles, previously named according to decisions in taken in 2002, to be renamed in a single numerical series, hence DPB1*0102 will become DPB1*100:01. The decision was also taken to remove the 'w' from the HLA-C allele names, but to still require this when reporting HLA-C antigens, to prevent confusion with complement factor nomenclature, hence Cw*0102 will become C*01:02, whereas Cw1 will remain Cw1.

Full details of the HLA Nomenclature are made available both on the IMGT/HLA Database website[39, 40] and also on the HLA Nomenclature website "hla.alleles.org" which in addition to providing static HLA sequence alignments, is a reference website for HLA Nomenclature. The current release of the IMGT/HLA Database, version 2.27.0 includes over 4000 HLA allele sequences from 34 HLA genes, and includes details on over 7400 cells that have been sequenced for one or more HLA alleles. Since 2000 the IMGT/HLA Sequence Database and the work of the HLA Nomenclature Committee has been supported by the generous donations of a number of commercial companies, immunogenetic organizations and bone marrow registries, for which we are grateful.

The value of a systematic nomenclature and a database of HLA alleles sequences to the user communities in transplantation, research and clinical practice, is critically dependant on the quality and accuracy of the information it contains. Even single nucleotide errors in transcribing and reporting sequences cannot be tolerated if the data is to be relied on. The job of maintaining and curating the database is thus of vital importance and necessarily requires meticulous attention to detail. However, the IMGT/HLA Sequence Database now goes well beyond just providing a list of sequences and provides a whole range of linked information and incorporates many tools for data retrieval, analysis and submission of new data. With the completion of the Human Genome Project and the identification of many new polymorphic genes, the IMGT/HLA Sequence Database and the HLA Nomenclature, which has evolved over the past thirty years, is clearly a model of how this new polymorphic data can be managed.

Useful websites
HLA Nomenclature: http://hla.alleles.org
IMGT/HLA Homepage: http://www.ebi.ac.uk/imgt/hla/

ACKNOWLEDGMENTS

I would like to thank all the members of the WHO Nomenclature Committee for Factors of the HLA System for the input into the HLA Nomenclature, and in particular Peter Parham for his helpful discussions. Thanks go to James Robinson, Kavita Mistry, Matthew Waller, and Sylvie Fail for their work on the IMGT/HLA Database: Rodrigo Lopez, Hamish McWilliam, Peter Stoehr, and colleagues at the EBI for their continued support of the database. I would like to acknowledge the support of the following organizations for the IMGT/HLA Database: Histogenetics, Abbot, One Lambda, Biotest, Invitrogen, Olerup SSP, Gen-Probe, BAG Health care, Innogenetics, the American Society for Histocompatibility and Immunogenetics, the European Federation of Immunogenetics, the Anthony Nolan Trust, Be the Match Foundation, and the National Marrow Donor Program (NMDP).

REFERENCES

1. Marsh SGE. HLA nomenclature and the IMGT/HLA Sequence Database. In: Bock G, Goode J, eds. Immunoinformatics: Bioinformatic Strategies for Better Understanding of Immune Function - No 254. London: Novartis Foundation Symposium 2003;165-76.
2. Bruning JW, van Leeuwen A, van Rood JJ. Leucocyte Antigens. In: Amos B, van Rood JJ, eds. Histocompatibility Testing 1965. Copenhagen, Denmark: Munksgaard 1965;275-83.
3. Nomenclature-Committee. Nomenclature: HL-A. In: Curtoni ES, Mattiuz PL, Tosi RM, eds. Histocompatibility Testing 1967. Copenhagen, Denmark: Munksgaard 1967;449.
4. Amos DB. Human Histocompatibility Locus HL-A. Science 1968;159:659-60.
5. Amos DB. Why "HLA". In: Hahn AB, Rodey GE, eds. ASHI: The First 25 Years (1974-1999): American Society for Histocompatibility and Immunogenetics 1999:64-6.
6. Walford RL. First meeting WHO Leukocyte Nomenclature Committee, New York, September 1968. In: Terasaki PI, ed. History of HLA: Ten Recollections. Los Angeles: UCLA Tissue Typing Laboratory 1990:121-49.
7. WHO Nomenclature Committee. Nomenclature for Factors of the HL-A System. Bull Wld Hlth Org 1968;39:483-6.
8. WHO Nomenclature Committee. WHO Terminology Report. In: Terasaki PI, ed. Histocompatibility Testing, 1970. Copenhagen: Munksgaard, 1970:49.
9. WHO Nomenclature Committee. WHO Terminology Report. Bull Wld Hlth Org 1972;47:659-62.
10. WHO IUIS Terminology Committee. Nomenclature for Factors of the HLA System. Bull Wld Hlth Org 1975;52:261.
11. WHO Nomenclature Committee. Nomenclature for Factors of the HLA System, 1977. Bull Wld Hlth Org 1978;56:461-5.
12. WHO Nomenclature Committee. Nomenclature for Factors of the HLA System, 1980. In: Terasaki PI, ed. Histocompatibility Testing, 1980. Los Angeles: UCLA Tissue Typing Laboratory 1980;18-20.
13. WHO Nomenclature Committee. Nomenclature for factors of the HLA system 1984. In: Albert ED, Baur MP, Mayr WR, eds. Histocompatibility Testing, 1984. Berlin: Springer-Verlag 1985:4-8.
14. Bodmer WF, Albert E, Bodmer JG, et al. Nomenclature for factors of the HLA system, 1987. In: Dupont B, ed. Immunobiology of HLA. New York: Springer-Verlag 1989:72-9.
15. Bodmer JG, Marsh SGE, Parham P, et al. Nomenclature for factors of the HLA system, 1989. Tissue Antigens 1990;35:1-8.
16. Marsh SGE, Bodmer JG. HLA Class II Sequence Databank. Human Immunology 1993;36:44.
17. Zemmour J, Parham P. HLA class I nucleotide sequences, 1991. Tissue Antigens 1991;37:174-80.
18. Zemmour J, Parham P. HLA class I nucleotide sequences, 1992. Tissue Antigens 1992;40:221-8.
19. Arnett KL, Parham P. HLA class I nucleotide sequences, 1995. Tissue Antigens 1995;46:217-57.
20. Mason PM, Parham P. HLA class I region sequences, 1998. Tissue Antigens 1998;51:417-66.
21. Marsh SGE, Bodmer JG. HLA-DRB nucleotide sequences, 1990. Immunogenetics 1990;31:141-4.
22. Marsh SGE, Bodmer JG. HLA class II nucleotide sequences, 1991. Tissue Antigens 1991;37:181-9.
23. Marsh SGE, Bodmer JG. HLA class II nucleotide sequences, 1992. Tissue Antigens 1992;40:229-43.
24. Marsh SGE, Bodmer JG. HLA class II region nucleotide sequences, 1994. Eur J Immunogenet 1994;21:519-51.
25. Marsh SGE, Bodmer JG. HLA class II region nucleotide sequences, 1995. Tissue Antigens 1995;46:258-80.
26. Marsh SGE. HLA class II region sequences, 1998. Tissue Antigens 1998;51:467-507.
27. Marsh SGE. Nomenclature for Factors of the HLA System, Update January 1995. Tissue Antigens 1995;45:220-2.
28. Robinson J, Malik A, Parham P, Bodmer JG, Marsh SGE. IMGT/HLA database—a sequence database for the human major histocompatibility complex. Tissue Antigens 2000;55:280-7.
29. Robinson J, Waller MJ, Parham P, Bodmer JG, Marsh SGE. IMGT/HLA Database—a sequence database for the human major histocompatibility complex. Nucleic Acids Res 2001;29:210-3.
30. Bodmer JG, Marsh SGE, Albert E, et al. Nomenclature for factors of the HLA system, 1990. Tissue Antigens 1991;37:97-104.
31. Bodmer JG, Marsh SGE, Albert E, et al. Nomenclature for factors of the HLA system, 1991. In: Tsuji T, Aizawa M, Sasazuki T, eds. HLA 1991. Oxford: Oxford University Press 1992:17-31.
32. Bodmer JG, Marsh SGE, Albert E, et al. Nomenclature for factors of the HLA system, 1994. Tissue Antigens 1994;44:1-18.

33. Bodmer JG, Marsh SGE, Albert E, et al. Nomenclature for factors of the HLA system, 1995. Tissue Antigens 1995;46:1-18.
34. Bodmer JG, Marsh SGE, Albert ED, et al. Nomenclature for factors of the HLA system, 1996. Tissue Antigens 1997;49:297-321.
35. Bodmer JG, Marsh SGE, Albert ED, et al. Nomenclature for factors of the HLA system, 1998. Tissue Antigens 1999;53:407-46.
36. Marsh SGE, Bodmer JG, Albert ED et al. Nomenclature for factors of the HLA system, 2000. Tissue Antigens 2001;57:236-83.
37. Marsh SGE, Albert ED, Bodmer WF, et al. Nomenclature for factors of the HLA system, 2002. Tissue Antigens 2002;60:407-64.
38. Marsh SG, Albert ED, Bodmer WF, et al. Nomenclature for factors of the HLA system, 2004. Tissue Antigens 2005;65:301-69.
39. Robinson J, Waller MJ, Fail SC, et al. The IMGT/HLA database. Nucleic Acids Res 2009;37:D1013-7.
40. Robinson J, Waller MJ, Fail SC, Marsh SGE. The IMGT/HLA and IPD databases. Hum Mutat 2006;27:1192-9.

Chapter 6

HLA Molecules of the Major Histocompatibility Complex

James McCluskey, Stephanie Gras, Mandvi Bharadwaj,
Lars Kjer-Nielsen, Whitney Macdonald,
Philippa Saunders, Jamie Rossjohn

INTRODUCTION

The adaptive immune response is regulated by HLA molecules of the major histocompatibility complex (MHC) through their interaction with clonally distributed Antigen (Ag)-specific αβ T-cell receptors expressed on T-cells. Antigen-specific T-cell responses are driven by the recognition of HLA-peptide complexes presented by the classical HLA class I and class II molecules at the surface of antigen presenting cells (APC). This chapter discusses the pathway of Ag loading, the structural features of HLA molecules and the principles governing antigen recognition by classical αβ T-cell receptors.

HLA MOLECULES

Classical HLA molecules are encoded by 6 distinct, yet homologous loci (HLA-A, B, Cw, DR, DQ and DP) linked on the short arm of human chromosome 6 (Klein, 1987). This region is called the major histocompatibility complex reflecting the historical discovery of this gene complex as the major cluster of gene loci that control organ allograft rejection or acceptance (Amos et al, 1955; Snell, 1957; Snell and Higgins, 1951; Strominger, 2002). This aspect of HLA-biology is extremely important clinically but complicates understanding the actual function and evolutionary importance of these genes and their proteins. Understanding the biology of the MHC from the perspective of transplantation is generally very confusing for newcomers such as medical students and young scientists. Its more cogent to consider the HLA genes of the MHC as the traditional 'immune response genes' (IR genes) that mandate antigen-specific immunity. Thus, at about the time they were recognized as controlling allograft acceptance versus rejection, the IR genes were independently discovered for their control of immune responsiveness to defined antigens [for review of the history see (McDevitt et al, 1972)]. HLA molecules are also known to be important genetic determinants of autoimmunity, tumor immunity, allergic responses including drug hypersensitivity and protection against infectious disease (Chessman et al, 2008; Hill, 2001; Larsen and Alper, 2004; Mallal et al, 2002; Martin et al, 2004; Segal and Hill, 2003; Thorsby, 1997; Undlien et al, 2001; Carrington and O'Brien, 2003). The mechanism by which these molecules exert this enormous influence is directly related to their three-dimensional structure that is designed to capture peptide fragments of catabolised pathogen proteins, Figure 6.1. Equally important to their structure/function is their extraordinarily high level of polymorphism in human populations. Accordingly, we first review the structure and function of HLA molecules and the conventional αβ T-cell receptors that recognize them during Ag-specific T-cell responses.

HLA CLASS I STRUCTURE

The HLA class I molecules comprise the polymorphic class Ia, HLA-A, B and C molecules and the relatively non-polymorphic class Ib, HLA-E, F, G and Hfe (HLA-H) molecules. HLA-A, B and C molecules comprise a single heavy chain complexed to a smaller molecule known as β2microglobulin (Bjorkman et al, 1987a, b), Figure 6.1A. The heavy chain is anchored in the membrane and has a short cytoplasmic tail. Although the gene structure of *HLA-A, B* and *C* loci and the overall shape of the respective molecules is similar, the primary amino acid structure of these molecules differ from each other significantly. The HLA-A, B and C class I heavy chains all associate non-covalently with a single molecule of β2 microglobulin, which is non-polymorphic and encoded on chromosome 17, Figure 6.1A. An excess of β2 microglobulin is produced by most cell types providing sufficient light chain for assembly of all the class Ia and class Ib molecules expressed by the cell. It is estimated that there are between 10^4 and 10^6 class I molecules on most nucleated cell types with all three locus products expressed in a co-dominant fashion (i.e. the products of both maternal and paternal MHC loci are simultaneously expressed by all cells). However, the levels of surface expression of most HLA-C molecules tend to be lower than the HLA-A and HLA-B products.

The three-dimensional structure of a class I molecule is ideally suited to capture short peptides for presentation to T-cells. The Antigen binding cleft of the heavy chain (residues 1-180) contains a central groove about 25Å long, within which are a series of pockets suited to accommodate amino acid side chains from the peptide (Bjorkman et al, 1987b; Garrett et al, 1989), Figures 6.1A and 6.2A and B. The outermost domains $α_1$ and $α_2$ comprise two long α-helices separated by the Ag-binding cleft, the floor of which is composed of β-pleated sheet, Figure 6.1A. HLA-A, HLA-B and HLA-C are all highly polymorphic as well as being the products of different loci, Figure 6.3. The major site of the structural polymorphism in HLA class I and class II molecules is in the region of the antigen binding cleft (Bjorkman and Parham, 1990; Margulies and McCluskey, 2003), Figure 6.3. The distinct pockets of the HLA class I antigen-binding cleft, designated pocket A, B, C, D, E, and F respectively (Fig. 6.2B), vary in their chemical properties from one allotype to another according to polymorphisms in these pockets (Garrett et al, 1989). The same principle applies to the HLA class II molecules although the pocket nomenclature is different. The polymorphic amino acid side chains in the MHC (Fig. 6.3) alter the electrostatic surface charge, hydrophobicity, size and shape of HLA antigen pockets according to the specific side chain chemistry of the amino acids lining each pocket. The polymorphisms within the HLA cleft have the effect of altering the peptide binding properties of allelic class I molecules so that each of them will bind a unique repertoire of peptides. The length of class I-bound peptides is usually between 8 and 10 amino acids reflecting the fact that the ends of bound peptide are tucked in to the cleft where they are ligated by a network of h-bonds between conserved heavy chain residues and the free amino- and carboxyl-terminus of the peptide, Figure 6.4A. This

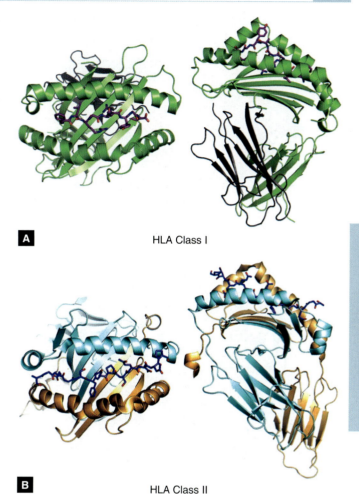

Figs 6.1A and B: The three-dimensional structure of HLA molecules. (A) The class I molecule HLA-B8 seen from above (left panel) and from the side (right panel) as a ribbon diagram. The class I heavy chain is in green and the light chain, β2 m is in dark grey. The peptide FLRGRAYGL is derived from the Epstein-Barr virus EBNA 3A antigen (Kjer-Nielsen et al, 2002a) and represented in purple stick. (B) The class II molecule HLA-DQ8 is shown complexed to a foreign peptide derived from wheat gluten (represented in blue stick). The α and β chains are shown in pale cyan and pale orange respectively. View from the top (left panel) and side-on (right panel). Note that the peptide extends beyond the antigen-binding cleft

property of HLA class I allows peptides with different sequences at their termini to be bound in the same way by different class I allotypes. This is not the case for HLA class II-bound peptides that are generally longer than those captured by class I molecules, and therefore overhang the cleft. The conserved binding of peptide termini by class I molecules restricts the canonical length of most bound peptides to 8-10 amino acids allowing dominant anchor residues to be discerned by sequencing pools of heterogeneous peptides eluted from a given class I allotype. The energy of binding of class I peptides is shared between the dominant anchor sites, minor anchor sites and the h-bonding network at the peptide termini. Nonetheless, peptides longer than 8-10 amino acids can occasionally bind class I molecules (estimated to be approximately 5% of class I epitopes) and these are not accommodated in the current algorithm-based methods for predicting T-cell determinants as discussed below and tabulated in Table 6.2 (Burrows et al, 2006). Hence these longer ligands are not as easily predicted. The termini of longer peptides (>10 residues) generally remain tucked into the cleft such that the central part of the peptide bulges upwards from the Antigen-binding cleft to accommodate the extra residues (Archbold et al, 2009; Bell et al, 2009; Green et al, 2004; Robbins et al, 1995; Speir et al, 2001; Tynan et al, 2005a; Tynan et al, 2007), Figures 6.4B and C. HLA class I-peptide complexes are sometimes abbreviated as pMHC-I or pHLA-I.

The relatively conserved structure of the membrane-proximal α3 domain of the class I molecule interacts with CD8 co-receptor molecules on T-cells via a flexible loop of the α3 domain (residues 223-229) that is clamped

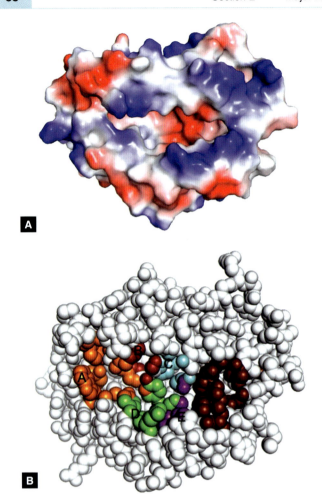

Figs 6.2A and B: The antigen binding cleft of class I molecules contains 6 major pockets (A-F) that determine the specificity of peptide binding. (A) The cleft of a mouse class I molecule with the peptide removed revealing the shape and charge of the empty specificity pockets. Electronegative, red; electropositive, blue. Adapted with permission from ref 176. (B) Space filling model of a human class I molecule depicting the antigen-binding cleft, with those residues occupying the major specificity pockets coloured A, orange; B, red; C, cyan; D, green; E, purple; F, brown

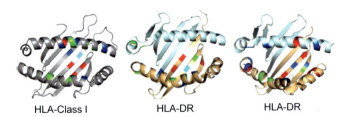

Fig. 6.3: Location of polymorphisms in the antigen-binding cleft of HLA molecules. The residues that are most polymorphic are colored such that red>blue>green. Note the α-chain of DR is essentially monomorphic so the polymorphism in DR is centred in one half of the cleft. Adapted with permission from ref.176

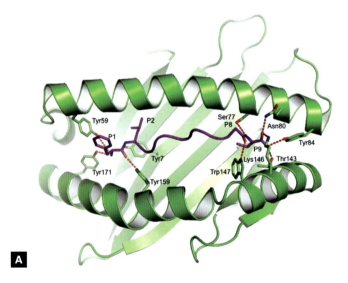

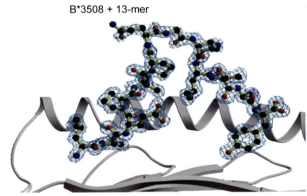

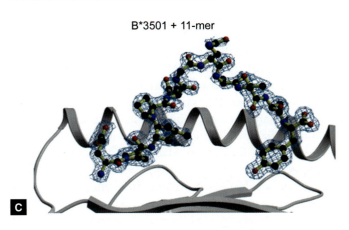

Figs 6.4A to C: (A) A network of highly conserved bonds ligates bound peptide to the N-terminus (left) and to the C-terminus (right) of the class I molecule. The α-carbon backbone and side chains of the intervening residues of the peptide are shown as a simple coil. Sidechains of amino acids that participate in conserved h-bonds and that are conserved in all class I molecules are shown. Peptides longer than 10 amino acids can also bind HLA-class I molecules but their termini remain tucked into the cleft so the peptide bulges as for (B) a 13-mer peptide from Epstein-Barr virus bound the HLA-B*3508 and (C) an 11-mer peptide from Epstein-Barr virus bound the HLA-B*3501. Fig. 6.4B is adapted with permission from reference 282 and Fig. 6.4C is reproduced with permission from reference 189

between the complementarity-determining region (CDR)-like loops of the CD8 molecule (Gao et al, 1997). Notably, some HLA-class I allotypes, such as HLA-A68, lack the appropriate residues in this region of the α3 domain and cannot interact with CD8, yet still function as antigen receptors for stimulation of killer T-cells. This region of the α3 domain is sometimes mutated on purpose to reduce non-specific binding of MHC-I tetramers when staining CD8+ T-cells.

HLA Class I Peptide-binding Motifs

The unique set of peptides bound by any given class I allotype tends to share a preferred sequence 'motif' determined by the spacing of amino acid side chains in the peptide antigen that form dominant anchor sites for binding to each unique HLA cleft (Falk et al, 1991; Marsh et al, 2000; Rammensee et al, 1993a; Rotzschke et al, 1990). Table 6.1 gives the canonical peptide-binding motif for peptides that preferentially bind to selected HLA class I allotypes. More extensive databases of MHC ligands have been compiled by various groups (Brusic et al, 1998; Rammensee et al, 1995). A number of databases use bioinformatic algorithms to analyze protein sequences of interest for determinants predicted to bind HLA molecules. These include SYFPEITHI (Rammensee et al, 1999), MHCPEP (Brusic et al, 1998) and the NIAID, Bioinformatics and Molecular Analysis Section algorithm that ranks potential 8-mer, 9-mer, or 10-mer peptides based on a predicted half-time of dissociation (BIMAS) (Parker et al, 1995). Useful websites that include peptide-ligand databases and predictive algorithms are shown in Table 6.2. Peptide-binding motifs are not absolute predictors of whether or not a given peptide will bind to a class I allotype and nor do they account for all peptides that do bind to particular class I molecules. Ligands that deviate from empirically determined binding motifs represent up to 30 percent of bound peptides where the energetics of Ag binding are complex and do not conform to predictable binding parameters. Algorithms for predicting class I epitopes have been further refined by taking into account the impact of proteasomal cleavage on the generation of antigenic peptides (Hakenberg et al, 2003; Kesmir et al, 2002; Kuttler et al, 2000).

Canonical peptide-binding motifs generally contain two or three preferred primary anchor residues whose amino acid side chains fit well into distinct pockets within the class I cleft where they provide significant energy of binding (Rammensee et al, 1993a). Dominant anchor sites usually occupy the B-pocket and F-pocket of class I molecules, Figures 6.5A and B. For example, HLA-B27 prefers peptides with a sequence X<u>R</u>XXXXXX<u>Y</u> where the preferred anchor residues are arginine at position 2 (P2) and tyrosine at position 9 (P9) (Buxton et al, 1992; Jardetzky et al, 1991; Rotzschke et al, 1994). The B-pocket has a number of different chemical architectures controlled principally by the heavy chain side chains at position 45 that can favor peptide anchor residues with long side chains containing either a positive charge (e.g. B*2705; P2-Arg) (Buxton et al, 1992) or a negative charge (B*4405; P2-Glu) (DiBrino et al, 1995) depending on the HLA counter charge at the base of the pocket, Figure 6.5A. Alternatively some class I molecules have a shallow or constricted B-pocket (Menssen et al, 1999) and select residues like Proline at position 2 (e.g. B*3501; P2-Pro) (Falk et al, 1993), Figure 6.5A. The F-pocket accommodates the carboxyl terminus of bound peptide (PΩ) and can select residues with aromatic sidechains (e.g. B*4405; PΩ- Tyr/Phe) (Zernich et al, 2004), charged side chains (A*1101; PΩ-Lys) (Levitsky et al, 2000) or hydrophobic residues (e.g. A*0201; PΩ-Leu/Ile) (Hunt et al, 1992), depending upon the chemical properties of the pocket, Figure 6.5B.

The intervening residues (denoted as 'X') between dominant anchor sites are much more varied in their sidechains, however the peptide often contains secondary anchor sites that contribute to HLA-binding (Deres et al, 1993). These secondary sites are usually more degenerate in the side chains they will accommodate and yet still support strong binding, see Table 6.1. For instance HLA-

Table 6.1: Peptide-binding motifs of some HLA class I molecules

HLA allotype	2	3	5	8	9
A*01		D/E			Y
A*02	L/M				V/L
A*03	L/V/M				K/Y/F
A*11					K
A*24	Y/F				F/W/I/L
A*26	V/T/I/F/L				Y/F
A*29	E/M				Y/L
A*31					R
A*33					R
A*68	V/T				R
A*69	V/T				V/L
B*07	P				L/F
B*08		K/R	K/R		
B*14	R,		R		L
B*15	Q				Y/F
B*18	E				
B*27	R/Q				Y
B*35	P				Y
B*37	D			F/M/L	I/L
B*38					F/L
B*39	R/H				L
B*40	E				L
B*44	E				Y/F
B*46					Y/F
B*48	Q/K				L
B*51					F/I
B*52				I/V	I/V
B*53	P				
B*54	P				
B*55	P				
B*56	P				
B*57	A/T/S				F/W
B*58	A/T/S				W/F
B*67	P				
B*73	R				P
B*78	P/A/G				
C*01		P			L
C*03	A				L/M
C*04	Y/P				L
C*06					L

The dominant anchor sites are shown for residue positions 2, 3, 5, 8 and 9.

by a multi-catalytic protease known as the proteasome (Schubert et al, 2000). The major source of these proteins are so-called DRIPs, or defective ribosomal products, that are thought to derive from poorly folded nascent proteins

B8 contains three dominant anchor sites (Reid et al, 1996). This is shown in the structure of B8 complexed to the viral peptide FLRGRAYGL (single letter amino acid nomenclature) in which P3-Arg, P5-Arg, and P9-Leu make crucial contacts with the HLA molecule (Kjer-Nielsen et al, 2002a), Figure 6.5C. In addition, some of the non-anchor amino acids will not play any direct role in class I binding but instead will protrude above the cleft where they are available for interaction with the Ag-specific αβ T-cell receptor. Closely related class I subtypes can have significant differences in peptide repertoire as well as in the structural conformation with which the same peptide is bound (Macdonald et al, 2003; Rojo et al, 1993; Rotzschke et al, 1992; Sesma et al, 2002; Villadangos et al, 1995). These differences can impact on T-cell selection and differential recognition of these allotypes. However, in considering vaccine design, Sette and colleagues have grouped HLA-A and B allotypes into 9 supertypes that share common peptide binding motifs potentially accounting for most HLA-A and B polymorphism (Sette and Sidney, 1999), Table 6.3. However, it remains unclear whether this approach really can predict peptides that can be presented across multiple supertypes. Rammensee has reported little overlap (<5%) in the natural peptides bound to disparate members of the B44 supertype suggesting limited utility of this approach in predicting authentic ligands shared by members of the same supertype (Hillen et al, 2008).

MHC Class I Peptides

Peptides bound by class I molecules are constitutively derived from endogenous self and foreign proteins so they are being physiologically presented continuously (Rammensee et al, 1995) and might comprise as many as 20,000 different peptides being simultaneously presented by any one MHC-I allotype on the cell surface, e.g. HLA-A2 (Hunt et al, 1992). Peptides can be recovered from cell surface HLA molecules by immuno affinity purification of the HLA proteins, elution of the peptides (usually by low pH) and their subsequent separation by several rounds of reverse phase HPLC (Rammensee et al, 1993b). Heterogeneous mixtures of endogenous HLA class I-bound peptides can be sequenced as a pool to reveal dominant anchor amino acids that are over-represented at P2 and P8/9, and sometimes at a third anchor residue generally P3 [e.g. HLA B8 (Reid et al, 1996; Kjer-Nielsen et al, 2002a)]. As mentioned earlier, this is possible because the amino-terminus of the peptide is tucked into the cleft (Fig. 6.4A) allowing a clean start to

Table 6.2: Useful Websites related to HLA structure, polymorphism and peptide binding

American Society for Histocompatibility and Immunogenetics	http://www.ashi-hla.org/	HLA Sequences; archives; Useful contact numbers. Professional Information
Australasian and South East Asian Tissue Typing Society	http://www.aseatta.org.au/	HLA Sequences Professional information
European Federation for Immunogenetics	http://www.efiweb.eu/	Professional information
British Society for Histocompatibility and Immunogenetics	http://www.bshi.org.uk/	Sequence alignments, EFI Testing standards
Anthony Nolan HLA Informatics	http://www.anthonynolan.org.uk/ http://www.anthonynolan.org.uk/research/hlainformaticsg roup/	HLA Sequence data nomenclature updates
Sanger Centre Home Page	http://www.sanger.ac.uk/	Human Genome Project Chromosome 6 maps; clones
Immunogenetics (IMGT) database	http://www.ebi.ac.uk/imgt/hla/	HLA Sequence data nomenclature updates, TCR and Ig databases
NIAID, Bioinformatics and Molecular Analysis Section	http://bimas.dcrt.nih.gov/molbio/hla_bind/	HLA peptide binding prediction
SYFPEITHI	http://www.syfpeithi.de/	Peptide binding prediction

Table 6.3: HLA class I binding motifs cluster into 9 major[1] supertypes

Supertype	Position 2	C-terminus
A1	TI or LVMS	FWY
A2	AILMVT	LIVMAT
A3	AILMVST	RK
A24	YF or WIVLMT	FI or YWLM
B7	P	AILMVFWY
B44	E or D	FWYLIMVA
B27	RHK	FYL or WMI
B62	QL or IVMP	FWY or MIV
B58	ATS	FWY or LIV

[1] A supertype represents a number of HLA class I allotypes with shared peptide binding motifs (Sette and Sidney, 1999)

A1 supertype : A*0101, A*0102, A*2501, A*2601, A*2602, A*2604, A*3201, A*3601, A*4301, A*8001

A2 supertype : A*0201, A*0202, A*0203, A*0204, A*0205, A*0206, A*0207, A*6802, A*6901

A3 supertype : A*0301, A*1101, A*3101, A*3301, A*6801

A24 supertype : A*2301, A*2402, A*2404, A*3001, A*3002, A*3003

B7 supertype : B*0702, B*0703, B*0704, B*0705, B*1508, B*3501, B*3502, B*3503, B*51, B*5301, B*5401, B*5501, B*5502, B*5601, B*5602, B*6701

B44 supertype : B*18, B*3701, B*4402, B*4403, B*4001, B*4006

B27 supertype : B*1401, B*1402, B*1503, B*1509, B*1510, B*1518, B*3801, B*3802, B*3901, B*3902, B*3903, B*3904, B*4801, B*4802, B*7301, B*2701-08

B62 supertype : B*4601, B*52, B*1501 (B62), B*1502 (B75), B*1513 (B77)

the sequence which is not possible when peptides of differing lengths overhang at their amino-terminus, as is the case for HLA class II-bound peptides. Individual peptide species can be sequenced from pools by mass spectrometry methods especially in less complex peptide mixtures present in discrete RP-HPLC fractions (Engelhard et al, 1993; Huczko et al, 1993; Hunt et al, 1992; Purcell and Gorman, 2001; Purcell et al, 2001). Experiments of this nature have identified many self-peptides that are constitutively presented by class I molecules. The repertoire of class I-bound peptides includes housekeeping proteins, receptors, MHC molecules themselves and proteins from all parts of the cell. Class I molecules generally capture endogenous peptides created in the cytoplasm however specialized dendritic cells (DCs) can capture intact Ag from exogenous sources (Heath and Carbone, 2001b) and this can be processed and presented through TAP-dependent and TAP-independent mechanisms (Ackerman et al, 2003; Lehner and Cresswell, 2004; Rock et al, 2004; Shen et al, 2004). This process is known as cross-presentation and is important in presenting determinants from viruses that do not infect DCs (and therefore the viral proteins that are not synthesized in DCs responsible for priming of immune responses)(Carbone and Heath, 2003). Cross presentation is also important in tolerising against self-Ag that may not be synthesized in DCs (Heath and Carbone, 2001a). However, in most cell types the peptides presented by class I molecules are apparently derived from endogenously translated proteins that are degraded

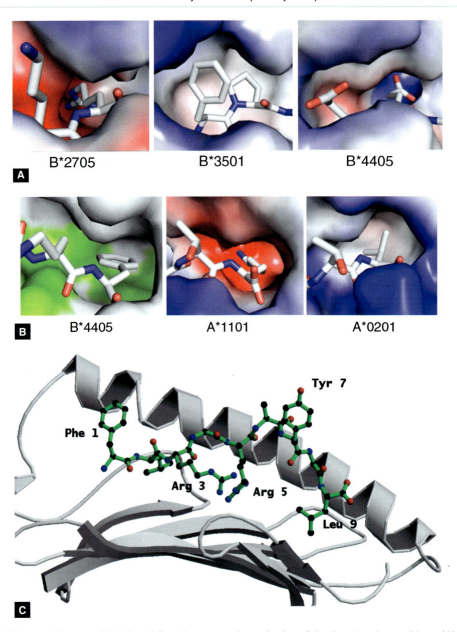

Figs 6.5A to C: The differing architecture of the B and F pockets governing selection of dominant anchor residues. (A) The electronegative B pocket of HLA-B*2705 contrasts with the occluded B pocket of HLA-B*3501, and the electropositive B pocket of HLA-B*4405. (B) The hydrophobic F pocket of HLA-B* 4405 selects different side chains to the electronegative F pocket of HLA-A*1101 and neutral F pocket of HLA-A*0201. Electronegative, red; electropositive, blue; neutral, white; green, aromatic. (C) the nonamer peptide FLRGRAYGL bound to HLA-B*0801 showing the three anchor residues P3Arg, P5Arg and P9 Leu. The peptide is shown as a ball and stick in green. HLA-B*0801 alpha-1 helix and cleft floor in grey. The alpha-2 helix has been removed to show the peptide. Fig. 6.5C is adapted with permission from reference 145

comprising a high proportion of all newly translated products in living cells (Princiotta et al, 2003; Schubert et al, 2000; Yewdell et al, 1999; Yewdell et al, 2001). Many of these polypeptides are ubiquitinated and thus marked out for degradation by the proteasome (Hershko and Ciechanover, 1998; Pamer and Cresswell, 1998). Since these peptides are largely derived from molecules synthesized within the cell, the peptide loading of HLA class I molecules on most cell types requires infection of host cells or gene transcription leading to cytoplasmic translation of proteins for presentation to the immune system.

The peptides presented by class I molecules are recognized by antigen specific T-cells of the CD8 phenotype. Thus class I molecules are mostly used to present antigens to cytotoxic T-cells (CTL).

Ag Processing in the Class I Pathway

Assembly of class I molecules with antigenic peptides requires coordination of multiple processes to firstly create peptides then to transport and load them into the cleft of nascent class I molecules in the endoplasmic reticulum (ER) (Heemels and Ploegh, 1995; Williams et al, 2002). The major source of peptides for class I presentation is thought to derive from processing of peptides in the cytoplasm by the proteasome (Shastri et al, 2002). The proteasome is an evolutionarily ancient barrel-like structure that degrades polypeptides into 8 to 17 amino acid long peptides (Lehner and Cresswell, 1996; Rivett and Hearn, 2004). The proteasome is comprised of 14 subunits, two of which, known as LMP2 and LMP7 are encoded within the Class II region of the major histocompatibility complex (Pamer and Cresswell, 1998). These MHC-linked subunits are not part of the constitutive proteasome but are induced during immune responses by cytokines such as IFN-γ thus creating the 'immunoproteasome'. Peptides created by the proteasome have a very short half-life in the cytoplasm unless they are protected from further degradation (Reits et al, 2003). A small fraction (~1%) of degraded polypeptides are actively transported across the membrane of the endoplasmic reticulum and into the lumen where empty class I molecules reside (Fruci et al, 2003). This transport is facilitated by a dimeric molecular pump known as the TAP molecule (TAP = transporter of antigenic peptides or sometimes transporter associated with antigen processing) (Momburg and Hammerling, 1998). The TAP genes are also encoded within the Class II region of the major histocompatibility complex, closely linked to the genes encoding LMP2 and LMP7 (McCluskey et al, 2004). The TAP gene products belong to the ABC (ATP-binding cassette) family of transporters that includes the multidrug resistance-like pump. This observation suggests coevolution of the linked genes controlling the creation of peptides in the cytoplasm (immunoproteasome LMP2 and 7), their capture and transport into the ER (TAP1/2) and their presentation to T-cells (class I molecules). The linkage of these genes might allow their coordinated regulation by cytokines (McCluskey et al, 2004) which might benefit from open chromatin or shared promoter elements, such as in the intergenic region between TAP1 and LMP2 (Seliger et al, 2002). Another explanation for MHC-linkage of the TAP loci could involve selection of favorable combinations of TAP alleles with alleles of the immunoproteasome to customise peptide specificities for polymorphic class I molecules. However, specific patterns of linkage disequilibrium that fit this design have not been observed in humans. Instead, hTAP selects peptides that are generally well suited to the binding preferences of polymorphic HLA class I molecules which suggests co-evolution of these genes has become independent of their linkage even though their co-regulation in cells might be advantaged by this linkage.

The TAP associates with peptides on the cytoplasmic side of the ER membrane and with class I molecules on the lumenal surface and so is capable of delivering peptides directly to the class I molecules (McCluskey et al, 2004). Peptides between 8 and 40 amino acids in length can bind the TAP but peptides of 8-10 amino acids are most efficiently translocated commensurate with the optimal length of peptides that bind class I molecules (Momburg et al, 1994b). Human TAP translocates peptides created by the proteasome and thus containing hydrophobic or basic carboxyl termini well suited to binding most human class I molecules (Uebel and Tampe, 1999; van Endert et al, 1995). In contrast mouse TAP predominantly translocates peptides with hydrophobic termini (Momburg et al, 1994a). Peptides that are translocated into the ER may be protected by heat shock proteins that facilitate Ag loading and presentation (Lammert et al, 1997). Frequently, peptides longer than 8-10 aa are translocated into the ER and these can be trimmed to their optimal length by amino-terminal peptidases that then create the N-terminus of the peptide (Fruci et al, 2001; Rock et al, 2004; Serwold et al, 2002).

The TAP-associated glycoprotein called tapasin is also encoded in the MHC and functions to facilitate peptide loading of class I molecules in the ER (Cresswell et al, 1999). Tapasin bridges HLA class I molecules to the TAP molecules in association with the chaperone calreticulin and the thiol oxidoreductase ERp57 that together form the peptide loading complex (Cresswell et al, 1999; Williams et al, 2002). Tapasin stabilizes the empty class I dimer retaining it in the ER until peptide loading by the peptide loading complex. Optimization of the class I peptide cargo (Williams et al, 2002) involves transient disulphide bond formation with ERp57 (Wearsch and Cresswell, 2007) perhaps to protect the MHC-I alpha 2 disulfide bond against reduction and thus to maintain the binding groove in a peptidereceptive state (Dick et al, 2002; Dong et al, 2009; Kienast et al, 2007). HLA class I molecules show polymorphism in the extent of their tapasin-dependence for efficient peptide loading. For example, HLA-8 B*2705 and HLA-B*4405 are relatively tapasin-independent whereas HLA-B*4402 is very dependent upon tapasin for proper peptide loading and cell surface expression (Peh et al, 1998; Zernich et al, 2004). The repertoire of peptides bound by tapasin-dependent allotypes appears to be more efficiently optimised than the peptides bound by allotypes that are highly tapasin-independent such as HLA-B*4405 (Williams et al, 2002; Zernich et al, 2004).

MHC Class II Molecules

The class II molecules include HLA-DR, DQ and DP, each of which is encoded by a distinct genetic locus clustered in the class II region spanning ~2 megabases. The overall protein structure adopted by class II molecules is similar to class I, but this is achieved by the association of two membrane bound chains known as α and β (Germain et al, 1986; Madden, 1995), Figure 6.1B. The α and β chains assemble non-covalently to create an antigen binding cleft located above a conserved membrane proximal structure which can interact with CD4 on T-cells Figure 1B. The MHC class II α and β chains are each encoded by distinct loci, which are closely linked as pairs of α and β genes (i.e. *DRB1α/DRB1β; DQB1α/DQB1β* and *DPB1α/DPB1β*). The *HLA-DR, DQ* and *DP* loci are all highly polymorphic. The polymorphisms are confined largely to the antigen binding pocket of these molecules but in HLA-DR they are confined to the DR beta chain (DRB1, 3, 4 and 5 genes) with the DR alpha chain (*DRA* gene) being essentially monomorphic (Margulies and McCluskey, 2003), Figure 6.3. HLA-DP and DQ contain polymorphisms in both the alpha and beta chain genes (*DPA, DPB, DQA and DQB*). The number of alleles at each of these loci is growing steadily as high resolution HLA typing is applied to clinical testing and anthropological studies (Marsh et al, 2002; Marsh et al, 2000).

Class II Ag Presentation

The pathway of Ag processing and presentation by HLA class II molecules is fundamentally different from that of class I molecules (Cresswell, 1994; Unanue, 2002). HLA class II molecules mainly acquire peptides created in the endocytic compartment (including lysosomes) (Chicz et al, 1993; Chicz et al, 1992) but a significant fraction of these peptides are also derived from the cytoplasm (Brooks and McCluskey, 1993; Dongre et al, 2001). Endosomes are membrane bound vesicles that shuttle proteins between various vacuolar compartments of the cell and are separated from the cytoplasm by a lipid bilayer. Exogenous antigens are internalized by endocytosis and transported to lysosomes and other acidified compartments containing proteolytic enzymes (Nakagawa and Rudensky, 1999) so that many of the peptides presented by class II molecules are derived from exogenous antigens. Class II molecules assemble initially in the endoplasmic reticulum with a monomorphic protein known as the invariant chain (Ii). Each class II αβ/Ii complex is a nine-subunit transmembrane protein containing three alpha-beta heterodimers associated with an Ii chain homotrimer (Roche et al, 1991). The invariant chain prevents class II loading with peptides derived from the ER and also escorts newly synthesized molecules to a specialized endosomal compartment (MCII) through a sorting signal in its cytosolic tail. The MCII compartment is thought to be the site of most peptide loading for HLA class II molecules. Once this acidified endosomal compartment has been reached, the invariant chain is sequentially degraded by cathepsin-mediated proteolysis (Nakagawa and Rudensky, 1999) to generate CLIP, or class II-associated Invariant chain peptide (Riberdy et al, 1992) that binds the cleft of class II molecules in a manner almost indistinguishable from nominal peptide antigens (Ghosh et al, 1995; Zhu et al, 2003).

The loading of class II molecules with peptides generally requires a function carried out by the HLA-DM molecule (Morris et al, 1994). HLA-DM comprises two gene products HLA-DM A and B both of which are encoded in the class II region of the major histocompatibility complex. HLA-DM is believed to interact directly with class II molecules to catalyze the dissociation of CLIP and promote loading of peptide in both acidic endosomal and recycling compartments (Brocke et al, 2002; Denzin and Cresswell, 1995; Denzin et al, 1996; Sloan et al, 1995). This activity of HLA-DM can be modulated by a second class II-related molecule called HLA-DO which synergises with DM under some conditions but at some concentrations can disrupt DM function (Brocke et al, 2002). HLA-DO is mainly expressed in B cells suggesting it may play a role in augmenting presentation of specific (cognate) Ag by high affinity B cells rather than non-specific B cells. As well as acting as a peptide editor, HLA-DM may also alter the conformation of a given peptide loaded in different cellular compartments such that these alternate conformations can be distinguished by specific T-cells (Pu et al, 2004).

Most peptides that bind class II molecules are 8-15aa in length and are derived from the activity of endosome/

lysosome proteases, particularly the cathepsins (Nakagawa and Rudensky, 1999; Villadangos et al, 1999). Distinct cathepsins play different roles in thymic and peripheral APC (Nakagawa and Rudensky, 1999; Villadangos et al, 1999). In humans, a gamma interferon-inducible lysosomal thiol reductase (GILT) is also constitutively present in late endocytic compartments of APCs and appears to be crucial for breaking disulphide bonds that prevent efficient Ag processing by the cathepsins and related proteases (Maric et al, 2001).

The pathways of antigen presentation exploited by class II molecules means they can present both endogenously and exogenously derived antigenic peptides. Thus T-cell responses to toxins, phagocytosed material and non-infectious virions are all potentially available via the class II pathway. Antigen presentation by dendritic cells is highly regulated with maturation of class II molecules being tuned by inflammatory signals that shut down endocytosis and mobilize intracellular class II molecules and other components of the Ag presentation machinery to maximize presentation of the right Ags (Cella et al, 1997; Lanzavecchia and Sallusto, 2001). The T-cells that recognize class II molecules are generally CD4 positive T helper cells. The role of T helper cells is to augment macrophage function and to promote differentiation and proliferation of B cells and cytotoxic T-cells.

HLA Class II Structure and the Nature of Bound Peptides

Class II molecules bind longer peptides than those bound by class I molecules (Chicz et al, 1992; Stern et al, 1994) and MHC class II peptide binding motifs are less well characterized, Table 6.4. Peptides bind class II molecules in an extended conformation with about a third of the peptide surface being accessible to solvent and therefore available for interaction with the antigen receptor on T-cells (Brown et al, 1993; Jardetzky et al, 1994; Jardetzky et al, 1996; Murthy and Stern, 1997; Stern et al, 1994), Figure 6.1B. In a peptide complex of HLA-DR1, five of the thirteen side chains of an influenza matrix peptide were buried in pockets with extensive hydrogen bonding between conserved HLA-DR1 residues and the main chain of the peptide showing how this generic mode of binding can potentially ligate diverse peptides (Brown et al, 1993). Many of the peptides bound to class II molecules are derived from other MHC products (Chicz et al, 1993; Chicz et al, 1992). The termini of class II-bound peptides are not ligated by the same network of h-bonds that bind class I peptides and so they can hang over the end of the cleft and even form hair-pin bends that affect the structure of the class II molecule (Zavala-Ruiz et al, 2004), Figure 6.1B. The superantigens, such as the staphylococcal enterotoxins, bind class II as an intact

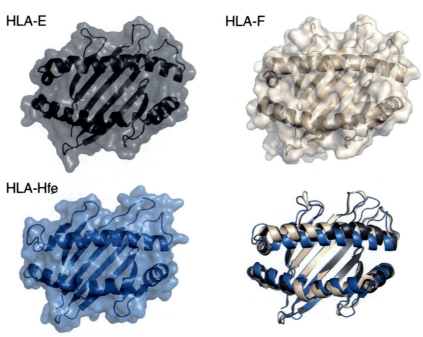

Fig. 6.6: Structure of the class Ib molecules HLA-E, HLA-F and Hfe. The molecules are shown as transparent space filling models with the ribbon of the α-carbon backbone evident. The cleft of Hfe is obtunded and apparently incapable of binding peptides. Bottom right shows an overlay of the three structures

protein outside the conventional peptide antigen-binding site explaining their lack of restriction to any particular class II alleles (Jardetzky et al, 1994).

Class Ib Molecules

The class Ib HLA-E, F, G and Hfe (HLA-H) molecules also associate with β2 microglobulin and are encoded by genes within the MHC telomeric to HLA-A (Sullivan et al, 2006). The class Ib molecules are much less polymorphic than classical class I molecules and bind a highly restricted set of peptides. In fact the Hfe molecule has relatively closed Ag binding cleft and therefore does not bind any peptides, instead being involved in iron metabolism through its interactions with the transferrin receptor. Oddly enough, Hfe has been reported to bind to T-cells but the general significance of this is not clear (Rohrlich et al, 2005). The structure of HLA-E, G and Hfe is shown in Figure 6.6.

The 8 alleles of HLA-E produce only 3 different proteins; the 20 alleles of HLA-F make 4 unique proteins, whereas HLA-G has 23 alleles that make 7 different proteins. Additional isoforms of HLA-G are expressed in many cells, including a soluble secreted form arising from alternate splicing (Pyo et al, 2006). The function of these isoforms is not clear though there is some evidence that soluble HLA-G may have biological activity (LeMaoult et al, 2003). The peptides that bind class Ib molecules generally have more primary anchor sites than peptides that bind class Ia molecules. This may be one reason for the narrow peptide repertoire of these molecules (Clements et al, 2005; O'Callaghan and Bell, 1998) noting that the repertoire of peptides that bind HLA-G peptides exceeds that for HLA-E (Ishitani et al, 2003; Lee et al, 1998; Lee et al, 1995).

Non-classical, class Ib molecules such as HLA-E (Braud et al, 1998; Brooks et al, 1999) and HLA-G (LeMaoult et al, 2003) serve as ligands for NK cells (Natural Killer) that normally function to eliminate cells that have lost expression of class I. By interacting with NK receptors these class I molecules turn off the NK cell signaling and thereby prevent lysis of HLA-expressing cells (Allan et al, 2002; Boyington et al, 2000; King et al, 2000). Some NK cells also recognize classical HLA molecules such as HLA-B and HLA-C directly (Lanier, 1998; Parham, 2005) or indirectly in the form of processed HLA signal sequence peptides presented by HLA-E molecules (Bland et al, 2003). Indeed the main source of peptides bound by HLA-E molecules is derived from the HLA class I signal sequence or leader peptide, including the HLA-G leader sequence (Braud et al, 1998; Brooks et al, 1999). Thus HLA-E molecules might be thought of as providing a quality control system that screens for altered Ag presentation by detection of HLA loss. This screening process is likely to be particularly important on tumor cells and virus-infected antigen presenting cells (APC) where class I loss is a common reason for escape from immune surveillance by CTL. Under these circumstances NK cells are thought to play a role in eliminating unwanted class I-negative cells. HLA-E is known to influence the activation of natural killer (NK) cells through its interactions with members of the CD94/NKG2 receptor group (Borrego et al, 1998; Vance et al, 1998). HLA-E and HLA-G are also present in the cells of the placental trophoblast where they may serve to interact with the large numbers of NK cells that infiltrate the uterine mucosa in early pregnancy (King et al, 2000; LeMaoult et al, 2003). HLA-G apparently regulates NK-cell activation through it role as a ligand for the killer-cell immunoglobulin (Ig)-like receptor (KIR) 2DL4, and by furnishing peptides that engender the cell-surface expression of HLA-E, particularly in the trophoblast (Ishitani et al, 2003; Rajagopalan et al, 2006). In addition, HLA-G interacts with the Ig-like transcript (ILT)2 and ILT4 receptors, which are expressed by a variety of cell types (Allan et al, 1999; Shiroishi et al, 2003). Moreover, HLA-G is thought to be a disulfide-linked dimer on the cell surface (Boyson et al, 2002). The function of HLA-F is not understood although it is also expressed in the NK-rich trophoblast tissue, consistent with a role in regulating NK cells.

Class Ib molecules can also direct T-cell responses to bacteria and viruses, in addition to tumors and self-antigens by presentation of peptide antigens in a class Ia-like fashion (for a recent review, see Rodgers and Cook, 2005; Sullivan et al, 2006). For instance, HLA-E drives CMV-specific CD8+ T-cell responses by recognizing a viral homologue of the class I leader-sequence peptides (Hoare et al, 2006; Pietra et al, 2003). This response is only seen in individuals whose HLA genotype lacks the particular leader sequence that is identical to the CMV homologue (Pietra et al, 2003). Those individuals with HLA allotypes that do contain the CMV sequence presumably tolerise these CMV-specific CD8+ T-cells.

HLA Polymorphism and Nomenclature

Within human populations HLA-A, B, C, DR, DQ and DP loci are highly polymorphic (Marsh et al, 2000) with a growing number of alleles recognized at each locus. HLA alleles at a given locus can differ from each other by 1-30 amino acid residues (Robinson et al, 2003). The nomenclature of HLA alleles and their loci is determined by the WHO Nomenclature Committee for Factors of the HLA System (Marsh et al, 2002). This committee oversees the naming of new alleles and publishes regular updates to the list of recognized HLA alleles. The IMGT/HLA database http://www.ebi.ac.uk/imgt/hla provides a centralized repository for the sequences of the alleles named by the nomenclature committee. This database also provides analytical tools for studying HLA sequences. The HLA sequences have also been extended to include intron sequences and the 3' and 5' untranslated regions in the alignments and also the inclusion of new genes such as MICA. The IMGT/MHC database (http://www.ebi.ac.uk/ipd/mhc/index.html) also provides a similar resource for the MHC of other species. Lists of newly described HLA alleles that are based on gene sequencing and have been ratified by the WHO Nomenclature Committee for Factors of the HLA System are published monthly in the journal *Tissue Antigens*. In addition, complete listings are published at 3-5 years intervals in journals such as *Tissue Antigens*, *Immunogenetics* and *Human Immunology*.

Table 6.4: Peptide-binding motifs of selected HLA- class II molecules

HLA allotypes	1	3	4	5	6	7	8	9	10	11
DPA1, DPB1	F/L/M			F/L			I/A			
DPA1, DPB1	Y/L/V/F/K		D/S/Q/T		Y/F/W/V			L/V/I		
DPA1, DPB1	F/L/Y/M					F/L/Y			V/Y/I	
DQA1*05/ DQB1*02	F/W/Y/I/L/V		D/E/L/V/I/H		P/D/E	E/D		F/Y/W/V/I/L/M		
DQA1*03/ DQB1*03		A/G/S/T		A/V/L/I						
DQA1*03/ DQB1*03	F/Y/I/M/L/V			V/L/I/M/Y		V/F/M/L/V/I				
DQA1*03/ DQB1*03	R/K				A/G			N/E/D		
DQA1*0101/ DQB1*05	L			Y/F/W						
DQA1*0102/ DQB1*06					L/I/V			A/G/S/T		
DRB1*0101	Y/F/W/L/I/M/V/A		L/M/A/I/V/N		A/G/S/T/C/P			L/A/I/V/N/F/Y/M/W		
DRB1*0102	I/L/V/M		A/L/M		A/G/S/T/C/P			I/L/A/M/Y/W		
DRB1*03	L/I/F/M/V		D		K/R		L	Y/L/F		
DRB1*04	F/L/V							N/QS/T		
HLA allotypes	**1**	**3**	**4**	**5**	**6**	**7**	**8**	**9**	**10**	**11**
DQB1*04/ DQB4*01	F/Y/W				S/T					
DRB1*07	F/I/L/V/Y				N/S/T					
DRB1*08	F/I/LV/Y			H/K/R						
DQB1*09/ DQB4*01	Y/F/W/L		A/S							
DRB1*11	Y/F		L/V/M/A/F/Y		R/K/H			A/G/S/P		
DQB1*11/ DQB3*02	Y/F				R/K		R/K			

Contd...

Contd...

	1	3	4	5	6	7	8	9	10	11
DRB1*12	I/L/F/Y	L/N/M			V/Y			Y/F/M		
DRB1*13	I/V/F		Y/W/L/V/A/M		R/K		Y/F/A/S/T			
DQB1*13/ DQB3*01	I/L/V				R/K			Y		
HLA allotypes	**1**	**3**	**4**	**5**	**6**	**7**	**8**	**9**	**10**	**11**
DRB1*15	L/V/I		F/Y/I			I/L/V/M/F				
DQB1*15/ DQB5*01	I/L/V									H/K/R
DRB3*02	Y/F/I/L		N		A/S/P/D/E			L/V/I/S/G		
DRB3*03	I/L/V		N		A/S/P/D/E			I/L/V		
DRB5*01	F/Y/L/M		Q/V/L/M					R/K		

The dominant anchor sites are shown for peptide positions 1-11.

Antigen Recognition in T Cell Immunity

HLA molecules are now understood to be receptors for peptides derived from self and foreign antigens that are captured within the cleft of the HLA molecules and presented to T cells. Thus, T cells, through their specific antigen receptors, are designed to constantly scrutinize the array of different HLA-peptide complexes that are continuously presented on cellular surfaces (Garcia, 1999; Garcia et al, 1999; Hennecke and Wiley, 2001; van der Merwe and Davis, 2003). There are two distinct families of genes encoding either αβ or γδ T-cell receptors. The αβ T-cell receptors are expressed on about 95 percent of all T-cells and show greater variability than the γδ T-cell receptors. This review of TCR interactions will concentrate on αβ receptors. Variability in αβ TCRs arises from the random gene rearrangements, combinatorial diversity and N-region deletions/additions that occur among the different segments of TCR genes that are rearranged during development in the thymus (Davis and Bjorkman, 1988), Figure 6.7. The TCR β-chain genes comprise a cluster of multiple V-regions, Diversity segments and Joining regions that randomly create different VDJ combinations further diversified by untemplated nucleotide additions and deletions at the VDJ junctions, so-called N-region diversity. The TCR α-chain genes comprise a cluster of multiple V-regions and Joining regions that also create different VJ combinations that are further diversified by N-region diversity (Davis, 1990). Estimates of the potential repertoire of unique T-cell receptors (10^{15}) (Davis and Bjorkman, 1988) vastly exceed the actual number of T-cells in humans (10^{11}-10^{12}) and the naturally expressed repertoire of TCR diversity is even smaller (~10^7-10^8), particularly in the memory compartment (Arstila et al, 1999), Figure 6.7.

Peptide antigens alter the HLA molecule by occupying the antigen-binding cleft thereby changing the molecular display scrutinized by T-cells through the antigen-specific αβ T-cell receptor. This concept was first understood by Zinkernagel and Doherty whose studies of anti-viral T-cell recognition (Doherty and Zinkernagel, 1975; Zinkernagel and Doherty, 1974, 1997) led to their award of the Nobel prize for Medicine in 1996. Once an appropriate ligand is identified, TCRs become incorporated into a higher order structure, perhaps involving oligimerization of the TCRs and their incorporation into the immunological synapse (Bromley et al, 2001; Grakoui et al, 1999). The mechanism leading from antigen ligation into T-cell signaling remains unclear. Recent evidence links Ag-ligation with a conformational change in the constant domain of the TCR alpha chain (Beddoe et al, 2009) potentially positioned to alter the conformation of the signaling component of the TCR, known as the CD3 complex. A conformational change in the CD3 complex is associated with recruitment of the cytoplasmic adaptor protein, Nck to CD3 epsilon and subsequent TCR signaling (Collins et al, 2002; Martinez-Martin et al, 2009). The atomic detail of the TCR interactions with major histocompatibility complex-peptide (MHCp) complexes has been illuminated

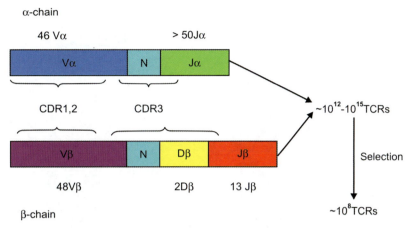

Fig. 6.7: Generation of diversity in T-cell receptor genes. Combinatorial diversity is generated by random rearrangement of any one of multiple Vβ genes with any one of multiple D-segments and any one of multiple J-segments. Similar random rearrangements occur between Vα and Jα segments. Further variation is introduced by small deletions and addition of untemplated nucleotides at the junctions of rearranged genes (N-region diversity). The potential repertoire of unique TCRs is estimated to be between 10^{12}-10^{15} (Arstila et al, 1999). These rearranged genes are transcribed with exons encoding the constant regions, Cβ and Cα. The Complementarity Determining Regions, CDR1 and 2 are encoded within the V-genes and the CDR3 regions are encoded by the VDJ and VJ segments

recently, permitting several generalizations about this interaction (Degano et al, 2000; Ding et al, 1999; Ding et al, 1998; Garboczi et al, 1996; Garcia et al, 1998; Garcia et al, 1996; Hennecke et al, 2000; Kjer-Nielsen et al, 2003; Luz et al, 2002; Reinherz et al, 1999; Reiser et al, 2003; Reiser et al, 2000; Reiser et al, 2002; Rudolph et al, 2006; Speir et al, 1998; Stewart-Jones et al, 2003; Archbold et al, 2009; Feng et al, 2007; Gras et al, 2009; Maynard et al, 2005; Nicholson et al, 2005; Tynan et al, 2007). Firstly, TCR recognition of the MHCp complex occurs by the loops of CDRs 1, 2 and 3, Figures 6.8A and B. The CDR1 and 2 are encoded in the V-region exons of TCR genes whereas the CDR3 is derived from the VDJ junction and associated N regions that generate the most variable part of the TCR, Figure 6.7.

Secondly, MHCp binding often occurs via an approximate diagonal docking mode, noting that this varies by up to 75° among different TCR-MHCp complexes. The basis of diagonal TCR-MHCp binding is unknown but might be dictated by the need for simultaneous CD4/CD8 co-receptor ligation or intracellular signaling (Garcia et al, 1999; Hennecke and Wiley, 2001; Rudolph and Wilson, 2002), Figure 6.9A. Thirdly, within this docking mode, the relative role of each CDR loop can vary significantly. While the CDR 1 and CDR2 loops of the TCR often contact the MHCα helices and the hypervariable CDR3 regions frequently interact with the peptide (Rudolph et al, 2006) there are many exceptions to this simplification. Thus, peptide contacts can be mediated by the CDR1 and CDR2 loops while the CDR3 loops can interact with HLA residues (Ely et al, 2005; Godfrey et al, 2008; Gras et al, 2008; Kjer-Nielsen et al, 2003), Figure 6.9B.

Structural analyzes of TCRs have been complemented by biophysical studies of the TCR/MHCp interaction. Such studies, using surface plasmon resonance and calorimetry approaches, have shown the TCR/MHCp interaction to be dominated by weak intermolecular interactions (low µM range), with slow association rates and fast dissociation rates (van der Merwe and Davis, 2003). The slow association rates are consistent with the conformational plasticity of the CDR loops often observed upon MHCp engagement. The CDR loops of the TCR are inherently flexible but are stabilized upon MHCp ligation (Boniface et al, 1999; Krogsgaard et al, 2003; Willcox et al, 1999). The CDR loops can also be rigid in their conformation before and after ligation as for the NKT TCR interaction with CD1d-alpha galactosyl ceramide complex and the ELS4 TCR interaction with a bulged viral peptide bound to HLA-B*3501 (Tynan et al, 2007), where even the CDR3 loops are largely rigid in their conformation (Borg et al, 2007). The biological outcome of TCR engagement is considered to be related to the half-life and heat capacity changes upon complexation (Boniface et al, 1999; Kersh et al, 1998; Krogsgaard et al, 2003; Krummel et al, 2000; Willcox et al, 1999).

A two-step mechanism of TCR recognition of MHCp has been postulated, whereby the TCR is initially guided to interact with the MHC α-helices via its relatively rigid CDR1 and CDR2 loops, subsequently followed by

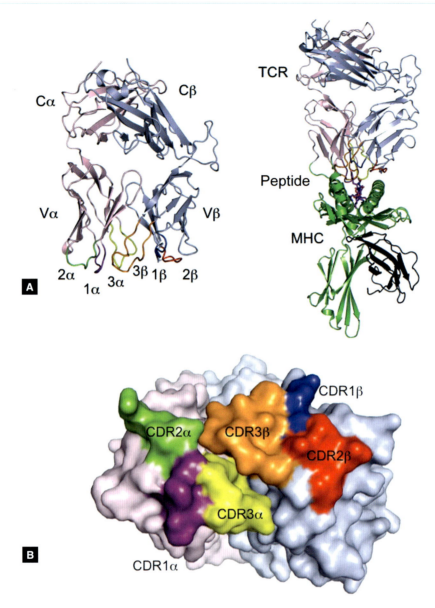

Figs 6.8A and B: Overall landscape of TCR structure and HLA-peptide ligation. (A) The crystal structures of the TCR alone (left panel) showing the loops of CDR1, 2 and 3 from both the Vα and Vβ chains (numbered). This TCR is shown in complex with HLA-class I/peptide complex (right panel). The CDR loops of the TCR form the ligand-binding surface that interacts with the exposed residues of the HLA-peptide complex. (B) Space-filling model of the ligand-binding surface of the TCR with the CDR regions individually labeled and coloured to show the juxtaposition of the CDR3α (yellow) and CDR3β (orange). In this particular receptor CDR3β is highly involved in peptide-MHC recognition (Gras et al., 2009)

induced fit of the CDR3 loops over the peptide (Wu et al, 2002). This model has the appeal that it predicts a stereotypic footprint for the TCR on MHC α-helices (Garboczi and Biddison, 1999). Indeed, one of the great mysteries of T-cell recognition is that even though the TCR is immunoglobulin-like, antigen recognition is highly restricted to MHCp ligands. There is some evidence that MHC reactivity is inherent in the germline-encoded portions of the TCR (Zerrahn et al, 1997) consistent with subtle biases in V-region usage for MHC class I versus class II-restricted T-cell selection (Sim et al, 1996; Sim et al, 1998a; Sim et al, 1998b). This is also consistent with the notion that MHC restriction is guided by docking onto a mixture of conserved and polymorphic residues at the MHCp interface (Garboczi and Biddison, 1999). Conserved sites for CDR1/2 docking onto HLA molecules have been observed in a number of recent structural studies. Thus, in navigating the prominent

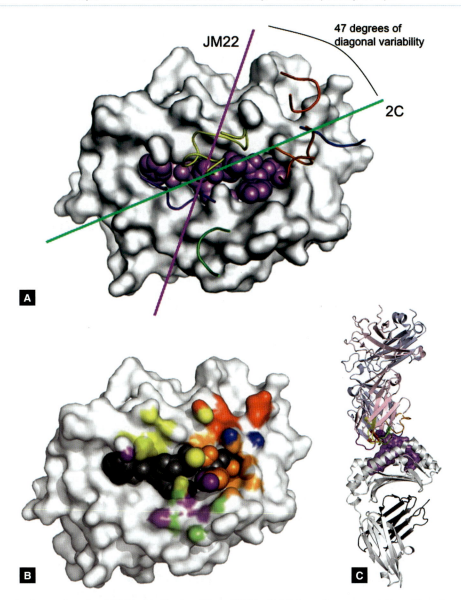

Figs 6.9A to C: A broadly diagonal mode of MHCp-binding by different TCRs. (A) Schematic representation of two diagonal variations in MHCp class I – TCR complexes, the almost orthogonally oriented JM22 (Stewart-Jones et al., 2003) and the more diagonal 2C (Garcia et al., 1996). Variation can be up to 75° in the TCR orientation over the MHCp complex. CDR loops are colored CDR1α purple; CDR1β blue; CDR2α green blue; CDR2β red; CDR3α yellow; CDR3β orange. (B) The footprint of the CDR loops of a class I-restricted TCR, LC13, docking onto HLA-B8-peptide complex (Kjer-Nielsen et al, 2003). The CDR contact surface is color coded, (HLA-B8, white space filling; peptide, grey sphere). (C) TCR recognition of a bulged peptide. In this case the 13-mer peptide described also in Figure 6.4B is interacting with the TCR (colored) from a cytolytic T-cell clone. The TCR makes a minimal footprint on the HLA-B*3508 molecule (grey) involving residues 65, 69 and 155 and many contacts with peptide residues (purple)

bulge of a 13-mer peptide, a T-cell receptor from a killer T-cell makes only a few HLA contacts suggesting a "minimal" footprint for HLA-restriction involving residues 65, 69 and 155 (Tynan et al, 2005b), Figure 6.9C. When all the TCR-pMHC-I structures solved by X-ray crystallography to date are examined, MHC-I residues 65, 69 and 155 virtually all make contacts with the TCR suggesting these represent a "restriction triad" that facilitates docking of the TCR onto MHC molecules (Tynan et al, 2005b). A different study of a number of Vβ8.2 TCR-MHC-II complexes revealed the use of identical TCR β-chain residues ("interaction codons") making MHC-II alpha-helical contacts (Feng et al, 2007). Cross-reactive T-cells have also been observed to use fixed residues in making contacts with different MHC class II molecules (Dai et al, 2008). The notion that germline-encoded interaction codons might provide a bias for TCR-MHC interactions has also been supported in transgenic systems that show defective positive selection *in vivo* when interactions of this kind made by the TCR CDR2 residues are impaired (Scott-Browne et al, 2009). These contacts might be TCR Vβ-specific and MHC stereotypic. Indeed, Garcia and colleagues have suggested that each TCR variable-region gene product engages particular MHC allotypes through a 'menu' of structurally coded recognition motifs that have arisen through co-evolution (Garcia et al, 2009). Nonetheless, TCR promiscuity, and therefore the capacity to engage different HLA allotypes, also appears dependent upon inherent plasticity in binding dictating significant degeneracy in the TCR-MHC footprint, perhaps facilitated by contacts made by interaction codons and engagement of the accessory molecules CD4 and CD8 (Archbold et al, 2008; Ely et al, 2008; Ely et al, 2005). Indeed, this plasticity is not confined to the TCR itself. In recognizing a bulged 11-mer viral peptide, a TCR from a killer T-cell is able to maximize the contacts made with the HLA class I molecule because the protruding peptide is able to crumple upon ligation with the TCR (Tynan et al, 2007). Moreover, single residue polymorphism among three HLA-B44 allotypes altered the mode of binding and dynamics of a bound viral epitope such that peptide flexibility was a critical parameter in enabling preferential TCR engagement with HLA-B* 4405 in comparison to HLA-B*4402 or B*4403 (Archbold et al, 2009).

T Cell Allorecognition

Given that T cells are MHC-restricted it is difficult to understand why they should ever recognize a foreign HLA type. However in practise they do and at very high frequency such that between 1/10 and 1/1000 clonally distinct T cells are capable of recognizing any random allogeneic HLA molecule. Given the number of T cells in the human lymphoid system, this represents a striking tendency for T cells which are normally restricted to recognizing self HLA molecules complexed to foreign peptides, to cross react on allogeneic HLA molecules. Allorecognition by T cells can be the result of direct recognition of an allogeneic MHCp complex. Alternatively, T cell allorecognition can also occur indirectly, when peptides derived from the allogeneic HLA molecules are presented as nominal antigens by host HLA moecules after processing by the host Ag-presenting cells (Lechler et al, 1990).

The molecular basis of direct T cell allorecognition has been a conundrum for over 50 years (Sherman and Chattopadhyay, 1993). If T cell receptors are inherently biased towards recognition of MHC structures then allorecognition may be thought of as a predictable cross-reaction aided by random peptides presented by the alloantigen (Heath et al, 1991). This cross-reaction can arise from direct recognition of the allogeneic MHC-peptide complex that usually depends on the peptide antigen. Since the endogenous peptides selected for presentation by allogeneic HLA molecules are likely to be quite distinct from those presented by syngeneic HLA molecules, the array of unfamiliar ligands expressed by allograft cells is highly diverse, amplifying opportunities for alloreaction. However, in some cases of T-cell alloreactivity, the allogeneic HLA molecule itself might be the major focus of the TCR interaction (Lechler et al, 1990). The structure of an allogeneic TCR/MHCp complex from a mouse system (2CLd/QL9) reveals the allogeneic class I molecule L^d is recognized in a very different manner to the cognate class I molecule K^b (Colf et al, 2007). $H2K^b$ and $H2L^d$ have 31 amino acid differences and there is no sequence similarity between the $H2K^b$-restricted octamer self-peptide, dEV8, and the $H2L^d$-restricted nonamer allopeptide, QL9. The two TCR footprints were not unusual for TCR-pMHC-I structures but were very distinct from each other including in their docking geometry, complementarity and chemistry. Thus, of 16 $H2K^b$ contact residues conserved in $H2L^d$, only 6 were contacted by 2C in both complexes, and only 4 of these used the same residues on 2C (Colf et al, 2007), Figure 6.10. The direct T-cell allorecognition by the 2C receptor ends up being a combination of both peptide-centric and MHC-centric interactions, but with a heavy bias towards the MHC (Rossjohn and McCluskey, 2007).

Another study solved the crystal structure of a complex involving a TCR and a naturally processed octapeptide bound to the allogeneic murine H-$2K^b$ MHC class I molecule (Reiser et al, 2000). In this allospecific TCR, the CDR3 of the alpha chain folded away from the peptide binding groove making no contact with the bound peptide, which instead was contacted by the CDR3β of the TCR. This study further emphasizes how a peptide-specific alloreactive TCR interacts with allo-MHCp in a manner analogous to self-MHC molecules (Reiser et al, 2000).

Recent structural studies on the basis of human T-cell alloreactivity have been reported on a commonly used antiviral T-cell receptor (LC13 TCR) found in

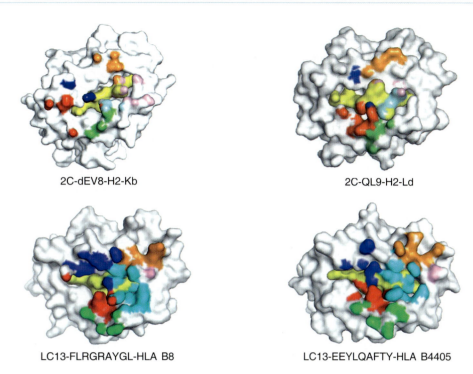

Fig. 6.10: Direct T cell allorecognition of disparate cognate and allogeneic peptide-HLA complexes can be mediated either by distinct binding modes (non-mimicry) or essentially identical modes of binding to cognate and allogeneic ligands (molecular mimicry). The TCR footprint of the CDR loops of the 2C (Garcia et al, 1996; Colf et al., 2008) and LC13 (Kjer-Nielsen et al., 2003; Macdonald et al., 2009) T cell receptors are shown on their cognate and allogeneic pMHC-I ligands. The footprints demonstrate non-mimicry of the 2C allorecognition and mimicry of the LC13 allorecognition. The 2C TCR cognate ligand H2K^b bound to dev8 (top left); 2C alloligand, H2L^d bound to QL9 (top right); LC13 TCR cognate ligand, HLA-B*0801-FLR (bottom left) and LC13 alloligand, HLA-B*4405-EEY (bottom right). Space filling models of MHC-I shown in grey, peptide in yellow and CDR contact sites coloured separately for each CDR

B*0801+ individuals. In addition to this antiviral specificity, the LC13 CTL also alloreact through their TCR with certain subtypes of the common B44 allotype, HLA-B*4402 and HLA-B*4405 bound to an endogenous self-peptide. The cognate (self) HLA-B* 0801 and the allogeneic B44 allotypes vary substantially in their amino acid sequence, with 24-25 amino acid differences. Despite these polymorphic HLA differences, and the disparate sequences of the viral and allopeptides, the LC13 TCR engaged the different self and allogeneic peptide-HLA complexes in a virtually identical fashion (Macdonald et al, 2009), Figure 6.10. This interaction involves molecular mimicry of the viral peptide by the allopeptide, as well as mimicry of HLA-B*0801 by B*4402 and B*4405. Surprisingly, the LC13 T-cells alloreact against HLA-B*4402 but not HLA-B*4403. The single residue polymorphism between HLA-B*4402 and HLA-B*4403 affected the capacity of the allopeptide to alter its conformation upon TCR ligation (Macdonald et al, 2009). Although the allopeptide binding to B*4403 was less efficient than for B*4402 and B*4405, the endogenous allopeptide is apparently still naturally presented and recognized with physiological consequences for the developing T-cell repertoire in HLA-B*4403/B*0801 heterozygotes. Such individuals lack the dominant LC13 TCR and instead select T-cells that react with the same cognate B*0801-restricted viral determinant but without alloreactivity on B*4402 or B*4405 (Burrows et al, 1997). T-cells from heterozygous individuals focussed on the polymorphic differences between HLA-B*0801 and HLA-B44, shifting the footprint from peptide residues towards the carboxyl terminus to residues near the amino terminal part of the viral peptide ligand (Gras et al, 2009). This shift in specificity of the antiviral response to the same viral determinant allows immunological tolerance towards the HLA-B*4402 and B*4405 molecules.

Taken together, allorecognition of disparate cognate and allogeneic peptide-HLA complexes can be mediated by distinct modes of cognate and allogeneic binding (non-mimicry) as well as near identical modes of cognate and allogeneic binding (molecular mimicry). The relative importance of mimicry versus non-mimicry remains to be determined. Whatever, the dominant rules that dictate the mode of direct T-cell allorecognition, it is clear that some alloantigens are more important than others in exciting alloreactivity and graft rejection (Doxiadis et al, 1996). For instance HLA-B allotypes are generally more potent alloantigens than HLA-A, but even within this generalization there are sub-hierarchies of alloantigen potency without a clear explanation (Mifsud et al, 2008). This observation presents the transplant community with a challenge to unlock the principles that might underpin rational selection of more permissible mismatches in organ transplantation.

Biased T Cell Receptor Usage

The phenomenon of TCR bias of the V gene segments, preferred V-region usage or T cell receptor immunodominance, has been observed in the CTL response to a number of different viral infections (Callan and McMichael, 1999) including Epstein-Barr virus (Argaet et al, 1994; Callan et al, 1998; Callan et al, 2000; Miles et al, 2005), measles (Mongkolsapaya et al, 1999), influenza (Callan et al, 1995; Kedzierska et al, 2004) and HIV-1 (Wilson et al, 1998). For example, in unrelated HLA-B8+ individuals, an immunodominant CTL response, of which LC13 is the prototypic CTL, is generated against the Epstein-Barr virus peptide, FLRGRAYGL (Argaet et al, 1994; Callan et al, 1998). The crystal structure of HLA-B8-FLRGRAYGL complexed to 1.8Å resolution (Kjer-Nielsen et al, 2002a), the crystal structure of the non-liganded immunodominant TCR to 1.5Å resolution (Kjer-Nielsen et al, 2002b) and the crystal structure of the LC13/HLA-B8-FLR complex have been resolved to 2.5Å resolution (Kjer-Nielsen et al, 2003). These studies reveal that residues encoded by each of the highly selected V, D, N and J gene sequences of this immunodominant TCR were critical to the antigen specificity of the receptor. Moreover, upon recognizing antigen, the immunodominant TCR underwent extensive conformational changes in the complementarity determining regions (CDRs), including the disruption of the canonical structures of the germline-encoded CDR1α and CDR2α loops to produce an enhanced fit with the HLA-peptide complex. These changes were energetically dependent upon the highly selected V-D-N-J residues in the TCR, suggesting that the basis of immunodominance in this example relies upon the exquisite specificity of the TCR for MHCp. In another study of an immunodominant HLA-A2-restricted TCR recognizing influenza virus a conserved arginine-serine-serine sequence in complementarity determining region 3 (CDR3) of the Vβ segment dominates the response. In the structure of the HLA-A2-peptide complex only main chain atoms of the peptide were visible to the TCR thus offering a rather bland or "vanilla" peptide to the T-cell (Davis, 2003). The resulting orientation of the TCR Vαβ was orthogonal to the peptide-binding groove of HLA-A2, facilitating insertion of the conserved arginine in Vβ CDR3 into a notch in the surface of the HLA-A2-peptide complex. This unique mode of binding mode appears to underly the immunodominant T-cell response in this example driven mainly by Vβ interactions (Stewart-Jones et al, 2003; Ishizuka et al, 2008). Turner and colleagues have reviewed the structural constraints that determine the binding of a TCR to its ligand and the persistence of certain TCRs in an immune repertoire concluding that immunodominance in TCR selection is explicable on structural grounds (Gras et al, 2008; Turner et al, 2006).

HLA and Disease Associations

Although polymorphic HLA class I molecules present pathogen-derived peptides to killer T-cells mediating protective immunity, particular MHC-I allotypes are much more strongly associated with inflammatory, autoimmune-like diseases than they are with protective immunity phenotypes in infectious disease (Margulies et al, 2008), Table 6.5. Thus, certain MHC-I allotypes are associated with inflammatory diseases like ankylosing spondylitis [odds ratio>150 (Brown et al, 1996; Ramos and Lopez de Castro, 2002)], Behçet's disease [odds ratio~10 (Kotter et al, 2001; Shiina et al, 1999)] and Birdshot Retinopathy [odds ratio> 200 (Feltkamp, 1990; Levinson et al, 2004)] however, the reason for these associations are not understood (Margulies et al, 2008). Even stronger HLA associations are emerging with certain drug hypersensitivity reactions, Table 6.6. These associations potentially provide a specific trigger to assist unraveling the mechanism of MHC-I disease associations. Hypersensitivity to the reverse transcriptase inhibitor abacavir has been strongly associated with HLA-B*5701 (Mallal et al, 2002; Mallal et al, 2008). HLA-B*1502 is strongly associated with carbamazepine-induced Stevens-Johnson syndrome and toxic epidermal necrolysis (SJS/TEN; odds ratio >1000 in Han Chinese) (Chung et al, 2004). Allopurinol-induced severe cutaneous adverse reactions are strongly linked to HLA B*5801(Hung et al, 2005). Notably, these drugs are ring compounds with reactive groups that might interact with endogenous polypeptides. The resultant genetic associations are sufficiently strong that the US Federal Drug Authority has recommended HLA-B*1502 testing before Carbamazepine is prescribed and baseline testing for HLA-B*5701 is recommended before starting abacavir therapy

Table 6.5: Some HLA-associations with disease

Disease	HLA association	Reference
Addison's disease	DR3	(Maclaren and Riley, 1986)
HIV associated AIDS progression	A29, B22- rapid progression B14, C8 - nonprogression B27, B57, C14- protective C16, B35- susceptible	(Carrington and O'Brien, 2003; Hendel et al., 1999)
Ankylosing spondylitis	B27	(Brewerton et al., 1973)
Behçet's disease	B51	(Ohno et al., 1982)
Birdshot retinopathy	A29	(Tabary et al., 1990)
Celiac disease–gluten-sensitive enteropathy	DQ2	(Karell et al., 2003)
Cerebral Malaria	B53- protective	(Hill et al., 1992)
Chronic active hepatitis	B8, DR3	(Mackay, 2008)
De Quervain's thyroiditis	Bw35	(Nyulassy et al., 1977)
Dermatitis herpetiformis	Dw3	(Solheim et al., 1977)
Graves' disease	DRB1*03/DRB3*0101, DRB3*0202	(Chen et al., 1999)
Hemochromatosis	A3, B7, B14 Hfe	(Barton et al., 2005) (Beutler, 2006)
Insulin-dependent diabetes mellitus (Type 1)	A1, B8, DR3, B39	(Price et al., 1999) (Nejentsev et al., 2007) (Todd et al., 1988)
IgA nephropathy	B35	(Alamartine et al., 1991)
Juvenile rheumatoid arthritis	B27, DR5, DR8	(Berntson et al., 2008)
Late onset adrenal hyperplasia with hirsutism	Aw33/B14	(Kuttenn et al., 1985)
Myasthenia gravis	A1, A3, B8, DR3;	(Degli-Esposti et al., 1992)
Narcolepsy	DQB1*0602- susceptibility	(Pelin et al., 1998)
Pemphigus vulgaris	HLA-DR4	(Wucherpfennig et al., 1994; Wucherpfennig and Strominger, 1995)
Primary progressive Multiple sclerosis	DR2, DRB1*1501, DQB1*0602 - progression DRB1*1501-severe morbidity	(Vasconcelos et al., 2009)
Psoriasis	Cw6	(Griffiths and Barker, 2007)
Psoriatic arthritis	B27	(Winchester, 1995)
Reiter syndrome or reactive arthritis	B27	(Ebringer and Wilson, 2000)
Rheumatoid arthritis	DR4	(Gao et al., 1991; Gao et al., 1990; Stastny et al., 1988)
Salmonella arthritis	B27	(Ebringer and Wilson, 2000)
Sjögren's syndrome	DR3, B8	(Hietaharju et al., 1992)
Lupus erythematosus	DR2, DR3	(Graham et al., 2007)
Takayasu's disease	B52, DR4	(Flores-Dominguez et al, 2002)
Tumor immunity (reduced risk of chronic myeloid leukemia)	B8	(Posthuma et al., 1999)

(Mallal et al, 2008). Multiorgan reactions to abacavir occur in approximately 2-8 percent of patients with HIV-1 infection (Mallal et al, 2002; Mallal et al, 2008). Indeed, initial evidence for an immunological basis to abacavir hypersensitivity syndrome was reflected in the presence of infiltrating CD8+ T-cells in the skin of patients with a rash (Phillips et al, 2002) and the induction of elevated TNFα and IFNγ in patient whole blood and/or mononuclear cells exposed to abacavir *in vitro* (Martin et al, 2007). For immunologically confirmed abacavir hypersensitivity syndrome in the PREDICT-1 clinical trial, *HLA-B*5701* was associated with a positive predictive value of 47.9 percent and a negative predictive value of 100 percent (Mallal et al, 2008). The prevalence of abacavir hypersensitivity varies according to the genetic background of the population, probably because of ethnic

Table 6.6: HLA associations with drug reactions

Drug	Toxicity	HLA association	Reference
Abacavir	HS	B*5701	(Hetherington et al., 2002; Mallal et al., 2002; Martin et al., 2004)
Allopurinol	SJS/TEN and HS	B*5801	(Hung et al., 2005)
Aminopenicillin	HS	A2, DRw52	(Romano et al., 1998)
Aspirin	Asthma	DPB1*0301	(Kim et al., 2005;
	Urticaria	DRB1*1302-DQB1*0609	Kim et al., 2008)
Carbamazepine	HS and SJS/TEN	B*1502	(Chung et al., 2004; Hung et al., 2006)
Clozapine (Clozaril)	Agranulocytosis	B38, DR4 DR2	(Hummer et al., 1994; Yunis et al., 1995)
d-penicillamine	Proteinuria	B8, DR3, DR1	(Wooley et al., 1980)
Flucloxacillin	Hepatitis	B*5701	(Daly et al., 2009)
Gold Sodium thiomalate	Proteinuria,	B8, DR3	(Wooley et al., 1980)
Hydralazine	Systemic lupus erythematosus	DR4	(Batchelor et al., 1980)
Levamisole	Agranulocytosis	B27	(Schmidt and Mueller-Eckhardt, 1977)
Nevirapine	Skin rash in Thai	B*3505	(Chantarangsu et al., 2009)
	HS in Italian	Cw8-B14	(Littera et al., 2006)
	HS in Japanese population	Cw8	(Gatanaga et al., 2008)
	Rash-associated hepatitis	DRB1*0101	
NSAIDs	Anaphylactoid reaction	DR11	(Quiralte et al., 1999)
Oxicam	SJS/TEN	A2, B12	(Roujeau et al., 1987)
Phenytoin	SJS/TEN	B*1502	(Man et al., 2007)
Sulfamethoxazole	Fixed drug eruptions	A30, B13, Cw6	(Ozkaya-Bayazit and Akar, 2001)
Sulfonamides	TEN	A29, B12, DR7	(Roujeau et al., 1986)
Ximelagatran	Hepatitis (elevated alanine aminotransferase)	DRB1*07, DQA1*02	(Kindmark et al., 2008)

HS- Hypersensitivity syndrome, SJS- Stevens-Johnson syndrome, TEN-toxic epidermal necrolysis, NSAIDs- Nonsteroidal anti-inflammatory drugs.

variation in the phenotypic frequency of HLA-B*5701 in some populations (Mallal et al, 2008). For instance abacavir hypersensitivity is less common in African Americans who are known to have higher frequency of HLA-B*5801 and HLA-B*5702/03 subtypes and a correspondingly lower frequency of HLA-B*5701 than patients of European descent. Accurate clinical assignment of the hypersensitivity is essential to avert confounding the association with HLA-B*5701, especially where this allotype is present at a low frequency. Accordingly, it is now normal practice to carry out HLA-B*5701 genotyping to prevent abacavir hypersensitivity (Mallal et al, 2008). Systemic reactions to abacavir appear to be driven by drug-specific activation of cytokine-producing, cytotoxic CD8+ T-cells (Chessman et al, 2008). Recognition of abacavir requires conventional Ag presentation and is uniquely restricted by HLA-B*5701 and not closely related HLA allotypes with polymorphisms in the Ag-binding cleft. Hence, the strong association of HLA-B*5701 with abacavir hypersensitivity reflects specificity through creation of a novel ligand as well as HLA-restricted Ag presentation (Chessman et al, 2008). The mechanism of abacavir hypersensitivity suggests two layers of specificity operate to single out HLA-B*5701 as a genetic determinant of this drug hypersensitivity. The first level of specificity occurs during drug-protein targeting which is likely to significantly reduce the pool of potential ligands available for host class I molecules. The second layer of specificity occurs through selective binding and presentation of ligands by MHC-I molecules due to the polymorphic nature of the Ag-binding cleft. Perhaps the strong association of ankylosing spondylitis with HLA-B27, birdshot retinopathy with

HLA-A29 or Beçhet's disease with HLA-B51 also reflects more than one level of specificity. Thus, pathogen derived small molecules (or enzymes) may interact with, or modify specific peptides which are then subject to further selection by particular MHC-I allotypes creating pathogenic ligands of highly refined specificity.

HLA class II allele associations with disease are much more common than class I associations but there are few examples in which the mechanism is well understood (Jones et al, 2006). Perhaps the best example is Celiac disease, a common T-cell mediated disease caused by dietary gluten that occurs almost exclusively in association with HLA-DQ2 or HLA-DQ8, either alone or in combination. HLA-DQ8 without HLA-DQ2 is present in only 6 percent of patients with celiac disease while both HLA-DQ2 and HLA-DQ8 together are present in approximately 10 percent of patients (Karell et al, 2003). By contrast, around 95 percent of patients have HLA-DQ2 and consequently much more is known about HLA-DQ2-associated celiac disease than HLA-DQ8-associated disease. In HLA-DQ2-associated celiac disease, intestinal T-cell lines and clones are almost exclusively HLA-DQ2-restricted and recognize a variety of peptides derived from each of the sub-fractions of wheat gluten as well as homologous sequences in rye secalins and barley hordeins (Anderson et al, 2000; Arentz-Hansen et al, 2000; Arentz-Hansen et al, 2002; Vader et al, 2003). Pre-treatment of wheat gliadin with transglutaminase (TG2) increases γ-interferon (gamma-IFN) secretion and proliferation of HLA-DQ2-restricted gliadin-specific intestinal T-cells (Molberg et al, 1998; van de Wal et al, 1998). Fine mapping of HLA-DQ2-restricted epitopes has identified a preference for glutamate at anchor positions P4 or P6, and occasionally P7, corresponding to glutamine residues susceptible to deamidation by TG2 *in vitro* (Arentz-Hansen et al, 2000; Arentz-Hansen et al, 2002; Molberg et al, 1998; Qiao et al, 2005; Vader et al, 2003; van de Wal et al, 1998). Nevertheless, most T-cell reactivity in HLA-DQ2-associated celiac disease is directed towards the immunodominant wheat gluten T-cell epitopes (DQ2-a-I; PFPQPELPY, and DQ2-a-II: PQPELPYPQ) that are contained within a single, protease-resistant α-gliadin peptide (Anderson et al, 2000; Arentz-Hansen et al, 2002).

Moreover, these epitopes are highly dependent upon only a single Gln→Glu deamidation at P4 or P6 for optimal T-cell reactivity. Notably, the low affinity interaction between the unmodified DQ2-a-I peptide and HLA-DQ2 is substantially enhanced when the P4 Gln is deamidated, improving T-cell recognition by many T-cell clones, presumably because of better MHC-II binding of the peptide (Kim et al, 2004). T helper 1 responses in HLA-DQ8–associated celiac pathology are predictably HLA-DQ8–restricted and recognize multiple gliadin peptides (Tye-Din and Anderson, 2008). Although these determinants are mostly deamidated, some are not. Moreover DQ8-restricted gliadin peptides are commonly located in protease-sensitive sites of gliadin. Together, these aspects of DQ8-gliadin determinants contrast with the more absolute deamidation-dependence and relative protease-resistance of the dominant gliadin peptide in DQ2-mediated disease. The crystal structure of HLA-DQ8 has been solved in complex with a dominant gliadin epitope EGSFQPSQE containing deamidated Gln residues at P1 and P9 (Henderson et al, 2007).

The data in DQ2-and DQ8-related celiac disease establish distinct molecular mechanisms underlying the respective DQ associations. However, they also show that HLA-DQ8-mediated celiac disease is subtly different from the HLA-DQ2-mediated form of the disease suggesting a basis for the lower disease risk associated with HLA-DQ8.

It remains a challenge to determine the basis of HLA-associations with autoimmune diseases like Type 1 diabetes and multiple sclerosis. Perhaps these MHC-II associations, like the strong associations of drug hypersensitivity with certain MHC-I allotypes, depend on the preferential presentation of defined determinants from single autoantigens, thus shortening the odds for observing a HLA preference.

ACKNOWLEDGMENTS

We wish to thank The Roche Organ Transplantation Research Fund, NHMRC Australia, Australian Research Council and the Australian Research Council for research funding. JR is an ARC Federation Fellow.

This chapter has been substantially revised from a previously published chapter authored by James McCluskey in the "Immunobiology of the Human MHC. Proceedings of the 13th International Histocompatibility Workshop and Conference", IHWG Press, Seattle, 2007.

BIBLIOGRAPHY

1. Ackerman AL, Kyritsis C, Tampe R, Cresswell P. Early phagosomes in dendritic cells form a cellular compartment sufficient for cross presentation of exogenous antigens. Proc Natl Acad Sci USA 2003;100:12889-94.
2. Alamartine E, Sabatier JC, Guerin C, Berliet JM, Berthoux F. Prognostic factors in mesangial IgA

glomerulonephritis: An extensive study with univariate and multivariate analyses. Am J Kidney Dis 1991;18:12-19.
3. Allan DS, Colonna M, Lanier LL, Churakova TD, Abrams JS, Ellis SA, McMichael AJ, Braud VM. Tetrameric complexes of human histocompatibility leukocyte antigen (HLA)-G bind to peripheral blood myelomonocytic cells. J Exp Med 1999;189:1149-56.
4. Allan DS, Lepin EJ, Braud VM, O'Callaghan CA, McMichael AJ. Tetrameric complexes of HLA-E, HLA-F, and HLA-G. J Immunol Methods 2002;268:43-50.
5. Amos DB, Gorer PA, Mikulska ZB. An analysis of an antigenic system in the mouse (the H-2 system). Proc R Soc Lond B Biol Sci 1955;144:369-80.
6. Anderson RP, Degano P, Godkin AJ, Jewell DP, Hill AV. In vivo antigen challenge in celiac disease identifies a single transglutaminase-modified peptide as the dominant A-gliadin T cell epitope. Nat Med 2000;6: 337-42.
7. Archbold JK, Ely LK, Kjer-Nielsen L, Burrows SR, Rossjohn J, McCluskey J, Macdonald WA. T cell allorecognition and MHC restriction—A case of Jekyll and Hyde? Mol Immunol 2008;45:583-98.
8. Archbold JK, Macdonald WA, Gras S, Ely LK, Miles JJ, Bell MJ, Brennan RM, Beddoe T, Wilce MC, Clements CS, et al. Natural micropolymorphism in human leukocyte antigens provides a basis for genetic control of antigen recognition. J Exp Med 2009;206:209-19.
9. Arentz-Hansen H, Korner R, Molberg O, Quarsten H, Vader W, Kooy YM, Lundin KE, Koning F, Roepstorff P, Sollid LM, McAdam SN. The intestinal T cell response to alpha-gliadin in adult celiac disease is focused on a single deamidated glutamine targeted by tissue transglutaminase. J Exp Med 2000;191:603-12.
10. Arentz-Hansen H, McAdam SN, Molberg O, Fleckenstein B, Lundin KE, Jorgensen TJ, Jung G, Roepstorff P, Sollid LM. Celiac lesion T cells recognize epitopes that cluster in regions of gliadins rich in proline residues. Gastroenterology 2002;123:803-09.
11. Argaet VP, Schmidt CW, Burrows SR, Silins SL, Kurilla MG, Doolan DL, Suhrbier A, Moss DJ, Kieff E, Suclley TB, et al. Dominant selection of an invariant T cell antigen receptor in response to persistent infection by Epstein-Barr virus. J Exp Med 1994;180:2335-40.
12. Arstila TP, Casrouge A, Baron V, Even J, Kanellopoulos J, Kourilsky P. A direct estimate of the human alphabeta T cell receptor diversity. Science 1999;286:958-61.
13. Barton JC, Wiener HW, Acton RT, Go RC. HLA haplotype A*03-B*07 in hemochromatosis probands with HFE C282Y homozygosity: frequency disparity in men and women and lack of association with severity of iron overload. Blood Cells Mol Dis 2005;34:38-47.
14. Batchelor JR, Welsh KI, Tinoco RM, Dollery CT, Hughes GR, Bernstein R, Ryan P, Naish PF, Aber GM, Bing RF, Russell GI. Hydralazine-Induced systemic lupus erythematosus: influence of HLA-DR and sex on susceptibility. Lancet 1980;1:1107-09.
15. Beddoe T, Chen Z, Clements CS, Ely LK, Bushell SR, Vivian JP, Kjer-Nielsen L, Pang SS, Dunstone MA, Liu YC, et al. Antigen ligation triggers a conformational change within the constant domain of the alpha/beta T cell receptor. Immunity 2009;30(6):777-88.
16. Bell MJ, Burrows JM, Brennan R, Miles JJ, Tellam J, McCluskey J, Rossjohn J, Khanna R, Burrows SR. The peptide length specificity of some HLA class I alleles is very broad and includes peptides of up to 25 amino acids in length. Mol Immunol 2009;46(8-9):1911-17.
17. Berntson L, Damgard M, Andersson-Gare B, Herlin T, Nielsen S, Nordal E, Rygg M, Zak M, Fasth A. HLA-B27 predicts a more extended disease with increasing age at onset in boys with juvenile idiopathic arthritis. J Rheumatol 2008;35:2055-61.
18. Beutler E. Hemochromatosis: Genetics and pathophysiology. Annu Rev Med 2006;57:331-47.
19. Bjorkman PJ, Parham P. Structure, function, and diversity of class I major histocompatibility complex molecules. Annu Rev Biochem 1990;59:253-88.
20. Bjorkman PJ, Saper MA, Samraoui B, Bennett WS, Strominger JL, Wiley DC. Structure of the human class I histocompatibility antigen, HLA-A2. Nature 1987a;329:506-12.
21. Bjorkman PJ, Saper MA, Samraoui B, Bennett WS, Strominger JL, Wiley DC. The foreign antigen binding site and T cell recognition regions of class I histocompatibility antigens. Nature 1987b;329:512-18.
22. Bland FA, Lemberg MK, McMichael AJ, Martoglio B, Braud VM. Requirement of the proteasome for the trimming of signal peptide-derived epitopes presented by the nonclassical major histocompatibility complex class I molecule HLA-E. J Biol Chem 2003;278:33747-52.
23. Boniface JJ, Reich Z, Lyons DS, Davis MM. Thermodynamics of T cell receptor binding to peptide-MHC: Evidence for a general mechanism of molecular scanning. Proc Natl Acad Sci USA 1999;96:11446-51.
24. Borg NA, Wun KS, Kjer-Nielsen L, Wilce MC, Pellicci DG, Koh R, Besra GS, Bharadwaj M, Godfrey DI, McCluskey J, Rossjohn J. CD1d-lipid-antigen recognition by the semiinvariant NKT T cell receptor. Nature 2007;448:44-49.
25. Borrego F, Ulbrecht M, Weiss EH, Coligan JE, Brooks AG. Recognition of human histocompatibility leukocyte antigen (HLA)-E complexed with HLA class I signal sequence-derived peptides by CD94/NKG2 confers protection from natural killer cell-mediated lysis. J Exp Med 1998;187:813-18.
26. Boyington JC, Motyka SA, Schuck P, Brooks AG, Sun PD. Crystal structure of an NK cell immunoglobulin-like receptor in complex with its class I MHC ligand. Nature 2000;405:537-43.
27. Boyson JE, Erskine R, Whitman MC, Chiu M, Lau JM, Koopman LA, Valter MM, Angelisova P, Horejsi V, Strominger JL. Disulfide bond-mediated dimerization of HLAG on the cell surface. Proc Natl Acad Sci USA 2002;99:16180-85.

28. Braud VM, Allan DS, O'Callaghan CA, Soderstrom K, D'Andrea A, Ogg GS, Lazetic S, Young NT, Bell JI, Phillips JH, et al. HLA-E binds to natural killer cell receptors CD94/NKG2A, B and C. Nature 1998;391:795-99.
29. Brewerton DA, Hart FD, Nicholls A, Caffrey M, James DC, Sturrock RD. Ankylosing spondylitis and HL-A 27. Lancet 1973;1:904-07.
30. Brocke P, Garbi N, Momburg F, Hammerling GJ. HLA-DM, HLA-DO and tapasin: Functional similarities and differences. Curr Opin Immunol 2002;14: 22-9.
31. Bromley SK, Burack WR, Johnson KG, Somersalo K, Sims TN, Sumen C, Davis MM, Shaw AS, Allen PM, Dustin ML. The immunological synapse. Annu Rev Immunol 2001;19:375-96.
32. Brooks AG, McCluskey J. Class II-restricted presentation of a hen egg lysozyme determinant derived from endogenous antigen sequestered in the cytoplasm or endoplasmic reticulum of the antigen presenting cells. J Immunol 1993;150:3690-97.
33. Brooks AG, Borrego F, Posch PE, Patamawenu A, Scorzelli CJ, Ulbrecht M, Weiss EH, Coligan JE. Specific recognition of HLA-E, but not classical, HLA class I molecules by soluble CD94/NKG2A and NK cells. J Immunol 1999;162:305-13.
34. Brown JH, Jardetzky TS, Gorga JC, Stern LJ, Urban RG, Strominger JL, Wiley DC. Three-dimensional structure of the human class II histocompatibility antigen HLA-DR1. Nature 1993;364:33-39.
35. Brown MA, Pile KD, Kennedy LG, Calin A, Darke C, Bell J, Wordsworth BP, Cornelis F. HLA class I associations of ankylosing spondylitis in the white population in the United Kingdom. Ann Rheum Dis 1996;55:268-70.
36. Brusic V, Rudy G, Harrison LC. MHCPEP, a database of MHC-binding peptides: Update 1997. Nucleic Acids Res 1998;26:368-71.
37. Burrows SR, Rossjohn J, McCluskey J. Have we cut ourselves too short in mapping CTL epitopes? Trends Immunol 2006;27:11-16.
38. Burrows SR, Silins SL, Cross SM, Peh CA, Rischmueller M, Burrows JM, Elliott SL, McCluskey J. Human leukocyte antigen phenotype imposes complex constraints on the antigenspecific cytotoxic T lymphocyte repertoire. Eur J Immunol 1997;27:178-182.
39. Buxton SE, Benjamin RJ, Clayberger C, Parham P, Krensky AM. Anchoring pockets in human histocompatibility complex leukocyte antigen (HLA) class I molecules: Analysis of the conserved B ("45") pocket of HLA-B27. J Exp Med 1992;175:809-20.
40. Callan MF, McMichael AJ. T cell receptor usage in infectious disease. Springer Semin Immunopathol 1999;21:37-54.
41. Callan MF, Annels N, Steven N, Tan L, Wilson J, McMichael AJ, Rickinson AB. T cell selection during the evolution of CD8+ T cell memory in vivo. Eur J Immunol 1998;28:4382-90.
42. Callan MF, Fazou C, Yang H, Rostron T, Poon K, Hatton C, McMichael AJ. CD8(+) T cell selection, function, and death in the primary immune response in vivo. J Clin Invest 2000;106:1251-61.
43. Callan MF, Reyburn HT, Bowness P, Rowland-Jones S, Bell JI, McMichael AJ. Selection of T cell receptor variable gene-encoded amino acids on the third binding site loop: A factor influencing variable chain selection in a T cell response. Eur J Immunol 1995;25:1529-34.
44. Carbone FR, Heath WR. The role of dendritic cell subsets in immunity to viruses. Curr Opin Immunol 2003;15:416-20.
45. Carrington M, O'Brien SJ. The influence of HLA genotype on AIDS. Annu Rev Med 2003;54:535-51.
46. Cella M, Sallusto F, Lanzavecchia A. Origin, maturation and antigen presenting function of dendritic cells. Curr Opin Immunol 1997;9:10-16.
47. Chantarangsu S, Mushiroda T, Mahasirimongkol S, Kiertiburanakul S, Sungkanuparph S, Manosuthi W, Tantisiriwat W, Charoenyingwattana A, Sura T, Chantratita W, Nakamura Y. HLA-B*3505 allele is a strong predictor for nevirapine-induced skin adverse drug reactions in HIV-infected Thai patients. Pharmacogenet Genomics 2009;19:139-46.
48. Chen QY, Huang W, She JX, Baxter, F, Volpe R, Maclaren NK. HLA-DRB1*08, DRB1*03/DRB3*0101, and DRB3*0202 are susceptibility genes for Graves' disease in North American Caucasians, whereas DRB1*07 is protective. J Clin Endocrinol Metab 1999;84:3182-86.
49. Chessman D, Kostenko L, Lethborg T, Purcell AW, Williamson NA, Chen Z, Kjer-Nielsen L, Mifsud NA, Tait BD, Holdsworth R, et al. Human leukocyte antigen class I-restricted activation of CD8+ T cells provides the immunogenetic basis of a systemic drug hypersensitivity. Immunity 2008;28:822-32.
50. Chicz RM, Urban RG, Gorga JC, Vignali DA, Lane WS, Strominger JL. Specificity and promiscuity among naturally processed peptides bound to HLA-DR alleles. J Exp Med 1993;178:27-47.
51. Chicz RM, Urban RG, Lane WS, Gorga JC, Stern LJ, Vignali DA, Strominger JL. Predominant naturally processed peptides bound to HLA-DR1 are derived from MHC-related molecules and are heterogeneous in size. Nature 1992;358:764-68.
52. Chung WH, Hung SI, Hong HS, Hsih MS, Yang LC, Ho HC, Wu JY, Chen YT. Medical genetics: A marker for Stevens-Johnson syndrome. Nature 2004;428:486.
53. Clements CS, Kjer-Nielsen L, Kostenko L, Hoare HL, Dunstone MA, Moses E, Freed K, Brooks AG, Rossjohn J, McCluskey J. Crystal structure of HLA-G: A nonclassical MHC class I molecule expressed at the fetal-maternal interface. Proc Natl Acad Sci USA 2005;102:3360-65.
54. Colf LA, Bankovich AJ, Hanick NA, Bowerman NA, Jones LL, Kranz DM, Garcia KC. How a single T cell receptor recognizes both self and foreign MHC. Cell 2007;129:135-46.

55. Collins AV, Brodie DW, Gilbert RJ, Iaboni A, Manso-Sancho R, Walse B, Stuart DI, van der Merwe PA, Davis SJ. The interaction properties of costimulatory molecules revisited. Immunity 2002;17:201-10.
56. Cresswell P, Bangia N, Dick T, Diedrich G. The nature of the MHC class I peptide loading complex. Immunol Rev 1999;172:21-28.
57. Cresswell P. Assembly, transport, and function of MHC class II molecules. Annu Rev Immunol 1994;12:259-93.
58. Dai S, Huseby ES, Rubtsova K, Scott-Browne J, Crawford F, Macdonald WA, Marrack P, Kappler JW. Crossreactive T cells spotlight the germline rules for alphabeta T cell-receptor interactions with MHC molecules. Immunity 2008;28:324-34.
59. Daly AK, Donaldson PT, Bhatnagar P, Shen Y, Pe'er I, Floratos A, Daly MJ, Goldstein DB, John S, Nelson MR, et al. HLA-B*5701 genotype is a major determinant of drug-induced liver injury due to flucloxacillin. Nat Genet 2009;41:816-19.
60. Davis MM, Bjorkman PJ. T cell antigen receptor genes and T cell recognition. Nature 1988;334:395-402.
61. Davis MM. T cell receptor gene diversity and selection. Annu Rev Biochem 1990;59:475-96.
62. Davis MM. The problem of plain vanilla peptides. Nat Immunol 2003;4:649-50.
63. Degano M, Garcia KC, Apostolopoulos V, Rudolph MG, Teyton L, Wilson IA. A functional hot spot for antigen recognition in a superagonist TCR/MHC complex. Immunity 2000;12:251-61.
64. Degli-Esposti MA, Andreas A, Christiansen FT, Schalke B, Albert E, Dawkins RL. An approach to the localization of the susceptibility genes for generalized myasthenia gravis by mapping recombinant ancestral haplotypes. Immunogenetics 1992;35:355-64.
65. Denzin LK, Cresswell P. HLA-DM induces CLIP dissociation from MHC class II alpha beta dimers and facilitates peptide loading. Cell 1995;82:155-65.
66. Denzin LK, Hammond C, Cresswell P. HLA-DM interactions with intermediates in HLADR maturation and a role for HLA-DM in stabilizing empty HLA-DR molecules. J Exp Med 1996;184:2153-65.
67. Deres K, Beck W, Faath S, Jung G, Rammensee HG. MHC/peptide binding studies indicate hierarchy of anchor residues. Cell Immunol 1993;151:158-67.
68. DiBrino M, Parker KC, Margulies DH, Shiloach J, Turner RV, Biddison WE, Coligan JE. Identification of the peptide binding motif for HLA-B44, one of the most common HLA-B alleles in the Caucasian population. Biochemistry 1995;34:10130-138.
69. Dick TP, Bangia N, Peaper DR, Cresswell P. Disulfide bond isomerization and the assembly of MHC class I-peptide complexes. Immunity 2002;16:87-98.
70. Ding YH, Baker BM, Garboczi DN, Biddison WE, Wiley DC. Four A6-TCR/peptide/HLA-A2 structures that generate very different T cell signals are nearly identical. Immunity 1999;11:45-56.
71. Ding YH, Smith KJ, Garboczi DN, Utz U, Biddison WE, Wiley DC. Two human T cell receptors bind in a similar diagonal mode to the HLA-A2/Tax peptide complex using different TCR amino acids. Immunity 1998;8:403-411.
72. Doherty PC, Zinkernagel RM. H-2 compatibility is required for T cell-mediated lysis of target cells infected with lymphocytic choriomeningitis virus. J Exp Med 1975;141:502-507.
73. Dong G, Wearsch PA, Peaper DR, Cresswell P, Reinisch KM. Insights into MHC class I peptide loading from the structure of the tapasin-ERp57 thiol oxidoreductase heterodimer. Immunity 2009;30:21-32.
74. Dongre AR, Kovats S, deRoos P, McCormack AL, Nakagawa T, Paharkova-Vatchkova V, Eng J, Caldwell H, Yates JR, 3rd, Rudensky AY. In vivo MHC class II presentation of cytosolic proteins revealed by rapid automated tandem mass spectrometry and functional analyses. Eur J Immunol 2001;31:1485-94.
75. Doxiadis II, Smits JM, Schreuder GM, Persijn GG, van Houwelingen HC, van Rood JJ, Claas FH. Association between specific HLA combinations and probability of kidney allograft loss: The taboo concept. Lancet 1996;348:850-53.
76. Ebringer A, Wilson C. HLA molecules, bacteria and autoimmunity. J Med Microbiol 2000;49:305-11.
77. Ely LK, Burrows SR, Purcell AW, Rossjohn J, McCluskey J. T cells behaving badly: Structural insights into alloreactivity and autoimmunity. Curr Opin Immunol 2008;20:575-80.
78. Ely LK, Kjer-Nielsen L, McCluskey J, Rossjohn J. Structural studies on the alphabeta T cell receptor. IUBMB Life 2005;57:575-582.
79. Engelhard VH, Appella E, Benjamin DC, Bodnar WM, Cox AL, Chen Y, Henderson RA, Huczko EL, Michel H, Sakaguichi K, et al. Mass spectrometric analysis of peptides associated with the human class I MHC molecules HLA-A2.1 and HLA-B7 and identification of structural features that determine binding. Chem Immunol 1993;57:39-62.
80. Falk K, Rotzschke O, Grahovac B, Schendel D, Stevanovic S, Jung G, Rammensee HG. Peptide motifs of HLA-B35 and -B37 molecules. Immunogenetics 1993;38:161-62.
81. Falk K, Rotzschke O, Stevanovic S, Jung G, Rammensee HG. Allele-specific motifs revealed by sequencing of self-peptides eluted from MHC molecules. Nature 1991;351:290-96.
82. Feltkamp TE. HLA and uveitis. Int Ophthalmol 1990;14:327-33.
83. Feng D, Bond CJ, Ely LK, Maynard J, Garcia KC. Structural evidence for a germlineencoded T cell receptor-major histocompatibility complex interaction 'codon'. Nat Immunol 2007;8:975-83.
84. Flores-Dominguez C, Hernandez-Pacheco G, Zuniga J, Gamboa R, Granados J, Reyes PA, Vargas-Alarcon G. Alleles of the major histocompatibility system associated

with susceptibility to the development of Takayasu's arteritis. Gac Med Mex 2002;138:177-83.
85. Fruci D, Lauvau G, Saveanu L, Amicosante M, Butler RH, Polack A, Ginhoux F, Lemonnier F, Firat H, van Endert PM. Quantifying recruitment of cytosolic peptides for HLA class I presentation: impact of TAP transport. J Immunol 2003;170:2977-84.
86. Fruci D, Niedermann G, Butler RH, van Endert PM. Efficient MHC class I-independent amino-terminal trimming of epitope precursor peptides in the endoplasmic reticulum. Immunity 2001;15:467.
87. Gao GF, Tormo J, Gerth UC, Wyer JR, McMichael AJ, Stuart DI, Bell JI, Jones EY, Jakobsen BK. Crystal structure of the complex between human CD8alpha(alpha) and HLA-A2. Nature 1997;387:630-34.
88. Gao XJ, Brautbar C, Gazit E, Segal R, Naparstek Y, Livneh A, Stastny P. A variant of HLA-DR4 determines susceptibility to rheumatoid arthritis in a subset of Israeli Jews. Arthritis Rheum 1991;34:547-551.
89. Gao XJ, Olsen NJ, Pincus T, Stastny P. HLA-DR alleles with naturally occurring amino cid substitutions and risk for development of rheumatoid arthritis. Arthritis Rheum 1990;33:939-46.
90. Garboczi DN, Biddison WE. Shapes of MHC restriction. Immunity 1999;10: 1-7.
91. Garboczi DN, Ghosh P, Utz U, Fan QR, Biddison WE, Wiley DC. Structure of the complex between human T cell receptor, viral peptide and HLA-A2. Nature 1996;384:134-41.
92. Garcia KC, Adams JJ, Feng D, Ely LK. The molecular basis of TCR germline bias for MHC is surprisingly simple. Nat Immunol 2009;10:143-47.
93. Garcia KC, Degano M, Pease LR, Huang M, Peterson PA, Teyton L, Wilson IA. Structural basis of plasticity in T cell receptor recognition of a self peptide-MHC antigen. Science 1998;279:1166-72.
94. Garcia KC, Degano M, Stanfield RL, Brunmark A, Jackson MR, Peterson PA, Teyton L, Wilson IA. An alpha beta T cell receptor structure at 2.5 A and its orientation in the TCR-MHC complex. Science 1996;274:209-19.
95. Garcia KC, Teyton L, Wilson IA. Structural basis of T cell recognition. Annu Rev Immunol 1999;17:369-97.
96. Garcia KC. Molecular interactions between extracellular components of the T cell receptor signaling complex. Immunol Rev 1999;172:73-85.
97. Garrett TP, Saper MA, Bjorkman PJ, Strominger JL, Wiley DC. Specificity pockets for the side chains of peptide antigens in HLA-Aw68. Nature 1989;342:692-96.
98. Gatanaga H, Honda H, Oka S. Pharmacogenetic information derived from analysis of HLA alleles. Pharmacogenomics 2008;9:207-14.
99. Germain RN, Braunstein NS, Brown MA, Glimcher LH, Lechler RI, McCluskey J, Margulies DH, Miller J, Norcross MA, Paul WE, et al. Structure and function of murine class II major histocompatibility complex genes. Mt Sinai J Med 1986;53:194-201.
100. Ghosh P, Amaya M, Mellins E, Wiley DC. The structure of an intermediate in class II MHC maturation: CLIP bound to HLA-DR3. Nature 1995;378:457-62.
101. Godfrey DI, Rossjohn J, McCluskey J. The fidelity, occasional promiscuity, and versatility of T cell receptor recognition. Immunity 2008;28:304-14.
102. Graham RR, Ortmann W, Rodine P, Espe K, Langefeld C, Lange E, Williams A, Beck S, Kyogoku C, Moser K, et al. Specific combinations of HLA-DR2 and DR3 class II haplotypes contribute graded risk for disease susceptibility and autoantibodies in human SLE. Eur J Hum Genet 2007;15:823-30.
103. Grakoui A, Bromley SK, Sumen C, Davis MM, Shaw AS, Allen PM, Dustin ML. The immunological synapse: A molecular machine controlling T cell activation. Science 1999;285:221-27.
104. Gras S, Burrows SR, Kjer-Nielsen L, Clements CS, Liu YC, Sullivan LC, Bell MJ, Brooks AG, Purcell AW, McCluskey J, Rossjohn J. The shaping of T cell receptor recognition by self-tolerance. Immunity 2009;30: 193-203.
105. Gras S, Kjer-Nielsen L, Burrows SR, McCluskey J, Rossjohn J. T cell receptor bias and immunity. Curr Opin Immunol 2008;20:119-25.
106. Green KJ, Miles JJ, Tellam J, Van Zuylen WJ, Connolly G, Burrows SR. Potent T cell response to a class I-binding 13-mer viral epitope and the influence of HLA micropolymorphism in controlling epitope length. Eur J Immunol 2004;34:2510-19.
107. Griffiths CE, Barker JN. Pathogenesis and clinical features of psoriasis. Lancet 2007;370: 263-71.
108. Hakenberg J, Nussbaum AK, Schild H, Rammensee HG, Kuttler C, Holzhutter HG, Kloetzel PM, Kaufmann SH, Mollenkopf HJ. MAPPP: MHC class I antigenic peptide processing prediction. Appl Bioinformatics 2003;2:155-58.
109. Heath WR, Carbone FR. Cross-presentation in viral immunity and self-tolerance. Nat Rev Immunol 2001a;1:126-34.
110. Heath WR, Carbone FR. Cross-presentation, dendritic cells, tolerance and immunity. Annu Rev Immunol 2001b;19: 47-64.
111. Heath WR, Kane KP, Mescher MF, Sherman, LA. Alloreactive T cells discriminate among a diverse set of endogenous peptides. Proc Natl Acad Sci U S A 1991;88:5101-05.
112. Heemels MT, Ploegh H. Generation, translocation, and presentation of MHC class I restricted peptides. Annu Rev Biochem 1995;64:463-91.
113. Hendel H, Caillat-Zucman S, Lebuanec H, Carrington M, O'Brien S, Andrieu JM, Schachter F, Zagury D, Rappaport J, Winkler C, et al. New class I and II HLA alleles strongly associated with opposite patterns of progression to AIDS. J Immunol 1999;162:6942-46.
114. Henderson KN, Tye-Din JA, Reid HH, Chen Z, Borg NA, Beissbarth T, Tatham A, Mannering SI, Purcell AW, Dudek NL, et al. A structural and immunological basis

for the role of human leukocyte antigen DQ8 in celiac disease. Immunity 2007;27:23-34.
115. Hennecke J, Wiley DC. T cell receptor-MHC interactions up close. Cell 2001;104:1-4.
116. Hennecke J, Carfi A, Wiley DC. Structure of a covalently stabilized complex of a human alphabeta T- cell receptor, influenza HA peptide and MHC class II molecule, HLA-DR1. EMBO J 2000;19:5611-24.
117. Hershko A, Ciechanover A. The ubiquitin system. Annu Rev Biochem 1998;67:425-79.
118. Hetherington S, Hughes AR, Mosteller M, Shortino D, Baker KL, Spreen W, Lai E, Davies K, Handley A, Dow DJ, et al. Genetic variations in HLA-B region and hypersensitivity reactions to abacavir. Lancet 2002;359:1121-22.
119. Hietaharju A, Korpela M, Ilonen J, Frey H. Nervous system disease, immunological eatures, and HLA phenotype in Sjögren's syndrome. Ann Rheum Dis 1992;51:506-09.
120. Hill AV, Elvin J, Willis AC, Aidoo M, Allsopp CE, Gotch FM, Gao XM, Takiguchi M, Greenwood BM, Townsend AR, et al. Molecular analysis of the association of HLA-B53 and resistance to severe malaria. Nature 1992;360:434-39.
121. Hill AV. Immunogenetics and genomics. Lancet 2001;357:2037-41.
122. Hillen N, Mester G, Lemmel C, Weinzierl AO, Muller M, Wernet D, Hennenlotter J, Stenzl A, Rammensee HG, Stevanovic S. Essential differences in ligand presentation and T cell epitope recognition among HLA molecules of the HLA-B44 supertype. Eur J Immunol 2008;38:2993-3003.
123. Hoare HL, Sullivan LC, Pietra G, Clements CS, Lee EJ, Ely LK, Beddoe T, Falco M, Kjer-Nielsen L, Reid HH, et al. Structural basis for a major histocompatibility complex class Ibrestricted T cell response. Nat Immunol 2006;7:256-64.
124. Huczko EL, Bodnar WM, Benjamin D, Sakaguchi K, Zhu NZ, Shabanowitz J, Henderson RA, Appella E, Hunt DF, Engelhard VH. Characteristics of endogenous peptides eluted from the class I MHC molecule HLA-B7 determined by mass spectrometry and computer modeling. J Immunol 1993;151:2572-87.
125. Hummer M, Kurz M, Barnas C, Saria A, Fleischhacker WW. Clozapine-induced transient white blood count disorders. J Clin Psychiatry 1994;55:429-32.
126. Hung SI, Chung WH, Jee SH, Chen WC, Chang YT, Lee WR, Hu SL, Wu MT, Chen GS, Wong TW, et al. Genetic susceptibility to carbamazepine-induced cutaneous adverse drug reactions. Pharmacogenet Genomics 2006;16:297-306.
127. Hung SI, Chung WH, Liou LB, Chu CC, Lin M, Huang HP, Lin YL, Lan JL, Yang LC, Hong HS, et al HLA-B*5801 allele as a genetic marker for severe cutaneous adverse reactions caused by allopurinol Proc Natl Acad Sci USA 2005;102:4134-39.
128. Hunt DF, Henderson RA, Shabanowitz J, Sakaguchi K, Michel H, Sevilir N, Cox AL, Appella E, Engelhard VH. Characterization of peptides bound to the class I MHC molecule HLAA2.1 by mass spectrometry. Science 1992;255:1261-63.
129. Ishitani A, Sageshima N, Lee N, Dorofeeva N, Hatake K, Marquardt H, Geraghty DE. Protein expression and peptide binding suggest unique and interacting functional roles for HLAE, F, and G in maternal-placental immune recognition. J Immunol 2003;171:1376-84.
130. Ishizuka J, Stewart-Jones GB, van der Merwe A, Bell JI, McMichael AJ, Jones EY. The structural dynamics and energetics of an immunodominant T cell receptor are programmed by its Vbeta domain. Immunity 2008;28:171-82.
131. Jardetzky TS, Brown JH, Gorga JC, Stern LJ, Urban RG, Chi YI, Stauffacher C, Strominger JL, Wiley DC. Three-dimensional structure of a human class II histocompatibility molecule complexed with superantigen. Nature 1994;368:711-18.
132. Jardetzky TS, Brown JH, Gorga JC, Stern LJ, Urban RG, Strominger JL, Wiley DC. Crystallographic analysis of endogenous peptides associated with HLA-DR1 suggests a common, polyproline II-like conformation for bound peptides. Proc Natl Acad Sci USA 1996;93:734-38.
133. Jardetzky TS, Lane WS, Robinson RA, Madden DR, Wiley DC. Identification of self peptides bound to purified HLA-B27. Nature 1991; 353:326-29.
134. Jones EY, Fugger L, Strominger JL, Siebold C. MHC class II proteins and disease: A structural perspective. Nat Rev Immunol 2006;6:271-82.
135. Karell K, Louka AS, Moodie SJ, Ascher H, Clot F, Greco L, Ciclitira PJ, Sollid LM, Partanen J. HLA types in celiac disease patients not carrying the DQA1*05-DQB1*02 (DQ2) heterodimer: Results from the European Genetics Cluster on Celiac Disease. Hum Immunol 2003;64: 469-77.
136. Kedzierska K, Turner SJ, Doherty PC. Conserved T cell receptor usage in primary and recall responses to an immunodominant influenza virus nucleoprotein epitope. Proc Natl Acad Sci USA 2004;101:4942-47.
137. Kersh GJ, Kersh EN, Fremont DH, Allen PM. High- and low-potency ligands with similar affinities for the TCR: The importance of kinetics in TCR signaling. Immunity 1998;9:817-26.
138. Kesmir C, Nussbaum AK, Schild H, Detours V, Brunak S. Prediction of proteasome cleavage motifs by neural networks. Protein Eng 2002;15:287-96.
139. Kienast A, Preuss M, Winkler M, Dick TP. Redox regulation of peptide receptivity of major histocompatibility complex class I molecules by ERp57 and tapasin. Nat Immunol 2007;8:864-72.
140. Kim CY, Quarsten H, Bergseng E, Khosla C, Sollid LM. Structural basis for HLADQ2-mediated presentation of gluten epitopes in celiac disease. Proc Natl Acad Sci USA 2004;101:4175-79.

141. Kim SH, Choi JH, Lee KW, Shin ES, Oh HB, Suh CH, Nahm DH, Park HS. The human leucocyte antigen-DRB1*1302-DQB1*0609-DPB1*0201 haplotype may be a strong genetic marker for aspirin-induced urticaria. Clin Exp Allergy 2005;35,:339-44.

142. Kim SH, Hur GY, Choi JH, Park HS. Pharmacogenetics of aspirin-intolerant asthma. Pharmacogenomics 2008;9:85-91.

143. Kindmark A, Jawaid A, Harbron CG, Barratt BJ, Bengtsson OF, Andersson TB, Carlsson S, Cederbrant KE, Gibson NJ, Armstrong M, et al. Genome-wide pharmacogenetic investigation of a hepatic adverse event without clinical signs of immunopathology suggests an underlying immune pathogenesis. Pharmacogenomics J 2008;8:186-95.

144. King A, Allan DS, Bowen M, Powis SJ, Joseph S, Verma S, Hiby SE, McMichael AJ, Loke YW, Braud VM. HLA-E is expressed on trophoblast and interacts with CD94/NKG2 receptors on decidual NK cells. Eur J Immunol 2000;30:1623-31.

145. Kjer-Nielsen L, Clements CS, Brooks AG, Purcell AW, Fontes MR, McCluskey J, Rossjohn J. The structure of HLA-B8 complexed to an immunodominant viral determinant: peptide-induced conformational changes and a mode of MHC class I dimerization. J Immunol 2002a;169:5153-60.

146. Kjer-Nielsen L, Clements CS, Brooks AG, Purcell AW, McCluskey J, Rossjohn J. The 1.5 a crystal structure of a highly selected antiviral T cell receptor provides evidence for a structural basis of immunodominance. Structure (Camb) 2002b;10:1521-32.

147. Kjer-Nielsen L, Clements CS, Purcell AW, Brooks AG, Whisstock JC, Burrows SR, McCluskey J, Rossjohn J. A structural basis for the selection of dominant alphabeta T cell receptors in antiviral immunity. Immunity 2003;18,:53-64.

148. Klein J. The Natural History of The Major Histocompatibility Complex (New York: Wiley & Sons). 1987.

149. Kotter I, Gunaydin I, Stubiger N, Yazici H, Fresko I, Zouboulis CC, Adler Y, Steiert I, Kurz B, Wernet D, et al. Comparative analysis of the association of HLA-B*51 suballeles with Beçhet's disease in patients of German and Turkish origin. Tissue Antigens 2001;158:166-70.

150. Krogsgaard M, Prado N, Adams EJ, He XL, Chow DC, Wilson DB, Garcia KC, Davis MM. Evidence that structural rearrangements and/or flexibility during TCR binding can contribute to T cell activation. Mol Cell 2003;12:1367-78.

151. Krummel M, Wulfing C, Sumen C, Davis MM. Thirty-six views of T cell recognition. Philos Trans R Soc Lond B Biol Sci 2000;355:1071-76.

152. Kuttenn F, Couillin P, Girard F, Billaud L, Vincens M, Boucekkine C, Thalabard JC, Maudelonde T, Spritzer P, Mowszowicz I, et al. Late-onset adrenal hyperplasia in hirsutism. N Engl J Med 1985;313:224-31.

153. Kuttler C, Nussbaum AK, Dick TP, Rammensee HG, Schild H, Hadeler KP. An algorithm for the prediction of proteasomal cleavages. J Mol Biol 2000;298:417-29.

154. Lammert E, Arnold D, Nijenhuis M, Momburg F, Hammerling GJ, Brunner J, Stevanovic S, Rammensee HG, Schild H. The endoplasmic reticulum-resident stress protein gp96 binds peptides translocated by TAP. Eur J Immunol 1997;27:923-27.

155. Lanier LL. NK cell receptors. Annu Rev Immunol 1998;16:359-393.

156. Lanzavecchia A, Sallusto F. Regulation of T cell immunity by dendritic cells. Cell 2001;106:263-66.

157. Larsen CE, Alper CA. The genetics of HLA-associated disease. Curr Opin Immunol 2004;16:660-67.

158. Lechler RI, Lombardi G, Batchelor JR, Reinsmoen N, Bach FH. The molecular basis of alloreactivity. Immunol Today 1990;11:83-88.

159. Lee N, Goodlett DR, Ishitani A, Marquardt H, Geraghty DE. HLA-E surface expression depends on binding of TAP-dependent peptides derived from certain HLA class I signal sequences. J Immunol 1998;160:4951-60.

160. Lee N, Malacko AR, Ishitani A, Chen MC, Bajorath J, Marquardt H, Geraghty DE. The membrane-bound and soluble forms of HLA-G bind identical sets of endogenous peptides but differ with respect to TAP association. Immunity 1995;3:591-600.

161. Lehner PJ, Cresswell P, Recent developments in MHC-class-I-mediated antigen presentation. Curr Opin Immunol 2004;16:82-89.

162. Lehner PJ, Cresswell P. Processing and delivery of peptides presented by MHC class I molecules. Curr Opin Immunol 1996;8: 59-67.

163. LeMaoult J, Le Discorde M, Rouas-Freiss N, Moreau P, Menier C, McCluskey J, Carosella ED. Biology and functions of human leukocyte antigen-G in health and sickness. Tissue Antigens 2003;62:273-84.

164. Levinson RD, Rajalingam R, Park MS, Reed EF, Gjertson DW, Kappel PJ, See RF, Rao NA, Holland GN. Human leukocyte antigen A29 subtypes associated with birdshot retinochoroidopathy. Am J Ophthalmol 2004;138:631-34.

165. Levitsky V, Liu D, Southwood S, Levitskaya J, Sette A, Masucci MG. Supermotif peptide binding and degeneracy of MHC: peptide recognition in an EBV peptide-specific CTL response with highly restricted TCR usage. Hum Immunol 2000;61:972-84.

166. Littera R, Carcassi C, Masala A, Piano P, Serra P, Ortu F, Corso N, Casula B, La Nasa G, Contu L, Manconi PE. HLA-dependent hypersensitivity to nevirapine in Sardinian HIV patients. Aids 2006;20:1621-26.

167. Luz JG, Huang M, Garcia KC, Rudolph MG, Apostolopoulos V, Teyton L, Wilson IA. Structural comparison of allogeneic and syngeneic T cell receptor-peptide-major histocompatibility complex complexes: a buried alloreactive mutation subtly alters peptide presentation substantially increasing V(beta) Interactions. J Exp Med 2002;195:1175-86.

168. Macdonald WA, Chen W, Gras S, Archbold JA, Tynan FE, Clements CS, Bharadwaj M, Kjer-Nielsen L, Saunders P, Wilce MCJ, et al. T cell allorecognition due to molecular mimicry. Immunity (in press), 2009.
169. Macdonald WA, Purcell AW, Mifsud N, Ely LK, Williams DS, Chang L, Gorman JJ, Clements CS, Kjer-Nielsen L, Koelle DM, et al. A Naturally Selected Dimorphism within the HLA-B44 Supertype Alters Class I Structure, Peptide Repertoire and T cell Recognition. J Exp Med 2003;198:679-91.
170. Mackay IR. Historical reflections on autoimmune hepatitis. World J Gastroenterol 2008;14:3292-3300.
171. Maclaren NK, Riley WJ. Inherited susceptibility to autoimmune Addison's disease is linked to human leukocyte antigens-DR3 and/or DR4, except when associated with type I autoimmune polyglandular syndrome. J Clin Endocrinol Metab 1986;62:455-59.
172. Madden DR. The three-dimensional structure of peptide-MHC complexes. Annu Rev Immunol 1995;13:587-622.
173. Mallal S, Nolan D, Witt C, Masel G, Martin AM, Moore C, Sayer D, Castley A, Mamotte C, Maxwell D, et al. Association between presence of HLA-B*5701, HLA-DR7, HLA-DQ3 and hypersensitivity to HIV-1 reverse-transcriptase inhibitor abacavir. Lancet 2002;359:727-32.
174. Mallal S, Phillips E, Carosi G, Molina J-M, Workman C, Toma J, Jägel-Guedes E, Rugina S, Kozyrev O, Cid JF, et al. The PREDICT-1 study: A randomised, double blind trial to determine the clinical utility of HLA-B*5701 pharmacogenetic screening for abacavir hypersensitivity in HIV-infected patients (Study CNA106030). New England Journal of medicine 2008;358:568-579.
175. Man CB, Kwan P, Baum L, Yu E, Lau KM, Cheng AS, Ng MH. Association between HLA-B*1502 allele and antiepileptic drug-induced cutaneous reactions in Han Chinese. Epilepsia 2007;48:1015-18.
176. Margulies D, McCluskey J. The Major Histocompatibility Complex and its Encoded Proteins. In Fundamental Immunology, W. Paul, ed. (Philadelphia: Lippincott Williams & Wilkins), 2003.
177. Margulies DH, Rossjohn J, McCluskey J. The Major Histocompatibility Complex and its Encoded Proteins. In Fundamental Immunology, WE Paul, ed (New York: Lippincott-Raven) 2008.
178. Maric M, Arunachalam B, Phan UT, Dong C, Garrett WS, Cannon KS, Alfonso C, Karlsson L, Flavell RA, Cresswell P. Defective antigen processing in GILT-free mice. Science 2001;294:1361-65.
179. Marsh SG, Albert ED, Bodmer WF, Bontrop RE, Dupont B, Erlich HA, Geraghty DE, Hansen JA, Mach B, Mayr WR, et al. Nomenclature for factors of the HLA system, 2002. Tissue Antigens 2002;60:407-64.
180. Marsh SG, Parham P, Barber LD. The HLA Facts Book (London: Academic Press) 2000.
181. Martin AM, Almeida CA, Cameron P, Purcell AW, Nolan D, James I, McCluskey J, Phillips E, Landay A, Mallal S Immune responses to abacavir in antigen-presenting cells from hypersensitive patients. Aids 2007;21: 1233-44.
182. Martin AM, Nolan D, Gaudieri S, Almeida CA, Nolan R, James I, Carvalho F, Phillips E, Christiansen FT, Purcell AW, et al. Predisposition to abacavir hypersensitivity conferred by HLA-B*5701 and a haplotypic Hsp70-Hom variant. Proc Natl Acad Sci USA 2004;101:4180-85.
183. Martinez-Martin N, Risueno RM, Morreale A, Zaldivar I, Fernandez-Arenas E, Herranz F, Ortiz AR, Alarcon B. Cooperativity between T cell receptor complexes revealed by conformational mutants of CD3epsilon. Sci Signal 2, ra43, 2009.
184. Maynard J, Petersson K, Wilson DH, Adams EJ, Blondelle SE, Boulanger MJ, Wilson DB, Garcia KC. Structure of an autoimmune T cell receptor complexed with class II peptide-MHC: insights into MHC bias and antigen specificity. Immunity 2005;22:81-92.
185. McCluskey J, Rossjohn J, Purcell AW. TAP genes and immunity. Curr Opin Immunol 2004;16:651-59.
186. McDevitt HO, Deak BD, Shreffler DC, Klein J, Stimpfling JH, Snell GD. Genetic control of the immune response. Mapping of the Ir-1 locus. J Exp Med 1972;135:1259-78.
187. Menssen R, Orth P, Ziegler A, Saenger W. Decamer-like conformation of a nona-peptide bound to HLA-B*3501 due to non-standard positioning of the C terminus. J Mol Biol 1999;285:645-53.
188. Mifsud NA, Purcell AW, Chen W, Holdsworth R, Tait BD, McCluskey J. Immunodominance hierarchies and gender bias in direct T(CD8)-cell alloreactivity. Am J Transplant 2008;8:121-32.
189. Miles JJ, Elhassen D, Borg NA, Silins SL, Tynan FE, Burrows JM, Purcell AW, Kjer-Nielsen L, Rossjohn J, Burrows SR, McCluskey J. CTL Recognition of a Bulged Viral Peptide Involves Biased TCR Selection. J Immunol 2005;175:3826-34.
190. Molberg O, McAdam SN, Korner R, Quarsten H, Kristiansen C, Madsen L, Fugger L, Scott H, Noren O, Roepstorff P, et al. Tissue transglutaminase selectively modifies gliadin peptides that are recognized by gut-derived T cells in celiac disease. Nat Med 1998;4:713-17.
191. Momburg F, Hammerling GJ. Generation and TAP-mediated transport of peptides for major histocompatibility complex class I molecules. Adv Immunol 1998;68:191-256.
192. Momburg F, Neefjes JJ, Hammerling GJ. Peptide selection by MHC-encoded TAP transporters. Curr Opin Immunol 1994a;6:32-37.
193. Momburg F, Roelse J, Hammerling GJ, Neefjes JJ. Peptide size selection by the major histocompatibility complex-encoded peptide transporter. J Exp Med 1994b;179: 1613-23.
194. Mongkolsapaya J, Jaye A, Callan MF, Magnusen AF, McMichael AJ, Whittle HC. Antigen-specific expansion of cytotoxic T lymphocytes in acute measles virus infection. J Virol 1999;73:67-71.
195. Morris P, Shaman J, Attaya M, Amaya M, Goodman S, Bergman C, Monaco JJ, Mellins E. An essential role for HLA-DM in antigen presentation by class II major histocompatibility molecules. Nature 1994;368:551-54.

196. Murthy VL, Stern LJ. The class II MHC protein HLA-DR1 in complex with an endogenous peptide: implications for the structural basis of the specificity of peptide binding. Structure 1997;5:1385-96.
197. Nakagawa TY, Rudensky AY. The role of lysosomal proteinases in MHC class IImediated antigen processing and presentation. Immunol Rev 1999;172:121-29.
198. Nejentsev S, Howson JM, Walker NM, Szeszko J, Field SF, Stevens HE, Reynolds P, Hardy M, King E, Masters J, et al. Localization of type 1 diabetes susceptibility to the MHC class I genes HLA-B and HLA-A. Nature 2007;450:887-92.
199. Nicholson MJ, Hahn M, Wucherpfennig KW. Unusual features of self-peptide/MHC binding by autoimmune T cell receptors. Immunity 2005;23: 351-60.
200. Nyulassy S, Hnilica P, Buc M, Guman M, Hirschova V, Stefanovic J. Subacute (de Quervain's) thyroiditis: Association with HLA-Bw35 antigen and abnormalities of the complement system, immunoglobulins and other serum proteins. J Clin Endocrinol Metab 1977;45:270-74.
201. O'Callaghan, CA, Bell JI. Structure and function of the human MHC class Ib molecules HLA-E, HLA-F and HLA-G. Immunol Rev 1998;163:129-38.
202. Ohno S, Ohguchi M, Hirose S, Matsuda H, Wakisaka A, Aizawa M. Close association of HLA-Bw51 with Beçhet's disease. Arch Ophthalmol 1982;100:1455-58.
203. Ozkaya-Bayazit E, Akar U. Fixed drug eruption induced by trimethoprimsulfamethoxazole: Evidence for a link to HLA-A30 B13 Cw6 haplotype. J Am Acad Dermatol 2001;45:712-17.
204. Pamer E, Cresswell P. Mechanisms of MHC class I—restricted antigen processing. Annu Rev Immunol 1998;16:323-58.
205. Parham P. MHC class I molecules and KIRs in human history, health and survival. Nat Rev Immunol 2005;5:201-14.
206. Parker KC, Shields M, DiBrino M, Brooks A, Coligan, JE. Peptide binding to MHC class I molecules: implications for antigenic peptide prediction. Immunol Res 1995;14:34-57.
207. Peh CA, Burrows SR, Barnden M, Khanna R, Cresswell P, Moss DJ, McCluskey J. HLA-B27-restricted antigen presentation in the absence of tapasin reveals polymorphism in mechanisms of HLA class I peptide loading. Immunity 1998;8:531-42.
208. Pelin Z, Guilleminault C, Risch N, Grumet FC, Mignot E. HLA-DQB1*0602 homozygosity increases relative risk for narcolepsy but not disease severity in two ethnic groups. US Modafinil in Narcolepsy Multicenter Study Group. Tissue Antigens 1998;51:96-100.
209. Phillips EJ, Sullivan JR, Knowles SR, Shear NH. Utility of patch testing in patients with hypersensitivity syndromes associated with abacavir. Aids 2002;16: 2223-25.
210. Pietra G, Romagnani C, Mazzarino P, Falco M, Millo E, Moretta A, Moretta L, Mingari MC. HLA-E-restricted recognition of cytomegalovirus-derived peptides by human CD8+ cytolytic T lymphocytes. Proc Natl Acad Sci USxA 2003;100:10896-901.
211. Posthuma EF, Falkenburg JH, Apperley JF, Gratwohl A, Roosnek E, Hertenstein B, Schipper RF, Schreuder GM, D'Amaro J, Oudshoorn M, et al. HLA-B8 and HLA-A3 coexpressed with HLA-B8 are associated with a reduced risk of the development of chronic myeloid leukemia. The Chronic Leukemia Working Party of the EBMT. Blood 1999;93:3863-65.
212. Price P, Witt C, Allcock R, Sayer D, Garlepp M, Kok CC, French M, Mallal S, Christiansen F. The genetic basis for the association of the 8.1 ancestral haplotype (A1, B8, DR3) with multiple immunopathological diseases. Immunol Rev 1999;167:257-74.
213. Princiotta MF, Finzi D, Qian SB, Gibbs J, Schuchmann S, Buttgereit F, Bennink JR, Yewdell JW. Quantitating protein synthesis, degradation, endogenous antigen processing. Immunity 2003;18:343-54.
214. Pu Z, Lovitch SB, Bikoff EK, Unanue ER. T cells distinguish MHC-peptide complexes formed in separate vesicles and edited by H2-DM. Immunity 2004;20: 467-76.
215. Purcell AW, Gorman JJ. The use of post source decay in matrix assisted laser desorptionionisation mass spectrometry to delineate T cell determinants. J Immunol Methods 2001;249:17-31.
216. Purcell AW, Gorman JJ, Garcia-Peydro M, Paradela A, Burrows SR, Talbo GH, Laham N, Peh CA, Reynolds EC, Lopez De Castro JA, McCluskey J. Quantitative and qualitative influences of tapasin on the class I peptide repertoire. J Immunol 2001;166:1016-27.
217. Pyo CW, Williams LM, Moore Y, Hyodo H, Li SS, Zhao LP, Sageshima N, Ishitani A, Geraghty DE. HLA-E, HLA-F, HLA-G polymorphism: genomic sequence defines haplotype structure and variation spanning the nonclassical class I genes. Immunogenetics 2006;58: 241-51.
218. Qiao SW, Piper J, Haraldsen G, Oynebraten I, Fleckenstein B, Molberg O, Khosla C, Sollid LM. Tissue transglutaminase-mediated formation and cleavage of histamine-gliadin complexes: biological effects and implications for celiac disease. J Immunol 2005;174: 1657-63.
219. Quiralte J, Sanchez-Garcia F, Torres MJ, Blanco C, Castillo R, Ortega N, de Castro FR, Perez-Aciego P, Carrillo T. Association of HLA-DR11 with the anaphylactoid reaction caused by nonsteroidal anti-inflammatory drugs. J Allergy Clin Immunol 1999; 103:685-89.
220. Rajagopalan S, Bryceson YT, Kuppusamy SP, Geraghty DE, van der Meer A, Joosten I, Long EO. Activation of NK cells by an endocytosed receptor for soluble HLA-G. PLoS Biol 4, e9, 2006.
221. Rammensee H, Bachmann J, Emmerich NP, Bachor OA, Stevanovic S. SYFPEITHI: Database for MHC ligands and peptide motifs. Immunogenetics 1999;50:213-19.

222. Rammensee HG, Falk K, Rotzschke O. Peptides naturally presented by MHC class I molecules. Annu Rev Immunol 1993a;11:213-44.
223. Rammensee HG, Friede T, Stevanoviic S. MHC ligands and peptide motifs: first listing. Immunogenetics 1995;41:178-228.
224. Rammensee HG, Rotzschke O, Falk K. MHC class I-restricted antigen processing—lessons from natural ligands. Chem Immunol 1993b;57:113-33.
225. Ramos M, Lopez de Castro JA. HLA-B27 and the pathogenesis of spondyloarthritis. Tissue Antigens 2002;60:191-205.
226. Reid SW, McAdam S, Smith KJ, Klenerman P, O'Callaghan CA, Harlos K, Jakobsen BK, McMichael AJ, Bell JI, Stuart DI, Jones EY. Antagonist HIV-1 Gag peptides induce structural changes in HLA B8. J Exp Med 1996;184:2279-86.
227. Reinherz EL, Tan K, Tang L, Kern P, Liu J, Xiong Y, Hussey RE, Smolyar A, Hare B, Zhang R, et al. The crystal structure of a T cell receptor in complex with peptide and MHC class II. Science 1999;286:1913-21.
228. Reiser JB, Darnault C, Gregoire C, Mosser T, Mazza G, Kearney A, van der Merwe PA, Fontecilla-Camps JC, Housset D, Malissen B. CDR3 loop flexibility contributes to the degeneracy of TCR recognition. Nat Immunol 2003;4:241-47.
229. Reiser JB, Darnault C, Guimezanes A, Gregoire C, Mosser T, Schmitt-Verhulst AM, Fontecilla-Camps JC, Malissen B, Housset D, Mazza G. Crystal structure of a T cell receptor bound to an allogeneic MHC molecule. Nat Immunol 2000;1:291-97.
230. Reiser JB, Gregoire C, Darnault C, Mosser T, Guimezanes A, Schmitt-Verhulst AM, Fontecilla-Camps JC, Mazza G, Malissen B, Housset D. A T cell receptor CDR3beta loop undergoes conformational changes of unprecedented magnitude upon binding to a peptide/MHC class I complex. Immunity 2002;16:345-54.
231. Reits E, Griekspoor A, Neijssen J, Groothuis T, Jalink K, van Veelen P, Janssen H, Calafat J, Drijfhout JW, Neefjes J. Peptide diffusion, protection, degradation in nuclear and cytoplasmic compartments before antigen presentation by MHC class I. Immunity 2003;18:97-108.
232. Riberdy JM, Newcomb JR, Surman MJ, Barbosa JA, Cresswell P. HLA-DR molecules from an antigen-processing mutant cell line are associated with invariant chain peptides. Nature 1992;360:474-77.
233. Rivett AJ, Hearn AR. Proteasome function in antigen presentation: immunoproteasome complexes, Peptide production, and interactions with viral proteins. Curr Protein Pept Sci 2004;5:153-61.
234. Robbins PA, Garboczi DN, Strominger JL. HLA-A*0201 complexes with two 10-Mer peptides differing at the P2 anchor residue have distinct refolding kinetics. J Immunol 1995;154:703-09.
235. Robinson J, Waller MJ, Parham P, de Groot N, Bontrop R, Kennedy LJ, Stoehr P, Marsh SG. IMGT/HLA and IMGT/MHC: Sequence databases for the study of the major histocompatibility complex. Nucleic Acids Res 2003;31:311-14.
236. Roche PA, Marks MS, Cresswell P. Formation of a nine-subunit complex by HLA class II glycoproteins and the invariant chain. Nature 1991;354:392-94.
237. Rock KL, York IA, Goldberg AL. Post-proteasomal antigen processing for major histocompatibility complex class I presentation. Nat Immunol 2004;5: 670-77.
238. Rodgers JR, Cook RG. MHC class Ib molecules bridge innate and acquired immunity. Nat Rev Immunol 2005;5:459-71.
239. Rohrlich PS, Fazilleau N, Ginhoux F, Firat H, Michel F, Cochet M, Laham N, Roth MP, Pascolo S, Nato F, et al. Direct recognition by alphabeta cytolytic T cells of Hfe, a MHC class Ib molecule without antigen-presenting function. Proc Natl Acad Sci USA 2005;102:12855-60.
240. Rojo S, Garcia F, Villadangos JA, Lopez de Castro JA. Changes in the repertoire of peptides bound to HLA-B27 subtypes and to site-specific mutants inside and outside pocket B. J Exp Med 1993;177:613-20.
241. Romano A, De Santis A, Romito A, Di Fonso M, Venuti A, Gasbarrini GB, Manna R. Delayed hypersensitivity to aminopenicillins is related to major histocompatibility complex genes. Ann Allergy Asthma Immunol 1998;80:433-37.
242. Rossjohn J, McCluskey J. How a home-grown T cell receptor interacts with a foreign landscape. Cell 2007;129:19-20.
243. Rotzschke O, Falk K, Deres K, Schild H, Norda M, Metzger J, Jung G, Rammensee, HG. Isolation and analysis of naturally processed viral peptides as recognized by cytotoxic T cells. Nature 1990;348:252-54.
244. Rotzschke O, Falk K, Stevanovic S, Gnau V, Jung G, Rammensee HG. Dominant aromatic/aliphatic C-terminal anchor in HLA-B*2702 and B*2705 peptide motifs. Immunogenetics 1994;39:74-77.
245. Rotzschke O, Falk K, Stevanovic S, Jung G, Rammensee HG. Peptide motifs of closely related HLA class I molecules encompass substantial differences. Eur J Immunol 1992;22:2453-56.
246. Roujeau JC, Bracq C, Huyn NT, Chaussalet E, Raffin C, Duedari N. HLA phenotypes and bullous cutaneous reactions to drugs. Tissue Antigens 1986;28:251-54.
247. Roujeau JC, Huynh TN, Bracq C, Guillaume JC, Revuz J, Touraine R. Genetic susceptibility to toxic epidermal necrolysis. Arch Dermatol 1987;123: 1171-73.
248. Rudolph MG, Wilson IA. The specificity of TCR/pMHC interaction. Curr Opin Immunol 2002;14:52-65.
249. Rudolph MG, Stanfield RL, Wilson IA. How TCRs bind MHCs, peptides, and coreceptors. Annual Review of Immunology 2006;24:419-66.
250. Schmidt KL, Mueller-Eckhardt C. Agranulocytosis, levamisole, and HLA-B27. Lancet 1977;2:85.
251. Schubert U, Anton LC, Gibbs J, Norbury CC, Yewdell JW, Bennink JR. Rapid degradation of a large fraction of newly synthesized proteins by proteasomes. Nature 2000;404:770-74.

252. Scott-Browne JP, White J, Kappler JW, Gapin L, Marrack P. Germline-encoded amino acids in the alpha beta T-cell receptor control thymic selection. Nature 2009;458: 1043-46.
253. Segal S, Hill AV. Genetic susceptibility to infectious disease. Trends Microbiol 2003;11:445-48.
254. Seliger B, Bock M, Ritz U, Huber C. High frequency of a non-functional TAP1/LMP2 promoter polymorphism in human tumors. Int J Oncol 2002;20:349-53.
255. Serwold T, Gonzalez F, Kim J, Jacob R, Shastri N. ERAAP customizes peptides for MHC class I molecules in the endoplasmic reticulum. Nature 2002;419:480-83.
256. Sesma L, Montserrat V, Lamas JR, Marina A, Vazquez J, Lopez de Castro JA. The peptide repertoires of HLA-B27 subtypes differentially associated to spondyloarthropathy (B*2704 and B*2706) differ by specific changes at three anchor positions. J Biol Chem 2002;277:16744-49.
257. Sette A, Sidney J. Nine major HLA class I supertypes account for the vast preponderance of HLA-A and -B polymorphism. Immunogenetics 1999;50:201-12.
258. Shastri N, Schwab S, Serwold T. Producing nature's gene-chips: the generation of peptides for display by MHC class I molecules. Annu Rev Immunol 2002;20: 463-93.
259. Shen L, Sigal LJ, Boes M, Rock KL. Important role of cathepsin S in generating peptides for TAP-independent MHC class I crosspresentation in vivo. Immunity 2004;21:155-65.
260. Sherman LA, Chattopadhyay S. The molecular basis of allorecognition. Annu Rev Immunol 1993;11:385-402.
261. Shiina T, Tamiya G, Oka A, Takishima N, Inoko H. Genome sequencing analysis of the 1.8 Mb entire human MHC class I region. Immunol Rev 1999;167:193-99.
262. Shiroishi M, Tsumoto K, Amano K, Shirakihara Y, Colonna M, Braud VM, Allan DS, Makadzange A, Rowland-Jones S, Willcox B, et al. Human inhibitory receptors Ig-like transcript 2 (ILT2) and ILT4 compete with CD8 for MHC class I binding and bind preferentially to HLAG. Proc Natl Acad Sci U S A 2003;100:8856-61.
263. Sim BC, Aftahi N, Reilly C, Bogen B, Schwartz RH, Gascoigne NR, Lo D. Thymic skewing of the CD4/CD8 ratio maps with the T-cell receptor alpha-chain locus. Curr Biol 1998a;8:701-04.
264. Sim BC, Lo D, Gascoigne NR. Preferential expression of TCR V alpha regions in CD4/CD8 subsets: class discrimination or co-receptor recognition? Immunol Today 1998b;19:276-82.
265. Sim B-C, Zerva L, Greene MI, Gascoigne NRJ. Control of MHC restriction by TCR Va CDR1 and CDR2. Science 1996;273:963.
266. Sloan VS, Cameron P, Porter G, Gammon M, Amaya M, Mellins E, Zaller DM. Mediation by HLA-DM of dissociation of peptides from HLA-DR. Nature 1995;375:802-06.
267. Snell GD, Higgins GF. Alleles at the histocompatibility-2 locus in the mouse as determined by tumor transplantation. Genetics 1951;36:306-10.
268. Snell GD. The genetics of transplantation. Ann N Y Acad Sci 1957;69:555-60.
269. Solheim BG, Albrechtsen D, Thorsby E, Thune P. Strong association between an HLADw3 associated B cell alloantigen and dermatitis herpetiformis. Tissue Antigens 1977;10:114-18.
270. Speir JA, Garcia KC, Brunmark A, Degano M, Peterson PA, Teyton L, Wilson IA. Structural basis of 2C TCR allorecognition of H-2Ld peptide complexes. Immunity 1998;8:553-62.
271. Speir JA, Stevens J, Joly E, Butcher GW, Wilson IA. Two different, highly exposed, bulged structures for an unusually long peptide bound to rat MHC class I RT1-Aa. Immunity 2001;14:81-92.
272. Stastny P, Ball EJ, Khan MA, Olsen NJ, Pincus T, Gao X. HLA-DR4 and other genetic markers in rheumatoid arthritis. Br J Rheumatol 27 Suppl 1988;2:132-38.
273. Stern LJ, Brown JH, Jardetzky TS, Gorga JC, Urban RG, Strominger JL, Wiley DC. Crystal structure of the human class II MHC protein HLA-DR1 complexed with an influenza virus peptide. Nature 1994;368:215-21.
274. Stewart-Jones GB, McMichael AJ, Bell JI, Stuart DI, Jones EY. A structural basis for immunodominant human T cell receptor recognition. Nat Immunol 2003;4:657-63.
275. Strominger JL. Human histocompatibility proteins. Immunol Rev 2002; 185:69-77.
276. Sullivan LC, Hoare HL, McCluskey J, Rossjohn J, Brooks AG. A structural perspective on MHC class Ib molecules in adaptive immunity. Trends Immunol 2006;27:413-20.
277. Tabary T, Lehoang P, Betuel H, Benhamou A, Semiglia R, Edelson C, Cohen JH. Susceptibility to birdshot chorioretinopathy is restricted to the HLA-A29.2 subtype. Tissue Antigens 1990;36:177-79.
278. Thorsby E. Invited anniversary review: HLA associated diseases. Hum Immunol 1997;53:1-11.
279. Todd JA, Acha-Orbea H, Bell JI, Chao N, Fronek Z, Jacob CO, McDermott M, Sinha AA, Timmerman L, Steinman L, et al. A molecular basis for MHC class II—associated autoimmunity. Science 1988;240:1003-09.
280. Turner SJ, Doherty PC, McCluskey J, Rossjohn J. Structural determinants of T-cell receptor bias in immunity. Nat Rev Immunol 2006;6:883-94.
281. Tye-Din J, Anderson R. Immunopathogenesis of celiac disease. Curr Gastroenterol Rep 2008;10:458-65.
282. Tynan FE, Borg NA, Miles JJ, Beddoe T, El-Hassen D, Silins SL, van Zuylen WJ, Purcell AW, Kjer-Nielsen L, McCluskey J, et al. The high resolution structures of highly bulged viral epitopes bound to the major histocompatability class I: Implications for T-cell receptor engagement and T-cell immunodominance. J Biol Chem 2005a;280(25):23900-09.
283. Tynan FE, Burrows SR, Buckle AM, Clements CS, Borg NA, Miles JJ, Beddoe T, Whisstock JC, Wilce MC, Silins

SL, et al. T cell receptor recognition of a 'super-bulged' major histocompatibility complex class I-bound peptide. Nat Immunol 2005b;6:1114-22.
284. Tynan FE, Reid HH, Kjer-Nielsen L, Miles JJ, Wilce MC, Kostenko L, Borg NA, Williamson NA, Beddoe T, Purcell AW, et al. A T cell receptor flattens a bulged antigenic peptide presented by a major histocompatibility complex class I molecule. Nat Immunol 2007;8:268-76.
285. Uebel S, Tampe R. Specificity of the proteasome and the TAP transporter. Curr Opin Immunol 1999;11:203-08.
286. Unanue ER. Perspective on antigen processing and presentation. Immunol Rev 2002;185:86-102.
287. Undlien DE, Lie BA, Thorsby E. HLA complex genes in type 1 diabetes and other autoimmune diseases. Which genes are involved? Trends Genet 2001;17:93-100.
288. Vader LW, Stepniak DT, Bunnik EM, Kooy YM, de Haan W, Drijfhout JW, Van Veelen PA, Koning F. Characterization of cereal toxicity for celiac disease patients based on protein homology in grains. Gastroenterology 2003;125:1105-13.
289. van de Wal Y, Kooy Y, van Veelen P, Pena S, Mearin L, Papadopoulos G, Koning F. Selective deamidation by tissue transglutaminase strongly enhances gliadin-specific T cell reactivity. J Immunol 1998;161:1585-88.
290. van der Merwe PA, Davis SJ. Molecular interactions mediating T cell antigen recognition. Annu Rev Immunol 2003;21:659-84.
291. van Endert PM, Riganelli D, Greco G, Fleischhauer K, Sidney J, Sette A, Bach JF. The peptide-binding motif for the human transporter associated with antigen processing. J Exp Med 1995;182:1883-95.
292. Vance RE, Kraft JR, Altman JD, Jensen PE, Raulet DH. Mouse CD94/NKG2A is a natural killer cell receptor for the nonclassical major histocompatibility complex (MHC) class I molecule Qa-1(b). J Exp Med 1998;188:1841-48.
293. Vasconcelos CC, Fernandez O, Leyva L, Thuler LC, Alvarenga RM. Does the DRB11501 allele confer more severe and faster progression in primary progressive multiple sclerosis patients? HLA in primary progressive multiple sclerosis. J Neuroimmunol 2009;214(1-2):101-3.
294. Villadangos JA, Bryant RA, Deussing J, Driessen C, Lennon-Dumenil AM, Riese RJ, Roth W, Saftig P, Shi GP, Chapman HA, et al. Proteases involved in MHC class II antigen presentation. Immunol Rev 1999;172:109-20.
295. Villadangos JA, Galocha B, Garcia F, Albar JP, Lopez de Castro JA. Modulation of peptide binding by HLA-B27 polymorphism in pockets A and B, and peptide specificity of B*2703. Eur J Immunol 1995;25:2370-77.
296. Wearsch PA, Cresswell P. Selective loading of high-affinity peptides onto major histocompatibility complex class I molecules by the tapasin-ERp57 heterodimer. Nat Immunol 2007;8:873-81.
297. Willcox BE, Gao GF, Wyer JR, Ladbury JE, Bell JI, Jakobsen BK, van der Merwe PA. TCR binding to peptide-MHC stabilizes a flexible recognition interface. Immunity 1999;10:357-65.
298. Williams A, Peh CA, Elliott T. The cell biology of MHC class I antigen presentation. Tissue Antigens 2002;59: 3-17.
299. Wilson JD, Ogg GS, Allen RL, Goulder PJ, Kelleher A, Sewell AK, O'Callaghan CA, Rowland-Jones SL, Callan MF, McMichael AJ. Oligoclonal expansions of CD8(+) T cells in chronic HIV infection are antigen specific. J Exp Med 1998;188:785-90.
300. Winchester R. Psoriatic arthritis. Dermatol Clin 1995;13: 779-92.
301. Wooley PH, Griffin J, Panayi GS, Batchelor JR, Welsh KI, Gibson TJ. HLA-DR antigens and toxic reaction to sodium aurothiomalate and D-penicillamine in patients with rheumatoid arthritis. N Engl J Med 1980; 303:300-02.
302. Wu LC, Tuot DS, Lyons DS, Garcia KC, Davis MM. Two-step binding mechanism for T-cell receptor recognition of peptide MHC. Nature 2002;418: 552-56.
303. Wucherpfennig KW, Strominger JL. Molecular mimicry in T cell-mediated autoimmunity: Viral peptides activate human T cell clones specific for myelin basic protein. Cell 1995;80:695-705.
304. Wucherpfennig KW, Sette A, Southwood S, Oseroff C, Matsui M, Strominger JL, Hafler DA. Structural requirements for binding of an immunodominant myelin basic protein peptide to DR2 isotypes and for its recognition by human T cell clones. J Exp Med 1994;179:279-90.
305. Yewdell J, Anton LC, Bacik I, Schubert U, Snyder HL, Bennink JR. Generating MHC class I ligands from viral gene products. Immunol Rev 1999;172:97-108.
306. Yewdell JW, Schubert U, Bennink JR. At the crossroads of cell biology and immunology: DRiPs and other sources of peptide ligands for MHC class I molecules. J Cell Sci 2001;114:845.

Chapter 7

Immunogenetic Databases

D Middleton, F Gonzalez

"While the individual man is an unsolvable puzzle, in the aggregate he becomes a mathematical certainty"

SUMMARY

This chapter describes the vast polymorphism of immunogenetic genes with special reference to HLA and killer cell immunoglobulin-like receptors (KIR). Having discussed how this polymorphism may have arisen and what it means to the health of individuals and populations, we describe a database available on the website www.allelefrequencies.net to disseminate information on the frequency data of these genes.

INTRODUCTION

The Major Histocompatibility Complex (MHC) is the most polymorphic region in the human genome. Situated on the short arm of chromosome (6p21.3), the MHC covers 7.6Mb and is densely packed with immunological genes, including HLA genes. The HLA genes encode a set of transmembrane proteins that present peptides to specific antigen receptors on T cells. This extensive polymorphism explains the basis of tissue rejection in transplantation and defines the repertoire of antigenic determinants to which each individual is capable of responding. It is also one explanation of the MHC linkage to many autoimmune diseases, in that particular HLA molecules are required to mediate the presentation of autoantigens to autoreactive T cells. The human MHC is associated with more than 100 diseases, most of which are immune mediated. Because of the application of HLA typing to clinical transplantation, there is a great amount of knowledge known on the population genetics of the human MHC.

At the last release (2.25.2) from the IMGT/HLA Database 3,528 in 2.25.2 there were 3,634 (3,528 reported and the rest 106 were kept as confidential). In the future what would you prefer for the website?, to keep all 3,634 even if some of them might be discarded after their confirmation at Anthony Nolan? human leukocyte antigen (HLA) alleles had been described.[1] The number of alleles is constantly increasing. When HLA typing started in the 1960s, polymorphisms were detected using antisera which contained antibodies to specific HLA antigens. At that time, and for many years, there were only a few determinants to recognize. Signs that the MHC had more polymorphism began when some of the antigens were shown to have "splits" or subtypes. In other words, antigens like HLA-A9 were found to be subdivided into HLA-A23 and HLA-A24. These subtypes were characteristically found in populations originating from different geographical regions. However, a vast explosion in finding new polymorphisms has come with the advent of molecular techniques enabling laboratories to sequence new alleles. These alleles are given a name on submission to the IMGT/HLA Database (see Chapter 23). As the original HLA antigens were determined using cells and antisera primarily from individuals of European ancestry, the molecular techniques allowed definition of alleles in non-European populations. Antigens previously typed by serology as identical in different ethnic groups, were found to be coded by different alleles using molecular techniques. In the days of serology, many sera which did not react with all individuals who had a particular HLA antigen were discarded. Presumably some of these sera were reacting against individual alleles of that antigen.

Population Studies

In the early days of serology it was known that HLA antigens varied in frequency according to ethnicity of the population tested, to the extent that some antigens were found in one ethnic group but not in another. With the advent of molecular techniques this variability was shown to be even more profound, to the extent that many alleles have only been found in one individual/family. This knowledge has led to the use of HLA allele frequency rivalling that of mitochondria and Y chromosome markers in anthropological studies. In order to do a proper anthropological study the population being tested requires to be of a sufficient number. Increasing the sample size increases the probability of finding an HLA allele in that population. For example, the probability of missing an allele which is present at a frequency of 1 percent in the population is 0.134 when the number of individuals tested in the population is 100. It is also important to define the demographics of the population being studied. The individuals need to be unrelated and to be normal, healthy and to be from the same ethnicity, speak the same language, have grandparents from the same area and to be in Hardy-Weinberg equilibrium.

Selection of HLA Alleles

When knowledge of the function of HLA molecules (presenting peptides to the T cell Receptor of the immune system) became available several theories on selection of HLA alleles to explain the vast polymorphism were proposed. Substitutions occur throughout the coding region of the HLA molecule but there are more substitutions leading to changes in amino acids in the region where the peptide is bound and where interaction with the T cell receptor occurs. This differential variation cannot be explained by mutation and random drift as these effects would equally apply to all regions of a gene, regardless of their functional significance. Chapter 23 gives greater detail of the process used in naming the HLA alleles but suffice to say that those alleles that differ in the first four digits will differ in amino acid content, although some will have the same amino acid sequence in the binding region of the molecule. Individuals who have two alleles at a particular locus (heterozygous) will presumably have the ability to bind more peptides than those with one allele (homozygous). However, similarities in binding properties of the molecular will occur when the two alleles are similar, i.e. from the same allele lineage, (such alleles have the same first two digits) than when the two alleles are more divergent. Thus selection (overdominate selection) may occur to increase divergence between alleles and favor new or low frequency alleles to give a greater repertoire of peptide binding properties. However, HLA homozygotes are generally healthy indicating that the benefits of HLA polymorphism are subtle and not always present.

A further broad category of selection is frequency dependent selection. Microorganisms can adapt to their host by mutation of the peptide bound by the HLA molecule. This is likely to be directed at HLA alleles previously frequent and successful in the population. Thus the host that has rare alleles gains an advantage. For example, HLA-B* 5301 has been shown to give an advantage in protection against malaria compared to the more common allele HLA-B*3501, from which it is derived.[2] However, this advantage could be lost once the malarial parasite adapts to evade peptide presentation by HLA-B*5301.

As the HLA loci are closely linked, an allele selected for will result, by linkage equilibrium, in the whole haplotype increasing in frequency. However, this tight linkage disequilibrium especially between HLA-DR and HLA-DQ loci decreases the phenotypically observed polymorphism. High levels of polymorphism may also be maintained through balancing selection in which alleles disadvantageous for one disease are advantageous for another.

The origin of the extensive HLA polymorphism has been the subject of considerable controversy and speculation and the reader is referred to the review by Meyer and Thomson on how selection has shaped variation of the HLA system. This review concludes that several modes of selection are probably acting simultaneously.[3]

Generation of New Alleles

Different mechanisms generate new alleles. Some alleles are formed by insertion of sequences usually small, from another allele, termed conversion. Usually this interchange of sequences will be between alleles of the same locus, but interchange of sequences between alleles of different loci, although not common, has occurred. For example, HLA-B*4601 is the product of conversion between HLA-B*1501 and HLA-Cw*0102. Less frequent are alleles formed by point mutations. However, some of these single substitutions occur in other alleles, so they too could be recombination products. Some of the substitutions are silent, not leading to a change in amino acid, and are thus the result of genetic drift. The peptide loading abilities of the HLA alleles can be tremendously altered by one or a few substitutions of amino acids. Conversion alone will not generate diversity but will increase substantially the divergence once new alleles have been formed by point mutations.

Comparisons of MHC of humans, chimpanzees and gorillas show that none of the HLA class I alleles have been preserved over a five million year period, despite the structured similarities between class I alleles in these species and the lack of species specific substitutions. This contrasts with the sharing of amino acid sequences in other proteins in these species. During the 150,000 years that modern humans have existed, there is a tendency for new alleles to replace older alleles. For HLA-DRB1, it would appear that, whereas most of the allelic lineages pre-date the separation of the hominoid species, most of the HLA-DRB1 alleles have been generated after the separation of human and chimpanzee species. These replacements could be brought about by changing antigen environment, illustrated by the differences in alleles between North and South America. Whereas nearly all HLA-A and -B alleles in North America are identical to alleles brought by the original migrants from the Old World, there are many new alleles in South America, probably due to the biologically diverse environment of South America. These new alleles may also have arisen because of frequency dependency in these small populations, with low numbers of alleles to start with.[4,5] There was only one new allele common to the three Amerindian populations studied and all new HLA-B alleles had substitutions in the peptide binding regions. Interestingly, in a study showing that populations with increased HLA diversity lived in areas of high pathogen diversity, the HLA-B locus was shown as being under stronger selection pressure than HLA-A or HLA-C.[6]

Despite the formation of new alleles in these indigenous populations there will be a much larger number of alleles in large urban populations brought about by admixture from individual populations. Ultimately, the modern large scale movement in populations will lead to populations having large number of alleles and possibly a reduction of allele formation due to frequency dependency.

HLA and Transplantation

The application of HLA matching in stem cell transplantation has produced many new alleles. A potential recipient has a one in four chances of finding an HLA identical sibling. Many Stem Cell Registries have been set up to hold information on HLA typed unrelated potential donors. Whereas the majority of these donors are initially typed at the 2-digit level, they are typed at the 4-digit level when it appears that they might be a suitable donor for a recipient who has also been typed at the 4-digit level. Thus, knowledge of which geographical region/county an HLA allele may be found is important for "search" strategy. Increasingly more importance is being placed on the determination of alleles at 4-digit resolution. T cell mediated rejection in stem cell transplantation appears to have been instigated by a single amino acid substitution between alleles of the HLA-B*44 family.[7] Laboratories providing a clinical service for the HLA antibody screening in prospective renal transplant recipients are finding antibodies to one allele of a HLA family in patients whose HLA type includes an allele of the same family.

HLA and Disease

Many studies have been conducted on HLA in disease associations. The diseases may be infectious or autoimmune based. The differences between individuals and populations in their HLA repertoire lead to differences in their response to foreign and autologous antigens. History abounds with information on indigenous populations being decimated by the introduction of new pathogens from the influx of individuals from other continents. However, few of the many HLA disease studies have led to the introduction of HLA typing to aid diagnosis, with the obvious exceptions of ankylosing spondylitis, narcolepsy and celiac diseases. When an association is found in a disease it may be that the HLA allele in question is involved in the disease or the association may be due to strong linkage disequilibrium with a neighbouring gene. For example, the ancestral haplotype 8.1 (HLA-A*01, -B*08, -DRB1*01,-DQB1*02, -DQA1*05) is associated with many autoimmune diseases. Whereas it appears that some of the HLA genes present on this haplotype are involved in type 1 diabetes and celiac disease, in other diseases the susceptible gene is unknown. Worth mentioning in this context is the MHC Haplotype Consortium formed to generate sequence data of MHC reference haplotypes.[8]

Association of the same allele in different ethnic populations suggests that the allele itself is involved in the mechanism of the disease. One problem with the emphasis of determining HLA allele associations in a disease is that it is not necessarily the allele that may have an association, but an epitope or amino acid within that allele. This epitope or amino acid could also be shared by other alleles. Thus, we believe that discerning epitope/amino acid association should be the goal in such studies and we have sought to help the situation by introducing an analysis— See Section "Online Bioinformatic Analysis Tool"

Part of the problem in determining HLA associations with a disease is the interplay in various factors of the immune response, including HLA, natural killer (NK) cells and cytokines. This presents difficulties in determining clear associations with polymorphisms of any of these factors in a disease. It is also a reason why we have sought to include polymorphisms of NK receptors and cytokines in the database described in this chapter. For example, as part of the ancestral haplotype 8.1, the tumor necrosis factor (TNF) alleles which regulate the expression of that cytokine have been much studied in autoimmunity. Other problems relating to disease association studies are differences in study design, ethnicity of the population study, appropriate controls, and a disease being thought of as a single entity, when, in fact, it is composed of several diseases. Consideration of the function of the HLA molecule would highlight the importance of the same strain of an organism being taken into account in association studies. These problems are described in a review of hepatitis B and C infections but equally apply to other diseases.[9]

A relatively new infectious disease, for example, HIV, may show stronger genetic associations because there has been insufficient time for deleterious alleles to be eliminated by selection. HLA-B*27 and –B*57 are associated with an improved prognosis whereas some alleles of HLA-B*35 lead to poorer prognosis, even those differing by one amino acid from HLA-B*35 alleles which are not deleterious.[10] Whereas the HLA-DRB1*1302 allele is associated with spontaneous clearance of hepatitis B, it is the HLA-DRB1*1101-DQB1*1302 haplotype which is associated with clearance of hepatitis C.[11]

The introduction of pharmacogenetics has led to HLA typing of individuals to assess risk prior to giving of drugs. For example, the association of HLA-B*5701 with sensitivity to Abacavir, a drug used in the treatment of HIV patients.[12]

HLA and Vaccination

Reliance on epitope sharing and similar peptide binding properties of alleles will be important in vaccine developments. Here again HLA studies in various ethnic populations will be important to examine suitability of vaccine provision. Fortunately, from the aspect of vaccination a large percentage of HLA class I and possibly class II can be grouped (so called HLA supertypes) by overlapping peptide binding repertoires.

KIR Receptors

Recently, another very polymorphic region has gained much interest in the field of immunogenetics. The Killer-cell Immunoglobulin-like Receptor (KIR) complex, because of the variability of its gene content and of the alleles of each gene contained therein, has been shown to rival the MHC in the extent of its polymorphism. Natural killer (NK) cells not only have a role in pathogen control but also in pregnancy and therefore may be genes undergoing natural selection. Although the KIR genes and their HLA ligands are inherited on different chromosomes there is evidence for their co-evolution. Strong negative correlations have been shown between presence of activating KIR genes and their corresponding ligands and weak positive relationships between the inhibitory genes and their ligands, the negative correlation between KIR2DL2 and the HLA-C1 group being the exception.[13] This initial result has been confirmed in a 15th International Histocompatibility Workshop project in 23 global populations (submitted for publication). Significant correlations were observed between KIR2LD2 and KIR2DL3 and their ligand HLA-C1 group. These two KIR genes are allelic and so while KIR2DL2 frequencies are negatively correlated with HLA-C1 group, a strong positive correlation existed between KIR2DL3 homozygous frequencies and HLA-C1 group. Previous results have shown that this combination results in increased viral killing in NK cells[14] and the KIR2DL3 receptor, which has a weaker affinity for its ligand HLA-C1 than its allele KIR2DL2, has a beneficial prognosis in hepatitis C infection in the absence of KIR2DL1.[15] KIR diversity has also been shown to moderate the NK response to a diverse array of microbial pathogens and may influence susceptibility to many different infections.[16] Moreover, Single and colleagues found a negative correlation between distance from East Africa and frequency of activating KIR genes and their corresponding ligands, concluding that this was a balance between selection on HLA and KIR loci.[13] Norman and colleagues have shown that two lineages of KIR3DL1 have co-evolved with different groups of HLA-Bw4 allotypes and that they have been maintained by balancing selection throughout global movement of population from Africa.[17] Non-random associations have also been found in the Japanese population, several associations being limited to females supporting the view that reproduction is a strong selective pressure acting on KIR genes.[18]

Allele Frequency Database

As mentioned in the previous sections, there is a tremendous amount of data available on the frequencies in populations of the aforementioned alleles. To have frequency data of Histocompatibility and Immunogenetic genes in a readily available format would be a valuable resource. Greater knowledge of the distribution of HLA and other immunogenetic gene alleles in human populations will aid matching of donors and recipients in stem cell transplantation and facilitate tracing of the history and origins of human populations. With this in mind, a database as an electronic central source to contain frequencies in normal worldwide populations of alleles in polymorphic immunogenetic genes has been developed over the last few years.[19] Initially, data was collected for the HLA class I (A, B, C) and class II (DRB1, DRA1, DQB1, DQA1, DPB1, DPA1) classical genes, but more recently the database has been expanded to contain data from non-classical HLA (E, G), Killer-cell Immunoglobulin-like Receptor (KIR), Cytokine and MHC class I related gene A and B [MICA, MICB]. In addition, a component on the rarity of HLA alleles has been added. Moreover, the data has been expanded to include not only allelic but also haplotype and genotype information. The data can be accessed through a website (http://www.allelefrequencies.net) which is freely available to all individuals. In this section, we describe how the website is constructed, what can be performed on the website and the data contained therein.

During the last year, the website has been revamped and reconstructed to make it more user-friendly. We have organised the website allocating searching tools, breakdowns, etc. according to existing stored polymorphisms (Fig. 7.1). A registration process has been introduced. This is not to make it difficult for an investigator to search the website – the data is freely available to all. It is only a means whereby the interests of the person using the site can be ascertained, giving an indication of areas in which the website can be improved. An individual registers on the first visit to the site and thereafter only enters name and password that she/he decided at registration. This information is stored confidentially and converged globally rather than individually.

Organization and Content

Presently, the Allele Frequency Database contains data in allele, haplotype and genotype format depending on the polymorphism of interest. The database is based on a relational database model system utilizing MySQL as the database management system (DBMS), which operates under GNU General Public License. The website can be accessed utilizing any of the most common browsers (IE®, Firefox®, Safari®, Opera®, Google

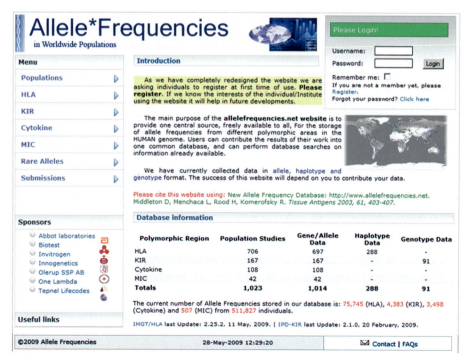

Fig. 7.1: Allele frequencies website (http://www.allelefrequencies.net)

Chrome®, etc.) giving the facility to the user to access data without the need to install a package.

Population Demographic Data

An important aspect of the website is that demographic details of the population are known. The population is given a name which aptly describes it, using the following if applicable; country, region, ethnicity, tribe and polymorphic region examined. When a new population is submitted which cannot be given a name different from a population already on the website, the new population is numbered to give differentiation e.g. Japan pop 1, Japan pop 2, etc. A list of populations is given under the "Populations Section". Regardless of what search is performed, clicking on the population name will give demographic details of that population. This information will include, number of individuals and ethnicity of the population, whether the population is urban, rural, urban and rural or unknown, whether it is known if the grandparents or parents of the individuals came from the same region, which technique was used to determine the data and the source (the reason why the population was typed). Additionally, coordinates for latitude and longitude are entered giving the facility to produce visual population comparisons. There is no requirement that data from the population has been published in a peer-reviewed population, but if it has, the reference is given. For some populations it is necessary to add notes to give an explanation to the data. This could be, for example, those populations that do not have the same number of individuals typed for each locus, or in those instances when a pair of alleles cannot be distinguished, that the frequency data is given under one of the alleles. The email address of the contributor of the data is given in the event that an individual searching the data would like to contact the contributor.

Submission of Data

The original idea of submitting the data to the website was that the contributor would submit the demographic data online and then be issued with a spreadsheet in which she/he would enter the frequency data. However, this has now changed to asking the contributor to send the data directly to the website, in the manner most convenient to them. In essence, the majority of the data (demographic and frequency) has been entered by ourselves taking the data from publications in peer-reviewed journals. Allele frequencies are entered in a three decimal format and phenotype frequency (number of individuals with the gene/allele) as a percentage. The original intention was to indicate an allele that could be determined in a laboratory, but which was not found in that population as zero, thus distinguishing that allele from alleles that could not be determined. However, this information is seldom given in publications.

From the start, the intention was to collect frequency data for HLA alleles, i.e. at 4-digit resolution. However, as this was not possible, the contributor was given the opportunity to enter data at the 2-digit level. This was particularly important in those instances where a contributor had some data at the allele level and some data at the allele lineage level (2-digit). Bearing in mind that many HLA alleles have been expanded from 4-digit to 6-digit and even 8-digit, it was quickly realised that to limit data to only allele frequency would lead to very limited data. An automatic allele catalogue is generated when a new release is announced by the IMGT/HLA or IPD-KIR Group (1, 20) providing allele length for 2, 4, 6 and 8 digits for HLA, and 3, 5 and 7 digits for MIC and KIR. For the sake of clarity in this chapter, we hereafter refer to data as being from allele even in those instances where it refers to allele lineage data.

Data Available

Data has now been submitted from 1,023 populations. These populations are composed of 706 HLA populations, 167 KIR populations, 108 Cytokines populations and 42 MIC populations from a total of 511,827 individuals. Table 7.1 indicates the HLA populations available, grouped by the number of individuals in the population and by resolution of data, with the understanding that a population may be typed for several loci and different levels of resolution. For instance, a population from Northern Ireland has frequencies for A*01 (2 digits) and A*0101, A*0102 (4 digits). At present, a high percentage of the data is only available at 2-digit. However, as techniques improve and are implemented into laboratories, the percentage of populations with higher resolution will improve. Data may be filtered to only show data at certain degrees of resolution. Similar numbers of individuals have been typed at each of the different levels of resolution for HLA-A, -B, -DRB1. This is because many of the populations submitted have been typed for all three loci (Table 7.2). Table 7.3 shows data available by geographical region for each polymorphic region. Asia has the highest number of populations twice that of any other region, typed for HLA.

Chapter 7 ■ Immunogenetic Databases

Table 7.1: HLA populations on website by locus and level of resolution

Locus	Total		2 digits		4 digits		6 digits		8 digits	
	Pops	Indiv	Pops	Indiv	Pops	Indiv	Pops	Indiv	Pops	Indiv
HLA-A	338	414,183	215	388,927	222	107,194	159	91,808	46	6,694
HLA-B	344	414,582	223	387,446	221	109,321	72	9,220*	10	1,902
HLA-C	229	67,814	136	46,352	174	31,866	67	8,542	4	824
HLA-DMA	2	292			2	292				
HLA-DMB	2	292			2	292				
HLA-DPA1	51	4,696	19	1,997	46	4,444	36	3,348		
HLA-DPB1	203	21,989	7	1,387	203	21,989	66	5,427		
HLA-DQA1	225	27,079	93	12,156	221	26,636	26	3,029		
HLA-DQB1	347	68,684	122	35,376	321	46,782	85	8,364		
HLA-DRB1	488	442,625	249	341,250	403	135,839	237	96,257		
HLA-E	4	230			4	230	2	88	1	60
HLA-G	10	815			10	815	7	453		

Some populations have data which differ in resolution according to the allele tested; *USA Caucasian Pop 1 (n=61,655) was typed for few alleles at 6 digits resolution for HLA-A and -DRB1 but not for -B.

Table 7.2: Number of populations by number of loci typed

Number of loci typed	Number of pops	A	B	C	DPA1	DPB1	DQA1	DQB1	DRB1
8	3	3	3	3	3	3	3	3	3
7	23	23	23	21	4	23	23	22	22
6	39	39	39	32	1	21	25	38	39
5	70	58	57	41	12	15	30	67	70
4	108	59	59	40	12	49	45	68	100
3	245	127	127	75	2	31	89	116	168
2	101	21	29	8	17	36	7	31	49
1	108	8	7	9	1	26	4	2	37
	697	338	344	229	52	204	226	347	488

9 populations had only haplotype data which were not included in this table; 232 populations containing typing for A, B and DRB1 were found in this analysis.

Table 7.3: Populations available by geographic region

Region	HLA	KIR	Cytokines	MIC	Total
Asia	234	39	16	13	302
Australia	7	2	-	-	9
Eastern Europe	41	10	17	-	68
Middle East	32	7	8	2	49
North Africa	23	1	1	1	26
North America	46	15	23	5	89
Pacific	47	9	-	-	56
South and Central America	113	33	11	8	165
Sub-Saharan Africa	48	18	3	3	72
Western Europe	115	33	29	10	187
Total	706	167	108	42	1,023

Searching for Data

The following search mechanisms can be equally applied to frequency data from any of the genes on the website. Figure 7.2 shows the screen shown when an individual wishes to make a search. For HLA a search is performed by locus. There is a facility to have a starting and ending allele or one or a number of individual alleles can be selected to perform a search. A search can be performed based on all populations or a specific population(s), by geographic region, ethnicity or year in which data was determined. Data from the more recent years is more likely to be of higher resolution and possibly more accurate. Additionally, an individual can exclude populations that do not satisfy an optimal sample size by selecting populations with sample size equal to or more than 50, 100, 500, 1000 individuals. Moreover, an investigator can include the source of data by filtering information on whether the population was derived from an anthropology study, a stem cell donor registry, controls for disease study, blood donors, or solid organ unrelated donors, etc. "Distribution" enables the data to be shown on a global map. As an example of this we have shown the distribution of HLA-A*0201 (Fig. 7.3). There are several ways to retrieve and show frequencies. Data can be shown each allele at a time, with the populations being either in alphabetical order or in ascending order of frequency of the allele in question. Data may also be shown giving all data for one population before moving to the next population. In this case, alleles may be in chronological order or in ascending order of frequency of data. On many occasions the data searched for will be available on several pages and the investigator can move from page to page. However, it is possible to print out all data at one time. As part of interaction among different databases an individual is able to retrieve this information through Extensible Markup Language (XML) files to facilitate a further computation.

A list with all coincidences that match with the criteria is displayed giving information for the name of the allele or gene, name of the population where the allele or gene was found, the phenotype or allele frequency, the number of individuals tested for that allele or gene. A link to the IMGT/HLA Database is provided to consult the sequence and further information on a particular allele. In addition, users can filter results for positive (frequencies over 0.0) or negatives (0.0) values if they are interested in only populations where the allele or gene was found.

Haplotype Data

The HLA data can be searched by haplotypes. Data submitted to the website is on haplotypes that occur at 1 percent or greater in the population. The haplotypes may contain one or several of the following loci; HLA-A,-B,-C,-DRB1,-DPA1,-DPB1,-DQA1,-DQB1. Haplotype data

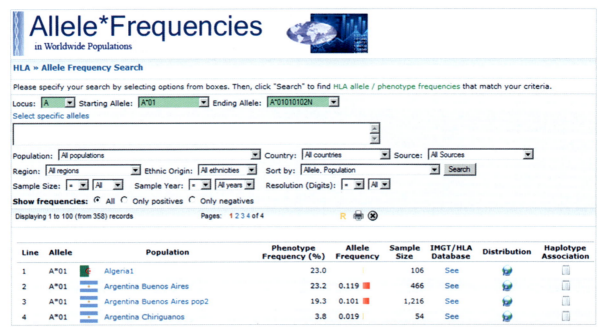

Fig. 7.2: Example of a HLA allele frequency search

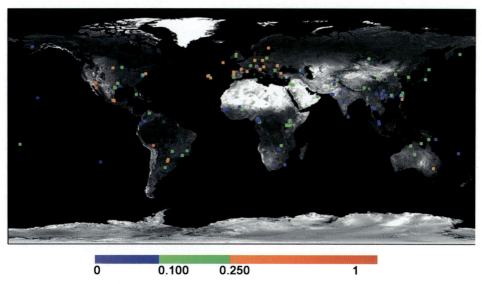

Fig. 7.3: Worldwide allele frequency incidence of the HLA-A*0201 allele

is searched by entering one or more alleles, at different loci, and ascertaining the frequencies of haplotypes which contain those alleles. There is also a facility to search for MICA and HLA-B haplotypes. If the haplotype does not exist on the database a message will be displayed. Results can be sorted by haplotype order, population name or from the highest to the lowest frequency value.

KIR

It is believed that the combination of presence/absence of KIR genes is very important in ascertaining the overall inhibitory/activating natural killer cell profile of an individual. Thus, the facility of entering and being able to search for KIR genotypes (i.e. presence/absence of KIR genes in an individual) in a population has been developed. The genotypes have been numbered (Genotype ID) and we would encourage individuals to use this number in their publication. A new ID number is assigned in consecutive numeric order each time a new genotype is reported to the website.

KIR genotypes were initially differentiated into 'A' and 'B' haplotypes by the absence/presence respectively of a 24 kb HindIII fragment on Southern blotting.[21] The A haplotype has one activating KIR gene (KIR2DS4) which may or may not be functional due to a deletion, whereas the B haplotype has several activating genes (See Chapter 3). Thus, it is simple to define whether a person has an A or a B haplotype and consequently, to define an individual genotype as AA. The difficulty arises in differentiating AB from BB haplotypes. A study on KIR gene and allele determination using 77 families was able to define if one or two copies of a KIR gene were present.[22] As a result of this, an A haplotype was defined as one that had all the following genes present; KIR2DL1, KIR2DL3, KIR2DS4, KIR3DL1, in addition to the framework genes KIR2DL4, KIR3DL2, KIR3DL3, KIR2DP1. Initially, the genotypes on the website were differentiated into AA, AB, and BB haplotypes using this definition. However, we have now reverted to naming the genotypes as AA or Bx where x may indicate an A or B haplotype because of new evidence (P. Parham personal communication).

On some occasions a contributor has not defined all genes, but rather than lose this data the genotype has been entered with a box indicating that the gene may be present or absent. In these instances, the genotype has not been designated as unique if it only differed from known genotypes in some genes not tested. We have also introduced a facility whereby if an individual enters a genotype which has not previously been reported the genotype(s) closest in context will be shown. Figure 7.4 gives an example of a genotype search. An individual can retrieve information by filtering by population(s), country, genotype ID, and haplotype group. She/he can also select only the most common genotype by searching for genotypes that only occur in a specific number of populations.

Interestingly, this compilation of genotypes has resulted in 337 genotypes in 91 populations on which genotype information was provided. Table 7.4 shows how often these genotypes occur in populations and in individuals. Many of the genotypes have been reported

Table 7.4: Number of KIR genotypes in populations and in individuals

Genotypes	Number of populations	Individuals
166*	1	189*
37	2	101
34	3	154
15	4	96
6	5	46
37	6-10	601
34	11-50	1,626
8	>50	6,641
337		9,454

*150 genotypes in 1 individual 12 genotypes in 2 individuals
2 genotypes in 3 individuals 1 genotype in 4 individuals
1 genotype in 5 individuals

in one population and indeed in one individual. At present, it is difficult to know if some of these genotypes may have been reported in error. It is worth noting from the previous KIR family study that when genotypes are determined at the allele level, 90 percent of individuals have a different genotype.[22] Noteworthy is that this study was performed in a very homogeneous Caucasian population of 1.5 million with very little immigration. This vast polymorphism in the KIR region has previously been discussed.[23]

An important aspect of our endeavors has been to present the data in a graphical manner. We have included two figures to show examples of the KIR data available. Figures 7.5 and 7.6 show examples of the incidence of KIR gene and allele frequencies in worldwide populations. The variability of all available KIR gene frequencies in worldwide populations is shown in Figure 7.7. Not all populations have been tested for all KIR genes – hence the difference in the total number of populations tested for each KIR gene. Despite KIR2DL4, KIR3DL2 and KIR2DL3 being thought to be present in all populations, there is information on absence of these genes in some individuals in certain populations (Fig. 7.8). KIR genotype and allele data on International Histocompatibility and Immunogenetic Workshop (IHW) cell lines is also available on the website.

As an extension to the data provided by the Allele Frequencies Database the aim is to include haplotype estimation from phenotype data, using algorithms compiled from simulation data from a previous study in KIR populations.[24] Moreover, we wish to add

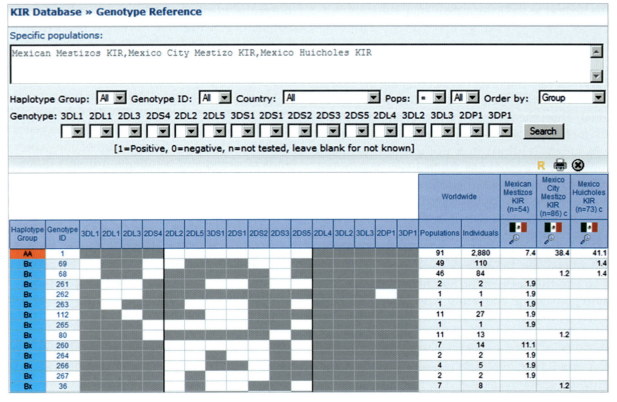

Fig. 7.4: Example of the KIR genotype frequency search

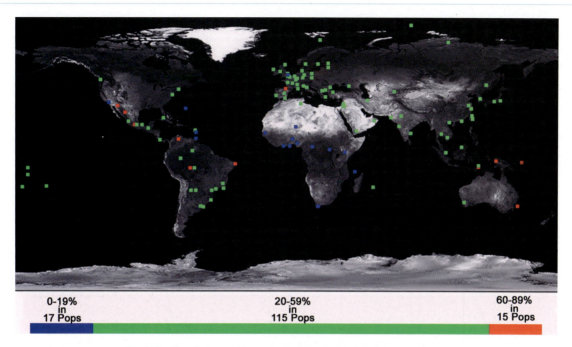

Fig. 7.5: Populations with varying levels of KIR2DS1 gene frequency

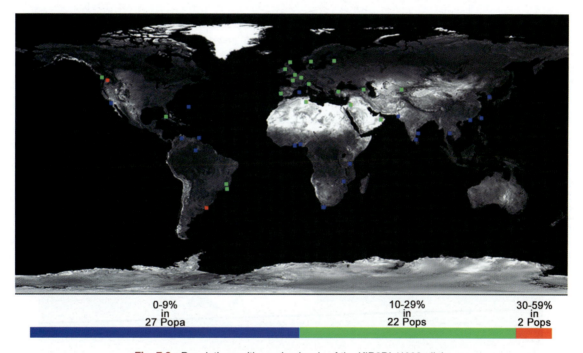

Fig. 7.6: Populations with varying levels of the KIR3DL1*002 allele

information concerning relationships between KIR gene and HLA ligands in worldwide populations and incorporate data from KIR disease studies. This would include reports of negative associations of KIR and disease which, with the bias of publishing positive findings, are too often ignored.

Rare Alleles

A page on the website has recently been developed to contain data on rare HLA alleles. As mentioned previously many of the HLA alleles have been reported in only one individual. The percentage of alleles from Release 2.25.2

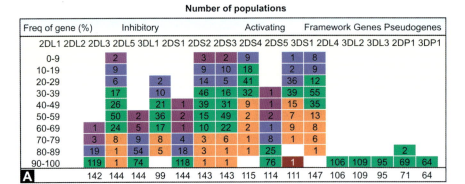
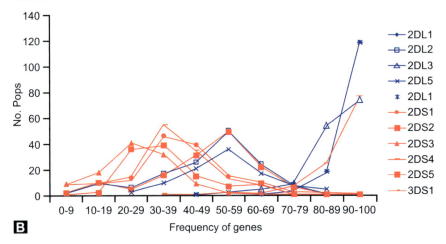

Figs 7.7A and B: Variability of KIR genes in worldwide populations

Gene	Individuals	Populations
2DL4 NEG	3	3
3DL2NEG		5
3DL3NEG	7	4

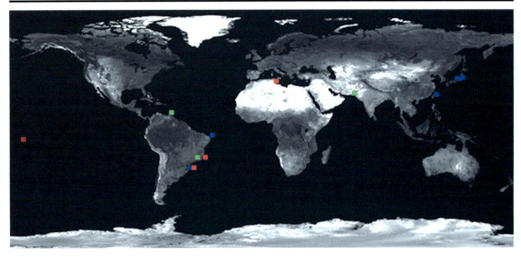

Fig. 7.8: Absence of KIR2DL4, KIR3DL2, KIR3DL3 in worldwide populations from a total of 91 populations and 9,536 individuals

found in the Northern Ireland population was 3.9 percent, 4.2 percent, 5.2 percent, 5.3 percent for HLA-A, -B, -C, -DRB1 respectively. At present the website does not have frequencies of rare alleles, merely whether they have been found or not after their initial sequencing. Using different sources we have sought to ascertain, whether the alleles have been found after the initial reporting to and naming by the IMGT/HLA Database.[1] The sources used are as follows; confirmation of the sequence to IMGT/HLA, the website www.allelefrequencies.net, National Marrow Donor Program (NMDP) and the results from a project of the 15th IHIWS (Fig 7.9).[25] As part of this project, a list of HLA alleles which at that time had only been found on three or less occasions using the previously mentioned sources was produced. The 20 participating laboratories in this IHIWS project were asked if they had found any of these alleles in their population. If they had, information on the ethnicity of the individual, the population the individual belonged to and the haplotype containing the allele, or if not available, the phenotype, was obtained. All sources of data were then analysed to examine rarity of the HLA alleles. In nearly all HLA loci, approximately 40 percent of alleles had been found on only one occasion, the initial sequence submission to IMGT/HLA.[1]

All data is now available to search on the website. The investigator can The investigator can decide based on the criteria she/he uses, which alleles might be rare. They can introduce these criteria to the individual sources of data or to the combined sources. Figure 7.10 shows an example of this search. Information is also provided as to whether the rare allele has an equivalent allele identical in exons 2 and 3 for HLA class I or exon 2 for HLA class II, or a synonymous allele, i.e. one not differing in amino acid content.

Recently, we have included a simplified online form where individual laboratories can submit data reporting whether an allele was found in their laboratory typing. The database is updated with all new releases from IMGT/HLA through an automatic mechanism that is executed when a new release is made available.

The information being collected is open-ended and it will never be possible to state with complete assurance whether an allele is rare but we hope that information provided will go some way to giving some appreciation of how rare the alleles are. It is our belief that some rationale needs to be introduced in the requirements for testing of these alleles. A similar project to ours was commenced at the same time in USA populations[26] and work is on-going to combine the two sets of data. Indeed, on the website a designation given to each allele in the USA study uses the acronym C for common and WD for well documented.

Accessing Information from an External Source

Although the Allele Frequency Database cannot be completely downloaded, individuals are allowed to access the data by setting a link where specifications need

	IMGT/HLA	Allele Frequencies Website			IMGT/HLA					NMDP							Other Labs					ASHI
	Allele	Pops with allele in website	See lower resolution	See sequences identical over exons 2 + 3'	Allele initially sequenced in population	Sequence confirmed	Cells	Groups	Length	Total	AFA	API	CAU	HIS	NAM	OTH	Total	BLA	CAU	MES	HIS	OTH	Conf
1	A*01010101	3	A*0101, A*010101	A*01010102N, A*010101, A*0122N, A*0132, A*0134N	Caucasoid - England, Europe; Caucasoid- Southern Africa	Confirmed	5	5	Full	-							-						C WD
2	A*01010102N	0	A*0101, A*010101	A*01010101N, A*0104N, A*0122N, A*0132, A*0134N	Caucasoid - Spain, Europe	Unconfirmed	1	1	Full	-							0						
3	A*010102	0	A*0101		Mixed-American Indian/Caucasoid	Unconfirmed	1	1	Partial	-							0						
4	A*010103	0	A*0101		Unknown	Unconfirmed	2	1	Partial	-							0						
5	A*010104	0	A*0101		Unknown	Unconfirmed	1	1	Partial	-							0						
6	A*010105	0	A*0101		Caucasoid - Germany, Europe	Unconfirmed	1	1	Partial	-							0						
7	A*0102	20			Black-Unknown Africa:Black- Unknown, North America	Confirmed	2	2	Full	>5							-						C
8	A*0103	8			Black - Ethopia North Africa; Black - Somalia, Africa; Caucasoid - Unknown	Confirmed	6	3	Partial	>5							-						

Fig. 7.9: Sources of data for rare alleles

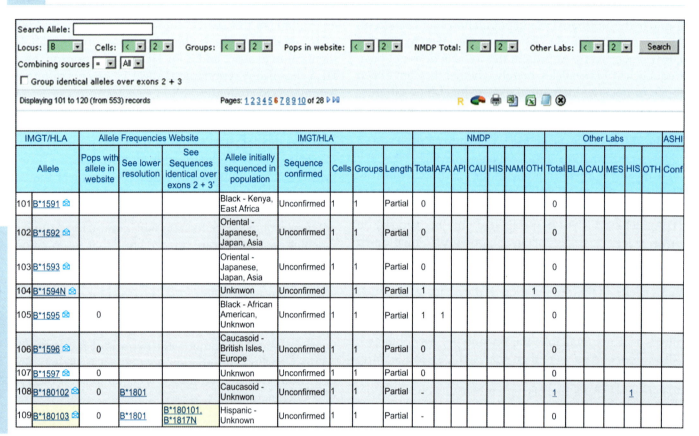

Fig. 7.10: Example of rare allele search

to be described. Presently, this tool is available for all allele searches. More information on specifications for accessing information from an external source can be found in online documentation on the website.

Online Bioinformatic Analysis Tools

An analysis tool has been introduced whereby frequency data on HLA alleles can be converted to the corresponding frequency data of amino acids. We believe it makes more sense to compare the frequency of amino acids in a population to other populations, especially in the context of a disease association study. Obviously, only those populations with 4 digits minimum resolution can be used for this tool. It is thus possible, knowing the frequency of the allele in a population, to ascertain and sum the frequencies of amino acid at each of the variable positions of the HLA molecule in that population (Fig. 7.11).

CONCLUSION

We trust that we have provided a facility that is of benefit to the histocompatibility and immunogenetic community—the website receives on average 40 hits per day. We wish to expand the website; adding more data to the existing polymorphic regions, introducing new polymorphic regions, e.g. data on HLA minor antigens and providing tools to analyse the data directly on the website. However, for this venture to continue successfully individuals/laboratories need to provide data and to suggest improvements to the website.

From the outset, we have been concerned on the accuracy of data. We are now working towards examining data submitted with analysis tools to clarify this issue. Under the auspices of a COST grant 'HLA-NET',[27] we intend in the future to ask for the raw data of individuals in the population provided and the sequences of primers/probes, etc. used in the technique. This will enable us to analyse the data. We also will provide tools on the website for analysis of new data and comparison of that data with existing data. Under the banner of 'HLA-NET', we are investigating the possibility of initiating a new open-access journal to carry population data in a set format.

OTHER DATABASES

- *Bone Marrow Donors Worldwide*
  Bone Marrow Donors Worldwide (BMDW) is the continuing effort to collect the HLA phenotypes of

Allele	Freq (%)	9	17	43	44	58	62	63	65	66	67	70	73	74	76	77	79	80	80	82	83
A*0205	2.40	Y	R	R	R	G	G	E	R	K	V	H	T	H	V	D	G	T	L	R	G
A*0302	0.30	F	R	Q	R	G	Q	E	R	N	V	Q	T	D	V	D	G	T	L	R	G
A*2301	2.70	S	R	Q	R	G	E	E	G	K	V	H	T	D	E	N	R	I	A	L	R
A*24020101	12.00	S	R	Q	R	G	E	E	G	K	V	H	T	D	E	N	R	I	A	L	R
A*2409N	0.10	S	R	Q	R	G	E	E	G	K	V	H	T	D	E	N	R	I	A	L	R
A*2502	0.10	Y	R	Q	R	G	R	N	R	N	V	Q	T	D	E	S	R	I	A	L	R
A*2608	0.10	Y	R	Q	R	G	R	N	R	N	V	H	T	D	A	N	G	T	L	R	G
A*3004	0.10	S	S	Q	R	R	Q	E	R	N	V	H	T	D	E	N	G	T	L	R	G
A*310102	5.10	T	R	Q	R	R	Q	E	R	N	V	H	T	I	D	V	D	G	T	L	R	G
A*3301	1.30	T	R	Q	R	G	R	N	R	N	V	H	T	I	D	V	D	G	T	L	R	G
A*3402	0.10	Y	R	Q	R	G	R	N	R	N	V	Q	T	D	V	D	G	T	L	R	G
A*6601	0.20	Y	R	Q	R	G	R	N	R	N	V	Q	T	D	V	D	G	T	L	R	G
A*680101	1.30	Y	R	Q	R	G	R	N	R	N	V	Q	T	D	V	D	G	T	L	R	G
A*680102	3.90	Y	R	Q	R	G	R	N	R	N	V	Q	T	D	V	D	G	T	L	R	G

Position	9	17	43	44	56	62	63	65	66	67	70	73	74	76	77	79	80	81	82	83
Frequency by Protein (%)	S=14.9 Y=8.1 T=6.4 F=0.3	R=29.6 S=0.1	Q=27.3 R=2.4	R=29.7	G=24.5 R=5.2	E=14.8 R=7 Q=5.5 G=2.4	E=22.7 N=7	R=14.9 G=14.8	K=17.2 N=12.5	V=29.7	H=23.8 Q=5.9	T=23.3 I=6.4	D=27.3 H=2.4	E=15 V=14.6 A=0.1	N=15 D=14.6 S=0.1	R=14.9 G=14.8	I=14.9 T=14.8	A=14.9 L=14.8	L=14.9 R=14.8	R=14.9 G=14.8

Fig. 7.11: Population alleles by frequency data of amino acids

volunteer bone marrow donors and cord blood units, and for the coordination of their worldwide distribution. http://www.bmdw.org

- *dbMHC Anthropology*
  HLA and related loci and their relationship to health/disease/anthropology. Standardization and support of DNA typing, data transfer and interpretation. http://www.ncbi.nlm.nih.gov/gv/mhc/ihwg.cgi?cmd=page&page=AnthroMain

- *The IMGT/HLA Database*
  The official database of the WHO Nomenclature Committee for factors of the HLA System. http://www.ebi.ac.uk/imgt/hla/

- *The IPD-KIR Database*
  The official database of the KIR Nomenclature Committee. http://www.ebi.ac.uk/ipd/kir/

- *Immune Epitope Database*
  The Immune Epitope Database (IEDB) and Analysis Resource contain data related to antibody and T cell epitopes for humans, non-human primates, rodents, and other animal species. http://www.immuneepitope.org/home.do

- The Leucocyte Receptor Complex (LRC) Haplotype Project
  Framework and resource for LRC- and KIR linked association studies. The LRC haplotype project aims to provide information for this interaction by sequencing common LRC haplotypes. http://www.sanger.ac.uk/HGP/Chr19/LRC/

OTHER APPLICATIONS

- *PyPop*
  PyPop is an environment developed by the Thomson lab for doing large-scale population genetic analyses including: Conformity to Hardy-Weinberg expectations, tests for balancing or directional selection; estimates of haplotype frequencies (and their distributions) and measures and tests of significance for linkage disequilibrium (LD). http://www.pypop.org/

- *Arlequin*
  Arlequin is an exploratory population genetics software environment able to handle large samples of molecular data (RFLPs, DNA sequences, microsatellites), while retaining the capacity of analyzing conventional genetic data (standard multi-locus data or mere allele frequency data). http://lgb.unige.ch/arlequin/

- *PHYLIP*
  PHYLIP is a free package of programs for inferring phylogenies. It is distributed as source code, documentation files, and a number of different types of executables. http://evolution.genetics.washington.edu/phylip.html

- *Clustal X*
  Clustal X is a new windows interface for the ClustalW multiple sequence alignment program. It provides an integrated environment for performing multiple sequence and profile alignments and analysing the results. http://bips.u-strasbg.fr/fr/Documentation/ClustalX/

ACKNOWLEDGMENTS

We are indebted to the following sponsors whose help has made this project viable: Abbott, Biotest, Innogenetics, Invitrogen, Olerup SSP, One Lambda, and Tepnel Lifecodes and to Ralph Komerofsky who produced the technical aspects of the first version of the website.

REFERENCES

1. Robinson J, Malik A, Parham P, Bodmer JG, Marsh SGE. IMGT/HLA - A sequence database for the human major histocompatibility complex. Tissue Antigens 2000;55: 280-7.
2. Hill AV.HIV and HLA: Confusion or complexity? Nature Med 1996;2:395-6.
3. Meyer D, Thomson G. How selection shapes variation of the human major histocompatibility complex: A review. Am Hum Genet 2001;65:1-26.
4. Belich MP, Madrigal JA, Hildeband WH, et al. Unusual HLA-B alleles in two tribes of Brazilian Indians. Nature 1992;357:326-9.
5. Watkins DI, McAdams SN, Liu X et al. New recombinant HLA alleles in a tribe of South American Amerindians indicates rapid evolution of MHC class I loci. Nature 1992;357:329-33.
6. Prugnolle F, Manica A, Charpentier M. Guegan JF, Guernier V, Balloux F. Pathogen-driven selection and worldwide HLA class I diversity. Current Biology 2005;15:1022-7.
7. Fleischhauer K, Kernan NA, O'Reilly RJ, Dupont B, Yang SY. Bone marrow allograft rejection by T lymphocytes recognising a single amino acid difference in HLA-B44. New Engl J Med 1990;323:1818-21.
8. Horton R, Gibson R, Coggill P, et al. Variation analysis and gene annotation of eight MHC haplotypes: The MHC Haplotype Project. Immunogenetics 2008; 60:1-18.
9. Singh R, Kaul R, Kaul A, Khan K. A comparative review of HLA associations with hepatitis B and C viral infections across global populations. World J Gastroenterology 2007;13:1770-87.
10. Gao X, Nelson GW, Karachi P, et al. Effect of a single amino acid change in MHC class I molecules on the rate of progression to AIDS. N Engl J Med 2001; 344:1668-75.
11. Thursz M. MHC and the viral hepatitides. Quart J Med 2001;94:287-91.
12. Mallai S, Nolan D, Witt C, et al. Association between the presence of HLA-B*5701, HLA-DR7 and HLA-DQ3 and hypersensitivity to HIV-1 reverse-transcriptase inhibitor abacavir. Lancet 2002;359:727-32.
13. Single RM, Martin MP, Gas X, et al. Global diversity and evidence of coevolution of KIR and HLA. Nature Genetics 2007;39:1114-9.
14. Ahlenstiel G, Martin MP, Gao X, Carrington M, Rehermann B. Distinct KIR/HLA compound genotypes affect the kinetics of human antiviral natural killer cell responses. J Clin Invest 2008;118:1017-26.
15. Kaloo S, Thio CL, Martin MP et al. HLA and NK cell inhibitory receptor genes in resolving hepatitis C virus infection. Science 2004;305:872-4.
16. Korbel DS, Normal PJ, Newman KC, et al. Killer Ig-like receptor (KIR) genotype predicts the capacity of human KIR-positive $CD56^{dim}$ NK cells to respond to pathogen-associated signals. J Immunol 2009;182:6426-34.
17. Norman PJ, Abi-Rached L, Gendzekhadze K, et al. Unusual selection on the KIR3DL1/S1 natural killer cell receptor in Africans. Nature Genetics 2007; 39:1092-9.
18. Yawata M, Yawata N, Draghi M, Little A-M, Partheniou F, Parham P. Roles for HLA and KIR polymorphisms in natural killer cell repertoire selection and modulation of effector function. JEM 2005;203:633-45.
19. Middleton D, Menchaca L, Rood H, Komerofsky R. New allele frequency database. Tissue Antigens 2003;61:403-7.
20. Robinson J, Waller MJ, Stoher P, Marsh SGE. IPD - the Immuno Polymorphism Database. Nucleic Acids Research 2005;331:D523-6.
21. Uhrberg M, Valiante NM, Shum BP, et al. Human diversity in killer cell inhibitory receptor genes. Immunity 1997;7:753-63.
22. Middleton D, Meenagh A, Gourraud PA. KIR haplotype content at the allele level in 77 Northern Irish families. Immunogenetics 2007;59:145-58.
23. Middleton D, Gonzalez F, Meenagh A, Gourraud PA. Diversity of KIR genes, alleles and haplotypes. (In press).
24. Gourraud PA, Gagne K, Bignon JD, Cambon-Thomsen A, Middleton D. Preliminary analysis of a KIR haplotype estimation algorithm: A simulation study. Tissue Antigen 2007;69:96-100.
25. Middleton D, Gonzalez F, Fernandez-Vina M, et al. A bioinformatic approach to ascertaining the rarity of HLA alleles. Submitted for publication.
26. Cano P, Klitz W, Mack SJ, et al. Common and well documented HLA alleles. Hum Immunol 2007;60:392-417
27. www.cost.esf.org European Cooperative in science and technology (COST). A European Network of the HLA diversity for histocompatibility, clinical transplantation, epidemiology and population genetics (HLA-NET). Biomedicine and Molecular Biosciences (BMBS) Action BM0803.

Chapter 8

Complement Genes in the Central Region of the MHC

Ágnes Szilágyi, Márton Doleschall, George Füst

INTRODUCTION

The complement system is one of the major plasma enzyme systems, with an important role in the defense against bacterial and fungal infections, in the elimination of potentially pathogenic immune complexes, and in the generation of adaptive immune response as well as protective inflammation. Complement activation is, however, a 'double-edged sword': it also has a major role in the pathomechanism of several diseases, such as autoimmune disorders, myocardial infarction or stroke. It comprises 20 proteins, which activate each other in a cascade-like manner. Activation is controlled by several membrane and soluble regulatory proteins. Similar to other plasma enzyme systems, the main mechanism of complement activation is *limited proteolysis* that is, the proteolytic cleavage of a single peptide bond, which results in the generation of two fragments, usually unequal in size.

The complement system can be activated via three pathways (Fig. 8.1). The *classical pathway* (CP) is started by intramolecular events within the first component of complement, C1. One C1 molecule consists of one molecule of C1q, as well as two C1r and two C1s molecules ($C1q(r_2s_2)$). The main activators of the classical pathway are antigen-antibody complexes, but it can be activated by bacteria, viruses and many other substances as well. Binding of the 'heads' of C1q leads to conformational changes in the molecule acting on the ring-like $C1r_2$-$C1s_2$ complex and this results in sequential activation of C1r and C1s by limited proteolysis. Activated C1s or C1 esterase is a potent trypsin-like proteolytic enzyme, which has two substrates, C4 and C2. First, C4 is activated by the generation of two fragments, the smaller C4a and the much bigger C4b, which – in its nascent form – can attach to molecules on cell surfaces or soluble proteins through covalent bonds (Fig. 8.2 top insert). C4b then binds C2, which is similarly cleaved by the C1 esterase enzyme into two fragments, i.e. C2b and C2a. C2a – which has enzymatic activity – remains loosely attached to C4b and forms the CP C3-cleaving enzyme or C3 convertase (C4b2a). Since C3 is the most abundant and functionally most important complement protein, its activation by proteolytic cleavage is the most significant event of complement activation. Similar to C4, C3 is also cleaved to a small fragment, C3a, which – by acting through its receptor – has potent anaphylatoxic properties (e.g. it increases the permeability of blood vessels, causes mastocyte degranulation resulting in histamine generation, along with the contraction of smooth muscles). Again, and similarly to C4b (the two parent proteins have similar structure), the bigger fragment, C3b in its nascent form can covalently bind to molecules on cells or soluble proteins. C3b fragments can be further cleaved into different fragments, some of which remain covalently attached and serve as ligands for various complement receptors. These processes are most important in the opsonization of bacteria and fungi, which is an indispensable step for antimicrobial defense. The uncleaved C3b is a constituent of the CP C5-cleaving enzyme or C5 convertase (C3b2a4b) beside C4b and C2a, of which C2a is the enzymatically active fragment. One of the central steps of complement activation is the proteolytic cleavage of C5 into two fragments by C5 convertase. The small fragment of C5, C5a is a highly potent biologically active material. In addition to its anaphylatoxin-like activity which is similar to that of C3a, C5a acts on

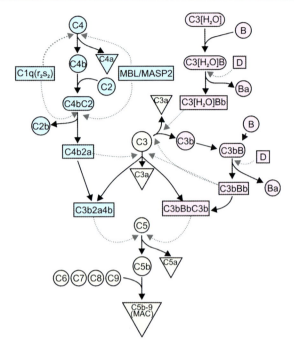

Fig. 8.1: Schematic representation of complement system and its three pathways. Classical and lectin pathways are indicated by blue, alternative pathway by pink and common complement components by yellow. The complement components and complexes having proteolytic activities are represented by square shapes, while the components having effector functions by triangles. The generation of complement products and the assembly of complement complexes are indicated by black arrows, and the proteolytic cleavage by intermittent gray arrows

polymorphonuclear leukocytes as well: attracts, activates and aggregates them, as well as increases their attachment to the endothelial cells. The bigger fragment itself cannot attach to the cells covalently; nevertheless, its binding is followed by an interaction (known as the 'common terminal pathway') of the late acting proteins of complement activation that is, of C5, C6, C7, C8 and several molecules of C9. A doughnut-like structure, the 'membrane attack complex (MAC)' or C5b-9 is generated within the cell membrane. MAC generation may lead to osmotic lysis of erythrocytes, some bacteria, and tumor cells. In the case of nucleated cells, however, a rather different process occurs: generation of MAC within the membrane of these cells results in activation of the arachidonic acid pathways of leukotriene, prostaglandin and cytokine formation. These events are indispensable for the generation of protective and pathogenic inflammation. Complement activation is regulated by complement regulatory proteins that comprise a couple of factors acting on the level of C3/C5 convertases. These include the decay accelerating factor (DAF) that promotes the dissociation of convertases and the membrane cofactor protein (MCP) that acts as a cofactor for cleavage inactivation of convertases by factor I, whereas complement receptor type 1 (CR1) has both decay-accelerating and cofactor-like activity.

Another activation pathway, the *alternative pathway* (AP) is usually activated by bacteria and viruses, as well as by several other substances (Fig. 8.1). It begins with the autoactivation of C3 molecules in the plasma, which leads to the formation of the C3b-like C3 ($C3(H_2O)$). This molecule has the capacity to bind one molecule of factor B (Bf), which is then activated by an enzymatically active protein, factor D (Df) (Fig. 8.2). Cleavage of Bf results in the formation of Ba, which – to our knowledge – has no major biological activity, and of Bb, which remains attached to the C3b-like C3 and forms an unstable fluid-phase C3 convertase ($C3(H_2O)Bb$). This enzyme cleaves C3, and similar to the process described above for CP, nascent C3b covalently binds to cell surfaces, then Bf is bound and cleaved by Df resulting in C3bBb complex, which is the definite AP C3-cleaving enzyme. When two adjacent C3b protein molecules are present on the cell surface, Bb assumes the ability to cleave C5 as the AP C5 convertase (C3bBbC3b). Half-life of the C3bBb and C3bBbC3b complexes can be elevated by the binding of another complement protein, properdin, whereas dissociation of the AP C3/C5 convertases can be induced by regulatory proteins, including the same molecules as in the case of CP (DAF, MCP, and CR1, respectively) and the complement factor H (Hf). The later possesses both decay-accelerating and cofactor-like activity and therefore, it prevents fluid-phase activation of the alternative pathway.

The third pathway, *the lectin pathway* (LP) is activated by surfaces containing certain carbohydrates such as mannose, which are able to bind MBL that is, mannose-binding lectin (Figs 8.1 and 8.2 top insert). This binding is followed by the activation of another complement protein, MASP2, which is thus enabled to cleave C4 into the same fragments as those produced by C1s. The subsequent process (i.e. C3-cleaving, followed by generation of the C5 convertase) is the same as in the case of CP activation.

Three complement proteins, C4, C2 and Bf are encoded in the class III region of the major histocompatibility complex (MHC). As it was shown above, together with C3, these important proteins are the constituents of the two proteolytic enzyme complexes indispensable for the most important steps of complement activation that is, for the cleavage and activation of C3 and C5. Separated from each other by

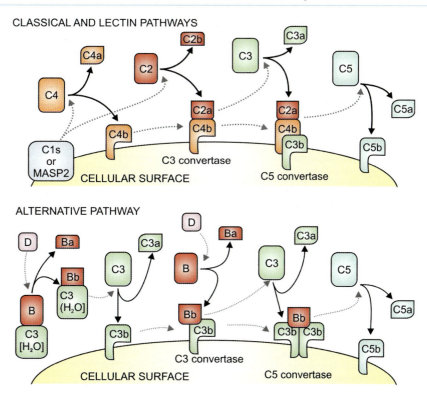

Fig. 8.2: Assembly of complement convertases in classical/lectin and alternative pathways. The generation of complement products by cleavage is indicated by black arrows, the assembly of complexes by intermittent black arrows, and the proteolytic cleavage by intermittent gray arrows

only 421 bases, the loci of C2 and factor B are in close proximity and reside approximately 30 kb telomerically to the genes encoding the two isoforms of C4, C4A and C4B (Fig. 8.3). These four genes are the hallmarks of the MHC complement gene cluster (MCGC), a tightly linked gene-dense region, characterized by extreme complexity as regards polymorphisms and variations in gene size and copy number. C2 and factor B share extensive protein sequence and functional homology, just as does C4A and C4B, and therefore, these two sets of genes are supposed to have arisen by gene duplication from common ancestors.[1] These MHC-linked complement genes are usually inherited as a single linkage group, also known as a complotype that characterizes their main polymorphic variants.[2] Complotypes are designated in arbitrary order as C2, Bf, C4A and C4B variants.[3]

Complement Component C2

Protein Structure and Physiology of Complement Component C2

The second component of human complement is a 100 kDa, single-chain glycoprotein that provides the catalytic subunit of the C3/C5 convertases of the classical and lectin pathways (Figs 8.1 and 8.2). This protein, mainly synthesized by the liver, circulates in the blood as a serine protease zymogen, present in a concentration of 11-35 µg/ml.[4] Proteolytically inactive C2 is able to associate with a C4b molecule bound to surface of cellular or protein antigens in an Mg^{2+}- and Ca^{2+}-dependent manner. Upon binding, C2 is cleaved by C1s to release a small inactive fragment (C2b) into the fluid phase, while the larger C2a fragment remains bound on the surface and initiates the formation of C4b2a and C4b2a3b complexes. In the case of the other complement components, the larger cleavage product is termed as 'b' and the smaller one as 'a', but designation is reversed in the case of C2 for historical reasons.

C2 protein belonging to the peptidase S1 family is synthesized as a proenzyme of 752 amino acid residues including a leader peptide of 20 amino acids. Post-translational modification of the polypeptide involves the formation of several disulfide bonds and glycolyzation; 15.9 percent of the mature glycoprotein is carbohydrate composed of fucose, galactose, mannose, N-acetylglucosamine and N-acetylneuraminate.[5] The

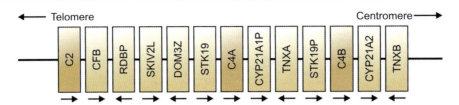

Fig. 8.3: Schematic representation of MHC complement gene cluster (MCGC). The arrow below each gene indicates the direction of gene transcription

trilobular structure of the protein consists of an N-terminal domain comprising three complement control protein (CCP) modules (amino acids 22-206), a von Willebrand factor type A (vWFA) domain (amino acids 254-452), and a C-terminal serine protease (SP) domain (amino acids 464-752) separated by short connecting segments (Fig. 8.4A).[6, 7] The three CCP modules (also known as short consensus repeats (SCR) or Sushi domains) contribute structural elements for the initial binding of the molecule to C4b.[8] In addition to these CCP modules, the cleaved product of C2b contains the seven N-terminal residues of vWFA along with the linker segment between these two domains. Interestingly, mutations described in the connecting regions (S189F in the CCP/vWFA and G444R in the vWFA/SP segment, see the description below at type II deficiency) interfere with C2 secretion, confirming that these linkers are essential for correct folding and/or appropriate conformation of the peptide.[9] The vWFA domain mediates ligand-binding through its Mg^{2+}-coordinating residues. The serine protease domain of the molecule exhibits catalytic activity against its targets but only in the context of the C4b2a complex, otherwise it assumes an inactive zymogen-like conformation.[10]

The Gene of Complement Component C2 and its Regulation

The gene of the complement component C2 is the most telomeric constituent of the MHC complement gene cluster (Fig. 8.3) that lies at a distance of approximately 600 kb from the 5' end of the *HLA-B* gene.[11, 12] The *C2* gene spans 18 kb of genomic DNA and comprises 18 exons. Intron 3 of the gene contains a human-specific SINE (short interspersed sequence)-type retroposon, SINE-R.C2, apparently derived from a human endogenous retrovirus, HERV-K10.[13] A number of studies reported the presence of multiple *C2* gene transcripts in various cell lines arising from the deletion of one or two exons.[14, 15]

C2 expression in response to an acute-phase stimulus is regulated predominantly by IFNγ, with cell-specific differences in the response.[16, 17] Several transcription initiation sites were described in the 5' flanking region of the *C2* gene; however, their role in the constitutive and tissue-specific expression of *C2* has not been fully characterized yet.[18, 19] Termination of C2 transcription is strongly regulated by the binding of a zinc finger protein that protects the promoter of factor B from transcriptional interference, as it is separated by only 421 bp from the *C2* polyadenylation site.[20]

Deficiency of Complement Component C2

Deficiency of C2 (C2D) is the most common genetic defect of the complement system in individuals of European descent; the estimated frequency of the null allele (C2*Q0) is about 1 percent.[21] This recessive trait can result from two different molecular mechanisms. In type I deficiency, no detectable C2 protein is synthesized, mainly because of a 28-bp deletion beginning 9 base pairs upstream of the 3'-end of exon 6. This mutation involves the 5'-splice site of intron 6 that causes skipping of the preceding exon (exon 6) during RNA processing resulting in a shift of the reading frame and generation of a premature termination codon. Hence, although some C2 mRNA is produced, no stable C2 protein is generated.[22] This type of C2 deficiency is in linkage disequilibrium with the extended haplotype 18.1, characterized by HLA-A25, -Cw12, -B18, BfS, C4A4, C4B2 and HLA-DR15.[23, 24] A case report has later described another mutation causing type I deficiency that is, a two base-pair deletion in exon 2 of the *C2* gene linked to HLA-A3, -B35, BfF, C4A3,2, C4B0, HLA-DR4 alleles, resulting in frame shift and immediate stop codon.[25]

In type II deficiency, a C2 polypeptide is synthesized, but it is retained intracellularly, because a missense mutation resulting in critical amino acid substitution in the C2 protein structure prevents its secretion. Molecular heterogeneity of this deficiency was demonstrated by Wetsel et al,[9] who have isolated two type II C2*Q0 genes that contained different mutations at highly conserved residues. One of these is a G/A substitution at nucleotide 1930, leading to a glycine to arginine change at codon

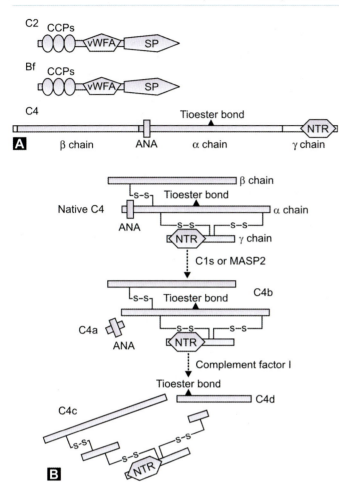

Figs 8.4A and B: (A) Schematic representation of the protein structures of complement component C2 (C2), complement factor B (Bf) and complement component C4 (C4). Abbreviations: ANA—anaphylatoxin domain; CCP—complement control protein module; NTR—netrin domain; SP—serine protease domain; vWFA—von Willebrand factor type A domain. (B) Schematic representation of the C4 activation and degradation

444 of the mature protein that is a part of the extended haplotype containing HLA-A2, -B5, C2Q0, BfS, C4A3, C4B1, HLA-DR4. The other missense mutation (nucleotide 566 C→T) – causing an amino acid change from serine to phenylalanine at residue 189 – is tightly linked to the haplotype HLA-A11, -B35, C2Q0, BfS, C4A0, C4B1, HLA-DR1.[9] A subsequent study has described another type II mutation associated with the HLA-A28, -B58, -DR12 haplotype that is, a G to A transition at nucleotide 392, resulting in a cysteine to tyrosine substitution at codon 111.[26] Each type II amino acid change produces a mutant, full-length C2 precursor, the progression of which through the normal C2 secretory pathway is delayed.

Variations of Complement Component C2

In addition to the most common structural form (C2C or C2(1)), a rare basic (C2B or C2(2)) and a rare acidic allotype (C2A) of the protein have been identified in humans by gel electrophoresis. Moreover, several rare acidic and basic variants have been recognized by isoelectric focusing, followed by western blotting and immunofixation. These variants occur in all major races; however, their overall prevalence is less than 5 percent.[27] In order to elucidate the functional differences among structural variants, the hemolytic ability of sera was compared among individuals with different C2 allotypes, in an early study. Comparing sera bearing C2C/C2C, C2B/C2C or C2B/C2B allotypes, no significant differences were found in the mean functional activity or in the rates at which they caused lysis of sensitized red blood cells.[28] In agreement with this result, another study revealed no differences in the activities of C2C homozygote and C2B/C2C heterozygote type sera or sera bearing a rare variant (C2A′) in heterozygote form (C2A′/C2C). However, the hemolytic activity of sera obtained from C2A/C2C heterozygote individuals was significantly higher, than that of C2C homozygotes or C2B/C2C heterozygotes.[29] Varga et al have measured complement-mediated precipitation inhibiting activity of different C2 type sera. Decreased inhibition by sera from individuals homozygous for the C2B allotype compared to C2C homozygotes suggested that C2B has a lesser ability than C2C to mediate the interaction between immune complexes and the complement system.[30]

Apart from these protein allotypes determined by phenotyping over the past decades, only a few variations have been described at the DNA level. A recent study sequencing the coding and the adjacent intronic regions of the C2 gene did not found any substantial variability at this locus.[31] The authors pointed out two polymorphisms (E318D, IVS10), found to be associated with age-related macular degeneration both separately, and as a part of particular haplotypes of the region containing the genes of C2 and factor B (for details, see the section '*Disease associations of the complement components encoded in the central MHC region*'). The causative role of these SNPs has not been confirmed yet; however, their utility as haplotype tagging markers of this region is of great importance.

Other polymorphisms of the C2 gene have also been described including a variable number of tandem repeats (VNTR) located within intron 3 of the gene, as a part of the SINE-R.C2 retroposon.[13, 32] The locus contains a sequence of 41 bp average length, which is repeated 23 and 17 times in the two most common alleles. This VNTR gives rise to a multiallelic *Sst*I restriction fragment length polymorphism (RFLP) of the *C2* gene. RFLPs are variations in the DNA sequence that can be detected by cleaving DNA into pieces with the appropriate restriction enzymes and analyzing the size of the resulting fragments by gel electrophoresis.

Qualitative and Quantitative Methods for the Measurement of Complement Component C2

The essential role of complement component C2 in CP and LP warrants accurate measurement of its functional capacity and the determination of its variant forms with diverse functional and chemical properties. Enzyme-linked immunosorbent assay (ELISA) is appropriate for measuring the concentration of the complement component C2 in various biological fluids;[33] however, this method is rarely used in diagnostic laboratories. The ELISA technique affords quantization of an unknown amount of proteins by attaching them to a surface, followed by binding of a specific antibody linked to an enzyme. In the final step, a substrate of the enzyme is added, resulting in the generation of detectable signal, the intensity of which is proportional to the quantity of the bound protein. In the case of complement C2, the ability of the molecule to fulfill its biological function is more important as regards human disease, than its exact quantity and therefore, determination of its functional activity is more widely used. The most commonly applied functional assay is a hemolytic test, involving molecular titration of C2 in the tested serum in order to evaluate its ability to restore the hemolytic activity of human serum selectively deficient in C2.[34]

Different allotypes of the functional C2 protein can be determined with the method described by Alper et al.[27] First, isoelectric focusing of serum proteins is performed on polyacrylamide gel, followed by overlaying the gel with agarose-containing gelatin, Mg^{2+}, Ca^{2+}, antibody-sensitized sheep erythrocytes, and homozygous C2-deficient serum. After solidification, the bands corresponding to the hemolytically active C2 isoforms appear. By interpreting the results of this method beside the pattern revealed in the sera of homozygote C2C carriers, acidic or basic bands – compared to the common ones – can be detected in individuals bearing rare allotypes. Slightly modified or improved methods applying direct immunofixation or immunoblotting with a specific anti-human-C2 antibody following isoelectric focusing have also been described.[35-38]

A number of variations of the complement *C2* gene – that modify the restriction pattern of different enzymes (such as *Taq*I, *Bam*HI and *Sst*I) and therefore, create biallelic and multiallelic restriction fragment length polymorphisms – have also been identified.[13, 39-41] Genotyping of these variations can be performed by separating the restriction digests of genomic DNA with agarose gel electrophoresis. Fragments of different lengths are then transferred to nitrocellulose membranes, followed by hybridization with radioactively labeled C2-specific DNA probes and detection by exposure to X-ray film.[32, 42] This technique affords straightforward determination of different alleles at the DNA level, based on the differences in the sizes of resulting fragments corresponding to the different regions of the *C2* gene.

Complement Factor B

Protein Structure and Physiology of Complement Factor B

Complement factor B (Bf), a single polypeptide chain plasma glycoprotein with a molecular mass of 90 kDa, plays an indispensable role in the alternative complement pathway by providing the proteolytic component of C3/C5 convertases (Figs 8.1 and 8.2). The average serum concentration of Bf, synthesized mainly by the liver, is about 180 μg/ml with a wide range from 74 to 286 μg/ml as determined by sensitive radioassays.[4] Alternative activation of the complement system leads to the cleavage of Bf and subsequent assembly of C3b with the proteolytically active Bb in the presence of Mg^{2+}. As the formation of the C4b2a complex in CP/LP requires the presence of both Mg^{2+} and Ca^{2+} ions, this enables distinguishing between the two complement activation pathways in functional studies, by adding different chelating agents to the sera. *In vitro* experiments demonstrated that, besides its role in the activation of the alternative pathway, Bf is a cofactor in antibody-independent monocyte-mediated cytotoxicity,[43] macrophage spreading,[44] cleavage and activation of plasminogen,[45] and proliferation of B lymphocytes.[46-48]

Factor B protein, a member of the peptidase S1 family, is synthesized as a pro-enzyme that consists of 764 residues including a 25 amino acid signal peptide. After the formation of disulfide bonds and glycosylation, the mature protein contains 8.6 percent carbohydrate, comprising the same molecules as C2 (fucose, galactose, mannose, N-acetylglucosamine and N-acetyl-neuraminate, respectively), but in a different molar ratio.[5] Differences in the rate and content of glycosylation are likely to account for the difference between the molecular masses of the two mature proteins (Bf: 90 kDa vs C2: 100 kDa). The structure of Bf is very similar to that of the C2 molecule. It consists of – starting from the N-terminus – three CCP modules (amino acids 35-220), a short connecting segment, a vWFA module (amino acids 270-469), a short connecting segment and an SP domain (amino acids 477-757) (Fig. 8.4A). Transmission electron micrography visualization of the molecule supports a trilobular conformation, corresponding to the three domains of the protein.[6] The structure and function of each domain are similar to that of the C2 domains; however, the quantity and type of the amino acid residues constituting the modules may be different.

The Gene of Complement Factor B and its Regulation

Complement factor B is encoded by a 6-kb gene (*CFB*), located immediately 3' to the *C2* gene in the same transcriptional orientation (Fig. 8.3). These two closely related genes have very similar exon-intron structures, both comprise 18 exons and share 42 percent identity.[49] The main difference between them is their size (18 kb vs 6 kb of *C2* and *CFB*, respectively), principally resulting form the difference between the sizes of their intronic sequences. Transcription of *CFB* is under independent control in hepatic and extrahepatic cells through a number of *cis*-acting elements, some of which extend into the 3' region of the *C2* gene.[50] Expression of *CFB* was widely studied and found to be induced by a broad array of proinflammatory cytokines (IFN-γ, IL-1β, IL-6, TNF-α)[51-55] and hormones[56,57] in a tissue and cell type-specific manner, whereas cytokine-enhanced expression can be inhibited with different growth factors.[58,59]

Deficiency of Complement Factor B

Inherited complement factor B deficiency has not yet been described in humans; hence, many suggested that this state would likely be lethal. Surprisingly, however, factor B deficient mice were found to be viable and exhibited no overt phenotypic abnormalities in spite of the complete absence of the alternative pathway function.[60]

Variations of Complement Factor B

CFB is known to encode more than 30 protein variants that can be identified by gel electrophoresis and/or isoelectric focusing. The combined frequency of the two most common allotypes, BfS and BfF – named after their mobility (i.e. slow and fast, respectively) – is more than 95 percent. Both the mean level and the hemolytic capacity was reported to show correlation with the particular Bf phenotype in the order of BfF/BfF > BfF/BfS > BfS/BfS *in vitro*; however, a considerable variation was observed within the types.[61,62] The BfF isoform has two subtypes: BfFA and BfFB. These three alleles (BfS, BfFA, and BfFB, respectively) differ from each other at the DNA level in non-synonymous substitutions of nucleotides 94 and 95, resulting in the change of the seventh amino acid of the mature protein. Residue 7, corresponding to the 32nd amino acid of the premature polypeptide, contains arginine (CGG) in BfS, glutamine (CAG) in BfFA, and tryptophan (TGG) in BfFB. This amino acid change is responsible for the difference in the electrophoretic mobility of the proteins, as the F variants carry more positively charged amino acids and thus move faster toward the anode.[63,64] In addition to these common substitutions residing in the small Ba fragment of the molecule, structural variations of the Bb fragment were also described.[65] Besides, a number of apparently non-expressing factor B allotypes have been identified and denoted as "QL", referring to the relatively low concentration of the protein in sera.[66] However, a study by Siemens et al[67] revealed that these alleles encode hypomorphic, but functionally active proteins and therefore, cannot be considered Bf*Q0 variants.

Screening for additional variations in the *CFB* gene at the DNA level allowed the identification of novel polymorphisms, although only a couple of these exhibited considerable diversity in healthy individuals.[31] One of these is a T to A transversion at nucleotide 26, resulting in a leucine to histidine change at residue 9 (L9H) of the signal peptide that has been fairly much studied recently, as a haplotype-tagging variation associated with particular diseases (see the section *'Disease associations of the complement components encoded in the central MHC region'* for details).[68,69]

A recent study[70] has revealed two gain-of-function mutations in Bf, causing increased AP activation. Both reside in the vWFA module, a region that is critical for the interaction between C3b and Bf. Formation of the C3bBb complex is enhanced in the presence of the mutant allele of F286L that carries a leucine instead of phenylalanine at codon 286. C3 convertase enzymes containing a mutant Bf resulting from a lysine to glutamic acid change at residue 323 (K323E) are more resistant to decomposition by DAF or Hf, that results in increased enzyme activity *in vivo*.

Qualitative and Quantitative Methods for the Measurement of Complement Factor B

The complement factor B content of sera is commonly measured by ELISA- the principle of which corresponds to that of C2 - or radial immunodiffusion. In the radial immunodiffusion or Mancini technique, a specific antibody is incorporated into an agarose gel, followed by the addition of the samples containing an unknown amount of factor B into preformed wells of the antibody-containing gel. Reaction of the protein with Bf-specific antibody produces a ring of precipitation that will appear at the point, where the antigen and antibody have reached equivalence that allows the quantization of Bf in the tested sera.[71, 72]

For phenotyping the different structural forms of factor B, serum or plasma samples are separated by high-voltage gradient thin-layer agarose electrophoresis, using a Ca^{2+}-containing buffer. This is followed by immunofixation with a monospecific antiserum layered on to the gel surface and visualization with a protein stain.[34, 65, 73] The electrophoretic mobility difference of the allotypes allows characterization of the common Bf forms, S and F along with a number of rare variants (e.g. S07, F1). Subtypes of the F allotype (FA and FB) are detectable by a modification of the buffer system[74] or by isoelectric focusing in polyacrylamide gel, followed by immunofixation with anti-factor B.[75, 76]

Genotyping methods for common and rare variations of *CFB* at the DNA level have also been developed including polymerase chain reaction (PCR), followed by RFLP based on the restriction patterns of the *Msp*I and *Bsl*I enzymes (to distinguish S from F and FA from FB, respectively)[77, 78] and sequence-specific primer-based polymerase chain reaction assays.[79]

Complement Component C4

Protein Structure and Physiology of Complement Component C4

Complement component C4 functions as the non-enzymatic subunit of the C3 and C5 convertases for the classical and the lectin activation pathways of the complement system (Figs 8.1 and 8.2).[80] The C4 protein (204 kDa) is synthesized mainly in the liver, as a single chain of 1744 amino acids. It belongs to the alpha-2 macroglobulin protein family, but has acquired two specific modules during evolution, namely an anaphylatoxin domain (702-736 amino acids) mediating proinflammatory effects and a netrin domain (1595-1742 amino acids) with unknown physiological role.[81] The single-chain C4 protein undergoes post-translational modification, which results in a disulfide-linked heterotrimer consisting of α (680-1449 amino acids, 93 kDa), β (20-675 amino acids, 75 kDa) and γ (1454-1744 amino acids, 33 kDa) chains (Fig. 8.4A). Besides the formation of the heterotrimer structure, an internal thioester bond, a characteristic feature of alpha-2 macroglobulin protein family, is formed between the sulfhydryl group of Cys1010 and the carbonyl group of Gln1013.[82] Additional post-translational modifications include glycosylation and tyrosine sulfation.[83] Following secretion into the plasma, where its concentration is about 0.5 mg/ml, a 22 residue peptide (1428-1449 amino acids) is removed from the C-terminus of the α chain.[84] In the plasma, native C4 is proteolytically cleaved in the classical pathway by C1s and in the lectin pathway by MASP2, producing an anaphylatoxin, C4a (680-756 amino acids) and a modulatory subunit, C4b (Fig. 8.4B). After the release of the C4a peptide, the thioester bond between Cys1010 and Gln1013, which is hidden in the native protein, becomes exposed upon activation. The carbonyl group of Gln1013 in this activated subunit initiates nucleophilic attack to its antigenic target molecules, to bind C4b to the surface of cellular and protein antigens through covalent ester or amide linkage. Bound C4b is a modulatory subunit of C3 convertase (C4b2a) and C5 convertase (C3b4b2a); C2a can cleave and activate C3 and C5 along with the downstream processes only following the binding of C4b.[85, 86] In addition to the formation of MAC, the release of C3a and C5a anaphylatoxins, and the opsonization of immune complexes, further consequences of C4 activation include the generation of C4a with a weak anaphylatoxic activity.[87] Complement activation is regulated on the level of C4, by a series of CCP module-containing soluble and membrane factors such as CR1, DAF, and MCP, through the dissociation of C3/C5 convertases or the degradation of C4,[88] when C4b is cleaved to C4c and C4d (957-1336 amino acids) by complement factor I, whereby it looses all of its functional interaction sites.

Isotypes of Complement Component C4

There are two isotypes of C4 protein, C4A and C4B, distinguished from each other by four amino acids between positions 1120 to 1125 (PCPVLD for C4A and LSPVIH for C4B) that are responsible for the structural and functional differences.[89] The binding efficiency of Gln1013 depends on the C4 isotype and the nature of the antigen or antibody molecules. The C4b fraction from the C4A preferentially binds to amino groups of proteins such as immune complexes, whereas C4b from C4B forms ester bonds, using hydroxyl groups of protein and carbohydrate antigens such as the bacterial cell wall. The isotypes differ from each other not only in their preference for acceptor nucleophiles, but also in the mechanism of transacylation.[90] The names of the two isotypes are derived from their electrophoretic mobilities: C4A migrates faster in the agarose gel at alkaline pH because the protein is acidic; whereas C4B migrates slower, because the protein is basic.[91] Moreover, their serologic and hemolytic activities, binding properties towards complement receptors and antibody aggregates, as well as the half-lives of their C4b fragments are also different.[92]

The Gene and the Genetic Module of Complement Component C4 and its Regulation

The *C4* gene encodes a 5.4-kb transcript, assembled from 41 exons, and the amino acid residues for the C4A/C4B isotypes are located in exon 26.[93] Each *C4* gene may be short form (S, a length of 14.6 kb) or long form (L, a length of 21.0 kb), caused by the integration of an endogenous retrovirus HERV-K (a length of 6.4 kb) into intron 9.[94, 95] The short and long *C4* gene can encode either a C4A or a C4B protein, although more of the *C4A* genes are long and in parallel, more of the *C4B* genes are short. Three quarters of the *C4* genes in East Asian, Indian and White populations have the retrovirus integrated and one quarter do not, but the frequency of short *C4* genes is 40 percent in Blacks.[96-98] The size of *C4* genes influences total C4 protein plasma concentration and the short form is related to higher C4 concentration.[99] Consistently with the higher frequency of short *C4* genes in Blacks, C4B serum concentration is higher in Blacks as compared to Whites and the same holds true for total C4 concentration because of the increased levels of C4B.[100]

The *C4* gene resides in MHC III region linked tightly to three neighboring genes: serine/threonine kinase 19 (*STK19*, also known as *RP1*) steroid 21-hydroxylase (*CYP21A2*), and tenascin-X (*TNXB*) (Fig. 8.3).[101] This region is designated as **RCCX,** reflecting the names of constituent genes in order *STK19* (*RP1*)-*C4*-*CYP21A2*-*TNXB* and has modular structure with copy number variation (Fig. 8.5A). Accordingly, the number of RCCX modules may vary from one to three (very rarely four), creating mono-, bi- or trimodular (very rarely quadrimodular) structures on a chromosome.[102] About one-tenth of the chromosomes from human subjects – regardless of their racial ancestry – have monomodular RCCX comprising the four genes in the above-mentioned sequence. There is a bimodular RCCX region in about three quarters of the chromosomes: the first module from the direction of the telomere contains an intact *STK19* gene, an intact *C4* gene that encodes either *C4A* or *C4B*, an inactive pseudogene of steroid 21-hydroxylase (*CYP21A1P*) gene, and a truncated tenascin-X gene (*TNXA*). The second module is composed of a truncated serine/threonine kinase 19 gene (*STK19P*), an intact *C4A* or *C4B* gene, an intact *CYP21A2* gene, and an intact *TNXB* gene (Fig. 8.5A).[97] The breakpoint of segmental duplication is positioned at exon 7 of the *STK19* gene and intron 32 of the *TNX* gene.[103] The structure of the trimodular RCCX region, with a prevalence of about 10% is similar to that of the bimodular one. In summary, all the *C4* genes are active, but only one of the repeated copies is active in the case of *STK19*, *TNX*, and *CYP21* – all the others are inactive pseudogenes independently on the number of RCCX modules. The monomodular haplotype harbors a short or a long *C4* gene; the bimodular haplotype can be LL or LS; and the LLL, LSL or LSS haplotypes occur in the trimodular structure (Fig. 8.5B). The prevalences of haplotypes are generally similar and reflect the frequencies of short and long *C4* genes in populations with different ethnic background, but the monomodular S haplotype is much less frequent in East Asians and Indians, than in Whites.[96, 98]

From another point of view, the gene frequency of *C4A* is slightly higher, than that of *C4B*.[104] The number of *C4* genes present in a diploid genome varies between two and six in healthy subjects, and the total number of *C4A* and *C4B* genes varies from zero to five and from zero to four, respectively.[105] About half of the individuals have four *C4* genes; almost the entire other half possesses three or five genes, whereas two or six genes occur only rarely. As expected, individuals with a higher copy number of total *C4*, *C4A* or *C4B* genes express an elevated amount of total C4, C4A or C4B proteins in their blood, whereas lower copy number leads to decreased C4, C4A or C4B protein levels.[96] Most of the individuals with four *C4* genes have two *C4A* and two *C4B* genes – resulting in equal plasma levels of the two C4 isotypes, but one-third of the individuals have a lower level of either the C4A or the C4B protein, because of the lack of the *C4A* or the *C4B* gene on either or both of the chromosomes, referred to as heterozygote or homozygote C4A*Q0 and C4B*Q0 carriers, respectively.[106] The copy number variation of RCCX modules generates qualitative and quantitative diversity of complement C4, which in turn mediates inter-

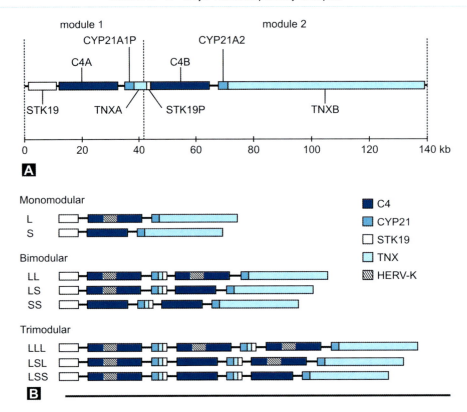

Figs 8.5A and B: (A) Scale representation of bimodular RCCX region with two long C4 genes. (B) Schematic representation of monomodular, bimodular and trimodular RCCX considering short and long C4 genes

individual differences in the strength of immune effector systems to respond to diverse challenges.[97] The modular structure of RCCX may also promote gene conversion or non-allelic homologous recombinations during meiosis.[107]

The principal site of C4 synthesis is the liver; however, C4 genes are also expressed in a variety of tissues and cell types. IFNγ can induce the transcription of C4 in a dose-dependent manner in many different cell lines.[108] The influence of other cytokines on transcription is limited to particular cell lines only and there is some evidence from hepatoma-derived cell lines for the unequal expression of C4A and C4B.[109,110] A TATA-less core promoter, responsible for the transcriptional regulation of C4 contains Sp1 binding sites for constitutive and E-box for IFNγ-induced transcription.[111, 112]

Deficiency of the Complement Component C4

The lack of C4A or C4B protein – occurring in a subset of subjects carrying C4A*Q0 or C4B*Q0 – does not cause a serious pathological condition directly, but it is associated with the risk of contracting several diseases (see the section 'Disease associations of the complement components encoded in the central MHC region' for details). Non-expression of the active C4 protein is extremely rare, but most of the deficient individuals have systemic lupus erythematosus, increased susceptibility to infections[113] or suffer from certain other diseases.[114] C4 deficiencies arise from the deletion of complete genes along with the RCCX module or the presence of defective genes expressing incorrect transcripts and inactive protein products.[115] A defective C4A gene often results from a CT insertion in exon 29, as this leads to a frame shift mutation, an early stop codon in exon 30, and a truncated transcript.[116] This mutation can transfer into the C4B gene probably by gene conversion, to generate a C4B pseudogene.[117]

Variations of C4A and C4B

In addition to the C4A and C4B isotypes exhibiting most important functional differences, about 40 polymorphic allotypes of C4 have been identified, based mainly on gross charge differences in electrophoretic mobilities and in hemolytic activity. Within an isotype, allotypes are given numbers in increasing order of their anodal migration. The two most common allotypes in all ethnic groups are C4A3 and C4B1; other frequent allotypes for C4A are A2, A4, A6, A1, whereas for C4B these include B2, B3, and B5.[118]

Besides the four isotype-specific amino acid residues distinguishing C4A from C4B, four further amino acids define the serological antigenic determinants of human C4, known as Chido (Ch) and Rodgers (Rg).[119, 120] The Ch and Rg blood groups are formed by the deposition of the polymorphic C4d fragments on the membranes of erythrocytes. Alloantibodies against Rg and Ch antigens can develop in blood transfusion recipients with C4A or C4B deficiency and can agglutinate the transfused erythrocytes. Six Ch (Ch1–Ch6) and two Rg (Rg1 and Rg2) antigens are defined from a battery of alloantibodies against C4. Through molecular cloning and sequencing of the corresponding genomic DNA from human subjects with normal and reversed serologic antigenicities, it has been found that the Chido antigenic determinants reside at amino acid positions of 1207, 1210 for Ch1 (A and R), at 1053, 1101–1106 for Ch2 (G and LSPVIH), at 1176 and 1188–1191 for Ch3 (S, A and R), at 1120–1125 for Ch4 (LSPVIH), at position of 1073 for Ch5 (G), and at 1176 for Ch6 (S), while the Rodgers antigenic determinants are located at 1207, 1210 for the Rg1 (V and L), and at 1176, 1207, 1210 for Rg2 (N, V and L). Rg1, Rg2, Ch1, Ch4, Ch5 and Ch6 are linear sequence determinants, whereas Ch2 and Ch3 are conformational determinants.[121] Most C4A are associated with Rg and C4B with Ch, but reverse associations of C4A with Ch and C4B and Rg are also well documented.[122, 123]

Apart from isotype-specific residues, amino acid interchanges are without physiological consequences in most cases, but C4A6 allotype – being in strong linkage disequilibrium with HLA-B17 – is an exception. The Arg477 residue in C4A6 is replaced by Trp and this eliminates the binding site for C5 and thereby almost completely abolishes hemolytic activity.[124, 125] This observation was further substantiated by the characterization of a hemolytically inactive C4B1 allotype – associated with the haplotype characterized by HLA-A28, -Cw4, -B35, C4A3, C4B1 and HLA-DR6 – carrying the P459L substitution, which is located adjacent to the polymorphic site on C4A6.[126]

Qualitative and Quantitative Methods for the Measurement of Complement Component C4

The need for determining both of the level of plasma C4 protein and the genetic diversity of C4 genes (derived from copy number variation and polymorphic variants) has been generated by studies into the associations with certain disorders or disease risk. Naturally, independent methods are required to check and confirm their presence as well as the accuracy of their measurement; ideally, these methods are used in combination.

Standard immunochemical methods, such as ELISA and radial immunodiffusion are valuable tools for measuring C4 protein level. The methods commonly used to determine C4 not only measure the native proteins, but also their major soluble C4b ore C4c fragments formed during activation and degradation. Apart from the examination of C4 as a marker of whole complement activation, functional activities of C4 proteins need to be measured when a non-functional or dysfunctional variant is suspected.[127]

There are a number of methods for studying the genetic diversity of *C4* genes. For several decades, the number of *C4A* and *C4B* genes was determined from the relative plasma levels of the proteins they encode. Allotyping of the two isotypes is performed jointly, by high voltage agarose gel electrophoresis (HVAGE) of EDTA plasma, followed by immunofixation. The principle of C4 allotyping is based on the marked differences in the electric charge of *C4A* and *C4B* gene products (C4A and C4B proteins), as this leads to different electrophoretic mobility. In order to suppress post-translational glycosylation and incomplete proteolysis, plasma samples must be pretreated with neuraminidase and carboxypeptidase B. The allotypes are determined by their relative positions after electrophoresis and then, the relative (or in some cases absolute) copy number of *C4A* and *C4B* is estimated. When no band is present in the C4A or C4B region of a subject, this means that there is no functional *C4A* or *C4B* gene and the individual may be considered a homozygous C4A*Q0 or C4B*Q0 carrier. The drawback of this method is that the absolute number of *C4A/C4B* genes can not be determined accurately – notwithstanding this, it is still an important technique for the determination of C4 allotypes.[91, 128]

Clearly, straightforward methods for direct counting of *C4A/C4B* copy numbers are of utmost importance. A comprehensive technique, applying the genomic restriction fragment length polymorphism (RFLP) method in combination with Southern blot was developed by Yu and coworkers[104, 107] to determine the accurate number of *C4A* and *C4B* genes. Briefly, genomic DNA is digested with the appropriate restriction enzymes and the resulting fragments are separated by electrophoresis, blotted, and then hybridized with labeled probes. Relative band intensities, which are proportional to relative gene quantity, can be estimated. Based on the *Taq*I and *Psh*AI polymorphic pattern of the *STK19, C4, CYP21,* and *TNX* loci, not only the accurate number of the corresponding genes (*STK19* and *STK19P, C4A* and *C4B, CYP21A1P* and *CYP21A2, TNXA* and *TNXB,* respectively), but the ratio of short and long *C4* genes can be determined, along with the number of RCCX modules on a chromosome. Besides, a further advantage of RFLP analysis is that gene rearrangements such as insertions and deletions can be detected in the modular structure. Nevertheless, the method has several disadvantages: it is quite laborious and time consuming, it requires large amounts of undegraded genomic DNA, as well as the employment of radioisotopes.[92]

As the adaptation of PCR seemed promising to overcome these problems, a number of PCR methods using sequence-specific primers were designed to determine gene copy numbers, polymorphisms, and arrangement in RCCX.[129-134] However, being a semiquantitative assay, conventional PCR combined with gel electrophoresis became widely used only for rapid *C4A* and *C4B* deletion screening. A multiplex PCR and capillary gel electrophoresis (CGE) based, high-throughput approach for *C4A* and *C4B* gene dosage determination was developed.[135] This elaborate method has proven highly time- and cost-effective, hence it is an attractive alternative to the low-throughput, labor-intensive techniques used previously. However, the need for strict compliance with reaction parameters and technology requirements limited the widespread adaptation of this methodology.

Highly sensitive quantitative real-time PCR (qPCR) is one of the most preferred techniques among up to date methods for DNA quantification. It allows for continuous tracking of the accumulating PCR product during the reaction; hence, no subsequent post-PCR analysis is required. Recently, two quantitative real-time polymerase chain reaction (qPCR) approaches have been developed for determining the gene copy number of *C4A* and *C4B*.[105,136] In this approach, fluorescence is generated proportionally to the amount of the PCR product amplified with *C4A* or *C4B* specific primers and probes, and real-time measured fluorescence reaches a pre-specified threshold after a given number of PCR cycles. The number of cycles needed to reach the threshold is highly proportional to the copy number of *C4* genes.

More recently, a novel multiplex ligation-dependent probe amplification (MLPA) assay has been developed with three synthetic probe parts.[137] For MLPA, only small amounts of DNA are required and within one multiplex assay, not only *C4A* and *C4B* gene copy numbers can be determined, but also Chido and Rodgers alleles can be distinguished. Moreover, the assay detects the HERV-K insertion in intron 9 and a silencing CT insertion in exon 29.

Disease Associations of the Complement Components Encoded in the Central MHC Region

Complement Proteins as Marker Alleles of Extended Ancestral Haplotypes in the MHC Region

Conserved extended haplotypes (CEH) or ancestral haplotypes (AH) are characteristic features of the major histocompatibility complex.[138,139] CEHs – genetically fixed units shared by many unrelated individuals – extend over the three main classes of MHC, from class I (*HLA-Cw, -B*) to class II (*HLA-DRB1, -DQB1*), including gene variants (SNPs, microsatellites, copy number polymorphisms) encoded in the central (class III) MHC region. These CEHs consist of continuous sequences at least between *HLA-B* and *-DRB1-DQB1* genes, although some of them extend to *HLA-A* or even beyond, until the olfactory receptor cluster in telomeric direction or to the *HLA-DP* alleles in centromeric direction. Many of these CEHs are closely linked to human – mostly autoimmune – diseases; their existence, however, hinders precise localization of the genes associated with the given disease. CEHs were first defined when the existence of complotypes (consisting of specific variants of the complement protein encoding genes *C2, CFB, C4A* and *C4B* located in the central MHC region) and their strong linkage to some *HLA-B, -Cw* and *-DRB1* alleles were described.[140] Initially, these associations were recognized during pedigree analysis of data obtained in families affected by autoimmune or other diseases, and of control haplotypes occurring in unaffected individuals.[141,142] Later, the existence of these CEHs was confirmed by direct analysis of cell lines from individuals carrying homozygous MHC regions, collected at International Histocompatibility Workshops, Centre d'Etude de Polymorphisme Humain (CEPH) or other sources.[143,144] Eight of these haplotypes were recently sequenced in the framework of the MHC Haplotype Project.[145]

When the two largest registers[144,146] of conserved, extended haplotypes are considered, it seems that most CEHs contains one *C4A* and one *C4B* gene, the majority of which are C4A3 and C4B1, respectively. Specifically, out of the 37 CEHs enlisted in the paper of Dorak et al,[144] 22 had one *C4A* and *C4B* gene each, whereas 13 of them were C4A3, C4B1. The C4A*Q0 variant occurred in only three CEHs, while C4B*Q0 was found much frequently, in 9 extended haplotypes. Duplicated *C4A* and *C4B* genes were detected in three and two extended haplotypes respectively, usually along with the Q0 variant of the other *C4* gene. *C2* was not identified in all haplotypes; however, all but three of the characterized ones had the most common C variant, one extended haplotype contained a C2*Q0 variant, and 2 CEHs contained the C2B variant. Out of the 37 CEHs, 27 had the most common S form of the Bf protein, whereas F, F1 and F3 variants were present in 4, 3 and 3 haplotypes, respectively.

Therefore, when considered individually, complement alleles are markers of a few haplotypes. However, considering them together revealed that the most common complotype (C2C,BfS,C4A3,C4B1) is rare, as it was present in only in 6/37 CEHs,[144] while complotypes of the other CEHs exhibited high variability. When studying disease association with the MHC-encoded complement genes, it is very important to consider the haplotype(s) to which they belong.

Association of the C4A*Q0 Carrier State with Autoimmune Diseases

Clearly, this is the case of an association between SLE or type 1 diabetes and a low copy number of the *C4A* gene (Table 8.1). This is the earliest-recognized and very strong MHC-disease association for both SLE[147-149] and type 1 diabetes.[150, 151] This association was further confirmed by a recent study, in which the copy numbers of *C4A* and *C4B* genes were determined.[152, 153] The authors studied 1241 Caucasian Americans including SLE patients, their first-degree relatives, and healthy controls. In comparison with healthy subjects, patients with SLE were found to carry a low copy number of *C4A* (none or just a single copy), while high (>2) copy number was found to be protective.

However, soon it became clear that C4A*Q0 is a major constituent of the so-called 8.1 ancestral haplotype (HLA-A1, -Cw7, -B8, TNFABa2b3, TNF2, C2C, BfS, C4A*Q0, C4B1, HLA-DRB1 0301,-DRB3 0101, -DQA1 0501, -DQB1 0201).[144, 146, 149, 154] By contrast, in collaboration with N. Mehra and his coworkers, we found a segregation between low copy number of the *C4A* gene and an Indian HLA-DR3-B8 haplotype tightly associated with type 1 diabetes: This haplotype contains the *C4A* gene.[155] This Indian haplotype contained BfF instead of BfS in the Caucasian ancestral haplotype 8.1 and a subtype of it (BfFB) was overrepresented in Asian Indian type 1 diabetic patients.[79] Therefore, it cannot be excluded that the strong association found in Caucasian populations between the low copy number of *C4A* (i.e. 0 or 1 copy) and autoimmune diseases is due to other constituent alleles of the 8.1 ancestral haplotype. Since, it is well known that the 8.1 AH is associated with both a significant prevalence of immune complexes and higher titers of antinuclear antibodies, it is not surprising that carriers of this haplotype are at an increased risk for SLE, type 1 diabetes, and other autoimmune diseases.[156]

Association between C2 and C4 Deficiency and Autoimmune Diseases

Similar to the deficiency of other CP proteins (such as C1q, C1r and C1s), homozygous C2 deficiency, the most frequent (its prevalence is 1/10000 to 1/30000 in Caucasian populations) form of the hereditary deficiency of CP proteins is associated with SLE in 10-30 percent of cases (Table 8.1).[157, 158] CP deficiency states are the strongest known susceptibility factors for development of SLE.[159] As it was detailed above, the most common defect is a deletion in intron 6, which results in a premature stop codon in exon 7 and thereby leading to an arrest of protein synthesis. According to initial descriptions, SLE associated with C2D is generally a mild variant of the disease with predominantly skin and joint manifestations, but without development of severe symptoms including serositis, neuropsychiatric alterations or renal involvement.[160, 161] However, a more recent study performed in a relatively large cohort of 45 patients with homozygous C2D, found no significant difference in disease severity between patients who carry or do not carry homozygous C2 deficiency.[158] According to this study, SLE in C2D starts usually in adulthood, at a mean age of onset of 37 years.[158] There are marked differences between the autoantibody profiles of SLE patients with and without C2D: In the former group, ANA (antinuclear antibodies) and anti-DNA antibodies occur only rarely.[158, 161, 162] By contrast, Jonsson et al[158] found increased levels of anti-phospholipid and anti-C1q antibodies in C2D-SLE. In addition to SLE, an increased susceptibility for mixed-type connective tissue disease and vasculitis was also described for C2D patients.[158] In contrast to homozygous C2D, no increased risk for autoimmune diseases was reported in heterozygous C2 deficiency, which occurs at a 1-2 percent frequency in Caucasians.

Complete C4 deficiency that is, the absence of functional *C4A* and *C4B* genes in both chromosomes, is extremely rare (about 25 cases were reported so far) and is associated with SLE in three-quarter of cases.[163]

Table 8.1: Diseases frequently associated with variations or deficiencies of the complement proteins encoded in the MHC region

	Associated disease	Mechanism
Homozygous C2 deficiency	SLE	Impaired capacity for handling immune complexes, disturbances of cellular waste (apoptotic cell debris)-disposal, aberrant tolerance-induction, abnormality of cytokine regulation
Homozygous C2 deficiency	Increased risk of infections with encapsulated bacteria	Abnormal antibody and complement mediated defense
Variations and mutations in the CFB gene	Age-related macular degeneration (AMD), atypical hemolytic uremic syndrome (HUS)	Increased activation of the alternative pathway
Low copy number of the C4A gene	Different autoimmune diseases	Unknown, linked to the 8.1 ancestral haplotype
Low copy number of the C4B gene	Increased risk of morbidity in cardiovascular diseases, high risk of short-term mortality after acute myocardial infarction	Unknown, may be associated with abnormal function of the 21-hydroxylase enzyme encoded by the CYP21A2 gene next to the C4B gene

Although deficiencies of the CP proteins are present in only a minor subset (about 1%) of SLE patients, explaining the causes of this association is most important, also for a better understanding of the pathomechanism of the disease.[164] On the other hand, C2 and C4 levels are very low during acute exacerbations of SLE and this acquired deficiency may trigger mechanisms similar to those activated by congenital deficiencies. There are various explanations for the strong association between the deficiency of CP proteins and SLE or SLE-like diseases.[164,165] It can result from impaired capacity for handling immune complexes, disturbances of cellular waste-disposal due to overloading of clearance mechanism by apoptotic cell debris, aberrant tolerance-induction, or the abnormality of cytokine regulation.

Association of C2 Deficiency with Infections

C2D is associated not only with SLE, but with an increased susceptibility to certain infections as well (Table 8.1). About 25 percent of C2-deficient homozygotes have increased susceptibility to severe bacterial infections.[166] Predominant pathogens include *S. pneumoniae*, *H. influenzae* and *N. meningitidis* in these patients.[167] In a Swedish study performed in 40 C2D subjects, 57 percent of the patients had a history of invasive infection caused by encapsulated bacteria, mainly *S. pneumoniae*.[168] According to a recent review,[166] C2D subjects had significantly lower serum levels of IgG2, IgG4, and IgD – albeit significantly higher levels of IgA and IgG3 – whereas their serum levels of IgG1 and IgM were similar to those of the controls. C2D patients with an increased susceptibility to bacterial infection had significantly lower mean levels of IgG4 and IgA, than those without infections and with a higher-than-normal mean IgA level. Of 13 C2-deficient homozygotes with infections, 85 percent had IgG4 deficiency, compared to 64 percent of 25 subjects without infections.

Association of the C4B*Q0 Carrier State with Cardiovascular and Other Diseases

As we detailed in a recent review article,[106] our group made original observations almost 20 years ago, while studying the age-dependent distribution of different phenotypic MHC-linked complement allotypes. First, polymorphisms of *C2*, *CFB*, and *C4A/C4B* genes were determined in plasma samples from healthy individuals of different ages. Elderly individuals participating in this and subsequent studies met the criteria of the so-called SENIEUR Protocol[169] that is, could be considered perfectly healthy. Comparing 252 healthy 'young' (<45 years old), and 482 healthy 'old' (61-90 years old) individuals revealed a marked age-related decrease of C4B*Q0-carrier frequency in the 'old' group.[170] This decrease in frequency was dramatic among men (<45, 61-90: 0.176, and 0.0278, respectively), but less marked in women (0.146 vs. 0.068). The frequency of C4B*Q0 carriers found in the 'young' group was in agreement with frequency values reported from several other laboratories, and this suggested that the findings in the 'old' group may be representative also for populations in other countries. Similar findings were obtained, when the study was repeated in another Caucasian population, in Iceland. It turned out, however, that the age-dependent decrease in the percentage of C4B*Q0 carriers was restricted to regular smokers only.[171,172] This finding indicates that C4B*Q0 carrier state (i.e. a 0 or 1 copy of the *C4B* gene in the diploid genome) is associated with a shortened life expectancy in current smokers, as well as this higher risk of premature mortality can be reversed by quitting smoking (Table 8.1).

Having made these observations, we assumed that early elimination of C4B*Q0 carriers from the population of healthy individuals is due to their increased susceptibility to a disease or several diseases with a high mortality rate, as well as that even the survivors can not be considered healthy any longer. If this assumption is true, there should be an increased percentage of C4B*Q0 carriers among patients with these diseases, as compared to age-matched, healthy controls. We found indeed a significantly ($p<0.0001$) higher C4B*Q0 carrier frequency among elderly (>60 years old) Hungarian patients with acute myocardial infarction (AMI),[173] ischemic stroke or transient ischemic attack,[174] and in patients with severe coronary artery disease.[175]

Later, when it had become clear that the selection of C4B*Q0 carriers out of the healthy Icelandic population is dependent on their smoking habits, we also examined smoking status during the comparisons of C4B*Q0 carriers among cardiovascular patients and healthy controls. This study was performed first in Iceland, followed by a confirmatory investigation undertaken in Hungary.[172] Comparing Icelandic and Hungarian AMI patients with Hungarian and Icelandic healthy controls of matching age, revealed a highly significant ($p<0.0001$) increase in the frequency of C4B*Q0 carriers among smokers in both populations, whereas no significant difference was observed among non-smokers. In the same study,[172] we also found a significant ($p=0.005$) increase in the percentage of C4B*Q0 carriers among smoking Icelandic patients with angina pectoris, compared to smoking healthy controls of the same age. Recently, these findings were confirmed by the results of a group from Finland,[176] showing that smokers who carry C4B*Q0 together with HLA-DRB1-01 are at an increased risk for cardiovascular disease.

Finally, we also demonstrated repeatedly, in both countries[173, 177] that short-term mortality after AMI is much higher in C4B*Q0 carriers, than in non-carriers The Icelandic study was performed in 142 AMI patients, followed up for 12 months. Significant differences occurred only for the carrier state of a low *C4B* copy number.[177] The mortality of patients who carried a low (zero or one) *C4B* copy number (C4B*Q0) was significantly ($p=0.003$) higher, than that of those with at least two copies of *C4B*. This association was also found to be limited to regularly smoking patients.[177] As regards the association between high short-term mortality and low *C4B* gene copy number, our results reflect a relationship, which is comparable to – or even stronger than – the other genetic associations reported so far. The hazard ratio of C4B*Q0 carriers for an early death after myocardial infarction was estimated at 4.65 (1.47-14.71) by multiple logistic regression. Mortality after myocardial infarction or after an acute coronary event in general has been found to be associated with polymorphisms in the *IL6* gene (−174 G>C SNP; hazard ratio 3.89 [1.71-8.86]),[178] the insulin-like growth factor-I promoter (hazard ratio 1.49 [1.20-2.10])[179] and, in Orientals, the *LTA* gene (252 A>G SNP; hazard ratio 2.46 [1.24-4.86]).[180]

At present, we cannot provide a definitive explanation for both the increased susceptibility for AMI and the increased risk of early post-AMI mortality, observed in smokers who carry C4B*Q0. Theoretically, three different, but not mutually exclusive explanations are possible: a) Low levels of *C4B* lead to an impaired ability for the safe elimination of immune complexes. This explanation does not seem probable, as no strong association has been described between any homozygous complement deficiency and cardiovascular diseases. b) Since *C4A/C4B* copy number variations are encoded in the MHC region known to be rich in extended ancestral haplotypes, it cannot be excluded that the lack of *C4B* gene is linked to one of these haplotypes. However, according to the literature data presented above and as shown by a recent family study, C4B*Q0 is not significantly linked to any of the extended haplotypes. c) Low *C4B* copy number – that is, the lack of the *C4B* gene in one or both chromosomes – may be linked to impaired function of the neighboring *CYP21A2* gene. This impairment, if it exists, may entail serious consequences (including abnormalities of steroid metabolism) and an increase by indirect mechanisms, such as enhanced IL-6 synthesis,[181] may lead to an excessive risk of cardiovascular disease and increased short-term mortality.

If a link between C4B*Q0 and impaired 21-hydroxylase function can be demonstrated, a reasonable and testable hypothesis for a C4B*Q0-associated increase in cardiovascular disease morbidity/mortality can be formulated. Our group is currently studying the mechanism of this linkage, using different techniques.

In addition to cardiovascular diseases, additional human pathologies were also reported to occur more frequently in carriers of C4B*Q0. Interestingly, a positive association (increased risk) was found with two behavioral disorders, i.e. attention deficit hyperactivity disorder[182] and autism.[183-185] The strong association reported between Henoch-Schönlein purpura – a vasculitis of unknown etiology – and C4B*Q0 carrier state is explained by the deficient handling of immune complexes in carriers of low *C4B* copy numbers.[186] Two infection-related pathological conditions, erythema nodosum in leprosy[187] and familiar HCV-related liver cirrhosis[188] were also reported to be linked to a low *C4B* gene copy number.

The Role of Bf and C2 in Two Complement-mediated Diseases: Age-related Macular Degeneration and Atypical Hemolytic Uremic Syndrome

The relationship of age-related macular degeneration (AMD) – the leading cause of blindness in industrialized countries affecting 30-50 million elderly individuals globally – and the complement system was described by several groups concomitantly, in 2005 (Table 8.1).[189-191] This initial observation was repeated in Caucasian and other populations by several other groups (reviewed by [192]). AMD is a degenerative disorder, mainly affecting the central macular region of the retina. It is characterized by the formation of drusen, pigment epithelial changes and choroidal neovascularization. The etiology of the disease is complex and susceptibility is influenced by both environmental (e.g. cigarette smoking) and genetic factors. Variants (especially Y402H) and haplotypes of the complement factor H gene (*CFH*) on chromosome 1q32 were found to be strongly associated with the disease. The rare allele of the Y402H polymorphism, involving a tyrosine to *histidine* change at codon 402, impairs the affinity of the factor H molecule to retinal/macular surfaces, and this leads to a less effective inhibition of local complement activation. Interestingly enough, different complement activation products were detected recently in the blood of AMD patients, indicating that systemic complement activation had occurred.[193] The levels of complement activation products were correlated to *CFH* haplotypes. Mutation in the *CFH* gene is now considered responsible for a substantial portion of genetic risk: some variants and haplotypes of the gene increase, whereas others decrease the susceptibility for AMD. Complement proteins are present in the drusen and furthermore, factor H – being an important regulator of the alternative pathway – may markedly influence the intraocular events leading to AMD.

Since, other complement proteins are also involved in the functioning or the regulation of the alternative pathway, it seemed reasonable to study, whether their variants may also be connected with the disease. Two complement proteins encoded in the central MHC region, Bf and C2 were also found associated with AMD risk by Gold et al.[31] These authors conducted a study in two independent cohorts of approximately 900 individuals with AMD and approximately 400 matched controls. Haplotype analyses identified a statistically significant, common risk haplotype (H1) and two protective haplotypes. The L9H variant of *CFB* and the E318D variant of *C2* (H10), as well as the R32Q variant of *CFB* (encoding the BfFA subtype of BfF) and a variant in intron 10 of *C2* (H7), confer a significantly reduced risk of AMD (odds ratio = 0.44 (0.33-0.60), $p=8.45 \times 10^{-8}$ and 0.36 (0.23-0.56), $p=4.14 \times 10^{-6}$, respectively). Combined analysis of the *C2* and *CFB* haplotypes and *CFH* variants shows that 56 percent of unaffected controls harbor at least one protective CFH or C2/BF haplotype, whereas 74 percent of AMD patients lack any protective haplotype. The authors concluded[31] that the modified risk of AMD is confined to the *C2*/*CFB* region, because the disease-associated haplotypes did not exhibit any significant linkage disequilibrium to class III or class II antigens. This important observation was replicated almost immediately in both case-control and family studies by several groups.[68, 194] but could not be reproduced in a study performed in a Chinese population.[77] In a very recent multilocus analysis,[195] Age-related Eye Disease Study cohorts subjects were genotyped among others for SNPs of *CFH*, *C2*, *CFB*, *C3* genes. One of the two studied SNPs in *CFB*, rs4151667 conferred a significantly decreased (OR: 0.36 (0.19-0.70) $p=0.002$) risk of AMD to carriers. A similar risk could be attributed to two SNPs of *C2*, but these were in significant linkage disequilibrium with the rs4151667 SNP of *CFB*. Interestingly enough, the authors found an interaction between one SNP of *CFB* and Y402H of *CFH*, indicating that variant Bf effectively cancels the aberrant activity of a mutated Hf protein, to that of the wild-type phenotype. According to the study of Montes et al,[196] the functional basis of the protection against AMD conferred by a common polymorphism of Bf is its decreased potential to form AP C3 convertase and amplify complement activation.

Recently, the connection between Bf and another complement-mediated disease – atypical hemolytic uremic syndrome (HUS) – was also described (Table 8.1).[70] HUS is a disease characterized by thrombocytopenia, Coombs-negative hemolytic anemia, and acute renal failure. Most cases of HUS (typical form) evolve after prodromal diarrhea and are associated with *E. coli* infection. Five to ten percent of the cases (atypical HUS), however, are not associated with infection and have the poorest prognosis. Atypical HUS was found related to mutations or polymorphisms of several complement regulator proteins, such as Hf,[197] membrane cofactor protein,[198] and factor I.[199] Goicoechea de Jorge et al[70] identified a subgroup of atypical HUS patients, showing persistent AP activation and found within this subgroup two families carrying a mutation in the Bf gene. Both were gain-of-function mutations resulting in enhanced formation of AP C3-cleaving enzyme (C3bBb) or an increased resistance to inactivation by complement regulators. This finding further supports the critical role of the alternative complement pathway in the pathogenesis of atypical HUS.

CONCLUSION

The three complement proteins, C2, Bf and C4 – encoded by four genes (*C2*, *CFB*, *C4A* and *C4B*) in the central part of MHC – have major physiological functions. Being key factors in the activation of complement system, these proteins are indispensable for the most important steps of complement activation, i.e. the cleavage and activation of C3 and C5 molecules. Complement is part of the innate immune system. The alternative pathway (AP) is one of the phylogenetically oldest immune mechanisms. By contrast, the classical pathway (CP) is one of the most important effector mechanisms of the acquired humoral immune response. Interestingly enough, the precursors of enzymatically active complement proteins of the AP and CP (Bf and C2, respectively) have very similar functions, indicating that they were generated by gene duplication. The consequences of the deficiency of the two genes, however, are quite different. C2 deficiency is the commonest complement defect, which has no direct causal role in any disease, but can be associated with an increased risk of autoimmune disease or bacterial infections. By contrast, not a single case of Bf deficiency has yet been described, indicating that this is presumably a lethal mutation.

Recently, two severe diseases, i.e. age-related macular degeneration and atypical hemolytic uremic syndrome were recognized as at least partially complement-mediated entities. The hallmark of these diseases is increased AP activation. It is not surprising therefore, that particular polymorphisms of Bf are protective against AMD, whereas a gain-of function mutation of the same protein was found to increase the risk of atypical HUS.

The *C4* genes are encoded in a peculiar part of the central MHC and together with three other types of genes, they constitute the so-called RCCX module. *C4* genes exhibit several different types of polymorphisms (they are among the most polymorphic genes in the human genome) including module variations (the RCXX modules may be present in 1, 2, 3 and rarely 4 copies), resulting in copy number variations of the *C4* genes. In addition, *C4* genes may be short or long (due to an insertion of a retrovirus), and can be either *C4A* or *C4B*, encoding two isoforms with different functions of the C4 protein. Both C4A and C4B proteins have many different allotypes as well. Due to this high degree of polymorphism, it is not surprising that the imbalance of *C4* genes, mainly low copy number of the *C4A* and *C4B* genes, is associated with an increased risk of several serious disorders, such as different autoimmune or cardiovascular diseases.

KEY ISSUES AND FUTURE DIRECTIONS

One of the most important obstacles for the evaluation of diseases related to the MHC region is the very strong linkage disequilibrium existing within this region. Since many extended haplotypes (associated with severe autoimmune diseases including multiple sclerosis or systemic lupus erythematosus) contain deficient complement genes (such as the ancestral haplotype 8.1 lacking *C4A*, the 18.1 carrying C2*Q0 or a lot of others that do not harbor *C4B* genes), it would be justified to re-evaluate systematically the role of the complement genes in disease associations.

The proteins encoded in the MHC region participate – along with other complement proteins – not only in physiological complement activation, but also in pathological complement activation leading to several serious and common diseases (such as acute myocardial infarction or stroke). In view of the foregoing and of the new approach of therapeutic interventions, complement activation-inhibiting therapy can be expected to appear in clinical practice soon. Apparently, the inhibition of the steps of complement activation (C3 and C5 cleavage and activation), in which MHC-encoded complement proteins participate, are the primary targets of such interventions. A monoclonal antibody inhibiting C5 cleavage has already been used with success in paroxysmal nocturnal hemoglobinuria and coronary bypass operations; therefore, many other applications of this agent can be expected in the near future.

TAKE-HOME MESSAGES

- The three complement proteins (C2, Bf, C4) encoded in the central MHC region have major functions in the activation of the classical/lectin and alternative complement pathways, as the constituents of C3 and C5 convertase enzymes.
- Genes of C2 and Bf have similar organization and the two encoded proteins are structurally and functionally very similar as well.
- C4 protein exists in two isoforms, C4A and C4B that differ in several functions. The two forms are encoded by two genes, *C4A* and *C4B*, both of which exhibit copy number variation.
- Homozygous deficiency of C2 is the most common complement defect and it is associated with increased risk of SLE and certain bacterial infections.
- Low copy number of the *C4B* gene is associated with an increased risk of cardiovascular diseases and high short-term mortality after acute myocardial infarction.
- Both C2 and Bf have a significant modifying effect on a mainly complement-mediated disease, age-related macular degeneration, which is the most frequent cause of blindness in the industrial world.

REFERENCES

1. Milner CM, Campbell RD. Genetic organization of the human MHC class III region. Front Biosci 2001;6:D914-26.
2. Yu CY. Molecular genetics of the human MHC complement gene cluster. Exp Clin Immunogenet. 1998;15:213-30.
3. Alper CA, Awdeh ZL, Yunis EJ. Complotypes, extended haplotypes, male segregation distortion, and disease markers. Hum Immunol 1986;15:366-73.
4. Oglesby TJ, Ueda A, Volanakis JE. Radioassays for quantitation of intact complement proteins C2 and B in human serum. J Immunol Methods 1988;110:55-62.
5. Tomana M, Niemann M, Garner C, Volanakis JE. Carbohydrate composition of the second, third and fifth components and factors B and D of human complement. Mol Immunol 1985;22:107-11.
6. Smith CA, Vogel CW, Muller-Eberhard HJ. MHC Class III products: An electron microscopic study of the C3 convertases of human complement. J Exp Med 1984;159:324-9.
7. Bentley DR. Primary structure of human complement component C2. Homology to two unrelated protein families. Biochem J 1986;239:339-45.
8. Xu Y, Volanakis JE. Contribution of the complement control protein modules of C2 in C4b binding assessed by analysis of C2/factor B chimeras. J Immunol 1997;158:5958-65.
9. Wetsel RA, Kulics J, Lokki ML, et al. Type II human complement C2 deficiency. Allele-specific amino acid substitutions (Ser189 → Phe; Gly444 → Arg) cause impaired C2 secretion. J Biol Chem 1996;271:5824-31.
10. Krishnan V, Xu Y, Macon K, Volanakis JE, Narayana SV. The crystal structure of C2a, the catalytic fragment of classical pathway C3 and C5 convertase of human complement. J Mol Biol 2007;367:224-33.
11. Carroll MC, Katzman P, Alicot EM, et al. Linkage map of the human major histocompatibility complex including the tumor necrosis factor genes. Proc Natl Acad Sci USA 1987;84:8535-9.
12. Dunham I, Sargent CA, Trowsdale J, Campbell RD. Molecular mapping of the human major histocompatibility complex by pulsed-field gel electrophoresis. Proc Natl Acad Sci USA 1987;84:7237-41.
13. Zhu ZB, Hsieh SL, Bentley DR, Campbell RD, Volanakis JE. A variable number of tandem repeats locus within the human complement C2 gene is associated with a retroposon derived from a human endogenous retrovirus. J Exp Med 1992;175:1783-7.
14. Cheng J, Volanakis JE. Alternatively spliced transcripts of the human complement C2 gene. J Immunol 1994;152:1774-82.
15. Perlmutter DH, Cole FS, Goldberger G, Colten HR. Distinct primary translation products from human liver mRNA give rise to secreted and cell-associated forms of complement protein C2. J Biol Chem 1984;259:10380-5.
16. Gerritsma JS, Gerritsen AF, De Ley M, van Es LA, Daha MR. Interferon-gamma induces biosynthesis of complement components C2, C4 and factor H by human proximal tubular epithelial cells. Cytokine 1997;9:276-83.
17. Lappin DF, Guc D, Hill A, McShane T, Whaley K. Effect of interferon-gamma on complement gene expression in different cell types. Biochem J 1992;281 (Pt 2):437-42.
18. Sullivan KE, Wu LC, Campbell RD, Valle D, Winkelstein JA. Transcriptional regulation of the gene for the second component of human complement: promoter analysis. Eur J Immunol 1994;24:393-400.
19. Sullivan KE. Four conserved promoter motifs regulate transcription of the gene encoding human complement component C2. J Immunol 1997;158:5868-73.
20. Ashfield R, Patel AJ, Bossone SA, et al. MAZ-dependent termination between closely spaced human complement genes. Embo J 1994;13:5656-67.
21. Alper CA. Inherited deficiencies of complement components in man. Immunol Lett 1987;14:175-81.
22. Johnson CA, Densen P, Hurford RK, Jr., Colten HR, Wetsel RA. Type I human complement C2 deficiency. A 28-base pair gene deletion causes skipping of exon 6 during RNA splicing. J Biol Chem 1992;267:9347-53.
23. Fu SM, Kunkel HG, Brusman HP, Allen FH, Jr., Fotino M. Evidence for linkage between HL-A histocompatibility genes and those involved in the synthesis of the second component of complement. J Exp Med 1974;140:1108-11.

24. Clavijo OP, Delgado JC, Awdeh ZL, et al. HLA-Cw alleles associated with HLA extended haplotypes and C2 deficiency. Tissue Antigens 1998;52:282-5.
25. Wang X, Circolo A, Lokki ML, Shackelford PG, Wetsel RA, Colten HR. Molecular heterogeneity in deficiency of complement protein C2 type I. Immunology 1998;93:184-91.
26. Zhu ZB, Atkinson TP, Volanakis JE. A novel type II complement C2 deficiency allele in an African-American family. J Immunol 1998;161:578-84.
27. Alper CA. Inherited structural polymorphism in human C2: Evidence for genetic linkage between C2 and Bf. J Exp Med 1976;144:1111-5.
28. Raum D, Glass D, Carpenter CB, Schur PH, Alper CA. Mapping of the structural gene for the second component of complement with respect to the human major histocompatibility complex. Am J Hum Genet 1979;31:35-41.
29. Tokunaga K, Araki C, Juji T, Omoto K. Genetic polymorphism of the complement C2 in Japanese. Hum Genet 1981;58:213-6.
30. Varga L, Alper CA, Zam Z, Fust G. Decreased inhibition of immune precipitation by sera with the C2 B allotype. Clin Immunol Immunopathol 1991;59:65-71.
31. Gold B, Merriam JE, Zernant J, et al. Variation in factor B (BF) and complement component 2 (C2) genes is associated with age-related macular degeneration. Nat Genet 2006;38:458-62.
32. Zhu ZB, Volanakis JE. Allelic associations of multiple RFLPs of the gene encoding complement protein C2. Am J Hum Genet. 1990;46:956-62.
33. Greffard A, Bourgarit JJ, le Maho S, Lambre CR. Determination of the complement component C2 by ELISA in human serum and bronchoalveolar lavage fluids. Immunol Lett 1987;15:145-51.
34. Varga L, Fust G. Assays for complement proteins encoded in the class III region of human MHC. Curr Protoc Immunol 2005;Chapter 13:Unit 13 7.
35. Meo T, Atkinson JP, Bernoco M, Bernoco D, Ceppellini R. Structural heterogeneity of C2 Complement protein and its genetic variants in man: A new polymorphism of the HLA region. Proc Natl Acad Sci USA 1977;74:1672-5.
36. Doxiadis G, Doxiadis I, Grosse-Wilde H. Polymorphism of human C2 detected by immunoblotting. Hum Genet 1985;70:355-8.
37. Segurado OG, Arnaiz-Villena A. Simultaneous detection of allotypes in native and activated human C2 by isoelectric focusing and silver staining. J Immunol Methods 1989;117:9-15.
38. Uring-Lambert B, Gas S, Goetz J, et al. Detection of the genetic polymorphism of human C2 (native protein and C2a fragment) by immunoblotting after polyacrylamide gel isoelectric focusing. Complement 1985;2:185-92.
39. Woods DE, Edge MD, Colten HR. Isolation of a complementary DNA clone for the human complement protein C2 and its use in the identification of a restriction fragment length polymorphism. J Clin Invest 1984;74:634-8.
40. Cross SJ, Edwards JH, Bentley DR, Campbell RD. DNA polymorphism of the C2 and factor B genes. Detection of a restriction fragment length polymorphism which subdivides haplotypes carrying the C2C and factor B F alleles. Immunogenetics 1985;21:39-48.
41. Bentley DR, Campbell RD, Cross SJ. DNA polymorphism of the C2 locus. Immunogenetics 1985;22:377-90.
42. Ratanachaiyavong S, Campbell RD, McGregor AM. Enhanced resolution of the SstI polymorphic variants of the C2 locus: Description of a new size class. Hum Immunol 1989;26:310-20.
43. Hall RE, Blaese RM, Davis AE, 3rd, et al. Cooperative interaction of factor B and other complement components with mononuclear cells in the antibody-independent lysis of xenogeneic erythrocytes. J Exp Med 1982;156:834-43.
44. Gotze O, Bianco C, Cohn ZA. The induction of macrophage spreading by factor B of the properdin system. J Exp Med 1979;149:372-86.
45. Sundsmo JS, Wood LM. Activated factor B (Bb) of the alternative pathway of complement activation cleaves and activates plasminogen. J Immunol 1981;127:877-80.
46. Kolb WP, Morrow PR, Tamerius JD. Ba and Bb fragments of factor B activation: Fragment production, biological activities, neoepitope expression and quantitation in clinical samples. Complement Inflamm 1989;6:175-204.
47. Peters MG, Ambrus JL, Jr., Fauci AS, Brown EJ. The Bb fragment of complement factor B acts as a B cell growth factor. J Exp Med 1988;168:1225-35.
48. Praz F, Ruuth E. Growth-supporting activity of fragment Ba of the human alternative complement pathway for activated murine B lymphocytes. J Exp Med 1986;163:1349-54.
49. Campbell RD, Bentley DR, Morley BJ. The factor B and C2 genes. Philos Trans R Soc Lond B Biol Sci 1984;306:367-78.
50. Wu LC, Morley BJ, Campbell RD. Cell-specific expression of the human complement protein factor B gene: Evidence for the role of two distinct 5'-flanking elements. Cell 1987;48:331-42.
51. Huang Y, Krein PM, Muruve DA, Winston BW. Complement factor B gene regulation: Synergistic effects of TNF-alpha and IFN-gamma in macrophages. J Immunol 2002;169:2627-35.
52. Huang Y, Krein PM, Winston BW. Characterization of IFN-gamma regulation of the complement factor B gene in macrophages. Eur J Immunol 2001;31:3676-86.
53. Perlmutter DH, Goldberger G, Dinarello CA, Mizel SB, Colten HR. Regulation of class III major histocompatibility complex gene products by interleukin-1. Science 1986;232:850-2.
54. Perlmutter DH, Colten HR, Adams SP, May LT, Sehgal PB, Fallon RJ. A cytokine-selective defect in interleukin-1 beta-mediated acute phase gene expression in a subclone

of the human hepatoma cell line (HEPG2). J Biol Chem 1989;264:7669-74.
55. Ripoche J, Mitchell JA, Erdei A, et al. Interferon gamma induces synthesis of complement alternative pathway proteins by human endothelial cells in culture. J Exp Med 1988;168:1917-22.
56. Hasty LA, Brockman WW, Lambris JD, Lyttle CR. Hormonal regulation of complement factor B in human endometrium. Am J Reprod Immunol 1993;30:63-7.
57. Lappin DF, Whaley K. Modulation of complement gene expression by glucocorticoids. Biochem J 1991;280 (Pt 1):117-23.
58. Circolo A, Welgus HG, Pierce GF, Kramer J, Strunk RC. Differential regulation of the expression of proteinases/antiproteinases in fibroblasts. Effects of interleukin-1 and platelet-derived growth factor. J Biol Chem 1991;266:12283-8.
59. Circolo A, Pierce GF, Katz Y, Strunk RC. Anti-inflammatory effects of polypeptide growth factors. Platelet-derived growth factor, epidermal growth factor, and fibroblast growth factor inhibit the cytokine-induced expression of the alternative complement pathway activator factor B in human fibroblasts. J Biol Chem 1990;265:5066-71.
60. Matsumoto M, Fukuda W, Circolo A, et al. Abrogation of the alternative complement pathway by targeted deletion of murine factor B. Proc Natl Acad Sci USA 1997;94:8720-5.
61. Lokki ML, Koskimies SA. Allelic differences in hemolytic activity and protein concentration of BF molecules are found in association with particular HLA haplotypes. Immunogenetics 1991;34:242-6.
62. Mortensen JP, Lamm LU. Quantitative differences between complement factor-B phenotypes. Immunology 1981;42:505-11.
63. Davrinche C, Abbal M, Clerc A. Molecular characterization of human complement factor B subtypes. Immunogenetics 1990;32:309-12.
64. Campbell RD. The molecular genetics and polymorphism of C2 and factor B. Br Med Bull 1987;43:37-49.
65. Alper CA, Boenisch T, Watson L. Genetic polymorphism in human glycine-rich beta-glycoprotein. J Exp Med 1972;135:68-80.
66. Geserick G, Abbal M, Mauff G, Siemens I. Factor B (BF) nomenclature statement. Complement Inflamm 1990;7:255-60.
67. Siemens I, Brenden M, Mauff G, et al. Apparently non-expressed alleles of factor B (BF) code for hypomorphic proteins. Immunogenetics 1992;37:24-8.
68. Maller J, George S, Purcell S, et al. Common variation in three genes, including a noncoding variant in CFH, strongly influences risk of age-related macular degeneration. Nat Genet 2006;38:1055-9.
69. Richardson AJ, Islam FM, Guymer RH, Baird PN. Analysis of rare variants in the complement component 2 (C2) and factor B (BF) genes refine association for age-related macular degeneration (AMD). Invest Ophthalmol Vis Sci 2009;50:540-3.
70. Goicoechea de Jorge E, Harris CL, Esparza-Gordillo J, et al. Gain-of-function mutations in complement factor B are associated with atypical hemolytic uremic syndrome. Proc Natl Acad Sci USA 2007;104:240-5.
71. Mancini G, Carbonara AO, Heremans JF. Immuno-chemical quantitation of antigens by single radial immunodiffusion. Immunochemistry 1965;2:235-54.
72. Giclas PC. Alternative pathway evaluation. Curr Protoc Immunol. 2001; Chapter 13:Unit 13 2.
73. Alper CA, Johnson AM. Immunofixation electrophoresis: A technique for the study of protein polymorphism. Vox Sang 1969;17:445-52.
74. Suzuki K, Harumoto T, Ito S, Matsumoto H. Subtyping of Factor-B by Agarose-Gel Electrophoresis. Electrophoresis 1987;8:481-5.
75. Geserick G, Patzelt D. Factor B (BF) subtyping by isoelectric focusing: methods, nomenclatures, genetics and forensic application. Electrophoresis 1988;9:418-21.
76. Teng YS, Tan SG. Subtyping of properdin factor B (Bf) by isoelectrofocusing. Hum Hered 1982;32:362-6.
77. Chu J, Zhou CC, Lu N, Zhang X, Dong FT. Genetic variants in three genes and smoking show strong associations with susceptibility to exudative age-related macular degeneration in a Chinese population. Chin Med J (Engl) 2008;121:2525-33.
78. Jahn I, Mejia JE, Thomas M, et al. Genomic analysis of the F subtypes of human complement factor B. Eur J Immunogenet 1994;21:415-23.
79. Kumar N, Kaur G, Tandon N, Mehra NK. Allotyping human complement factor B in Asian Indian type 1 diabetic patients. Tissue Antigens 2008;72:517-24.
80. Campbell RD, Law SK, Reid KB, Sim RB. Structure, organization, and regulation of the complement genes. Annu Rev Immunol 1988;6:161-95.
81. Martinez OP, Longman-Jacobsen N, Davies R, et al. Genetics of human complement component C4 and evolution the central MHC. Front Biosci 2001;6:D904-13.
82. Law SK, Lichtenberg NA, Levine RP. Covalent binding and hemolytic activity of complement proteins. Proc Natl Acad Sci USA 1980;77:7194-8.
83. Chan AC, Atkinson JP. Oligosaccharide structure of human C4. J Immunol 1985;134:1790-8.
84. Hortin G, Chan AC, Fok KF, Strauss AW, Atkinson JP. Sequence analysis of the COOH terminus of the alpha-chain of the fourth component of human complement. Identification of the site of its extracellular cleavage. J Biol Chem 1986;261:9065-9.
85. Dodds AW, Ren XD, Willis AC, Law SK. The reaction mechanism of the internal thioester in the human complement component C4. Nature 1996; 379:177-9.
86. Takata Y, Kinoshita T, Kozono H, et al. Covalent association of C3b with C4b within C5 convertase of the classical complement pathway. J Exp Med 1987;165:1494-507.

87. Hugli TE, Kawahara MS, Unson CG, Molinar-Rode R, Erickson BW. The active site of human C4a anaphylatoxin. Mol Immunol 1983;20:637-45.
88. Dierich MP, Schulz TF, Eigentler A, Huemer H, Schwable W. Structural and functional relationships among receptors and regulators of the complement system. Mol Immunol 1988;25:1043-51.
89. Finco O, Li S, Cuccia M, Rosen FS, Carroll MC. Structural differences between the two human complement C4 isotypes affect the humoral immune response. J Exp Med 1992;175:537-43.
90. Law SK, Dodds AW. The internal thioester and the covalent binding properties of the complement proteins C3 and C4. Protein Sci 1997;6:263-74.
91. Awdeh ZL, Alper CA. Inherited structural polymorphism of the fourth component of human complement. Proc Natl Acad Sci USA 1980;77:3576-80.
92. Wu YL, Yang Y, Chung EK, et al. Phenotypes, genotypes and disease susceptibility associated with gene copy number variations: Complement C4 CNVs in European American healthy subjects and those with systemic lupus erythematosus. Cytogenet Genome Res 2008;123:131-41.
93. Belt KT, Carroll MC, Porter RR. The structural basis of the multiple forms of human complement component C4. Cell 1984;36:907-14.
94. Carroll MC, Alper CA. Polymorphism and molecular genetics of human C4. Br Med Bull 1987;43:50-65.
95. Chu X, Rittner C, Schneider PM. Length polymorphism of the human complement component C4 gene is due to an ancient retroviral integration. Exp Clin Immunogenet 1995;12:74-81.
96. Saxena K, Kitzmiller KJ, Wu YL, et al. Great genotypic and phenotypic diversities associated with copy-number variations of complement C4 and RP-C4-CYP21-TNX (RCCX) modules: A comparison of Asian-Indian and European American Populations. Mol Immunol 2009;46:1289-303.
97. Yu CY, Chung EK, Yang Y, et al. Dancing with complement C4 and the RP-C4-CYP21-TNX (RCCX) modules of the major histocompatibility complex. Prog Nucleic Acid Res Mol Biol 2003;75:217-92.
98. Yu CY, Whitacre CC. Sex, MHC and complement C4 in autoimmune diseases. Trends Immunol 2004;25:694-9.
99. Yang Y, Chung EK, Zhou B, et al. Diversity in intrinsic strengths of the human complement system: Serum C4 protein concentrations correlate with C4 gene size and polygenic variations, hemolytic activities, and body mass index. J Immunol 2003;171:2734-45.
100. Moulds JM, Warner NB, Arnett FC. Quantitative and antigenic differences in complement component C4 between American blacks and whites. Complement Inflamm 1991;8:281-7.
101. Horton R, Wilming L, Rand V, et al. Gene map of the extended human MHC. Nat Rev Genet 2004;5:889-99.
102. Yang Z, Mendoza AR, Welch TR, Zipf WB, Yu CY. Modular variations of the human major histocompatibility complex class III genes for serine/threonine kinase RP, complement component C4, steroid 21-hydroxylase CYP21, and tenascin TNX (the RCCX module). A mechanism for gene deletions and disease associations. J Biol Chem 1999;274:12147-56.
103. Shen L, Wu LC, Sanlioglu S, et al. Structure and genetics of the partially duplicated gene RP located immediately upstream of the complement C4A and the C4B genes in the HLA class III region. Molecular cloning, exon-intron structure, composite retroposon, and breakpoint of gene duplication. J Biol Chem 1994;269:8466-76.
104. Blanchong CA, Zhou B, Rupert KL, et al. Deficiencies of human complement component C4A and C4B and heterozygosity in length variants of RP-C4-CYP21-TNX (RCCX) modules in caucasians. The load of RCCX genetic diversity on major histocompatibility complex-associated disease. J Exp Med 2000;191:2183-96.
105. Wu YL, Savelli SL, Yang Y, et al. Sensitive and specific real-time polymerase chain reaction assays to accurately determine copy number variations (CNVs) of human complement C4A, C4B, C4-long, C4-short, and RCCX modules: Elucidation of C4 CNVs in 50 consanguineous subjects with defined HLA genotypes. J Immunol 2007;179:3012-25.
106. Szilagyi A, Fust G. Diseases associated with the low copy number of the C4B gene encoding C4, the fourth component of complement. Cytogenet Genome Res 2008;123:118-30.
107. Chung EK, Yang Y, Rennebohm RM, et al. Genetic sophistication of human complement components C4A and C4B and RP-C4-CYP21-TNX (RCCX) modules in the major histocompatibility complex. Am J Hum Genet 2002;71:823-37. Epub 2002 Sep 11.
108. Volanakis JE. Transcriptional regulation of complement genes. Annu Rev Immunol 1995;13:277-305.
109. Blanchong CA, Chung EK, Rupert KL, et al. Genetic, structural and functional diversities of human complement components C4A and C4B and their mouse homologues, Slp and C4. Int Immunopharmacol 2001;1:365-92.
110. Falus A, Kramer J, Walcz E, et al. Unequal expression of complement C4A and C4B genes in rheumatoid synovial cells, human monocytoid and hepatoma-derived cell lines. Immunology 1989;68:133-6.
111. Ulgiati D, Subrata LS, Abraham LJ. The role of Sp family members, basic Kruppel-like factor, and E box factors in the basal and IFN-gamma regulated expression of the human complement C4 promoter. J Immunol 2000;164:300-7.
112. Vaishnaw AK, Mitchell TJ, Rose SJ, Walport MJ, Morley BJ. Regulation of transcription of the TATA-less human complement component C4 gene. J Immunol 1998;160:4353-60.
113. Hauptmann G, Tappeiner G, Schifferli JA. Inherited deficiency of the fourth component of human complement. Immunodefic Rev 1988;1:3-22.
114. Samano ES, Ribeiro Lde M, Gorescu RG, Rocha KC, Grumach AS. Involvement of C4 allotypes in the

pathogenesis of human diseases. Rev Hosp Clin Fac Med Sao Paulo 2004;59:138-44.
115. Braun L, Schneider PM, Giles CM, Bertrams J, Rittner C. Null alleles of human complement C4. Evidence for pseudogenes at the C4A locus and for gene conversion at the C4B locus. J Exp Med 1990;171:129-40.
116. Barba G, Rittner C, Schneider PM. Genetic basis of human complement C4A deficiency. Detection of a point mutation leading to nonexpression. J Clin Invest 1993;91:1681-6.
117. Lokki ML, Circolo A, Ahokas P, Rupert KL, Yu CY, Colten HR. Deficiency of human complement protein C4 due to identical frameshift mutations in the C4A and C4B genes. J Immunol 1999;162:3687-93.
118. Mauff G, Luther B, Schneider PM, et al. Reference typing report for complement component C4. Exp Clin Immunogenet 1998;15:249-60.
119. O'Neill GJ, Yang SY, Tegoli J, Berger R, Dupont B. Chido and Rodgers blood groups are distinct antigenic components of human complement C4. Nature 1978;273:668-70.
120. Tilley CA, Romans DG, Crookston MC. Localization of Chido and Rodgers determinants to the C4d fragment of human C4. Nature 1978;276:713-5.
121. Giles CM, Uring-Lambert B, Goetz J, et al. Antigenic determinants expressed by human C4 allotypes; a study of 325 families provides evidence for the structural antigenic model. Immunogenetics 1988;27:442-8.
122. Yu CY, Belt KT, Giles CM, Campbell RD, Porter RR. Structural basis of the polymorphism of human complement components C4A and C4B: Gene size, reactivity and antigenicity. Embo J 1986;5:2873-81.
123. Yu CY, Campbell RD, Porter RR. A structural model for the location of the Rodgers and the Chido antigenic determinants and their correlation with the human complement component C4A/C4B isotypes. Immunogenetics 1988;27:399-405.
124. Anderson MJ, Milner CM, Cotton RG, Campbell RD. The coding sequence of the hemolytically inactive C4A6 allotype of human complement component C4 reveals that a single arginine to tryptophan substitution at beta-chain residue 458 is the likely cause of the defect. J Immunol 1992;148:2795-802.
125. Kinoshita T, Dodds AW, Law SK, Inoue K. The low C5 convertase activity of the C4A6 allotype of human complement component C4. Biochem J 1989;261:743-8.
126. McLean RH, Niblack G, Julian B, et al. Hemolytically inactive C4B complement allotype caused by a proline to leucine mutation in the C5-binding site. J Biol Chem 1994;269:27727-31.
127. Mollnes TE, Jokiranta TS, Truedsson L, Nilsson B, Rodriguez de Cordoba S, Kirschfink M. Complement analysis in the 21st century. Mol Immunol 2007;44: 3838-49.
128. Sim E, Cross SJ. Phenotyping of human complement component C4, a class-III HLA antigen. Biochem J 1986;239:763-7.
129. Barba GM, Braun-Heimer L, Rittner C, Schneider PM. A new PCR-based typing of the Rodgers and Chido antigenic determinants of the fourth component of human complement. Eur J Immunogenet 1994;21:325-39.
130. Chung EK, Yang Y, Rupert KL, et al. Determining the one, two, three, or four long and short loci of human complement C4 in a major histocompatibility complex haplotype encoding C4A or C4B proteins. Am J Hum Genet 2002; 71:810-22.
131. Grant SF, Kristjansdottir H, Steinsson K, et al. Long PCR detection of the C4A null allele in B8-C4AQ0-C4B1-DR3. J Immunol Methods 2000;244:41-7.
132. Lee HH, Chang SF, Tseng YT, Lee YJ. Identification of the size and antigenic determinants of the human C4 gene by a polymerase chain-reaction-based amplification method. Anal Biochem 2006;357:122-7.
133. Man XY, Luo HR, Li XP, Yao YG, Mao CZ, Zhang YP. Polymerase chain reaction based C4AQ0 and C4BQ0 genotyping: Association with systemic lupus erythematosus in South West Han Chinese. Ann Rheum Dis 2003;62:71-3.
134. Tseng YT, Lee HH, Lee YJ. An investigation of the C4 gene arrangement in ethnic Chinese (Taiwanese). Int J Immunogenet 2008;35:323-9.
135. Szilagyi A, Blasko B, Ronai Z, Fust G, Sasvari-Szekely M, Guttman A. Rapid quantification of human complement component C4A and C4B genes by capillary gel electrophoresis. Electrophoresis 2006;27:1437-43.
136. Szilagyi A, Blasko B, Szilassy D, Fust G, Sasvari-Szekely M, Ronai Z. Real-time PCR quantification of human complement C4A and C4B genes. BMC Genet 2006;7:1.
137. Wouters D, van Schouwenburg P, van der Horst A, et al. High-throughput analysis of the C4 polymorphism by a combination of MLPA and isotype-specific ELISA's. Mol Immunol 2009;46:592-600.
138. Dawkins R, Leelayuwat C, Gaudieri S, et al. Genomics of the major histocompatibility complex: Haplotypes, duplication, retroviruses and disease. Immunol Rev 1999;167:275-304.
139. Alper CA, Larsen CE, Dubey DP, Awdeh ZL, Fici DA, Yunis EJ. The haplotype structure of the human major histocompatibility complex. Hum Immunol 2006;67: 73-84.
140. Awdeh ZL, Raum D, Yunis EJ, Alper CA. Extended HLA/complement allele haplotypes: Evidence for T/t-like complex in man. Proc Natl Acad Sci USA 1983;80:259-63.
141. Dawkins RL, Christiansen FT, Kay PH, et al. Disease associations with complotypes, supratypes and haplotypes. Immunol Rev 1983;70:1-22.
142. Alper CA, Awdeh Z, Yunis EJ. Conserved, extended MHC haplotypes. Exp Clin Immunogenet 1992;9:58-71.
143. Traherne JA, Horton R, Roberts AN, et al. Genetic analysis of completely sequenced disease-associated MHC haplotypes identifies shuffling of segments in recent human history. PLoS Genet 2006;2:e9.

144. Dorak MT, Shao W, Machulla HK, et al. Conserved extended haplotypes of the major histocompatibility complex: Further characterization. Genes Immun 2006;7:450-67.
145. Horton R, Gibson R, Coggill P, et al. Variation analysis and gene annotation of eight MHC haplotypes: The MHC Haplotype Project. Immunogenetics 2008;60:1-18.
146. Yunis EJ, Larsen CE, Fernandez-Vina M, et al. Inheritable variable sizes of DNA stretches in the human MHC: Conserved extended haplotypes and their fragments or blocks. Tissue Antigens 2003;62:1-20.
147. Christiansen FT, Dawkins RL, Uko G, McCluskey J, Kay PH, Zilko PJ. Complement allotyping in SLE: Association with C4A null. Aust N Z J Med 1983;13:483-8.
148. Reveille JD, Arnett FC, Wilson RW, Bias WB, McLean RH. Null alleles of the fourth component of complement and HLA haplotypes in familial systemic lupus erythematosus. Immunogenetics 1985;21:299-311.
149. Howard PF, Hochberg MC, Bias WB, Arnett FC, Jr, McLean RH. Relationship between C4 null genes, HLA-D region antigens, and genetic susceptibility to systemic lupus erythematosus in Caucasian and black Americans. Am J Med 1986;81:187-93.
150. McCann VJ, McCluskey J, Kelly H, et al. Thyrogastric autoimmunity and MHC associated alleles at the C4 locus in patients with type 1 (insulin-dependent) diabetes. Diabetologia 1984;27 Suppl:124-5.
151. Skanes V, Larsen B, Sampson-Murphy L, Farid NR. Polymorphism of the fourth component of complement in Graves' disease and type I diabetes mellitus. Clin Invest Med 1985;8:126-32.
152. Yang Y, Chung EK, Wu YL, et al. Gene copy-number variation and associated polymorphisms of complement component C4 in human systemic lupus erythematosus (SLE): Low copy number is a risk factor for and high copy number is a protective factor against SLE susceptibility in European Americans. Am J Hum Genet 2007;80:1037-54.
153. Yang YL, Chu JY, Luo ML, et al. Amplification of PRKCI, located in 3q26, is associated with lymph node metastasis in esophageal squamous cell carcinoma. Genes Chromosomes Cancer 2008;47:127-36.
154. Candore G, Modica MA, Lio D, et al. Pathogenesis of autoimmune diseases associated with 8.1 ancestral haplotype: A genetically determined defect of C4 influences immunological parameters of healthy carriers of the haplotype. Biomed Pharmacother 2003;57:274-7.
155. Kaur G, Kumar N, Szilagyi A, et al. Autoimmune-associated HLA-B8-DR3 haplotypes in Asian Indians are unique in C4 complement gene copy numbers and HSP-2 1267A/G. Hum Immunol 2008;69:580-7.
156. Candore G, Lio D, Colonna Romano G, Caruso C. Pathogenesis of autoimmune diseases associated with 8.1 ancestral haplotype: Effect of multiple gene interactions. Autoimmun Rev 2002;1:29-35.
157. Barilla-LaBarca ML, Atkinson JP. Rheumatic syndromes associated with complement deficiency. Curr Opin Rheumatol 2003;15:55-60.
158. Jonsson G, Sjoholm AG, Truedsson L, Bengtsson AA, Braconier JH, Sturfelt G. Rheumatological manifestations, organ damage and autoimmunity in hereditary C2 deficiency. Rheumatology (Oxford) 2007;46:1133-9.
159. Tsao BP. An update on genetic studies of systemic lupus erythematosus. Curr Rheumatol Rep 2002;4:359-67.
160. Agnello V. Association of systemic lupus erythematosus and SLE-like syndromes with hereditary and acquired complement deficiency states. Arthritis Rheum 1978;21:S146-52.
161. Agnello V. Lupus diseases associated with hereditary and acquired deficiencies of complement. Springer Semin Immunopathol 1986;9:161-78.
162. Pickering MC, Botto M, Taylor PR, Lachmann PJ, Walport MJ. Systemic lupus erythematosus, complement deficiency, and apoptosis. Adv Immunol 2000;76:227-324.
163. Pickering MC, Walport MJ. Links between complement abnormalities and systemic lupus erythematosus. Rheumatology (Oxford) 2000;39:133-41.
164. Carneiro-Sampaio M, Liphaus BL, Jesus AA, Silva CA, Oliveira JB, Kiss MH. Understanding systemic lupus erythematosus physiopathology in the light of primary immunodeficiencies. J Clin Immunol 2008;28 Suppl 1:S34-41.
165. Truedsson L, Bengtsson AA, Sturfelt G. Complement deficiencies and systemic lupus erythematosus. Autoimmunity 2007;40:560-6.
166. Alper CA, Xu J, Cosmopoulos K, et al. Immunoglobulin deficiencies and susceptibility to infection among homozygotes and heterozygotes for C2 deficiency. J Clin Immunol 2003;23:297-305.
167. Figueroa JE, Densen P. Infectious diseases associated with complement deficiencies. Clin Microbiol Rev 1991;4:359-95.
168. Sjoholm AG, Jonsson G, Braconier JH, Sturfelt G, Truedsson L. Complement deficiency and disease: An update. Mol Immunol 2006;43:78-85.
169. Ligthart GJ, Corberand JX, Fournier C, et al. Admission criteria for immunogerontological studies in man: The SENIEUR protocol. Mech Ageing Dev 1984;28:47-55.
170. Kramer J, Fulop T, Rajczy K, Nguyen AT, Fust G. A marked drop in the incidence of the null allele of the B gene of the fourth component of complement (C4B*Q0) in elderly subjects: C4B*Q0 as a probable negative selection factor for survival. Hum Genet 1991;86:595-8.
171. Arason GJ, Bodvarsson S, Sigurdarson ST, et al. An age-associated decrease in the frequency of C4B*Q0 indicates that null alleles of complement may affect health or survival. Ann N Y Acad Sci 2003;1010:496-9.
172. Arason GJ, Kramer J, Blasko B, et al. Smoking and a complement gene polymorphism interact in promoting cardiovascular disease morbidity and mortality. Clin Exp Immunol 2007;149:132-8.
173. Kramer J, Rajczy K, Hegyi L. C4B*Q0 allotype as a risk factor for myocardial infarction. British Medical Journal 1994;309:313-4.

174. Kramer J, Harcos P, Prohaszka Z, et al. Frequencies of certain complement protein alleles and serum levels of anti-heat-shock protein antibodies in cerebrovascular diseases. Stroke 2000;31:2648-52.
175. Szalai C, Fust G, Duba J, et al. Association of polymorphisms and allelic combinations in the tumour necrosis factor-alpha-complement MHC region with coronary artery disease. J Med Genet 2002;39:46-51.
176. Palikhe A, Sinisalo J, Seppanen M, Valtonen V, Nieminen MS, Lokki ML. Human MHC region harbors both susceptibility and protective haplotypes for coronary artery disease. Tissue Antigens 2007;69:47-55.
177. Blasko B, Kolka R, Thorbjornsdottir P, et al. Low complement C4B gene copy number predicts short-term mortality after acute myocardial infarction. Int Immunol 2008;20:31-7.
178. Antonicelli R, Olivieri F, Bonafe M, et al. The interleukin-6 -174 G>C promoter polymorphism is associated with a higher risk of death after an acute coronary syndrome in male elderly patients. Int J Cardiol 2005;103:266-71.
179. Yazdanpanah M, Rietveld I, Janssen JA, et al. An insulin-like growth factor-I promoter polymorphism is associated with increased mortality in subjects with myocardial infarction in an elderly Caucasian population. Am J Cardiol 2006;97:1274-6.
180. Mizuno H, Sato H, Sakata Y, et al. Impact of atherosclerosis-related gene polymorphisms on mortality and recurrent events after myocardial infarction. Atherosclerosis 2006;185:400-5.
181. Fantidis P, Perez De Prada T, Fernandez-Ortiz A, et al. Morning cortisol production in coronary heart disease patients. Eur J Clin Invest 2002;32:304-8.
182. Odell JD, Warren RP, Warren WL, Burger RA, Maciulis A. Association of genes within the major histocompatibility complex with attention deficit hyperactivity disorder. Neuropsychobiology 1997;35:181-6.
183. Warren RP, Singh VK, Cole P, et al. Increased frequency of the null allele at the complement C4b locus in autism. Clin Exp Immunol 1991;83:438-40.
184. Odell D, Maciulis A, Cutler A, et al. Confirmation of the association of the C4B null allele in autism. Hum Immunol 2005;66:140-5.
185. Sweeten TL, Odell DW, Odell JD, Torres AR. C4B null alleles are not associated with genetic polymorphisms in the adjacent gene CYP21A2 in autism. BMC Med Genet 2008;9:1.
186. Stefansson Thors V, Kolka R, Sigurdardottir SL, Edvardsson VO, Arason G, Haraldsson A. Increased frequency of C4B*Q0 alleles in patients with Henoch-Schönlein purpura. Scand J Immunol 2005;61:274-8.
187. de Messias IJ, Santamaria J, Brenden M, Reis A, Mauff G. Association of C4B deficiency (C4B*Q0) with erythema nodosum in leprosy. Clin Exp Immunol 1993;92:284-7.
188. Pasta L, Pietrosi G, Marrone C, et al. C4BQ0: A genetic marker of familial HCV-related liver cirrhosis. Dig Liver Dis 2004;36:471-7.
189. Edwards AO, Ritter R, 3rd, Abel KJ, Manning A, Panhuysen C, Farrer LA. Complement factor H polymorphism and age-related macular degeneration. Science 2005;308:421-4.
190. Haines JL, Hauser MA, Schmidt S, et al. Complement factor H variant increases the risk of age-related macular degeneration. Science 2005;308:419-21.
191. Hageman GS, Anderson DH, Johnson LV, et al. A common haplotype in the complement regulatory gene factor H (HF1/CFH) predisposes individuals to age-related macular degeneration. Proc Natl Acad Sci USA 2005;102:7227-32.
192. Jakobsdottir J, Conley YP, Weeks DE, Ferrell RE, Gorin MB. C2 and CFB genes in age-related maculopathy and joint action with CFH and LOC387715 genes. PLoS ONE 2008;3:e2199.
193. Scholl HP, Charbel Issa P, Walier M, et al. Systemic complement activation in age-related macular degeneration. PLoS ONE 2008;3:e2593.
194. Spencer KL, Hauser MA, Olson LM, et al. Protective effect of complement factor B and complement component 2 variants in age-related macular degeneration. Hum Mol Genet 2007;16:1986-92.
195. Bergeron-Sawitzke J, Gold B, Olsh A, et al. Multilocus analysis of age-related macular degeneration. Eur J Hum Genet 2009.
196. Montes T, Tortajada A, Morgan BP, Rodriguez de Cordoba S, Harris CL. Functional basis of protection against age-related macular degeneration conferred by a common polymorphism in complement factor B. Proc Natl Acad Sci USA 2009;106:4366-71.
197. Caprioli J, Bettinaglio P, Zipfel PF, et al. The molecular basis of familial hemolytic uremic syndrome: Mutation analysis of factor H gene reveals a hot spot in short consensus repeat 20. J Am Soc Nephrol 2001;12:297-307.
198. Noris M, Brioschi S, Caprioli J, et al. Familial haemolytic uraemic syndrome and an MCP mutation. Lancet 2003;362:1542-7.
199. Fremeaux-Bacchi V, Dragon-Durey MA, Blouin J, et al. Complement factor I: A susceptibility gene for atypical haemolytic uraemic syndrome. J Med Genet 2004;41:e84.

Chapter 9

HLA-G, -F and -E: Polymorphism, Function and Evolution

Pablo Gomez-Prieto, Carlos Parga-Lozano, Diego Rey,
Enrique Moreno, Antonio Arnaiz-Villena

INTRODUCTION

HLA-G

HLA-G is a nonclassical HLA class I molecule that has tolerogenic functions and acts on cells of both innate and adaptive immunity.[1,2] The molecular mechanisms leading to tolerance involve interaction between HLA-G and receptors that are expressed at the surface of NK- or T cytotoxic cells.[3,4] The inhibitory effects of HLA-G are mediated through direct binding to inhibitory receptors NK (ILT2, ILT4, KIR2DL4), T (CD8) and antigen presenting (via ILT-4) cells.[1] HLA-G is expressed in fetal extravillous trophoblast, adult thymic epithelial cells, cornea and nail matrix (immune privileged sites). Along with its isoforms, it induces allograft acceptance, probable autoimmunity[5] and may help infections and tumors to escape from immune system surveillance.[1,6] An HLA-G study on apes shows how a deletion in intron 2 is specific for Old World but not for New World primates[6-9] and how a relatedness dendrogram shows HLA-E closer primary DNA sequence similarity to MHC-G New World monkeys.[8,10]

HLA-F

The HLA-F was characterized in 1990 as a nonclassical class I gene;[11] its protein shows a short cytoplasmic tail since exon 7 is not present in mature transcripts. HLA-F has conserved the residues cysteine pairs 101 and 164,[12] which are crucial to conform its tri-dimensional structure and the important N-linked glycosylation site (Asn 86); it has cytoplasmic domains shorter than those of classical HLA molecules and has also conserved most of the key residues at the CD8-binding domain. The expression of HLA-F is restricted to B cells and lymphoid tissues such as thymus, spleen, tonsil and fetal liver. It is also expressed only in the cytoplasm of trophoblast cells (weekly during the first 3 months of pregnancy). HLA-F expression increases and moves to the cell surface with the progression of pregnancy from the second trimester onwards.[13,14] The gene seems to associate with beta 2-microglobulin, transporter associated (TAP) with antigen processing and calreticulin inside the cell.[13] It is not yet known whether HLA-F is able to associate with peptide or other small organic molecules in order to present antigens for starting an immune response. HLA-F has also been observed on the surface of Epstein-Barr virus-transformed lymphoblastoid cell lines and on some monocyte cell lines.[15] The function of this nonclassical class I gene is unknown; however, its primary structure is conserved in primates (bonobo, gorilla and orangutan), particularly key residues that conform three dimensional peptide binding region of classical class I presenting cells.[16] The peptide binding region synonymous and nonsynonymous substitutions do not significantly differ from other nonclassical class I molecule regions.[17]

HLA-E

HLA-E is a nonclassical class I gene with a low polymorphism. It has been mapped between HLA-C and HLA-A loci on the short arm of the chromosome 6.[18] RNA transcripts of this gene are expressed in cytoplasm and surface of extravillous cytotrophoblast cells in the last part of pregnancy[19] and the level of expression can be augmented upon stimulation with interferon gamma.[20,21] This protein is implicated in the presentation of intracellular derived peptides, exclusively from other

HLA class I signal sequence proteins.[19] to the cytotoxic T cells and is present in all nucleated cells.[22] HLA-E is expressed on trophoblast, where it interacts with NK receptor CD94-NK2GA and its leader peptide may be presented by HLA-G molecules expressed on the cell surface and interact with NK cells.[23] In the present report, exons 2, 3, 4, and all introns are used for both DNA and protein MHC-E polymorphism description.

DETECTION OF ALLELISM

Peripheral blood lymphocytes are used to extract DNA. Different methodologies exist for both HLA-G, HLA-E and HLA-F typing.[24] Newly appearing alleles can be detected similarly by using allele specific oligonucleotides or primers.

HLA-G Polymerase Chain Reaction (PCR)—Single Specific Oligonucleotide (SSO) Typing

PCR Amplification

Genomic DNA is amplified using PCR. In order to obtain the complete exon 2, intron 2 and exon 3 HLA-G sequences, a specific 5′ primer (G-25′: TCCATGAGGTATTTCAGCGC) and a specific 3′ primer (G-33′: GGTACCCGCGCGCTGCAGCA) are used.[25] PCR reactions include 10x PCR buffer, 125 mM dNTP mix, 1 mM of each primer and 0.025 U/µl Taq Polymerase (Perkin Elmer) in a final volume of 100 µl. The PCR conditions consist of 30 cycles of 96°C, 15 s; 55°C, 15 s; and 72°C, 1 min in a programmable heat block (9600 Perkin Elmer). The PCR products obtained are electrophoresed in a 2 percent agarose and detected by staining with ethidium bromide.

Oligonucleotide Labelling

Specific oligonucleotides for HLA-E are labeled with dig-ddUTP (Boehringer Mannheim, Germany) following the manufacturer's recommendations (see Table 2 in Ref. 24). Other oligonucleotides may be used for new alleles by studying genomic DNA specific differences.

Dot/Slot Blotting

PCR products are blotted onto a nylon membrane (Amersham, UK) as follows: i) for denaturation, 80 µl of the amplification reaction is taken, and 320 µl of NaOH 0.5 M is added to it. This is mixed well and maintained at room temperature for 10 min. 400 µl of ammonium acetate 2 M is added, and this is mixed well and put in ice; ii) 50 µl of this final mixture is transferred to a spot of the nylon membrane previously soaked in ammonium acetate 1 M. Once the sample had passed through the membrane, 500 µl of ammonium acetate 1 M is added. The membrane is air dried at room temperature and further dried to completion at 80°C for 2 h (Baking), or illuminated with a 254 nm ultraviolet (UV) lamp for 5 min. Alternatively, PCR products can be blotted directly onto the membrane (1 µl) which is then dried at room temperature. With constant gentle agitation, the membranes are made wet with 0.4 M NaOH for 10 min and then equilibrated with ammonium acetate 2 M. The membranes are dried as described above.

Hybridization

Each membrane is placed into a 50 ml tube with TMAC solution (10 ml) as hybridization buffer containing the dig-ddUTP-labeled oligonucleotide probe. It is incubated with rotation for 3 h at 54°C.

Washing

With constant gentle agitation, the membrane is rinsed in 100 ml per membrane of 2x SSPE, 0.1 percent SDS at room temperature for 5 min, twice. The membrane is washed first in 100 ml of TMAC solution [50 mM Tris-HCl (pH 8.0), 3 M TMAC, 0.5 M EDTA, 0.1% SDS] at room temperature for 10 min followed by 100 ml of preheated TMAC solution at 60°C for 15 min, twice. These are then hybridized with oligoprobes G2.2, G3.2 and G3.6, washed with preheated TMAC solution at 63°C for 15 min followed by washing in 100 ml of 2x SSPE.

Chemiluminescent Detection

The following washes are done at room temperature, with constant shaking. The wash volume is approximately 100 ml per 100 cm^2 of membrane. This is washed immediately in buffer 1 (100 mM Tris-HCl, pH 7.2, 150 mM NaCl) for 5 min, buffer 2 (buffer 1 containing 1% blocking reagent, Boehringer) for 30 min and then incubated in buffer 1 containing AP-antibody anti-dig (75 mU/ml, dilution 1:10,000) for 30 min. Next, the membrane is washed twice in buffer 1 for 15 min each and then in buffer 3 (100 mM Tris-HCl, pH 9.5, 100 mM NaCl, 50 mM MgCl$_2$) for 5 min. Following this, it is incubated in buffer 3 for 5 min, made wet with the CDP-star substrate solution (Phototope-star Detection kit for nucleic acids, New England Biolabs, UK) and then dried briefly (but not completely) and exposed with an X-ray film for a variable time (5 min or more).

Color Development for Alkaline Phosphatase

This is the same as the chemiluminescent protocol but using buffer 3 containing nitroblue tetrazolium choloride (NBT) solution (30 µl of NBT stock per 10 ml of buffer 3) and X-Phosphate (30 µl of X-Phosphate stock per 10 ml of buffer 3) (Boehringer Manhein, Germany) instead of CPD-star substrate. NBT stock: 100 mg/ml nitroblue tetrazolium salt in 70 percent dimethyl formamide. X-Phosphate stock: 50 mg/ml 5-Bromo-4-chloro-3-indodyl phosphate in dimethyl formamide. Incubation is done in complete darkness. The color is developed in a few minutes and is completed in one day (do not shake). The membrane is washed in 50 ml of TE 10:1, pH 8.0, to stop the color development.

HLA-G PCR-Restriction Fragment Length Polymorphism (RFLP)—DNA Typing

PCR Amplification

Genomic DNA is amplified using PCR. To obtain exon 2 and exon 3 HLA-G sequences separately, two specific primer sets, G-25': TCCATGAGGTATTTCAGCGC: G-23': CTGGGCCGGAGTTACTCACT and G-35': CACACCCTCCAGTGGATGAT: G-33': GGTACC-CGCGCGC TGCAGCA, are respectively used.[25] PCR reactions include 10x PCR buffer, 125 mM dNTP mix, 1 mM of each primer and 0.025 U/µl Taq Polymerase (Perkin Elmer) in a final volume of 100 µl. The PCR conditions consist of 30 cycles of 96°C, 15 s; 55°C, 15 s; and 72°C, 1 min in a programmable heat block (9600 Perkin Elmer).

Digestion

Following the HLA-G exon 2 or exon 3 amplification, aliquots (10 µl) of the reaction mixture are digested with the restriction endonucleases as follows: i) exon 2 amplifications are digested using MspI, HinfI, AsuI and ApaI, and ii) exon 3 with AcyI, PpuMI and BseRI following the manufacturers' recommendations. The digestion products are size-resolved in a 6 percent acrylamide gel or 2 percent Nusieve agarose and detected by staining with ethidium bromide. Interpretations of the possible results are given in Table 2, see Ref. 24.

HLA-E PCR-SSO Typing

PCR Amplification

Genomic DNA from peripheral blood mononuclear cells is amplified by using the PCR. In order to obtain the complete exon 2, intron 2 and exon 3 HLA-E sequences, a specific 5' primer (E25': TGTGAATTCTCT ACCGGGAGTAGAGAGG) and a specific 3' primer (E33': AGCCCTGT GGACCCTCTT) are used (26). PCR reactions include 10x PCR buffer (10 mM Tris-HCl pH 8.4 at 24 °C, 50 mM KCl, 0.1 mg/ml gelatin, 0.02% NP40, 1.5 mM $MgCl_2$, final concentrations), 125 mM 2% deoxyribonucleoside-5' triphosphate (dNTP) mix, 1 mM of each primer and 0.025 U/µl Taq Polymerase (Perkin Elmer) in a final volume of 100 ml. The PCR conditions consist of 30 cycles of 94 °C, 30 s; 65 °C, 1 min; and 72°C, 1 min in a programmable heat block (9600 Perkin Elmer). The PCR products obtained are electrophoresed in a 2% agarose gel and detected by staining with ethidium bromide. Specific oligonucleotides for HLA-E are labeled with dig-ddUTP as described above. Also, Dot/slot-blot is the same as that used for HLA-G typing.

Prehybridization

Each membrane is placed in a 50-ml tube with hybridization buffer (6x SSPE, 5x Magic Denhardt, 0.1% Lauryl sarcosine, 0.02% SDS, 0.2 ml/cm²) for 30 min at 42°C.

Hybridization

The hybridization solution used in prehybridization is removed, and the hybridization solution (0.2 ml/cm²) containing the dig-ddUTP-labeled oligonucleotide probe is added. This is incubated for 3 hour at 42°C.

Washing

This process is done as follows: With constant gentle agitation, the membrane is rinsed in 100 ml per membrane of 2x SSPE, 0.1% SDS at room temperature for 5 min, twice. The membrane is washed in 100 ml of tetramethylammonium chloride (TMAC) solution (50 mM Tris-HCl (pH 8.0), 3 M TMAC, 0.5 M EDTA, 0.1% SDS) at room temperature for 10 min. It is further washed twice in 100 ml of preheated TMAC solution at 50°C for 15 min and then washed in 100 ml of 2x SSPE. The detection steps are the same as described above.

HLA-E and -G Sequence-Based Typing (SBT)

HLA-E and -G PCR products from both chromosomes comprising exon 2, intron 2 and exon 3 sequences are identified by differential migration in 2 percent agarose gel electrophoresis and purified with a Qiaquick gel extraction kit (Qiagen, Hilden, Germany). Double-stranded DNA templates are sequenced using the Sanger's dideoxy chain terminator method, with dye-labeled dideoxy terminators. DNA samples are analyzed in a Perkin Elmer (Foster City, CA) 373A automated DNA sequencer as described previously.[27] HLA-E and -G amplification primers are also used as sequencing primers. Due to relatively low genetic polymorphism, SBT can be applied for HLA-E and -G typing because ambiguous positions are assigned correctly.

HLA-F Typing

cDNA typing from EBV cell lines are used for cDNA sequencing.[16]

RNA Extraction, Reverse Transcription and cDNA Amplification

RNA is extracted from eight cell lines (two common chimpanzees: Puddin and Suzanne; two bonobos: Jill and Matata; two gorillas: Sinsing and Rok and two orangutans: Kichil and Molec) using the nonidet P (NP)-40 protocol.[33] Cells (10^7 per line) are pelleted and dissolved in 250 ml of lysis buffer (10 mM Tris pH 8.6, 140 mM NaCl, 1.5 mM $MgCl_2$, 0.5% NP-40) with RNAsin 1000 U/ml (final concentration) (Promega, Madison, WI). The mixture is incubated for 1 min at 4°C. The lysates are centrifuged and supernatants transferred to 250 ml of proteinase K (PK) buffer x2 (200 mM Tris pH 7.5, 25 mM ethylenediaminetetraacetic acid, 300 mM NaCl, 2% sodium dodecyl sulfate) containing 200 mg of proteinase K. Samples are further incubated for 30 min at room temperature. A standard phenol-chloroform extraction is done in order to obtain whole RNA. cDNA synthesis is performed using a Reverse Transcription System (Promega) according to the manufacturer's protocols. In order to amplify the MHC-F cDNA from EBVlymphocyte RNA, a 40-cycle round of polymerase chain reaction is used. The sequences of primers used are F1-50: 50-TCC CAG ACG CGG AGG TTG C; CR-30: 50-CAA GTG CAA TTC TGC TAC ATT G. These primers are located in the 5'UT (base -40 to base -22) and 3'UT (base 1006 to base 1027) regions, respectively.

cDNA Sequencing

cDNA-amplified HLA-F fragments are identified by 0.7% agarose gel electrophoresis and purified by vacuum-propelled minicolumns (Magic Minipreps, Promega). The purified fragments are inserted into the pMOS T vector. Ligation, transformation and identification of recombinant colonies are carried out following the manufacturer's recommendations. Double-stranded DNA templates are sequenced using the Sanger's dideoxy chain terminator method. The cDNA samples are analyzed in a Perkin Elmer (Foster City, CA) 373 A Automated DNA sequencer.[34]

POLYMORPHISM

HLA-G

The relatively low polymorphism seen in the nonclassical HLA molecules till date could be attributed to a general lack of investigations in this area. The available information on genetic polymorphism in HLA-E,-F and -G is summarized in Figures 9.1, 9.2 and 9.3 respectively.

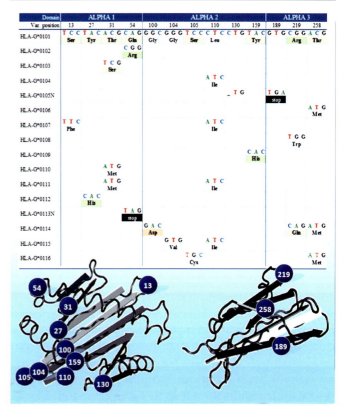

Fig. 9.1: HLA-G proteins and their polymorphism. Protein alleles (n=16, including two null alleles); α-1, α-2 and α-3 domains of human leukocyte antigen-G protein. Probably HLA-G*0113N is not expressed; alpha-1 domain of HLA-G*0105N may be expressed. Variable amino acidic positions are indicated in table (codons) and in blue circles. See also[28-30]

HLA-F

HLA-F protein polymorphism	
Alleles = 5 (1 null)	Variable sites = 4

Domain	5'-UTR	α-1	α-2	α-3
Var.position	-9	50	118	251
HLA-F*0101	G C C Ala	C C G Pro	T A C Tyr	T C T Ser
HLA-F*0102	G T C Val			
HLA-F*0103				C C T Pro
HLA-F*0104		C A G Gln		
HLA-F*Nu11			T A A stop	

Fig. 9.2: HLA-F protein and its polymorphism in α-1, α-2 and α-3 domains of the HLA-F protein. Variable amino acidic positions are indicated in table (codons) and in green circles. See also[30]

HLA-E

HLA-E protein polymorphism	
Alleles = 3 (0 null)	Variable sites = 2

Domain	α-2	
Var.position	107	157
HLA-E*0101	A G G Arg	A G A Arg
HLA-E*0103	G G G Gly	
HLA-E*0104	G G G Gly	G G A Gly

Fig. 9.3: Protein HLA-E and its polymorphic alleles (n= 3) in α-1 and α-2 domains. Variable amino acidic positions are indicated in table (codons) and in purple circles. See also[30]

FUNCTION

HLA-G, -F, and -E molecules are believed to be Immune supressors.

HLA-G

HLA-G and immune system
Reduced expression → immune system stimulation
Increased expression → immune system suppression
Antigen presenting by HLA-G itself?
HLA-G and immune system

HLA-G and Immune System

Figure 9.4 summarizes the postulated functions of HLA-G based on recent publications describing biological and clinical benefits.[1] These effects are nevertheless criticized, mainly because of a lack of availability of internationally standardized reagents, specifically anti-HLA-G monoclonal antibodies.[31] A concerted international effort similar to the one used for the classical HLA loci (HLA-A,B,C) is required to validate monoclonal HLA-G antibodies in free intergroup exchanges. This would help immensely in understanding the role of HLA-G in immune response.

Identification of healthy human individuals who lack the full HLA-G molecule,[28, 29] and the finding of a 'null' allele HLA-G*0113N (Fig. 9.1), which may not even transcribe HLA-G α-1 protein domain in homozygosis, cast doubts about the necessity of an HLA-G full molecule for life. Also, *Cercopithecinae* apes do not express full MHC-G molecule either.[32] Hence immune redundant mechanisms may exist to substitute HLA-G function in certain situations.

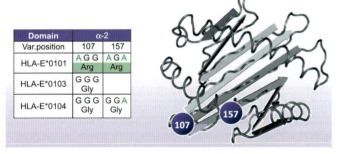

	NK lymphocytes	co-receptor	T Lymphocytes	co-receptor	Antigen-presenting cells	co-receptor
−	Cytolysis	ILT-2	Cytotoxic function	ILT-2	DC maturation	ILT-4
−	Transendothelial migration	ILT-2	Supressive T cells		Antigen presentation	ILT-4
+	Supressive NK cells	ILT-2	Secretion of Th2 cytokines		DC trafficking	ILT-4
+	Secretion of proangiogenic factors	KIR2DL4			Tolerogenic APC	
−	Proliferation	ILT-2		ILT-2, ILT-4		
−	Apoptosis	CD8		CD8		
+	Inhibitory receptors					

Fig. 9.4: HLA-G and immune system, DC: Dendritic cells

HLA-G and Immunopathology

HLA-G and immunopathology
Tumors: Reduced immune response by surface HLA-G expression
Transplants and pregnancy: Avoid rejection by HLA-G expression
Autoimmune and inflammatory diseases: Modulated by HLA-G surface expression
Viral infections: Reduced immune response by inducing HLA-G expression

HLA-F

HLA-F function
Expressed on B lymphocytes? On cytotrophoblast?
Expression and function not clarified yet

The HLA-F gene is known to bind β2-microglobulin.[11] The protein is shorter than the typical HLA class I molecule due to the lack of exon 7 from the mature HLA-F mRNA, resulting in a protein with a short cytoplasmatic domain. No specific peptide binding to native HLA-F has been found, and tertiary structure of HLA-F protein has been obtained only for heavy chain and β2-m.

A monoclonal antibody has been described,[33] that detects HLA-F only in the cytoplasm of peripheral blood B lymphocytes and B cell lines. Since no surface expression is detected, HLA-F exists as an empty heterodimer without a peptide. IFN-γ treatment has been shown to increase the expression of HLA-F mRNA and HLA-F protein, but not cell surface expression. Using recombinant HLA-F protein bound to β2-m without peptide, Lepin et al recently described an antibody.[34] HLA-F expression was detected in tonsil, spleen and thymus tissue with this reagent and again, no cell surface protein was expressed. On the other hand, other researchers found HLA-F surface expression in vivo.[15, 23] Further, HLA-F protein was found expressed in certain tissues and cell lines, including bladder, skin and liver cell lines. Other tissues or cell lines showed no surface expression, except for EBV-transformed lymphoblastoid cell lines and some monocyte cell lines.

No surface expression on normal B cells or on any peripheral blood lymphocytes could be detected with these latter monoclonal antibodies. Although these results are contradictory; however, the studied cell lines express HLA-F on their surface. Again, a multicenter study for validating HLA-F-detecting antibodies, as well as for validating anti-HLA-E and -G antibodies could help resolve the issue.[31, 34] It has been shown that HLA-F tetramers bind to peripheral blood monocytes and B cells as well as cells transfected with the inhibitory NK receptors, ILT2 and ILT4. However, the relevance of this interaction to in vivo function is questionable since all HLA class I show a similar interaction through the α-3 domain.[23] Cytotrophoblast also seems to express HLA-F.[14, 19]

HLA-E

HLA-E function
Pregnancy - Switching off NK lymphocytes - Modulating adequate T cell response
It could act synergistically with HLA-G

HLA-E binds nonamer peptides derived from other HLA class I signal sequences with restricted repertoire.[35] Interestingly, this showed that peptide binding to HLA-E is dependent on TAP. It has been suggested that HLA-E peptide binding and surface expression is strictly regulated by the expression of other HLA class I molecules.

A role of HLA-E in human pregnancy is postulated.[14,19] Fetal cells (trophoblast) invade into the decidua, and fuse with and open up maternal uterine arteries in order to facilitate an adequate supply of blood to the developing fetus through an interaction with decidual NK cells. Trophoblast invading maternal decidua only expresses HLA-E, -F and -G,[23] and HLA-C,[36] but no other class I or class II MHC molecule. HLA-E binds signal peptide derived from HLA-G and HLA-C, because HLA-E cannot bind peptides derived from HLA-F.[37] The HLA-E/G peptide complex interacts very strongly with CD94/NKG2A or NKG2C NK receptors relative to other HLA-E/class I. Trophoblasts avoid maternal NK cell surveillance to father allogenic proteins. This must be through soluble HLA-G protein,[23, 38, 39] and HLA-E bound to HLA-G signal peptide.[40-43]

Also, placental interface about 10% of leukocytes are T cells[44] which have characteristics of being more activated than peripheral blood lymphocytes.[45] T cell activation is triggered by fetal antigens, which are also found in maternal blood,[46] and could be important for trophoblast invasion. These T cells consist of αβ T and γδ T cells, with the number of γδ T cells increasing during the course of pregnancy while their numbers are very low in normal peripheral blood. Th1 and Th2 γδ T lymphocytes have been observed, and some of them may respond to HLA-E[47] to produce cytokines without cytotoxicity to trophoblast via CD94/NKG2 receptors in order to facilitate placentation.

EVOLUTION

HLA-G evolution
• Restricted polymorphism • Different for each Old and New World ape species • A few healthy humans only express alpha-1 HLA-G protein domain

The most extensive characterized members of the HLA class I gene family are the HLA-A,-B and -C loci products. Cloning studies made it possible to characterize new class I genes; some of them are complete genes, and have been called non classical HLA class I genes.[48-52] HLA-G is one of the three nonclassical human major histocompatibility complex (MHC) class I genes (HLA-E,-F,-G)[53] and is located telomeric to HLA-A locus on human chromosome 6p showing a high degree of sequence similarity at the nucleotide and amino acid levels with HLA-A2.[54] HLA-G has been widely studied because of its postulated role in the maternal-fetal relationship[55] and the following characteristics have been found:

1. HLA-G shows a relatively restricted polymorphism.[9,25,28,56,57] The sixteen HLA-G alleles (Fig. 9.1) found up until now[9,30] show a strong linkage disequilibrium with HLA-A alleles in different populations.[25,58-60]

2. HLA-G is expressed preferentially on extravillous trophoblast cells at the materno-fetal interface;[31] this preferential expression suggests that HLA-G products may play an important role in the immune tolerance of the semi-allogeneic fetus by the mother.[61] Some authors find a more extensive tissue expression,[1] and others doubt of extensive tissue HLA-G expression.[31] Recent work has shed light on the function of HLA-G and has suggested that the expression of HLA-G on target cells protects them from natural killer (NK) cell-mediated lysis through immunoglobulin NK inhibitory receptors ILT-2, ILT-4 and KIR2DL4.[1]

3. There are at least six major alternatively spliced forms of HLA-G mRNA:[55] HLA-G1, G2, G3 and G4, which encode membrane-bound proteins containing 3, 2,1 and 2 external domains, respectively and two HLA-G soluble forms (-G5 and -G6). The latter are encoded by mRNA molecule(s), -G1 and -G2 which retain intron 4 that is partially translated.[62,63]

4. MHC-class I genes of a New World primate (cotton-top tamarin: Saguinus oedipus, which separated from the Old World primates lineage 38 million years ago) seem to share more sequence homologies with human HLA-G gene than with classical HLA class I genes,[64,65] (Fig. 9.5). Thus, it has been proposed that HLA-G could be the ancestral MHC class I gene, and that MHC classical class I genes of the cotton top tamarin could be homologous to human HLA-G locus. Others have suggested that HLA-E may be more similar to cotton-top tamarin MHC[10,66] (Fig. 9.6).

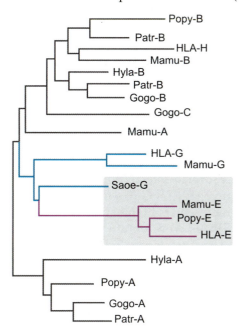

Fig. 9.6: Cotton-top Tamarins (Saoe) DNA sequence. MHC-G is more closely related to primate MHC-E than to primate MHC-G sequence in the NJ tree (shown) and also in DNA base percentage similarity (not shown). HLA: human MHC; Patr: chimpanzee MHC; Gogo: gorilla MHC; Popy: orangutan MHC; Hyla: gibbon MHC

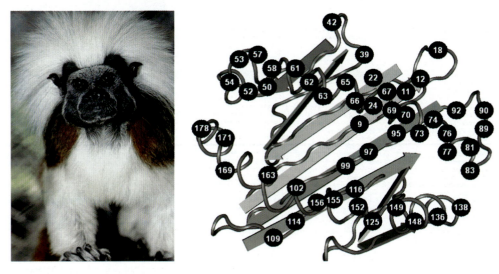

Fig. 9.5: Saeo (Cotton-top Tamarins) MHC-G clusters in relatedness dendrograms with other primates MHC-E (see also Fig. 9.10)

5. HLA-G intron 2 sequences show conserved motifs in all species studied so far, particularly a 23 base pair (bp) deletion between positions 161 and 183 which seem to be locus specific.[32] However, the cotton-top tamarin-G intron 2 does not bear this deletion[39] (Fig. 9.7).

New World Primates

The New World monkeys lineage separated about 38 million years ago, at least from the lineage that was going to give rise to Old World and from the anthropoid monkeys. Cotton-top Tamarins (Saoe) inhabit the Central-South American continent (Costa Rica, Panamá, Colombia) and are found to have functional MHC-G-like genes instead of MHC-A and -B genes;[64] MHC-C sequences have been detected in these Saoe[67] (Fig. 9.8), which may strongly interact with killer immunoglobulin-like receptors (KIR).[10] G-like molecules are assumed to be antigen presenters in this species.

Both alleles were obtained from three different monkeys. The characteristic 23 bp deletion between bases 161 and 183 does not appear in tamarins which is surprising since this deleted intron 2 sequence is present in all MHC-G primate alleles studied so far,[68] (Fig. 9.7). The two most feasible explanations for this phenomenon could be that:

1. The MHC-G like sequences in S. oedipus described do not give rise to the Old World monkey and human MHC-G alleles; and
2. The 23 bp intron 2 deletion (Fig. 9.7) most likely occurred after separation of the New World: Old World monkey lineages about 38 million years ago.

The first hypothesis is more favored, since eluted peptides from Cotton-top Tamarin MHC-G like molecules are not typical of MHC-G (G. Rammansee, personal communication).[69]

On the other hand, S. oedipus give birth to monozygotic twins after 4-5 months of pregnancy and, thereafter, are taken care of by their fathers who carry them until they are weaned and only give them to their mother for feeding.[70] Whether this peculiar pregnancy

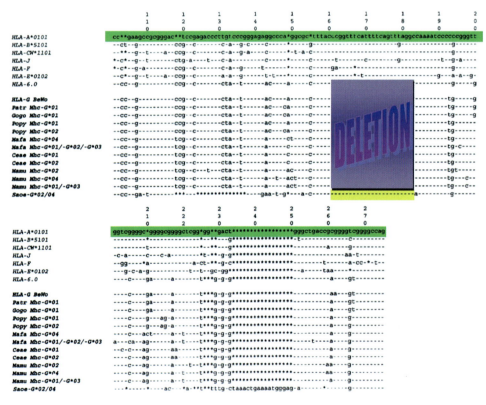

Fig. 9.7: MHC-G intron 2 nucleotide sequences compared to other MHC sequences (see also[32, 68]) Shaded sequences correspond to the 23 bp deletions observed in all introns 2 from MHC-G sequences. Cotton-top Tamarins (Saoe) do not show this typical deletion and this further casts doubts whether majority of the MHC alleles described in cotton-top tamarins belong to the MHC-G lineage. Otherwise, this deletion may have appeared in the Old World monkeys lineage. Saoe intron 2 sequence belongs to Saoe-G*02 and -G*04 alleles which have been sequenced in three different monkeys. Identity between residues is indicated by a dash (—) and deletions are denoted by an asterisk (*)

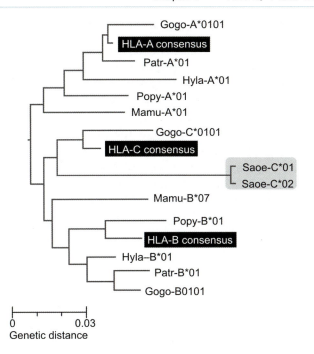

Fig. 9.8: New World monkeys. The Cotton-top Tamarin (Saguinus oedipus, Saoe) MHC-C. Two different MHC-C sequences have been reported (GenBank accession numbers AF005217 and AF005218), which cluster with other primates MHC-C. This is represented in a NJ dendogram (For specific primate Latin abbreviations names, see also Figure 9.6 legend)

and it is not known whether this is translated into protein.[10, 67]

Old World Primates (Cercopithecinae Subfamily)

This group of monkeys lives in Eurasia and Africa. Their pregnancy lasts for 5 months and they usually deliver one monkey. *M. mulatta* (Mamu, rhesus monkey), *M. fascicularis* (Mafa, cynomolgous monkey) and *C. aethiops* (Ceae, green monkey) MHC-G alleles all bear stop codons at a very restricted area of exon 3 (at codon 164, some alleles also show stop signals at 133, and at 118, and others at 176 codons,[32] (Fig. 9.9). The α-1 domain of the molecule is always preserved in all studied species and may suffice for MHC-G function in Cercopithecinae. Considering the postulated role of MHC-G in preserving the fetus from maternal NK cell attack and also that the pregnancies are normal and usually bearing one fetus in these monkeys, MHC-G molecules may exist in these species lacking α-2 domains. Otherwise, the existence of reading-through stop codon mechanisms might be present; these have also been found in certain mammalian genes.[71-73]

A total of 43 *Cercopithecinae* individuals were tested for a stop codon at position 164 and all of them were found to be positive. This is a general feature of this subfamily and may have occurred before speciation within the group precursors (at least 30 million years ago, when they separated from higher primates, Hylobates and Pongidae). Stop base triplets have also been reported in humans at codons 107 and the cysteins 101 and 164 that are crucial to maintain the overall molecule tertiary structure have also been found substituted by another amino acid.[32] All these anomalies have been observed in a heterozygous form. Mothers in these species are

is related to their peculiar MHC-G system is not known. Due to the high polymorphism found in Saoe-G molecules (11 alleles) at NK, TCR and antigen binding site (Fig. 9.5), it is possible that these G molecules are classical antigen presenting molecules in New World monkeys, since no other class I MHC molecules are found—except another one which seems to be MHC-C,

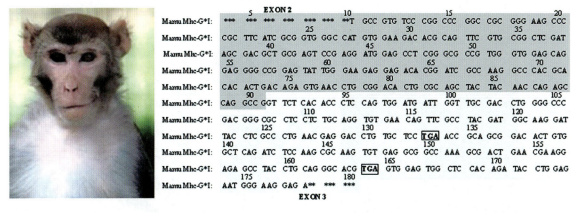

Fig. 9.9: Macaca mulatta. MHC-G exon 2 and exon 3 sequence, which shows two stop codon positions at exon 3 (TGA) (five individuals were studied). Macaca fascicularis (four individuals) and Cercopithecus aethiops (five individuals) also showed stop codons at MHC-G exon 3. All of these monkeys belong to Cercopithecinae family and show one stop codon at the 164 position. Some other Macaca species (43 individuals were studied) show additional stop codons at 118, 133, and 176 exon 3 residues[32]

exposed to relatively few allogeneic fetuses, since 92% of pregnancies have the α-male as a father.[70]

Polymorphism in Pongidae

Gorilla and chimpanzee (Figs 9.10 and 9.11) do not seem to have high polymorphism. However, more individuals need to be studied to ensure the existence of a low polymorphism in these two species. The almost non-existence of alleles parallels the relatively low polymorphism seen in humans (see also Fig. 9.1).[68] Mothers show relatively high exposure to allogeneic fetuses -polygamy.[70] However, the orangutan (Fig. 9.12) shows five protein alleles that affect both the TcR and antigen binding site. Thus, the very low MHC-G polymorphism may only have appeared 15 million years ago, when the orangutan diverged from the human lineage. Orangutan may show long lasting male-female relationship, that exposes the mother to relatively few allogeneic fetuses.[70]

Polymorphism in Humans

While low polymorphism needs to be further established in the gorilla and chimpanzee, in human there is comparatively (to other HLA loci) low polymorphism with 16 protein alleles. Many Negroid, Caucasoid and Mongoloid individuals have been studied.[60, 68] The allelism does not affect either the TCR, NK or antigen binding site suggesting that there must be a strong selective pressure for invariancy. Nevertheless, humans bearing null alleles in homozygosity have been found in the α3 domain,[74] (see Fig. 9.1). HLA-G*0113N has not been found in homozygosity. Polygamy in primitive societies (and to some extent in todays) is a human characteristic.

HLA-G as a Peptide-presenting Molecule

It was initially postulated that HLA-G molecules do not present antigens and may send negative signals from fetal cytotrophoblast to maternal NK cells in order to avoid

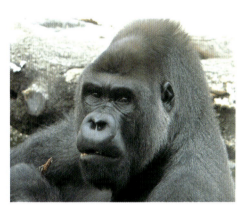
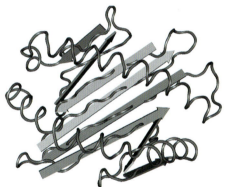

Fig. 9.10: Gorilla gorilla. Only one MHC-G allele was found in gorilla

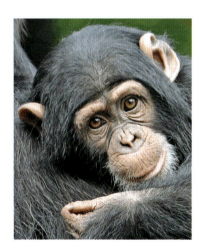
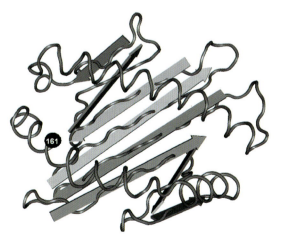

Fig. 9.11: Pan troglodytes. One variable position and two different MHC-G alleles were found in chimpanzee

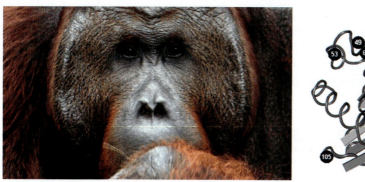
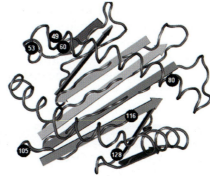

Fig. 9.12: Pongo pygmaeus. Five orangutan MHC-G alleles were found in variable positions

fetal rejection.[55] Indeed, relatively low polymorphism is detected in HLA-G molecules in most world populations.[60] Figure 9.1 which apparently does not affect either the antigen or the T cell receptor binding sites[68] supports the idea that HLA-G is not an antigen presenting molecule. In addition, it does not show the three hypervariable regions at the peptide binding site like other HLA presenting molecules. In fact, HLA-G mostly binds endogenous peptides which may help the molecule reach the cell surface.[75] However, while it seems established that HLA-G has a highly restricted peptide repertoire,[31] little contradiction has been drawn from the Rammensee solid work showing that HLA-G molecules are classical peptide presenters.[69]

Conclusions on HLA-G Evolution

The following conclusions can be drawn from the phylogenetic study of MHC DNA sequences:
1. An orthologous gene, Qa-2, occurs in mice.[76]
2. Many G-like alleles exist in primate species that separated from the human lineage at least 38 million years ago, particularly the Cotton-top Tamarin which lives in Central and South America. These alleles are polymorphic at TCR, NK receptor and antigen binding sites. It is likely that the MHC-G function in these New World monkeys is similar to classical HLA class I presenting molecules.
3. Only postulated isoforms not bearing α2 HLA-G domain are found in *Cercopithecinae* monkeys, due to the existence of stop codons in homozygosis mainly at position 164 (other stop codon positions are observed). These mutations appeared in the *Cercopithecinae* common ancestors after the separation of human and *Pongidae* lineage, about 35 million years ago. Either α2-lacking MHC-G isoforms may suffice for function or stop codons reading through mechanisms are present in protein translation and all isoforms are then possible (see above).
4. Orangutans (separated from human lineage about 15 million years ago) show more MHC-G alleles than gorillas and chimpanzees with variability at TCR, NK, and antigen binding sites.
5. Gorilla and chimpanzee MHC-G allelisms seem to be low, but more data are necessary to confirm it.
6. Humans have fourteen productive alleles (proteins) which represents a relatively low polymorphism. This indicates that there must be a strong selective pressure for invariance at the HLA-G molecules in humans.
7. All findings are consistent with the hypothesis that MHC-G proteins may be tolerogenic molecules either at the TCR -inflammation,[5] graft rejection[1,77] - or NK cell, and other immune system levels,[1] switching off cells which usually attack foreign (including fetus) or self (autoimmune) antigens.
8. The peculiarities of MHC-G genes in primates (not following a lineal evolutionary pattern) suggest that within species behavior peculiarities give rise to particular fetal maternal relationships that may shape MHC-G evolution. For instance, Cotton-top Tamarins always give birth to monozygotic twins, which thereafter cling to the father and are born to long-lasting monogamous couples. All other primates (including humans) are polygamous (with further within-species peculiarities) and mothers are in contact with many different fetuses regarding MHC antigens. However, *Cercopithecinae* and orangutan (less exposed species to allogeneic fetuses) are the most polymorphic at the MHC level.[70] A hypothesis may be put forward that a mechanism avoiding a high MHC-G allelism has been developed for the polygamous species (Old World and anthropoid monkeys and humans). This would protect the

mother against frequently MHC incompatible trophoblast aggression (as is seen in some pregnancy related tumors) and, on the other hand, would confer the mother with a simple nonpolymorphic system to switch off fetal NK and other immune system cells.[1]

MHC-G, KIR, HLA-G

MHC-G/MHC-C interactions
• KIR (immunoglobulin-like receptors) ↔ Interaction with MHC-G and -C
• NK (natural killer lymphocytes)

Human leukocyte antigen G (HLA-G) has been shown to be a tolerogenic molecule for the immune response, particularly against the maternal immune system by fetal cytotrophoblast.[1] It gives negative signals for natural killer (NK) and T cells.[78, 79] In addition, lack of HLA-G has been shown to be associated with inflammatory and autoimmune diseases[1, 5] and its presence in tumors to activate an immune tumor escape mechanism.[1] Viral infections also activate HLA-G synthesis and promote infections.[1] Some alleles have been shown to be linked to disease.[1] Also, HLA-G is important for predicting graft rejection and for avoiding it by enhancing HLA-G in situ synthesis.[1] However, some aspects of HLA-G need to be further studied, particularly the MHC-G molecule evolution within primates evolving 40 million years ago (from New to Old World primates).[80] This natural "experiment" may provide us clues to MHC function and physiopathology.

On the other hand, NK immunoglobulin-like receptors (KIR) receive negative signals for cytotoxicity from HLA-G (KIR2DL4),[81] and HLA-C inhibitory KIR response is one of the strongest NK lymphocyte inhibition signals.[82] In fact, MHC class I genes and KIR-like receptor genes are thought to have coevolved in primates.[80, 83] All KIR stem from KIR3DL and KIRDX, which diverged about 135 million years ago and have coevolved with MHC-G and MHC-C as well as other MHC genes.[84] However, this coevolution shows atypical features:

1. MHC-G molecules have a different kind of molecule for each primate species;[66]
2. MHC-C molecules have been found in orangutans (Pongo pygmaeus) but not in all individuals—which does not mean they do not have it.[85]

Because New World monkeys separated from Old World monkeys about 40 million years ago[80] and NK KIR have existed since about 135 million years ago, it is striking that no New World monkey MHC-C equivalent has been found. This unusual species-specific evolution of MHC-G molecules related to MHC-C and NK lymphocyte inhibition is considered below.

Conjoint KIR and MHC Class I Evolution

KIR have been present in species since at least 135 million years ago.[84] The coevolution with MHC-C and -G, in particular, must have been parallel. MHC-C has been demonstrated to be the strongest inhibitory signal to KIR+ NK lymphocytes, as all individuals can combine at least one HLA-C epitope with its cognate KIR,[84] and MHC-G is also an inhibitory molecule for KIR.[1]

Humans, chimpanzees, gorillas, and orangutans have all been shown to have both MHC and KIR molecules.[85] Recently, KIR have also been found in New World monkeys.[86] Cotton-top Tamarins show an MHC molecule that seems to be a classical antigen presenter (Fig. 9.5) according to its polymorphism and distribution, However, it is not orthologous to G, not intron 2 deletion, closer to HLA-E in DNA sequence,[66] although it was assigned as MHC-G (Fig. 9.7).[64] In addition, two different MHC-C molecules have been found with a primary DNA sequence similar to MHC-C[87] in Cotton-top Tamarins, which may interact with a putative KIR system that has existed since 135 million years ago at least[85] and also in other New World monkeys.[86] This could be the first-described MHC-C molecules with an inhibitory function in New World monkeys.[87] Four different Saguinus oedipus individuals were analyzed with a total of 23 clones; one of them was heterozygous for the two MHC-C sequences, suggesting the existence of at least one locus with two alleles.[10, 87]

Thus, the MHC-C locus seems to exist in New World monkeys. This observation suggests that all these species may have a KIR system that existed at least since 135 million years ago.[84,86] Because New World monkeys separated from the Old World line of apes and this from orangutan[85] (last attested with MHC-C molecules) about 40 million years ago, it is likely that all New World monkeys also have a KIR/MHC-C immune regulation system. More studies to characterize the KIR system in New World monkeys are under way and information from all these will help to sort out relationships between two adaptive immune systems: that of NK cells and T lymphocytes.[10,88]

1.	Standardization of antibodies	Need validation of MHC-G, -F, -E monoclonal antibodies through International workshop
2.	Function	Whether MHC-G presents or does not present peptides to elicit immune response.
3.	Evolution	New World primates: MHC-E or MHC-G? Classical presenters; relationship with KIR system; relationship with MHC-C Old World primates: Cercopithecinae and some healthy humans do not have full HLA-G molecule Population studies of MHC-G alleles.
4.	Immunopathology	Linkage of HLA-G and disease Does HLA-G in tumors suppress immune responses, therapeutics? Does HLA-G in transplants suppress immune response, therapeutics? Do viral infections suppress immune response through HLA-G expression, therapeutics? What is the exact physiopathology of MHC-F and -E?

Fig. 9.13: Unsolved issues concerning MHC-G, F and E loci

Finally, KIR evolution may be more complicated than is apparent. This system has only recently been discovered in human beings. According to the geographic gradient, while the activating KIR genes (KIR DS and also haplotype B) occur in worldwide populations, the inhibitory KIRs (DL or haplotype A) do not. This may be because of a more pronounced HLA driven coevolution of stimulant KIR receptors,[88] as HLA is a powerful genetic marker to relate human populations according to geography.[89]

KEY ISSUES FOR FUTURE RESEARCH

MHC-G, -F, -E Questions

There are some unsolved issues concerning MHC-G, and many physiopathological questions need to be answered about MHC-F and -E genes/proteins. These are briefly presented in Figure 9.13.

ACKNOWLEDGMENTS

This work is supported in part by grants from the Spanish Ministry of Health (FISS PI051039 and PI080838), Spanish Ministry of Foreign Affairs (A/9134/07 and A/17727/08) and three different Mutua Madrileña Automovilista grants.

REFERENCES

1. Carosella ED, Moreau P, LeMaoult J, Rouas-Freiss N. HLA-G: From biology to clinical benefits. Cell Trends Immunol 2008;29:125-32.
2. Favier B, LeMaoult J, Carosella ED. Functions of HLA-G in the Immune System. Tissue Antigens 2007;69:150-52.
3. Rouas-Freiss N, Marchal RE, Kirszenbaum M, Dausset J, Carosella ED. The alpha1 domain of HLA-G1 and HLA-G2 inhibits cytotoxicity induced by natural killer cells: Is HLA-G the public ligand for natural killer cell inhibitory receptors? Proc Natl Acad Sci U S A 1997;94:5249-54.
4. Le Gal FA, Riteau B, Sedlik C, et al. HLA-G-mediated inhibition of antigen-specific cytotoxic T lymphocytes. Int Immunol 1999;11:1351-56.
5. Castro M, Morales P, Catálfamo M, et al. Lack of HLA-G soluble isoforms in Graves-Basedow thyrocytes and complete cDNA sequence of the HLA-G*01012 allele. European Journal of Immunogenetics 1998;25:311-15.
6. Arnaiz-Villena A, Martinez-Laso J, Castro MJ, et al. The evolution of the MHC-G gene does not support a functional role for the complete protein. Immunological Reviews 2001;183:65-75.
7. Arnaiz-Villena A, Martinez-Laso J, Serrano-Vela JI, Reguera R, Moscoso J. HLA-G polymorphism and evolution. Tissue Antigens 2007;69:156-59.
8. Morales P, Martinez-Laso J, Castro MJ, et al. An evolutionary overview of the MHC-G polymorphism: Clues to the unknown function(s). In: Springer-Verlag, ed. Major Histocompatibility Complex Evolution, Structure, and Function. Tokyo 2000;463-79.
9. Arnaiz-Villena A, Martinez-Laso J, Moscoso J, et al. HLA-G and HLA-E alleles: A worldwide study. In: Hansen AJ, ed. Immunobiology of the Human MHC, Proceedings of the 13th International Histocompatibility Workshop and Conference. Seattle: International Histocompatibility Working Group Press, 2006;220-21.
10. Parga-Lozano C, Reguera R, Gomez-Prieto P, Arnaiz-Villena A. Evolution of major histocompatibility complex G and C and natural killer receptors in primates. Human Immunology 2009; In press:
11. Geraghty DE, Wei XH, Orr HT, Koller BH. Human leukocyte antigen F (HLA-F). An expressed HLA gene composed of a class I coding sequence linked to a novel transcribed repetitive element. J Exp Med 1990;171:1-18.

12. Grossberger D, Parham P. Reptilian class I major histocompatibility complex genes reveal conserved elements in class I structure. Immunogenetics 1992;36:166-74.
13. Allan DS, Lepin EJ, Braud VM, O'Callaghan CA, McMichael AJ. Tetrameric complexes of HLA-E, HLA-F, and HLA-G. J Immunol Methods 2002'268:43-50.
14. Shobu T, Sageshima N, Tokui H, et al. The surface expression of HLA-F on decidual trophoblasts increases from mid to term gestation. Journal of Reproductive Immunology 2006;72:18-32.
15. Lee N, Geraghty DE. HLA-F surface expression on B cell and monocyte cell lines is partially independent from tapasin and completely independent from TAP. J Immunol 2003;171:5264-71.
16. Rojo R, Castro MJ, Martinez-Laso J, et al. MHC-F DNA sequences in bonobo, gorilla and orangutan. Tissue Antigens 2005;66:277-83.
17. O'Callaghan CA, Bell JI. Structure and function of the human MHC class Ib molecules HLA-E, HLA-F and HLA-G. Immunol Rev 1998;163:129-38.
18. Koller BH, Geraghty D, Orr HT, Shimizu Y, DeMars R. Organization of the human class I major histocompatibility complex genes. Immunol Res 1987;6:1-10.
19. Ishitani A, Sageshima N, Hatake K. The involvement of HLA-E and -F in pregnancy. J Reprod Immunol 2006;69:101-13.
20. Mizuno S, Trapani JA, Koller BH, Dupont B, Yang SY. Isolation and nucleotide sequence of a cDNA clone encoding a novel HLA class I gene. J Immunol 1988;140:4024-30.
21. Koller BH, Geraghty DE, Shimizu Y, DeMars R, Orr HT. HLA-E. A novel HLA class I gene expressed in resting T lymphocytes. J Immunol 1988;141:897-904.
22. Zinkernagel RM, Doherty PC. MHC-restricted cytotoxic T cells: studies on the biological role of polymorphic major transplantation antigens determining T-cell restriction-specificity, function, and responsiveness. Adv Immunol 1979;27:51-177.
23. Ishitani A, Sageshima N, Lee N, et al. Protein expression and peptide binding suggest unique and interacting functional roles for HLA-E, F, and G in maternal-placental immune recognition. J Immunol 2003;171:1376-84.
24. Gomez-Casado E, Martinez-Lasot J, Castro MJ, et al. Detection of HLA-E and -G DNA alleles for population and disease studies. Cell Mol Life Sci 1999;56:356-62.
25. Morales P, Corell A, Martinez-Laso J, et al. Three new HLA-G alleles and their linkage disequilibria with HLA-A. Immunogenetics 1993;38:323-31.
26. Ohya K, Kondo K, Mizuno S. Polymorphism in the human class I MHC locus HLA-E in Japanese. Immunogenetics 1990;32:205-9.
27. Arnaiz-Villena A, Timon M, Corell A, Perez-Aciego P, Martin-Villa JM, Regueiro JR. Brief report: Primary immunodeficiency caused by mutations in the gene encoding the CD3-gamma subunit of the T-lymphocyte receptor. N Engl J Med 1992;327:529-33.
28. Suarez MB, Morales P, Castro MJ, et al. A new HLA-G allele (HLA-G*0105N) and its distribution in the Spanish population. Immunogenetics 1997;45:464-65.
29. Castro MJ, Morales P, Rojo-Amigo R, et al. Homozygous HLA-G*0105N healthy individuals indicate that membrane-anchored HLA-G1 molecule is not necessary for survival. Tissue Antigens 2000;56:232-39.
30. The Anthony Nolan Trust. URL:http://www.anthony-nolan.org.uk
31. Apps R, Gardner L, Moffett A. A critical look at HLA-G. Trends in Immunology 2009;29:313-21.
32. Castro MJ, Morales P, Fernandez-Soria V, et al. Allelic diversity at the primate Mhc-G locus: Exon 3 bears stop codons in all Cercopithecinae sequences. Immunogenetics 1996;43:327-36.
33. Wainwright S, Biro P, Holmes C. HLA-F is a predominantly empty, intracellular, TAP-associated MHC class Ib protein with a restricted expression pattern. J Immunol 2000;164:319-28.
34. Lepin EJ, Bastin J, Allan D, et al. Functional characterization of HLA-F and binding of HLA-F tetramers to ILT2 and ILT4 receptors. Eur J Immunol 2000;30:3552-61.
35. Lee N, Goodlett D, Ishitani A, Marquardt H, Geraghty D. HLA-E surface expression depends on binding of TAP-dependent peptides derived from certain HLA class I signal sequences. J Immunol 1998;160:4951-60.
36. King A, Burrows T, Hiby S, et al. Surface expression of HLA-C antigen by human extravillous trophoblast. Placenta 2000;21:376-87.
37. Lee N, Llano M, Carretero M, et al. HLA-E is a major ligand for the natural killer inhibitory receptor CD94/NKG2A. Proc Natl Acad Sci USA 1998;95:5199-204.
38. Morales P, Pace J, Platt J, et al. Placental cell expression of HLA-G2 isoforms is limited to the invasive trophoblast phenotype. J Immunol 2003;171:6215-24.
39. Solier C, Aguerre-Girr M, Lenfant F, et al. Secretion of pro-apoptotic intron 4-retaining soluble HLA-G1 by human villous trophoblast. Eur J Immunol 2002;32:3576-86.
40. Cooper M, Fehniger T, Turner S, et al. Human natural killer cells: A unique innate immunoregulatory role for the CD56bright subset. Blood 2001;97:3146-51.
41. Ashkar A, Black G, Wei Q, et al. Assessment of requirements for IL-15 and IFN regulatory factors in uterine NK cell differentiation and function during pregnancy. J Immunol 2003;171:2937-44.
42. Saito S, Nishikawa K, Morii T, et al. Cytokine production by CD16-CD56 bright natural killer cells in the human early pregnancy decidua. Int Immunol 1993;5:559-63.
43. Higuma-Myojo S, Sasaki Y, Miyazaki S, Sakai M, Siozaki A, Miwa N. Cytokine profile of natural killer cells in early human pregnancy. Am J Reprod Immunol 2005;54:21-29.
44. Trundley A, Moffet A. Human uterine leukocytes and pregnancy. Tissue Antigens 2004;63:1-12.
45. Saito S. Cytokine network at the feto-maternal interface. J Reprod Immunol 2000;47:87-103.

46. Van Rood J, Claas F. Both self and non-inherited maternal HLA antigens influence the immune response. Immunol Today 2000;21:269-73.
47. Barakonyi A, Kovacs K, Miko E, Szereday L, Varga P, Szekeres-Bartho J. Recognition of nonclassical HLA class I antigens by gamma delta T cells during pregnancy. J Immunol 2002;168:2683-88.
48. Koller BH, Geraghty DE, DeMars R, Duvick L, Rich SS, Orr HT. Chromosomal organization of the human major histocompatibility complex class I gene family. J Exp Med 1989;169:469-80.
49. Geraghty DE, Pei J, Lipsky B, et al. Cloning and physical mapping of the HLA class I region spanning the HLA-E-to-HLA-F interval by using yeast artificial chromosomes. Proc Natl Acad Sci USA 1992;89:2669-73.
50. Schmidt C, Orr H. A physical linkage map of HLA-A, -G, 7.5p and -F. Human Immunology 1991;31:180-85.
51. Chimini G, Boretto J, Marguet D. Molecular analysis of the human MHC class I region using yeast artificial chromosome clones. Immunogenetics 1990;32: 419-26.
52. Ragoussis J, Bloemer K, Pohla H, Messer G, Weiss E, Ziegler A. A physical map including a new class I gene (cda 12) of the human major histocompatibility complex (A2:B13 haplotype) derived from a monosomy 6 mutant cell line. Genomics 1989;4:301-8.
53. Geraghty DE, Koller BH, Orr HT. A human major histocompatibility complex class I gene that encodes a protein with a shortened cytoplasmic segment. Proc Natl Acad Sci USA 1987;84:9145-9.
54. Kirist M, Kunz H, Gill T. Analysis of the sequence similarities of classical and nonclassical class I genes. In: Tsuji M, Aizawa M, Sasuzuki T, eds. HLA 1991. Oxford: Oxford University Press 1991;1021-30.
55. Carosella ED, Dausset J, Kirszenbaum M. HLA-G revisited. Immunology Today 1996;17:407-9.
56. Pook MA, Woodcock V, Tassabehji M, et al. Characterization of an expressible nonclassical class I HLA gene. Human Immunology 1991;32:102-9.
57. Yamashita T, Fujii T, Watanabe Y, et al. HLA-G gene polymorphism in a Japanese population. Immunogenetics 1996;44:186-91.
58. Karhukorpi J, Ikáheimo I, Silvennoinen-Kassinen S, Tiilikainen A. HLA-G polymorphism and allelic association with HLA-A in a Finnish population. Eur J Immunogenetics 1996;23:153-55.
59. Alegre R, Moscoso J, Martinez-Laso J, et al. HLA genes in Cubans and detection of Amerindian alleles. Mol Immunol 2007;44:2426-35.
60. Arnaiz-Villena A, Chandanayingyong D, Chiewsilp P, Diaz-Campos N. Non classical HLA class I antigens: HLA-E. genetic diversity of HLA: Functional and Medical implications. In: auchet R, et al (Eds). Workshop reports. Sevres, France: EDK, 1997.
61. King A, Loke Y. On the nature and function of human uterine granular lymphocytes. Immunol Today 1991;12:432-35.
62. Pistoia U, Morandi F, Wang X, Ferrone S. Soluble HLA-G: Are they clinically relevant? Semin Cancer Biol 2007;17:469-79.
63. Rebmann V, LeMaoult J, Rouas-Freiss N, Carosella ED, Grosse-Wilde H. Quantification and Identification of certain Soluble HLA-G Molecule Structures. Tissue Antigens 2006. In press:
64. Watkins DI, Chen ZW, Hughes AL, Evans MG, Tedder TF, Letvin NL. Evolution of the MHC class I genes of a New World primate from ancestral homologues of human nonclassical genes. Nature 1990;346:60-63.
65. Watkins D, Letvin N, Hughes A, Tedder T. Molecular cloning of cDNA that encode MHC class I molecules from a new world primate (Saguinus oedipus). Natural selection acts a positions that may affect peptide presentation to T cells. J Immunol 1990;144:1136-43.
66. Arnaiz-Villena A, Morales P, Gomez-Casado E, et al. Evolution of MHC-G in primates: A different kind of molecule for each group of species. J Reprod Immunol 1999;43:111-25.
67. Alvarez-Tejado M, Martinez-Laso J, Garcia-Torre C. Description of a new kind of MHC DNA sequence in Saguinus oedipus (cotton-top tamarin). Eur J Immunogenet 1998;25:287-92.
68. Arnaiz-Villena A, Martinez-Laso J, Alvarez M, et al. Primate Mhc-E and -G alleles. Immunogenetics 1997;46:251-66.
69. Diehl M, Munz C, Keilholz W. Nonclassical HLA-G molecules are classical peptide presenters. Curr Biol 1996;6:305-14.
70. Burton F. The multimedia guide to the non-human primates. Scarborough. Prentice Hall, 1995.
71. Peltola M, Chiatayat D, Peltonen L, Jalanko A. Characterization of a point mutation in aspartyl glucosaminidase gene: Evidence for a readthrough of a translational stop codon. Hum Mol Genet 1994;3:2237-42.
72. Howard M, Frizzell R, Bedwell D. Aminoglycoside antibiotics restore CFTR function by overcoming premature stop mutations. Nat Med 1996;2:467-69.
73. Fernandez-Soria V, Morales P, Castro M. Transcription and weak expression of HLA-DRB6: A gene with anomalies in exon 1 and other regions. Immunogenetics 1998;48:16-21.
74. Ober C, Aldrich C, Rosinsky B, et al. HLA-G1 protein expression is not essential for fetal survival. Placenta 1998;19:127-32.
75. Rammensee HG. Chemistry of peptides associated with MHC class I and class II molecules. Curr Opin Immunol 1995;7:85-96.
76. Le Bouteiller P, Blascitz A. The functionality of HLA-G is emerging. Immunol Rev 1999;167:233-44.
77. Paul P, Rouas-Freiss N, Khalil-Daher I, et al. HLA-G expression in melanoma: A way for tumor cells to escape from immunosurveillance. Proc Natl Acad Sci U S A 1998;95:4510-15.

78. Carosella ED, Moreau P, Le Maoult J, Le Discorde M, Dausset J, Rouas-Freiss N. HLA-G molecules: From maternal-fetal tolerance to tissue acceptance. Adv Immunol 2003;81:199-252.
79. Le Rond S, Azema C, Krawice-Radanne I, et al. Evidence to Support the Role of HLA-G5 in Allograft Acceptance through Induction of Immunosuppressive/Regulatory T Cells. J Immunol 2006;176:3266-76.
80. Castro MJ, Morales P, Martínez-Laso J, et al. Evolution of MHC-G in humans and primates based on three new 3'UT polymorphisms. Human Immunology 2000;61:1157-63.
81. Rouas-Freiss N, Goncalves RM, Menier C, Dausset J, Carosella ED. Direct evidence to support the role of HLA-G in protecting the fetus from maternal uterine natural killer cytolysis. Proc Natl Acad Sci U S A 1997;94: 11520-5.
82. Valiante N, Uhrberg M, Shilling H, et al. Functionally and structurally distinct NK cell receptor repertoires in the peripheral blood of two human donors. Immunity 1997;7:739-51.
83. Hao L, Nei M. Rapid expansion of killer cell immunoglobulin-like receptor genes in primates and their coevolution with MHC Class I genes. Gene 2004; 347:149-59.
84. Moesta A, Abi-Rached L, Norman P, Parham P. Chimpanzees use more varied receptors and ligands than humans for inhibitory killer cell Ig-like receptor recognition of the MHC-C1 and MHC-C2 epitopes. The Journal of Immunology 2009;182:3628-37.
85. Guethlein L, Flodin L, Adams EJ, Parham P. NK cell receptors of the orangutan (Pongo pygmaeus): A pivotal species for tracking the coevolution of killer cell Ig-like receptors with MHC-C. The Journal of Immunology 2002;169:220-29.
86. Cadavid L, Lun C. Lineage-specific diversification of killer cell Ig-like receptors in the owl monkey, a New World primate. Immunogenetics 2009;61:27-41.
87. Alvarez-Tejado M, Martínez-Laso J, García-de-la-Torre C, et al. Description of two Mhc-C-related sequences in the New World monkey Saguinus oedipus. European Journal of Immunogenetics 1998;25:409-17.
88. Middleton D, Meenagh A, Serrano-Vela JI, Moscoso J, Arnaiz-Villena A. Different Evolution of Inhibitory and Activating Killer Immunoglobulin Receptors (KIR) in Worldwide Human Populations. The Open Immunology Journal 2008;1:42-50.
89. Moscoso J, Crawford MH, Vicario JL, et al. HLA genes of Aleutian Islanders living between Alaska (USA) and Kamchatka (Russia) suggest a possible southern Siberia origin. Molecular Immunology 2008;45:1018-26.

Chapter 10

HLA Typing Technologies

Linda Smith, Samantha Fidler

HLA typing was first performed using serological techniques based on the complement-dependent cytotoxicity assay. Since the 1980s, there has been an enormous growth in the use of DNA technology in the field, starting with Restriction Fragment Length Polymorphism (RFLP) techniques, followed by several PCR (Polymerase Chain Reaction) based assays, including various forms of Sequence-Specific Oligonucleotide probe (SSO), Sequence-Specific Primer amplification (SSP), Single-Strand Conformation Polymorphism (SSCP), sequence-based typing (SBT) and microarray applications. Even with the best of these techniques, complete discrimination of all possible ambiguous allele combinations is not guaranteed. Due to the complexity of HLA nomenclature, terms have evolved to describe the level of discrimination obtained. The accepted terms are low, medium and high resolution. Generally, low resolution is the equivalent of serological typing, whereas high resolution results unambiguously state the alleles detected at a particular locus for that individual.

A combination of methods is often required to achieve adequate definition of an individual's HLA type and may include the use of serology to prove protein level expression of those alleles demonstrated by molecular methods. Such expression of alleles is often important in donor-recipient matching for hematopoietic stem cell transplantation.

SEROLOGY

Following the development in 1964 of the microcytotoxicity assay by Terasaki and McLelland, serological typing became the mainstay of HLA typing until the development of recombinant DNA technology in the 1980s. Although routine, high volume HLA typing by serological methods has now been superseded, many histocompatibility laboratories still employ this technique in certain circumstances.

The Complement-dependant Lymphomicrocytotoxicity Test—Principles

Separated lymphocytes (see section 1.3) of an individual to be HLA typed are incubated with a set of HLA specific alloantisera and/or monoclonal antibodies. If the specific HLA antigen is present on the cell, the antibody binds. Rabbit serum, used as a source of complement, is added. If antibody is bound to HLA antigen on the cell surface it activates the complement through the classical pathway which via the membrane attack complex damages the cell membrane making it permeable to vital stains. Results are visualized by adding a dye, usually a fluorochrome such as ethidium bromide. If a reaction has taken place, ethidium bromide enters the cell and binds to the DNA (Fig. 10.1). Double staining is normally used to help distinguish between live and dead cells. For example, ethidium bromide used to stain dead cells and acridine orange or carboxyfluoroscein diacetate (CFDA) which stain all cells, quenched using bovine hemoglobin, are used to visualize both living and dead cells simultaneously. The cells can be read on an inverted fluorescent microscope, results usually recorded as a percentage of dead cells.

Alloantisera

The HLA system is highly polymorphic, and each HLA molecule carries a number of specific polymorphic epitopes. The antibodies used for typing (alloantisera) react with these polymorphic epitopes. As antigenic

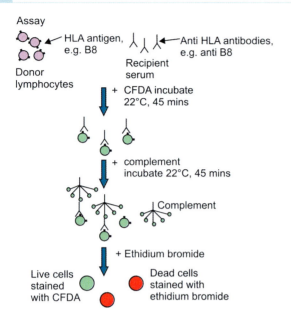

Fig. 10.1: Diagrammatic representation of complement dependent cytotoxicity assay

determinants (epitopes) are shared between different HLA antigens, one antibody can react with a number of different HLA antigens. For these reasons, alloantisera have to be carefully selected and screened for typing purposes. Alloantisera from multiparous women or multi-transfused individuals are the traditional source of typing sera. As they may contain multiple antibodies each reacting with different epitopes, extensive screening is required to fully characterise these sera. Additionally, HLA class II sera generally require platelet absorption to remove reactivity with class I antigens. For this reason, most individual laboratories no longer find their own alloantisera and commercially available monoclonal antibodies are increasingly popular in laboratories still performing typing by CDC. Although monoclonal antibodies react with a single epitope, they may not be operationally monospecific (reactive with a single HLA antigen) due to the sharing of epitopes by HLA antigens and they still require extensive quality checks and assessment to determine their specificity.

Methods for Isolating Lymphocytes

Ficoll Gradient Centrifugation

Viable peripheral blood lymphocytes are obtained by density gradient centrifugation using Ficoll. Diluted whole blood is layered over Ficoll-Hypaque that has a specific gravity corresponding to the density of lymphocytes. Centrifugation allows the isolation of mononuclear cells consisting primarily of lymphocytes at the Ficoll interface. The denser erythrocytes and granulocytes settle to the bottom of the tube, platelets remain floating in the uppermost layer (Fig. 10.2). Other sources of lymphocytes, such as spleen or lymph nodes, may also be used for typing.

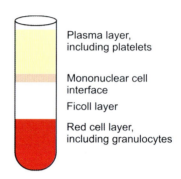

Fig.10. 2: Ficoll gradient after centrifugation

The isolated lymphocytes consist of a mixture of T and B cells. HLA class I typing can be performed readily using the isolated lymphocytes as HLA class I antigens are expressed on both T and B cells. HLA class II antigens are expressed primarily on B cells. Therefore, for HLA class II typing enrichment or purification of B lymphocytes is required. A number of techniques are available for T and B cell separation.

Nylon Wool Columns

Nylon wool columns or straws were first used to separate T and B cells in the 1970s. Peripheral blood lymphocytes are incubated in a nylon wool column at 37°C for one hour. Nonadherent T cells are collected by washing through the column. Subsequently, adherent B cells can easily be recovered by sharply tapping the column to release the B cells followed by washing through the column.

Neuraminidase Treated Sheep Erythrocytes

Peripheral blood lymphocytes are incubated with neuraminidase treated sheep erythrocytes. The sheep erythrocytes selectively bind to and form rosettes with human T lymphocytes. After Ficoll gradient centrifugation, rosetted T cells pellet at the bottom of the tube and B cells remain at the gradient interface. The T cells can be recovered by incubating the pellet at 37°C, and lysing the sheep red cells with ammonium chloride solution.

Magnetic Beads

Peripheral blood lymphocytes or whole blood are incubated with polystyrene microspheres with a magnetizable core coated with monoclonal antibody specific for non-HLA markers present on particular lymphocyte subsets (e.g. CD8 for T cells, and CD19 for B cells). The cells form rosettes with the beads, which can subsequently be isolated and washed by use of a magnet. The beads do not affect cell viability, and the cell preparation can be used with the beads still attached.

Complement

Rabbit serum is used as a source of complement. Complement batches must be carefully screened as the amount of complement and naturally occurring antibodies that react nonspecifically with human lymphocytes can vary significantly. Serum pooled from multiple rabbits is usually used to minimize these problems.

Pros and Cons of Serological Typing

Pros   Easy to perform
        No expensive equipment
        Relatively fast results – approximately 1 to 3 hours to perform
        Low level resolution – with good antisera reliable results
        Detects protein expression
        Can use cell preparations required for crossmatching

Cons   Large volume of blood required
        Requires viable lymphocytes
        Difficult to find good alloantisera for rare antigens
        Requires detailed evaluation of sera reactivity and interpretation of complex–reactivity patterns to determine HLA antigens present
        Usually not capable of high resolution typing

DNA-BASED METHODS

Restriction Fragment Length Polymorphism (RFLP)

Early molecular typing methods used restriction fragment length polymorphism (RFLP) applications. Genomic DNA is cut with a restriction enzyme, whose restriction site corresponded to a polymorphism characteristic of a particular allele. Therefore, DNA fragments of differing sizes are obtained depending on whether or not the polymorphic restriction site is present and thus whether the DNA is cut by the enzyme. The resulting DNA fragments were size-fractionated by agarose gel electrophoresis and transferred to a nylon membrane for probing with locus-specific probes. Unfortunately, not all alleles can be discriminated using this technique. In more recent times, a combination of PCR and RFLP has been applied to avoid the need for blotting and probing. However, it is a not a technique that can be easily employed in a high throughput laboratory and is not widely used.

Reference Strand Conformational Analysis (RSCA)

This assay is not commonly used. Single stranded DNA from the sample to be HLA typed is annealed to reference DNA strands followed by capillary electrophoresis in a nondenaturing polyacrylamide gel. Nucleotide mismatches between the test DNA and reference DNA results in the heteroduplex DNA adopting a conformation that is dependent on the mismatches. The HLA type is assigned on the basis of accurate measurement of mobility of the DNA in the gel, i.e. the DNA mobility is shape or conformation dependant in polyacrylamide gel electrophoresis. The method relies on excellent reference standards, conformational data and is a complex and difficult assay.

PCR Based Methods

The emergence of Polymerase Chain Reaction (PCR) in the mid 1980s had an immediate impact on HLA typing. PCR is used to amplify specific regions of an HLA gene using exon and locus-specific primers (oligonucleotides).

There are 3 steps in the PCR reaction which together are referred to as one cycle:

1. *Denaturing* of double stranded test DNA by heating to 94-96 °C, which causes separation of the two strands by disrupting the hydrogen bonds between complementary bases of the DNA strands thereby exposing the primer binding site.
2. *Annealing* (binding) of the primers to the targeted gene sequence. Two primers, often termed "upstream" and "downstream" or "forward" and "reverse" or " 5' and 3' ", which anneal at each end of the target region, are used. The nucleotide composition of the primers determines the temperature required to ensure specificity of binding for this step, which is usually between 45-68 °C.
3. *Extension* of the annealed primers to form new DNA strands by incorporation of free dNTP's (deoxy-Nucleoside-Tri-Phosphates) by the thermostable enzyme Taq polymerase, usually at 72°C. The

polymerase synthesizes a new strand complementary to the DNA template strand in the 5' to 3' direction. The time of this cycle is dependent on the length of the target DNA, as well as the type of Taq polymerase being utilized. The above process is repeated for 25-35 cycles resulting in an exponential increase in the number of copies of double stranded target DNA.

The ongoing addition of new alleles to the HLA databases can influence the reliability of any molecular typing system. New alleles may contain polymorphisms in the PCR primer annealing sites, which will then fail to amplify with the current PCR primers. Internet accessible databases such as the IMGT database (http://www.ebi.ac.uk/imgt/hla/) should be checked for new alleles on a regular basis to ensure that the primer specificities still amplify all HLA alleles.

SSO (Sequence Specific Oligohybridization)

Target DNA can undergo PCR amplification using exon and locus-specific probes. In early versions of this method, the PCR amplicon was then immobilised, for example on nylon membranes, and ^{32}P-labelled allele-specific oligonucleotide probes were allowed to hybridize to the immobilized DNA. For each allele-specific probe used, a separate membrane is required. This is followed by washing steps at various temperatures to ensure the specificity of binding for each oligo probe. The oligo probes will remain bound only to their complementary sequence in the amplicon providing the washing temperatures are optimized. Nowadays, most SSO assays are so-called reverse-SSO assays, where the allele-specific oligos are immobilized and the PCR amplicon, which has been biotin-labelled by the use of biotinylated PCR primers, is allowed to hybridize to the immobilized oligos. The labelled target DNA amplicons bound to specific probes are detected via streptavidin-horseradish peroxidase (HRP) and a chromogenic substrate, which generates a blue "line" at the position of the positive probe (Fig. 10.3). There are many commercially available reverse SSO kits, where multiple probes are bound in a ladder format to nylon strips. Reactivity patterns can be interpreted manually using charts included in the kits, or using genotyping software.

The initial traditional method is more suited to high-throughput laboratories than the reverse-SSO method, as many samples can be amplified and spotted onto a series of membranes followed by probing. The reverse SSO applications are better suited to laboratories with a low throughput and for the one-off typing of individual

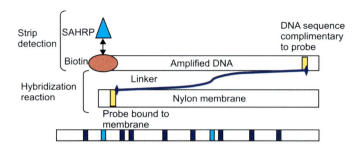

Fig. 10.3: Schematic representation of Reverse Line blot SSO

samples. However, in the latter, as all probes are on the one membrane, the melting temperature of all probes must be similar.

A more recent development using SSO-oligo hybridization is Luminex® xMAP technology. Each of a series of SSO-probes is immobilized on a different colored microspheres (beads). Hybridization of the biotinylated PCR-amplified DNA to those beads carrying a specific probe is detected using streptavidin-conjugated phycoerythrin (Fig. 10.4). The different colored beads and fluorescent signals are detected using the Luminex® compact flow cytometer. Lasers excite the internal dye which uniquely identifies each bead, and also any captured reporter fluorescence. More than 100 individual beads (and therefore greater than 100 different probes) are available for each assay, which results in a relatively high resolution typing result. The PCR and hybridization process takes place in a single 96-well PCR plate, so that up to 96 samples can be processed at one time. This makes this method more suitable for a higher throughput situation than some of the alternative SSO methods. Results generally provide medium resolution HLA typing, although high resolution results are often obtained, depending on the allele combinations present.

PCR-SSP (Sequence Specific Primer)

In this method, many different PCR primer pairs are used in multiple small-scale PCR reactions, where each reaction is specific for an allele or group of alleles present in the target DNA within the HLA locus of interest. It is based on the principle that a completely matched primer will amplify more efficiently than a primer with one or more mismatches. In this way, each PCR reaction is specific for the presence of the complementary sequence in the target DNA. The base at the 3' end of the primer confers specificity of hybridization, where an exact match is required for hybridization to enable synthesis of a new strand of DNA in the PCR reaction. Each reaction also

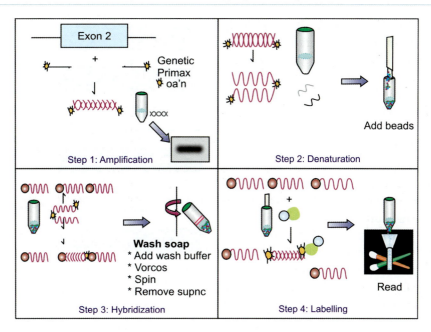

Fig. 10.4: Principle of the OneLambda LABType Reverse SSO method

contains an additional pair of primers targeting a nonpolymorphic (or "housekeeping") gene, which act as an internal control for the PCR reaction and to confirm that a negative reaction is not, in fact, a failed PCR. Melting temperature optimization of the primer pairs is necessary to allow successful PCR amplification for all primer pairs under the same thermal cycling conditions within a single thermal cycler. The presence of amplification products is detected by agarose electrophoresis and ethidium bromide staining of the DNA (Fig. 10.5). Depending on the number of primer sets used, low, medium or high resolution results can be obtained. Some primers will amplify multiple alleles, so specificity is determined by the pattern of positive and negative reactions. This can be done manually, or using specific software packages for each kit. There are multiple commercial kits available on the market. They vary in composition to suit many different applications. For example, there are kits which enable low resolution HLA-A, B, DRB1 typing of a sample on a single plate.

The major advantage of this system is that it is the fastest of the molecular methods. It has become the method of choice for those laboratories performing DNA based typing for cadaveric donor HLA typing. However, it is an expensive method, requires relatively large amounts of DNA and is not particularly suited to high throughput applications.

In some laboratories, the SSP assay is used as a supplement to serology by using subsets of primers for the more difficult to define serological specificities. It can also used to detect the presence or absence of HLA-B*27 for the diagnosis of ankylosing spondylitis, and its application for single allele-specific assays is increasing as certain drug hypersensitivity reactions are being linked to particular HLA alleles. For example, HLA-B*5701 and abacavir hypersensitivity, HLA-B*1502 and carbamazepine sensitivity.

Note: The presence of a second band in lanes 1 and 3 indicates a positive result for that primer pair. The band common to all lanes is the internal positive control band.

PCR-Single Strand Conformation Polymorphism (SSCP)

Under certain physical conditions, double stranded DNA will form secondary structures. The pattern of "loops" and "hairpins" which form are dependent on the nucleotide sequence. If two alleles have different sequences, the types and placements of secondary structures should differ. A small amount of amplified and denatured DNA is electrophoresed under

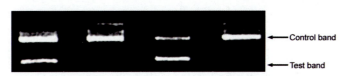

Fig. 10.5: Electrophoresis of SSP products

nondenaturing conditions, followed by silver staining. The secondary structure formed by different alleles can be differentiated by the migration patterns in the gel matrix. This method is somewhat complex for routine HLA typing, but can be used in donor-recipient matching, particularly for HLA class II genes.

Sequencing Based Typing (SBT)

HLA typing by SBT began as a tool for resolving ambiguities arising from other molecular methods. One of the disadvantages of SSO and SSP methods is that they are unlikely to detect a new undefined allele, unless the variation occurs at the specific site detected by the probe or primer, resulting in unexpected or unique reaction patterns. The advantage of SBT is that it determines the complete nucleotide sequence of the alleles present. The introduction of dye-labelled primers and automated fluorescent sequence techniques has allowed wider acceptance and use of sequencing techniques in HLA laboratories. In addition, the replacement of "slab-gel" sequencers with capillary based systems has increased the efficiency and decreased the cost of sequencing.

The principle of these systems is as follows:
1. PCR amplification of the polymorphic region of the HLA loci (most commonly exon 2 for Class II, and exons 2+3 for Class I). Unincorporated nucleotides and primers are removed by one of a number of purification systems (e.g. columns, magnetic beads)
2. The PCR product is then sequenced using multiple sequencing primers covering the length of the template in separate sequencing reactions (Fig. 10.6).

Principles of Dye Terminator Cycle Sequencing

The sequencing reaction contains a combination of DNA template, sequencing primer, DNA polymerase, deoxynucleotides (dNTP's) and dye-labelled dideoxynucleotides (ddNTP's). In the sequencing PCR reaction, the extension product increases in length by the formation of a phosphodiester bridge between the 3'- hydroxyl group and the end of the primer and the 5'- phosphate group of the incoming deoxynucleotide. In the dideoxy method of DNA sequencing (Sanger, et al 1977), the incorporation of a dideoxynucleotide results in termination of the extending sequence due to the lack of a 3'-hydroxyl group on the dideoxynucleotide. Four dyes are used to label and thus specifically identify the A, C, G and T extension products. All four colors emit a different wavelength and can therefore be combined in a single lane or capillary injection. (Earlier methods

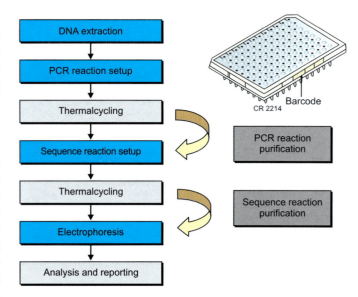

Fig. 10.6: Outline of sequencing based typing workflow

utilizing radio-labelled ddNTP's required 4 separate reactions and lanes on a polyacrylamide gel.) Successive PCR rounds of denaturation, annealing and extension in a thermal cycler generate a series of fragments of increasing size with a dye-labelled nucleotide in the final position. Following cycling, the extension products are purified by either ethanol precipitation or magnetic beads. The fragments are then passed through polyacrylamide gels or capillaries and are separated according to size, with the smaller fragments migrating faster than the larger fragments. The fluorescent label on each fragment is excited as it passes by a scanning laser beam. The light emitted by the excitation of the dyes is recorded by CCD camera, then recorded and processed by data collection software and stored as a gel image (Figs 10.7 and 10.8). Data from the gel image is analyzed by sequence analysis software that identifies each base and displays the DNA sequence in an electropherogram (Fig. 10.9).

Further analysis (editing) of the DNA sequence by specialized allele assignment software, (e.g. Assign SBT, SBT Engine, AccuType, HLA SequiTyper) which compares the sample sequence to a library of currently identified alleles to finally determine the HLA type present.

Assay Design

The initial PCR can be designed in a number of ways. PCR primers can be located within the exon of interest, in the flanking intron, or in the adjacent exon. Situating

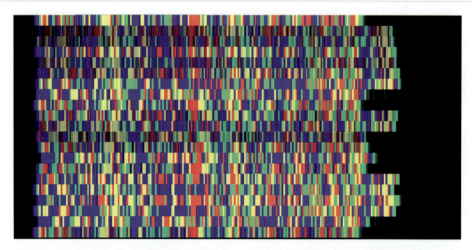

Fig. 10.7: Gel image from a sequence run on an Applied Biosystems 3730

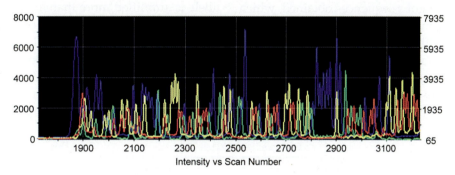

Fig. 10.8: Expanded raw data view from a single capillary

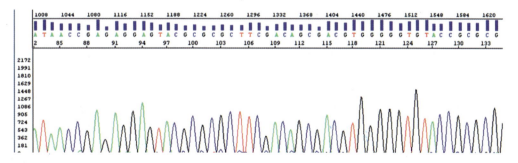

Fig. 10.9: Analyzed data file

primers within the exon of interest will result in incomplete exon sequence, as portions of the exon outside the PCR primer sites are not amplified (Fig. 10.10). However, the primers are easier to design as the exons are well characterized and the sequence data for all identified alleles is available.

The advantage of using primers located in the introns (Figs 10.12 and 10.13) is that it will result in complete exon sequence data, however, the lack of published intronic sequence data limits this approach. There is also a risk of allele "dropout" due to unidentified polymorphisms in the primer site resulting in a lack of amplification. PCR primers may be designed to be locus specific for the region of interest in which all alleles at this locus are amplified; or allele/group specific, where only those specific alleles or groups of alleles are

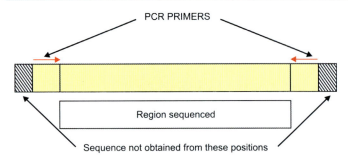

Fig. 10.10: PCR primer location

amplified (Fig. 10.11). The PCR reactions for each set of primers are generally performed in separate tubes, resulting in the two alleles present in a heterozygous sample being amplified in separate tubes. This reduces the number of heterozygous sequences obtained, which makes the allele assignment process far simpler. Allele- or group-specific amplification is particularly suitable for the HLA-DRB1 locus, where designing locus-specific primers that amplify only one of the genes present, without simultaneously amplifying additional loci (such as DRB3, DRB4, etc.), can be difficult.

However, the use of allele or group-specific primers requires that there is either prior knowledge of the alleles present to enable the selection of the appropriate primer paries (e.g. from serological typing), or that multiple PCRs are performed and each checked by gel electrophoresis to determine which primer pairs have resulted in the generation of products to be sequenced. This limits the use of such a strategy as a first pass typing method. An alternative approach is to mix the primers together in one reaction tube, known as multiplexing (Fig. 10.14), although this requires a great deal of optimisation of the PCR conditions and primer concentrations in order to ensure that all primers are equally efficient at the same conditions. Without this, "preferential amplification" can be observed, where one allele is amplified more than another, sometimes to the extent that the presence of the second allele is undetected.

Several options are available when considering the design of sequencing primers. One of the most commonly used approaches is to add "universal tags" to the PCR primers (as shown in the Class II strategy diagram Fig. 10.13), which then act as targets for complementary

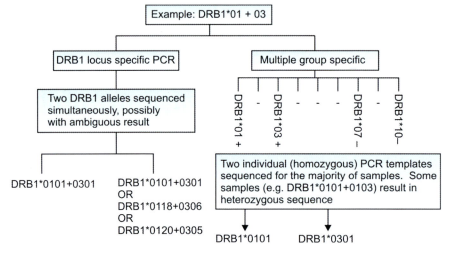

Fig. 10.11: Locus specific vs Group specific PCR amplification prior to sequencing

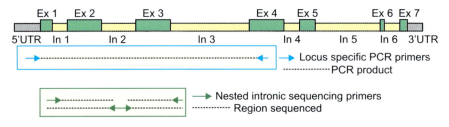

Fig. 10.12: Example of Class I PCR and Sequencing strategy

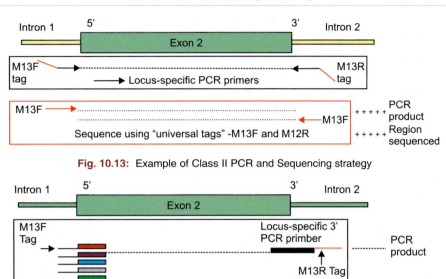

Fig. 10.13: Example of Class II PCR and Sequencing strategy

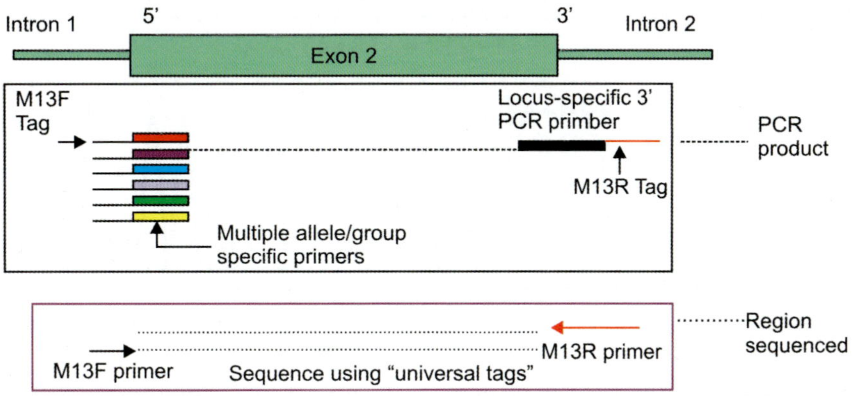

Fig. 10.14: Example of Multiplex Group/Allele specific PCR strategy for Class II

sequencing primers. The PCR primer hybridizes to the target DNA, but the tag does not. Alternatively, "nested" sequencing primers, which are internal to the PCR primers, can be used. These may be either in the introns (as shown in the Class I strategy diagram Fig. 10.12) or exons. In the majority of situations, sequencing in both directions is necessary, particularly for heterozygous templates in order to confirm any areas of sequence where the bases are not clear, either due to poor sequence quality, or to confirm heterozygote positions.

Analysis

The significant advantage of Sequence Based Typing is that it will often result in high resolution typing results. However, in some cases the sequence obtained does not discriminate between certain allele combinations. For example HLA-DRB1*0101+0301 has the same heterozygous nucleotide sequence as DRB1*0118+0306 and DRB1*0120+0305, as shown in Figure 10.11 above. The location and specificity of the PCR primers used will determine the number of ambiguous combinations obtained. Ambiguous allele combinations arise because multiple allele combinations have the same combined nucleotide sequence over the region amplified. There are three kinds of ambiguity:

1. Multiple alleles that have the same nucleotide sequence in the region sequenced but differ in exons outside the region sequenced. These may be resolved by amplifying and sequencing the additional exons. Included within this group are alleles where the differences result in altered gene expression, which may not need to be resolved, depending on the clinical situation. The use of serological methods can be invaluable in clarifying these ambiguities.

2. Those due to cis/trans ambiguities, (e.g. HLA-B*350101+380101 or 530101+3905). In this case, the alleles share the same sequence motifs, but in different combinations (Fig. 10.15). These ambiguities can be resolved by the use of additional group or allele-specific PCR reactions designed to amplify individual alleles present followed by further sequencing of these additional PCR products. A more efficient approach is to use additional sequencing primers (often known as Group Specific Primers – GSPs, or Sequence Specific Primers – SSPs) which anneal to only one of the alleles present, thus allowing exclusion of one or more of the possible combinations. In some cases, where there are differences in both exon 2 and 3, more than one of these primers may be required to completely resolve the ambiguity.

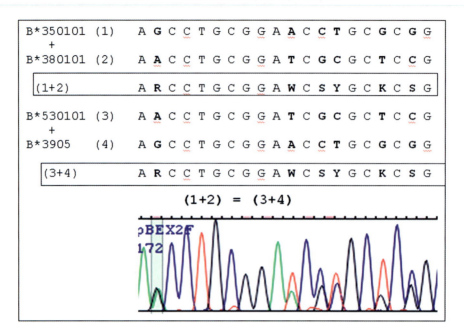

Fig. 10.15: Example of cis/trans ambiguity – B350101+380101 have the same consensus sequence as B*530101+3905

3. Silent substitutions, where subtypes of an allele may differ at the nucleotide level but not in the expressed protein. These ambiguities do not need resolving for most clinical purposes.

Summary of PCR and Sequence Assay Design

A summary of the advantages and disadvantages of the different approaches to assay design are shown in the below (Table 10.1).

Microarrays

The use of Microarray technology is a relatively recent development in HLA typing. Microarrays can be used to distinguish between DNA sequences that differ by as little as a single nucleotide. Microarrays have the capability of being a high throughput HLA typing application as they are capable of performing thousands of hybridizations in a single experiment, and have the added attraction of requiring very little DNA.

The principle of the assay is as follows:
1. DNA probes complementary to the sequence motifs present in most HLA alleles are bound to a solid substrate (usually glass, but can be silicon chips or nylon membranes). Thousands of probes are placed in known locations on a single DNA microarray.
2. DNA is amplified by PCR using fluorescently labelled primers, and is then hybridized to the immobilized complementary probes. The sample DNA will only anneal to the oligo probes that match it perfectly, a single mismatch is sufficient to prevent hybridization under appropriate conditions.
3. Hybridized targets are detected using a laser detection system.
4. HLA typing is determined by assessing the pattern of hybridization of the ordered set of oligos, using specialized software.

Microarrays can be fabricated using a variety of technologies, including printing with fine pins, inkjet printing or electrochemistry. Some of these methods can be used by laboratories to manufacture their own microarrays. This allows the design of oligos to be customized, as compared to purchasing more expensive commercial arrays. (Manufacturers include Affymetrix, Agilent, Nimblegen, and Illumina.) Both the oligo design and data analysis components of this technology are highly complex and, as such, may not be readily applicable in many routine HLA typing laboratories, while commercial systems are expensive.

Next-Generation Sequencing

Recently emerging sequencing platforms are capable of producing massive amounts of sequence data per run. Instruments from Illumina/Solexa (Genome Analyzer), Roche/454 (FLX) and Applied Biosystems (SOLiD), are capable of producing millions of bases of sequence in a single run, and have the potential to significantly change the approach to HLA typing. A major advantage of these

Table 10.1: Summary of assay design approaches

Assay Stage	Approach	Advantage	Disadvantage
PCR	Intronic Primers	Complete exon sequence obtained	Hard to design due to lack of available data
	Exonic Primers	Easier to design	Loss of sequence data at exon boundaries
	Locus specific	Only one locus amplified	Not always one suitable site, may require multiple primers (then difficult to optimise)
Ambiguity Resolution	Heterozygous amplification	Less PCR reactions	Cis/Trans ambiguities
	Group/Allele specific	Sequences generally unambiguous	Multiple initial PCRs
Sequencing	Intronic Universal Tags	Single primer for all	Requires specific PCR template
	Exonic nested primers	Easy to design, locus specific	Loss of sequence at exon boundaries
	Intronic nested primers	Locus specific	Difficult to design, multiple primers may be required

approaches is that because sequences are generated from single molecules, there are none of the complications of cis/trans ambiguities.

The platforms acquire sequence data from amplified single DNA fragments, although the processes differ between the three manufacturers. For example, in the Roche 454 GS/FLX system, small fragments of DNA (e.g. sheared DNA or PCR products) are bound to adaptors, which then allow them to be captured on beads (one fragment per bead). The term "library" is often used to describe the solution of DNA fragments, regardless of whether they are generated by DNA shearing or PCR amplification. A water-in-oil emulsion containing PCR reagents and one bead per droplet is created which is then used to allow the amplification of each fragment individually in its droplet. After amplification, the water-in-oil emulsion is broken, beads not carrying any DNA are removed, and the beads with their single amplified DNA fragment, are distributed into the wells of a fibre optic slide called a PicoTiterPlate. The size of the well is designed to fit only one bead. Following the distribution of beads to the plate, Pyrosequencing is performed. This is a "sequencing-by-synthesis" method where a successful nucleotide incorporation event is detected as emitted photons. Polymerase and one exclusive dNTP per cycle are flowed across the plate, generating one or more incorporation events, and the emitted light is proportional to the number of incorporated nucleotides. Photons are detected by a CCD camera. Excess reagents from each round are removed by enzyme containing wash solutions. The use of this technology from Roche 454 allows greater read lengths (up to 400bp) when compared to the other two platforms, which generate read lengths of less than 100bp. With each plate having approximately 1.2 million successful reads of up to 400bp, 500Mb of data can be generated per run. The development of barcode-like identifying oligo "tags" which can be attached to the DNA fragments before they are ligated to the beads allows multiple samples to be processed in the one reaction run. The sequence data generated by each sample can by identified and segregated by the unique "oligo tag" it carries.

However, there are currently some factors that make the routine use of this technology in HLA typing an expensive exercise. For locus-specific PCR-based approaches, library preparation methods are costly, time- and labour-intensive and impractical for projects involving large numbers of individuals. For any one individual, the amplicons need to be purified and quantitated, before any of the sequence-specific primer ligation and library preparation steps are undertaken. Given the need to multiply this process by the number of patients who are studied in parallel, the magnitude of the problem becomes apparent. However, some cost reduction can be obtained by dividing the PicoTiterPlate into smaller segments, and in addition using the "barcode" type oligo "tags" to the DNA of each individual so as to allow DNA from multiple individuals to be pooled for sequencing. An alternative approach to the PCR amplification of the region of interest is "target enrichment". This process uses microarray to capture the target regions from samples which have been size selected. Probes are designed at relatively short intervals across the region of interest and bound to the sequence capture array. Fragmented DNA is hybridized to the array, and unbound DNA is washed away. The DNA is then eluted from the chip and amplified using Ligation Mediated PCR. This is a PCR technique applied to DNA molecules where the sequence of only one end of the template is known. The PCR products obtained from this procedure then ready for amplification and sequencing.

Processing the huge amounts of sequence data resulting from a NextGen run to produce a HLA type will require significant development of specialized software. Such software will need to identify the individual sequences belonging to each sample, align the overlapping sequences from each sample to generate a complete consensus sequence, and compare this sequence to the reference database to assign the alleles. One of the advantages of this technology, however, is that the issue of ambiguous allele combinations will not arise as each sequence is generated from clonally amplified single molecules.

Choice of Method

Each laboratory will have different requirements that determine the choice of techniques employed for HLA typing. The clinical application and urgency need to be balanced against the number of samples, availability of equipment, staff skills and budget. The need for low or high resolution typing also influences the choice of method. For example, solid organ transplant candidates do not generally require high resolution HLA typing, whereas for bone marrow transplantation it is essential.

Since DNA can be isolated from cells long after they are viable for serological testing, typing by molecular methods has a distinct advantage. Molecular typing is superior to serological methods for determining allele group subtypes, however, these methods can still produce ambiguous results. While the use of serological HLA typing methods may be declining, they still have a valuable contribution in confirming the expression of alleles on the cell surface. For these reasons, many laboratories employ a combination of serological and molecular methods.

BIBLIOGRAPHY

Serology

1. Amos DB, et al. A simple microcytotoxicity test. Transplantation 1969;7:220.
2. Terasaki PI, McClelland JD. Microdroplet assay of human serum cytotoxins. Nature 1964.
3. Dynal beads (Dynabeads R) Technical Tips manual.
4. UniSorb nylon wool column technical data sheet. (Novamed Ltd).
5. Weiner MS, Bianco C, Nussenzweig V. Enhanced binding of neuraminidase-treated sheep erythrocytes to human T lymphocytes. Blood 1973;42:939-46.

PCR

6. Saiki R, et al. Enzymatic amplification of β-globin Genomic sequences and restriction site analysis for diagnosis of sickle cell anemia. Science 1985;230(4732):1350-54.
7. Mullis KB, Faloona F. Specific synthesis of DNA *in vitro* via a polymerase catalysed chain reaction. Meth Enzymol 1987;155:355-450.
8. Saiki RK et al. Primer directed enzymatic amplification of DNA with a thermostable DNA polymerase. Science 1988;239:487-91.

RFLP

9. Inoko H, Ota M. PCR-RFLP. In: Hui KM, Bidwell JL, eds. Handbook of HLA Typing Techniques. Boca Raton, FL: CRC Press, Inc; 1993.

RSCA

10. Turner DM, et al. HLA-A typing by reference strand-mediated conformation analysis (RSCA) using a capillary-based semi-automated genetic analyser. Tissue Antigens 1999;54:400-04.

SSCP

11. Carrington M, et al. Typing of HLA-DQA1 and DQB1 using DNA single-strand conformation polymorphism. Hum Immunol 1992;33:208-12.

SSP

12. Olerup O, Zetterquist H. HLA-DR typing by PCR amplification with sequence-specific primers (PCR SSP) in 2 hours: An alternative to serological DR typing in clinical practice including donor-recipient matching in cadaveric transplantation. Tissue Antigens 1992;39:225-35.
13. Olerup O, Zetterquist H. HLA-DR typing of polymerase chain reaction amplification with sequence-specific primers (PCR-SSP). In: Hui KM, Bidwell JL, Eds. Handbook of HLA Typing Techniques. Boca Raton, FL: CRC Press, Inc 1993;149-74.
14. Tonks, S, March SG, Bunce M, Bodmer JM. Molecular typing for HLA class I using ARMS-PCR: further developments following the 12th International Histocompatibility Workshop. Tissue Antigens 1999;53:175-83.

SSOP

15. Wordsworth P. Techniques used to define human MHC antigens: polymerase chain reaction and oligonucleotide probes. Immunol Lett 1991;29:37-39.
16. Tiercy J M, et al. A comprehensive HLA-DRB,-DQB, and –DPB oligotyping procedure by hybridisation with sequence-specific oligonucleotide probes. In: Hui KM, Bidwell JL Eds. Handbook of HLA typing Techniques, Boca Raton, FL: CRC Press, Inc 1993;p:99-116.
17. Cao K, Chapek M, FernandeZ-Vina MA. High and intermediate resolution DNA typing systems for class I HLA-A,B, C genes by hybridisation with sequence-specific oligonucleotide probes (SSOP).

Sequence Based Typing

18. Cereb N, et al. Locus-specific amplification of HLA class I genes from genomic DNA: Locus-specific sequences in the first and third introns of HLA-A, -B, and -C alleles. *Tissue Antigens* 1995 Jan;45(1):1–1.
19. Lee KW, Steiner N, Hurley CK. Clarification of HLA-B serologically ambiguous types by automated DNA sequencing. Tissue Antigens 1998;51:536-40.
20. Kotsch K, Wehling J, Blasczyk R. Sequencing of HLA class II genes based on the conserved diversity of the noncoding regions: Sequencing based typing of HLA-DRB genes. Tissue Antigens 1999, 53:486-97.
21. Kurz B, et al. New high resolution typing strategy for HLA-A locus alleles based on dye terminator sequencing of haplotypic group-specific PCR-amplicons of exon 2 and exon 3. Tissue Antigens 1999;53:81-96.
22. Sayer D, et al. HLA-DRB1 DNA sequencing based typing: An approach suitable for high throughput typing including unrelated bone marrow registry donors. Tissue Antigens 2001;57:46-54.

Microarray

23. Guo Z, Hood L, Petersdorf EW. Oligonucleotide arrays for high resolution HLA typing. Rev Immunogenet 1999;1(2):220-30.
24. Fortina P, et al. Simple two-color array-based approach for mutation detection. Eur J Hum Genet 2000;8:884-94.
25. Zhang F, et al. Oligonucleotide microarray for HLA-DRB1 genotyping: Preparation and clinical evaluation. Tissue Antigens 2005 May;65(5):467-73.
26. Zhang F, Hu SW, Huang J, Wang H, Wen Z, Yongyao G, Wang S. Development and clinical evaluation of oligonucleotide microarray for HLA-AB genotyping. Pharmacogenomics 2006;7:973–85.

NextGen

27. Schuster SC. Next generation sequencing transforms today's biology. Nature Methods 2008;5(1): 16-18.
28. Wold B, Myers, RM. Sequence census methods for functional genomics. Nature Methods 2008; 5(1): 19-21.
29. Pettersson E, Lundeberg J, Ahmadian A. Generations of sequencing technologies. Genomics 2009; 93:105-11.

General

30. Mallal S, et al. HLA-B*5701 screening for hypersensitivity to abacavir. N Engl J Med 2008 Feb 7;358(6):568-79.
31. Hung SI, et al. Genetic susceptibility to carbamazepine-induced cutaneous adverse drug reactions. Pharmacogenet. Genomics 2006;16(4):297-306.
32. Middleton D. HLA typing from Serology to Sequencing Era. Iran J Allergy, Asthma, Immunol 2005 June;4(2): 53-66.
33. Gerlach JA. Human Lymphocyte Antigen molecular typing: How to identify the 1250+ alleles out there. Arch Pathol Lab Med 2002;126:281-84.
34. Hui KM, Bidwell JL Eds. Handbook of HLA typing Techniques, Boca Raton, FL: CRC Press, Inc;1993.
35. Bidwell JL, Navarrete C (Eds). Histocompatibility Testing. Imperial College Press 2001.
36. ASHI Laboratory Manual Fourth Edition 2000.

Chapter 11

Computer Programs for the Development of SBT for HLA

David Charles Sayer

INTRODUCTION

No other human genetic system has been the subject of such intense typing technology development as the HLA genes (and gene products). This chapter describes the evolution of DNA sequencing for HLA typing and the sequence analysis software developments that have taken DNA sequencing from an impractical, inefficient and expensive HLA test to the high throughput, routine test now used in many laboratories worldwide.

As has been the trend for other HLA typing technologies, SBT now no longer provides the typing accuracy it was once able to provide and a new technology breakthrough is required. The new breakthrough is likely to be one of the so-called Next Generation Sequencing (NGS) technologies. Despite the relative recent emergence of NGS, the HLA typing community, as it was with "conventional" sequencing, has been quick to seize on NGS' potential to provide unparalleled typing accuracy. This chapter will also discuss NGS based HLA typing (NGSBT) developments to date.

DNA SEQUENCING—THE EARLY YEARS

The first practical methods for sequencing the order of bases in a DNA molecule were described by Sanger[1,2] and Maxam and Gilbert.[3] The methods were similar in that they identified the terminal base of radiolabeled DNA fragments following electrophoretic separation. However, the methods differed in the way the DNA fragments were generated. DNA fragments generated by the Maxam-Gilbert method relied on the cleavage of radiolabeled DNA at sequence specific sites following chemical treatment. These experiments were performed in different tubes and resulted in one tube containing fragments that terminated in G, one containing fragments that terminated in a purine (either A or G), one containing fragments terminating in a pyrimidine (either C or T) and one containing fragments terminating in C. The contents of each tube were fractionated in adjacent lanes in a polyacrylamide gel and the sequence was read by determining the order of electrophoretic migration.

In contrast, the Sanger method generated DNA fragments following enzymatic DNA synthesis from an oligonucleotide primer using DNA polymerase in the presence of deoxynucleotides (deoxys) and chain terminating dideoxynucleotides (dideoxys). The incorporation of deoxys enabled continuing DNA chain extension. Dideoxys contain a hydrogen molecule (H) on the 3' carbon instead of a hydroxyl group (OH) and, when incorporated, prevented further chain extension resulting in the generation of DNA fragments that differed in length by a single base. The sequencing reactions were performed in four different tubes with each tube containing a different dideoxy (A,C,G and T). The contents of each tube were also fractionated in adjacent lanes in a polyacrylamide gel and the sequence was read in the same manner as the method of Maxam-Gilbert.

With the exception of the Next Generation sequencing technologies, it is the chain termination method of Sanger that is used by almost all laboratories that perform DNA sequencing today. However, there have been a number of technological improvements that have taken a tedious, time consuming method that generated up to 100 bases of sequence over a few days to the automated sequencing instruments of today that can generate tens of thousands of bases in a single day. Despite the technological improvements, and the substantial improvements in throughput, the basic principles have not changed.

TOWARDS HIGH THROUGHPUT SANGER SEQUENCING

The major technological advances in DNA sequencing, following the initial descriptions in 1977, were driven by accuracy and throughput requirements of the Human Genome Project.

The first major technological advance was to dye label oligonucleotide primers and the subsequent birth of the automated sequencing era in 1986.[4] Instead of labeling DNA with hazardous radiolabels, oligonucleotide sequencing primers were labeled with one of four different fluorescent dyes for each of the different bases. Sequencing reactions were performed in 4 separate tubes (one for each dye/base) and then pooled before fractionation in a single lane of a polyacrylamide gel. The gel was mounted into an automated DNA sequencer that had a laser which scanned the bottom of an electrophoresis plate and excited the DNA fragments as they migrated through the gel. Detectors collected the emission intensities of the excited dyes and software converted the emission data into an electropherogram consisting of a series of peaks of four colors representing the four bases in sequence order reading from left to right. The peak heights reflected to the number of DNA fragments with a terminal dideoxy. The ability to pool DNA fragments into a single lane enabled four times the amount of sequencing to be performed. The introduction of dye-labeled dideoxys, described in 1987[5] represented a significant breakthrough for two major reasons. The first was that it enabled the sequencing reaction to be performed in a single tube increasing throughput potential by reducing the number of sequencing reactions from 4 to 1 per sample, but more importantly it enables DNA sequencing to be performed with any sequencing primer without the need for the primer to be dye labeled.

CYCLE SEQUENCING

Essentially, cycle sequencing is a PCR but with a single (sequencing) primer, Prior to the introduction of cycle sequencing DNA Sanger sequencing was performed on relative large amounts of DNA with a heat labile polymerase. For cycle sequencing, smaller amounts of DNA are required and the high temperatures of the PCR result in increased specificity thereby improving sequence data quality and increasing sequence read lengths.

In cycle sequencing the DNA template exists as a pool of many DNA molecules. Multiple sequencing primer molecules simultaneously create new DNA molecules from the DNA template. During the extension phase Taq polymerase incorporates either a di-deoxy or a deoxy at each position within the extending DNA chain. The rate at which Taq incorporates deoxys/dideoxys varies from one position in the template to the next. This resulted in dramatic variation in peak heights seen in the sequence electropherograms. At a position where the rate of incorporation of dideoxys is high compared to the rate of incorporation of deoxys more fragments will terminate at this position and the sequence peak will be high. In some cases the incorporation rate of dideoxys is too low and a peak may be generated that is not able to be discriminated from background, resulting in an increased risk of sequence errors made by the automated base calling software. Sequencing with thermolabile polymerase, such as T7 polymerase, incorporates deoxys/dideoxys at a consistent rate and as a result peak heights are less variable and fewer sequencing errors are made. The variation in the nucleotide incorporation rate between Taq and T7 was shown to be the result of a single residue within the active site of the Taq and T7.[6] Thermolabile polymerase, such as T7, cannot be used for cycle sequencing, thus to combine the benefits of cycle sequencing and the even incorporation rates of T7 polymerase, the T7 component critical for even incorporation of di-deoxys site was introduced into Taq polymerase.

The enzyme modifications, and subsequent improvements in dye technology with the introduction of "Big Dyes"[7] have resulted in partial improvements in base call accuracy and sequence read lengths but the variability in peak heights still remain today and have implications for sequencing PCR products containing heterozygous sequence.

DNA SEQUENCING AS A METHOD FOR HLA TYPING

Early sequencing studies demonstrated that HLA diversity is generated by the inter-allelic and inter-locus exchange of DNA motifs and HLA alleles exist as a patchwork of variable regions interspersed with conserved sequences.[8] This feature led to the development of typing techniques directed to the variable regions using PCR and sequence specific oligonucleotide probes (SSO)[9] and sequence specific primers (SSP).[10] HLA types were assigned from the pattern of sequence motifs inferred by primer and probe reactivity. This indirect method of partial gene sequencing began to reveal the extent of HLA diversity resulting in an explosion in the rate of identification of novel alleles. Novel alleles were identified as a result of unexpected reactivity with probes and primers, usually because the novel allele contained a variable region found in other alleles. The novel alleles were then characterized by DNA sequencing.

Whilst improving the accuracy of HLA typing, SSO and SSP did not provide information in the so-called conserved regions. Furthermore SSO and SSP approaches require constant updating as new alleles are described. A method was required that interrogated all nucleotides amplified in the PCR, without prejudice and would not need updating with the description of new alleles. Such an approach is DNA sequencing based HLA typing (SBT).

The HLA genes, in comparison to many other genes, lend themselves perfectively to be genotyped by DNA sequencing. For example, HLA class I is only a little over 3kb in length, there are a relatively small number of exons that are sufficiently small enough so that they can be completely sequenced with a single sequencing reaction. Exons 2 and 3 of the HLA Class I genes encode the molecules' peptide binding region, are the most polymorphic exons and are 270 and 276 bp in length respectively. Similarly, exon 2 of the DRB1, DQB1 and DPB1 encodes the class II peptide binding region, and are also less than 300 bp in length. The read lengths required for sequencing these exons are well within the capabilities of conventional Sanger sequencing. However the down side to sequencing HLA genes is that each gene is a member of a multi gene family with high sequence homology to other genes, pseudogenes and gene fragments, requiring that PCR amplification procedures are designed for high specificity. Designing appropriate PCR assays for HLA SBT presented a significant challenge. However Malcolm McGinnis, Pete Krausa and Jason Stein whilst at Applied Biosystems (Foster City, USA) and later at Forensic Analytical (South San Francisco USA), and Atria Genetics (South San Francisco, USA), began commercially manufacturing SBT assays for all classical HLA loci. They used a locus specific amplification approach where each locus is amplified in a single tube PCR. The assays included exons 2, 3 and 4 for HLA-A and -B and exons 2 and 3 for HLA-C. The class II assays were directed to exon 2 with the DRB1 assay being based on the innovative development that came out of Royal Perth Hospital.[11,12] The SBT kits manufactured by McGinnis et al included PCR primers, polymerase, PCR reaction purification reagents, sequencing primers, sequence reaction mix and sequence reaction cleanup reagent. This standardized approach guaranteed high quality sequence data on a consistent basis but data analysis and assigning an HLA type from a DNA sequence became the bottleneck that prevented SBT from being a routine procedure.

SEQUENCE ANALYSIS SOFTWARE REQUIREMENTS FOR HLA SBT

Whilst the sequencing technology and standardized kits enabled high throughput SBT the bottle neck was sequence analysis. The SBT procedure includes a sequencing reaction in both directions for each amplified exon. At a minimum the sequence analysis software was required to align forward and reverse sequences, perform base calling, concatenate sequence from different exons, create a consensus sequence and compare the final sequence against a library of sequences from HLA alleles to determine which allele(s) have the same sequence as the test sequence. Given that HLA alleles may differ by a single base sequencing accuracy is critical for accurate typing. Hemizygous sequence from cloned DNA derives the accuracy from sequencing many clones that cover the same region, a procedure that is impractical for HLA and, furthermore, HLA is complicated by the level of polymorphism and the degree of heterozygosity. For locus specific PCR amplification approaches to HLA many samples, at least for HLA-A, -B –C and DRB1 will be heterozygous. Thus the most fundamental requirement for a sequence analysis software program for HLA is the ability to accurately base call heterozygous sequence. Amongst the first to tackle this issue were Erik Rozemuller and Marcel Tilanus at the University Hospital in Utrecht, The Netherlands. Accurate base calling of heterozygous sequence is not a trivial issue. Heterozygous sequence contains 2 peaks at one position and the sequence analysis software must be able to discriminate between artefact and what is a real heterozygous sequence. This problem is compounded by the variable incorporation rates of dye labeled deoxy/ dideoxys, discussed above, where heterozygous sequence is frequently represented as two peaks that are NOT identical in height (Fig. 11.1). The discrepancy in heights of two peaks at one position can be dramatic such that one, or both, peak(s) may only just be visible above background. Fortunately most SBT approaches include sequence of the same region in both directions. The reverse sequence is reversed and complimented by the software so that it aligns to the forward sequence, thus there is a "duplicate" representation of sequence at each position and given that the complimentary bases are

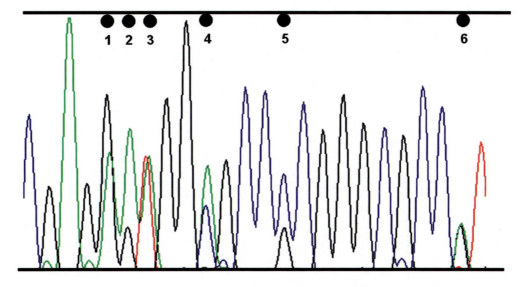

Fig. 11.1: *HLA Sequence analysis requires accurate base calling of heterozygous sequence*: An accurate base calling software for HLA sequencing based typing must be able to discriminate artifact and true signal in an environment of peak height variability, especially at "heterozygous" positions within the sequence, figure shows a region of HLA-DRB1 from a heterozygous sample. Heterozygous sequence contains 2 peaks representing each nucleotide inherited from the maternal and paternal haplotypes. However, the data is complex as a result of the variable incorporation rates of dye labeled di-deoxynucleotides and may be complicated further by the presence of noise artefacts. Heterozygous positions are indicated by a dot (●). Heterozygous position 1, contains two peaks that are higher than some of the homozygous peaks. Only the heterozygous positions 3 and 6 have heterozygous peaks identical to each other in height. The peaks at all other heterozygous positions differ in height, with a large difference in height seen for polymorphic positions 2 and 5. Homozygous peaks that are 2, 4, 11 and 20 from the left contain noise artefacts. An accurate base call software must discriminate homozygous peaks with noise artefacts and true heterozygous peaks

sequenced, the heterozygous sequence profile is usually different.

One remarkable feature of Sanger sequencing is the reproducibility of the rate of incorporation of dye labeled dideoxys/deoxys at each position within a sequence. This means that the relative peak heights, or the pattern of peak heights within the same region of sequence between samples is almost identical. Furthermore the rate of incorporation of nucleotides is quantitative, so that a heterozygous peak is smaller than a homozygous peak of the same sequence (Fig. 11.2). By applying this information to sequence electropherogram analysis it becomes possible to determine the difference between artefact and heterozygous sequence. Whilst this can be done by eye by a skilled operator, it was Erik Rozemullers' software, PolAll[13] that enabled this analysis to be performed automatically. PolAll performed a peak height analysis at each position within the sequence and called heterozygous peaks if it could be demonstrated that there were two peaks present, each of which was reduced in height compared to when each peak was present as a homozygote (Fig. 11.3). This approach required the simultaneous analysis of many samples that included both homozygous alternatives, in addition to heterozygous samples, in order to be able to accurately call the heterozygous sequence. This approach also indirectly provided valuable quality control information. PolAll produced a series of graphs at each position within the sequence that plotted the peak heights of each possible pair of bases regardless of the bases that were present. So for each position within the sequence there was a graph for the peak heights of A v G, A v C, A v T, C v G, C v T and G v T. Each point on each graph represented data from each sample and collectively the data enabled heterozygous positions to be easily identified as a cluster of points on the graph midway between the cluster of points for each of the alternative homozygous peaks. Furthermore, the software plotted any signal present and so background and poorly separated peaks were easily detected. Unfortunately the software was not commercially available and so the global implementation of DNA sequencing as a high throughput approach was still impeded by the sequence analysis bottleneck.

It was the development of the Assign-SBT sequence analysis software that heralded the start of DNA sequencing as high throughput, frontline tool for HLA typing. Assign-SBT was developed by Damian

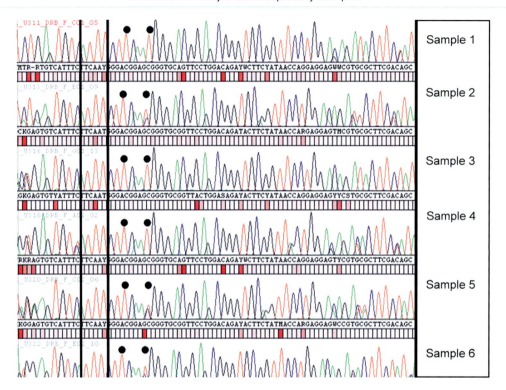

Fig. 11.2: *Sequence electropherogram data is reproducible between samples:* Figure shows the sequence electropherogram data in the same region for 6 different samples. This figure illustrates the reproducible nature of sequence electropherogram profiles. That is, the relative peak heights for identical sequence are almost identical between different samples. As an example a string of three T nucleotide peaks between all samples have been boxed. In each case the first T peak is lower in height than the second T peak by approximately the same amount. The second T peak is marginally greater than the third T peak for all samples. When a peak is present as a heterozygote, the peak is lower in height than when the peak is present for homozygous sequence. This is shown for the two T peaks with a black dot (●) above them. Each sample is homozygous T at the first position and samples 2, 5 and 6 are heterozygous T/C at the second position. In addition to an additional C peak, the T peak at the heterozygous positions are reduced in height compared to the homozygous T peak for samples 1, 3 and 4. The reproducible and quantitative nature of automated Sanger sequencing is exploited by sequence analysis software to enable accurate base calling and discrimination between artifact and heterozygous sequence

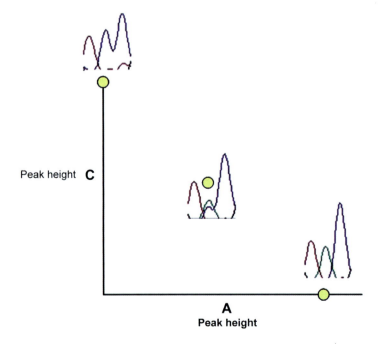

Fig. 11.3: This figure demonstrates the principles behind Rozemullers PolAll software and how PolAll is used to base call heterozygous sequence. PolAll is a multi-sequence analysis tool that creates several graphs each for one peak height of one peak v another for each combination of CvA, TvA, GvA, AvT, GvT, for every position within the region sequenced. Figure shows just one graph of the peak height of CvA. There are 3 points (●) on the graph representing sequence from three samples. Included on the graph (for illustration purposes only) is electropherogram data from which the graphs are created. The graphs represent the central peak(s). The point on the C axis indicates a peak that has high C signal and no A signal representing homozygous C sequence. The point on the A axis indicates A signal but no C signal representing homozygous A sequence and the point midway between the two points on the A and C axis indicates an A and C signal, each of which is reduced compared to the homozygous sequence

Goodridge and David Sayer whilst at the Department of Clinical Immunology and Biochemical Genetics (DCIBG) at Royal Perth Hospital in Western Australia. Assign-SBT was specifically designed to enable laboratories to perform all their HLA typing by sequencing. It performed throughput analysis, had an accurate and unique approach to base calling, especially for heterozygous sequence, it was simple to use and included unique quality control features appropriate for a clinical testing laboratory.

Assign-SBT took advantage of the reproducible nature reproducible nature of dideoxy incorporation rates by Taq polymerase and, therefore, sequence peak profiles and analyzed the data in a unique way. An algorithm was built into the Assign-SBT software that re-drew the sequence peaks normalized relative to the expected peak height for a homozygous peak at each position within the sequence. This results in each homozygous peak being the same height as each other and heterozygous peaks being approximately 50 percent the height of the homozygous peaks. Regardless of the size of the original homozygous peak, heterozygous peaks are usually close to 50 percent the height of the original peak. When base calling was performed on the normalized data heterozygous base calling accuracy was improved because the software no longer had to determine if small heterozygous peaks were "background" (Fig. 11.4). In addition to increasing heterozygous base call accuracy, analyzing the data in this way had additional quality control benefits. In suboptimal situations it is possible that one allele is amplified in greater quantities than the other allele in a heterozygous sample. In these situations, the heterozygous peaks will no longer be the same height as each other and the peaks from the over amplified allele will be greater than the peaks of the alternative allele. This is not easily detected on data that is not normalized.

With the development of Assign-SBT, DCIBG became one of, if not the first laboratory in the world to perform HLA typing for all HLA typing requests by DNA sequencing. This included solid organ transplant work up, bone marrow transplantation registry donors, transplant patients, disease association studies and other research applications.

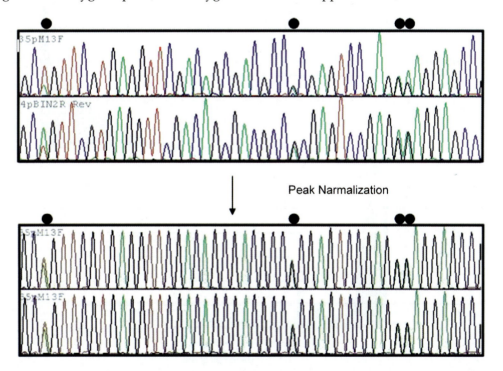

Fig. 11.4: *Normalization of sequence electropherogram data to improve heterozygous base calling accuracy:* The Assign software exploits the reproducible nature of automated Sanger sequencing, demonstrated in Figure 11.2, to improve heterozygous base calling. Assign contains an algorithm that re-draws the electropherogram peaks relative to their expected height for a homozygous peak for expected bases at each position. The result of this is that all homozygous peaks tend to be the same height and heterozygous peaks tend to be half the height of homozygous peaks. This is illustrated in figure. The top panel shows sequence in both the forward and reverse directions. Heterozygous positions are indicated by the black dots (●). The lower panels show the same sequence after normalization. Heterozygous peaks are easily recognizable. Assign performs base calling on this data resulting in improved heterozygous base calling accuracy

HLA SBT AND THE IMPORTANCE OF QUALITY CONTROL

Despite all the advances in technology and software that have occurred to date, DNA sequencing for HLA typing can only be high throughput if high quality data can be achieved on a consistent basis. Assign-SBT will not perform a base call error if the sequence quality is optimal (Fig. 11.5), and given that checking for base call errors and manually correcting base calls slows the SBT procedure significantly, and increases the cost, obtaining high quality data is an imperative.

SBT is a complex procedure requiring many steps that are required to be completed optimally in order to produce DNA sequence of the quality required for accurate base calling. There is no such thing as a perfect base calling software program because of the variability in DNA sequence quality. All base callers will produce base call errors on poor quality data resulting in the requirement for manual assessment of data and the correction of incorrect base calls or the removal of poor quality data from the analysis. Checking through sequence to identify base call errors can completely remove the high throughput capabilities and also run the risk of typing errors. Given the importance of data quality to the accuracy and cost of the test, quantitative assessment of data quality is critical.

Ewing and Green of the University of Washington included quality scoring of sequence peaks as part of the base calling algorithm in their genome sequence analysis software, Phred.[14] The Phred quality scores are a probability that a base call is an error based on the algorithm $QV = 10 * \log_{10}(PE)$, where PE is the probability that the base call is incorrect. Thus, a Phred score of 40 indicates that there is a 1 in 10,000 chance that the base call is incorrect.

Phred was designed for the analysis of hemizygous sequence from cloned DNA and when used to analyze

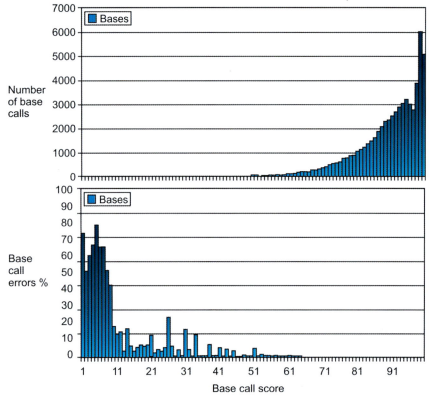

Fig. 11.5: Assign-SBT software performs a quantitative assessment of quality of each peak (called a Base Call Score) within the sequence which can then be used for quality control analysis. Figure shows data from 80 samples sequenced for HLA-A across exons 2,3 and 4. A total of 65,304 calls were available for analysis. The top graph in the figure shows the distribution of Base Call Scores (BCS) for each base call analyzed. The lower graph shows the percentage of base call errors for base calls with a particular BCS. The data shows that base call errors are only made on data with the lowest BCS. No base call errors have been on data with a BCS greater than 70. Thus, the greater the BCS the less the probability that base call changes (sequence edits) need to be made. Obtaining data of such high quality on a consistent basis removes the sequence analysis bottleneck when using Assign-SBT

sequence from PCR products from polymorphic genes it scored the heterozygous positions as it would call poor quality homozygous data. Phred was incorporated into Applied Biosystems (Foster City, USA) and other manufacturers' software to provide an instant guide as to sequence quality. The quality data above the sequence traces enabled the operator to review the quality of the data in combination with the trace data. Low Phred scores indicated low quality homozygous data or good quality heterozygous data, but it at least directed the operator to positions of interest or positions within the data where base call errors were likely to exist. Whilst the additional quality control information was valuable and a step forward, the Assign-SBT software took quality control analysis to a new level and enabled the application of traditional laboratory testing quality control practices to DNA sequencing, including the generation of longitudinal quality control graphs, the ability to assign quantitative quality targets and also the ability to assess inter laboratory DNA sequence quality variability.

Assign-SBT contains an alternative to Phred (Called a Base Call Score or BCS) where the quality score of heterozygous sequence is not penalised purely because it is heterozygous. This approach became the cornerstone of the analysis of DNA sequence using Assign-SBT.

According to the BCS algorithm, perfect sequence, or perfect peaks generated for base calling are symmetrical cones, separated completely from neighbouring peaks without underlying noise or background. Assign-SBT scores each peak according to how it fits to the ideal. Any step in the SBT procedure if not performed optimally will contribute adversely to these ideals. The maximum BCS is for a sequence peak is 50 BCS units and the more the peak deviates from the ideal the less the score. In SBT it is usually the consensus sequence from the forward and reverse strands that is analyzed against a library of allele sequences. The consensus sequence BCS is calculated by adding the BCS from sequence from each direction resulting in a consensus sequence BCS having a maximum score of 100 BCS units.

In order to be high throughput, it is important to remove the need to check the automatic base call at positions within the sequence. We have shown that there is an inverse correlation between base call score and base call error (Fig. 11.5) and based on the data shown in Figure 11.5 Assign SBT includes a BCS cut off that the sequence must exceed otherwise a manually inspected in order to eliminate a base call error. There is no need to manually check sequence base calls at positions where the BCS is high. If the BCS at all positions for a sample are high there is no need to check base calls for that particular sample and the sequence analysis component to SBT becomes negligible.

Given that a quantitative quality score is given for each base call, and sequence quality tends to affect the entire sequence read rather than individual sequence positions, the BCS system can be used in a much broader approach to quality control. For example, if we determine the mean BCS of adjacent positions within a sequence we can assign the mean BCS as the quality score for the region from which the mean was calculated. So a mean BCS for all bases within an exon of a gene represents a single quantitative quality score for the exon. Plotting the mean BCS across the same region between different samples enables an assessment of sample to sample variability and the generation of longitudinal quality control plots (Fig. 11.6). The user can then set performance expectations and monitor the graphs for deviations from quality expectations. The quality control functions within Assign-SBT are extensive and flexible so that a user can create a quality control program that suits their laboratory.

The overall affect of a focus on quality control is that the user builds quality into the system and ensures on going high quality data resulting in SBT being an efficient and effective high through-put approach to HLA typing.

Given the importance in data quality in the SBT procedure and the lack of a community quantitative standard for sequence quality we became concerned that the data accepted as being appropriate quality in one laboratory would be rejected as poor quality by another laboratory. Therefore as an exercise for the 14th International Histocompatibility Workshop in Melbourne, Australia, laboratories were requested to provide sequence data they considered typical from their laboratory, for an inter-laboratory assessment of quality using Assign-SBT. Given BCS is an assessment of peak quality regardless of the origin of the peak, doesn't matter if the peak is from different nucleotides, sequences or genes, the assessment of quality is the same.

The results of this inter-laboratory assessment of sequence quality were alarming.[15] There appeared to be substantial differences in laboratories' perception of quality, particularly for those laboratories that used in-house methods for SBT. The data suggested that what some laboratories considered good quality sequence would not be considered good quality by other laboratories. The reasons for the discrepancies were not

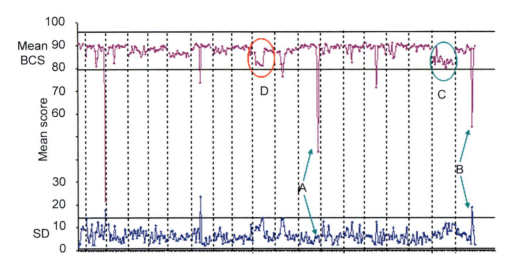

Fig. 11.6: The graph in figure demonstrates a sample to sample, longitudinal assessment of quality using the Base Call Scores. The points in the top part of the graph represent the mean base call score (BCS) of consensus sequence nucleotides within exon 2 of HLA for different samples. The consensus sequence is from forward and reverse sequence reads and the consensus BCS is calculated by adding the forward sequence BCS and the reverse sequence BCS. The maximum BCS for an individual sequence is 50 and therefore the maximum BCS for a consensus sequence from forward and reverse is 100. The points in the lower part of the graph represent the standard deviation (SD) of the same data for the same samples. The data between the vertical bars distinguish successive sequence runs, thus enabling a sample to sample and run to run assessment of quality. Both the mean and SD are used for the interpretation of quality control data. It is usual for the mean BCS to mirror the SD. Good quality sequence will have a high BCS with little variability and so a low SD. However the data indicated as A has a low mean BCS and a relatively low SD (<50), indicating the data across the exon is of the same but low quality. This is consistent with data being calculated from good quality data from a single direction only. In contrast the mean BCS from the data at B is greater than 50, and so must be from sequence from 2 directions, and the SD is relatively high. This is typical profile of poor quality data obtained from each direction indicating a problem with the starting template. None of the other samples sequenced on this run were of poor quality indicating that there is no specific problem with the PCR or sequencing run itself. The data at C represents data from a single run where each sample has a lower BCS relative to all other samples, indicating a problem with the PCR or sequencing run that affects all samples. The data at D is from a 2 separate PCR runs that were sequenced in the same run. The BCS from all samples from one PCR run are lower than those from the PCR from the other run. Checking for differences between the two different runs, such as change of reagents, will provide evidence for the reason for the change in quality. Note that despite the obvious difference in quality the data is still >80 BCS units and base call errors are unlikely

investigated in detail and a follow-up study has not yet been performed to determine if those laboratories with poor quality data have addressed this issue.

MEETING THE CHALLENGES OF AMBIGUITIES AND THE INCREASING COMPLEXITY OF MOLECULAR HLA TYPING

SBT has helped the discovery and characterization of new alleles and the increase in new alleles in recent years has resulted in increased numbers of ambiguous typings where the best result only indicates if one of several alternative genotypes is present. There are two main reasons for ambiguous typings by SBT; they can arise because two or more pairs of allele combinations result in identical heterozygous sequence (heterozygous ambiguities, or HA) or because alleles differ outside the region sequenced (genotype ambiguities, or GA).

There are two commonly used approaches to SBT. One approach separates alleles prior to sequencing using a panel of PCR primers to various allele groups.[16] The advantage here is that for many samples that are heterozygous the alleles are amplified independently and sequencing is performed on hemizygous template. As a result sequence analysis is simplified because fewer samples are heterozygous and there are fewer HA. The disadvantage of this approach is that many PCRs per sample are performed, and each has to be optimized, and more DNA is required. Furthermore, depending, on how many PCR primer sets are used some samples will contain a pair of unique alleles that are amplified with the same primer pair, resulting in heterozygous sequence and the possibility of HA. The alternative approach is to use a single PCR per locus. This can be performed using a single pair of primers to locus specific polymorphisms[17] or a pool of primers to several allele groups.[11,12] The advantage is that a single PCR is performed and less DNA is required. However, many samples will be heterozygous, there will be greater numbers of HA and sequence analysis requires accurate base calling of heterozygous sequence. Many class I SBT strategies sequence exons 2, 3 and 4. Alleles that are defined by polymorphisms in other exons and non-coding regions will be GA. The question as to whether there are functional differences between alleles characterized by polymorphisms outside of exons that encode the antigen recognition site (with the exception of expression variants), and whether such ambiguities need to be resolved will not be discussed here. Therefore, assuming all ambiguities are required to be resolved, achieving high resolution unambiguous HLA typing requires at least a two-step process where the result from the initial step guides the requirements of the second step. This is also the case for the allele group amplification approach because if many primer sets are used the assay resembles an SSP where the successful PCR products are sequenced, and if fewer primers are used, HA will exist which requires an additional step for their resolution.

Sequencing can be used for both the initial and subsequent steps to obtain to high resolution typing. HA occur as a result of the inter-allelic and inter-locus sharing of sequence motifs and is illustrated in Figure 11.7A. In order to determine which alleles of a HA are present the trans order of the appropriate motifs from at least one allele needs to be ascertained. This can be performed by sequencing the original PCR product with one or more allele specific sequencing primers, called HARPS (Heterozygous Ambiguity Resolving Primers), directed to motifs that discriminate the alleles involved in the HA (Fig. 11.7B). Sequencing with the HARP results in hemizygous sequence which is analyzed in Assign-SBT with the original sequence data to deduce the high resolution typing result.

There are two important software requirements for the HARPS system to work efficiently. The first is to determine which HARP or HARPS are required to resolve a specific ambiguity and the second is to be able

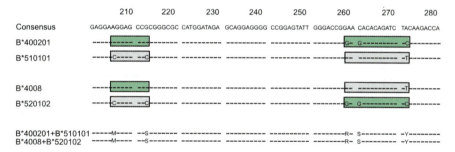

Fig. 11.7A: Heterozygous HLA Ambiguities occur as a result of inter- and intra-locus exchange of sequence motifs

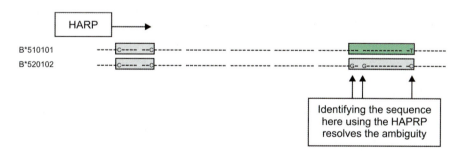

Fig. 11.7B: Figure 11.7A shows an example of an HLA-B heterozygous ambiguity where the sequence generated from a locus specific SBT for HLA-B*400201+B*510101 is identical to the sequence generated by B*4008 + B*520102. The critical polymorphic regions that result in this heterozygous ambiguity are shown. The alleles involved differ at critical positions at 205 and 213 and also at 259, 261 and 272. The alternative sequence motifs present at 259, 261 and 272 that are present on B*400201 and B*510101 are found on the B*520102 and B*4008 allele respectively. In order to determine the precise genotype of the sample by sequencing, one of the alleles needs to be sequenced independently of the other to determine the order of nucleotides at position 213 and 259. This is performed using a sequencing primer which is specific for one of the alleles. In this example the sequencing primer (or HARP, see text) is directed to the sequence motif at 205 and 213 (Fig. 11.7B). The Assign software contains the sequence information of the HARP and combines this information with the sequence at positions 259, 261 and 272 to determine the precise genotype of the sample

to combine the data from one or more HARPS to deduce the typing result.

Just as HLA allele frequencies differ between racial and ethnic groups and therefore laboratories, so do the frequency and types of HA. In some laboratories a large percentage of typings may be without ambiguity whilst the converse may be true in other laboratories. Furthermore one laboratory may resolve the majority of HA with a particular panel of HARPS and a completely different panel of HARPS may be required in another laboratory. Fortunately though, HARPS requirements do not change significantly as new alleles are described. This is because the motifs to which HARPS are designed are shared between alleles and loci and new alleles are made up of a patchwork of existing motifs arranged in a unique order. Providing that the HARPS panel has been carefully selected it is likely that new HA that have arisen as the result of the description of new alleles will not require the development of a new HARP.

Here at, Conexio Genomics Steve Hodges has developed a suite of software programs designed to facilitate optimum use of HARPS. One of the programs, HARPSFinder is available through the web (http://harpsfinder.conexio-genomics.com/). The program allows a user to enter an allele, or pair of alleles, the software will then list the HA associated with allele pair and provide a HARPS solution to resolve the HA. The software is updated quarterly with WHO nomenclature allele library updates. HARPS Finder works by assessing the sequence homology between available HARPS and the alleles of the heterozygous ambiguity and then by applying rules as to the likelihood that (1) the HARP will generate specific sequence (2) and the generated data sequences through appropriate regions to resolve the ambiguity, HARPSFinder will provide a list of HARPS that will most likely resolve the ambiguity.

The reported HARPS include a "HARPS score". The score summarizes the homology between the HARP and sequence of the alleles of the heterozygous ambiguity; the higher the score, the greater the probability that the HARP will be successful. This dynamic approach to selecting HARPS enables the maximum number of HA to be resolved with the minimum set of HARPS and is used successfully by scores of laboratories worldwide.

The suite of HARPS analysis software programs enables the user to perform a variety of analyzes to assist with individual laboratory's unique approaches to HLA typing. For example, we can define the most optimal set of HARPS for any laboratory based on the laboratory's allele frequency information, we can determine which HA cannot be resolved and we can also determine the HARPS required to get a high resolution typing result from a low resolution result that has been obtained by alternative typing technologies such as SSO and SSP.

The use of HARPS to resolve HA is an effective strategy to achieve high resolution typing. However technical limitations of conventional sequencing technology prevent some HA from being resolved. For example, readable sequence does not start until anywhere from 20-40 bp from the HARP so HA that include 2 sequence motifs that are less that 20-40 bp apart may not be resolvable in this way. The ability to sequence the first base after the sequencing primer is technically possible, however, the focus of sequence technology development has been to maximize sequence read lengths and the "cost" of this is the loss of sequence immediately after the sequencing primer. Despite improvements in sequence read length, sequencing from the start of exon 2 in HLA class I, through to the end of exon 3 cannot be performed reliably. Therefore HA that exist from motifs at the beginning of exon 2 and end of exon 3 may also be unresolvable.

SBT of PCR products with conventional sequencing technology, even with the use of HARPS, may not result in complete unambiguous HLA typing in all cases.

NEXT GENERATION SEQUENCING: THE PROMISE OF HIGH RESOLUTION UNAMBIGUOUS HLA TYPING

In SBT an HLA type is assumed if there is complete homology between the test sequence and allele sequences within the library. However the reference sequence library from the IMGT database (http://www.ebi.ac.uk/imgt/hla/) is a significant under-estimate of alleles seen in HLA laboratories. For example, the New York HLA service testing company, HistoGenetics, has reported that they have identified more new alleles for some HLA loci than have been described in the IMGT database. There are also many laboratories globally with new alleles that remain uncharacterized. Therefore it is possible that a heterozygous sequence with complete identity with an allele pair within the database may actually have resulted from a different pair of alleles, where one or both alleles do not exist in the library. Such cases have recently been described[18] and it is becoming dangerous to assign an HLA "type" based on sequence homology because of the limitations of the reference sequence library.

Recent advances in typing technology and analysis software have unravelled more complexity and pushed accurate HLA genotyping almost beyond the capabilities of the technology currently available. A typing breakthrough is required. The only way that complete unambiguous typing can be achieved is by sequencing the allele from the maternal and paternal chromosomes completely (including the 5' and 3' untranslated regions and all coding and other noncoding regions) and independently, thereby eliminating all genotype and HA. This cannot be achieved with conventional technology in an efficient manner.

The Next Generation sequencing (NGS) technology will undoubtedly provide the required solution. Of the 3 NGS systems (Life Technologies' SOLiD system, Illumina's Genetic Analyzer and Roche's 454 system) currently being used in genomic sequencing facilities, it is the 454 technology that is showing immediate promise as the NGS based HLA typing technology (NGSBT).

Sanger sequencing of PCR products results in a signal that represents the majority of DNA molecules amplified in the PCR. The presence of background may indicate that additional non-specific DNA fragments present in the PCR product have also been sequenced. Due to the sensitivity limitations of conventional DNA sequencing non-specific products will not be identified if they represent approximately <5% of total DNA molecules within the amplicon. In contrast, 454 can sequence each DNA molecule from a PCR product independently. The obvious attraction of 454 sequencing, given that each molecule is sequenced independently, is that the order of polymorphic motifs are determined thereby eliminating HA ambiguities. The other significant attraction, and also a considerable advantage over the other NGS technologies, is that the 454 can now generate sequence reads close to 300 bp, with reports that >400 bp is achievable and read lengths of increasing size are promised as the technology improves.

To put a read length of 300 bp into perspective for HLA typing; Exon 2 for DRB1 is 270 bp in length, Exon 1 for Class I is 270 bp and Exon 2 for Class I is 276 bp. These exon sizes are within the read length capabilities of 454, meaning that both alleles in a heterozygous PCR product can be sequenced completely independently without heterozygous ambiguity. There are additional advantages brought by the 454 sequencing approach. For Sanger sequencing PCR specificity is critical to avoid difficulties with base calling. This requirement for specificity requires strict PCR protocols. For 454 sequencing specificity is not necessarily required, in fact a lack of specificity may be a significant advantage to NGSBT. If additional HLA loci can be amplified in a single PCR, NGSBT can be performed simultaneously for several HLA loci, potentially without ambiguity.

As sequence read lengths increase new PCR strategies or other approaches to preparing DNA template for sequencing can be designed to optimize the advantages brought by 454 sequencing.

The use of 454 for NGSBT has been recently described[19] and several laboratories are now assessing this approach.

As was the case with Sanger sequencing the key to successful NGSBT is data analysis. The NGSBT issues though are completely different than those for Sanger sequencing. From a single PCR product, several hundred thousand sequences may be generated. These sequences represent most DNA molecules amplified in the PCR product, and as described above, will include sequences from co-amplified genes. At Conexio, Damian Goodridge has added NGSBT functionality to existing sequencing analysis software to create one of the most versatile sequence genotyping software currently available. Assign-ATF can analyze Sanger sequencing data from any automated DNA sequencer, it can perform genotyping of variant detection for any genetic system and can also analyze data from NGS technology. For NGSBT, the software imports all sequence text files, sorts them according to the sample, then sorts all identical sequences for the sample and compares them with the appropriate reference library to assign a genotype to each locus. Despite the large number of sequences per PCR product, the software can analyze data from multiple loci and multiple samples to ensure that the software remains high throughput. Similar to Assign-SBT the NGSBT analysis software is simple to use, and includes valuable quality control information.

CONCLUSION

For many patients the only treatment available to treat leukemia is hematopoitic stem cell transplantation. When a compatible donor cannot be found within the patients family, an unrelated donor is sought from an unrelated bone marrow donor registry. HLA matching of the donor and recipient is critical for a successful outcome following transplantation. It is this requirement that has driven the development of accurate methods for tissue typing and in doing so has revealed the incredible polymorphism of HLA genes. Most alleles are defined by polymorphisms in the region that encodes the peptide binding site and arise from the inter-allelic and inter-locus exchange of sequence motifs. However, as sequencing enables more of the HLA gene to be interrogated, alleles characterized by polymorphisms in non-coding regions and other exons have been described. The functional significance of polymorphisms outside of the peptide binding grove needs to be determined. Obtaining a high resolution result is becoming increasingly complicated and obtaining a completely unambiguous result may be beyond the capabilities of many laboratories. However, only a relatively small amount of the total number of possible alleles exist in any population, yet heterozygous ambiguities include alleles and allele combinations that may have only ever been seen in a single individual, or at best, are found at low frequencies in remote populations. Thus, the actual probability of an alternative genotype being present maybe greater than the probability that a typing error has been made. This issue has been addressed in a formal way by Cano et al, who defined alleles at all classical HLA loci as being rare, common or well defined.[20] The report stopped short of suggesting that genotypes should be excluded based on allele frequencies but did suggest a strategy for dealing with rare alleles when reporting to regulatory authorities.

Despite technological advances, particularly sequence analysis software advances, that have enabled HLA typing to be performed by DNA sequencing, it is now apparent that conventional automated Sanger sequencing as the sole typing technique is inadequate if a complete unambiguous HLA typing is to be obtained in an efficient manner. Locus specific assays must be at least a 2 step process where the first step determines what is required to determine high resolution. This includes which HARPS are required to resolve the heterozygous ambiguities, and if additional exons or non coding regions are required to be examined. The Next Generation sequencing technologies will no doubt be the next HLA typing breakthrough. Early studies using 454 technology has shown great promise but this technology is technically challenging and it is early days in its development. However, the HLA typing community has a history of adapting technology for which it wasn't designed in order to obtain highest possible HLA typing accuracy and it is likely that this precedent will continue with emerging technologies.

REFERENCES

1. Sanger F, Coulson AR. A Rapid method for determining sequences in DNA by primerd synthesis with DNA polymerase. J Mol Biol. 1975;94(3):441-8.
2. Sanger F, Nicklen S, Coulson AR. DNA Sequencing with chain terminating inhibitors. Proc Natl Acad Sci USA 1977; 74 (12):5463-7.
3. Maxam AM, Gilbert W. A new method for sequencing DNA. Proc Natl Acad Sci USA 1977; 74(2):560-4.
4. Smith LM, Sanders JZ, Kaiser RJ, Huges P, Dodd C, Connell CR, Heiner C, Kent SB, Hood LE. Fluorescence detection in automated DNA sequence analysis. Nature 1986; 321 (6071):674-9.
5. Prober JM, Trainer GL, Dam RJ, Hobbs FW, Robertson CW, Zagursky RJ, Cocuzza AJ, Jensen MA, Baumeister K. A system for rapid DNA sequencing with fluorescent chain-terminating dideoxynucleotides. Science 1987; 238(4825):336-41.
6. Tabor S, Richardson CC. A single residue in DNA polymerases of the Escherichia coli DNA polymerase I family is critical for distinguishing between deoxy- and dideoxyribonucleotides. Proc Natl Acad Sci USA. 1995; 92(14):6339-43.
7. Rosenblum BB, Lee LG, Spurgeon SL, Khan SH, Menchen SM, Heiner CR, Chen SM. New dye labeled terminators for improved DNA sequencing patterns. Nucleic Acids Res 1997; 25(22);4500-4.
8. Arnot D, Lillie JW, Auffray C, Kappes D, Strominger JL. Inter-locus and intra-allelic polymorphisms of HLA class I antigen gene mRNA Sequences that generates HLA diversity. Immunogenetics 1984;20(3):237-52.
9. Angelini G, de Preval C, Gorski J, Mach B. High-resolution analysis of the human HLA-DR polymorphism by hybridization with sequence-specific oligonucleotide probes. Proc Natl Acad Sci USA 1986;83(12):4489-93.
10. Zetterquist H, Olerup O. Identification of the HLA-DRB1*04, DRB1*07, and -DRB1*09 alleles by PCR amplification with sequence-specific primers (PCR-SSP) in 2 hours. Hum Immunol 1992;34(1):64-74.
11. Sayer D, Whidborne R, Brestovac B, Trimboli F, Witt C, Christiansen F.HLA-DRB1 DNA sequencing based typing: An approach suitable for high through-put typing including unrelated bone marrow registry donors.Tissue Antigens 2001;57(1):46-54.
12. Sayer DC, Whidborne R, De Santis D, Rozemuller E, Christiansen FT, Tilanus MG A multi centre evaluation demonstrates that single tube amplification protocols for sequencing based typing of HLA-DRB1 and DRB3,4 and 5. Tissue Antigens 2004; 63(5):412-23.
13. Rozemuller EH, Eliaou JF, Baxter-Lowe LA, Charron D, Kronick M, Tilanus MG. An evaluation of a multicenter study on HLA-DPB1 typing using solid-phase Taq-cycle sequencing chemistry. Tissue Antigens. 1995;46(2):96-103.
14. Ewing B, Green P. Base calling of automated sequencer traces using phred. II Error probabilities. Genome Res 8:186-194.
15. Sayer DC, Goodridge DM.Pilot study: Assessment of interlaboratory variability of sequencing-based typing DNA sequence data quality. Tissue Antigens 2007;69 Suppl 1:66-8.
16. Kotsch K, Wehling J, Kohler S, Blaszczyk R. Sequencing of HLA Class I genes based on conserved diversity of the

noncoding regions: Sequencing based typing of the HLA-A gene. Tissue Antigens 1997; 50(2):178-91.
17. Cereb N, Maye P, Lee S, Kong Y, Yang SY. Locus-specific amplification of HLA class I genes from genomic DNA: Locus-specific sequences in the first and third introns of HLA-A, -B, -C alleles. Tissue Antigens 1995; 45(1):1-11.
18. Danzer M, Polin H, Fae I, Fischer GF, Gabriel C. HLA-Cw*0740 a new allele mistyped by generic sequencing and identified by allelic separation. Tissue Antigens 2006;68(2): 177-8.
19. Bentley B, Higuchi R, Hoglund B, Goodridge D, Sayer D, Trachtenberg E and Erlich HA High-Resolution, High Through-put HLA Genotyping by Next Generation Sequencing Tissue Antigens in press.
20. Cano P, Klitz W, Mack SJ, Maiers M, Marsh SG, Noreen H, Reed EF, Senitzer D, Setterholm M, Smith A, Fernández-Viña M. Common and well-documented HLA alleles: Report of the Ad-Hoc committee of the american society for histocompatiblity and immunogenetics. Hum Immunol 2007;68(5):392-417. Epub 2007 Feb 15.

Section 3

MHC and Disease

Chapter 12

The Genetics of Type 1 Diabetes

Grant Morahan, Michael Varney

INTRODUCTION

Recent breakthroughs in understanding the genetic basis of Type 1 diabetes (T1D) present us with a timely opportunity to review the field. The approach and findings from the T1D genetics studies provide a model for other complex genetic diseases for which causative genes still await identification.

T1D is a disease in which the insulin-producing beta cells are destroyed as the result of an autoimmune process. Evidence that T1D has both a genetic and an environmental basis is very strong. For example, the concordance rate in identical twins is higher than for non-identical twins, and ranges up to 70 percent.[1] Family studies show the relative risk decreases with less genetic sharing with the proband (summarized by Harrison).[2] Even stronger evidence comes from the NOD mouse, which exhibits many characteristics of the human disease, and is the only inbred mouse strain to do so (see review by Leiter).[3]

Mapping studies in both humans and NOD mice showed that the major histocompatibility complex (HLA and H2, respectively) is the predominant susceptibility locus in both species. This was shown as early as 1974 in a canonical study by Nerup and colleagues, which showed that affected sib-pairs (ASPs) tended to inherit the same HLA genes from each parent.[4,5] In retrospect, this is unsurprising since autoimmunity involves mounting tissue-specific T-cell responses, and T-cells are restricted by antigen presented in the context of self-MHC. However, at the time T1D was not recognized as an autoimmune disease, and the phenomenon of MHC restriction was only just discovered from studies of antiviral responses in the mouse.[6]

The availability of the NOD mouse allowed more detailed genetic investigation, as well as the use of genetic modifications to explore in greater detail the role of individual genes. Following the recognition that the unusual class II alleles of the NOD mouse shared a common residue at position 57 with human class II susceptibility alleles,[7] a number of groups produced NOD mice transgenic for "normal" class II alleles. Such transgenic mice were protected from developing diabetes (see review by Slattery).[8]

The task of identification of susceptibility genes in complex genetic diseases has proven to be notoriously difficult. In response to this problem, a worldwide effort was launched to gather the resources to provide sufficient power for disease gene identification. The Type 1 Diabetes Genetics Consortium (T1DGC)[9] has now recruited and characterized over 4,000 ASP families, and has conducted the largest studies of both linkage[10] and genome-wide association of complex genetic diseases.[11] These studies have now revealed a tally of over forty genes that affect the risk of developing T1D; this number includes several T1D risk genes that were described from earlier reports. By far the most important gene influencing T1D susceptibility is *IDDM1*, mapping to the HLA complex. In this review, the role of HLA will be discussed in most detail owing to its importance. We will also describe the most recent advances in discovery of T1D susceptibility genes.

THE HLA COMPLEX

It is nearly forty years since the first observations that the frequency of certain HLA antigens named HL-W15[12] and HL-A8 and W15,[13] now known as HLA-B62 (B*1501) and B8 (B*0801), were increased in T1D compared to controls.[14] The subsequent discoveries that the HLA association was even greater with the new mixed lymphocyte reaction defined antigens Dw3 and Dw4[15] serologically defined as DR3 and DR4[16,17] has prompted an extensive investigation into the HLA antigens, alleles and haplotypes associated with T1D. Association studies in the HLA region are complicated by the presence of extensive linkage disequilibrium which makes identification of a single HLA gene difficult, as closely related genes are inherited simultaneously. This, together with under-powered or poorly controlled studies, can lead to incorrect assumptions about the role of individual HLA genes. The role of large collaborative association studies has therefore played an important part in the history of defining the genetic contribution of HLA genes to T1D susceptibility.

DR and DQ

The association with DR was confirmed in a large collaborative study that compared over 800 patient samples with controls; DR4 was associated in all populations (Caucasian, Black and Japanese), DR3 in most populations, HLA–B appeared secondary to DR and the relative risk of DR3,4 heterozygotes was higher than for DR3,3 and DR4,4 homozygotes.[18] The synergy between DR3 and DR4 helped exclude the model that diabetes was associated with a single recessive gene linked to HLA and clearly indicated a more complex mode of inheritance with multiple loci.[19] An antigen at the second HLA class II locus to be defined, HLA-DQ8, was observed in association with DR4 positive type 1 diabetics when detected serologically[20,21] or molecularly using restriction fragment length polymorphism.[22,23] Nucleotide sequencing of the DQB genes associated with diabetes suggested that the absence of a single amino acid, aspartate at DQ beta 57 was associated with protection from diabetes[24] and that differing residues at position 57 were associated with susceptibility.[25] However, it quickly became clear that DQ was not the only susceptibility loci and that DR and DQ contributed equally.[26,27] Many studies over the subsequent twenty years have identified that the DR and DQ loci, inherited as a DRB1-DQA1-DQB1 haplotype, contribute the pre-dominant genetic risk associated with T1D and that there is a hierarchy of risk associated with different haplotypes when compared to controls in different ethnic populations.[28-33] The use of the affected family based control (AFBAC) has helped overcome some of the ethic mismatching difficulties associated with direct association studies.[34] A hierarchy of risk associated with DR-DQ haplotypes is shown as a generalized summary in Table 12.1 which, for convenience, lists the haplotypes by DQ association.

Table 12.1: Hierarchy of risk associated with DR-DQ haplotypes

DQ,DR	DRB1-DQA1-DQB1	T1D Aassociation	Association risk
DQ8, DR4	0405-0301-0302	Susceptibility	High
DQ8, DR4	0401-0301-0302	Susceptibility	High
DQ8, DR4	0402-0301-0302	Susceptibility	Intermediate
DQ8, DR4	0407/08-????-0302	Susceptibility	Low
DQ8, DR4	0404-0301-0302	Susceptibility	Low
DQ8, DR4	0403-0301-0302	Protection	Low
DQ8, DR4	0406-????-0302	Protection	Low
DQ8, DR8	08??-????-0302	Susceptibility	Intermediate
DQ7, DR4	0408-????-0304	Susceptibility	High
DQ7, DR4	0401-0301-0301	Protection	Intermediate
DQ2, DR4	0405-0301-0201	Susceptibility	High
DQ2, DR9	0901-????-0201	Susceptibility	High
DQ2, DR3	0301-0501-0201	Susceptibility	Intermediate
DQ2, DR7	0701-0201-0201	Protection	Low
DQ4, DR4	0405-????-0401	Susceptibility	Low
DQ1,DR14	1401-0101-0503	Protection	High
DQ1,DR2	1501-0102-0602	Protection	High
DQ1,DR13	1301-0103-0603	Protection	Intermediate
DQ9,DR7	0701-0201-0303	Protection	High
DQ8, DR4	0405-0301-0302	Susceptibility	High
DQ8, DR4	0401-0301-0302	Susceptibility	High
DQ8, DR4	0402-0301-0302	Susceptibility	Intermediate
DQ8, DR4	0407/08-????-0302	Susceptibility	Low
DQ8, DR4	0404-0301-0302	Susceptibility	Low
DQ8, DR4	0403-0301-0302	Protection	Low
DQ8, DR4	0406-????-0302	Protection	Low
DQ8, DR8	08??-????-0302	Susceptibility	Intermediate
DQ7, DR4	0408-????-0304	Susceptibility	High
DQ7, DR4	0401-0301-0301	Protection	Intermediate
DQ2, DR4	0405-0201-0201	Susceptibility	High
DQ2, DR4	0401-0301-0201	Susceptibility	Low
DQ2, DR9	0901-????-0201	Susceptibility	High
DQ2, DR3	0301-0501-0201	Susceptibility	Intermediate
DQ2, DR7	0701-0201-0201	Protection	Low
DQ4, DR4	0405-????-0401	Susceptibility	Low
DQ4, DR4	0404-0301-0402	Susceptibility	Low
DQ4, DR8	0401-0401-0402	Susceptibility	Low
DQ1,DR14	1401-0101-0503	Protection	High
DQ1,DR2	1501-0102-0602	Protection	High
DQ1,DR13	1301-0103-0603	Protection	Intermediate
DQ9,DR7	0701-0201-0303	Protection	High

Abbreviated and three locus HLA haplotypes are shown with a generalized summary of T1D association and risk derived from the current literature.

The greatest risk is associated with DQ8 (DQB1*0302) positive haplotypes, e.g. DRB1*0405-DQA1*0301-DQB1*0302, yet the association is not complete as there are DQ8 positive haplotypes associated with protection, e.g. DRB1*0403-DQA1*0301-DQB1*0302. The DQ8 positive haplotypes appears to have a gradient of risk dependent upon the DRB1 allele, e.g. DRB1*0405-DQA1*0301-DQB1*0302 is associated with high risk whereas DRB1*0404-DQA1*0301-DQB1*0302 is associated with low risk. That DR contributes independent of DQ is illustrated by the observation that DRB1*0405 remains associated with susceptibility in the absence of DQ8. DQ2 is associated with susceptibility on the DQ2-DR3 haplotype but with protection on the DQ2-DR7 haplotype. This difference in risk is likely to reflect a different DQ2 molecule; DQA1*0501-DQB1*0201 (DR3) compared to DQA1*0201-DQB1*0202 (DR7) rather than a DR difference. This difference highlights the potential contribution of DQA1 in the haplotype and the progressive identification of HLA alleles that are highly similar in sequence. For example, DQB1*0201 (DR3) and DQB1*0202 (DR7) are associated with different DQA1 alleles and differ only at a single nucleotide position in codon 135 located in exon 3. DQ4 is the third DQ association which is observed at low frequency across most populations and is often found as a secondary association in relative predispositional analyzes in which the high risk genotypes are first removed.[35]

A comparison of closely related DR-DQ haplotypes that have significantly different susceptibility associations have suggested that the difference may be attributed to relatively few amino acid positions, e.g. DRB1*0401-DQA1*0301-DQB1*0302 (high risk) and DRB1*0404-DQA1*0301-DQB1*0302 (low risk) which differ only at codons 71 and 86. These differences may be sufficient to significantly alter the peptide-binding properties of the molecule and may result in a differential binding of a putative "diabetagenic" peptide. Perhaps the most striking association of an individual haplotype is not with susceptibility but with protection. The earliest observations also included an almost complete protection afforded by a DR2 positive haplotype defined as DRB1*1501-DQA1*0102-DQB1*0602.[36] Other protective haplotypes include DRB1*0701-DQA1*0201-DQB1*0303, DRB1*1403-DQA1*0101-DQB1*0503 and DRB1*1301-DQA1*0102-DQB1*0603. Protection from type one diabetes may be mediated by thymic deletion of high affinity putative diabetagenic peptides presented by class II molecules with similar structure[37] or by a gene in linkage disequilibrium with the DR-DQ haplotype. A recent analysis of DRB1*1501-DQA1*0102-DQB1*0602 haplotypes suggests that loss of protection is associated with sequence polymorphism in the DQA2 gene. DQA2 is the adjacent expressed gene to DQB1.[38]

Whilst a hierarchy of susceptibility and protection is associated with individual DR-DQ haplotypes the greatest susceptibility is associated with the heterozygote DR3, DR4-DQ8 genotype where the combined risk is greater than the individual components indicating a synergy between the two.[19,26] This synergy may result from the formation of DQ heterodimers formed by pairing in *trans* on the cell surface in addition to the heterodimers formed in *cis*;[39]

cis DQA1*0501-DQB1*0201   trans DQA1*0501/DQB1*0302
cis DQA1*0301-DQB1*0302   trans DQA1*0301/DQB1*0201

Other high-risk genotypes that may form a risk associated heterodimer include;

cis DQA1*0401-DQB1*0402   trans DQA1*0401/DQB1*0302
cis DQA1*0301-DQB1*0302

DQA1*0401 differs by a single amino acid substitution at position 75 and is structurally similar[40] and

cis DQA1*0501-DQB1*0201   trans DQA1*0301/DQB1*0201
cis DQA1*0301-DQB1*0303

observed in Taiwanese.[41] This *trans* haplotype has also been observed in *cis* as a lower risk susceptibility haplotype in Africans.[42]

Whilst the primary DR,DQ associations are not useful in disease diagnosis they do have a role in predictive and preventative medicine. Large scale population screening for the high risk DR3, DR4-DQ8 genotype in infants in two studies has identified that between 6.7 percent and 8 percent of the general population are at risk and of these 5.6 percent and 2.5 percent respectively were positive for two or more diabetes associated auto antibodies of which, in one study, 42 percent had progressed to diabetes.[43, 44]

DP

The contribution of the third HLA class II gene, DP, to T1D susceptibility has been problematic to ascertain due to the co-inheritance of the primary risk DR and DQ genes, inconsistent typing approaches and inadequately powered studies. Previous studies have identified multiple susceptibility and protective alleles in different ethnic populations.[45-52] The most reproducible associations are DPB1*0402 with protection and DPB1*0301 and *0202 with susceptibility. A recent large replication study using a highly reproducible genotyping system examined the role of DPA1-DPB1 haplotypes and confirmed the protective association of DPA1*0103-DPB1*0402, the susceptibility association DPA1*0103-DPB1*0301 and provided evidence for a susceptibility association with DPA1*0103-DPB1*0202. In addition DP haplotypes were found to only contribute to risk associated with DR4-DQ8 negative haplotypes and that individual DPA and DPB amino acid substitutions may contribute to susceptibility.[53]

HLA Class I and Extended HLA Haplotypes

Whilst the initial HLA association with T1D was found with class I antigens that were in linkage disequilibrium with class II antigens, subsequent analyzes have identified an independent role of class I. HLA-A24 is associated with accelerated beta cell destruction,[54] progression to disease[55] and individual A24 alleles with susceptibility (A*2402/03) and protection (A*2407).[56] HLA-B*3906 is associated with susceptibility and a younger age of onset[57] after adjustment for linkage disequilibrium. Independent associations for HLA A and B, in particular B*39, were validated in the most recent and largest analysis.[58]

The characterization of extended HLA haplotypes[59] which include T1D associated loci, that are largely conserved between HLA-A and DP highlights the difficulties of associating an individual locus or group of linked loci with susceptibility. For example, DR3 is observed on two extended haplotypes associated with T1D;

A*0101-B*0801-C*0701-DRB1*0301-DQA1*0501-DQB1*0201-DPA1*0103-DPB1*0101 (B8-DR3) and A*3002-B*1801-C*0501-DRB1*0301-DQA1*0501-DQB1*0201-DPA1*0103-DPB1*0202 (B18-DR3).

A comparison of the frequency of the two extended haplotypes suggests that the B18-DR3 haplotype predominates in Basques[60,61] and that the B8-DR3 haplotype confers lower risk[62] although differences at DPA1 may contribute to a differential risk for this haplotype.[53]

HLA, Age of Onset and Decade of Diagnosis

Following the initial association of T1D with class I antigens, a difference in age of onset of disease was also observed to be associated with different HLA antigens.[63] Subsequent studies have been inconclusive with the DR3, DR4-DQ8 genotype, the B18-DR3 haplotype, A*2402, C*0702 and B*3906 being associated with an early age of onset and the B8-DR3 haplotype and B*4403 with a later age of onset.[27,46,57,64,65] This is not surprising for a polygenic disease with an unknown environmental that has risen in incidence over the last eighty years.[66] The rising incidence is associated with a significant decrease in the proportion of patients with the high risk HLA genotype, DR3,DR4-DQ8[67,68] and an increase in the frequency of individuals with an intermediate risk genotype.[69] This suggests that environmental conditions are responsible for the increase in incidence and is accounted for by individuals with an intermediate HLA risk genotype who may previously not have been diagnosed with T1D. These observations have implications for the future predictive value of HLA genotyping.

HLA and T1D Autoantibodies

The clinical presentation of T1D is preceded by a variable asymptomatic in which the appearance of four autoantibodies directed against islet cells (ICA), insulin (IAA), glutamic acid decarboxylase (GAD65) and protein tyrosine phosphatase-related IA-2 (IA-2) have been shown to predict T1D.[70] Whilst neither autoantibody is an absolute predictor of diabetes, the HLA genotype may have a modifying effect on the generation of autoantibodies. DQ8 and/or DR4 are significantly associated with the presence of ICA and IAA autoantibodies and whereas DR3 and or DQ2 is associated with GAD65 autoantibodies.[71] IA-2 autoantibodies have been associated with DRB1*04 or *07 or *09.[72]

HLA SNPs

Finally, mention must be made of the most intensive study of the HLA complex. The T1DGC sponsored an investigation of over 3,000 SNPs and 60 microsatellites in the extended HLA region in 11,279 individuals from 2363 affected sib-pair families. Together with conventional HLA typing, the data was made widely available for researchers to analyze using a wide variety of analytical methods. The reports of these investigations were published in a special issue of Diabetes, Obesity and Metabolism.[73] Amongst the highlights from these analyzes were definition of certain SNPs that were preferentially inherited by HLA-identical, rather than HLA mismatched sibs. As these sibs did not differ in HLA-DR haplotypes, this suggested additional recessively acting gene(s) near the class II region.[74]

Barker et al showed that two SNPs (rs2040410 and rs7454108) could define the presence or absence of the

DR3/4-DQ8 genotype. This allows detection of the highest T1D risk HLA heterozygous genotype much more rapidly and economically than conventional HLA typing.[75]

NON-HLA T1D SUSCEPTIBILITY GENES

As discussed above, although the MHC is the major risk factor for T1D susceptibility, additional non-MHC genes are also required. Perhaps the most definitive evidence for this comes from studies of the NOD mouse.

The advantages of the NOD mouse model include that it excludes environmental effects such as diet, infection, etc; and that it allows directed breeding programs such that a strain may be derived which is genetically identical to NOD, except for a small chromosome region derived from a diabetes-resistant strain. Several groups around the world have searched for such genes, with over 30 loci currently mapped. Many of these loci are by themselves able to prevent T1D almost completely, even though the mice have a fully susceptible major histocompatibility complex; see for example, one such locus, *Idd11*.[76,77] These and similar studies hold the hope that identifying genes responsible for conferring resistance may provide clues for preventing disease in otherwise genetically susceptible subjects.

In humans, searches for non-HLA diabetes susceptibility genes have adopted one of two main strategies: testing variants in candidate genes for *association* with disease; or *linkage* studies, involving hypothesis-free searching for regions shared by sibs affected by T1D. Association studies require comparing genotype frequencies in large numbers of cases with controls; problems with these studies include recruiting sufficiently large samples, together with the adequacy of matching of the control samples. Linkage studies also require recruitment of large numbers of affected sib-pairs, and depend on these sibs inheriting from each parent common chromosome regions which could contain disease gene loci.

The T1DGC resources supported the most comprehensive linkage studies yet reported.[10,78] The results from these genome scans put beyond doubt the involvement of the HLA locus in T1D, generating a logarithm of the odds (LOD) score in excess of 200. However, the other outcome from these studies was disappointing: apart from the insulin locus, no other chromosome region attained a LOD>3. Suggestive evidence of linkage (LOD > or =2.2) was observed near *CTLA4* on chromosome 2q32.3 (LOD = 3.28). Some evidence for linkage was also detected at two regions on chromosome 19 (LOD = 2.84 and 2.54). Perhaps it is not surprising that no other significant loci were found, as the T1DGC families were recruited from diverse ethnic backgrounds and from very diverse environmental exposures.

By assembling sufficient resources for comprehensive linkage studies, the T1DGC was also able to support the largest genome-wide association study (GWAS) conducted.[11] The GWAS projects carried out by the Wellcome Trust Case Control Consortium[79] and by the T1DGC have proved to be the most successful in identifying T1D risk genes. Rather than giving a detailed historical overview of the field, this review will now focus on those genes which have been confirmed as playing a role in T1D susceptibility by these GWAS projects.

Genome-wide Association Studies of T1D

Until recently, association studies relied upon specific hypotheses for selection of candidate genes, and (more often that not) a small selection of SNPs or other genetic markers within those genes. The advent of high throughput genotyping methods has allowed determination of hundreds of thousands of SNPs in large numbers of DNA samples. This technical advance has made it feasible to conduct genome-wide association tests which make no prior assumptions about the nature of any susceptibility gene(s) other than that they will be tagged by SNPs whose allele frequencies differ between groups of cases and controls. GWAS projects obviously involve hundreds of thousands of comparisons, so P values necessary to obtain statistical significance must be lower than 10-6, translating to a nominal P <0.05. Since most common complex genetic diseases have individual gene effects with low odds ratios, these considerations mean that GWAS must compare thousands of cases with thousands of controls. The expense of recruiting and genotyping such large numbers of subjects effectively means that GWAS are out of the reach of most individual laboratories so must be conducted by consortia.

The first GWAS of T1D was reported by the Welcome Trust Case-Control Consortium as part of a larger study with six other common diseases.[79] In total, 14k cases and 3k controls drawn from the UK population were typed. Comparison of the T1D cases with controls allowed confirmation of 5 of 6 previously reported genes: *HLA, PTPN22, CTLA4, IL2RA* and *IFIH1*. Significant association with the INS gene was not found in this study. In addition, evidence was found for other genes on chromosomes 1p13, 4q27, 12q13, 12q24, 16p13 and 18q11.

In an independent GWAS of a Canadian cohort, with replication in T1DGC families and others, significant association was also found with SNPs on 12q24 (*ERBB3*) and 16p13 (*CLEC16A*).[80, 81]

Cooper, et al[82] extended the WTCCC study by combining its data with T1D cases from the GOKIND study and US controls. This meta-analysis found evidence for four previously unknown risk loci in chromosome regions 6q15, 10p15, 15q24 and 22q13. For possible candidate genes in these regions, see the discussion in these papers.

The T1DGC performed the largest ever GWAS analysis, typing a further set of cases and controls.[11] When combined with the previous datasets, this study compared over 7,700 cases and 9,000 controls. Any significant findings in this study were followed up in a further cohort of over 4,000 cases and 4,000 controls, as well as over 2,300 affected sib-pair families. In all, SNPs from a total of 42 distinct chromosome regions were identified that yielded P values less than 10^{-6}. Many of these SNPs, of course, defined genes that had been reported in the previous studies already cited. However, 28 regions were novel. Of these, 22 regions were confirmed in the replication study; sixteen strongly so. A further 6 regions were significant in the first cohort but not replicated in the independent study.

A summary of the GWAS outcomes is presented in Table 12.2, and some of the key genes are described in more detail below.

INS

A VNTR located 5′ of the Insulin gene was initially reported to be associated with T1D,[83] which was later confirmed by numerous studies. Consequently, fine mapping studies showed equally strong association to two SNPs (-23HphI and +1140AC), which cannot be significantly discriminated in Caucasian populations.[84,85] VNTR subsets, marked by specific haplotypes, may have variable strength of T1D association, as previously reported.[86]

PTPN22

PTPN22 (protein tyrosine phosphatase, nonreceptor type 22) confers the third highest risk for T1D[87] after *HLA-DR/DQ* and *INS*. This gene, on chromosome 1p13, encodes a lymphoid-specific phosphatase and is an excellent candidate for a role in T1D because it can down regulate T-cell activation.[88] The missense SNP *rs2476601* encodes a tryptophan substitution for arginine at codon 620; the R620W variant which was associated with T1D showed greater inhibition of T-cell receptor signaling.[87] The same variant was associated with to susceptibility other autoimmune diseases including rheumatoid arthritis[89] Graves' disease[90] and systemic lupus erythematosus.[91] The *PTPN22* SNP was also found to be associated with a risk for developing autoantibodies to GAD, which are predictive of T1D risk,[92] and was shown to affect the progression to clinical diabetes in ICA+ individuals who had tested for islet cell antibodies (ICA).[93] However, Asian and Indian T1D subjects did not show an association[94,95] and the 620W variant was absent or found at a low frequency in these populations.

CTLA4

While T-cell activation involves presentation of antigen by MHC molecules, various T-cells costimulatory molecules are also required, e.g. CD8 or CD4 for class I- and class II-restricted T-cells, respectively. Offsetting stimulatory signals is a function mediated by CTLA4, a member of the immunoglobulin superfamily.[96] CTLA4 is similar to the T-cell costimulatory CD28 and the genes for both these molecules are co-localized on chromosome 2q. Both molecules bind to ligands on antigen-presenting cells, but mediate different effects: CTLA4 transmits an inhibitory signal, whereas CD28 transmits a stimulatory signal to T-cells [see[96] for review]. Following linkage studies which showed sharing of susceptibility gene(s) on chromosome 2q, [see[78] for the largest such study] a number of groups examined association of *CTLA4* SNPs in T1D as well as other autoimmune diseases, particularly thyroiditis;[97-99] reviewed in.[100] While some studies were able to find and confirm increased transmission of the G allele of a 49A-G *CTLA4* variant with susceptibility[97, 98] others did not (e.g.[101]). Reasons for this inconsistency could include familiar problems: relatively small datasets, small numbers of SNPs tested, population heterogeneity. With the large samples sizes available for GWAS projects (see below) and the T1DGC, the issue of *CTLA4* in T1D could be evaluated and the consensus is that *CTLA4* is indeed a T1D risk gene. The T1DGC conducted a study of a full density SNP map over the *CTLA4* region in 2,000 families. This study indeed confirmed that variants in CTLA4 were associated with T1D risk.

Interleukin-2 Receptor (*IL2RA/CD25*)

IL-2 is a growth factor for T lymphocytes, which bind it via a receptor encoded by the *CD25* gene. Vella et al[102] conducted a systematic scan and were first to identify

Table 12.2: Most strongly associated confirmed genes and polymorphisms

Gene	Chr	Position	SNP	Combined P	Reference
HLA	6	32.7	rs9272346	5.5E-219	See text
INS	11	2.1	NA	NA	See text
PTPN22	1	114.2	rs2476601	1.3E-40	See text
C10orf59	10	90.0	rs10509540	1.3E-28	Barrett et al.
C12orf30	12	111.0	rs17696736	6.4E-18	WTCCC
LOC729980	22	28.9	rs5753037	2.6E-16	Barrett et al.
ERRB3	12	54.8	rs2292239; rs1701704	2.9E-16	WTCCC; Hakonarson et al.
CTRB2	16	73.8	rs7202877	3.1E-15	Barrett et al.
CTSH	15	77.0	rs3825932	3.2E-15	Cooper et al.
IL27	16	28.4	rs4788084	2.6E-13	Barrett et al.
C6orf173	6	126.7	rs9388489	4.2E-13	Barrett et al.
GSDML	17	35.3	rs2290400	5.5E-13	Barrett et al.
CLEC16A	16	11.1	rs12708716	7.3E-13	WTCCC, Hakonarson et al.
C14orf181	14	68.3	rs1465788	1.8E-12	Barrett et al.
BACH2	6	91.0	rs11755527	4.7E-12	Cooper et al.; Grant et al.
GLIS3	9	4.3	rs7020673	5.4E-12	Barrett et al.
Ubash3a	21	42.7	rs876498	6.4E-12	Concannon et al.; Grant et al.
SIRPG	20	1.6	rs2281808	1.2E-11	Barrett et al.
CD69	12	9.8	rs4763879	1.9E-11	Barrett et al.
PRKD2	19	51.9	rs425105	2.7E-11	Barrett et al.
CTLA4	2	204.4	rs231727	7.7E-11	WTCCC
intergenic	4	25.7	rs10517086	4.6E-10	Barrett et al.
SMARCE1	17	36.0	rs7221109	1.3E-09	Barrett et al.
IL10	1	205.0	rs3024505	1.9E-09	Barrett et al.
PRKCQ	10	6.4	rs947474	3.7E-09	Cooper et al.
intergenic	14	97.6	rs4900384	3.7E-09	Barrett et al.
SKAP2	7	26.9	rs7804356	5.3E-09	Barrett et al.
GAB3	X	153.6	rs2664170	7.8E-09	Barrett et al.
C1QTNF6	22	35.9	rs229541	2.0E-08	Cooper et al.
COBL	7	51.0	rs4948088	4.4E-08	Barrett et al.
UMOD	16	20.3	rs12444268	1.7E-07	Barrett et al.
PGM1	1	63.9	rs2269241	4.2E-07	Barrett et al.
DNAH2	17	7.6	rs16956936	5.3E-07	Barrett et al.
intergenic	2	12.6	rs1534422	2.1E-06	Barrett et al.
PTPN2	18	12.8	rs2542151	2.1E-06	WTCCC
IL2RA	10	6.1	rs12251307	2.3E-06	See text
ORF; PRM3; TNP2	16	11.3	rs416603	2.6E-06	Cooper et al.
intergenic	2	24.5	rs2165738	3.7E-06	Cooper et al.
IFIH1	2	162.9	rs3747517	2.3E-04	WTCCC

Chromosomal locations of genes or SNPs are indicated in megabases. SNPs shown are either those used in the cited study or near to the gene identified. In some cases, multiple genes are still candidates (e.g. *IL27* region; *TNP2* region). Combined P values calculated from both discovery and confirmation datasets. For genes found prior to the GWAS studies, P values were taken from Cooper et al.[82] NB The best SNP to detect the *INS* VNTR was not on the arrays used in the GWAS reports. Citations are to Barrett et al, 2009;[11] WTCCC;[79] Hakonarson et al 2008;[80] Cooper et al, 2008;[82] Concannon et al, 2008;[105] and Grant et al, 2009.[106]

significant association with T1D, and this was confirmed by subsequent studies[103, 104] as well as the T1DGC GWAS.

UBASH3A

As part of its linkage studies, the T1DGC had typed 2,496 multiplex families with over 6,000 SNPs. Although nowhere near as dense as a genome scan, analyses of this low-density genotyping nevertheless found that three of the top four markers corresponded to previously established T1D risk loci. The fourth SNP, rs876498, was confirmed by typing in independent sets of parent-affected child families and cases and controls thereby defining a new T1D risk gene.[105] The same gene was also identified in an independent GWAS.[106]

The gene indicated by this SNP is *UBASH3A*, which encodes the protein "Ubiquitin associated and SH3 domain containing protein 3A", also known as "Suppressor of T-cell signaling-2".[107, 108] It is expressed mainly in T-cells where it can interact with c-CBL to mediate down-regulation of protein tyrosine kinases such as ZAP70 that are activated upon T-cell receptor (TCR) stimulation.[107, 108] This functionality is similar to that of PTPN22 which also interacts with c-CBL and down regulates some of the same protein tyrosine.[109] Other functions of UBASH3A in T-cells such as participation in pro-apoptotic pathways[110] provide it with obvious ways in which it could contribute to the risk of autoimmunity and T1D.

IL12B

Although not significant in the T1DGC GWAS studies, the *IL12B* gene is nevertheless of some interest. The heterodimeric cytokines interleukin (IL) -12 and -23 (see refs 111, 112 for review) have diverse and important functions in regulating immune responses. These cytokines are formed by pairing of different alpha chains with a common p40 chain, which is encoded by the *IL12B* gene. IL-12 influences activated T-cells to secrete cytokines typical of inflammatory immune response, while IL-23 mediates recruitment and activation of cells required for the induction of chronic inflammation.[111,112] These or other of the functions mediated by these cytokines makes them, and consequently *IL12B*, ideal candidates for involvement in T1D. Indeed, IL-12 was shown to accelerate disease in the diabetes-prone NOD mouse[113] which shared a *Il12b* allele with other strains liable to autoimmune disease.[114] The *IL12B* gene contains no common missense polymorphisms,[115] suggesting that any role for this gene in disease would be due to variations in level of expression, rather than through the action of a protein variant.

IL12B was first implicated in playing a role in T1D susceptibility in a study of Australian and UK families in which sibs shared linkage to a region on chromosome 5q.[116] Alleles in the 3'UTR of the *IL12B* gene were differentially transmitted to affected offspring. These results were later confirmed in studies of T1D subjects from USA,[117] Japan,[118] and Spain[119] although, as is common for similar studies, others could not confirm an effect in different geographic regions and/or from other ethnic groups.

Despite this inconsistency, it is now clear that *IL12B* variants are indeed involved in predisposing to various diseases involve underlying immune dysregulation. These range from diseases such as dermatitis;[120, 121] to infections like cerebral malaria,[122-124] tuberculosis and leprosy;[125-127] to asthma[128, 129] and most recently to steroid-sensitive childhood nephrotic syndrome.[130] It is important to note that in these studies effects can be mediated by different polymorphisms within the *IL12B* gene. Thus, major effects have been attributable to the *rs3212227* SNP in the 3'UTR of *IL12B*, or polymorphisms in its promoter, or from a combination of both. An independent SNP, located 60 kb telomeric from *IL12B* itself, was also found to contribute independently to susceptibility in a major study of psoriasis.[131] In addition, the demonstration that polymorphisms in other genes can impact on *IL12B* expression and IL-12 production[132] emphasizes the complexity of regulation of this gene and its involvement in disease.

In the T1DGC affected sib-pair family collection, a set of SNPs within and flanking the *IL12B* gene were tested. No SNP showed individually significant association in the population as a whole. Nevertheless, subjects stratified according to genotype at the *IL12B* 3'UTR SNP showed small but significant differences in age of developing T1D. A common finding from the studies of *IL12B* in other diseases is that it seems not to be a susceptibility gene *per se*, but can exacerbate severity of the underlying disease. In the case of T1D, "severity" is measured by earlier onset. In this context, we conclude that the T1DGC findings are consistent. While there was no major effect of *IL12B* polymorphisms on T1D *risk* in the entire T1DGC group, they may have an impact on a subset of at risk individuals by increasing the effect of other genes, i.e. by reducing the age of onset. Whether this effect could be stronger in populations drawn from less diverse ethnic and environmental backgrounds remains to be determined.

CONCLUDING REMARKS

The GWAS discoveries mark the end of a long chapter in the type 1 diabetes story, but also indicate the start of another long phase of investigation. It is now clear that T1D genetics is much more complicated than we would have thought even a few years ago, with a large number of genes, each of which (apart from HLA) have a small overall effect.

There are many implications from these discoveries, but let us note the following important points:

1. Identification of the SNPs above is just the start of the next phase of discovery. These SNPs are unlikely to be the causative DNA variants in the autoimmune process. They are, however, in LD with such variants, so it will be possible for researchers to investigate LD blocks near each of these SNPs in order to identify the crucial changes which bring about increased susceptibility. This is particularly the case for SNPs such as on chromosome 10p, one of which in the T1DGC study was close to *ERBB3*, while in another study, the strongest SNP was closer to IKZF4.[80]
2. Once the genes have been identified, the role of the susceptibility allele in the disease process will have to be characterized. In some cases, the relevant SNP may change a protein sequence, leading to a change in function, as is the case for PTPN22, for example. In other cases, the SNP may affect a transcriptional control element leading to changes in expression of the gene. This appears to be the case for the *INS* VNTR and for the *IL12B* 3'UTR SNP. It is also possible that different haplotypes of SNPs may mediate different levels of susceptibility, as I seen at a large scale for the HLA complex itself.
3. Most of the genes implicated in T1D susceptibility encode molecules that are important in antigen presentation and T-cell activation. Genes which may act at the level of the Beta cell, e.g. *GLIS3*, are in the definite minority.
4. The small effect sizes for the identified SNPs/genes have been calculated from odds ratios determined by study of a very large number of subjects. That is their small effects are at a population level; at the level of the individual, the contribution of many or most of these genes is likely to be much larger.
5. The corollary of this observation is that preventative treatments may yet be developed to some of the genes already identified. However, whether these will only be effective in a small subset of cases is not known.
6. On the other hand, the evidence from the NOD mouse shows that blocking even a single susceptibility locus can almost completely prevent disease, so it may be possible that targeting a biological pathway may be effective even in individuals who would otherwise be susceptible.
7. Genetic epidemiology studies may now be conducted, to learn whether there are interactions of specific environmental factors with particular T1D susceptibility alleles. Perhaps these studies could begin with environmental influences that have yielded contradictory results, e.g. exposure to cow's milk or certain viruses.
8. Finally, the most successful GWAS in terms of T1D gene discovery was the T1DGC report, building on the WTCCC and other studies. It should be noted that the design of this study involved confirmation of the strongest associated SNPs from the WTCCC GWAS of ~2,000 UK T1D cases.[79] Thus, the strongest signals would have been contributed by T1D subjects from a population that would have been exposed to very different environmental factors than other populations. The population genetic structure is also likely to be different from that of other groups around the world. An independently conducted GWAS which did test a different population (mainly Canadian) but relied on smaller numbers of subjects, and whilst finding many of the same chromosome regions, was more limited in the number of genes discovered.[80] Whether there are population-specific T1D susceptibility alleles remains to be determined, but it is unlikely that many countries will be able to assemble the financial and material resources (i.e. 10,000 cases, 10,000 controls) to perform a GWAS on the same scale as the T1DGC's.

In summary, the last couple of years have seen remarkable progress in identification of susceptibility genes for T1D. Further characterization of these genes will enrich not only our understanding of this disease, but also of the architecture of complex genetic diseases.

ACKNOWLEDGMENTS

GM acknowledges support of the Diabetes Research Foundation of Western Australia, and grants #516700 and #513834 from the National Health and Medical Research Council of Australia. We also acknowledge the work of the Type 1 Diabetes Genetics Consortium in conducting the linkage scans, HLA genotyping, candidate gene testing and genome-wide association study cited in this review.

REFERENCES

1. Barnett AH, Eff C, Leslie RDG, Pyke DA. Diabetes in identical twins: A study of 200 pairs. Diabetologia 1981;20:87.
2. Harrison LC, Colman PG, Honeyman MC, Kay TWH. Type 1 diabetes - from pathogenesis to prevention. In: Turtle KT, Osata S (Eds), Diabetes in the New Millenium. Sydney: Pot Still Press, 1999.
3. Leiter EH. Nonobese diabetic mice and the genetics of diabetes susceptibility. Curr Diab Rep 2005;5:141-8.

4. Nerup J, Platz P, Andersen OO, et al. HL-A antigens and diabetes mellitus. Lancet. 1974;2:864-6.
5. Cudworth AG, Woodrow JC. Letter. HL-A antigens and diabetes mellitus. Lancet 1974;2:1153.
6. Zinkernagel RM, Doherty PC. Restriction of in vitro T-cell-mediated cytotoxicity in lymphocytic choriomeningitis within a syngeneic or semiallogeneic system. Nature 1974;248:701-2.
7. Morel PA, Dorman JS, Todd JA, McDevitt HO, Trucco M. Aspartic acid at position 57 of the HLA-DQ beta chain protects against type I diabetes: A family study. Proc Natl Acad Sci U S A. 1988;85:8111-5. Erratum in: Proc Natl Acad Sci U S A 1989;86:317.
8. Slattery RM, Miller JF. Influence of T lymphocytes and major histocompatibility complex class II genes on diabetes susceptibility in the NOD mouse. Curr Top Microbiol Immunol 1996;206:51-66.
9. Rich SS, Concannon P, Erlich H, et al. The Type 1 Diabetes Genetics Consortium. Ann N Y Acad Sci 2006;1079:1-8.
10. Concannon P, Chen WM, Julier C, et al. Genome-wide scan for linkage to type 1 diabetes in 2,496 multiplex families from the Type 1 Diabetes Genetics Consortium. Diabetes 2009;58:1018-22.
11. Barrett JC, Clayton DG, Concannon P, et al. Genome-wide association study and meta-analysis find that over 40 loci affect risk of type 1 diabetes. Nat Genet 2009 May 10 [Epub ahead of print].
12. Singal DP, Blajchman MA. Histocompatibility (HL-A) antigens, lymphocytotoxic antibodies and tissue antibodies in patients with diabetes mellitus. Diabetes 1973;22:429-32.
13. Nerup J, Andersen OO, Bendixen G, et al. Cell-mediated immunity in diabetes mellitus. Proc R Soc Med 1974;67:506-13.
14. Cudworth AG, Woodrow JC. Evidence for HL-A-linked genes in "juvenile" diabetes mellitus. Br Med J 1975;3:133-5.
15. Thomsen M, Platz P, Andersen OO, et al. MLC typing in juvenile diabetes mellitus and idiopathic Addison's disease. Transplant Rev 1975;22:125-47.
16. de Moerloose P JM, Bally C, Raffoux C, Pointel JP, Sizonenko P. HLA and DRW antigens in insulin-dependent diabetes. Br Med J 1978;1:823-4.
17. Farid NR, Sampson L, Noel P, Barnard JM, Davis AJ, Hillman DA. HLA-D—related (DRw) antigens in juvenile diabetes mellitus. Diabetes. 1979;28:552-7.
18. Svejgaard A, Platz P, Ryder LP. Insulin dependent diabetes mellitus. Histocompatibility 1980 (Ed), PC Terasaki 1980:638-56.
19. Rotter JI, Anderson CE, Rubin R, Congleton JE, Terasaki PI, Rimoin DL. HLA genotypic study of insulin-dependent diabetes the excess of DR3/DR4 heterozygotes allows rejection of the recessive hypothesis. Diabetes 1983;32:169-74.
20. Tait BD, Boyle AJ. DR4 and susceptibility to type I diabetes mellitus: Discrimination of high risk and low risk DR4 haplotypes on the basis of TA10 typing. Tissue Antigens 1986;28:65-71.
21. Schreuder GM, Tilanus MG, Bontrop RE, et al. HLA-DO polymorphism associated with resistance to type I diabetes detected with monoclonal antibodies, isoelectric point differences, and restriction fragment length polymorphism. J Exp Med 1986;164:938-43.
22. Festenstein H, Awad J, Hitman GA, et al. New HLA DNA polymorphisms associated with autoimmune diseases. Nature 1986;322:64-7.
23. Bohme J, Carlsson B, Wallin J, et al. Only one DQ-beta restriction fragment pattern of each DR specificity is associated with insulin-dependent diabetes. J Immunol 1986;137:941-7.
24. Todd JA, Bell JI, McDevitt HO. HLA-DQ beta gene contributes to susceptibility and resistance to insulin-dependent diabetes mellitus. Nature 1987;329:599-604.
25. Horn GT, Bugawan TL, Long CM, Erlich HA. Allelic sequence variation of the HLA-DQ loci: Relationship to serology and to insulin-dependent diabetes susceptibility. Proc Natl Acad Sci USA 1988;85:6012-6.
26. Sheehy MJ, Scharf SJ, Rowe JR, et al. A diabetes-susceptible HLA haplotype is best defined by a combination of HLA-DR and -DQ alleles. J Clin Invest 1989;83:830-5.
27. Caillat-Zucman S, Garchon HJ, Timsit J, et al. Age-dependent HLA genetic heterogeneity of type 1 insulin-dependent diabetes mellitus. J Clin Invest 1992;90:2242-50.
28. Noble JA, Valdes AM, Cook M, Klitz W, Thomson G, Erlich HA. The role of HLA class II genes in insulin-dependent diabetes mellitus: Molecular analysis of 180 Caucasian, multiplex families. Am J Hum Genet 1996;59:1134-48.
29. Park YS, She JX, Noble JA, Erlich HA, Eisenbarth GS. Transracial evidence for the influence of the homologous HLA DR-DQ haplotype on transmission of HLA DR4 haplotypes to diabetic children. Tissue Antigens 2001;57:185-91.
30. Kawabata Y, Ikegami H, Kawaguchi Y, et al. Asian-specific HLA haplotypes reveal heterogeneity of the contribution of HLA-DR and -DQ haplotypes to susceptibility to type 1 diabetes. Diabetes 2002;51:545-51.
31. Hermann R, Turpeinen H, Laine AP, et al. HLA DR-DQ-encoded genetic determinants of childhood-onset type 1 diabetes in Finland: An analysis of 622 nuclear families. Tissue Antigens 2003a;62:162-9.
32. Thomson G, Valdes AM, Noble JA, et al. Relative predispositional effects of HLA class II DRB1-DQB1 haplotypes and genotypes on type 1 diabetes: A meta-analysis. Tissue Antigens 2007;70:110-27.
33. Erlich H, Valdes AM, Noble J, et al. HLA DR-DQ haplotypes and genotypes and type 1 diabetes risk: Analysis of the type 1 diabetes genetics consortium families. Diabetes 2008;57:1084-92.

34. Thomson G. Mapping disease genes: Family-based association studies. Am J Hum Genet 1995;57:487-98.
35. Payami H, Joe S, Farid NR, et al. Relative predispositional effects (RPEs) of marker alleles with disease: HLA-DR alleles and Graves disease. Am J Hum Genet 1989;45:541-6.
36. Pugliese A, Kawasaki E, Zeller M, et al. Sequence analysis of the diabetes-protective human leukocyte antigen-DQB1*0602 allele in unaffected, islet cell antibody-positive first degree relatives and in rare patients with type 1 diabetes. J Clin Endocrinol Metab 1999;84:1722-8.
37. Cucca F, Lampis R, Congia M, et al. A correlation between the relative predisposition of MHC class II alleles to type 1 diabetes and the structure of their proteins. Hum Mol Genet 2001a;10:2025-37.
38. Husain Z, Kelly MA, Eisenbarth GS, et al. The MHC type 1 diabetes susceptibility gene is centromeric to HLA-DQB1. J Autoimmun 2008;30:266-72.
39. She JX. Susceptibility to type I diabetes: HLA-DQ and DR revisited. Immunol Today 1996;17:323-9.
40. Ronningen KS, Markussen G, Iwe T, Thorsby E. An increased risk of insulin-dependent diabetes mellitus (IDDM) among HLA-DR4,DQw8/DRw8,DQw4 heterozygotes. Hum Immunol 1989;24:165-73.
41. Chuang LM, Wu HP, Tsai WY, Lin BJ, Tai TY. Transcomplementation of HLA DQA1-DQB1 in DR3/DR4 and DR3/DR9 heterozygotes and IDDM in Taiwanese families. Diabetes Care 1995;18:1483-6.
42. Koeleman BP, Lie BA, Undlien DE, et al. Genotype effects and epistasis in type 1 diabetes and HLA-DQ trans dimer associations with disease. Genes Immun 2004;5:381-8.
43. Kukko M, Virtanen SM, Toivonen A, et al. Geographical variation in risk HLA-DQB1 genotypes for type 1 diabetes and signs of beta-cell autoimmunity in a high-incidence country. Diabetes Care 2004;27:676-81.
44. Baschal EE, Aly TA, Babu SR, et al. HLA-DPB1*0402 protects against type 1A diabetes autoimmunity in the highest risk DR3-DQB1*0201/DR4-DQB1*0302 DAISY population. Diabetes 2007;56:2405-9.
45. Balducci-Silano PL, Layrisse ZE. HLA-DP and susceptibility to insulin-dependent diabetes mellitus in an ethnically mixed population. Associations with other HLA-alleles. J Autoimmun 1995;8:425-37.
46. Tait BD, Harrison LC, Drummond BP, Stewart V, Varney MD, Honeyman MC. HLA antigens and age at diagnosis of insulin-dependent diabetes mellitus. Hum Immunol 1995;42:116-22.
47. Erlich HA, Rotter JI, Chang JD, et al. Association of HLA-DPB1*0301 with IDDM in Mexican-Americans. Diabetes 1996;45:610-4.
48. Nishimaki K, Kawamura T, Inada H, et al. HLA DPB1*0201 gene confers disease susceptibility in Japanese with childhood onset type I diabetes, independent of HLA-DR and DQ genotypes. Diabetes Res Clin Pract 2000;47:49-55.
49. Noble JA, Valdes AM, Thomson G, Erlich HA. The HLA class II locus DPB1 can influence susceptibility to type 1 diabetes. Diabetes 2000;49:121-5.
50. Cucca F, Dudbridge F, Loddo M, et al. The HLA-DPB1—associated component of the IDDM1 and its relationship to the major loci HLA-DQB1, -DQA1, and -DRB1. Diabetes 2001b;50:1200-5.
51. Al-Hussein KA, Rama NR, Ahmad M, Rozemuller E, Tilanus MG. HLA-DPB1*0401 is associated with dominant protection against type 1 diabetes in the general Saudi population and in subjects with a high-risk DR/DQ haplotype. Eur J Immunogenet 2003;30:115-9.
52. Cruz TD, Valdes AM, Santiago A, et al. DPB1 alleles are associated with type 1 diabetes susceptibility in multiple ethnic groups. Diabetes 2004;53:2158-63.
53. Varney MD Valdes AM, Carlson JA, et al. for the TIDGC. HLA-DP and Type 1 Diabetes Risk in the T1DGC. Diabetes (submitted) 2009.
54. Nakanishi K, Kobayashi T, Murase T, Naruse T, Nose Y, Inoko H. Human leukocyte antigen-A24 and -DQA1*0301 in Japanese insulin-dependent diabetes mellitus: Independent contributions to susceptibility to the disease and additive contributions to acceleration of beta-cell destruction. J Clin Endocrinol Metab 1999;84:3721-5.
55. Tait BD, Colman PG, Morahan G, et al. HLA genes associated with autoimmunity and progression to disease in type 1 diabetes. Tissue Antigens 2003;61:146-53.
56. Bugawan TL, Klitz W, Alejandrino M, et al. The association of specific HLA class I and II alleles with type 1 diabetes among Filipinos. Tissue Antigens 2002;59:452-69.
57. Valdes AM, Erlich HA, Noble JA. Human leukocyte antigen class I B and C loci contribute to Type 1 Diabetes (T1D) susceptibility and age at T1D onset. Hum Immunol 2005a;66:301-13.
58. Nejentsev S, Howson JM, Walker NM, et al. Localization of type 1 diabetes susceptibility to the MHC class I genes HLA-B and HLA-A. Nature 2007;450:887-92.
59. Dorak MT, Shao W, Machulla HK, et al. Conserved extended haplotypes of the major histocompatibility complex: Further characterization. Genes Immun 2006;7:450-67.
60. Bilbao JR, Villoslada P, Martin-Pagola A, Castano L. No evidence of pancreatic autoimmunity among patients with multiple sclerosis. Ann N Y Acad Sci 2004;1037:133-7.
61. Valdes AM, Wapelhorst B, Concannon P, Erlich HA, Thomson G, Noble JA. Extended DR3-D6S273-HLA-B haplotypes are associated with increased susceptibility to type 1 diabetes in US Caucasians. Tissue Antigens 2005b;65:115-9.
62. Baschal EE, Aly TA, Jasinski JM, et al. The frequent and conserved DR3-B8-A1 extended haplotype confers less diabetes risk than other DR3 haplotypes. Diabetes Obes Metab 2009;11 Suppl 1:25-30.
63. Schernthaner G, Ludwig H, Mayr WR. Juvenile diabetes mellitus: HLA-antigen frequencies dependent on the age of onset of the disease. J Immunogenet. 1976;3:117-21.

64. Deschamps I, Marcelli-Barge A, Poirier JC, et al. Two distinct HLA-DR3 haplotypes are associated with age related heterogeneity in type 1 (insulin-dependent) diabetes. Diabetologia 1988;31:896-901.
65. Valdes AM, Thomson G, Erlich HA, Noble JA. Association between type 1 diabetes age of onset and HLA among sibling pairs. Diabetes 1999;48:1658-61.
66. Gale EA. The rise of childhood type 1 diabetes in the 20th century. Diabetes 2002;51:3353-61.
67. Gillespie KM, Bain SC, Barnett AH, et al. The rising incidence of childhood type 1 diabetes and reduced contribution of high-risk HLA haplotypes. Lancet 2004;364:1699-700.
68. Hermann R, Knip M, Veijola R, et al. Temporal changes in the frequencies of HLA genotypes in patients with Type 1 diabetes—indication of an increased environmental pressure? Diabetologia 2003b;46:420-5.
69. Fourlanos S, Varney MD, Tait BD, et al. The rising incidence of type 1 diabetes is accounted for by cases with lower-risk human leukocyte antigen genotypes. Diabetes Care 2008;31:1546-9.
70. Knip M. Can we predict type 1 diabetes in the general population? Diabetes Care 2002;25:623-5.
71. Pihoker C, Gilliam LK, Hampe CS, Lernmark A. Autoantibodies in diabetes. Diabetes 2005;54 Suppl 2:S52-61.
72. Williams AJ, Aitken RJ, Chandler MA, Gillespie KM, Lampasona V, Bingley PJ. Autoantibodies to islet antigen-2 are associated with HLA-DRB1*07 and DRB1*09 haplotypes as well as DRB1*04 at onset of type 1 diabetes: The possible role of HLA-DQA in autoimmunity to IA-2. Diabetologia 2008; 51:1444-8.
73. Rich SS, Akolkar B, Concannon P, et al. Results of the MHC fine mapping workshop. Diabetes Obes Metab 2009;11 Suppl 1:108-9.
74. Morahan G, Mehta M, McKinnon E, James I. Effect of linkage status of affected sib-pairs on the search for novel type 1 diabetes susceptibility genes in the HLA complex. Diabetes Obes Metab 2009;11 Suppl 1:67-73.
75. Barker JM, Triolo TM, Aly TA, et al. Two single nucleotide polymorphisms identify the highest-risk diabetes HLA genotype: Potential for rapid screening. Diabetes 2008;57:3152-5.
76. Morahan G, McClive P, Huang D, Little P, Baxter A. Genetic and physiological association of diabetes susceptibility with raised Na+/H+ exchange activity. Proc Natl Acad Sci (USA) 1994;91:5898-902.
77. Brodnicki TC, Fletcher AL, Pellicci DG, et al. Localization of Idd11 is not associated with thymus and nkt cell abnormalities in NOD mice. Diabetes 2005;54:3453-7.
78. Concannon P, Erlich HA, Julier C, et al. Type 1 diabetes: Evidence for susceptibility loci from four genome-wide linkage scans in 1,435 multiplex families. Diabetes 2005;54:2995-3001.
79. Wellcome Trust Case Control Consortium. Genome-wide association study of 14,000 cases of seven common diseases and 3,000 shared controls. Nature 2007;447:661-78.
80. Hakonarson H, Grant SF, Bradfield JP, et al. A genome-wide association study identifies KIAA0350 as a type 1 diabetes gene. Nature 2007;448:591-4.
81. Hakonarson H, Qu HQ, Bradfield JP, et al. A novel susceptibility locus for type 1 diabetes on Chr12q13 identified by a genome-wide association study. Diabetes 2008;57:1143-6.
82. Cooper JD, Smyth DJ, Smiles AM, et al. Meta-analysis of genome-wide association study data identifies additional type 1 diabetes risk loci. Nat Genet 2008;40:1399-401.
83. Bell GI, Horita S, Karam JH. A polymorphic locus near the human insulin gene is associated with insulin-dependent diabetes mellitus. Diabetes 1984; 33:176-83.
84. Julier C, Lucassen A, Villedieu P, et al. Multiple DNA variant association analysis: Application to the insulin gene region in type I diabetes. Am J Hum Genet 1994;55:1247-54.
85. Barratt BJ, Payne F, Lowe CE, et al. Remapping the insulin gene/IDDM2 locus in type 1 diabetes. Diabetes 2004;53:1884-9.
86. Bennett S, Allen SJ, Olerup O, et al. Human leucocyte antigen (HLA) and malaria morbidity in a Gambian community. Trans R Soc Trop Med Hyg 1993;87:286-7.
87. Bottini N, Musumeci L, Alonso A, et al. A functional variant of lymphoid tyrosine phosphatase is associated with type I diabetes. Nat Genet 2004;36:337-8.
88. Cloutier JF, Veillette A. Cooperative inhibition of T-cell antigen receptor signaling by a complex between a kinase and a phosphatase. J Exp Med 1999;189:111-21.
89. Begovich AB, Carlton VE, Honigberg LA, et al. A missense single-nucleotide polymorphism in a gene encoding a protein tyrosine phosphatase (PTPN22) is associated with rheumatoid arthritis. Am J Hum Genet 2004;75:330-7.
90. Velaga MR, Wilson V, Jennings CE, et al. The codon 620 tryptophan allele of the lymphoid tyrosine phosphatase (LYP) gene is a major determinant of Graves' disease. J Clin Endocrinol Metab 2004;89:5862-5.
91. Kyogoku C, Langefeld CD, Ortmann WA, et al. Genetic association of the R620W polymorphism of protein tyrosine phosphatase PTPN22 with human SLE. Am J Hum Genet 2004;75:504-7.
92. Chelala C, Duchatelet S, Joffret ML, et al. PTPN22 R620W functional variant in type 1 diabetes and autoimmunity related traits. Diabetes 2007;56:522-6.
93. Hermann R, Lipponen K, Kiviniemi M, et al. Lymphoid tyrosine phosphatase (LYP/PTPN22) Arg620Trp variant regulates insulin autoimmunity and progression to type 1 diabetes. Diabetologia 2006;49:1198-208.
94. Baniasadi V, Das SN. No evidence for association of PTPN22 R620W functional variant C1858T with type 1 diabetes in Asian Indians. J Cell Mol Med 2008;12:1061-2.
95. Kawasaki E, Awata T, Ikegami H, et al. Systematic search for single nucleotide polymorphisms in a lymphoid tyrosine phosphatase gene (PTPN22): Association between a promoter polymorphism and type 1 diabetes in Asian populations. Am J Med Genet A 2006;140:586-93.

96. Noel PJ, Boise LH, Thompson CB. Regulation of T-cell activation by CD28 and CTLA4. Adv Exp Med Biol 1996;406:209-17.
97. Nistico L, Buzzetti R, Pritchard LE, et al. The CTLA-4 gene region of chromosome 2q33 is linked to, and associated with, type 1 diabetes. Belgian Diabetes Registry. Hum Mol Genet 1996;5:1075-80.
98. Marron M, Raffel L, Garchon H, et al. Insulin-dependent diabetes mellitus (IDDM) is associated with CTLA4 polymorphisms in multiple ethnic groups. Hum Mol Genet 1997;6:1275-82.
99. Ueda H, Howson JM, Esposito L, et al. Association of the T-cell regulatory gene CTLA4 with susceptibility to autoimmune disease. Nature 2003;423:506-11.
100. Gough SC, Walker LS, Sansom DM. CTLA4 gene polymorphism and autoimmunity. Immunol Rev 2005; 204:102-15.
101. Donner H, Seidl C, Braun J, et al. CTLA4 gene haplotypes cannot protect from IDDM in the presence of high-risk HLA DQ8 or DQ2 alleles in German families. Diabetes 1998;47:1158-60.
102. Vella A, Cooper JD, Lowe CE, et al. Localization of a type 1 diabetes locus in the IL2RA/CD25 region by use of tag single-nucleotide polymorphisms. Am J Hum Genet 2005;76:773-9.
103. Lowe CE, Cooper JD, Brusko T, et al. Large-scale genetic fine mapping and genotype-phenotype associations implicate polymorphism in the IL2RA region in type 1 diabetes. Nat Genet 2007;39:1074-82.
104. Qu HQ, Montpetit A, Ge B, Hudson TJ, Polychronakos C. Toward further mapping of the association between the IL2RA locus and type 1 diabetes. Diabetes 2007;56:1174-6.
105. Concannon P, Onengut-Gumuscu S, Todd JA, et al. A human type 1 diabetes susceptibility locus maps to chromosome 21q22.3. Diabetes 2008;57:2858-61.
106. Grant SF, Qu HQ, Bradfield JP, et al. Follow-up analysis of genome-wide association data identifies novel loci for type 1 diabetes. Diabetes 2009;58:290-5.
107. Carpino N, Turner S, Mekala D, et al. Regulation of ZAP-70 activation and TCR signaling by two related proteins, Sts-1 and Sts-2. Immunity 2004;20:37-46.
108. Wattenhofer M, Shibuya K, Kudoh J, et al. Isolation and characterization of the UBASH3A gene on 21q22.3 encoding a potential nuclear protein with a novel combination of domains. Hum Genet 2001;108:140-7.
109. Cohen S, Dadi H, Shaoul E, Sharfe N, Roifman CM. Cloning and characterization of a lymphoid-specific, inducible human protein tyrosine phosphatase, Lyp. Blood 1999;93:2013-24.
110. Collingwood TS, Smirnova EV, Bogush M, Carpino N, Annan RS, Tsygankov AY. T-cell ubiquitin ligand affects cell death through a functional interaction with apoptosis-inducing factor, a key factor of caspase-independent apoptosis. J Biol Chem 2007;282:30920-8.
111. Kastelein RA, Hunter CA, Cua DJ. Discovery and biology of IL-23 and IL-27: Related but functionally distinct regulators of inflammation. Annu Rev Immunol 2007;25:221-42.
112. Langrish CL, McKenzie BS, Wilson NJ, de Waal Malefyt R, Kastelein RA, Cua DJ. IL-12 and IL-23: Master regulators of innate and adaptive immunity. Immunol Rev 2004;202:96-105.
113. Trembleau S, Penna G, Bosi E, Mortara A, Gately M, Adorini L. Interleukin 12 administration induces T helper type 1 cells and accelerates autoimmune diabetes in NOD mice. J Exp Med 1995;181:817-21.
114. Ymer SI, Huang D, Penna G, et al. Polymorphisms in the Il12b gene affect structure and expression of IL-12 in NOD and other autoimmune-prone mouse strains. Genes Immun 2002;3:151-7.
115. Huang D, Cancilla M, Morahan G. Complete primary structure, chromosomal localisation, and definition of polymorphisms of the gene encoding the human Iinterleukin-12 p40 subunit. Genes and Immunity 2000;1:515-20.
116. Morahan G, Huang D, Ymer S, et al. Linkage disequilibrium of a Type 1 diabetes susceptibility locus with a regulatory IL12B allele. Nature genetics 2001;27:218-21.
117. Davoodi-Semiromi A, Yang JJ, She JX. IL-12p40 Is associated with type 1 diabetes in Caucasian-American families. Diabetes 2002;51:2334-6.
118. Yang JM, Nagasaka S, Yatagai T, et al. Interleukin-12p40 gene (IL-12B) polymorphism and Type 1 diabetes mellitus in Japanese: Possible role in subjects without having high-risk HLA haplotypes. Diabetes Res Clin Pract 2006;71:164-9.
119. Santiago JL, Martinez A, de La Calle H, Fernandez-Arquero M, de La Concha EG, Urcelay E. Th1 cytokine polymorphisms in spanish patients with type 1 diabetes. Hum Immunol 2005;66:897-902.
120. Tsunemi Y, Saeki H, Nakamura K, et al. Interleukin-12 p40 gene (IL12B) 3'-untranslated region polymorphism is associated with susceptibility to atopic dermatitis and psoriasis vulgaris. J Dermatol Sci 2002;30:161-6.
121. Capon F, Di Meglio P, Szaub J, et al. Sequence variants in the genes for the interleukin-23 receptor (IL23R) and its ligand (IL12B) confer protection against psoriasis. Hum Genet 2007;122:201-6.
122. Morahan G, Boutlis CB, Huang D, et al. A promoter polymorphism in the gene encoding interleukin-12 p40 (IL12B) is associated with mortality from cerebral malaria and with reduced nitric oxide production. Genes and Immunity 2002;3:414-8.
123. Boutlis CS, Lagog M, Chaisavaneeyakorn S, et al. Plasma interleukin-12 in malaria-tolerant papua new guineans: Inverse correlation with Plasmodium falciparum parasitemia and peripheral blood mononuclear cell nitric oxide synthase activity. Infect Immun 2003;71:6354-7.

124. Marquet S, Doumbo O, Cabantous S, et al. A functional promoter variant in IL12B predisposes to cerebral malaria. Hum Mol Genet 2008;17:2190-5.
125. Tso HW, Lau YL, Tam CM, Wong HS, Chiang AK. Associations between IL12B polymorphisms and tuberculosis in the Hong Kong Chinese population. J Infect Dis 2004;190:913-9.
126. Morahan G, Kaur G, Singh M, et al. Association of variants in the IL12B gene with leprosy and tuberculosis. Tissue Antigens 2007;69 Suppl 1:234-6.
127. Freidin MB, Rudko AA, Kolokolova OV, Strelis AK, Puzyrev VP. Association between the 1188 A/C polymorphism in the human IL12B gene and Th1-mediated infectious diseases. Int J Immunogenet 2006;33:231-2.
128. Morahan G, Huang D, Wu M, et al. Association of IL12B promoter polymorphism with severity of atopic and non-atopic asthma in children. Lancet 2002;360:455-9.
129. Randolph AG, Lange C, Silverman EK, et al. The IL12B gene is associated with asthma. Am J Hum Genet 2004;75:709-15.
130. Muller-Berghaus J, Kemper MJ, Hoppe B, et al. The clinical course of steroid-sensitive childhood nephrotic syndrome is associated with a functional IL12B promoter polymorphism. Nephrol Dial Transplant 2008.
131. Cargill M, Schrodi SJ, Chang M, et al. A large-scale genetic association study confirms IL12B and leads to the identification of IL23R as psoriasis-risk genes. Am J Hum Genet 2007;80:273-90.
132. Peng JC, Abu Bakar S, Richardson MM, et al. IL10 and IL12B polymorphisms each influence IL-12p70 secretion by dendritic cells in response to LPS. Immunol Cell Biol 2006;84:227-32.

Chapter 13

Genetic Determinants of Type 1 Diabetes—Immune Response Genes*

Neeraj Kumar, Gurvinder Kaur, Narinder K Mehra

SUMMARY

Type 1 diabetes (T1D) is a polygenic autoimmune disease. Susceptibility to T1D is strongly linked to a major genetic locus that is the Major Histocompatibility Complex (MHC) and several other minor loci including insulin, CTLA4, PTPN22, and others that contribute to diabetes risk in an epistatic way. We have observed that there are three sets of DR3+ve autoimmunity favoring haplotypes in the North Indian population that include B50-DR3, B58-DR3, and B8-DR3. The classical Caucasian autoimmunity favoring AH8.1 (HLA-A1 B8-DR3) is rare in the Indian population and has been replaced by a variant AH8.1v that differs from the Caucasian AH8.1 at several gene loci. Similarly, there are additional HLA-DR3 haplotypes A26-B8-DR3 (AH8.2), A24-B8-DR3 (AH8.3), A3-B8-DR3 (AH8.4) and A31-B8-DR3 (AH8.5) of which the AH8.2 is the most common. The fact that disease associated DR3+ve haplotypes show heterogeneity in different populations suggests that these might possess certain shared components that are involved in the development of autoimmunity.

Type 1 diabetes (T1D) is an autoimmune disease and is one of the most frequent chronic diseases of childhood. Although, the peak age of onset is 12-14 years, it may occur at any age. Recent epidemiological studies have shown that the incidence is comparable in adults.[1] It is the leading cause of blindness, amputations, end-stage renal disease and premature death. Enormous variations in the incidence of T1D in different populations have been observed. A child in Finland is almost 40 times more likely to develop T1D than a child in Japan and 400 times than that in China and Venezuela.[2] The incidence of T1D is constantly increasing in many countries. In most cases, T1D results from T lymphocyte dependent selective destruction of the insulin producing pancreatic islet β-cells, and the symptoms appear when the β-cell mass gets reduced by approximately 90 percent leaving to irreversible insulin deficiency. The disease is regulated by both genetic and environmental factors. The first degree relatives have been considered as the highest risk group. However, relatives account only for 10-15 percent of all newly diagnosed cases and therefore, may not be the real representative of the general population.[3] The human Major Histocompatibility complex or the human leukocyte antigen (HLA) region located on the short arm of chromosome 6 (6p21.3) contains the major disease locus referred to as insulin dependent diabetes mellitus-1 (IDDM1) gene.

IMMUNOLOGICAL MARKERS

In general, T1D is considered primarily a T-cell mediated disease, in which, the pancreatic islets show abundant infiltration by mononuclear cells that include dendritic cells, macrophages and T-cells resulting in an inflammatory reaction termed as "insulitits" leading to the loss of β-cell mass.[4] During the course of insulitis, β-cells undergo apoptosis probably induced by direct contact with activated macrophages and T-cells, and/or via soluble mediators secreted by these cells like cytokines, nitric oxide and oxygen free radicals.[5]

The disease process may take months to years during which there appear a number of immune related disease

---

*Reproduced with kind permission from Biomarkes Med 2009;3(2):153-73.

markers indicating the presence of ongoing β-cell damage, accompanied by a progressive decline of β-cell function.[6-8] This period is referred as "preclinical phase" and can be identified by the presence of autoantibodies in the serum of "at risk" individuals. Islet antibodies have been suggested as predictors of clinical diabetes in first degree relatives, which happens to be the highest risk group.[3] The islet-specific autoimmune process is also characterized by the appearance of circulating islet autoantibodies. Although, the presence of these antibodies are thought to be a sign of autoimmune response but these may not be considered as a cause of autoimmunity. A recent case report has shown the development of type 1 diabetes in a patient with X-linked agammaglobulinemia, suggesting that autoantibodies are not needed for either the initiation or progression of type 1 diabetes.[9]

Autoantibodies as Markers of Disease Risk

Although, islet β-cell damage is a T-cell mediated process, antibodies against self antigens have great significance in reaching accurate diagnosis and prediction of "at risk" individuals to develop T1D. In most cases, these autoantibodies appear many months or years before the onset of clinical disease suggesting that type 1 diabetes is not an acute but a long-term chronic disease. Studies using prospective and retrospective data have demonstrated that the presence of these autoantibodies could be used to predict individuals at risk of developing clinical disease. In this context, the number of autoantibodies, rather than their titer holds the key in predicting the development of disease. For example, a 10-year analysis on first degree relatives of diabetic patients showed that the likelihood of developing T1D was ~10 percent in the presence of one autoantibody, ~50 percent in the presence of two autoantibodies, and 60–80 percent in the presence of three autoantibodies (Fig. 13.1).[10] This suggests that individuals who are screened positive for two or more of these autoantibodies can be considered for an earlier therapeutic intervention trials long before their β-cell reserve is depleted. Interestingly, some people fail to develop disease even when autoantibodies are present, suggesting an important role of host determined factors.

Insulin Autoantibodies (IAA)

The first known β-cell protein to which an autoimmune response has been documented in T1D patients is insulin.[11] Nearly 70 percent of the newly diagnosed patients have been reported to have circulating antibodies to insulin.[12]

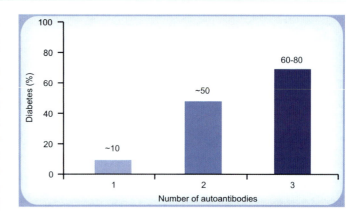

Fig. 13.1: Combination of islet autoantibodies (GAD65, IA2, IAA or others) predict Type 1 Diabetes in first degree relatives of patients in a 10-year follow-up study (based on the data from ref.10)

Glutamic Acid Decarboxylase-65 Autoantibodies (GADA)

GAD is the rate limiting enzyme required for the conversion of glutamic acid to γ-aminobutyric acid (GABA) and it exists in two forms, GAD65 (65kDa; 585 amino acids) and GAD67 (67kDa; 593 amino acids). Only the former is expressed in the β-cells of human islets. GAD is also expressed in the peripheral nervous systems, pancreatic islets, epithelial cells of the fallopian tube, and spermatozoa. Thus, unlike insulin, it is not a β-cell specific protein. Among Caucasians up to 70 percent of the new onset T1D patients have antibodies to GAD65, compared to 4 percent of healthy controls.[13] However, these antibodies have low prevalence in Indians, being ~14 percent in the North Indian T1D patients.[14] However, South Indian T1D patients follow the Caucasian pattern presenting 71.4 percent GAD65 positivity.[15]

Autoantibodies to Insulinoma-associated Protein 2 (IA-2)

Insulinoma-associated protein 2 (IA-2) is a member of the protein tyrosine phosphatase family. It is localized in the membrane of insulin secretory granules of islet β-cells. Initial studies have shown that 54-66 percent of Caucasian T1D patients have circulating antibodies to IA-2.[16,17] Among Indian T1D patients, the prevalence of these autoantibodies has been reported to be ~15 percent,[14] and ~37.4 percent South Indian patients.[15]

Autoantibodies to ICA12

ICA12 is a 622aa long β-cell antigen, also known as SOX-13.[18,19] Its gene shows homology to the SOX (SRY-related HMG box) family of transcription factors. Like GAD65 and IA-2, SOX proteins are not membrane bound but are intracellular proteins bound to chromatin.[20] ICA12 is present in pancreatic islets as well as exocrine pancreas. Caucasian population shows antibodies against this antigen in 10-30 percent of T1D patients vs 2-4 percent healthy controls.[21,22] However, T1D patients from North India showed a higher prevalence of ICA12 autoantibodies, 70-72 percent in T1D vs 4.2 percent in controls.[14,23]

Antibodies to Other Antigens

Studies involving estimation of autoantibodies in serum from recently diagnosed T1D patients and those with longer disease duration have led to the identification of several other antibody targets. For example, antibodies against autoantigens like heat shock protein (HSP)-60,[24] HSP-70,[25] HSP-90,[26] caboxypeptidase (CPE),[27] ICA69,[28] etc. have all been demonstrated in these patients.

Cellular Markers of T1D

T1D is caused by pathological T-cell responses that lead to the destruction of islet β-cells of pancreas. Several studies using nonobese diabetic (NOD) mice have shown that the MHC class II-restricted CD4+T-cells specific for peptides derived GAD65 play a crucial role in the initial phase of T1D.[29,30] GAD65-specific CD4+ T-cells have also been observed in recent-onset T1D patients and in relatives of T1D patients at risk to develop diabetes.[31] The presence of autoantibodies against different peptides of pancreatic islet β-cells suggests that MHC class II-restricted CD4+ T-cells identify the antigenic targets of the pathogenic β-cell. There is considerable overlap among the antigens, and even their specific epitopes, targeted by these cells. Soluble HLA-class II tetramers containing a peptide corresponding to an immunodominant epitope from human GAD65 have been used to analyze peripheral blood T-cells of newly diagnosed T1D patients and at-risk subjects.[32] These studies have led to the identification of human GAD65 peptides recognized by CD4+T-cells. Similar results have been obtained by using a combination of chromatography and mass spectrometry of GAD65 peptides bound by HLA-DR4 molecules.[33] These observations suggest that GAD65 may be one of the early CD4+T-cell targeted autoantigens. Additionally, other protein antigens including IA2,[34] HSP60,[35] ICA69,[36] etc. have been found to elicit CD4+ T-cell responses in recently onset T1D patients.

In addition to CD4+, CD8+ T-cells have also been shown to be involved in disease pathogenesis. Using adoptive transfer experiments in NOD mouse, it has been shown that the induction of diabetes requires both CD4+ and CD8+ T-cells.[37,38] This is further supported by another study showing contributions from both helper T-cells as well as β-cell specific cytotoxic T-cells in the disease pathogenesis.[39] Autoreactive cytotoxic T-cells recognize peptide epitopes displayed on the islet β-cell surface in the context of HLA class I molecules. These 8-10 amino acid epitopes are considered to be derived primarily from islet β-cell proteins. For the first time, Panina-Bordignon et al (1995)[40] have shown the presence of MHC class I HLA-A*0201-restricted CD8 + CTLs specific for a GAD peptide (GAD114-123) in the peripheral blood of subjects with recent-onset T1D and at high risk to develop T1D. However, GAD-specific CTLs were absent in healthy individuals expressing HLA-A*0201. In addition, CD8+T lymphocytes have been shown to be the predominant cells in the inflamed islets of an acutely diabetic patient.[41]

The islet β-cells, which express class I (but not class II) MHC molecules, can be directly recognized and killed by cytotoxic CD8+ T-cells specific for β-cell peptides. Several studies have shown that CD8+ T-cells are able to recognize the HLA class I associated peptide epitopes on insulin and proinsulin,[42,43] islet amyloid polypeptide (IAPP),[44] glutamic acid decarboxylase-65 (GAD65),[40] islet specific glucose-6-phsophatase catalytic subunit-related protein (IGRP)[45] and may be other proteins.

Models to Study Genetic Aspects of T1D

Various models have been generated and studied to understand the pathogenesis of T1D. The Copenhagen Model is an inflammatory model of the pathogenesis of T1D and explains the selective β-cell destruction. This model was first suggested by Nerup and co-workers (1988),[46] who further revised it in 1994,[47] and again in 2003.[48] According to this model, cytokines are considered to be the major effector molecules in the β-cell destruction. This model suggests that there are two phases in the pathogenesis of T1D (i) an initial cytokine-induced initiation phase, (ii) following phase of an antigen-dependent and lymphocyte-dependent amplification and perpetuation phase resulting in specific destruction of all β-cells. The possible sequence of the pathogenic events in the β-cell destruction has been studied *in vitro* and in animal models.

A number of animal models showing chemically or virally induced diabetes[49,50] have been used to enhance our understanding of the pathogenesis of T1D in humans. In addition to these, two animal models developing spontaneous diabetes have been widely used; the Non-Obese Diabetic (NOD) mice and the Bio-Breeding (BB) rat. Both of these are very useful as these are inbred strains that develop insulitis and diabetes closely resembling T1D in humans. Further, the animals can be biopsied, autopsied, and bred to study the genetic basis of T1D in humans. The genetic, immunological, and environmental components of the disease can be investigated under controlled conditions in these models.

NOD mouse exhibits susceptibility to spontaneous development of autoimmune diabetes and is an important model for dissecting tolerance mechanisms. The NOD and related strains were developed at Shionoi Research Laboratories in Aburahi (Japan) by Makino and colleagues and first reported in 1980.[51] Genetic loci associated with susceptibility to diabetes have been identified in these mice strains through the development of congenic strains and referred as insulin dependent diabetes (IDD) loci. NOD mice have polymorphisms in the IDD3 locus which are linked to IL-2 production. This cytokine promotes either immunity or tolerance in a concentration dependent fashion by acting on T-helper cells, cytotoxic T lymphocytes (CTLs) and natural killer (NK) cells. Low amounts of IL-2 in these mice may be needed to promote survival of Treg cells. Loss of IL-2 can thereby contribute to the development of autoimmunity in NOD mice.[52] Thus, autoimmune diabetes in these mice shares many similarities to type 1 diabetes (T1D) in humans including the presence of pancreas-specific autoantibodies, autoreactive CD4+ and CD8+ T-cells, and genetic associations to disease similar to that found in humans. NOD mice develop diabetes from 12 weeks with a higher prevalence in females (60-80%) than males (20-30%). For more than ten years, investigators have used a wide variety of tools to study these mice, including immunological reagents, transgenic and knockout strains;[53,54] these tools have tremendously enhanced the study of the fundamental disease mechanisms. In addition, investigators have recently developed a number of therapeutic interventions in this animal model that have now been translated into human therapies.[55-57]

Although NOD mice are commonly used than BB rats, two inbred lines of BB have also been used in several published studies.[58-60] These rats are designated as diabetes prone (DP-BB) and diabetes resistant (DR-BB). Diabetes in these models is multifactorial, involving MHC genes, but is not solely explained by effects of or alterations in MHC genes. The inbred NOD mice and BB rats represent genetic homogeneity, whereas in humans, T1D cases are genetically heterogeneous. This implies that observations made in spontaneous animal models inbred for dozens of generations might probably only be present in specific subgroups of T1D patients.[61]

Immunogenetic Markers

Almost a half of monozygotic twins of T1D patients go on to develop diabetes. There is a big difference between the concordance rates of monozygotic (50%) and dizygotic (~5%) twins suggesting the importance of genetic factors in the development of T1D. It may be noted that since the concordance rate of disease in monozygotic twins is not 100 percent, other factors including non germline (i.e. non inherited) genetic and environmental factors also play an important role in disease pathogenesis. Devendra and coworkers (2004) have suggested that a close interaction between genetic susceptibility and environmental factors (triggering or suppressive) is critical for the pathogenesis of T1D.[62] Compared to monozygotic twins, the risk for diabetes of a dizygotic twin is more or less similar to that of a first-degree relative of T1D patient (5%).[63] Thus the shared intrauterine environment does not seem to substantially enhance the development of diabetes. Similarly, the expression of anti-islet autoantibodies is much greater for monozygotic twins as compared to the dizygotic twins. The majority of monozygotic twins of T1D patients expressing anti-islet autoantibodies progress to diabetes.[63,64] Autoimmune diabetes in non-obese diabetic (NOD) mice and humans shares many genetic and pathophysiological characteristics. In both the species, the MHC and non-MHC genes contribute to disease susceptibility. However, the relative risk contributed by the MHC genes is much larger than that by non-MHC genes. Several T1D-associated alleles or genetic variants have been considered to provide either susceptibility to or protection from the disease.

Both association studies and linkage analysis using various analytical methods have been used to identify multiple susceptibility loci, and these are conventionally abbreviated as IDDM with a number, e.g. IDDM1, IDDM2, etc. with the number usually reflecting the order in which such loci were reported. Using the candidate gene approach, association studies dating about two decades ago provided evidence for the first two susceptibility loci, the HLA region (IDDM1)[65-67] and the insulin gene (INS) locus (IDDM2).[68-70] A comprehensive list of the currently known susceptibility loci (IDDM1 to IDDM 18) is shown in Table 13.1 with LOD scores from the 2005 T1DGC scan involving 1,435 families with 1,636 affected sibling pairs from the US, UK, and Scandinavia.[71] It may be noted that even though 18 IDDM genetic loci have been implicated, >50 percent of the genetic risk of developing diabetes is conferred by the HLA region.[72]

Major Histocompatibility Complex (MHC, IDDM1)

Worldwide, T1D has been reported to be strongly associated with HLA-DR3 or DR4 or both alleles, whereas HLA-DR15 has been found to be protective in North Indians and several other populations.[73-82] In addition, DQ2 (DQB1*0201-DQA1*0501) and DQ8 (DQB1*0302-DQA1*0301) which occur in strong linkage disequilibrium with DR3 and DR4 respectively are strongly associated with the disease in several Caucasian populations specially when present in DR3/DR4 heterozygous condition.[78-83] It has been suggested that DR3/DR4 heterozygosity exerts a synergistic effect and provide a much greater risk to T1D than DR3 homozygosity in most populations. The HLA-DR3-DQ2 and DR4-DQ8 are referred to as "high risk class II haplotypes" in this disease. However, Oriental population-like Japanese and Koreans have shown the

Table 13.1: Known susceptibility loci for type 1 diabetes and their genetic contribution expressed as LOD score

Locus	Chromosome	Candidate Genes	Markers	LOD
IDDM1	6p21.3	HLA-DR/DQ	TNFA	116.38
IDDM2	11p15.5	INSULIN VNTR	D11S922	1.87
PTPN22	1p13	PTPN22(LYP)	SNP=R620W	NR
IDDM3	15q26		D15S107	NR
IDDM4	11q13.3	MDU1, ZFM1, RT6, ICE, LRP5, FADD, CD3	FGF3, D11S1917 ESR, a046Xa9,	NR NR
IDDM5	6q25	SUMO4, MnSOD	SNP=M55VA allele 163 (G)	
IDDM6	18q12-q21	JK (Kidd), ZNF236	D18S487, D18S64	NR
IDDM7	2q31-33	NEUROD	D2S152, D251391	3.34
IDDM8	6q25-27		D6S281, D6S264, D6S446	NR
IDDM9	3q21-25		D3S1303, D3S1589, D3S3606	NR
IDDM10	10p11-q11	SDF-1	D10S565, D10S193	3.21
IDDM11	14q24.3-q31	ENSA, SEL-1L	D14S67	NR
IDDM12	2q33	CTLA-4	(AT)n 3' UTR, A/G Exon 1	3.34
IDDM13	2q34	IGFBP2, IGFBP5, NEUROD, HOXD8	D2S137, D2S164, D2S1471	NR
IDDM15	6q21		D6S283, D6S434, D6S1580	22.39
IDDM16	14q32	IGH		NR
IDDM17	10q25		D10S1750, D10S1773	NR
IDDM18	5Q31.1-33.1	IL12B	IL12B	NR
	1q42		D1S1617	NR
	16p12-q11.1		D16S3131	1.88
	16q22-q24		D16S504	2.64
	17q25			NR
	19q11			NR
	3p13-p14		D3S1261	1.52
	9q33-q34		D9S260	2.20
	12q14-q12		D12S375	1.66
	19p13.3-p.13.2		INSR	1.92

The IDDM14 denomination has not been assigned to any locus. According to the criteria of Lander and Kruglyak (1995) a LOD ≥ 3.6 is considered significant, NR= not reported in the 2005 T1DGC scan, which applies to loci that were not confirmed to have significant evidence for linkage in that study.

positive association of HLA-DRB1*09 with T1D.[84,85] Several studies have evaluated the effect of MHC haplotype associations on age at onset of T1D. For example, it has been reported that the DR3 association is observed predominantly in patients with younger ages (< 6 years) while there is no such similar analogy with DR4. Similarly, protective effects of alleles like HLA-DR15, DR5 or DR7 are also observed in early onset of disease.[86,87]

The peptide binding selectivity of HLA class II molecules has been shown to be influenced by the genetic polymorphism in these molecules. For example "P1 pocket" of the predisposing DQ2 and DQ8 molecules are much deeper than that of the protective DQ6.2 molecule.[88] In HLA-DR molecule "P4 pocket" plays an important role in peptide binding selectivity. On the contrary, this pocket in DQ2, DQ8 and DQ8.2 molecules has been reported to be similar suggesting no importance in determining susceptibility to diabetes.[88,89] Several studies have reported an increased occurrence of DQ8 in the patients of Caucasian origin.[78,82,90]

The "P9 Pocket" also plays an important role in peptide binding in autoimmune diseases, particularly T1D. In general, the protective HLA class II molecules (DQ6.2) carry an aspartate residue at position 57 in the β peptide chain (Aspβ57), whereas those that predispose to the disease carry an uncharged amino acid residue at this position (non-Aspβ57, carrying generally valine, alanine and serine), although there are some exceptions to this rule.[91] Residue β57 is located within P9 and plays an important role in determining the structure of this pocket. In HLA molecules which carry aspartate at position 57 in the β peptide chain, a salt bridge is formed between this negatively charged residue and a conserved positively charged residue (arginine) at position α76 (in DR molecules) or α79 (in DQ molecules).[89,92] This alters the shape of the P9 pocket relative to that seen in non-Aspβ57 molecules and hence alters the binding preference for corresponding anchor residues in the peptide. The non-Aspβ57 molecules preferentially bind to peptides with an acidic (negatively charged) residue at the P9 anchor point, because this residue can form a stabilizing salt bridge with the unopposed Arg α76 or Arg α79 residues.[89,93] However DQ2 molecule, which prefers large hydrophobic residues in P9, does not support this explanation. This could be attributed to the neighboring residues, which produce a larger P9 pocket than found in other non-Aspβ57 molecules like DQ8.[94,95] This shows the importance of the morphology of the entire pocket rather than the effect of a single residue. Nevertheless, the amino acid residue at β57 influences the peptide binding affinity and selectivity of DR and DQ molecules.[89,93,96]

Further it has been seen that HLA-DQB1 alleles that encode a nonaspartate amino acid (Ser, Ala, or Val) at position 57 in combination with HLA-DQA1 alleles with arginine at position 52, especially the DQA1*0301-DQB1*0201 heterodimer whether placed in trans (on DR3/DR4 haplotypes in most populations or DR3/DR9 haplotype in Chinese) or cis (DR7 haplotype in Blacks) configuration exhibit stronger positive association with T1D than DQB1 or DQA1 alone. This highlights the synergistic effect of DR3/DR4 heterozygosity in this disease. Our studies on the families of T1D patients from North India (unpublished data) have revealed the presence of three major HLA-DR3 haplotypes to be strongly associated with T1D (Fig. 13.2). These include B50-DR3, B58-DR3 and B8-DR3 in the decreasing order of relative risk (9.4, 7.3 and 4.5 respectively). This is quite in contrast to the Caucasians, in which only B8-DR3 {specially the A1-B8-DR3, ancestral haplotype, AH8.1} and additionally B18-DR3 in the western part of Europe have shown an association with T1D.[97-99]

Further analysis of the B8-DR3 set of haplotypes has shown that there are multiple B8-DR3 haplotypes included within this group that vary at the HLA-A locus. These haplotypes have been named as AH8.1v (A1-B8-DR3), AH8.2 (A26-B8-DR3), AH8.3 (A24-B8-DR3), AH8.4 (A3-B8-DR3) and AH8.5 (A31-B8-DR3).

It is interesting to note that the common Caucasian extended haplotype, namely AH 8.1 is rarely observed among the North Indians. Instead, it has been replaced by a unique haplotype AH 8.2 (HLA-A26-B8-DR3-DQ2) that occurs exclusively in India[74] and confers the relative risk similar to AH8.1 in Caucasians. The Indian and European diabetic conserved haplotypes share HLA-B*0801, DRB1*0301 and DQB1*02 but differ at several loci including the C locus, DRB3 and some microsatellite markers and SNPs interspersed in the HLA class I, class II, and class III regions.[74] Further, the B8-DR3 haplotypes in the North Indians also differ at the complotype, which is SC01 (Factor B*S-C2*C-C4A*0-C4B*1) in Caucasian AH8.1 and is FC11 among all Indian B8-DR3 carrying haplotypes (Table 13.2). We have reported earlier that the association of B8 and DR3 on two otherwise unrelated haplotypes might be coincidental.[100] The exact distribution of AH8.2 and its association with T1D in major population groups of India, the mechanism of its generation and its preference over AH8.1 have not been fully elucidated. We have earlier suggested that survival

Chapter 13 ■ Genetic Determinants of Type 1 Diabetes—Immune Response Genes*

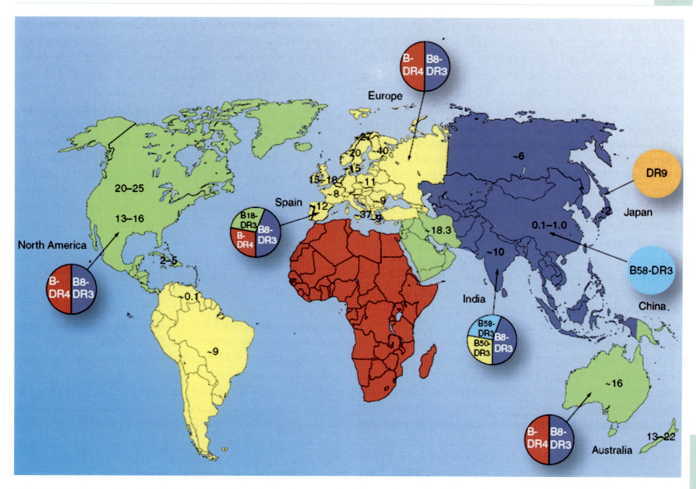

Fig. 13.2: Incidence (per 100,000/ year) of T1D and main disease susceptibility HLA alleles/ haplotypes in various parts of the world. Note three sets of disease conferring B-DR haplotypes in the Indian population: B8-DR3 similar to that observed in Caucasians, B58-DR3 as it occurs in the Chinese and B50-DR3 which occurs exclusively among Indians as a 'unique haplotype'. Also note that B18-DR3 also acts as the susceptibility haplotype in addition to B8-DR3 and B-DR4 among Spanish population

Table 13.2: Type 1 diabetes susceptibility conferring HLA-A-B-DR haplotypes in various population groups. Note the extensive diversity of HLA-DR3 haplotypes among North Indian subjects as compared to Caucasians and other population groups. Interestingly, the complotypes on B8-DR3 haplotypes vary among populations

Populations	Region	Haplotypes	Complotypes*	AH	Status
Caucasians	Northern Europe	A1-B8-DR3	SC01	8.1	Susceptible
		A-B-DR4	-	-	Susceptible
	Southern Europe	A1-B8-DR3	SC01	8.1	Susceptible
		A-B18-DR3	FC30	18.1	Susceptible
		A-B-DR4	-	-	Susceptible
Asian	North India	A1-B8-DR3	FC11	8.1v	Neutral
		A26-B8-DR3	FC11	8.2	Susceptible
		A24-B8-DR3	FC11	8.3	Susceptible
		A3-B8-DR3	FC11	8.4	Susceptible
		A31-B8-DR3	FC11	8.5	Susceptible
		A2-B50-DR3	S???	50.2	Susceptible
		A33-B58-DR3	SC01	58.1	Susceptible
	China	A33-B58-DR3	SC01	58.1	Susceptible

*Complotype denotes Factor B, C2, C4A, C4B   AH = ancestral haplotype

advantage of B8-DR3 haplotypes in north Indians as imposed by vigorous immune response to various pathogens may have led to the independent evolution of AH8.2 and other related haplotypes. Incidentally, the Indian AH8.1 is observed at a considerably reduced frequency and differs at several loci from the classical Caucasian AH8.1. Indeed it resembles more like the AH8.2 and therefore has been named as AH8.1v.[100] Among Indian T1D patients, additional disease conferring DR3+ve haplotypes namely AH8.3 (A24-B8-DR3), AH8.4 (HLA-A3-B8-DR3) and AH8.5 (HLA-A31-B8-DR3) have also been identified, all of whom are susceptibility conferring markers.

In addition to HLA-DR3, Caucasian diabetes patients usually show a strong association with HLA-DR4 and its two common molecular subtypes - DRB1*0401 and *0404.[81,82] However, our earlier studies indicate that while DR4 association in T1D is lacking among north Indian subjects,[73,75] patients from the Chennai region show positive association with DR4 family of alleles.[75]

Some studies have reported the modulatory effect of DPB1-alleles on the DQ-DR-associated risk of T1D. For example the DPB1*0301 is positively associated with Mexican-American T1D patients carrying high-risk DQ-DR genotypes, and this association is not due to a linkage disequilibrium between DP and DQ alleles.[101] Similarly, studies among Caucasian multiplex families from the US have shown a positive association of DPB1*0301 with T1D patients, who do not carry the DQ2-DR3/DQ8-DR4 genotypes.[102] Another study on T1D families from Sardinia and UK reported that DPB1*0402 conferred some protection.[103] Among Caucasians, the high risk associated with DPB1*0202 was indeed due to its strong linkage disequibrium with the predisposing B18-DR3 ancestral haplotype (AH18.2).[104] These studies suggest that susceptibility of the DP locus in T1D is conferred primarily by DPB1*0301 and DPB1*0202 alleles, and protection by DPB1*0402.

Tumor Necrosis Factor

The gene for tumor necrosis factor (TNF) resides in the central region (class III region) of human MHC flanked by a large number of other immunological genes. The locus for TNFα is located near the HLA-B locus. Several microsatellite and single nucleotide polymorphisms (SNPs) have been identified in the TNF gene region of which the most widely studied include -308 G to A and -238 G to A transitions. Allele -308A is a strong regulator of transcription and has been reported to be associated with an increased production of TNFα.[105-107]

In addition to the SNPs, six different microsatellites named TNFa to TNFf are also located in this region. Each of the microsatellites have variable number of alleles, for example TNFb (7 alleles), TNFc (2 alleles), TNFd (7 alleles) and TNFe (3 alleles) are comprised of (GA)n repeats, while TNFa (14 alleles) has (GT)n and TNFf (10 alleles) has (TG)n repeats.[108-112] It has been demonstrated that individuals with TNF -308*A-TNFa2 haplotypes are capable of producing high levels of TNF α cytokine.[113] The close location of TNFa to HLA-B and HLA-DR-DQ suggests that certain alleles are in linkage disequilibrium with each other. Therefore, TNFa could also serve as a marker for diseases with a known association with HLA-B-DR-DQ haplotypes.

Because TNFα is produced by activated cells of the immune system such as macrophages, monocytes and natural killer cells, it plays a very important role in immune function.[114] TNFα is known to induce the surface expression of HLA-DR and -DQ molecules,[115] and to modulate the activity of T and B lymphocytes.[114] Several studies have shown an association of TNFa microsatellites with Type 1 diabetes.[100,113,116] Furthermore, TNFa2 and TNFa9 have been reported to be increased among young T1D subjects in Japan suggesting that the TNFa polymorphism is associated with age at disease onset,[110] whereas no such association was observed among Italian.[117] Among various SNPs observed in the promoter region of TNFα, TNF-308G/A has been shown to be associated with several autoimmune diseases including T1D.[113,116] Some studies have also reported an association of TNFα-308A allele, which is linked to the haplotype HLA-A1-B8-DR3 (AH8.1) in the Caucasian populations with the overproduction of TNFα.[105]

MHC Class I Chain Related Gene A (MIC-A)

Sequence analysis of the MIC-A gene has revealed short tandem repeats of GCT. These (GCT)n microsatellite polymorphisms in the exon 5 code for polyalanine in the transmembrane (TM) region of MIC-A molecule.[118] In most populations, 5 MIC-A microsatellite alleles, each consisting of 4, 5, 6 and 9 repetitions of GCT and five repetitions of GCT with an additional nucleotide insertion (GCT → GGCT) have been identified[119] (Fig. 13.3). These alleles have accordingly been named A4, A5, A6, A9 and A5.1, and their sizes correspond to 179 bp, 182 bp, 185 bp, 194 bp, and 183 bp respectively. Additionally MIC-A7[120] and A10[121] have also recently been reported. There are not many studies describing the functional consequences of the exon 5 polymorphism

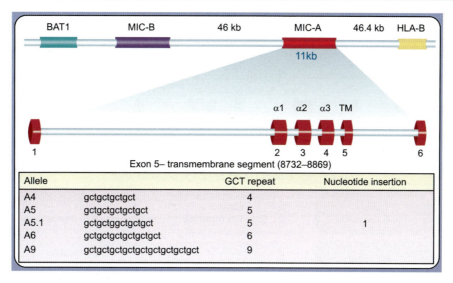

Fig. 13.3: Gene organization of MIC-A on chromosome 6p 21.3 with HLA-B oriented towards the telomeric side and MIC-B towards centromeric side. The trinucleotide GCT repeats are located within exon 5 that codes for transmembrane portion of MIC-A. Depending on the number of repeats, the MIC-A alleles are named as A4, A5, A5.1 (with one extra insertion of G nucleotide), A6 and A9

of MIC-A. It has been suggested that dihydrophobic Leu-Val tandem sequence at position 344-345 in the cytoplasmic tail of MIC-A is responsible for targeting the protein to the basolateral plasma membrane of the gut epithelial cells, which is the prime site of contact with effector NK and intraepithelial T-cells. In MIC-A5.1, an additional insertion of G creates a frame shift mutation resulting in a premature termination codon within the transmembrane region, as a result of which the MIC-A5.1 molecule is not translated till Leu-Val sequence at position 344-345. This MIC-A5.1 molecule is denied of Leu-Val sorting signal. This results in localization of MIC-A5.1 molecules to the apical plasma membrane region instead of the basolateral plasma membrane.[122]

The MIC-A gene also displays an unusual distribution of a number of variant amino acids in its extracellular domains α1, α2, and α3.[123] Comparison of allelic variants of MIC-A has revealed large differences in NKG2D binding that is associated with a single amino acid substitution at position 129 in the α2 domain. Varying affinities of MIC-A alleles for NKG2D may affect thresholds of NK-cell triggering and T-cell modulation.[124]

A number of studies have reported an association of MIC-A alleles with several autoimmune disorders, e.g. juvenile rheumatoid arthritis,[125] Addison's disease,[126] psoriasis and ankylosing spondylitis.[123] Similarly, reports have appeared describing associations of different MIC-A alleles with T1D in several populations. MIC-A9 has been shown to be positively associated with T1D in Chinese population,[127] whereas in Japanese[128] and Koreans,[129] MIC-A4 is positively associated and MIC-A6 is negatively associated. On the other hand, in Latvians[130] and Asian Indians,[15] MIC-A5 shows a positive association with T1D.

During the past two decades, a large number of genetic studies have been devoted to the search for additional T1D susceptibility loci, either by linkage or by association with candidate genes.

IDDM2: INSULIN-VNTR

IDDM2 locus maps to a variable number of tandem repeats (VNTR) located ~596 bases upstream of the transcription start site of insulin gene (*INS*) on chromosome 11p15.5[131] (Fig. 13.4). The IDDM2 locus contributes ~10 percent towards type 1 diabetes susceptibility.[131] Several studies have shown a strong association of the variable number of tandem repeat polymorphism in the insulin gene with type 1 diabetes.[68,77,132,133] Based on the number of tandem repeats of 14-15 bp G-rich sequences, these VNTR alleles are grouped into three classes: Class I alleles (20-63 repeats), Class II alleles (64-139 repeats) and Class III alleles (140-210 repeats). The short class I alleles are generally predisposing, especially in homozygous state, and they confer more than two fold relative risk for type 1 diabetes. On the other hand, class III alleles are associated with dominant protection.[131] However, there are some exceptions to this pattern of both class I and class III allelic association.[68] It is interesting to note that while class I alleles are the most common and occur at a frequency of nearly 80 percent in Caucasians, class III

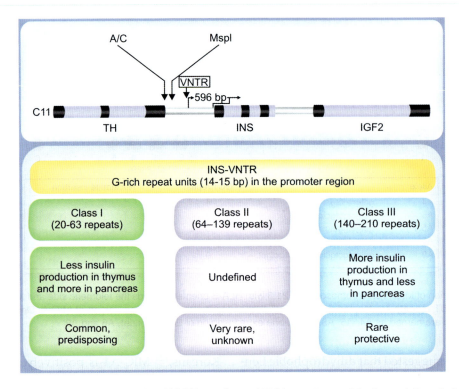

Fig. 13.4: **Insulin gene map.** Type 1 diabetes associated VNTRs are located 596 bp upstream of the transcription site in the promoter region of the gene. The lower half of the figure depicts a correlation between different classes of INS-VNTR alleles and insulin production thereby leading to susceptibility or resistance to T1D. The dark shaded boxes depict exons while light shaded boxes are intronic regions

alleles occur less common (nearly 20%) whereas class II alleles are most infrequent.[134]

The exact mechanism by which the insulin VNTR alleles influence the risk of type 1 diabetes is not well understood. Because the VNTR occurs in a non-coding region, its influence on diabetes risk cannot be attributed to an alteration of the protein sequence. Instead, the VNTR probably affects the transcription of the insulin gene in some way. These polymorphisms regulate the expression of two downstream genes: the insulin and insulin-like growth factor 2 (IGF2). These two growth factors play important roles in disease pathogenesis as insulin and its precursors are potential target autoantigens for β-cell destruction. Recent studies have shown a transcription of the insulin gene and other β-cell autoantigens, albeit at low levels in the thymus of mice[135] as well as in humans.[69,70] Indeed the allelic variations at the VNTR locus has been shown to influence the insulin mRNA expression level.[69] Whereas the increased transcription of the insulin gene in thymus is associated with protective class III alleles, the low levels of transcription are found in the case of predisposing class I alleles.

However, the situation is much the reverse in pancreas, i.e. higher insulin mRNA expression is associated with the class I alleles.[70] This suggests that negative selection of autoreactive thymocytes is dose dependent and raised concentrations of pre-proinsulin in the thymus may promote an efficient deletion of autoreactive T-cells for insulin and its precursors. This induces central immune tolerance to an important autoantigen in the pathogenesis of diabetes. This mechanism may explain the closer positive association of homozygous class I alleles having lower intrathymic insulin expression and higher expression in the pancreas thus increasing the risk to diabetes and dominant protective effect of class III alleles because of comparatively higher expression in the thymus and lower expression in pancreas.

The insulin growth factor 2 gene product (IGF-2) plays a critical role in T-cell development and thymic negative selection and therefore contributes towards IDDM2 associated susceptibility to diabetes. It has some homology to proinsulin;[136] therefore, it may also act as a selecting peptide for insulin reactive T-cells. It has been shown that the levels of IGF2 expression in thymus and pancreas are not associated with VNTR class I and class III alleles.[136,137] This suggests that the contributory role of IGF2 gene is independent of the insulin VNTR alleles. However, increased expression of IGF2 in the placenta is associated with class I alleles suggesting that it may influence intrauterine growth and birth size, which are risk factors for type 1 diabetes.[138,139]

IDDM 12: CYTOTOXIC T LYMPHOCYTE ASSOCIATED ANTIGEN-4 GENE

After MHC, the combined second most inheritable risk of ~15 percent to T1D is contributed by two candidate genes, namely insulin-VNTR and CTLA-4. Cytotoxic T lymphocyte associated antigen-4 (CTLA-4) along with CD28 and ICOS genes are located on chromosome 2 (2q31-35) in humans.[140-144] The 2q33 region is also referred to as IDDM12. Various polymorphisms in the 5'UTR, 3'UTR regulatory regions and exon 1 of CTLA-4 gene have been studied extensively in T1D and are shown in Figure 13.5.

CTLA-4 is a disulphide-linked homodimer expressed on the cell surface of activated cells that plays an important role in the regulation of T-cell function. It binds to ligands B7-1 (CD80) or B7-2 (CD86) expressed on the surface of antigen presenting cells and downregulates the alpha chain of IL-2 receptor (CD25) expression followed by decreased synthesis of IL-2.[145] CTLA-4 is also an important molecule by which CD4+CD25+ T regulatory cells exert their suppressive activity.[146] Given the function of CTLA-4 as a negative regulatory molecule of the immune system in general and that of HLA class II in the presentation of a specific antigen to initiate an immune response to the antigen, it is reasonable to speculate that a susceptible allele at CTLA-4 leads to autoimmunity, while the specific HLA haplotypes target the autoimmune attack to pancreatic islets through recruitment of specific CTLs and may be the natural killer (NK) cells. Two isoforms are known for CTLA-4: (i) the full-length transmembrane glycoprotein expressed transiently on the surface of activated CD4 and CD8 T-cells, also detected on B-cells, is the main isoform found in adult thymocytes and (ii) the soluble form (sCTLA-4). The latter is generated by alternative splicing of transmembrane domain and is mainly expressed by inactivated T-cells.[147] The full-length CTLA-4 receptor binds to the ligand B7 expressed on the surface of APCs having an antagonistic role of its counter receptor CD28. Its expression is up-regulated only 2-3

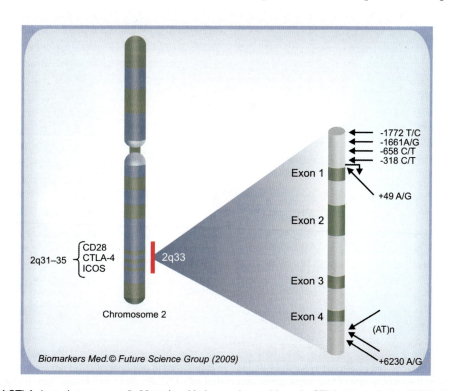

Fig. 13.5: Gene map of CTLA-4 on chromosome 2q33 region. Various polymorphisms in CTLA-4 gene in the 5'UTR, 3'UTR regulatory regions and exon 1 are shown in the map and have been studied extensively in T1D. The dark shaded boxes depict exons while light shaded boxes are intronic regions

days following T-cell activation and is merely a fraction of the expression level of constitutively expressed co-stimulator, CD28. Thus CTLA-4 is a low abundance but high avidity receptor on the surface of T-cells. Allelic variation at the CTLA-4 locus determines the levels of expression of the soluble CTLA-4 form. This may increase the inhibitory effects of CTLA-4 by competing CD28 for binding to the costimulatory B7-1 and B7-2 molecules on the antigen presenting cells. The ratio of sCTLA-4 to full-length CTLA-4 transcripts in unstimulated CD4 T-cells has been observed to be 50 percent lower in individuals with predisposing haplotype suggesting that the protective haplotype may be associated with higher levels of sCTLA-4 molecules. Therefore, the variation in the levels of CTLA-4, specially the soluble form, may affect the risk of developing autoimmune diseases including T1D. Because of its important role in the regulation of the immune response, CTLA-4 has emerged as a very strong candidate for association with autoimmune diseases including T1D.

CTLA-4 gene consists of four exons; the first encodes a V-like domain of 116 amino acids. An A to G substitution at nucleotide 49 in exon 1 results in an amino acid substitution (Thr/Ala) in the leader peptide. In addition to this, several CTLA-4 polymorphisms have been identified in humans, which have been used in genetic studies. These include polymorphisms in the 5' flanking promoter region, an (AT)n repeat in the 3' UTR, and a recently described A6230G SNP initially described as CT60 by Ueda et al 2003[144] outside the predicted CTLA-4 polyadenylation site.[148] The combined analysis of families from Finland, UK, US and other European populations revealed linkage with T1D and autoimmune thyroid disease in the 6.1kb region of CTLA4.[144] The +49G-CT60G haplotype was observed as a predisposing and +4949A-CT60A as the protective one. Susceptibility to T1D has been reported to be associated strongly with a SNP in the 5' end of CTLA-4 rather than polymorphism at the 3' UTR.[144]

PTPN22 Gene

Recently, it was discovered that after IDDM1, IDDM2 and IDDM12, the next gene which contributes the strongest risk towards susceptibility to T1D is PTPN22 (protein tyrosine phosphatase N22).[149-151] It alongwith other three major genes, e.g. IDDM1, IDDM2, and IDDM12 plays an important role in autoimmune response against the autoantigen- insulin (Fig. 13.6). The

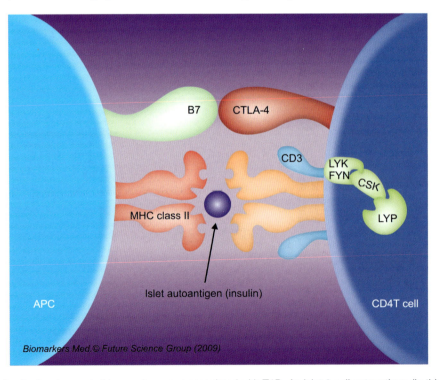

Fig. 13.6: Diagram showing the involvement of four major genes associated with T1D. An islet β-cell autoantigen (in this case peptide of insulin) is presented to CD4 T-cells by HLA class II molecules on antigen presenting cell (APC) leading to T-cell activation. Like CTLA-4, lymphoid tyrosine phosphatase (LYP) is also the inhibitor of T-cell activation and is encoded by PTPN22 gene. The LYP-CSK (C-terminal Src kinase) complex inhibits Lck signaling after HLA-peptide-TCR engagement

gene for PTPN22 is located on chromosome 1p13.2 and encodes a lymphoid-specific phosphatase known as Lyp. It performs the function of dephosphorylation of Lck, Fyn, and ZAP-10 proteins which are known to be important in T-cell signaling. Lyp binds to C-terminal Src kinase tyrosine kinase (Csk) resulting in the downregulation of activated T-cells, because Csk is an important suppressor of kinases that mediate T-cell activation. In addition, Lyp has been shown to play a negative regulatory role in T-cell signaling by binding to the adaptor molecule Grb2 (growth factor receptor-bound protein 2).[152]

Recently, positive association of a nonsynonymous SNP C1858T in codon 620 of PTPN22 gene has been reported with T1D from several populations including North America, UK, Italy and other countries.[149,150,153-156] The 1858T is a rare allele that changes the amino acid from arginine (R) to tryptophan (W) at position 620, resulting in disruption of the proline-rich binding motif 'PxxPxR', which is important for Lyp binding to both Csk and Grb2.[152,153] The reduced binding capacity of W620 Lyp (from 1858T allele) for Csk is supposed to disrupt the function of Csk as a downregulator of T-cell activation. T-cells lacking Lyp-Csk complex may result in a hyper immune response and therefore can lead to autoimmunity. It has been hypothesized that heterozygous individuals for the 1858T allele have reduced Lyp-Csk complexes, while the homozygous individuals have none.[153] The homozygous state is extremely rare which supports the above hypothesis, as lack of T-cell regulation leading to an immune assault may result in massive T-cell proliferation and ultimately to an autoimmune phenotype that could be potentially fatal. However, the fact that individuals do exist with such genotypes indicates that the Lyp-Csk interaction is not the only pathway leading to negative regulation of T-cell activation. Besides T1D, the 1858T allele has also been reported to be positively associated with other autoimmune diseases including rheumatoid arthritis and systemic lupus erythematosis.[157,158] However, a recent study could not show such an association of this T allele with T1D in India.[159]

FOXP3 Gene

FOXP3/ scurfin gene located on human chromosome Xp11.23 encodes a protein that is a member of the forkhead/wing-helix family of transcriptional regulators, and is specifically expressed in naturally occurring CD25+CD4+ regulatory T-cells.[160,161] Hori et al (2003)[161] have shown in a retroviral gene transfer experiment that the transfer of FOXP3 may convert naïve T-cells into a regulatory T-cell phenotype similar to the naturally occurring regulatory T-cells. These findings suggest that FOXP3 works as a master regulatory gene for the development of regulatory T-cells. Since an impaired T-cell activity can lead to an autoimmune disease,[162,163] the requirement of regulatory T-cells as important components in the homeostasis of the immune system can not be ignored. A mutation in the FOXP3 gene has also been reported to produce a rare recessive monogenetic disorder called IPEX (immune dysregulation, polyendocrinopathy including T1D, enteropathy and X-linked syndrome).[164] An autoimmune disease is supposed to develop as a result of misbalance between pro-inflammatory and anti-inflammatory cytokines indicating that the dysregulation of FOXP3/scurfin gene expression may lead to the development of autoimmune diabetes. Bassuny et al (2003)[165] have reported an association of a functional microsatellite polymorphism (GT)n in FOXP3 gene with susceptibility to T1D in the Japanese population. However similar studies conducted in other populations failed to confirm any such association.[166,167]

ICAM-1 Gene

The intercellular adhesion molecule-1 (ICAM-1) is a cell surface glycoprotein that is known to be expressed on macrophages, activated lymphocytes, thymic epithelial cells and vascular endothelial cells.[168] The gene of ICAM-1 is located on chromosome 19p13.2 and is a good candidate for T-cell mediated immune diseases because of the function of encoded protein. It is important for various leukocyte functions, e.g. antigen presentation and extravasation into lymphoid tissues and inflamed non-lymphoid tissues.[169,170] It functions as an adhesion receptor for the β integrins, LFA-1 and Mac-1 expressed on leucocytes.[171] Its engagement on antigen presenting cells and target cells by LFA-l expressed on T-cells provides a costimulatory signal for promoting T-cell activation.[168] Additionally, expression of ICAM-1 has been confirmed on pancreatic islet β-cells by electron microscopy[172] suggesting that it may be involved in the killer lymphocyte-mediated cytolysis of pancreatic islet β-cells. Therefore, this may be implicated in the pathogenesis of autoimmune diseases including T1D. Two single nucleotide polymorphisms (SNPs) have been described in exon 4 (G/A) and exon 6 (A/G), which change the amino acids G241R (glycine !arginine) and

K469E (lysine → glutamic acid) respectively.[173] Recent studies have shown an association of K469E polymorphism in ICAM-1 gene polymorphism with T1D[174] as well as age at onset of diabetes.[175]

Other Candidate Markers

Although, fine mapping of the intervals has not yet determined the identity of the putative diabetes susceptibility genes, certain intervals contain important candidate genes. For example, IDDM4 maps close to the galanin (GALN) and FAS-associated death domain (FADD) genes. GALN is a neuropeptide that may influence insulin secretion from the pancreas.[176] FADD is a cytoplasmic protein involved in the regulation of T-cell apoptosis, which may be an important mechanism in T1D.[176] Fine mapping and SNP-based fine mapping in T1D patients have narrowed the IDDM5 on chromosome 6q25 to ~212kb region containing only two genes, SUMO4 and TAB2.[177,178] A missense polymorphism 163A>G in SUMO4 gene leading M55V has been observed to be associated with T1D in several studies.[177]

IDDM7 maps close to the NeuroD/ BETA2 gene on chromosome 2q32. NeuroD/ BETA2, is an insulin gene transcription factor that plays an important role in the development of the pancreatic islet β-cells. Some studies have shown an association of heterozygosity for the Ala45Thr variant of this gene with type 1 diabetes[179,180] although, others have failed to confirm these findings.[181] It is reasonable to conclude that the effect of NeuroD/ BETA2, is independent of IDDM7.

IDDM13 is located on human chromosome 2 (2q35) close to the NRAMP1 gene, which is a host resistance gene. NRAMP1 is a divalent cation transporter that plays a key role in macrophage activation.[182] It affects the function of macrophages in a pleiotropic manner, which includes the expression of chemokines, IL-1β, TNF-α inducible nitric oxide synthetase and MHC class II molecules.[182] In the promoter region of NRAMP1, seven microsatellite alleles have been reported. An association of this polymorphism to infectious[182] and autoimmune diseases including T1D has been reported.[183] For example, while the allele 7 has been shown to be positively associated with T1D in the Japanese population,[184] allele 3 is associated with rheumatoid arthritis and also shows increased transmission to diabetic siblings with a first or second degree relative with rheumatoid arthritis. Interestingly, NRAMP1 does not show an association in those families which have sibs affected only with T1D.[185]

A susceptibility locus, IDDM18 close to IL12B gene, was reported and mapped to chromosome 5q31.1-q33.1.[186,187] IL12B encodes the p40 subunit of interleukin (IL) 12 and encodes T-cell response, and may therefore be important in T1D pathogenesis.[188] Linkage disequilibrium is confined to a 30kb region carrying IL12B, the only known gene. Several polymorphisms have been identified in IL12B[186,189] of which A allele of C1159A, shows a strong linkage disequilibrium with T1D in Australian and British diabetes families.[187] However, these results could not be corroborated.[190]

EXECUTIVE SUMMARY

- Type 1 diabetes is an organ specific, complex, polygenic autoimmune disease, in which both genetic as well as environmental factors contribute to its development.
- A number of gene loci referred to as IDDM1 to IDDM18 and others have been shown to confer risk to development of T1D. Among these, the locus IDDM1 represents the human Major Histocompatibility Complex (MHC), a locus that shows the strongest association and maximum risk.
- MHC is the most polymorphic complex in the human genome. The MHC haplotypes carrying DR3/DR4 are the most diabetogenic haplotypes followed by DR3/DR3 homozygous haplotypes in most Caucasian populations. Similarly, other haplotypes carrying DR5, DR7 or DR15 confer protection in most populations.
- In the Caucasian population, HLA-A1-B8-DR3 is the most common ancestral haplotype (AH8.1) that associates strongly with susceptibility to T1D and other autoimmune diseases.
- In contrast, the Indian population is characterized by the presence of three sets of DR3 positive haplotypes namely B50-DR3, B58-DR3 and B8-DR3, all of which show a positive association with the disease.
- Amongst the B8-DR3 group of haplotypes, the A1-B8-DR3 occurs with the least frequency (0.35%) in the Indian population and it differs from the classical European AH8.1 counterpart at several loci. It is therefore referred to as the variant form of AH8.1 (AH8.1v).
- In addition to AH8.1v, the Indian population has several other B8-DR3 haplotypes, which differ at HLA-A locus. These include AH8.2 (A26-B8-DR3), which is the most common followed by others like AH8.3 (A24-B8-DR3), AH8.4 (A3-B8-DR3) and AH8.5 (A31-B8-DR3).

- The multiple B8-DR3 haplotypes that occurs in the Indian population reveal extensive difference from the Caucasian ancestral haplotype AH8.1 spanning the whole extended MHC region except locus –B (B8) and DR3-DQ2 interval.
- The need for the occurrence of such extensive differences in the Indian population is not clear particularly since they are all disease associated. It is plausible to speculate these DR3+ve haplotypes share common regions that may be responsible for development of disease.
- It has been observed that the likelihood of developing of T1D increases with the coexistence of autoantibodies against GAD65, IA2, and IAA.
- In addition to MHC, there are other important loci, particularly those that code for insulin, CTLA4 and regulatory loci-like PTPN22 that also show strong associations with susceptibility to T1D. Like the MHC, these genes are also involved in regulating the immune homeostasis and effector functions and therefore influence immunopathogenesis of T1D.

FUTURE PERSPECTIVES

Population studies have revealed shared and distinct gene variants in multiple DR3+ve T1D favoring haplotypes that predispose an individual to disease. However, the underlying mechanism(s) that mediate this are not fully understood. Future studies could be designed to identify such shared genetic components in distinct population groups and thus narrow down to the region(s) of interest. One of the suggested regions is within and adjacent to the frozen DR3-DQ2 interval since this genetic segment remains well conserved in almost all the DR3+ve haplotypes across various populations. Similarly, information needs to be gathered for the predisposing DR4-DQ3 segment. It is known that certain DR4 subtypes, for example, DRB1*0403 exhibit dominant protection and thus suppress the otherwise predisposing ability of DR4-DQ3 haplotypes. Again, further studies focused on the kind of peptides bound by this subtype versus other DR4 subtypes could help unveil the specific underlying mechanistic differences. Such studies could be extended further to other protective alleles/haplotypes like the DR15, DR5 and DR7.

A major challenge that can be foreseen from above studies is the inherent characteristic of strong linkage disequilibrium within the MHC region. It is not easy to decipher the genetic marker(s) associated with T1D that are responsible for predisposition due to their direct role versus those that get highlighted due to their linkage with the actual yet unknown disease causing gene(s). Similarly, not much is known about the inter-regulatory functional networking between non MHC genes particularly transcription factors like PTPN22, FoxP3, and other immunomodulatory molecules like CTLA4, insulin, cytokines that lead to immunopathology rather than immunoprotection. It is also not clear what triggers the initiation of development of autoimmune response and factors that determine the age of disease onset.

Genetic studies like these have important implications in our understanding of disease pathogenesis, identification of high-risk individuals, disease diagnosis and management, and immunological therapeutic approaches.[191] For example, individuals with genetic propensities to autoimmunity and prevalence of multiple autoantibodies could be considered for an earlier therapeutic intervention and monitoring before their beta cell reserve is depleted.

REFERENCES

1. Molbak AG, Christau B, Marner B, Borch-Johnsen K, Nerup J. Incidence of insulin-dependent diabetes mellitus in age groups over 30 years in Denmark. Diabet. Med 1994;11:650-55.
2. Karvonen M, Viik-Kajander M, Moltchanova E, Libman I, LaPorte R, Tuomilehto J. Incidence of childhood type 1 diabetes worldwide. Diabetes Mondiale (DiaMond) Project Group. Diabetes Care 2000;23(10):1516-26.
3. Harrison LC. Risk assessment, prediction and prevention of type 1 diabetes. Pediatric Diabetes 2001;2:71-82.
4. Kloppel G, Lohr M, Habich K, Oberholzer M, Heitz PU: Islet pathology and the pathogenesis of type 1 and type 2 diabetes mellitus revisited. Surv. Synth. Pathol. Res 1985;4(2):110-25.
5. Eizirik DL Mandrup-Poulsen T. A choice of death- the signal transduction of immune-mediated beta cell apoptosis. Diabetologia 2001;44:2115-33.
6. Bonifacio E, Bingley PJ, Shattock M, et al. Quantification of islet-cell antibodies and prediction of insulin-dependent diabetes. Lancet 1990;335:147-49.
7. Riley WJ, Atkinson MA, Schatz DA, Maclaren NK. Comparison of islet autoantibodies in "pre-diabetes" and recommendations for screening. J Autoimmun 1990;3(Suppl)1:47-51.
8. Colman PG, McNair P, Margetts H et al. The Melbourne Pre-diabetes Study: Prediction of type 1 diabetes mellitus using antibody and metabolic testing. Med J Aust 1998;169(2):81-84.
9. Martin S, Wolf-Eichbaum D, Duinkerken G, et al. Development of type 1 diabetes despite severe hereditary B-lymphocyte deficiency. N Engl J Med 2001;345:1036-40.

10. Notkins AL, Lernmark A. Autoimmune type 1 diabetes: Resolved and unresolved issues. J Clin Invest 2001; 108:1247-52.
11. Palmer JP, Asplin CM, Clemons P, et al.: Insulin antibodies in insulin-dependent diabetics before insulin treatment. Science 1983;222:1337-39.
12. Yu J, Yu L, Bugawan TL, et al. Transient antiislet autoantibodies: Infrequent occurrence and lack of association with "genetic" risk factors. J. Clin. Endocrinol. Metab 2000;85(7):2421-28.
13. Hagopian WA, Michelsen B, Karlsen AE, Larsen F, Moddy A, Grubin CE: Autoantibodies in IDDM primarily recognize the 65,000-M(r) isoform of glutamic acid than the 67,000M(r) isoform of glutamic acid decarboxylase. Diabetes 1993;42(4):631-36.
14. Tandon N, Shtauvere-Brameus A, Hagopian WA, Sanjeevi CB. Prevalence of ICA-12 and other autoantibodies in north Indian patients with early-onset diabetes. Ann. N.Y. Acad. Sci 2002;958:214-17.
15. Sanjeevi CB, Kanungo A, Berzina L, Shtauvere-Brameus A, Ghaderi M, Samal KC. MHC class I chain-related gene a alleles distinguish malnutrition-modulated diabetes, insulin-dependent diabetes, and non-insulin- dependent diabetes mellitus patients from eastern India. Ann NY Acad Sci 2002;958:341-44.
16. Lampasona V, Bearzarro M, Genovese S, Bosi E, Ferrari M, Bonifacio E. Autoantibodies in insulin-dependent diabetes recognize distinct cytoplasmic domains of the protein tyrosine phosphatase-like IA-2 autoantigen. J Immunol 1996;157:2707-11.
17. Lan MS, Wasserfall C, Maclaren NK, Notkins AL. IA-2, a transmembrane protein of the protein tyrosine phosphatase family, is a major autoantigen in insulin-dependent diabetes mellitus. Proc. Natl. Acad Sci USA 1996;93:6367-70.
18. Rabin DU, Pleasic SM, Palmer-Crocker R, Shaphiro JA. Cloning and expression of IDDM-specific human autoantigens. Diabetes 1992;41:183-86.
19. Kasimiotis H, Myers M, Argentaro A. Sex determining region Y-related protein SOX13 is a diabetes autoantigen expressed in pancreatic islets. Diabetes 2000;49:555-61.
20. Penvy L, Lovell-Badge R. SOX genes find their feet. Curr Opin Genet Dev 1997;7:338-44.
21. Shtauvere-Brameus A, Hagopian W, Rumba I, Sanjeevi CB: Antibodies to new beta cell antigen ICA12 in Latvian diabetes patients. Ann. NY Acad Sci 2002;958:297-304.
22. Torn C, Shtauvere-Brameus A, Sanjeevi CB, Landin-Olsson M. Increased autoantibodies to SOX13 in Swedish patients with Type 1 diabetes. Ann. NY Acad Sci 2002;958:218-223.
23. Gupta M, Tandon N, Shtauvere-Brameus A, Sanjeevi CB. ICA12 autoantibodies are associated with Non-DR3/Non-DR4 patients with latent autoimmune diabetes in adults from Northern India. Ann. NY Acad Sci 2002;958:329-32.
24. Horvath L, Cervenak L, Oroszlan M, Prohaszka Z, Uray K, Hudecz F. Antibodies against different epitopes of heat-shock protein 60 in children with type 1 diabetes mellitus. Immunol Lett 2002;80:155-62.
25. Abulafia-Lapid R, Gillis D, Yosef O, Atlan H, Cohen IR. T-cells and autoantibodies to human HSP70 in Type 1 diabetes in children. J Autoimmun 2003;20:313-21.
26. Qin HY, Mahon JL, Atkinson MA, Chaturvedi P, Lee-Chan E, Singh B. Type 1 diabetes alters anti-hsp90 autoantibody isotype. J Autoimmun 2003;20:237-45.
27. Castano L, Russo E, Zhou L, Lipes MA, Eisenbarth GS. Identification and cloning of a granule autoantigen (carboxypeptidase-H) associated with type I diabetes. J Clin Endocrinol Metab 1991;73:1197-201.
28. Roep BO, Duinkerken G, Schreuder GM, Kolb H, de Vries RR, Martin S. HLA-associated inverse correlation between T-cell and antibody responsiveness to islet autoantigen in recent-onset insulin-dependent diabetes mellitus. Eur J Immunol 1996;26(6):1285-89.
29. Tisch R, Yang XD, Singer SM, Liblau RS, Fugger L, McDevitt HO. Immune response to glutamic acid decarboxylase correlates with insulitis in non-obese diabetic mice. Nature 1993;366:72-75.
30. Kaufman DL, Clare-Salzler M, Tian J, et al. Spontaneous loss of T-cell tolerance to glutamic acid decarboxylase in murine insulin-dependent diabetes. Nature 1993;366: 69-72.
31. Atkinson MA, Bowman MA, Cambell L, Darrow BL, Kaufman DL, Maclaren NK. Cellular immunity to a determinant common to glutamate decarboxylate and coxsackie virus in insulin-dependent diabetes mellitus. J Clin Invest 1994;94(5): 21-25.
32. Reijonen H, Novak EJ, Kochik S, Heninger A, Liu AW, Kwok WW. Detection of GAD65-specific T-cells by major histocompatibility complex class II tetramers in type 1 diabetic patients and at-risk subjects. Diabetes 2002; 51:1375-82.
33. Nepom GT, Lippolis JD, White FM, Masewicz S, Matro JA, Herman A. Identification and modulation of a naturally processed T-cell epitope from the diabetesassociated autoantigen human glutamic acid decarboxylase 65 (hGAD65). Proc Natl Acad Sci USA 2001;98:1763-68.
34. Durinovic-Bello I, Hummel M, Ziegler AG. Cellular immune response to diverse islet cell antigens in IDDM. Diabetes 1996;45:795-800.
35. Abulafia-Lapid R, Elias D, Raz I, Keren-Zur Y, Atlan H, Cohen IR. T-cell proliferative responses of type 1 diabetes patients and healthy individuals to human hsp60 and its peptides. J Autoimmun 1999;12:121-29.
36. Karges W, Hammond-McKibben D, Gaedigk R, Shibuya N, Cheung R, Dosch HM. Loss of self-tolerance to ICA69 in nonobese diabetic mice. Diabetes 1997;46:1548-56.
37. Bendelac A, Carnaud C, Boitard C, Bach JF. Syngeneic transfer of autoimmune diabetes from diabetic NOD mice to healthy neonates. Requirement for both L3T4+ and Lyt-2+ T-cells. J Exp Med 1987;166:823-32.
38. Yagi H, Matsumoto M, Kunimoto K, Kawaguchi J, Makino S, Harada M. Analysis of the roles of CD4+ and CD8+ T-

38. cells in autoimmune diabetes of NOD mice using transfer to NOD athymic nude mice. Eur J Immunol 1992;22: 2387-93.
39. Roep BO. The role of T-cells in the pathogenesis of Type 1 diabetes: From cause to cure. Diabetologia 2003;46: 305-21.
40. Panina-Bordignon P, Lang R, van Endert PM, Benazzi E, Felix AM, Pastore RM. Cytotoxic T-cells specific for glutamic acid decarboxylase in autoimmune diabetes. J Exp Med 1995;181:1923-27.
41. Bottazzo GF, Dean BM, McNally JM, MacKay EH, Swift PG, Gamble DR. In situ characterization of autoimmune phenomena and expression of HLA molecules in the pancreas in diabetic insulitis. NEJM 1985;313:353-60.
42. Wong FS, Karttunen J, Dumont C, Wen L, Visintin I, Philip IM. Identification of an MHC class I-restricted autoantigen in type 1 diabetes by screening an organspecific cDNA library. Nat Med 1999;5:1026-31.
43. Martinez NR, Augstein P, Moustakas AK, Augstein P, Moustakas AK. Papadopoulos GK. Disabling an integral CTL epitope allows suppression of autoimmune diabetes by intranasal proinsulin peptide. J Clin Invest 2003; 111:1365-71.
44. Panagiotopoulos C, Qin H, Tan R, Verchere CB. Identification of a beta-cell specific MHC class I restricted epitope in type 1 diabetes. Diabetes 2003;52:A46.
45. Lieberman SM, Evans AM, Han B, Takaki T, Vinnitakaya Y, Caldwell JA. Identification of the beta cell antigen targeted by a prevalent population of pathogenic CD8+ T-cells in autoimmune diabetes. Proc Natl Acad Sci USA 2003;100(14):8384-88.
46. Nerup J, Mandrup-Poulsen T, Molvig J, Helqvist S, Wogensen L, Egeberg J. Mechanisms of pancreatic β-cell destruction in type I diabetes. Diabetes Care 1988; 11(Suppl. 1):16-23.
47. Nerup J, Mandrup-Poulsen T, Helqvist S, et al. On the pathogenesis of IDDM. Diabetologia 1994;37 (Suppl. 2):S82-S89.
48. Bergholdt R, Heding P, Nielsen K, et al. Type 1 diabetes mellitus: An inflammatory disease of the islet. In Immunology of Type 1 Diabetes (Eisenbarth, GS (Ed) pp. 129–153, Eurekah.com and Kluwer Academic/Plenum Publishers, Amsterdam, The Netherlands, 2004.
49. Rossini AA, Handler ES, Mordes JP, Greiner DL. Animal models of human disease. Human autoimmune diabetes mellitus: Lessions from BB rats and NOD mice-Caveat emptor. Clin. Immunol. Immunopathol 1995;74:2-9.
50. Bone AJ. Animal models of type 1 diabetes. Curr. Opin. Oncol. Endocr. Metab. Invest. Drugs 2000;2:192-200.
51. Makino S, Kunimoto K, Muraoka Y, Mizushima Y, Katagiri K, Tochino Y. Breeding of a non-obese, diabetic strain of mice. Jikken. Dobutsu. 1980;29:1-13.
52. Tang Q, Adams JY, Penaranda C, et al. Central role of defective interleukin-2 production in the triggering of islet autoimmune destruction. Immunity 2008;28:687-97.
53. Delovitch TL, Singh B. The nonobese diabetic mouse as a model of autoimmune diabetes: Immune dysregulation gets the NOD. Immunity 1997;7:727-38.
54. King M, Pearson T, Shultz LD, et al. Development of new-generation HU-PBMC-NOD/SCID mice to study human islet alloreactivity. Ann NY Acad Sci 2007;1103:90-93.
55. Yang XD, Karin N, Tisch R, Steinman L, McDevitt HO. Inhibition of insulitis and prevention of diabetes in nonobese diabetic mice by blocking L-selectin and very late antigen 4 adhesion receptors. Proc Natl Acad Sci USA 1993; 90:10494-98.
56. Yang XD, Tisch R, Singer SM, et al. Effect of tumor necrosis factor alpha on insulin dependent diabetes mellitus in NOD mice. I. The early development of autoimmunity and the diabetogenic process. J Exp Med 1994;180:995-1004.
57. Fife BT, Guleria I, Gubbels Bupp M, et al. Insulin-induced remission in new-onset NOD mice is maintained by the PD-1-PD-L1 pathway. J Exp Med 2006; 203: 2737-47.
58. Mordes JP, Bortell R, Groen H, Geuberski D, Rossini AA, Greiner DL. Autoimmune Diabetes Mellitus in BB rats. In Frontiers in Animal Diabetes Research (Vol.2) (Sima AA and Shafrir E (Eds); 1-41, Harwood Academic Publishers, London, UK, 2001.
59. Mordes JP, Bortell R, Blankenhorn EP, Rossini AA, Greiner DL. Rat models of type 1 diabetes: Genetics, environment, and autoimmunity. ILARJ 2004;45:278-91.
60. Whalen BJ, Mordes JP, Rossini AA. The BB rat as a model of human insulin-dependent diabetes mellitus. Curr Protoc Immunol Chapter 15: Unit 15 13, 2001.
61. Greiner DL, Rossini AA, Mordes JP. Translating data from animal models into methods for preventing human autoimmune diabetes mellitus: Caveat emptor and primum non nocere. Clin Immunol 2001;100:134-43.
62. Devendra D, Liu E, Eisenbarth GS. Type 1 diabetes: Recent developments. BMJ 2004;328:750-54.
63. Redondo MJ, Rewers M, Yu L, et al. Genetic determination of islet cell autoimmunity in monozygotic twin, dizygotic twin, and non-twin siblings of patients with type 1 diabetes: Prospective twin study. BMJ 1999;13:318 (7185), 698-702.
64. Gottlieb PA, Eisenbarth GS. Human autoimmune diabetes. In: Molecular Pathology of Autoimmune Diseases. An Theofilopoulos, CA Bona (Eds), Taylor & Francis, New York, 2002;588-613.
65. Cudworth AG, Woodrow JC: Evidence for HL-A-linked genes in 'juvenile' diabetes mellitus. BMJ 1975;3:133-35.
66. Cudworth AG, Woodrow JC. Genetic susceptibility in diabetes mellitus: Analysis of the HLA association. BMJ 1976;2:846-48.
67. Deschamps I, Lestradet H, Bonaiti C, et al. HLA genotype studies in juvenile insulin-dependent diabetes. Diabetologia 1980;19:189-93.
68. Lucassen AM, Julier C, Beressi JP, Boitard C, Froguel P, Lathrop M. Susceptibility to insulin dependent diabetes mellitus maps to a 4.1kb segment of DNA spanning the insulin gene and associated VNTR. Nat Genet 1993;4: 305-10.
69. Pugliese A, Zeller M, Fernandez Jr A, Zalcberg LJ, Bartlett RJ, Ricordi C. The insulin gene is transcribed in the human thymus and transcription levels correlated with allelic

variation at the INS VNTR-IDDM2 susceptibility locus for type 1 diabetes. Nat Genet 1997;15:293-97.
70. Vafiadis P, Bennett ST, Todd JA, Nadeau J, Grabs R, Goodyer CG. Insulin expression in human thymus is modulated by INS VNTR alleles at the IDDM2 locus. Nat. Genet 1997;15:289-92.
71. Concannon P, Erlich HA, Julier C, et al. Type 1 diabetes: Evidence for susceptibility loci from four genome-wide linkage scans in 1,435 multiplex families. Diabetes 2005;54:2995-3001.
72. Noble JA, Valdes AM, Cook M, Klitz W, Thomson G, Erlich HA. The role of HLA class II genes in insulin-dependent diabetes mellitus: Molecular analysis of 180 Caucasian, multiplex families. Am J Hum Genet 1996;59:1134-48.
73. Mehra NK, Kaur G, Kanga U, Tandon N. Immunogenetics of autoimmune diseases in Asian Indians. Ann NY Acad Sci 2002;958:333-36.
74. Witt CS, Price P, Kaur G, Cheong K, Kanga U, Sayer D. The Common HLA-B8-DR3 haplotype in Northern India is different from that found in Europe. Tissue Antigens 2002;60:474-80.
75. Kanga U, Vaidyanathan B, Jaini R, Menon PS, Mehra NK. HLA haplotypes associated with type 1 diabetes mellitus in North Indian children. Hum. Immunol 2004;65:47-53.
76. Rani R, Sood A, Lazaro A, Stastny P. Associations of MHC class II alleles with insulin dependent diabetes mellitus (IDDM) in patients from North India. Hum Immunol 1999;60:524-31.
77. Rani R, Sood A, Goswami R. Molecular basis of predisposition to develop type 1 diabetes mellitus in North Indians. Tissue Antigens 2004;64:145-55.
78. Altobelli E, Blasetti A, Petrocelli R, et al. HLA DR/DQ alleles and risk of type I diabetes in childhood: A population-based case-control study. Clin Exp Med 2005;5:72-79.
79. Eller E, Vardi P, McFann KK, et al. Differential effects of DRB1*0301 and DQA1*0501-DQB1*0201 on the activation and progression of islet cell autoimmunity. Genes Immun 2007;8:628-33.
80. Guerin V, Leniaud L, Pedron B, Guilmin-Crepon S, Tubiana-Rufi N, Sterkers G. HLA-associated genetic resistance and susceptibility to type I diabetes in French North Africans and French natives. Tissue Antigens 2007;70:214-18.
81. Thomson G, Valdes AM, Noble JA, et al. Relative predispositional effects of HLA class II DRB1-DQB1 haplotypes and genotypes on type 1 diabetes: A meta-analysis. Tissue Antigens 2007;70:110-27.
82. Erlich H, Valdes AM, Noble J, et al. HLA DR-DQ haplotypes and genotypes and type 1 diabetes risk: Analysis of the type 1 diabetes genetics consortium families. Diabetes 2008;57:1084-92.
83. Kukko M, Virtanen SM, Toivonen A, et al. Geographical variation in risk HLA-DQB1 genotypes for type 1 diabetes and signs of beta-cell autoimmunity in a high-incidence country. Diabetes Care 2004;27(3):676-81.
84. Kawabata Y, Ikegami H, Kawaguchi Y, et al. Asian-specific HLA haplotypes reveal heterogeneity of the contribution of HLA-DR and –DQ haplotypes to susceptibility to type 1 diabetes. Diabetes 2002;51:545-51.
85. Ikegami H, Awata T, Kawasaki E, et al. The association of CTLA4 polymorphism with type 1 diabetes is concentrated in patients complicated with autoimmune thyroid disease: A multi-center collaborative study in Japan. J Clin Endocrin Metab 2005;91:1087-92.
86. Tait BD, Harrison LC, Drummond BP, Stewart V, Varney MD, Honeyman MC. HLA antigens and age at diagnosis of insulin dependent diabetes mellitus. Hum. Immunol. 1995;42(2):116-22.
87. Lambert AP, Gillespie KM, Thomson G, et al. Absolute Risk of Childhood-Onset Type 1 Diabetes Defined by Human Leukocyte Antigen Class II Genotype: A Population-Based Study in the United Kingdom. J Clin Endocrinol. Metab 2004;89:4037-43.
88. Cucca F, Lampis R, Congia M, Angius E, Nutland S, Bain SC. A correlation between the relative predisposition of MHC class II alleles to type 1 diabetes and the structure of their proteins. Hum Mol Genet 2001;10:2025-37.
89. Lee KH, Wucherpfennig KW, Wiley DC. Structure of a human insulin peptide–HLA-DQ8 complex and susceptibility to type 1 diabetes. Nat Immunol 2001;2:501-07.
90. Moghaddam PH, Zwinderman AH, de Knijff P. TNFa microsatellite polymorphism modulates the risk of IDDM in Caucasians with the high-risk genotype HLA DQA1*0501-DQB1*0201/ DQA1*0301- DQB1*0302. Belgian Diabetes Registry. Diabetes 1997;46:1514-15.
91. Awata T, Kuzuya T, Matsuda A, Iwamoto Y, Kanazawa Y, Okuyama M. High frequency of aspartic acid at position 57 of HLA-DQbchain in Japanese IDDM patients and non-diabetic subjects. Diabetes 1990;39:266-69.
92. Stern LJ, Brown JH, Jardetzky TS, Gorga JC, Urban RG, Strominger JL. Crystal structure of the human class II MHC protein HLA-DR1 complexed with an influenza virus peptide. Nature 1994;368:215-21.
93. Kwok WW, Domeier ME, Johnson ML, Nepom GT, Koele DM: HLA-DQB1 codon 57 is critical for peptide binding and recognition. J Exp Med 1996;183:1253-58.
94. Kwok WW, Domeier ME, Raymond FC, Byers P, Nepom GT. Allele-specific motifs characterize HLA-DQ interactions with a diabetes-associated peptide derived from glutamic acid decarboxylase. J Immunol 1996;156:2171–77.
95. Quarsten H, Paulsen G, Johansen BH, Thorpe CJ, Holm A, Buus S. The P9 pocket of HLA-DQ2 (non-Aspbeta57) has no particular preference for negatively charged anchor residues found in other type 1 diabetes-predisposing non-Aspbeta57 MHC class II molecules. Int Immunol 1998;10:1229-36.
96. Sato AK, Sturniolo T, Sinigaglia F, Stern LJ. Substitution of aspartic acid at b57 with alanine alters MHC class II peptide binding activity but not protein stability: HLA-DQ (a1*0201, b1*0302) and (a1*0201, b1*0303). Hum Immunol 1999;60:1227-36.

97. Segurado OG, Iglesias-Casarrubios P, Martinez-Laso J, Corell A, Martin-Villa JM, Arnaiz-Villena A. Auto-immunogenic HLA-DRB1*0301 allele (DR3) may be distinguished at the DRB1 non-coding regions of HLA-B8,DR3,Dw24 and B18,DR3,Dw25 haplotypes. Mol Immunol 1991;28:189-92.
98. Urcelay E, Santiago JL, de la Calle H, et al. Type 1 diabetes in the Spanish population: Additional factors to class II HLA-DR3 and -DR4. BMC Genomics 2005;6:56-62.
99. Noble JA, Valdes AM, Lane JA, Green AE, Erlich HA. Linkage disequilibrium with predisposing DR3 haplotypes accounts for apparent effects of tumor necrosis factor and lymphotoxin-alpha polymorphisms on type 1 diabetes susceptibility. Hum Immunol 2006;67:999-1004.
100. Mehra NK, Kumar N, Kaur G, Kanga U, Tandon N. Biomarkers of susceptibility to type 1 diabetes with special reference to the Indian population. Indian J. Med. Res 2007;125:321-44.
101. Erlich HA, Rotter JI, Chang JD, Shaw SJ, Raffel LJ, Klitz W. Association of HLA-DPB1*0301 with IDDM in Mexican-Americans. Diabetes 1996;45:610-14.
102. Noble JA, Valdes AM, Thomson G, Erlich HA. The HLA class II locus DPB1 can influence susceptibility to type 1 diabetes. Diabetes 2000;49:121-25.
103. Cucca F, Dudbridge F, Loddo M, Mulargia AP, Lampis R, Angius E. The HLA-DPB1-associated component of the IDDM1 and its relationship to the major loci HLA-DQB1-DQA1, and -DRB1. Diabetes 2001;50:1200-05.
104. Begovich AB, McClure GR, Suraj VC, Helmuth RC, Flides N, Bugawan TL. Polymorphism, recombination, and linkage disequilibrium within the HLA class II region. J Immunol 1992;148:249-58.
105. Wilson AG, Symons JA, McDowell TL, McDevitt HO, Duff GW. Effects of a polymorphism in the human tumor necrosis factor alpha promoter on transcriptional activation. Proc Natl Acad Sci USA 1997;94:3195-99.
106. Bouma G, Crusius JB, Oudkerk Pool M, et al. Ecretion of tumor necrosis factor alpha and lymphotoxin alpha in relation to polymorphisms in the TNF genes and HLA-DR alleles. Relevance for inflammatory bowel disease. Scand J Immunol 1996;43:456-63.
107. Koss K, Satsangi J, Fanning GC, Welsh KI, Jewell DP. Cytokine (TNF alpha, LT alpha and IL-10) polymorphisms in inflammatory bowel diseases and normal controls: Differential effects on production and allele frequencies. Genes Immun 2000;1(3):185-90.
108. Jongeneel CV, Briant L, Udalova IA, Sevin A, Nedospasov SA, Cambon-Thomsen A. Extensive genetic polymorphism in the human tumor necrosis factor region and relation to extended HLA haplotypes. Proc Natl Acad Sci USA 1991;88:9717-21.
109. Udalova IA, Nedospasov SA, Webb GC, Chaplin DD, Turetskaya RL. Highly informative typing of the human TNF locus using six adjacent polymorphic markers. Genomics 1993;16:180-86.
110. Obayashi H, Nakamura N, Fukui M, et al. Influence of TNF microsatellite polymorphisms (TNFa) on age-at-onset of insulin-dependent diabetes mellitus. Hum. Immunol 1999;60:974-78.
111. Nedospasov SA, Udalova IA, Kuprash DV, Turetskaya RL. DNA sequence polymorphism at the human tumor necrosis factor (TNF) locus. Numerous TNF/lymphotoxin alleles tagged by two closely linked microsatellites in the unstream region of the lymphotoxin (TNF-beta) gene. J Immunol 1991;147(3):1053-59.
112. Tsukamoto K, Ohta N, Shirai Y, Emi M. A highly polymorphic CA repeat marker at the human tumor necrosis factor alpha (TNFA alpha) locus. J Hum Genet 1998;43:278-79.
113. Pociot F, Briant L, Jongeneel CV. Association of tumor necrosis factor (TNF) and class II major histocompatibility complex alleles with the secretion of TNF-alpha and TNF-beta by human mononuclear cells: A possible link to insulin-dependent diabetes mellitus. Eur J Immunol 1993;23:224-31.
114. Makhatadze NJ. Tumor necrosis factor locus: Genetic organization and biological implications. Hum Immunol 1998;59:571.
115. Kim KA, Kim S, Chang I, et al. IFN gamma/TNF alpha synergism in MHC class II induction: Effect of nicotinamide on MHC class II expression but not on islet-cell apoptosis. Diabetologia 2002;45:385-93.
116. Monos DS, Kamoun M, Udalova IA. Genetic polymorphism of the human tumor necrosis factor region in insulin-dependent diabetes mellitus. Linkage disequilibrium of TNFab microsatellite alleles with HLA haplotypes. Hum Immunol 1995;44:70-79.
117. Gambelunghe G, Ghaderi M, Cosentino A, Falorni A, Brunetti P, Sajeevi CB. Association of MHC class I chain related gene-A (MIC-A) polymorphism with Type 1 diabetes. Diabetlogia 2000;43(4):507-14.
118. Mizuki N, Ota M, Kimura M, et al. Triplet repeat polymorphism in the transmembrane region of the MIC-A gene: A strong association of six GCT repetitions with Bachet disease. Proc Natl Acad Sci USA 1997;94(4):1298-1303.
119. Ota M, Katsuyama Y, Mizuki N, et al. Trinucleotide repeat polymorphism within exon 5 of the MICA gene (MHC class I chain-related gene A): Allele frequency data in the nine population groups Japanese, Northern Han, Hui, Uygur, Kazakhstan, Iranian, Saudi Arabian, Greek and Italian. Tissue Antigens 1997;49:448-54.
120. Rueda B, Pascual M, Lopez-Nevot MA, Gonzalez E, Martin J. A new allele within the transmembrane region of the human MIC-A gene with seven GCT repeats. Tissue Antigens 2002;60(6):526-28.
121. Perez-Rodriguez M, Corell A, et al. A new allele with ten alanine residues in the exon 5 microsatellite. Tissue Antigens 2000;55(2):162-65.
122. Suemizu H, Radosavljevic M, Kimura M, et al. A basolateral sorting motif in the MIC-A cytoplasmic tail. Proc. Natl. Acad Sci USA 2002;99(5):2971-76.
123. Bahram S. MIC genes: From genetics to biology. Adv. Immunol 2000;76:1-60.

124. Steinle A, Li P, Morris DL, Groh V, Lanier LL, Strong RK, Spies T. Interactions of human NKG2D with its ligands MIC-A, MIC-B and homologs of the mouse RAE-1 protein family. Immunogenetics 2001;53(4):279-87.
125. Nikitina-Zake L, Cimdina I, Rumba I, Dabadghao P, Sanjeevi CB. Major histocompatibility complex class I chain related (MIC) A gene, TNFα microsatellite alleles and TNFB alleles in juvenile idiopathic arthiritis patients from Latvia. Hum Immunol 2002;63(5):418-23.
126. Gambelunghe G, Falorni A, Ghaderi M, et al. Microsatellite polyorphism of the MHC class I chain related (MIC-A and MIC-B) genes marks the risk for autoimmune Addison's disease. J Clin Endocrinol Metab 1999;84(10): 3701-07.
127. Lee YJ, Huang FY, Wang CH, et al. Polymorphism in the transmembrane region of the MIC-A gene and type 1 diabetes. J Pediatr Endocrinol Metab 2000;13(5): 489-96.
128. Kawabata Y, Ikegami H, Kawaguchi Y, et al. Age-related association of MHC class I chain related gene A (MIC-A) with type (insulin-dependent) diabetes mellitus. Hum. Immunol. 2000;61(6):624-29.
129. Park Y, Lee H, Sanjeevi CB, Eisenbarth GS. MIC-A polymorphism is associated with Type 1 diabetes in the Korean population. Diabetes Care 2001;24(1):33-38.
130. Shtauvere-Brameus A, Ghaderi M, Rumba I, Sanjeevi CB: Microsatellite allele 5 of MHC class I chain related gene-A increases the risk for insulin-dependent diabetes mellitus in Latvians. Ann NY Acad Sci 2002;958:349-52.
131. Bennett ST, Lucassen AM, Gough SC, Powell EE, Undlien DE, Pritchard LE. Susceptibility to human type 1 diabetes at IDDM2 is determined by tandem repeat variation at the insulin gene minisatellite locus. Nat Genet 1995;9: 284-92.
132. Bell GI, Horita S, Karam JH. A polymorphic locus near the human insulin gene is associated with insulin-dependent diabetes mellitus. Diabetes 1984;33:176-83.
133. Bain SC, Prins JB, Hearne CM, Rodrigues NR, Rowe BR, Pritchard LE. Insulin gene region-encoded susceptibility to type 1 diabetes is not restricted to HLA-DR4-positive individuals. Nat Genet 1992;2:212-15.
134. Stead JD, Buard J, Todd JA, Jeffreys AJ. Influence of allele lineage on the role of the insulin minisatellite in susceptibility to type 1 diabetes. Hum Mol Genet 2000;9:2929-35.
135. Jolicoeur C, Hanahan D, Smith KM. T-cell tolerance toward a transgenic beta-cell antigen and transcription of endogenous pancreatic genes in thymus. Proc Natl Acad Sci USA 1994;9:16707-711.
136. Vafiadis P, Grabs R, Goodyer CG, Colle E, Polychronakos C. A functional analysis of the role of IGF2 in IDDM2-encoded susceptibility to type 1 diabetes. Diabetes 1998;47:831-36.
137. Vafiadis P, Bennett ST, Todd JA, Grabs R, Polychronakos C. Divergence between genetic determinants of IGF2 transcription levels in leukocytes and of IDDM2-encoded susceptibility to type 1 diabetes. J Clin Endocrinol Metab 1998;83:2933-39.
138. Dahlquist G, Bennich SS, Kallen B. Intrauterine growth pattern and risk of childhood onset insulin dependent (type 1) diabetes: Population based case-control study. BMJ 1996;313:1174-77.
139. Paquette J, Giannoukakis N, Polychronakos C, Vafiadis P, Deal C. The INS 5' variable number of tandem repeats is associated with IGF2 expression in humans. J Biol Chem 1998;273:14158-64.
140. Copeman JB, Cucca F, Hearne CM, Cornall RJ, Reed PW, Ronningen KS. Linkage disequilibrium mapping of a type 1 diabetes susceptibility gene (IDDM7) to chromosome 2q31–q33. Nat Genet 1995;9:80-85.
141. Morahan G, Huang D, Tait BD, Colman PG, Harrison LC. Markers on distal chromosome 2q linked to insulin-dependent diabetes mellitus. Science 1996;272:1811-13.
142. Nistico L, Buzzetti R, Pritchard LE, van der Auwera B, Giovannini C, Bosi E. The CTLA-4 gene region of chromosome 2q33 is linked to, and associated with, type 1 diabetes. Belgian Diabetes Registry. Hum Mol Genet 1996;5:1075-80.
143. Larsen ZM, Kristiansen OP, Mato E, Johannesen J, Puig-Domingo M, de Leiva A: IDDM12 (CTLA4) on 2q33 and IDDM13 on 2q34 in genetic susceptibility to type 1 diabetes (insulin-dependent). Autoimmunity 1999;31: 35-42.
144. Ueda H, Howson JM, Esposito L, et al. Association of the T-cell regulatory gene CTLA4 with susceptibility to autoimmune disease. Nature 2003;423:506-11.
145. Noel PJ, Boise LH, Thomson CB. Regulation of T-cell activation by CD28 and CTLA4. Adv Exp Med Biol 1996;406:209-17.
146. Paust S, Lu L, McCarty N, Cantor H. Engagement of B7 on effector T-cells by regulatory T-cells prevents autoimmune disease. PNAS 2004;101:10398-403.
147. Magistrelli G, Jeannin P, Herbault N et al. A soluble form of CTLA-4 generated by alternative splicing is expressed by nonstimulated human T-cells. Eur J Immunol 1999; 29:3596-3602.
148. Ling V, Wu PW, Finnerty HF, Agostino MJ, Graham JR, Chen S. Assembly and annotation of human chromosome 2q33 sequence containing the CD28, CTLA4, and ICOS gene cluster: analysis by computational, comparative, and microarray approaches. Genomics 2001;78:155-68.
149. Smyth D, Cooper JD, Collins JE, et al. Replication of an association between the lymphoid tyrosine phosphatase locus (LYP/PTPN22) with type 1 diabetes, and evidence for its role as a general autoimmunity locus. Diabetes 2004; 53:3020-23.
150. Onengut-Gumuscu S, Ewens KG, Spielman RS, Concannon P. A functional polymorphism (1858C/T) in the PTPN22 gene is linked and associated with type 1 diabetes in multiplex families. Genes Immun 2004;5: 678-80.
151. Santiago JL, Martinez A, de la Calle H, et al. Susceptibility to type 1 diabetes conferred by the PTPN22 C1858T polymorphism in the Spanish population. BMC Med Genet 2007;8:2350-54.

152. Hill RJ, Zozulya S, Lu YL, Ward K, Gishizky M, Jallal B. The lymphoid protein tyrosine phosphatase Lyp interacts with the adaptor molecule Grb2 and functions as a negative regulator of T-cell activation. Exp Hematol 2002;30:237-44.
153. Bottini N, Musumeci L, Alonso A, Rahmouni S, Nika K, Rostamkhani M. A functional variant of lymphoid tyrosine phosphatase is associated with type I diabetes. Nat. Genet 2004;36:337-38.
154. Criswell LA, Pfeiffer KA, Lum RF, et al. Analysis of families in the multiple autoimmune disease genetics consortium (MADGC) collection: The PTPN22 620W allele associates with multiple autoimmune phenotypes. Am J Hum Genet 2005;76(4):561-71.
155. Ladner MB, Bottini N, Valdes AM, Noble JA. Association of the single nucleotide polymorphism C1858T of the PTPN22 gene with type 1 diabetes. Hum Immunol 2005;66:60-64.
156. Saccucci P, Del Duca E, Rapini N, et al. Association between PTPN22 C1858T and type 1 diabetes: A replication in continental Italy. Tissue Antigens 2008;71(3): 234-37.
157. Kyogoku C, Langefeld CD, Ortmann WA, Lee A, Selby S, Carlton VE. Genetic association of the R620W polymorphism of protein tyrosine phosphatase PTPN22 with human SLE. Am. J. Hum Genet 2004;75:504-07.
158. McAllister LB, Jeffery DA, Lee AT, Batliwalla F, Remmers E, Criswell LA. A missense single-nucleotide polymorphism in a gene encoding a protein tyrosine phosphatase (PTPN22) is associated with rheumatoid arthritis. Am. J Hum Genet 2004;75:330-37.
159. Baniasadi V, Das SN. No evidence for association of PTPN22 R620W functional variant C1858T with type 1 diabetes in Asian Indians. J Cell Mol Med 2008;12: 1061-62.
160. Clark LB, Appleby MW, Brunkow ME, Wilkinson JE, Ziegler SF, Ramsdell F. Cellular and molecular characterization of the scurfy mouse mutant. J Immunol 1999;162:2546-54.
161. Hori S, Nomura T, Sakaguchi S. Control of regulatory T-cell development by the transcription factor Foxp3. Science 2003;299:1057-61.
162. Shevach EM. Regulatory T-cells in autoimmunity. Annu Rev Immunol 2000;18:423-49.
163. von Herrath MG, Harrison LC. Antigen-induced regulatory T-cells in autoimmunity. Nat Rev Immunol 2003;3:223-32.
164. Bennett CL, Christie J, Ramsdell F, Brunkow ME, Ferguson PJ, Whitesell L. The immune dysregulation, polyendocrinopathy, enteropathy, X-linked syndrome (IPEX) is caused by mutations of FOXP3. Nat Genet 2001;27:20-21.
165. Bassuny WM, Ihara K, Sasaki Y, Kuromaru R, Kohno H, Matsuura N. A functional polymorphism in the promoter/enhancer region of the FOXP3/Scurfin gene associated with type 1 diabetes. Immunogenetics 2003;55: 149-56.
166. Zavattari P, Deidda E, Pitzalis M, Zoa B, Moi L, Lampis R. No association between variation of the FOXP3 gene and common type 1 diabetes in the Sardinian population. Diabetes 2004;53:1911-14.
167. Sanchez E, Rueda B, Orozco G, Oliver J, Vilchez JR, Paco L. Analysis of a GT microsatellite in the promoter of the foxp3/scurfin gene in autoimmune diseases. Hum. Immunol 2005;66:869-73.
168. Lebedeva T, Dustin ML, Sykulev Y. ICAM-1 co-stimulates target cells to facilitate antigen presentation. Curr Opin Immunol 2005;17(5):251-58.
169. Dustin ML, Rothlein R, Bhan AK, Dinarello CA, Springer TA. Induction by IL1 and interferon-gamma: Tissue distribution, biochemistry, function of a natural adherence molecule (ICAM-1). J. Immunol 1986;137:245-54.
170. Springer TA. Adhesion receptors of the immune system. Nature 1990;346:425-34.
171. Diamond MS, Staunton DE, Marlin SD, Springer TA. Binding of the integrin MAC-1 (CD11b/CD18) to the third immunoglobulin-like domain of ICAM-1 (CD54) and its regulation by glycosylation. Cell 1991;65(6):961-71.
172. Yagi N, Yokono K, Amano K, Nagata M, Tsukamoto K, Hasegawa Y. Expression of intercellular adhesion molecule 1 on pancreatic β-cells accelerates β-cell destruction by cytotoxic T-cells in murine autoimmune diabetes. Diabetes 1995;44:744-52.
173. Vora DK, Rosenbloom CL, Beaudet AL, Cottingham RW. Polymorphisms and linkage analysis for ICAM-1 and the selectin gene cluster. Genomics 1994;21:473-77.
174. Nejentsev S, Guja C, McCormack R, et al. Association of intercellular adhesion molecule-1 gene with type 1 diabetes. Lancet 2003;362:1723-24.
175. Nishimura M, Obayashi H, Maruya E, et al. Association between type 1 diabetes age-at-onset and intercellular adhesion molecule-1 (ICAM-1) gene poloymorphism. Hum. Immunol 2000;61(5):507-10.
176. Eckenrode S, Marron MP, Nicholls R, Yang MC, Yang JJ, Guida Fonseca LC. Fine-mapping of the type 1 diabetes locus (IDDM4) on chromosome 11q and evaluation of two candidate genes (FADD and GALN) by affected sib pair and linkage-disequilibrium analyses. Hum Genet 2000;106:14-18.
177. Guo D, Li M, Zhang Y, et al. A functional variant of SUMO4, a new I kappa B alpha modifier, is associated with type 1 diabetes. Nat Genet 2004;36:837-41.
178. Owerbach D, Pina L, Gabbay KH. A 212-kb region on chromosome 6q25 containing the TAB2 gene is associated with susceptibility to type 1 diabetes. Diabetes 2004;53:1890-93.
179. Iwata I, Nagafuchi S, Nakashima H, Kondo S, Koga T, Yokogawa Y. Association of polymorphism in the NeuroD/BETA2 gene with type 1 diabetes in the Japanese. Diabetes 1999;48:416-19.
180. Hansen L, Jensen JN, Urioste S, Petersen HV, Pociot F, Eiberg F. NeuroD/BETA2 gene variability and diabetes: No associations to late-onset type 2 diabetes but an A45 allele may represent a susceptibility marker for type 1 diabetes among Danes. Diabetes 2000;49:876-78.

181. Dupont S, Dina C, Hani EH, Froguel P. Absence of replication in the French population of the association between beta2/NEUROD-A45T polymorphism and type 1 diabetes. Diabetes Metab 1999;25:516-17.
182. Searle S, Blackwell JM. Evidence for a functional repeat polymorphism in the promoter of the human NRAMP1 gene that correlates with autoimmune versus infectious disease susceptibility. J Med Genet 1999;36:295-99.
183. Bassuny WM, Ihara K, Matsuura N, Ahmed S, Kohno H, Kuromaru R. Association study of NRAMP1 gene promoter polymorphism and early onset type 1 diabetes. Immunogenetics 2002;54:282-85.
184. Takahashi K, Satoh J, Kojima Y, et al. Promoter polymorphism of SLC11A1 (formerly NRAMP1) confers susceptibility to autoimmune type 1 diabetes mellitus in Japanese. Tissue Antigens 2004;63:231-36.
185. Esposito L, Hill NJ, Pritchard LE, Cucca F, Muxworthy C, Merriman ME. Genetic analysis of chromosome 2 in type 1 diabetes: Analysis of putative loci IDDM7, IDDM12, and IDDM13 and candidate genes NRAMP1 and IA-2 and interleukin-1 gene cluster. IMDIAB Group. Diabetes 1998;47:1797-99.
186. Huang D, Cancill MR, Morahan G. Complete primary structure, chromosomal localisation, and definition of polymorphisms of the gene encoding the human interleukin-12p40 subunit. Genes Immun 2000;1:515-20.
187. Morahan G, Huang D, Ymer SI, et al. Linkage disequilibrium of a type 1 diabetes susceptibility locus with a regulatory IL12B allele. Nat Genet 2001;27:218-21.
188. Adorini L. Interleukin 12 and autoimmune diabetes. Nat Genet 2001;27:131-32.
189. Hall MA, McGlinn E, Coakley G, et al. Genetic polymorphism of IL-12 p40 gene in immune mediated disease. Genes Immun 2000;1:219-24.
190. Nerup J, Pociot F, European Consortium for IDDM studies. A genomwide scan for type 1-diabetes susceptibility in Scandinavian families identification of new loci with evidence of interactions. Am J Hum Genet 2001;69:1301-13.
191. Lander E, Kruglyak L. Genetic dissection of complex traits: Guidelines for interpreting and reporting linkage results. Nat Genet 1995;11:241-47.

Chapter 14

Genetics of Type 2 Diabetes

V Radha, S Kanthi Mathi, V Mohan

ABSTRACT

Type 2 diabetes is a complex condition characterized by elevated levels of plasma glucose, caused by impairment in both insulin secretion and insulin action. The etiopathogenesis of Type 2 Diabetes (T2D) involves interplay of both genetic and changing environmental factors. The genetics of T2D can be of two broad groups: Genetics of monogenic and polygenic forms of diabetes. In contrast to the rarer monogenic forms of diabetes like Maturity-Onset Diabetes of the Young (MODY) and neonatal diabetes, the more common T2D is a polygenic disorder. The individual susceptible and protective genes are more difficult to identify, given the limited individual impact of a single genetic locus. Indeed, a full understanding of the complex gene-gene and gene-environment interactions at play in this disease has proven quite challenging thus far. Two broad approaches have been used to define the genetic predisposition of T2D: (i) Candidate Gene approach which focuses on the search for an association between T2D and sequence variants in defined candidate genes which are chosen based on their known physiological function and (ii) Genome-Wide Association Studies (GWAS). Earlier, investigators have tried to unravel the role of genetics in T2D through epidemiological studies, candidate genes studies and family genetic linkage studies. While these approaches have provided important insights into some rare monogenic forms of diabetes, understanding the genetics of common T2D remains a major challenge. By examining the entire genome, it is possible to identify the genetic variations that are associated with specific diseases. Advances in genotyping techniques and the availability of large patient cohorts have made it possible to identify common genetic variants associated with T2D through GWAS. We are at an exciting time when improved understanding of gene–gene and gene–environmental interactions promise to unravel the etiopathogenesis of T2D.

Type 2 diabetes (T2D) is a complex heterogenous group of conditions characterized by elevated levels of plasma glucose, caused by impairment in both insulin secretion and insulin action. The etiopathogenesis of T2D involves interplay of both genetic and environmental factors. Although the recent increase in diabetes prevalence reflect the effects of changing environmental factors, multiple lines of evidence support the view that genetic factors are equally important:

- The prevalence of T2D varies widely among populations. The observation that the disease prevalence varies substantially among ethnic groups that share a similar environment supports the idea that genetic factors contribute to predisposition to the disease (Diamond, 2003).
- Familial aggregation of the disease is another source of evidence for a genetic contribution to the disease although admittedly families also share common environmental traits. The odds ratio for offspring of a single affected parent is 3.5 compared to those with no parental diabetes history and this increases to 6.1 if both parents are affected (Meigs et al., 2000; Radha and Mohan, 2007).
- The high concordance in monozygotic twins (over 80%) compared to 50% concordance in dizygotic twins provides compelling evidence for a genetic component in etiology of T2D (Vaag et al., 1995; Poulsen et al., 1999).
- Data from various studies are in support of a genetic basis for measures of both insulin sensitivity and insulin secretion (Gerich, 1998; Elbein et al., 1999).

The genetics of T2D can be considered under two broad groups: genetics of monogenic forms of diabetes, where a single gene is causal in the development of the disease and genetics of Polygenic forms of diabetes where a number of genes are responsible for the susceptibility of the disease.

Patterns of inheritance suggest that T2D is both polygenic and heterogeneous, that is, multiple genes are involved and different combinations of genes play a role in different subsets of individuals. Exactly how many genes are involved and what their relative contributions are, remain ambiguous.

Over the past two decades, four approaches have been used to unravel the genetics of T2D, each with some success. The first approach was to focus on forms of T2D transmitted with a Mendelian dominant pattern of inheritance and/or other specific clinical features, which resulted in the discovery of genes involved in Maturity Onset Diabetes of the Young (MODY), several syndromes of severe insulin resistance, neonatal diabetes, mitochondrial diabetes and other rare genetic syndromes. Together, these monogenic forms of T2D account for less than 5 percent of all forms of T2D (Duncan et al, 1998). The second was to search for genetic variants in candidate genes that might be associated with the common T2D (Hansen and Pedersen, 2005). In general, these studies have focused on functional candidate genes, i.e. genes whose products are known to play a role in glucose homeostasis, or positional candidate genes, i.e. genes located in chromosomal regions that had been identified in linkage studies. The third approach was to perform microarray gene expression analysis in an attempt to define genetic alterations in T2D. The fourth and more recent approach has been to perform high throughput – Genome Wide Association Studies (GWAS) which is expected to accelerate the speed of gene identification in T2D. In this chapter we first discuss the genetics of monogenic diabetes and later consider the more common polygenic forms of T2D.

MONOGENIC DIABETES

Some of the most compelling evidences that inherited variations can cause glycemic dysregulation comes from the clinical and genetic description of monogenic diabetes, including Maturity-Onset Diabetes of the Young (MODY), insulin resistance syndromes, mitochondrial diabetes, and neonatal diabetes. Although rare, these syndromes provide a framework for understanding and investigating the complex genetics of T2D.

Maturity-Onset Diabetes of the Young

MODY was first described in 1975 as a unique type of non-insulin-dependent, characterized by β-cell dysfunction, autosomal dominant diabetes in thin, young adults (usually <25 years of age) who are not prone to ketoacidosis (Tattersall and Fajans, 1975; Fajans et al, 2001). All patients clinically designated as MODY satisfied the following criteria of Tattersal and Fajans (1975):

a. Age at onset of diabetes is < 25 years.
b. Correction of hyperglycemia for a minimum period of 2 years without insulin.
c. Absence of ketonuria at any time
d. Evidence of autosomal dominant inheritance with three-generation transmission of diabetes.

This syndrome accounts for approximately 1-2 percent of diabetes cases worldwide, although MODY has been reported in as many as 5 percent of European diabetic cases (Hattersley et al., 1998). Six different MODY genes have been identified to date, although ~10 percent of MODY patients have no identifiable genetic mutation in any of them, possibly due to the presence of other undiscovered gene (s): the MODY "X".

- MODY 1 results from mutations in *HNF4A* on chromosome 20, which affects the development and function of human pancreatic β cells. MODY 1 is the third most common MODY subtype, with 31 mutations in 40 families described to date (Ellard and Colclough, 2006).
- MODY 2 results from mutations in the glucokinase gene (*GCK*) on chromosome 7p (Froguel et al., 1992; Hattersley et al., 1992) and accounts for ~20 percent of MODY cases. Inactivating mutations of *GCK* result in mild, stable, lifelong fasting hyperglycemia because those affected lack an effective glucose sensor. Drug treatment is rarely required, and microvascular disease is unusual (Frayling et al.,2001).
- MODY 3 results from mutations in *HNF1A* (*TCF1*), which impairs key steps of glucose transport, metabolism, and mitochondrial metabolism (Yamagata et al., 1996b). It is the most common MODY subtype, with more than 300 different mutations. Retinopathy and nephropathy are common in MODY 3; however, macrovascular disease is not (Bellanne-Chantelot et al., 2008; Ellard and Colclough, 2006).
- MODY 4 results from heterozygous mutations in the gene that encodes insulin promoter factor 1 (*IPF1* or *PDX1*), a transcription factor that regulates insulin gene transcription as well as islet and pancreatic

development. Homozygous mutations in exon 1 of *IPF1* give rise to pancreatic agenesis (Stoffers et al., 1997).

- MODY 5, a more common MODY variant than originally suspected, is unique in that it is associated with renal anomalies. *HNF1B* is highly expressed in the pancreas, liver, and kidney. Diabetes results from both hepatic insulin resistance and β cell loss. β cell dysfunction is more severe in MODY 5 than in MODY 3 and ketoacidosis has also been reported. These patients typically require insulin therapy and do not respond to sulfonylureas. *HNF1B* mutations have been associated with renal dysfunction, genitourinary problems, abnormal liver function, and hyperuricemia (Horikawa et al., 1997).
- MODY 6 has been shown to result from mutations in *NEUROD1 (BETA2)*, which is important for pancreatic development and insulin gene transcription. Patients develop moderately severe and progressive β cell dysfunction. MODY 6 is extremely rare, with only a few cases reported in the literature (Malecki et al., 1999).

MODY3 is the commonest form of MODY worldwide (Fajans et al., 2001). These patients are usually of normal Body Mass Index (BMI), often present with severe hyperglycemia, and have microvascular complications. The prevalence of MODY3 in patients with early-onset T2D varies from 2.5 to 36 percent (Kaisaki et al., 1997; Lehto et al., 1999; Aguilar-Salinas et al., 2001; Ng et al., 2001; Owen et al., 2003). The mutation P291fsinsC is found frequently in Caucasian MODY3 subjects and is known as a mutational "hotspot" (Kaisaki et al., 1997).

Common variation in *HNF-1A* gene have also been associated with impaired insulin secretion and I27L and A98V polymorphisms in the MODY3 gene (*TCF1*) are associated with increased risk of T2D in overweight individuals (Holmkvist et al., 2006). An association of Val 98 allele with south Indian patients presenting with MODY phenotype has been reported by (Shekhar et al, 2005). This allele was also associated with an earlier age at onset of T2D (Sahu et al., 2007). The I27L polymorphism thereby seems to increase future risk of T2D with an effect size similar to the novel T2D genes (Zeggini et al., 2007; Saxena et al., 2007; Scott et al., 2007; Sladek et al., 2007). An interaction between *HNF-4A* and peroxisome proliferator-activated receptor γ coactivator-1α (*PGC-1α*) is a prerequisite for induction of the gluconeogenesis genes Phosphoenolpyruvate Carboxykinase 1 (*PCK-1*) and Glucose 6 Phosphatase (*G6Pase*) (Rhee et al., 2003). SNPs rs4810424 and rs3212198 in the *HNF-4 A* gene showed a modest association with T2D in the combined sample. This is in line with findings from some previous studies (Love-Gregory et al., 2004; Silander et al., 2004). The –30G/A polymorphism in the *GCK* gene β-cell promoter has been associated with increased fasting plasma glucose (fPG) and reduced β-cell function (Stone et al., 1996). In addition, it has been shown to affect birth weight (Hattersley et al., 1998). Even though the –30G/A polymorphism has been associated with diabetes related traits, its contribution to T2D is less well known. However, in a recent meta analysis it was shown to have a modest but significant effect on T2D risk (Winckler et al., 2007).

A recent study showed that genetic variation in the *HNF-1A* and *HNF-4A* increase future risk of T2D. Carriers of the –30G/A polymorphism in the *GCK* gene have a sustained increase in fasting glucose concentrations which is not translated into an increased risk of future T2D. Taken together, the results indicate that common variants in the *HNF1A* and *HNF4A* genes are associated with a modestly increased risk of future T2D (Holmkvist et al., 2008).

Previous studies by Mohan et al (1985) reported a high prevalence of MODY in south Indians as defined using the clinical criteria of Tattersall and Fajans (1975). However, clinical criteria are no longer accepted for diagnosis of MODY (Hattersley et al., 2006). Recently, our work has revealed important insights into the genetics of MODY in south India. We identified 9 novel variants comprising 7 mutations (one novel mutation –538G → C at promoter region and six novel coding region mutations) and 2 polymorphisms in the *HNF1A* gene. Functional studies revealed reduced transcriptional activity of the *HNF1A* promoter for two of the promoter variants. One of the novel mutations Arg263His was identified in a family of 30 individuals. The mutation co-segregated with diabetes in this family and this mutation was not seen in non-diabetic members in the family, thus providing evidence for the mutation to be involved in causing MODY (Radha et al., 2009).

Neonatal Diabetes

Neonatal diabetes, which usually presents in the initial days or months of life, can be transient or permanent. The transient type of neonatal diabetes (TNDM), resolves at a median of 12 weeks, usually remits in childhood but is associated with an increased risk of T2D in adulthood. Permanent neonatal diabetes mellitus (PNDM), traditionally treated with insulin, are associated with activating mutations in the *KCNJ11* gene, which encodes the islet ATP-sensitive potassium channel Kir6.2 (Gloyn et al., 2004).

Activating mutations in *KCNJ11* result in constitutive opening of the inwardly rectifying potassium channel, hyperpolarization of the β cell membrane, and subsequent hypoinsulinemic diabetes. Conversely, loss-of-function polymorphisms have been associated with persistent hyperinsulinemia of infancy (Shyng et al., 1998). Several novel heterozygous missense activating mutations in *KCNJ11* have now been identified in TNDM. The severity of the mutation correlates with the clinical phenotype— some *KCNJ11* defects result in PNDM, and even more severe genetic mutations result in the DEND syndrome (developmental delay, epilepsy, neonatal diabetes) (Hattersley and Ashcroft, 2005). Mutations in this gene appear to be the most common cause of neonatal diabetes. It is interesting to note that the closely associated sulfonylurea receptor (*SUR1*) also plays an important role in neonatal diabetes. The dominant mutation results in neonatal hyperinsulinemia and subsequent hypoglycemia, and the heterozygous form may increase adult susceptibility to common T2D (Babenko and Bryan, 2003).

POLYGENIC TYPE 2 DIABETES

In contrast to the rarer monogenic forms of diabetes, as described above, the more common T2D is a polygenic disorder. The complex individual susceptible and protective genes are more difficult to identify, given the limited individual impact of a single genetic locus. Indeed, a full understanding of the complex gene-gene and gene-environment interactions at play in this disease has proven quite challenging thus far.

The susceptibility to complex forms of T2D is associated with changes in Single Nucleotide Polymorphisms (SNPs) that create amino acid variants in exons or influence the expression of genes in the regulatory pathways (McCarthy and Froguel, 2002). Alleles of these polymorphisms are present in both healthy individuals and T2D patients, although with statistically significant differences in the frequencies. The sequence variants are associated with an increase in the risk of developing the disease and are considered susceptibility variants, but not causative factors that unequivocally determine the disease.

Two broad approaches have been used to define the genetic predisposition of T2D. First is the candidate gene approach which focuses on the search for an association between T2D and sequence variants in or near biologically defined candidate genes which have been chosen based on their known physiological function. The importance of these variants or other nearby variants is tested by comparing the frequency in T2D patients and normal glucose tolerant subjects. A second approach is the genome-wide linkage scan strategy (Whittemore, 1996) in which regularly spaced markers are traced in families and sibling pairs for segregation with T2D. No prior knowledge of gene or gene effects is necessary, but the genetic locus must have sufficient impact on the disease susceptibility in order to be detectable.

The starting point for the candidate gene approach is the potential implications that either altered expression and/or function of a particular gene product (conferred by noncoding or coding genetic variants) may have on a biological function or on disease.

Extending the analysis of genes implicated in monogenic forms of diabetes has proved successful also for T2D as exemplified by *HNF4A*, *HNF1A* and *KCNJ11* genes. Common variants of *HNF4A* (MODY1) have been associated with T2D in both Finnish and Ashkenazi Jewish populations (Love-Gregory et al., 2004; Silander et al., 2004).

Our studies on *HNF4A* gene have revealed important insights into the role of its variants with the T2D. SNP rs4810424 and SNP rs736823 of the *HNF1A* gene were associated with T2D, whereas the Val255Met and SNP rs1884614 of *HNF1A* gene were shown to be protective. Further, in our study of a common polymorphism of the *HNF1A* gene, namely, the Ala 98 Val, clearly shows that in Asian Indians, the Ala98Val polymorphism of *HNF1A* gene is associated with MODY and with earlier age at onset of T2D (Anuradha et al., 2005). This association was also confirmed by another study (Sahu et al., 2007).

KCNJ11 Gene

The single nucleotide polymorphism (SNP) E23K of *KCNJ11* has now been convincingly shown to be associated with T2D. Although initial smaller studies failed to replicate the association of the E23K polymorphism with T2D, large scale studies and meta-analyzes have consistently associated the lysine variant with T2D, with an OR of 1.15 (Moore and Florez, 2008).

CAPN10 Gene

One of the earliest diabetes genes identified was *CAPN10*, which encodes an intracellular calcium-dependent cysteine protease that is ubiquitously expressed and can hydrolyze substrates important in calcium-regulated signaling pathways (Croall et al., 1991). Although subsequent studies have not produced a consistent relationship between variation in *CAPN10* and metabolic phenotypes, recent meta-analyzes indicate that variants in *CAPN10* may indeed confer a modest increase in T2D susceptibility. Interestingly, Calpain inhibitors increase insulin secretion and increase the metabolism of muscle glucose to glycogen in animal models (Moore and Florez, 2008). A recent study showed a positive correlation of calpain-10 expression on insulin secretory function in healthy human isolated pancreatic islets, whereas it may enhance lipotoxic activation of apoptosis in T2D islets effecting overall insulin secreting function (Ling et al., 2009).

PPAR-gamma Gene

One of the main candidate genes that is implicated in adipogenesis, insulin resistance and T2D is the Peroxisome Proliferator Activated Receptor-γ (*PPAR-γ*) gene. This is a transcription factor that is involved in adipogenesis and in regulation of adipocyte gene expression and glucose metabolism. Within a unique domain of *PPAR-γ 2* gene that enhances ligand-independent activation, a common Pro12Ala polymorphism has been identified (Altshuler et al., 2000). Deeb et al. (1998) reported that the Ala allele of this polymorphism was associated with increased insulin sensitivity and decreased risk of T2D in a Finnish and second generation Japanese cohort. Since this initial work, the preponderance of evidence has supported *PPARG*'s association with T2D, with an odds ratio (OR) of ~1.2 (Uusitupa et al., 2001). The risk of T2D conferred by this single nucleotide polymorphism (SNP) has been studied prospectively in the Finnish Diabetes Prevention Study and the larger Botnia Prevention Study. In the Finnish study, 500 subjects with impaired glucose tolerance, the relative risk of developing diabetes was doubled in alanine carriers, contradicting the prior evidence that the alanine allele was protective. In the larger Botnia study, comprising >2000 subjects, proline homozygotes were 1.7 times more likely to develop diabetes than alanine carriers (Lyssenko et al., 2005). In contrast we found that the Pro12Ala polymorphism of the *PPAR–γ* gene which is protective against diabetes of Caucasians does not offer protection in two cohorts of South Asians studied at Chennai, India and Dallas in US (Radha et al., 2006). If confirmed by larger studies, it may help us at least in part in understanding the increased susceptibility to insulin resistance (Sharp et al., 1987) and excessive risk for T2D observed in South Asians in general and Asian Indians in particular.

Plasma Cell Glycoprotein PC-1 Gene

The plasma cell glycoprotein 1 (*PC-1*) gene impairs insulin signaling at the insulin receptor level. The K121Q polymorphism of the *ENPP1/PC-1* gene is associated with insulin resistance/atherogenic phenotypes, including earlier onset of T2D and myocardial infarction (Bacci et al., 2005). The Q121 variant binds and inhibits insulin receptor more strongly than the K121 variant and is associated with insulin resistance and related metabolic abnormalities in the vast majority of studied populations. Prudente et al (2007) suggested that the Q121 allele is a gene variant with pleiotropic deleterious effects on insulin resistance, obesity and T2D. Other studies showed that the K121Q *PC-1* polymorphism has no significant impact on insulin sensitivity and is not a critical determinant for either diabetes or obesity (González-Sánchez et al., 2003; Seo et al., 2008). Our study in South Asians supports the hypothesis that *ENPP1* 121Q predicts genetic susceptibility to T2D in both South Asians and Caucasians (Abate et al., 2005).

PGC-1 Alpha Gene

Peroxisome proliferator-activated receptor-γ coactivator-1α (PGC-1α) is a cofactor involved in adaptive thermogenesis, fatty acid oxidation, and gluconeogenesis. Dysfunction of this protein is likely to contribute to the development of obesity and the metabolic syndrome. Franks and Loos (2006) showed that the *PGC-1* alpha sequence variation may interact with physical activity to modify diabetes risk via changes in oxidative energy metabolism. It has been observed that expression of PGC-1α is downregulated in muscles of Type 2 diabetic subjects. In addition, a common polymorphism of the *PGC-1α* gene (Gly482Ser), expressing reduced *PGC-1α* activity, has been linked to an increased risk of T2D. These observations suggest that either reduced levels or compromised activity of *PGC-1α* can be associated with the development of insulin resistance and T2D (Liang et al., 2006). In a study of seven *PGC1A* variants, only Gly482Ser polymorphism was associated with a 1.34 genotype relative risk of T2D in a European population (Ek et al., 2001). Our studies on Thr394Thr, Gly482Ser and +A2962G, of the peroxisome proliferator activated receptor-co-activator-1 alpha (*PGC-1A*) gene with T2D in Asian Indians showed that the Thr394Thr (G-A) polymorphism is associated with T2D and also with total, visceral and subcutaneous body fat (Vimaleswaran et al., 2005; 2006). A replication study from North India confirmed that the Thr394Thr and Gly482Ser variant genotypes are associated with T2D mellitus in two North Indian population groups thereby confirming our findings (Bhat et al., 2007).

Insulin Receptor Substrate-2 (IRS-2) Gene

Insulin receptor substrate (*IRS*)-2 plays an important role in insulin signaling and its disruption results in diabetes in mice. In humans, the *IRS-2* Gly1057Asp substitution was associated with lower risk of T2D in lean individuals, but with a higher risk in obese individuals. On similar lines *IRS-2* Asp1057 allele increases the risk of insulin resistance among obese individuals. Stefan et al (2003) suggest that the association of homozygosity for the Asp1057 allele in *IRS-2* with T2D in Pima Indians may be mediated by interaction of the polymorphism with obesity on several diabetes-related traits. In a Japanese study, Asp1057 allele and haplotype pairs were not associated with the risk of diabetes. However, type 2 diabetic patients, particularly obese patients, carrying the Asp1057 allele and the CA haplotype had increased insulin resistance. These results strongly suggest that the Gly1057Asp polymorphism in insulin receptor substrate-2 is not associated with β-cell dysfunction (Okazawa et al., 2003). Our study on insulin receptor substrate-2 (*IRS-2*) Gly1057Asp (G1057D) polymorphism in Asian Indians showed that the DD genotype increases susceptibility to T2D by interacting with obesity (Bodhini et al., 2007a).

Adiponectin Gene

Adiponectin, encoded by the *ADIPOQ* gene, is one of the adipocyte-expressed proteins that enhances insulin sensitivity and functions in regulating the homeostatic control of glucose, lipid and energy metabolism (Hu et al. 1996; Diez et al. 2003). Genome wide scans have mapped a susceptibility locus for T2D and obesity/metabolic syndrome to chromosome 3q27, where the ADIPOQ gene is located (Kissebah et al. 2000; Vionnet et al. 2000; Comuzzie et al. 2001; Lindsay et al. 2003). Single nucleotide polymorphisms (SNPs) of *ADIPOQ* gene have been genotyped in large datasets from various ethnic groups and several SNPs associated with hypoadiponectinemia, obesity and T2D have been identified (Menzaghi et al. 2002; Vasseur et al. 2003; Gibson et al. 2004; Berthier et al. 2005; Heid et al. 2006). Two single nucleotide polymorphisms (SNPs) in the adiponectin gene, a silent T to G substitution in exon 2 (+45T/G) and a G to T substitution in intron 2 (+276G/T), were significantly associated with T2D and adiponectin level in Japanese population and with insulin resistance in some Caucasian populations (Italy, Germany) (Hara et al., 2001; Menzaghi et al., 2002; Vasseur et al., 2002) and SNP 45 is associated with obesity in a German population (Stumvoll et al., 2002). In the proximal promoter region of the *APM1* gene: SNP-11426A/G and -11391A/-11377G haplotype predicted the associations with fasting plasma glucose, T2D and adiponectin levels (Menzaghi et al., 2002; Gu et al., 2004). Adiponectin has been associated with low diabetes risk. The metabolic effects of adiponectin are mediated by adiponectin receptors 1 (ADIPOR1) and 2 (ADIPOR2). A study on six polymorphisms in *ADIPOR1* and 16 polymorphisms in *ADIPOR2* a significant association between *ADIPOR1* haplotypes and diabetes risk was observed (Qi et al., 2007). Adiponectin is an adipose tissue specific protein that is decreased in subjects with obesity and T2D. Our study showed for the first time, that the +10211T → G polymorphism in the first intron of the adiponectin gene is associated with T2D, obesity and hypoadiponectinemia (Odds ratio 1.28; 95% CI 1.07–1.54; P = 0.008) in Asian Indian population (Vimaleswaran et al.,2008) thereby suggesting adiponectin to be a very important gene for obesity and T2D in Asian Indians.

TCF7L2 Gene

By far the strongest association with T2D till date is seen for SNPs in the gene encoding for *TCF7L2* gene (Grant et al., 2006). *TCF7L2* encodes for a transcription factor involved in Wnt signaling. Investigators at deCODE Genetics in Iceland first reported a strong association of a common T allele of rs7903146 in the gene of transcription factor 7–like 2 (*TCF7L2*) with an increased risk of T2D in three white populations (Grant et al., 2006). These results have subsequently been replicated and confirmed in multiple ethnic groups including Asian Indians (Zhang et al., 2006; Groves et al., 2006; Florez et al., 2006; Chandak et al., 2007; Horikoshi et al., 2007, Sanghera et al., 2008a). All of these studies demonstrate robust and convincing statistical evidence of association with diabetic risk and consistent effect sizes. The effect of the risk allele appears to be additive; one allele confers ~40 percent risk whereas two copies confer 80 percent risk of diabetes. The *TCF7L2* risk allele may result in a defective or poorly expressed protein that leads to decreased insulin secretion and consequent hyperglycemia (Moore and Florez, 2008). Our *TCF7L2* study showed the association of the rs12255372 and rs7903146 polymorphisms of the gene with T2D in southern India (Bodhini et al., 2007b). The 'T' allele of both rs12255372 and rs7903146 polymorphisms was associated with T2D. Further, the 'T' allele of these SNPs have shown association with T2D in the non obese subjects. The result of this study adds to the rapidly expanding body of evidence that implicates *TCF7L2* as an important risk factor for T2D in multiple ethnic groups (Bodhini et al., 2007b).

FTO Gene

A recent genome wide association (GWA) study for T2D in a UK population revealed a novel locus associated with body mass index (BMI)—the Fat Mass and Obesity Associated (*FTO*) gene on chromosome 16 (Frayling et al., 2007). The representative SNP rs9939609 was confirmed to be associated with elevated BMI after replication in over 38,000 study participants of European ancestry. In addition, adiposity appeared to mediate the association between *FTO* variant and the risk of T2D (Scott et al., 2007; Zeggini et al., 2007). Several other studies have also observed associations between *FTO* variants and obesity related traits in various populations (Dina et al., 2007, Chang et al., 2008). Earlier studies on rs9939609 T→A and rs7193144 C→T variants of the intron 1 of the *FTO* gene showed an association with T2D which was independent of BMI in Asian Indians (Yajnik et al., 2009). Our recent association study showed that rs8050136 C→A variant is associated with both generalized and central obesity among south Indians. This is the first study in an Asian Indian population that has looked at the association of the variant rs8050136 C→A of *FTO* gene in the intron 1 with several measures of obesity (BMI and waist circumference) as well as with T2D. The rs8050136 C/A polymorphism was associated with generalized obesity. The odds ratio (OR) for obesity for the CA genotype was significant even after adjustment for age, sex and diabetes [OR: 2.0 (95% CI: 1.57 –2.76), p < 0.0001]. This study demonstrated that there is no independent association of rs8050136 C→A with T2D as its association with T2D appears to be linked through obesity (Ramya et al., 2009) (Table 14.1).

Table 14.1: Summary of recent genetic studies in type 2 diabetes

1.	*PPAR g* gene (Pro12Ala)	Lyssenko et al., 2005	Pro12Ala polymorphism protective in Caucasians
2.	*PPAR g* gene (Pro12Ala)	Radha et al., 2006	Pro12Ala polymorphism not protective in south Asians
3.	*PGC-1 α* gene (Thr394Thr, Gly482Ser)	Bhat et al., 2007	Associated with type 2 diabetes
4.	*PGC-1 α* gene (Thr394Thr)	Vimaleswaran et al., 2005; 2006	Associated with type 2 diabetes and with body fat.
5.	*PGC-1 α* gene (Gly482Ser)	Liang et al., 2006	Associated with the development of insulin resistance and T2D
6.	*PGC-1 α* gene (Gly482Ser)	Ek et al., 2001	Associated with relative risk of type 2 diabetes in a European population
7.	*PC-1* gene (K121Q)	Bacci et al., 2005	Associated with insulin resistance/atherogenic phenotypes
8.	*PC-1* gene (K121Q)	Abate et al., 2005	Associated with type 2 diabetes
9.	*PC-1* gene (K121Q)	González-Sánchez et al., 2003	Has no significant impact on insulin sensitivity
10.	*IRS-2* gene (Gly1057Asp)	Bodhini et al., 2007a	D1057D genotype susceptible to diabetes by interacting with obesity
11.	*IRS-2* gene (Gly1057Asp)	Okazawa et al., 2003	It is not associated with β-cell dysfunction
12.	*TCF7L2* gene (rs7903146)	Sanghera et al., 2008a	Associated with type 2 diabetes in Asian Indians
13.	*TCF7L2* gene (rs7903146)	Chandak et al., 2007	Associated with type 2 diabetes
14.	*TCF7L2* gene (rs12255372; rs7903146)	Bodhini et al., 2007b	Associated with type 2 diabetes in Asian Indians
15.	*TCF7L2* gene (rs7903146)	Grant et al., 2006	T allele of rs7903146 associated with an increased risk of T2D
16.	Adiponectin gene	Vimaleswaran et al., 2008	+10211T→G Associated with type 2 diabetes
17.	Adiponectin gene	Stumvoll et al., 2002	SNP 45 is associated with obesity in a German population
18.	Adiponectin gene (+45T/G; +276G/T)	Hara et al., 2001; Menzaghi et al., 2002; Vasseur et al., 2002	Significantly associated with T2D and adiponectin level in Japanese population and with insulin resistance in some Caucasian populations
19.	*FTO* gene	Yajnik et al., 2009	Associated with type 2 diabetes in south Asian Indians
20.	*FTO* gene	Frayling et al., 2007	Associated with body mass index
21.	*FTO* gene	Dina et al., 2008, Chang et al., 2008	Associated with obesity related traits
22.	*CAPN10 gene*	Ling et al., 2009	Associated with insulin secreting function

GWA Studies for T2D Genes

For decades, investigators have worked to unravel the role of genetics in T2D through epidemiological studies, studies of candidate genes, and genetic linkage in families. While this has provided important insights into some rare monogenic forms of diabetes, understanding the genetics of common T2D remains a major challenge. By examining the entire genome, it is possible to identify, in an unbiased manner, the genetic variation that is associated with specific diseases. Over the past year, a number of exciting articles have been published based on high-throughput genome wide association (GWA) studies. GWAS is a hypothesis-free study and it has to be validated through replication studies. Further functional analysis and various tests are necessary to understand its function or characterization.

The results of five independent GWA screens for T2D genes have been published (Sladek et al., 2007; Zeggini et al., 2007; Scott et al., 2007; Saxena et al., 2007; Steinthorsdottir et al., 2007), and these were followed by five smaller GWA studies (Salonen et al., 2007; Rampersaud et al., 2007; Hayes et al., 2007; Florez et al., 2007; Hanson et al., 2007). The five large studies were all conducted using a two-stage strategy consisting of a GWA screen in an initial cohort of unrelated cases and controls followed by replication of the most significant findings in additional sets (Sanghera et al., 2008b; 2009).

Advances in genotyping techniques and the availability of large patient cohorts have made it possible to identify common genetic variants associated with T2D through genome-wide association studies (GWAS). So far, genetic variants on 19 loci have been identified (Lyssenko and Leif, 2009). The GWA studies suggest that from a genetic perspective, T2D represents a very large number of different disorders.

Implications of GWA Studies

The GWA association studies continue to open our eyes to the broad nature of molecules that might contribute to the pathogenesis of T2D. Clearly many of the genes identified in both GWA and positional cloning studies would not be considered typical "candidate" genes. It is especially important to keep in mind that most of the observed associations are in large domains of strong linkage disequilibrium in noncoding regions of the genome (Vavouri et al., 2006; Carroll et al., 2005; Birney et al., 2007). Thus, the true T2D genes may be placed at some distance from the association signals.

With this knowledge, it is interesting to note that several of the genes placed in the proximity of GWA signals are expressed in β cells. This, together with the findings of association with glucose-stimulated insulin secretion (Steinthorsdottir et al., 2007; Florez et al., 2006a; Sladek et al., 2007), has led some to conclude that β cell defects have a more primal role in the etiology of T2D than insulin resistance. The focus of the GWA studies on overt T2D favored finding genes marking a limitation of β cell function, since ultimately all forms of diabetes could be viewed as having relative insulin deficiency. The identification of variants predisposing to diabetes through effects on insulin sensitivity will require other study designs, such as ones based on association between insulin sensitivity and genotype in the prediabetic state, i.e. before the onset of overt hyperglycemia. Another factor clouding the discovery of potential insulin resistance genes in GWA studies may be the very strong environment-gene interactions for insulin resistance with body weight, physical activity, and other factors, as compared to the potentially purer manifestation of genetic control on insulin secretion.

With regard to prediction of disease, most of the single loci identified by GWA mark only a 10-20 percent increase in risk of disease, and even the strongest single association, *TCF7L2*, represents only about a doubling of disease risk in its homozygous state. Higher relative risks can be generated by combining multiple markers together. Indeed, about 97 percent of the population carry between 9 and 20 risk alleles at the 15 T2D loci identified thus far (Cauchi et al., 2008b). Thus, at present, even a panel of multiple genes has uncertain usefulness in genetic prediction and the more complete identification of markers need to be done to understand its usefulness.

As far as the therapeutic implications, these risk alleles do point to a number of previously uninvestigated pathways that might alter β cell function, insulin action, or metabolism. Even for variants that have a small effect on T2D risk, it is conceivable that the activity of the cellular pathways in which these are placed can be modulated by drugs to a much larger extent than what is observed as the consequence of natural variation. On the other hand, some of these pathways, such as the Wnt and cell-cycle pathways, are so central to normal cellular growth and function that finding a selective drug target may be difficult.

Future Prospects

Dissecting the genetics of T2D is still a complicated task but by no means the nightmare that it used to be (Neel,

1976). The last 10 years, particularly the last two, have brought about tangible breakthroughs and we can now list at least eighteen genes that have consistently been shown to increase the risk of T2D. Yet, these new findings should be considered only as a starting point. There is little doubt that additional T2D loci and genes will be identified through follow-up of "hot spots" in the existing scans (Zeggini et al., 2008) and GWA scans focused on certain ethnic groups and specific clinical or pathophysiological phenotypes of T2D. As the effect of these genetic variants becomes increasingly established, attention needs to be focused on gene-gene and gene-environment interactions.

BIBLIOGRAPHY

1. Abate N, Chandalia M, Satija P, Huet BA, Grundy SM, Sandeep S, Radha V, Deepa R, Mohan V. ENPP1/ Pc-1 K121Q polymorphism and genetic susceptibility to type 2 diabetes. Diabetes 2005;54:1207-13.
2. Aguilar-Salinas CA, Reyes-Rodriguez E, Ordonez-Sanchez ML, Torres MA, Ramirez-Jimenez S, Dominguez-Lopez A, Martinez-Francois JR, Velasco- Perez ML, Alpizar M, Garcia-Garcia E, Gomez-Perez F, Rull J, Tusie-Luna MT. Early-onset type 2 diabetes: Metabolic and genetic characterization in the Mexican population. J Clin Endocrinol Metab 2001;86:220-26.
3. Altshuler D, Hirschhorn JN, Klannemark M, Altshuler D, Hirschhorn JN, Klannemark M, Lindgren CM, Vohl MC, Nemesh J, Lane CR, Schaffner SF, Bolk S, Brewer C, Tuomi T, Gaudet D, Hudson TJ, Daly M, Groop L, Lander ES. The common PPAR-gamma Pro12Ala polymorphism is associated with decreased risk of Type 2 diabetes. Nat Genet 2000;26:76-80.
4. Anuradha S, Radha V, Deepa R, Hansen T, Carstensen B, Pederson O, Mohan V. A prevalent amino acid polymorphism at Codon 98 (Ala98Val) of the Hepatocyte Nuclear Factor-1a is associated with maturity onset diabetes of the young and younger age at onset of Type 2 diabetes in Asian Indians. Diabetes Care 2005;28:2430-35.
5. Bacci S, Ludovico O, Prudente S, Zhang YY, Di Paola R, Mangiacotti D, Rauseo A, Nolan D, Duffy J, Fini G, Salvemini L, Amico C, Vigna C, Pellegrini F, Menzaghi C, Doria A, Trischitta V. The K121Q polymorphism of the ENPP1/PC-1 gene is associated with insulin resistance/atherogenic phenotypes, including earlier onset of type 2 diabetes and myocardial infarction. Diabetes 2005;54(10):3021-25.
6. Babenko AP, Bryan J. SUR domains that associate with and gate KATP pores define a novel gatekeeper. J Biol Chem 2003;278:41577-80.
7. Bellanne-Chantelot C, Carette C, Riveline JP, Valero R, Gautier JF, Larger E, Reznik Y, Ducluzeau PH, Sola A et al. The type and the position of HNF1A mutation modulate age at diagnosis of diabetes in patients with maturity-onset diabetes of the young (MODY)-3. Diabetes 2008;57:503-08.
8. Berthier MT, Houde A, Cote M, Paradis AM, Mauriege P, Bergeron J, Gaudet D, Despres JP, Vohl MC. Impact of adiponectin gene polymorphisms on plasma lipoprotein and adiponectin concentrations of viscerally obese men. J Lipid Res 2005;46:237-44.
9. Bhat A, Koul A, Rai E, Sharma S, Dhar MK, Bamezai RNK. PGC-1α Thr394Thr and Gly482Ser variants are significantly associated with T2DM in two North Indian populations: A replicate case-control study. Hum Genet 2007;121:609-14.
10. Birney E, Stamatoyannopoulos JA, Dutta A, Guigo R, Gingeras TR, Margulies EH, Weng Z, Snyder M, Dermitzakis ET, et al. Identification and analysis of functional elements in 1% of the human genome by the ENCODE pilot project. Nature 2007;447:799-816.
11. Bodhini D, Radha V, Deepa R, Ghosh S, Majumder PP, Rao MR, Mohan V. The G1057D polymorphism of IRS-2 gene and its relationship with obesity in conferring susceptibility to type 2 diabetes in Asian Indians. (CURES-19). International Journal Obesity 2007a;31:97-102.
12. Bodhini D, Radha V, Monalisa Dhar, Narayani N, Mohan V. The rs12255372 (G/T) and rs7903146(C/t) polymorphisms of the TCF7L2 gene are associated with type 2 diabetes mellitus in Asian Indians. Metabolism Clinical and Experimental 2007b;56:1174-78.
13. Carroll JS, Liu XS, Brodsky AS, Li W, Meyer CA, Szary AJ, Eeckhoute J, Shao W, Hestermann EV, et al. Chromosome- wide mapping of estrogen receptor binding reveals long-range regulation requiring the forkhead protein FoxA1. Cell 2005;122:33-43.
14. Cauchi S, Meyre D, Durand E, Proenca C, Marre M, Hadjadj S, Choquet H, De Graeve F, Gaget S, et al.(2008b) Post genomewide association studies of novel genes associated with T2D show gene-gene interaction and high predictive value. PLoS ONE 3, e2031.
15. Chandak GR, Janipalli CS, Bhaskar S, Kulkarni SR, Mohankrishna P, Hattersley AT, Frayling TM, Yajnik CS. Common variants in the TCF7L2 gene are strongly associated with type 2 diabetes mellitus in the Indian population. Diabetologia 2007;50:63-67.
16. Chang YC, Liu PH, Lee WJ, Chang TJ, Jiag YD, Li HY, et al. Common variation the fat mass and obesity-associated (FTO) gene centers risk of obesity and modulates BMI in Chinese population. Diabetes 2008;57:2245-52.
17. Comuzzie AG, Funahashi T, Sonnenberg G, Martin LJ, Jacob HJ,Black AE, Maas D, Takahashi M, Kihara S, Tanaka S, Matsuzawa Y, Blangero J, Cohen D, Kissebah A. The genetic basis of plasma variation in adiponectin, a global endophenotype for obesity and the metabolic syndrome. J Clin Endocrinol Metab 2001;86:4321-25.
18. Croall DE, DeMartino GN. Calcium-activated neutral protease (calpain) system: Structure, function, and regulation. Physiol Rev 1991;71:813-47.

19. Deeb SS, Fajas L, Nemoto M, Pihlajamäki J, Mykkänen L, Kuusisto J, Laakso M, Fujimoto W, Auwerx J. A Pro12Ala substitution in PPAR-gamma2 associated with decreased receptor activity, lower body mass index and improved insulin sensitivity. Nat Genet 1998;20:284-87.
20. Diamond J. The double puzzle of diabetes. Nature 2003;423:599-602.
21. Diez JJ, Iglesias PB. The role of the novel adipocyte-derived hormone adiponectin in human disease. Eur J Endocrinol 2003;148:293-300.
22. Dina C, Meyre D, Gallina S, Durand E, Korner A, Jacobson P, Carlsson LM, Kiess W, Vatin V, et al. Variation in FTO contributes to childhood obesity and severe adult obesity. Nat. Genet 2007;39:724–26.
23. Duncan SA, Navas MA, Dufort D, Rossant J, Stoffel M. Regulation of a transcription factor network required for differentiation and metabolism. Science 1998;281:692-95.
24. Ek J, Andersen G, Urhammer SA, Gaede PH, Drivsholm T, Borch-Johnsen K, Hansen T, Pedersen O. Mutation analysis of peroxisome proliferator-activated receptor-g coactivator-1 (PGC-1) and relationships of identified amino acid polymorphisms to Type II diabetes mellitus. Diabetologia 2001;44:2220-26.
25. Elbein SC, Hasstedt SJ, Wegner K, Kahn SE. Heritability of pancreatic beta-cell function among nondiabetic members of Caucasian familial type 2 diabetic kindreds. J Clin Endocrinol Metab 1999;84:1398-1403.
26. Ellard S, Colclough K. Mutations in the genes encoding the transcription factors hepatocyte nuclear factor 1 alpha (HNF1A) and 4 alpha (HNF4A) in maturity-onset diabetes of the young. Hum Mutat 2006;27(9):854-69.
27. Fajans SS, Bell GI, Polonsky KS. Molecular mechanisms and clinical pathophysiology of maturity-onset diabetes of the young. N Engl J Med 2001;345:971-80.
28. Florez JC, Manning AK, Dupuis J, McAteer J, Irenze K, Gianniny L, Mirel DB, Fox CS, Cupples LA, Meigs JB. A 100K genome-wide association scan for diabetes and related traits in the Framingham Heart Study: Replication and integration with other genome-wide datasets. Diabetes 2007;56:3063-74.
29. Florez JC, Jablonski KA, Bayley N, Pollin TI, de Bakker PI, Shuldiner AR, Knowler WC, Nathan DM, Altshuler D. TCF7L2 polymorphisms and progression to diabetes in the Diabetes Prevention Program. N Engl J Med 2006a;355:241-50.
30. Florez JC, Jablonski KA, Bayley N, Pollin TI, de Bakker PI, Shuldiner AR, Knowler WC, Nathan DM, Altshuler D. TCF7L2 polymorphisms and progression to diabetes in the Diabetes Prevention Program. N Engl J Med 2006; 355:241-50.
31. Franks PW, Loos RJ. PGC-1alpha gene and physical activity in T2D mellitus. Exerc Sport Sci Rev 2006;34(4):171-5.
32. Frayling TM, Timpson NJ, Weedon MN, Zeggini E, Freathy RM, Lindgren CM, Perry JR, Elliott KS, Lango H, et al. A common variant in the FTO gene is associated with body mass index and predisposes to childhood and adult obesity. Science 2007;316:889-94.
33. Frayling TM, Evans JC, Bulman MP, Pearson E, Allen L, Owen K, Bingham C, Hannemann M, Shepherd M, Ellard S, Hattersley AT. Beta-cell genes and diabetes: Molecular and clinical characterization of mutations in transcription factors. Diabetes 2001;50(Suppl 1):S94-100.
34. Froguel P, Vaxillaire M, Sun F, Velho G, Zouali H, Butel MO, Lesage S, Vionnet N, Clement K, et al. Close linkage of glucokinase locus on chromosome 7p to early-onset non-insulin-dependent diabetes mellitus. Nature 1992;356:162-64.
35. González-Sánchez JL, Martínez-Larrad MT, Fernández-Pérez C, Kubaszek A, Laakso M, Serrano-Ríos M. K121Q PC-1 Gene Polymorphism Is Not Associated with Insulin Resistance in a Spanish Population. Obesity Research 2003;11:603–05.
36. Gerich JE. The genetic basis of type 2 diabetes mellitus: impaired insulin secretion versus impaired insulin sensitivity. Endocr Rev 1998;19:491–503.
37. Gloyn AL, Pearson ER, Antcliff JF, et al. Activating mutations in the gene encoding the ATP-sensitive potassium-channel subunit Kir6.2 and permanent neonatal diabetes. N Engl J Med 2004;350:1838-49.
38. Grant SF, Thorleifsson G, Reynisdottir I, Benediktsson R, Manolescu A, Sainz J, Helgason A, Stefansson H, Emilsson V, et al. Variant of transcription factor 7-like 2 (TCF7L2) gene confers risk of type 2 diabetes. Nature Genetics 2006;38(3):320-20.
39. Groves CJ, Zeggini E, Minton J, Frayling TM, Weedon MN, Rayner NW, Hitman GA, Walker M, Wiltshire S, Hattersley AT, McCarthy MI. Association analysis of 6,736 UK. Subjects provides replication and confirms TCF7L2 as a type 2 diabetes susceptibility gene with a substantial effect on individual risk. Diabetes 2006;55:2640-44.
40. Gibson F, Froguel P. Genetics of the ADIPOQ locus and its contribution to Type 2 diabetes susceptibility in French Caucasians. Diabetes 2004;53:2977-83.
41. Gu HF, Abulaiti A, Ostenson CG, Humphreys K, Wahlestedt C, Brookes AJ, Efendic S. Single nucleotide polymorphisms in the proximal promoter region of the adiponectin (APM1) gene are associated with type 2 diabetes in Swedish caucasians. Diabetes 2004;53 (Suppl 1): S31-5.
42. Hansen L, Pedersen O. Genetics of type 2 diabetes mellitus: Status and perspectives. Diabetes Obes Metab 2005;7:122-35.
43. Hanson RL, Bogardus C, Duggan D, Kobes S, Knowlton M, Infante AM, Marovich L, Benitez D, Baier LJ, Knowler WC. A search for variants associated with young-onset type 2 diabetes in American Indians in a 100K genotyping array. Diabetes 2007;56:3045-52.
44. Hara K, Mori Y, Dina C, Yasuda K, Tobe K, Yamauchi T, Okada T, Kadowaki H, Hagura R, Akanuma Y, Ito C, Kouichi M, Taniyama M, Motoro T, Froguel P, Kadowaki T. Genetic variation in the gene encoding adiponectin is associated with increased risk of type 2 diabetes. Diabetes 2001;50 (Suppl. 1):A244.
45. Hattersley A, Bruining J, Shield J, Njølstad P, Donaghue K. International Society for Pediatric and Adolescent

Diabetes (ISPAD) Clinical Practice Consensus Guidelines 2006-2007. The diagnosis and management of monogenic diabetes in children. Pediatric Diabetes 2006;7:352-60.

46. Hattersley AT, Ashcroft FM. Activating mutations in kir6.2 and neonatal diabetes: New clinical syndromes, new scientific insights, and new therapy. Diabetes 2005;54: 2503-13.

47. Hattersley AT, Beards F, Ballantyne E, Appleton M, Harvey R, Ellard S. Mutations in the glucokinase gene of the fetus result in reduced birth weight. Nature Genetics 1998;19:268-70.

48. Hattersley AT, Turner RC, Permutt MA, Patel P, Tanizawa Y, Chiu KC, O'Rahilly S, Watkins PJ , Wainscoat JS. Linkage of T2D to the glucokinase gene. Lancet 1992;339:1307-10.

49. Hayes MG, Pluzhnikov A, Miyake K, Sun Y, Ng MC, Roe CA, Below JE, Nicolae RI, Konkashbaev A., Bell GI, et al. Identification of type 2 diabetes genes in Mexican Americans through genome-wide association studies. Diabetes 2007;56:3033-44.

50. Heid IM, Wagner SA, Gohlke H, Iglseder B, Mueller JC, Cip P, Ladurner G, Reiter R, Stadlmayr A, Mackevics V, Illig T,Kronenberg F, Paulweber B. Genetic architecture of the APM1 gene and its inXuence on adiponectin plasma levels and parameters of the metabolic syndrome in 1,727 healthy Caucasians. Diabetes 2006;55:375-84.

51. Holmkvist J, Almgren P, Lyssenko V, Lindgren CM, Eriksson KF, Isomaa B, Tuomi T, Nilsson P, Groop L. Common variants in maturity-onset diabetes of the young genes and future risk of type 2 diabetes. Diabetes 2008;57(6):1738-44.

52. Holmkvist J, Cervin C, Lyssenko V, Winckler W, Anevski D, Cilio C, Almgren P, Berglund G, Nilsson P, Tuomi T, Lindgren CM, Altshuler D, Groop L. Common variants in HNF-1_ and risk of type 2 diabetes. Diabetologia 2006;49:2882-91.

53. Horikawa Y, Iwasaki N, Hara M, Furuta H, Hinokio Y, Cockburn B, Lindner T, Yamagata K, Ogata M, et al. Mutation in hepatocyte nuclear factor-1b gene (TCF2) associated with MODY. Nature Genetics 1997;17:384-85.

54. Horikoshi M, Hara K, Ito C, Nagai R, Froguel P, Kadowaki T. A genetic variation of the transcription factor 7-like 2 gene is associated with risk of T2D in the Japanese population. Diabetologia 2007;50:747-51.

55. Hu E, Liang P, Spiegelman BM. AdipoQ is a novel adipose-specific gene dysregulated in obesity. J Biol Chem 1996;271:10697-703.

56. Kaisaki PJ, Menzel S, Lindner T, Oda N, Rjasanowski I, Sahm J, Meincke G, Schulze J, Schmechel H, Petzold C, LedermannHM,Sachse G, Boriraj VV, Menzel R, Kerner W, Turner RC, Yamagata K, Bell GI. Mutations in the hepatocyte nuclear factor-1_ gene in MODY and early-onset NIDDM. Evidence for a mutational hotspot in exon 4. Diabetes 1997;46:528-35.

57. Kissebah AH, Sonnenberg GE, Myklebust J, Goldstein M, Broman K, James RG, Marks JA, Krakower RG, Jacob HW, Weber J, Martin L, Blangero J, Comuzzie AG. Quantitative trait loci on chromosomes 3 and 17 inXuence phenotypes of the metabolic syndrome. Proc Natl Acad Sci USA 2000;97:14478-83.

58. Lehto M, Wipemo C, Ivarsson SA, Lindgren C, Lipsanen-Nyman M, Weng J, Wibell L, Widen E, Tuomi T, Groop L. High frequency of mutations in MODY and mitochondrial genes in Scandinavian patients with familial early-onset diabetes. Diabetologia 1999;42:1131-37.

59. Liang H, Ward WF. PGC-1: A key regulator of energy metabolism. Adv Physiol Educ 2006;30:145-51.

60. Lindsay RS, Funahashi T, KrakoV J, Matsuzawa Y, Tanaka S, Kobes S, Bennett PH, Tataranni PA, Knowler WC, Hanson RL. Genome-wide linkage analysis of serum adiponectin in the Pima Indian population. Diabetes 2003;52:2419-25.

61. Ling C, Groop L, Guerra SD, Lupi R. Calpain-10 Expression Is Elevated in Pancreatic Islets from Patients with Type 2 Diabetes. Plosone 2009;4(8):e6558.

62. Love-Gregory LD, Wasson J, Ma J, et al. A common polymorphism in the upstream promoter region of the hepatocyte nuclear factor-4α gene on chromosome 20q is associated with T2D and appears to contribute to the evidence for linkage in an Ashkenazi Jewish population. Diabetes 2004; 53:1134-40.

63. Lyssenko V, Almgren P, Anevski D, Orho-Melander M, Sjögren M, et al. Genetic Prediction of Future T2D. PLoS Med 2005;2(12):e345.

64. Lyssenko V, Leif G. Genome-wide association study for T2D: Clinical applications. Current Opinion in Lipidology 2009;20 (2):87-91.

65. Malecki MT, Jhala US, Antonellis A, Fields L, Doria A, Orban T, Saad M, Warram JH, Montminy M , Krolewski AS. Mutations in NEUROD1 are associated with the development of T2D mellitus. Nature Genetics 1999;23(3): 323-28.

66. McCarthy MI, Froguel P. Genetic approaches to the molecular understanding of T2D. Am J Physiol Endocrinol. Metab 2002;283:E217-25.

67. Meigs JB, Cupples LA, Wilson PW. Parental transmission of T2D: The Framingham Offspring Study. Diabetes 2000;49:2201-07.

68. Menzaghi C, Ercolino T, Di Paola R, Berg AH, Warram JH, Scherer PE, Trischitta V, Doria A. A haplotype at the adiponectin locus is associated with obesity and other features of the insulin resistance syndrome. Diabetes 2002;51:2306-12.

69. Mohan V, Ramachandran A, Snehalatha C, Mohan R, Bharani G, Viswanathan M. High prevalence of Maturity Onset Diabetes of the Young (MODY). Diabetes Care 1985;8:371-74.

70. Moore A F, Florez JC. Genetic Susceptibility to T2D and Implications for Antidiabetic Therapy Annual Review of Medicine 2008;59:95-111.

71. Neel JV. In: The Genetics of Diabetes Mellitus, W. Creutzfeldt, J Köbberling, JV Neel (Eds). (Springer, Berlin 1976), 1-11.

72. Ng MC, Lee SC, Ko GT, Li JK, So WY, Hashim Y, Barnett AH, Mackay IR, Critchley JA, Cockram CS, Chan JC. Familial early-onset type 2 diabetes in Chinese patients: Obesity and genetics have more significant roles than autoimmunity. Diabetes Care 2001;24:663-71.
73. Okazawa K, Yoshimasa Y, Miyamoto Y, Takahashi-Yasuno Y, Miyawaki T, Masuzaki H, Hayashi T, Hosoda K, Inoue G, Nakao K. The haplotypes of the IRS-2 gene affect insulin sensitivity in Japanese patients with T2D. Diabetes Res Clin Pract 2005;68(1):39-48.
74. Owen KR, Stride A, Ellard S, Hattersley AT. Etiological investigation of diabetes in young adults presenting with apparent type 2 diabetes. Diabetes Care 2003;26:2088-93.
75. Poulsen P, Kyvik KO, Vaag A, Beck-Nielsen H. Heritability of type II (non-insulin-dependent) diabetes mellitus and abnormal glucose tolerance—A population-based twin study. Diabetologia 1999;42:139-45.
76. Prudente S, Chandalia M, Morini E, Baratta R, Dallapiccola B, Abate N, Frittitta L, Trischitta V. The Q121/Q121 Genotype of ENPP1/PC-1 Is Associated with Lower BMI in Non-diabetic Whites. Obesity 2007;15:1-4.
77. Qi L, Doria A, Giorgi E, Hu FB. Variations in adiponectin receptor genes and susceptibility to T2D in women: A tagging-single nucleotide polymorphism haplotype analysis. Diabetes 2007;56(6):1586-91.
78. Radha V, Ek J, Anuradha S, Hansen T, Pedersen O, Mohan V. Identification of novel variants in the hepatocyte nuclear factor 1 alpha gene in South Indian patients with maturity onset diabetes of young. J Clin Endocrine & Metabolism, March 31, doi:10.1210/jc. 2009;2008-2371.
79. Radha V, Mohan V. Genetic predisposition to type 2 diabetes among Asian Indians. Indian J Med Res 2007;125:259-74.
80. Radha V, Vimaleswaran KS, Babu HNS, Abate N, Chandalia M, Satija P, Grundy SM, Ghosh S, Majumder PP, Deepa R, Rao SMR, Mohan V. Role of genetic polymorphism peroxisome proliferator – Activated Receptor – 2 Pro 12Ala on ethnic susceptibility to diabetes in south Asian and Caucasian subjects. Diabetes Care 2006;29:1046-51.
81. Rampersaud E., Damcott, CM, Fu M, Shen H, McArdle P, Shi X, Shelton J, Yin J, Chang YP, et al. Identification of novel candidate genes for type 2 diabetes from a genome-wide association scan in the Old Order Amish: Evidence for replication from diabetes-related quantitative traits and from independent populations. Diabetes 2007;56:3053-62.
82. Ramya K, Radha V, Mohan V. FTO gene polymorphism rs8050136 is associated with obesity but not type 2 diabetes in south Indians. Submitted to Metabolism, 2009.
83. Rhee J, Inoue Y, Yoon JC, Puigserver P, Fan M, Gonzalez FJ, Spiegelman BM. Regulation of hepatic fasting response by PPARgamma coactivator-1alpha (PGC-1): Requirement for hepatocyte nuclear factor 4alpha in gluconeogenesis. PNAS 2003;100:4012-17.
84. Sahu RP, Aggarwal A, Zaidi G, Shah A, Modi K, Kongara S, Aggarwal S, Talwar S, Chu S, Bhatia V, Bhatia E. Etiology of Early-Onset Type 2 Diabetes in Indians: Islet Autoimmunity and Mutations in Hepatocyte Nuclear Factor 1A and Mitochondrial Gene Journal of Clinical Endocrinology and Metabolism 2007;92(7):2462-67.
85. Sanghera DK, Been L, Ortega L, Wander GS, Mehra NK, Aston CE, Mulvihill JJ, Ralhan S. Testing the association of novel meta-analysis-derived diabetes risk genes with type II diabetes and related metabolic traits in Asian Indian Sikhs. Journal of Human Genetics 2009;54:162-68.
86. Sanghera DK, Nath SK, Ortega L, Gambarelli M, Kim-Howard X, Singh JR, Ralhan SK, Wander GS, Mehra NK, Mulvihill JJ, Kamboh MI. TCF7L2 polymorphisms are associated with T2D in Khatri Sikhs from North India: Genetic variation affects lipid levels. Ann Hum Genet 2008a;72(4):499-509.
87. Sanghera DK, Ortega L, Han S, Singh J, Ralhan SK, Wander GS, Mehra NK, Mulvihill JJ, Ferrell RE, et al. Impact of nine common type 2 diabetes risk polymorphisms in Asian Indian Sikhs: PPARG2 (Pro12Ala), IGF2BP2, TCF7L2 and FTO variants confer a significant risk. BMC Med Genet 2008b;9:59.
88. Salonen JT, Uimari P, Aalto JM, Pirskanen M, Kaikkonen J, Todorova B, Hypponen J, Korhonen VP, Asikainen J, et al. T2D whole-genome association study in four populations: the DiaGen consortium. Am. J. Hum. Genet 2007;81: 338-45.
89. Saxena R, Voight BF, Lyssenko V, Burtt NP, de Bakker PI, Chen H, Roix JJ, Kathiresan S, Hirschhorn JN, et al. Genome-wide association analysis identifies loci for type 2 diabetes and triglyceride levels. Science 2007;316: 1331-36.
90. Scott LJ, Mohlke KL, Bonnycastle LL, Willer CJ, Li Y, Duren WL, Erdos MR, Stringham HM, Chines PS, et al. A genome-wide association study of T2D in Finns detects multiple susceptibility variants. Science 2007;316:1341-45.
91. Seo HJ, Kim SG, Kwon OJ. The K121Q Polymorphism in ENPP1 (PC-1) Is Not Associated with T2D or Obesity in Korean Male Workers. J Korean Med Sci 2008;23:459-64.
92. Sharp PS, Mohan V, Levy JC, Mather HM, Kohner EM. Insulin resistance in patients of Asian Indian and European origin with non-insulin dependent diabetes. Horm Metab Res 1987;129:84-85.
93. Shekher A, Venkatesan R, Raj D, Torben H, Bendix C, Oluf P, MohanV. A prevalent amino acid polymorphism at codon 98 (Ala98Val) of the hepatocyte nuclear factor-1_ is associated with maturity-onset diabetes of the young and younger age at onset of type 2 diabetes in Asian Indians. Diabetes Care 2005;28:2430-35.
94. Shyng SL, Ferrigni T, Shepard JB, Nestorowicz A, Glaser B, Permutt MA, Nichols CG. Functional analyses of novel mutations in the sulfonylurea receptor 1 associated with persistent hyperinsulinemic hypoglycemia of infancy. Diabetes 1998;47:1145-51.
95. Silander K, Mohlke KL, Scott LJ, Peck EC, Hollstein P, Skol AD, Jackson AU, Deloukas P, Hunt S, et al. Genetic variation near the hepatocyte nuclear factor-4alpha gene predicts susceptibility to T2D. Diabetes 2004;53:1141-49.

96. Sladek R., Rocheleau G, Rung J, Dina C, Shen L, Serre D, Boutin P, Vincent D, Belisle A, et al. A genome-wide association study identifies novel risk loci for T2D. Nature 2007;445:881-85.
97. Stefan N, Kovacs P, Stumvoll M, Hanson RL, Lehn-Stefan A, Permana PA, Baier LJ, Tataranni PA, Silver K, Bogardus C. Metabolic effects of the Gly1057Asp polymorphism in IRS-2 and interactions with obesity. Diabetes 2003;52(6):1544-50.
98. Steinthorsdottir V, Thorleifsson G, Reynisdottir I, Benediktsson R, Jonsdottir T, Walters GB, Styrkarsdottir U, Gretarsdottir S, Emilsson V, et al. A variant in CDKAL1 influences insulin response and risk of T2D. Nat Genet 2007;39:770-75.
99. Stoffers DA, Ferrer J, Clarke WL, Habener JF. Early-onset type-II diabetes mellitus (MODY4) linked to IPF1. Nature Genetics 1997;17:138-39.
100. Stone L, Kahn S, Fujimoto W, Deeb S, Porte D. A variation at position -30 of the betacell glucokinase gene promoter is associated with reduced beta-cell function in middle-aged Japanese-American men. Diabetes 1996;45:422-28.
101. Stumvoll M, Tschritter O, Fritsche A, Staiger H, Renn W, Weisser M, Machicao F, Haring H. Association of the T-G polymorphism in adiponectin (exon 2) with obesity and insulin sensitivity: Interaction with family history of type 2 diabetes. Diabetes 2002;51:37-41.
102. Tattersall RB, Fajans SS. A difference between the inheritance of classical juvenile-onset and maturity-onset type diabetes of young people. Diabetes 1975;24:44-53.
103. Uusitupa M, Lindi V, Lindström J, Louheranta A, Laakso M, Tuomilehto J. Impact of Pro12Ala polymorphism of the PPAR-γ gene on body weight and diabetes incidence in the Finnish diabetes prevention study. Int J Obesity 2001;25:S5.
104. Vaag A, Henriksen JE, Madsbad S, Holm N, Beck-Nielsen H. Insulin secretion, insulin action, and hepatic glucose production in identical twins discordant for non-insulin-dependent diabetes mellitus. J Clin Invest 1995;95:690-98.
105. Vasseur F, Lepretre F, Lacquemant C, Froguel P. The genetics of adiponectin. Curr Diab Rep 2003;3:151-58.
106. Vasseur F, Helbecque N, Dina C, Lobbens S, Delannoy V, Gaget S, Boutin P, Vaxillaire M, Lepretre F, Dupont S, Hara K, Clement K, Bihain B, Kadowaki T, Froguel P. Single-nucleotide polymorphism haplotypes in the both proximal promoter and exon 3 of the APM1 gene modulate adipocyte-secreted adiponectin hormone levels and contribute to the genetic risk for type 2 diabetes in French Caucasians. Hum Mol Genet 2002;11:2607-14.
107. Vavouri T, McEwen GK, Woolfe A, Gilks WR, Elgar G. Defining a genomic radius for long-range enhancer action: Duplicated conserved non-coding elements hold the key. Trends Genet 2006;22:5-10.
108. Vimaleswaran KS, Radha V, Ramya K, Babu HN, Savitha N, Roopa V, Monalisa D, Deepa R, Ghosh S, Majumder PP, Rao MR, Mohan V. A novel association of a polymorphism in the first intron of adiponectin gene with T2D, obesity and hypoadiponectinemia in Asian Indians. Human Genetics 2008;123(6):599-605.
109. Vimaleswaran KS, Radha V, Anjana M, Deepa R, Ghosh S, Majumder PP, Rao MRS, Mohan V. Effect of polymorphisms in the PPARGC1A gene on body fat in Asian Indians. International Journal of Obesity 2006;30:884-91.
110. Vimaleswaran KS, Radha V, Ghosh S, Majumder PP, Deepa R, Babu HNS, Rao MRS, Mohan V. Peroxisome proliferators-activated receptor- co-activator -1 (PGC-1) gene polymorphisms and their relationship to T2D in Asian Indians. Diabetic Medicine 2005;22:1516-21.
111. Vionnet N, Hani EH, Dupont S, Gallina S, Francke S, Dotte S, De Matos F, Durand E, Leprêtre F, Lecoeur C, Gallina P, Zekiri L, Dina C, Froguel P. Genomewide search for T2D susceptibility genes in French Whites: Evidence for a novel susceptibility locus for early-onset diabetes on chromosome 3q27–qter and independent replication of a T2D locus on chromosome 1q21-q24. Am J Hum Genet 2000;67:1470-80.
112. Whittemore AS. Genome scanning for linkage: An overview. Am J Hum.Genet 1996;59:704-16.
113. Winckler W, Weedon MN, Graham RR, McCarroll SA, Purcell S, Almgren P, Tuomi T, Gaudet D, Bostrom KB, Walker M, Hitman G, Hattersley AT, McCarthy MI, Ardlie KG, Hirschhorn JN, Daly MJ, Frayling TM, Groop L, Altshuler D. Evaluation of Common Variants in the Six Known Maturity-Onset Diabetes of the Young (MODY) Genes for Association With Type 2 Diabetes. Diabetes 2007;56:685-93.
114. Yajnik CS, Janipalli CS, Bhaskar S, Kulkarni SR, Freathy RM, Prakash S, Mani KR, Weedon MN, Kale SD, Deshpande J, Krishnaveni GV, Veena SR, Fall CH, McCarthy MI, Frayling TM, Hattersley AT, Chandak GR. FTO gene variants are strongly associated with T2D in South Asian Indians. Diabetologia 2009;52(2):247-52.
115. Yamagata K, Oda N, Kaisaki PJ, Menzel S, Furuta H, Vaxillaire M, Southam L, Cox RD, Lathrop GM, Boriraj VV, Chen X, Cox NJ, Oda Y, Yano H, Le Beau MM, Yamada S, Nishigori H, Takeda J, Fajans SS, Hattersley AT, Iwasaki N, Pedersen O, Polonsky KS, Turner RC, Velho G, Chevre J-C, Froguel P, Bell GI. Mutations in the hepatic nuclear factor 1alpha gene in maturity-onset diabetes of the young (MODY3). Nature 1996b;384:455-58.
116. Zeggini E, Scott LJ, Saxena R, Voight BF, Marchini JL, Hu T, de Bakker PI, Abecasis GR, Almgren P, et al. Meta-analysis of genome-wide association data and large-scale replication identifies additional susceptibility loci for type 2 diabetes. Nat. Genet 2008;40:638-45.
117. Zeggini E, Weedon MN, Lindgren CM, Frayling TM, Elliott KS, Lango H, Timpson NJ, Perry JR, Rayner NW, et al. Replication of genome-wide association signals in UK samples reveals risk loci for T2D. Science 2007;316:1336-41.
118. Zhang C, Qi L, Hunter DJ, Meigs JB, Manson JE, van Dam RM, Hu FB. Variant of transcription factor 7-like 2 (TCF7L2) gene and the risk of T2D in large cohorts of US women and men. Diabetes 2006;55:2645-48.

Chapter

15

Immunogenetic Mechanisms of Celiac Disease

Sophie Caillat-Zucman

Celiac Disease (CD) is a complex disorder of the small intestine caused by an inappropriate immune response to ingested gluten wheat, and similar proteins of rye and barley. The triggering role of cereal storage proteins was recognized in the 1950s by W Dicke, a young Dutch pediatrician who linked the onset of CD symptoms to the consumption of wheat bead and cereals, and proposed the first and still unique treatment of the disease, the gluten-free diet. It is characterized clinically by a malabsorption syndrome and histologically by villous atrophy, crypt hyperplasia and lymphocyte infiltrates of the epithelium and lamina propria, which in turn lead to nutrient malabsorption and/or chronic diarrhea. Its estimated prevalence is high (about 1%),[1] and its only current treatment is a lifelong exclusion of gluten from the diet (for review, see[2]).

CD has a strong genetic component, as illustrated by a concordance rate of nearly 90 percent in monozygotic twins compared to 20 percent in dizygotic twins and 10 percent in 1st-degree relatives.[3] A significant proportion of the genetic predisposition comes from HLA genes which are estimated to account for about 40 percent of the genetic risk. This susceptibility is primarily associated with specific MHC class II alleles. Thus, 90-95 percent of CD patients express the HLA-DQ2 molecule, formed by an α chain encoded by HLA-DQA1*0501 and a β chain encoded by DQB1*0201. These alleles can be inherited in *cis* (i.e. when present on the same parental chromosome) as in the case of the DR3 haplotype, or in *trans* (when the α and β chains are encoded by the different chromosomes from each parent, for instance DQA1*0501 on the DR11 haplotype from one parent and DQB1*0201 on the DR7 haplotype from the other parent) (Fig. 15.1). The remaining 5-10 percent CD patients express DQ8, encoded by DQA1*0301 and DQB1*0302 on certain DR4 haplotypes. Since most DQ2- or DQ8-positive individuals in the general population remain healthy, it appears that HLA-DQ2 and HLA-DQ8 are necessary, but there are not sufficient to predispose to CD. A large number of non-HLA genes (detailed below) likely contribute to the pathogenesis of CD, but the participation of a single predisposing non-HLA gene might be quite modest.

The strong association of CD with HLA class II alleles is in accordance with a central role for CD4 T cells in disease pathogenesis. Indeed, gluten-specific CD4 T cells can be isolated from the mucosa of CD patients but not from healthy individuals, and these cells are restricted by HLA-DQ2 or DQ8 molecules.[4] The principal disease-triggering component of wheat gluten belongs to a family of closely related proline- and glutamine-rich proteins called gliadins. In sharp contrast with virtually all other dietary proteins, gliadins—due to their high proline content—are strongly resistant to proteolysis by gastric, pancreatic and intestinal brush border membrane enzymes. Thus, intact long gliadin peptides can build up to high concentrations in the lumen of the small intestine. For unknow reasons, in CD patients, but not in healthy individuals, such undigested gliadin fragments present in the intestinal lumen can be transported across the epithelium and released in an intact form in the lamina propria. In genetically predisposed individuals, these gliadin epitopes can be processed by antigen presenting cells (APC) from the lamina propria, and presented by HLA-DQ2 or DQ8 molecules to gliadin-specific CD4 T cells which then proliferate and produce IFNγ. Among these gliadin peptides, a 33-mer peptide of α2-gliadin (p56-88 LQLQPFPQPQLPYP QPQLPY PQ

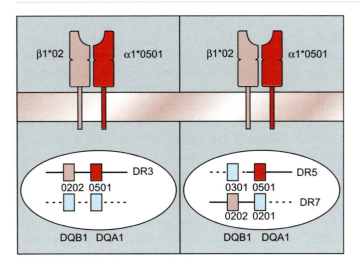

Fig. 15.1: HLA-DQ2 dimers in celiac disease

PQ LPYPQPQPF), which is generated under physiological conditions and is extremely resistant to gastrointestinal digestion due to its rich proline content, is the most powerful immunodominant gliadin peptide.[5] Of note, this 33-mer peptide is not present in other cereal proteins that do not cause celiac disease. How this long peptide can be transported across the intestinal epithelium begins to be understood: The transferrin receptor CD71 is responsible for its apical to basal retrotranscytosis, a process during which the peptide is protected from degradation, allowing its release in an intact form in the mucosa, where it triggers an immune response and perpetuates intestinal inflammation.[6]

Our understanding of the molecular basis for HLA association in CD has been elucidated recently, when it was shown that DQ2 and DQ8 molecules can only bind gliadin peptides if they have been enzymatically modified by a multifunctional enzyme, tissue transglutaminase (TG2). This pleiotropic enzyme, present in many organs including the small intestine, catalyzes an ordered deamidation of certain glutamine residues, the most abundant amino acid in gluten, by converting neutral glutamine into negatively charged glutamic acid.[7,8] Because both DQ2 and DQ8 share peptide binding motif preferences for peptides that contain many negatively charged residues,[9-12] it appears that TG2 has the capability to convert glutamine-rich gliadin peptides into highly immunogenic epitopes (reviewed in.[13] Thus, deamidation by TG2 is likely a crucial event in the generation of gluten-specific HLA-DQ2 or -DQ8-restricted CD4 T cell responses in CD. Only particular glutamine residues, however, are modified by TG2. Indeed, the spacing between glutamine and proline plays an essential role in the specificity of deamidation, and TG2 activity is particularly efficient on glutamine-X-proline motifs frequently found in gliadins.[14]

Altogether, these results establish the central role of adaptive immunity in CD, provided the two main environmental (gliadin) and genetic (HLA-DQ2 or DQ8) factors are present (Fig. 15.2). The major role of these two

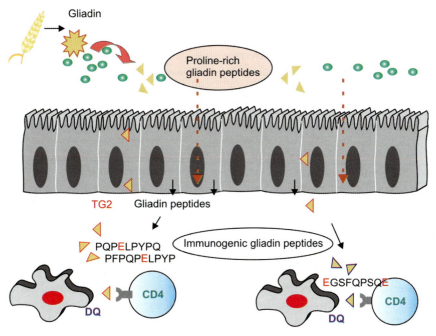

Fig. 15.2: The DQ2- or DQ8-restricted CD4 T cell response to gluten in celiac disease

factors is emphasized by the evidence of an HLA-DQ2 gene dose effect. Indeed, the risk of developing CD is fivefold higher in HLA-DQ2 homozygous than heterozygous individuals. This observation is correlated with the capacity of APCs from homozygous individuals to elicit stronger gliadin-specific CD4 T cell responses than APCs from heterozygous subjects, a property ascribed to the higher density of HLA-DQ2 molecules at their surface.[15] Moreover, the frequency of HLA-DQ2 homozygosity is higher in patients with severe CD that become refractory to gluten-free diet (Malamut GastroE 2009) compared to patients with uncomplicated CD (65% vs 40%). Conversely, the frequency of HLA-DQ2 homozygosity is lower (17%) in CD patients who spontaneously return to latency (= healthy condition) with no symptoms under normal diet (Matysiak Gut 2007).

Interestingly, experiments using intestinal gluten-specific CD4 T cell clones,[16] and analysis of X-ray crystal structure of DQ2 and DQ8 molecules[17,18] have demonstrated that HLA-DQ2 and DQ8 molecules employ different rules for selection of deamidated gliadin epitopes for CD4 T cell presentation. Hence, although DQ2- and DQ8-restricted T cells can recognize the same gliadin peptides in exactly the same registers (for instance peptides that share the core sequence QQPQQPFPQ), these peptides have been deamidated at different positions: Deamidation at position P4 or P6 is mandatory for recognition by DQ2-restricted T cells, whereas deamidation at positions P1 and/or P9 is critical for DQ8-restricted recognition. In addition, most of the characterized DQ2-restricted gliadin T cell epitopes have proline residues at P1, whereas DQ8 is unlikely to tolerate a proline at P1 and so selects other sequences that are more likely to be sensitive to proteases, in particular aminopeptidases. The X-ray structure of DQ2 complexed with gliadin peptides provides an explanation of why DQ2 is able of binding these proline-rich gluten peptides with high affinity.[18] In most HLA class II molecules (including DQ8), there is a hydrogen bond between the amide nitrogen of the P1 residue and the backbone carbonyl of residue $\alpha 53$.[17] This appears not to be the case for DQ2: A deletion of the $\alpha 53$ residue of DQA1*0501 possibly prevents the establishment of a hydrogen bond to the P1 amide, and therefore, a proline residue can be accommodated at this position without penalty.[19] These epitopes would likely be unavailable for binding to DQ8 in the same binding register. This may be the reason why DQ2 is predisposing to CD by its unique ability to bind Pro-rich gluten peptides that harbor many negatively charged residues, and is a stronger susceptibility determinant for CD than DQ8.

To summarize, highly antigenic gluten epitopes must share several properties: They are physiologically generated, are located in proline-rich regions protected from gastrointestinal proteolysis, are preferred substrates for TG2 that converts them in immunogenic peptides, and occur within the context of long, multivalent peptides such as the 33-mer peptide that contributes most, if not all, of the gliadin's antigenic properties. These different characteristics reflect successive steps of epitope selection at the levels of digestive and antigen-presenting cell processing, transglutaminase-mediated deamidation, and peptide binding to DQ2 and/or DQ8 molecules.[20] However, even when these successive steps occur, the requirements for immune destruction of intestinal epithelium are not encountered. This is exemplified by the observation that mice engineered to express HLA-DQ8 together with human CD4 molecule can generate strong CD4 T cell responses when fed with gluten, but do not develop enteropathy.[21] This indicates that complementary mechanisms contribute to breaking mucosal tolerance to gluten in CD.

Since over 60 percent of familial clustering of CD remains unexplained by HLA genes, the identification of additional genetic loci has been important to gain insights into the disease pathogenesis. Genome wide association studies have supported the idea that multiple gene variants, each with small effect, contribute to disease susceptibility. Eight chromosome regions outside the HLA region have been identified as being associated with CD: RGS1 on chromosome 1q31, IL18RAP on chromosome 2q12, CCR3 on chromosome 3p21, IL12A on chromosome 3q25, LPP on chromosome 3q28, IL2-IL21 on chromosome 4q27, TAGAP on chromosome 6q25, and SH2B3 on chromosome 12q24.[22] Interestingly, several of these eight identified regions harbor genes coding for proteins with known immune functions, such as cytokines or cytokine receptors, chemokines. It is possible that the presence of such variants might influence the quality or the intensity of the immune response.

Altogether, these data not only further increase our understanding of the molecular basis for genetic predisposition to CD, but also have significant interest in clinical practice. First, HLA-DQ2 and DQ8 are such strong disease risk factors that their absence has a negative predictive value for CD close to 100 percent. Therefore, HLA-DQ typing may help a physician to eliminate a CD diagnosis in the case of atypical clinical presentation of the disease (lack of typical symptoms, absence of anti-gliadin antibodies, doubtful histological lesions...). Second, the possibilities for future therapeutic strategies in CD patients through the use of agents that selectively destroy immunogenic gluten peptides may directly arise from the fine characterization of these epitopes. A bacterial prolyl endopeptidase treatment was shown to abolish the antigenicity of the 33-mer gliadin peptide in DQ2 individuals, and was also predicted to have comparable effects on other proline-rich putatively immunotoxic peptides identified from other polypeptides within the gluten proteome.[5] By contrast, the DQ8 molecule, which does not tolerate a proline at P1, can select other gluten sequences that are more likely to be sensitive to proteases such as aminopeptidases, but not to prolyl endopeptidase.[23] Thus, possible strategies for generating non-toxic varieties of gluten will differ in DQ2 and DQ8 patients. Finally, observations made in celiac disease are relevant for type 1 diabetes (T1D), another frequent autoimmune disease which is also associated with the DQ2 and DQ8 molecules, in particular when they are present together in heterozygous individuals. It was recently shown that genetic susceptibility to both CD and type 1 diabetes shares common alleles, in addition to HLA class II.[24] It is therefore likely that there is a common genetic background with respect to autoimmunity and inflammation in these two diseases, and that further combinations of other gene variants, together with epigenetic and environmental factors, determine the final disease onset.

REFERENCES

1. Maki M, Mustalahti K, Kokkonen J, Kulmala P, Haapalahti M, Karttunen T. Ilonen J, Laurila K, Dahlbom I, Hansson T, Hopfl P, Knip M. Prevalence of Celiac disease among children in Finland. N Engl J Med 2003;348:2517-24.
2. Sollid LM. Coeliac disease: Dissecting a complex inflammatory disorder. Nat Rev Immunol 2002;2:647-55.
3. Greco LR, I Romino. Coto N Cosmo Di, Percopo S, Maglio M, Paparo F, Gasperi V, Limongelli MG, Cotichini R, Agate CD', Tinto N, Sacchetti L, Tosi R, Stazi MA. The first large population based twin study of coeliac disease. Gut 2002;50:624-28.
4. Lundin KE, Scott H, Hansen T, Paulsen G, Halstensen TS, Fausa O, Thorsby E, Sollid LM. Gliadin-specific, HLA-DQ(alpha 1*0501,beta 1*0201) restricted T cells isolated from the small intestinal mucosa of celiac disease patients. J Exp Med 1993;178:187-96.
5. Shan L, Molberg O, Parrot I, Hausch F, Filiz F, Gray GM, Sollid LM, Khosla C. Structural basis for gluten intolerance in celiac sprue. Science 2002;297:2275-79.
6. Matysiak-Budnik T, Moura IC, Arcos-Fajardo M, Lebreton C, Menard S, Candalh C, Ben-Khalifa K, Dugave C, Tamouza H, G van Niel, Bouhnik Y, Lamarque D, Chaussade S, Malamut G, Cellier C, Cerf-Bensussan N, Monteiro RC, Heyman M. Secretory IgA mediates retrotranscytosis of intact gliadin peptides via the transferrin receptor in celiac disease. J Exp Med 2008; 205:143-54.
7. Dieterich W, Ehnis T, Bauer M, Donner P, Volta U, Riecken EO, Schuppan D. Identification of tissue transglutaminase as the autoantigen of celiac disease. Nat Med 1997;3: 797-801.
8. Molberg O, Mcadam SN, Korner R, Quarsten H, Kristiansen C, Madsen L Fugger, Scott H, Noren O, Roepstorff P, Lundin KEA, Sjostrom H, Sollid LM. Tissue transglutaminase selectively modifies gliadin peptides that are recognized by gut-derived T cells in celiac disease. Nature Medicine 4:713-17.
9. Johansen BH, Vartdal F, Eriksen JA, Thorsby E, Sollid LM. Identification of a putative motif for binding of peptides to HLA-DQ2. Int Immunol 1996;8:177-82.
10. van de Wal Y, Kooy YM, Drijfhout JW, Amons R, Koning F. Peptide binding characteristics of the coeliac disease-associated DQ(alpha1*0501, beta1*0201) molecule. Immunogenetics 1996;44:246-53.
11. Kwok WW, Domeier ML, Raymond FC, Byers P, Nepom GT. Allele-specific motifs characterize HLA-DQ interactions with a diabetes-associated peptide derived from glutamic acid decarboxylase. J Immunol 1996; 156:2171-77.
12. Godkin A, Friede T, Davenport M, Stevanovic S, Willis A, Jewell D, Hill A, Rammensee HG. Use of eluted peptide sequence data to identify the binding characteristics of peptides to the insulin-dependent diabetes susceptibility allele HLA-DQ8 (DQ 3.2). Int Immunol 1997;9:905-11.
13. Koning F. Celiac disease: Caught between a rock and a hard place. Gastroenterology 2005;129:1294-1301.
14. Vader LW, A de Ru, van der Wal Y, Kooy YM, Benckhuijsen W, Mearin ML. Drijfhout JWP. van Veelen, F Koning. Specificity of tissue transglutaminase explains cereal toxicity in celiac disease. J Exp Med 2002;195: 643-49.
15. Vader W, D Stepniak JW, Kooy Y, Mearin L, Thompson A, JJ van Rood, Spaenij L, Koning F. The HLA-DQ2 gene dose effect in celiac disease is directly related to the magnitude and breadth of gluten-specific T cell responses. Proc Natl Acad Sci USA 2003;100:12390-95.
16. Tollefsen S, H Arentz-Hansen, Fleckenstein B, Molberg O, Raki M, Kwok WW, Jung G, Lundin KE, Sollid LM. HLA-DQ2 and -DQ8 signatures of gluten T cell epitopes in celiac disease. J Clin Invest 2006;116:2226-36.
17. Lee KH, Wucherpfennig KW, Wiley DC. Structure of a human insulin peptide- HLA-DQ8 complex and susceptibility to type 1 diabetes. Nat Immunol 2001;2: 501-07.
18. Kim CY, Quarsten H, Bergseng E, Khosla C, Sollid LM. Structural basis for HLA-DQ2-mediated presentation of gluten epitopes in celiac disease. Proc Natl Acad Sci USA 2004;101:4175-79.
19. Bergseng E, Xia J, Kim CY, Khosla C, Sollid LM. Main chain hydrogen bond interactions in the binding of proline-rich gluten peptides to the celiac disease-

associated HLA-DQ2 molecule. J Biol Chem 2005; 280:21791-96.

20. Arentz-Hansen H, McAdam SN, Molberg O, Fleckenstein B, Lundin KE, Jorgensen TJ, Jung G, Roepstorff P, Sollid LM. Celiac lesion T cells recognize epitopes that cluster in regions of gliadins rich in proline residues. Gastroenterology 2002;123:803-09.

21. de Kauwe AL, Chen Z, Anderson RP, Keech CL, Price JD, Wijburg O, Jackson DC, Ladhams J, Allison J, McCluskey J. Resistance to celiac disease in humanized HLA-DR3-DQ2-transgenic mice expressing specific anti-gliadin CD4+ T cells. J Immunol 2009;182:7440-50.

22. Hunt KA, Zhernakova A, Turner G, Heap GA, Franke L, Bruinenberg M, Romanos J, Dinesen LC, Ryan AW, Panesar D, Gwilliam R, Takeuchi F, McLaren WM, Holmes GK, Howdle PD, Walters JR, Sanders DS, Playford RJ, Trynka G, Mulder CJ, Mearin ML, Verbeek WH, Trimble V, Stevens FM, Morain C O', Kennedy NP, Kelleher D, Pennington DJ, Strachan DP, McArdle WL, Mein CA, Wapenaar MC, Deloukas P, McGinnis R, McManus R, Wijmenga C, van Heel DA. Newly identified genetic risk variants for celiac disease related to the immune response. Nat Genet 2008;40:395-402.

23. Henderson KN, Tye-Din JA, Reid HH, Chen Z, Borg NA, Beissbarth T, Tatham A, Mannering SI, Purcell AW, Dudek NL, van Heel DA, McCluskey J, Rossjohn J, Anderson RP. A structural and immunological basis for the role of human leukocyte antigen DQ8 in celiac disease. Immunity 2007;27:23-34.

24. Smyth DJ, Plagnol V, Walker NM, Cooper JD, Downes K, Yang JH, Howson JM, Stevens H, McManus R, Wijmenga C, Heap GA, Dubois PC, Clayton DG, Hunt KA, van Heel DA, Todd JA. Shared and distinct genetic variants in type 1 diabetes and celiac disease. N Engl J Med 2008;359: 2767-77.

Chapter 16

HLA and Spondyloarthropathies

Muhammad Asim Khan

INTRODUCTION

The year 1973 was a very memorable one for science because of the discovery of a remarkable association of HLA-B27 with ankylosing spondylitis (AS), one of the strongest between an MHC molecule and a disease.[1,2] This association holds true worldwide and also extends to rheumatic diseases related to AS that are grouped together under the term "Spondyloarthropathies" (SpA).[3-7] HLA-B27 is the primary disease susceptibility gene for AS, but not a prerequisite because the disease also affects individuals who do not possess this gene.[4,8-10] It so happens that I myself have suffered from AS for 53 years, and it was in 1973 that my first child was born who had inherited my HLA-B27 gene.[4-6] Despite intense studies during all these years, the precise biological explanation for the remarkable association still remains elusive.[4,5,7] But I have enjoyed reviewing this subject over the years; and the current chapter is based on many of those publications.[4,5,8-23]

DISCOVERY OF HLA-B27

Erik Thorsby from Norway first described HLA-B27; he detected it by using an antibody that was produced by "planned immunization", a method that was being used at that time by several investigators.[24] He had immunized a colleague, FJH, with a skin transplant and cells from a healthy HLA identical donor because Erik assumed that the donor might possess a hitherto undetected HLA antigen. The recipient produced an antibody which detected a "new" antigen, which he named TH-FJH, and this antigen was later given the name HLA-B27.

Erik once communicated to me that subsequently when he tested his own family, he noticed that one family member who carried this new antigen had AS, while another had questionable AS.[5] However, since most of his family members who carried the new antigen were completely healthy, he discarded this finding as being caused by chance. He stated that he has ever since regretted that he did not pursue this possible association by testing some other patients who suffered from AS. Had he done so he would have been the very first to detect an association between an HLA antigen and a disease!

CLINICAL DESCRIPTION OF ANKYLOSING SPONDYLITIS AND RELATED SPONDYLOARTHROPATHIES

They are chronic systemic inflammatory rheumatic diseases that show a predilection for involvement of the axial skeleton (sacroiliac joints, spine, chest wall and hip and shoulder girdles), but may also present with peripheral joint involvement, enthesitis (inflammation of sites of bony attachments of tendons and ligaments), and/or extra-articular features, such as inflammation of the eyes (acute anterior uveitis), psoriasis or psoriasiform skin lesions, and chronic inflammatory bowel disease (ulcerative colitis or Crohn's disease).[4,21,25-27] This group of diseases also includes reactive arthritis that is triggered by infection with *Chlamydia* and by certain Gram-negative enteric infections[28] (Fig. 16.1 and Table 16.2). In general, most of the patients with AS and related SpA, tend to follow a chronic progressive disease course with variable disease activity. The patients with axial skeletal involvement usually present with chronic inflammatory back pain and stiffness, associated with slowly progressive impairment of spinal mobility that can finally result in spinal fusion (spondylitis) over many years.

AS is the predominant member or prototype of SpA and can often be the main final outcome (Fig. 16.1). The salient features of AS are listed in Table 16.1. It is a little more common and tends to be more severe in men. The mean age of onset is about 23 years of age, but it can also have a juvenile onset; and it is very unusual for the symptoms to begin after age 45. The term "primary AS" is used when there is no associated disease (and this is the most common form of AS), while "secondary AS" implies that it is accompanied by psoriasis, ulcerative colitis, Crohn's disease or reactive arthritis.[4,21,25,27]

Radiographic evidence of sacroiliac joint involvement (sacroiliitis) has been on is one of the hallmarks of AS. However, radiographic sacroiliitis is not easy to detect during early stage of the disease and especially in children and adolescents. Magnetic resonance imaging (MRI) has become a very helpful tool in detecting "pre-radiographic" sacroiliitis, especially in children, adolescents and young women because it can distinguish normal growth changes of sacroiliac joints from changes resulting from inflammation, and it does not involve any exposure to radiation.[4]

The term "undifferentiated SpA" is used when the patient has a limited form or early stage of the disease that does not meet the criteria for AS or the so-called "differentiated" forms of SpA.[29-32] It encompasses HLA-B27-associated disorders such as isolated oligoarthritis predominantly of the lower extremities, enthesitis or dactylitis or acute anterior uveitis (also called acute iritis), but without radiographic evidence of sacroiliitis or of

Table 16.1: The salient clinical features of AS

- The symptoms usually start in late teens and early twenties (mean age of onset is 23 but is younger in many developing parts of the world) as chronic back pain and stiffness of insidious onset in late adolescence and early adulthood; these symptoms worsen with prolonged rest or physical inactivity, but are eased on physical activity. It is very uncommon for the symptoms to begin after age 45.
- Generally good symptomatic response to anti-inflammatory dose of non-steroidal anti-inflammatory drugs (NSAIDs) and regular physical exercise.
- Tendency for inflammation at sites of bony insertions for tendons and ligaments (enthesitis), with adjacent subchondral bone edema (osteitis) and adjacent synovitis.
- Characteristic radiographic sacroiliitis and variable progression to spondylitis.
- Gradually progressive limitation of spinal mobility and later even chest expansion.
- Increased risk of anterior ocular inflammation (acute anterior uveitis).
- Increased familial incidence.
- Strong association with HLA-B27, but strength of this association varies appreciably among various racial and ethnic groups.
- No association with rheumatoid factor and antinuclear antibodies.
- Sometimes association with psoriasis, ulcerative colitis, Crohn's disease, and reactive arthritis.
- Occasional extraskeletal manifestations include aortitis, heart block, apical pulmonary fibrosis, or cauda equina syndrome.

spondylitis, or clinical evidence, psoriasis or gastrointestinal or genitourinary tract involvement. The undifferentiated form is also observed among children, and may begin with enthesitis causing pain in the heels and other bony sites, or lower extremity arthritis of one (especially the knee or ankle) or a few joints, without any other features; and these patients can gradually progress to AS over several years.[30]

HLA-B27 DISEASE ASSOCIATION

The strength of the association of HLA-B27 with AS and related SpA varies among the various SpA and also among the various ethnic and racial groups worldwide.[2-5,33-36] The data shown in Tables 16.2 and 16.3 pertain only to populations of north-western European extraction, and differ markedly from some of the other ethnic and racial groups worldwide; e.g., only up to 50 percent of African-American patients with primary AS posses HLA-B27 versus 95 percent of Scandinavian patients.[10-13,33-36]

HLA-B27 HOMOZYGOSITY AND DISEASE ASSOCIATION

HLA-B27 homozygosity increases the likelihood for developing AS by a factor of more than three; it was first

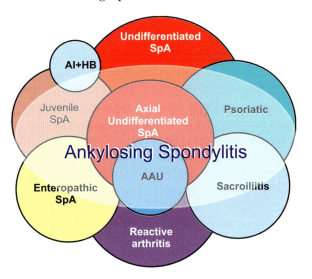

Fig. 16.1: Venn diagram showing overlapping features of AS and related SpA. AAU = acute anterior uveitis. AI+HB = Aortic incompetence with heart block [Adopted from: Elyan M, Khan MA. Diagnosing ankylosing spondylitis. *J Rheumatol* Suppl 2006; Sep;78:12-23.]

Table 16.2: Clinical comparison of AS and related SpA

Characteristics	AS	Reactive arthritis	Juvenile SpA	Psoriatic arthritis	Enteropathic SpA
Usual age at onset	Young adult age < 40	Young to middle-aged	Ages 8 to 16 years	Young to middle age	Adult
Sex ratio	2x more common in males	Predominantly males	Predominantly males	Equal	Equal
Usual type of onset	Gradual	Acute	Variable	Variable	Gradual
Sacroiliitis or spondylitis	Virtually 100%	<50%	<50%	>20%	<20%
Symmetry of sacroiliitis	Symmetric	Asymmetric	Variable	Asymmetric	Symmetric
Peripheral joint involvement	<15%	~90%	~90%	~95%	15% to 20%
HLA-B27 (in Whites)	~90%	~5%	~85%	~50%‡	~50%‡
Anterior eye inflammation§	25 to 40%	~50%	~20%	~20%	≤ 15%
Cardiac involvement	1% to 4%	5% to 10%	Rare	Rare	Rare
Skin or nail involvement	None	<40%	Uncommon	Virtually 100%	Uncommon
Role of infectious triggers	Unknown	Yes	Unknown	Unknown	Unknown

‡ In those with spondylitis or sacroiliitis.   §More often conjunctivitis in reactive arthritis

Table 16.3: Association of spondyloarthropathies with HLA-B27 in Euro-Caucasians

Disease	Approximate Prevalence of HLA-B27, %
Primary ankylosing spondylitis	90
Reactive arthritis	40–80
Juvenile spondyloarthropathy	70
Enteropathic spondyloarthritis	35–75
Psoriatic spondyloarthritis	40–50
Undifferentiated spondyloarthropathy	70
Acute anterior uveitis (acute iritis)	50
Aortic incompetence with heart block	80

- These data pertain to persons of north-western European extraction; the prevalence of HLA-B27 in the general healthy populations is approximately 8%.
- The association in South-Asians, Chinese, and Koreans is equally strong.
- However, the strength of this association is much weaker in some other populations; for example only up to 50% of African-American patients with primary AS possess HLA-B27.

reported in 1978.[37] This aspect was not thoroughly pursued by other investigators since then, but in 2006 this observation was finally confirmed.[38] Why is it that homozygous individuals with HLA-B27 are at least three times more likely to get the disease as opposed to heterozygous individuals? There are many possible explanations for this. These include, for example, possible increased cell surface expression of HLA-B27 or potentially increased effect of linked genes that may have influence on disease process or occurrence.

HLA-B27 PREVALENCE

The prevalence of HLA-B27 varies markedly in the various population groups in the world (see Table 16.4, and Figure 16.2; and speaking in general terms, the prevalence of AS roughly correlates with the prevalence of HLA-B27, but with certain glaring exceptions.[4,15,23,33-36,39,40] For example, HLA-B27 is present in West African countries, such as Senegal and Gambia, but it is very difficult to find any cases of AS among them.[23] There is no good explanation for this geographic distribution of HLA-B27, and a

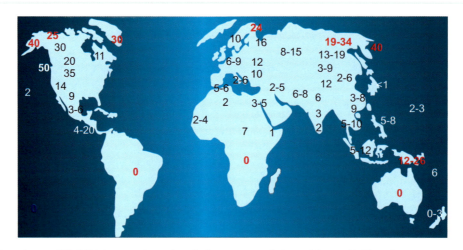

Fig. 16.2: Prevalence of HLA-B27 among the various indigenous populations of the world. Thus, for example, the prevalence of HLA-B27 in Australia is shown as zero because the native of the land do not possess this gene [Adopted from: Khan MA. Spondyloarthropathies: Editorial overview. Curr Opin Rheumatol 1995; 7: 263-9.]

Table 16.4: The prevalence of HLA-B27 in some population groups*	
Population groups	HLA-B27 prevalence (%)
Caucasoid population groups	
Ugro-Finnish	12-18
Northern Scandinavians	10-16
Slavic populations	7-14
Western Europeans	6-9
Southern Europeans	2-6
Sardinians	5
Basques	9-14
Turks	7-14
Arabs**, Jews, Armenians, and Iranians	3-5
Pakistanis	6-8
Indians (Asian)	2-6
North American native populations	
Eskimo-Aleut	25-40
Na-Dene (Haida Tlingit Dogrib Navajo)	20-50
Amerind	
North American	7-26
Mexicans-Mestizo	3-6
South American native populations	0
Asian population groups	
Chukchic	19-40
Uralic	8-24
Siberians	6-19
Japanese	< 1
Ainu (Native Japanese)	4
Koreans	3-8
Mongolians	3-9
Uygurs, Kazakhs, Turkic, Uzbek	3-8
Chinese	2-9

(Contd.)

(Contd.)

Population groups	HLA-B27 prevalence (%)
Tibetans	12
Southeast Asians	4-12
Micronesians (Nauru, Guam)	2-5
Melanesians (Papua New Guinea [5], Fiji, etc.)	4-53
Polynesians	0-3
Australian Aborigines	0
African population groups	
North Africans	3-5
West Africans (Mali, Gambia, and Senegal)	2-10
Pygmies	7-10
Bantu (Nigeria, Southern Africa)	0
San (Bushmen)	0

* The numbers are rounded off for simplicity, and indicate percentage prevalence in the general population. Table adapted from reference.[2]
** Prevalence of B27 may be much lower (closer to 1%) in the United Arab Emirates and adjacent parts of Saudi Arabia, and among Lebanese Maronite Christian Arabs.

hypothesis proposes that *Plasmodium falciparum* may have exerted a negative selection on this gene, and that the same selective pressure(s) that has contributed to reduce the HLA-B27 frequency in some regions has/have favored the fixing of newly generated B27 subtypes included in more advantageous HLA haplotypes.[41]

HLA-B27 POSITIVE VERSUS NEGATIVE DISEASE

The SpA can occur in the absence of HLA-B27 because there are additional, some as yet undiscovered, disease predisposing genetic factors. Presence of genetic heterogeneity of AS was first clearly exemplified by the difference between HLA-B27-positive and HLA-B27-negative patients.[8,27,42] For example, although there are many similarities, HLA-B27-negative AS is later in its onset; is significantly less often complicated by acute anterior uveitis, and more frequently accompanied by psoriasis, ulcerative colitis, and Crohn's disease; and it less often shows familial aggregation when compared with HLA-B27-positive AS.[8,27,42]

CLINICAL UTILITY OF HLA-B27 TYPING AS AN AID TO DIAGNOSIS

Chronic back pain is a very common condition in the general population and overwhelming majority of such individuals (approximately 95%) do not suffer from AS or related SpA. Back pain and stiffness due to AS can often precede unequivocal radiographic signs of sacroiliitis by several years.[43,44] Therefore, the status of the sacroiliac joints on a pelvic radiograph is not always easy to interpret in the early phase of the disease, particularly in adolescents, although MRI, a relatively costly technique, can help to detect early sacroiliitis in this clinical situation and without any gonadal radiation.[45-47] An overwhelming majority of individuals born with HLA-B27 never suffer from AS or related SpA.[23] Moreover, many patients can develop these diseases in the absence of this gene, especially in certain populations. For example, among the African-American population HLA-B27 is present in only about 50 percent of patients with primary AS versus 90 percent of those with northern European descent.[4,9-11,27,34-36]

Therefore, in the true sense HLA-B27 typing cannot be thought of as a routine, diagnostic, confirmatory, or screening test for AS in patients presenting with back pain or arthritis.[4,48-51] Typing for HLA-B27 is a relatively inexpensive test and it does not need to be repeated (unless for technical/laboratory error). But as a laboratory test in clinical medicine it is imperfect because it is neither 100 percent sensitive nor 100 percent specific. Although HLA-B27 typing can define the population at higher risk of AS and related SpA, it is of very limited practical value for that purpose in the general population because of the following reasons: no effective means of prevention is currently available, and most individuals with HLA-B27 never develop AS or a related SpA. The risk of development of AS or any type of SpA, even among B27-positive first-degree relatives of a B27-positive patient with AS, is only 20 percent at the most; and it is very much lower in the general public with HLA-B27.[52]

As a rule, if the history and physical examination findings suggest AS but the imaging findings do not permit this diagnosis to be made (X-rays and or MRI are normal or equivocal), resulting in a "toss-up situation" (the pretest probability is approximately 50 percent (toss-up) or in the range of 30 to 70 percent, typing for HLA-B27 may allow the presumptive diagnosis of AS to be accepted or rejected with greater certainty.[49-51] In patients with back pain or arthritis in whom the clinical history, physical examination and imaging findings do not suggest AS, testing for HLA-B27 will be inappropriate because a positive test result would still not permit the diagnosis of AS to be made.

The clinical utility of the test has to be interpreted in light of the *a priori* clinical likelihood of the disease in the subject in whom the test was ordered, because the value of HLA-B27 typing as an aid to diagnosing AS depends on the individual probability of the disease when the test is ordered.[49,51] Moreover, the prevalence of HLA-B27 in the general population and the strength of its association with AS and related SpA differ markedly among the various ethnic and racial groups worldwide (Fig. 16.2 and Table 16.4).[23,49,51] So the clinical utility of the test result has to also be based on the patient's ethnicity and race. As mentioned earlier, approximately 50 percent of African American patients with primary AS possess HLA-B27 (sensitivity of B27 test = 50%) versus 3 percent among the general population (specificity = 100 − 3 = 97%). In contrast, HLA-B27 is present in approximately 90 percent of primary AS patients of northern European descent (sensitivity = 90%) versus 8 percent of the general population (specificity = 100 − 8 = 92%).[49,51] The likelihood ratio of a positive test is the sensitivity divided by (100 - specificity). So it is 50/3 = 17 for African American and 90/8 = 11 for individuals of northern European descent. The likelihood ratio of a negative test is (100 - sensitivity) divided by the specificity. So it is 50/97 = 0.5 for African American and 10/92 = 0.1 for individuals of northern European descent. Thus a negative test in African Americans is clinically not helpful in lowering the pretest probability of AS, but a positive test is more helpful as an aid to diagnosis (positive likelihood ratio = 17) than in individuals of northern European descent (positive likelihood ratio = 11).[49,51]

The HLA-B27 test is very much more useful in Japanese patients in this clinical situation because of strong association with AS (sensitivity ≈ 80%) and a less than 1 percent prevalence of HLA-B27 in the general Japanese population (specificity = 100 − 1 = 99%);

resulting in positive likelihood ratio of >80) and negative likelihood ratio of $20/99 \approx 0.2$. Thus a test of very high specificity, for example the HLA-B27 test for AS in Japanese and to a lesser extent in African Americans, would give a relatively large positive likelihood ratio even if the sensitivity of the test is relatively lower when compared to, for example, individuals of northern European descent. Those interested in this subject of Bayesian analysis are referred to my prior publications on this subject.[49-51]

HLA-B27 is associated with acute anterior uveitis (acute iritis); therefore, this test may help ophthalmologists to better classify patient presenting with unilateral acute anterior uveitis and to refer those who possess this gene to rheumatologists, especially those patient who have associated musculoskeletal symptoms, because more than 75 percent of B27-positive patients will either already have or will develop AS or a related SpA.[31,53-55]

POLYMORPHISM OF HLA-B27

The HLA-B27 gene has remarkable polymorphism with 69 alleles based on nucleotide sequence differences, but some of these mutations are located within introns and thus are silent, or they occur in exons but do not cause amino acid changes. Thus at the translated protein level the number of subtypes of HLA-B27 (based on amino acid sequence differences) is smaller and can be encompassed by the numbering system HLA-B*2701 to HLA-B*2759, according to data published in the international ImMunoGeneTics database (IMGT, release 2.24.0)[56] (Table 16.5).

The worldwide distribution of the various subtypes of HLA-B27 is extremely variable; Table 16.6 lists the HLA-B27 subtype frequencies (%) of only the first 14 subtypes (except B*2710) among individuals possessing HLA-B27; the other more recent subtypes are much more rare and detailed data are unavailable.[22,23,57-62]

B*2705 (specifically the *B*27052* allele) is the most widespread subtype throughout the world and from which other subtypes seem to have evolved mostly from changes in exons 2 and 3 (which encode the alpha 1 and alpha 2 domains, respectively)[22,23] (Tables 16.7 and 16.8). Figure 16.3 describes the structure of HLA-B27 based on the crystallographic structure of HLA-B27;[63,64] it is a heterodimer composed of the HLA-B alpha (heavy) chain (encoded in the MHC Class I region) non-covalently linked with beta 2-microglobulin. It has a peptide-binding cleft (formed by the alpha 1 and alpha 2 domains of the alpha chain) that has six side-pockets (designated by the letters A through F) that accommodate the side chains of the amino-acids of the bound nonamer peptides.

Table 16.5: Currently identified HLA-B27 subtypes

B*2701		B*2710	B*2728	B*2744
B*2702		B*2711	B*2729	B*2745
B*2703		B*2712	B*2730	B*2746
B*2704		B*2713	B*2731	B*2747
B*2705	B*270502	B*2714	B*2732	B*2748
	B*270503	B*2715	B*2733	B*2749
	B*270504	B*2716	B*2734	B*2750
	B*270505	B*2717	B*2735	B*2751
	B*270506	B*2718	B*2736	B*2752
	B*270507	B*2719	B*2737	B*2753
	B*270508	B*2720	B*2738	B*2754
	B*270509	B*2721	B*2739	B*2755
	B*270510	B*2723	B*2740	B*2756
	B*270511	B*2724	B*2741	B*2757
B*2706	B*270512	B*2725	B*2742	B*2758
B*2707		B*2726	B*2743	
B*2759N				
B*2708		B*2727		
B*2709				

Note that HLA-B*2722 is not listed as this designation was withdrawn when subsequent studies should that it was identical to HLA-B*2706.

Worldwide studies indicate that the common subtypes B*2705, B*2704 and HLA-B*2702 are strongly associated with AS. Among the other subtypes, most of which are relatively uncommon, occurrence of AS in at least one patient with the following alleles has been reported, but needs association studies: B*2701, B*2703, B*2707, B*2708, B2710, B*2714, B*2715, B*2719 and B*2724.[22,23,57-62] HLA-B*2715 is observed in Asian populations, and it differs from B*2704 by only one amino acid, at heavy-chain residues 163 (Glu in B*2704 and Thr in B*2715)[60] (Table 16.8). Whether this difference impacts its association with AS is currently not known, but all 5 Chinese AS patients with B*2715 had juvenile onset of their disease.[60]

One of the strongest reasons to study the HLA-B27 subtypes is to learn the effects of the sequence variations on the peptide-binding specificity of the molecule. Among these peptides may be the putative arthritogenic peptide(s). It is also important to investigate whether certain subtypes show any preferential association with some of the clinical features or forms of AS and related SpA among the various ethnic/racial populations and geographic regions of the world. This may provide clues as to the mechanism of disease association, and may help to identify the polymorphic positions of HLA-B27 that may have a disease-predisposing role. There may exist a hierarchical ranking of strength of disease associations of some of the B27 subtypes, at least in some population groups, which may also result, at least in part, from

Table 16.6: HLA-B27 subtype frequencies (%) of only the first 14 subtypes (except B*2710) among individuals possessing HLA-B27; the other more recent subtypes are much more rare and detailed data are unavailable

Populations	*2701	*2702	*2703	*2704	*2705	*2706	*2707	*2708	*2709	*2711	*2713	*2714
North. Europe		10			90							
Siberia		14			84							2
Northern Spain		7			91		1				1	
Spain (Galicia)		18			80			3				
Sardinia		3			77				20			
Italy		30			65		2		3			
Greece		34	8		50		8					
Cyprus (Greeks)		52			32		17					
Azores				7	86		7					
Turkey	7	30			43		14	5				
Lebanon		24	12		35		30					
Israel (Jews)		48		3	38		13					
Northern India				33	61		6					
Western India				34.	34		18	12				2
Japan					82	18						
China		2			66	31		2				
Singapore (Chinese)					89	2	9					
Taiwan	0.05	0.5	3		87	4	7	2	0.02	0.02		
Taiwan (Han-Chinese)					94	6						
Taiwan (Aborigines)					100							
Indonesian Chinese					38		62					
Indonesian Native					6	6	89					
Malaysia					19	6	72	3				
Thailand					42	5	53					
Maoris					36	64						
Brazil		10	6		80			3			<1	
North Africa		50			50							
West Africa			32		68							

Note: The numbers are rounded off for simplicity.

Table 16.7: HLA-B27 subtype amino acid sequence variations

	HLA-B27 alpha1 domain amino acid variations												
	59	63	67	69	70	71	72	74	77	80	81	82	83
B*270502	Y	E	C	A	K	A	Q	D	D	T	L	L	R
B*2701	-	-	-	-	-	-	-	Y	N	-	A	-	-
B*2702	-	-	-	-	-	-	-	-	N	I	A	-	-
B*2703	H	-	-	-	-	-	-	-	-	-	-	-	-
B*2704	-	-	-	-	-	-	-	-	S	-	-	-	-
B*2706	-	-	-	-	-	-	-	-	S	-	-	-	-
B*2707	-	-	-	-	-	-	-	-	-	-	-	-	-
B*2708	-	-	-	-	-	-	-	-	S	N	-	R	G
B*2709	-	-	-	-	-	-	-	-	-	-	-	-	-
B*2710	-	-	-	-	-	-	-	-	-	-	-	-	-

(Contd.)

(Contd.)

	HLA-B27 alpha1 domain amino acid variations											
	59	63	67	69	70	71	72	74	77	80	81	82	83
B*2711	-	-	-	-	-	-	-	-	S	-	-	-	-
B*2712	-	-	-	T	N	T	-	-	S	N	-	R	G
B*2713	-	-	-	-	-	-	-	-	-	-	-	-	-
B*2714	-	-	-	-	-	-	-	-	-	-	-	-	-
B*2715	-	-	-	-	-	-	-	-	S	-	-	-	-
B*2716	-	-	-	T	N	T	-	-	-	-	-	-	-
B*2717	F	-	-	-	-	-	-	-	-	-	-	-	-
B*2718	-	-	S	T	N	T	-	Y	S	-	-	R	G
B*2719	-	-	-	-	-	-	-	-	-	-	-	-	-
B*2720	-	-	-	-	-	-	-	-	S	-	-	-	-
B*2721	-	-	-	-	-	-	-	-	S	-	-	-	-
B*2723	-	N	F	T	N	T	-	Y	S	-	-	-	-
B*2724	-	-	-	-	-	-	-	-	S	-	-	-	-
B*2725	-	-	-	-	-	-	-	-	S	-	-	-	-
B*2726	-	-	-	-	Q	-	-	-	S	-	-	R	G
B*2727	-	-	-	-	-	-	-	-	-	-	-	-	-
B*2728	-	-	-	-	-	-	-	-	-	-	-	-	-
B*2729	-	-	S	T	N	T	Y	-	-	-	-	-	-
B*2730	-	-	-	-	-	-	-	N	-	I	A	-	-
B*2731	-	-	-	-	Q	-	-	-	S	-	-	-	-
B*2732	-	-	-	-	-	-	-	-	-	-	-	-	-
B*2733	-	-	-	-	-	-	-	-	S	-	-	R	G
B*2734	-	-	-	-	-	-	-	-	-	-	-	-	-
B*2735	-	-	-	-	-	-	-	-	-	-	-	-	-
B*2736	-	-	-	-	-	-	-	-	S	-	-	-	-
B*2737	-	-	-	-	-	-	-	-	-	-	-	-	-
B*2738	-	-	-	-	-	-	-	-	-	-	-	-	-
B*2739	-	-	-	-	-	L	-	-	-	-	-	-	-
B*2740	-	-	-	-	-	-	-	-	S	N	-	R	G
B*2741	-	-	-	-	-	-	-	-	-	-	-	-	-
B*2742	-	-	-	-	-	-	-	-	-	N	-	R	G
B*2743	-	-	-	-	-	-	-	-	-	-	-	-	-
B*2744	-	-	-	-	-	-	-	Y	S	N	-	R	G
B*2745	-	-	-	-	-	-	-	-	-	-	-	-	-
B*2746	-	-	-	-	-	-	-	-	-	-	-	-	-
B*2747	-	-	-	-	-	-	-	-	-	-	-	-	-
B*2748	-	-	-	-	-	-	-	-	-	-	-	-	-
B*2749	-	-	-	-	-	-	-	-	-	-	-	F	-
B*2750	-	-	-	-	-	-	-	-	-	-	-	-	-
B*2751	-	-	-	-	-	-	-	-	-	-	-	-	-
B*2752	-	-	-	-	-	-	-	-	-	-	-	-	-
B*2753	-	-	-	-	-	-	-	-	-	I	A	-	-
B*2754	-	-	-	-	-	-	-	-	-	-	-	-	-
B*2755	-	-	-	-	-	-	-	-	-	-	-	-	-
B*2756	-	-	-	-	-	-	-	-	-	-	-	-	-
B*2757	-	-	-	-	-	-	-	-	-	N	I	A	-	-
B*2758	-	-	-	-	-	-	-	-	-	-	-	-	-
B*2759N	-	-	-	-	-	X	-	-	-	-	-	-	-

HLA-B*2737 has H to Y substitution at position 10 that is not shown in this Table.
HLA-B*2722 was withdrawn because it was found to be identical to HLA-B*2706.
HLA-B*2713 signal peptide has a single amino acid E to A substitution; however, the B*2713 molecule as expressed at the cell surface is identical to B*2705.

Table 16.8: HLA-B27 subtype amino acid sequence variations

	\multicolumn{14}{c}{HLA-B27 alpha 2 domain amino acid variations}
	94	95	97	103	105	113	114	116	131	152	156	163	167	171
B*270502	T	L	N	V	P	Y	H	D	S	V	L	E	W	Y
B*2701	-	-	-	-	-	-	-	-	-	-	-	-	-	-
B*2702	-	-	-	-	-	-	-	-	-	-	-	-	-	-
B*2703	-	-	-	-	-	-	-	-	-	-	-	-	-	-
B*2704	-	-	-	-	-	-	-	-	-	E	-	-	-	-
B*2706	-	-	-	-	-	-	D	Y	-	E	-	-	-	-
B*2707	-	-	S	-	-	H	N	Y	R	-	-	-	-	-
B*2708	-	-	-	-	-	-	-	-	-	-	-	-	-	-
B*2709	-	-	-	-	-	-	-	H	-	-	-	-	-	-
B*2710	-	-	-	-	-	-	-	-	-	E	-	-	-	-
B*2711	-	-	S	-	-	H	N	Y	R	-	-	-	-	-
B*2712	-	-	-	-	-	-	-	-	-	-	-	-	-	-
B*2713	-	-	-	-	-	-	-	-	-	-	-	-	-	-
B*2714	W	T	-	L	-	-	-	-	-	-	-	-	-	-
B*2715	-	-	-	-	-	-	-	-	-	E	-	T	-	-
B*2716	-	-	-	-	-	-	-	-	-	-	-	-	-	-
B*2717	-	-	-	-	-	-	-	-	-	-	-	-	-	-
B*2718	-	-	-	-	-	-	-	-	-	E	-	-	-	-
B*2719	I	I	R	-	-	-	-	-	-	-	-	-	-	-
B*2720	-	-	-	-	-	H	N	Y	R	E	-	-	-	-
B*2721	-	-	R	-	-	-	D	Y	-	E	-	-	-	-
B*2723	-	-	-	-	-	-	-	-	-	-	-	-	-	-
B*2724	-	-	S	-	-	H	N	Y	R	E	-	-	-	-
B*2725	-	-	-	-	-	-	-	-	-	E	W	L	-	-
B*2726	-	-	-	-	-	-	-	-	-	-	-	-	-	-
B*2727	-	-	-	-	-	H	N	Y	-	-	-	-	-	-
B*2728	-	-	-	-	-	-	-	-	-	-	-	T	-	H
B*2729	-	-	-	-	-	-	-	-	-	-	-	-	-	-
B*2730	-	-	-	-	-	-	-	-	-	-	-	-	-	-
B*2731	-	-	-	-	-	-	-	-	-	-	-	-	-	-
B*2732	-	-	S	-	-	-	-	-	-	-	-	-	-	-
B*2733	-	-	S	-	-	H	N	-	R	-	-	-	-	-
B*2734	-	-	S	-	-	H	D	-	R	-	-	-	-	-
B*2735	-	-	-	-	-	-	N	-	-	-	-	-	-	-
B*2736	-	-	-	-	-	-	-	-	-	-	-	-	-	-
B*2737	-	-	-	-	-	-	-	-	-	-	-	-	-	-
B*2738	-	-	-	-	-	-	-	-	-	-	-	L	-	-
B*2739	-	-	-	-	-	-	-	-	-	-	-	-	-	-
B*2740	-	-	-	-	-	-	-	-	-	E	-	-	-	-
B*2741	-	-	-	-	-	H	D	S	-	-	-	-	-	-
B*2742	-	-	-	-	-	-	-	-	-	-	-	-	-	-
B*2743	-	-	S	-	S	H	N	Y	R	-	-	-	-	-
B*2744	-	-	-	-	-	-	-	-	-	-	-	-	-	-
B*2745	-	-	-	-	-	-	-	-	-	-	R	-	-	-
B*2746	-	-	-	-	-	-	-	Y	-	-	-	-	-	-
B*2747	-	-	-	-	-	-	-	-	-	-	D	L	S	-
B*2748	-	-	-	-	-	-	-	-	-	-	-	-	-	-
B*2749	-	-	-	-	-	-	-	-	-	-	-	-	-	-
B*2750	-	-	-	-	-	-	-	-	-	-	-	-	S	-
B*2751	-	-	-	-	-	-	-	-	-	-	-	-	-	-
B*2752	-	-	-	-	-	-	-	-	-	-	-	-	-	-
B*2753	-	-	-	-	-	-	-	-	-	-	-	-	-	-
B*2754	-	-	-	-	-	-	-	-	-	E	-	-	-	-
B*2755	-	-	-	-	-	-	-	-	-	-	-	-	-	-
B*2756	-	-	-	-	-	-	-	-	-	-	-	-	-	-
B*2757	-	-	-	-	-	-	-	-	-	-	-	-	-	-
B*2758	-	-	-	-	-	-	-	-	-	-	-	-	-	-
B*2759N														

HLA-B*2722 was withdrawn because it was found to be identical to HLA-B*2706.

HLA-B*2713 signal peptide has a single amino acid E to A substitution; however, the B*2713 molecule as expressed at the cell surface is identical to B*2705.

differences in other co-inherited genetic factors, or due to environmental factors. For example, B*2705 is clearly disease-associated throughout the world, but not among the West Africans of Senegal and Gambia.[65,66]

HLA-B*2704 and HLA-B*2706 show an ethnically restricted distribution in Asia; e.g., B*2704 is a very common subtype in China and is strongly disease associated, whereas B*2706 is rare in Chinese people. There was only one report in 1997 of two Chinese AS patients carrying B*2706, but it has not been further substantiated.[60-62] On the other hand, B*2706 is a very prevalent subtype in Southeast Asian countries, such as Thailand and Indonesia, and it lacks any association with AS in those countries.[61,67] HLA-B*2706 has two changes relative to B*2704 at residue 114 (His to Asp) and 116 (Asp to Tyr) in the pockets D/E (Table 16.8 and Fig. 16.3). It is of interest that another HLA-B27 allele B*2709, that is present among Italian living on the island of Sardinia, also seems not to predispose to AS. B*2709 differs from the disease associated subtype B*2705 by only one amino acid, at heavy-chain residue 116 (Asp in HLA-B*2705; His in HLA-B*2709) in the F pocket that accommodates the peptide C-terminus (Table 16.8 and Fig. 16.4). It is very likely that both B*2706 and B*2709 subtypes neither predisposes to AS nor do they prevent the occurrence of this disease if the individual happens to co-inherit disease predisposing gene(s).[67-70]

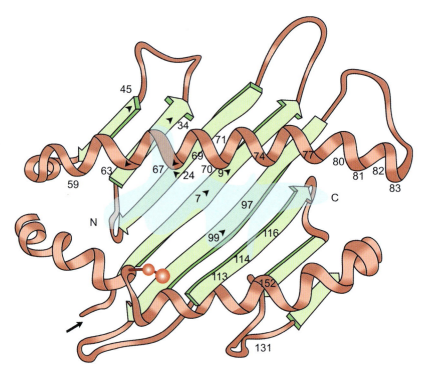

Fig. 16.3: A schematic ribbon diagram of the antigen-binding cleft of HLA-B27 with a nonameric (nine amino acid-long) antigenic peptide bound in its antigen-binding cleft. The view is from above, as seen from the viewpoint of a T-cell receptor. The middle portion of the bound peptide has an upward projecting central hump (not shown) that interacts with the T-cell receptor of the CD8 (+) T cells. The letters N and C indicate the amino (N) and carboxy (C) termini of the bound peptide. The dark arrow indicates the amino-terminus of the alpha (heavy) chain of the HLA-B27 molecule. The floor of the antigen-binding cleft is formed by the beta strands (broad arrows pointing away from the amino-terminus), and the margins are formed by alpha-helices shown as helical ribbons. The top alpha helix and the four beta strands to the left are from the alpha-1 domain of the heavy chain and the bottom alpha helix and the four beta strands to the right are from the alpha-2 domain. The disulfide bond is shown as two connecting spheres. Not marked are the six side pockets (assigned the letters A, B, C, D, E, and F) on the surface of the antigen-binding cleft. Pockets A and F are highly conserved deep pockets at the two ends of the antigen-binding cleft. The residues that form pocket B are marked by black arrowheads (at positions 7, 9, 24, 34, 45, 63, 67, and 99). The side chain of the second amino acid of the bound peptide is shown anchored into pocket B. The sites of amino acid substitutions that differentiate HLA-B*2705 from the first 12 variants are marked; they are residues 59, 69, 70, 71, 74, 77, 80, 81, 82, 83, 97, 113, 114, 116, 131, and 152. The two subtypes of HLA-B27 that seem to lack association with AS, that is, B*2706 and B*2709, differ from the disease associated subtypes B*2704 and B*2705 at residues 114 and 116, primarily affecting the conformation of pocket C/F. See Table to find how all of the currently known variants differ from each other (Adapted from: Khan MA. Spondyloarthropathies: editorial review. Curr Opin Rheumatol. 1994; 6:351-3; and modeled on the report by Madden DR, Gorga JC, Strominger JL, Wiley DC. The three-dimensional structure of HLA-B27 at 2.1 A resolution suggests a general mechanism for tight peptide binding to MHC. Cell. 1992;70:1035–48.)

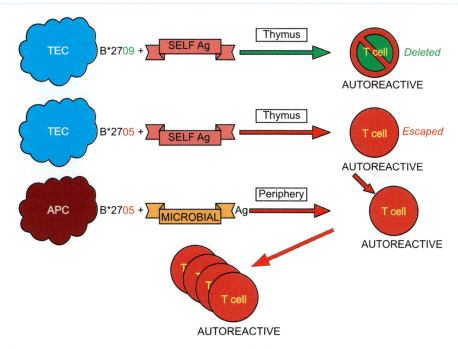

Fig. 16.4: Illustration of the hypothesis for the pathogenetic role of HLA-B*2705 molecule in the development of AS. The 'canonical' or 'non-canonical' conformation of a self-peptide p;resented by B*2709 or B*2705 molecules, may be critical in determining respectively deletion or escape from negative selection of autoreactive T cells in the thymus. Persistence of autoreactive T cells in the adults in B*2705 positive subjects may lead to cross-reaction with a homologous microbial antigen. Ag: antigen; APC: antigen presenting cell; TEC: thymic epithelial cell [Adopted from: Khan MA, Mathieu A, Sorrentino R, Akkoc N. The pathogenic role of HLA-B27 and its subtypes in ankylosing spondylitis. Autoimmunity Reviews 2007; 6(3):183-9.]

HYPOTHESES TO EXPLAIN THE PATHOGENIC ROLE OF HLA-B27

There is a very strong genetic predisposition to AS and related SpA dominated by HLA-B27, but how it results in disease has eluded researchers for more than 36 years.[5,22,71,72] None of the proposed theories have as yet satisfactorily explained the underlying mechanism and the differential association of HLA-B27 subtypes with AS. HLA-B27 binds and presents peptides to CD8+ T cells with high efficiency and is associated with comparatively better protection from certain viral diseases, than other HLA alleles. For example, HLA-B27 is strongly associated with spontaneous viral clearance of HCV, which has been mechanistically linked to a dominant CD8+ T cell epitope, and also has a protective role in HIV infection, indicated by its association with slow disease progression. In both human infections, HIV and HCV, a clear association between HLA-B27 and protection has been described, and it has been linked to a single epitope in each case.[73]

Therefore, it seems logical to concentrate in the antigen presenting properties of HLA-B27 in order to understand its possible role in disease pathogenesis.[74-75] According to the "arthritogenic" peptide hypothesis, HLA-B27 presents a microbial-derived "arhritogenic" peptide(s) for AS to develop. But no such peptide has yet been identified; and if there is an arthritogenic peptide then the CD8+ T cells is expected to play a role because MHC restriction indicates that CD8+ T-cells conventionally interact with MHC class I molecules and CD4+ T-cells interact with MHC class II molecules. But the evidence is mounting that the CD8+ T cells may not be the cells that are involved, at least in the B27 transgenic model that has been studied.[76]

In the frame of the "arthritogenic" peptide hypothesis, as discussed in an earlier review,[22] HLA-B*2705 positive patients with AS possess precursor T cells specific for a well-defined self peptide pVIPR (from the vasoactive intestinal peptide receptor 1) encoded by the VPAC1 gene mapping on chromosome 3, whereas B*2709 positive individuals lacked such a reactivity.[77] X-ray crystallography has shown that the B*2705 molecules bind the pVIPR peptide in two distinct conformations, whereas B*2709 molecules present the same peptide in only one of the two conformations, suggesting that the dual conformation in the B*2705 molecules could be responsible for a less efficient negative selection in B*2705 positive individuals.[77] Interestingly, a viral peptide pLMP2 (derived from latent membrane protein 2 of Epstein-Barr virus) is presented by B*2705 and B*2709 in two drastically deviating conformations.[78] Most interestingly, pLMP2 when bound to B*2705 molecules, displays a conformation very similar to that unique to the B*2705/pVPAC1. Thus molecular mimicry between a microbial and a self-peptide could trigger a cross-reactive cytotoxic T cell response activating those clonotypes which have not been eliminated during ontogenesis in the thymus[22] (Fig. 16.4). Further hypotheses are reviewed by the author elsewhere.[22] For example, it has also been proposed that HLA-B27 itself could become autoantigenic due to its sequence homology with certain microbial proteins, or that it may modify intracellular microbial handling or killing of the putative arthritogenic organisms that can result in aberrant or impaired immune response that leads to AS or related SpA, such as reactive arthritis.

A recent crystallographic and functional study investigated whether the exchange of arginine to citrulline (as a result of inflammatory processes that are accompanied by the post-translational modification of certain arginine residues within proteins to yield citrulline) affects the display of a peptide by HLA-B*2705 and HLA-B*2709.[79] A modified self-peptide, pVIPR-U5 (RRKWURWHL; U=citrulline), is presented by the two HLA-B27 molecules in distinct conformations. These binding modes differ not only drastically from each other but also from the conformations exhibited by the non-citrullinated peptide in a given subtype. The resultant differential reactivity of HLA-B27-restricted cytotoxic T cells with modified or unmodified pVIPR shows that the presentation of citrullinated peptides has the potential to influence immune responses.

In the past few years the research focus has shifted from the peptide-presenting function of HLA-B27 to include ideas based on aberrant aspects of its immunobiology.[5,22,71,72] For example, HLA-B27 molecules folds slowly and also has a tendency to misfold in the endoplasmic reticulum and lead to pathogenic immune responses. An excess of misfolded B27 proteins in the endoplasmic reticulum may activate an unfolded protein response that can trigger inflammation. In a rat model of SpA, an activation of the unfolded protein response in macrophages has been reported to correlate with the inflammatory disease.[72]

HLA-B27 can also form covalent heavy chain homodimers on the cell surface that are amenable to recognition by leukocyte receptors, and that might result in disease through immunomodulation of both innate and adaptive responses to arthritogenic pathogens.[80] CD4+ T-cells have been isolated from 3 HLA-B27 positive patients with AS that interact with HLA-B27, but are not present in B27 positive healthy individuals, thus breaking the conventional rules of MHC restriction.[81] These CD4+ T-cells appear to recognize non-conventional forms of HLA-B27, specifically B27 heavy chain homodimers that might mimic MHC class II molecules. It is possible that continual interaction between the two could trigger off T-cell effector functions that may initiate the disease process. In conclusion, the precise explanation of the role of HLA-B27 in disease causation has thus far eluded everybody; this may be because HLA-B27 may not work through one mechanism in every case. If this is so and one looks for an answer that will explain every case, then one will have a problem.[19]

ADDITIONAL DISEASE PREDISPOSING GENES BESIDES HLA-B27

A: Within MHC

HLA-B60 (*B*4001*) has been reported to increase the risk for AS three-fold, independent of HLA-B27 status, but there is no clear explanation for this effect.[82-84] Association of another HLA Class I molecule HLA-B*1403 with AS has been reported from Togo, a West African nation. It is of interest that HLA-B*1403 shows the B27 "supertype" motif, and it has been suggested that it may exert an effect on AS susceptibility according to the arthritogenic peptide model.[40] There is strong evidence, however, that HLA-B27 itself rather than B27-related class I haplotypes contributes to AS susceptibility.[85]

B: Non-MHC Genetic Contribution

More than 90 percent of the risk of developing AS is determined genetically, and recent studies, including linkage analyzes as well as candidate gene and genome-wide association studies, indicate prominent non-MHC genetic contribution,[86-88] and that multiple genes interact with nongenetic (environmental) factors to lead to immune-mediated mechanisms that result in the release of proinflammatory cytokines such as TNF-α, and contribute to disease occurrence. For example, the gene for the interleukin-23 receptor (IL-23R), which is located on chromosome 1p31.3 has recently been found to contribute roughly 9 percent of the population-attributable genetic risk for AS in Caucasians.[87,89]

IL-23R is a key factor in the regulation of a newly defined proinflammatory effector T-cell subset, Th17 cells, and interestingly IL-23 is selectively over-expressed in subclinical intestinal inflammation sites in patients with AS at levels similar to those seen in patients with Crohn's disease. Sequence variants in the IL-23R gene and its ligand have also been found to play a role in psoriasis. Successful treatment of Crohn's disease and psoriasis has been reported with a human anti-IL-12p40 monoclonal antibody ustekinumab, which blocks both IL-12 and IL-23, as these cytokines share the IL-12p40 chain.[90,91] Altogether, these recent findings indicate that genes participating in IL-23 signaling may be playing a prominent role in the pathogenesis of the chronic epithelial inflammation observed in AS, Crohn's disease, and psoriasis.

Another gene, ERAP1 (also called ARTS1 and ERAAP), which is located on chromosome 5q15 and encodes a transmembrane aminopeptidase with diverse immunologic functions and is located on chromosome 5, shows a strong association with AS, contributing roughly 23 percent of the population-attributable genetic risk for AS among Caucasian populations.[87,88,92] ERAP1 is involved in trimming peptides to the optimal length in the endoplasmic reticulum for presentation by MHC class I proteins, and that includes HLA-B27. It also cleaves cell surface receptors for the proinflammatory cytokines IL-1 (IL-1R2), IL-6 (IL-6R-α), and TNF (TNFR1), thereby downregulating their signaling. It is possible that genetic variants of ERAP1 could have proinflammatory effects through this mechanism.

Several variations (polymorphisms) in one of the members of the IL-1 gene (clustered on chromosome 2q12.1), IL1A have been found to influence the risk of AS.[93] Each of these variations changes a single protein building block (amino acid) in interleukin-1 alpha. It is an important modulator of the Th1 response but it is unclear how these variations contribute roughly 5 percent of the population-attributable genetic risk for AS among Caucasian populations.

Thus, the population-attributable genetic risks for HLA-B27 (40%), ERAP1 (23%), IL23R (9%), and IL1A (5%) add up, and there are ongoing genome-wide association studies of larger number of AS patients to find additional genes.[87,88] There are also functional studies underway of these candidate genes that have thus far been identified to better understand the pathogenesis of AS and related SpA and provide insight into potential new therapeutic approaches and/or disease prevention.

Regions on some of the other chromosomes are also being studied to see if they harbor additional susceptibility or severity genes that contribute to AS and its extra-articular manifestations.[94] Recent studies of chromosome 9q31-34 region has lead to the identification within SPA2 locus of a haplotype located near to TNFSF15, one of the major candidate genes in this region, that is strongly associated with predisposition to SpA.[86]

Non-genetic (Environmental) Triggers

Among the possible environmental triggers for AS onset, infections have long been suspected. It has been speculated that AS may be triggered by gut infection with *Klebsiella* bacteria. However, the evidence is circumstantial, based on the observation by some, but not all, investigators of elevated levels of antibodies against *Klebsiella pneumoniae* in the blood of patients with active disease. More convincing proof has been lacking. Thus, the environmental triggers for AS remain unknown, but the close relationships between AS and psoriasis and clinical and asymptomatic forms of Crohn's disease suggest the potential involvement of an immune reaction in the gut or skin that may be influenced by reactions to microbial infections. In many patients with reactive arthritis enteric infections with certain Gram-negative microbes (such as *Salmonella*, *Yersinia*, *Shigella*, and *Campylobacter*) as well as genitourinary infections with *Chlamydia*, which is often occult, are the triggering factors.[28,75] Moreover, in some patients with chronic undifferentiated SpA, chlamydial infection, may also be playing a role.[32]

Disease Heterogeneity

Heterogeneity of AS has been known for more than 31 years; it was first exemplified by the difference between HLA-B27-positive and HLA-B27-negative patients.[8-14] Although there are many similarities, HLA-B27-negative AS is later in its onset; is significantly less often complicated by acute anterior uveitis and more frequently accompanied by psoriasis, ulcerative colitis, and Crohn's disease; and it less often shows familial aggregation.[8,12,95-97] In fact, it is unusual to observe families among people of northern European extraction with two or more first-degree relatives affected with HLA-B27-negative AS in the absence of psoriasis, ulcerative colitis, or Crohn's disease in the family. A recent genetic study supports the existence of an HLA-B27-independent common link between gut inflammation and AS.[98] It is now well established that there are multiple genes involved in predisposing to AS and related SpA, and there is also heterogeneity of potential triggering factors (clearly established for many patients with reactive arthritis). These factors therefore can account for disease heterogeneity at the individual level and also account for worldwide racial, ethnic, and regional differences.[99,100]

REFERENCES

1. Brewerton DA, Hart FD, Nicholls A, Caffrey M, James DC, Sturrock RD. Ankylosing spondylitis and HL-A 27. Lancet 1973; Apr 28;1(7809): 904-7.
2. Schlosstein L, Terasaki PI, Bluestone R, Pearson CM. High association of an HL-A antigen, W27, with ankylosing spondylitis. N Engl J Med 1973; Apr 5;288(14):704-6.
3. Brewerton DA. Discovery: HLA and disease. Curr Opin Rheumatol. 2003;15(4):369–73.
4. Khan MA. Ankylosing Spondylitis. Oxford University Press, New York, 2009.
5. Khan MA. HLA-B27 and its pathogenic role. J Clin Rheumatol 2008; 14(1):50-2.
6. Khan MA. Patient-doctor. Ann Intern Med 2000;133: 233-5.
7. Taurog J. The mystery of HLA-B27: if it isn't one thing, it's another. Arthritis Rheum. 2007; 56(8):2478–81.
8. Khan MA, Kushner I, Braun WE. Comparison of clinical features of HLAB27 positive and negative patients with ankylosing spondylitis. Arthritis Rheum 1977; 20:909-12.
9. Khan MA, Braun WE, Kushner I, Grecek DE, Muir WA, Steinberg AG. HLAB27 in ankylosing spondylitis: Differences in frequency and relative risk in American Blacks and Caucasians. J Rheumatol 1977; 4(Suppl. 3): 39-43.
10. Khan MA. Racerelated differences in HLA association with ankylosing spondylitis and Reiter's disease in American Blacks and Whites. J Natl Med Assoc 1978; 70: 41-2.
11. Khan MA, Askari AD, Braun WE, Aponte CJ. Low association of HLAB27 with Reiter's syndrome in Blacks. Ann Intern Med 1979; 90: 202-3.
12. Khan MA, Kushner I, Braun WE. Genetic heterogeneity in primary ankylosing spondylitis. J Rheumatol. 1980; 7:383–6.
13. Mehra NK, Khan MA, Vaidya MC, Malaviya AN, Batta RK. HLA antigens in acute anterior uveitis and spondyloarthropathies in Asian Indians and their comparison with American Whites and Blacks. J Rheumatol 1983; 10: 981-4.
14. Khan MA. Ankylosing spondylitis and heterogeneity of HLAB27. Semin Arthritis Rheum 1988; 18: 134-41.
15. Khan MA. HLA-B27 and its subtypes in world populations. Curr Opin Rheumatol 1995; 7: 263-9.
16. Feltkamp TE, Khan MA, Lopez de Castro JA. The pathogenic role of HLA-B27. Immunology Today 1996; 17:5-7.
17. Khan MA. Spondyloarthropathies: Editorial overview. Curr Opin Rheumatol 1998; 10: 279-81.
18. Ball EJ, Khan MA. HLA-B27 polymorphism. Bone Joint Spine 2001, 68:378-82.
19. Khan MA and Ball EJ. Genetic aspects of ankylosing spondylitis. Best Pract Res Clin Rheumatol 2002; 16: 675-90.
20. Granfors K, Märker-Hermann E, De Keyser P, Khan MA, Veys EM, Yu DT. The cutting edge of spondyloarthropathy research in the millennium. Arthritis Rheum 2002;46:606-13.
21. Khan MA. Update on spondyloarthropathies. Ann Intern Med 2002;136:896-907.
22. Khan MA, Mathieu A, Sorrentino R, Akkoc N. The pathogenic role of HLA-B27 and its subtypes in ankylosing spondylitis. Autoimmunity Reviews 2007; 6(3):183-9.
23. Akkoc N, Khan MA. Epidemiology of ankylosing spondylitis and related spondyloarthropathies. In: Weisman MH, Reveille JD, van der Heijde D. (Eds.), Ankylosing Spondylitis and the Spondyloarthropathies: A Companion to Rheumatology. London, Mosby:-Elsevier: 2006;117-31.
24. Thorsby E, Kissmeyer-Nielsen: F. HL-A antigens and genes. III. Production of HL-A typing antisera of desired specificity. Vox Sang 1969; 17: 102-11.
25. Braun J, Sieper J. Ankylosing spondylitis. Lancet. 2007; Apr 21;369(9570):1379-90.
26. Khan MA. Ankylosing spondylitis and related Spondyloarthropathies. Spine: State of the Art Reviews, Philadelphia, Hanley and Belfus, Inc., September 1990.
27. Khan MA. Spondyloarthropathies. In Hunder G, ed. Atlas of Rheumatology, 4th ed. Philadelphia: Current Medicine 2005;151–80.
28. Khan MA, Sieper J. Reactive arthritis. In: Koopman WJ and Moreland LW (Editors). ARTHRITIS AND ALLIED CONDITIONS. (15th Edition), Lippincott Williams and Wilkins 2004;1335-55.
29. Zeidler H, Mau W, Khan MA. Unidifferentiated spondyloarthropathies. Rheum Dis Clin N Am 1992;18:187-202.
30. Kumar A, Bansal M, Srivastava DN, et al. Long-term outcome of unidifferentiated spondyloarthropathy. Rheumatol Int 2001; 20(6):221-4.
31. Munoz-Fernandez S, de Miguel ER, Cobo-Ibanez T, et al. Enthesis inflammation in recurrent acute anterior uveitis without spondylarthritis. Arthritis Rheum 2009 Jun 29;60(7):1985-90.
32. Carter JD, Gerard HC, Espinoza LR, et al. Chlamydiae as etiologic agents in chronic undifferentiated spondylarthritis. Arthritis Rheum 2009 May; 60(5): 1311-6.
33. Walsh B, Yocum D, Khan MA: Arthritis and HLA-B27 in North American tribes. Curr Opin Rheumatol 1998; 10: 319-325-34.
34. Khan MA. B27 and ankylosing spondylitis in different races. In Dawkins RL, Christiansen FT and Zilko PJ (Eds.): IMMUNOGENETICS IN RHEUMATOLOGY, Amsterdam, Excerpta Medica 1982;188-90.

35. Khan MA. Spondyloarthropathies in nonCaucasians. In Calin A (Ed.): SPONDYLARTHROPATHIES, New York, Grune and Stratton, 1984;265-77.
36. Khan MA. Spondyloarthropathies in nonCaucasian populations of the world. In: Ziff M, Cohen SB (Eds.): THE SPONDYLOARTHROPATHIES (ADVANCES IN INFLAMMATION RESEARCH, VOL. 9), New York, Raven Press, 1985;91-9.
37. Khan MA, Kushner I, Braun WE, Zachary AA, Steinberg AG. HLAB27 homozygosity in ankylosing spondylitis: relationship to risk and severity. Tissue Antigens 1978;11:434- 8.
38. Jaakkola E, Herzberg J, Laiho K, et al. Finnish HLA studies confirm the increased risk conferred by HLA-B27 homozygosity. Ann Rheum Dis 2006; 65: 775-80.
39. Mijiyawa M, Oniankitan O, Khan MA. Spondyloarthropathies in sub-Saharan Africa. Curr Opin Rheumatol 2000;12:281-6.
40. Lopez-Larrea C, Mijiyawa M, Gonzalez S, et al. Association of ankylosing spondylitis with HLA-B*1403 in a West African population. Arthritis Rheum 2002;46(11):2968-71.
41. Mathieu A, Cauli A, Fiorillo MT, Sorrentino R. HLA-B27 and ankylosing spondylitis geographic distribution as the result of a genetic selection induced by malaria endemic? A review supporting the hypothesis. Autoimmun Rev 2008;7(5):398-403.
42. Feldtkeller E, Khan MA, van der Linden S, van der Heijde D, Braun J. Age at disease onset and diagnosis delay in HLA-B27 negative vs. positive patients with ankylosing spondylitis. Rheumatol Int 2003; 23:61-6.
43. Khan MA. Ankylosing spondylitis: Clinical features. In: Hochberg M, Silman A, Smolen J, Weinblatt M, Weisman M (Editors). RHEUMATOLOGY, (3rd Edition). London, Mosby: A Division of Harcourt Health Sciences Ltd. 2003; 1161-81.
44. Khan MA, van der Linden SM, Kushner I, Valkenburg HA, Cats A. Spondylitic disease without radiological evidence of sacroiliitis in relatives of HLAB27 positive patients. Arthritis Rheum 1985; 28: 40-3.
45. Rudwaleit M, Khan MA, Sieper J. The challenge of diagnosis and classification in early ankylosing spondylitis: Do we need new criteria? Arthritis Rheum 2005; 52:1000-8.
46. Elyan M, Khan MA. Diagnosing ankylosing spondylitis. J Rheumatol Suppl 2006;78:12-23.
47. Rudwaleit M, van der Heijde D, Khan MA, Braun J, Sieper J. How to diagnose axial spondyloarthropathy early? Ann Rheum Dis 2004; 63:535-43.
48. Khan MA: Clinical application of HLAB27 test in rheumatic diseases: A current perspective. Arch Intern Med 1980;140: 177-80.
49. Khan MA, Khan MK. Diagnostic value of HLAB27 testing in ankylosing spondylitis and Reiter's syndrome. Ann Intern Med 1982;96: 70-6.
50. Khan MA. How the B27 test can help in the diagnosis of spondyloarthropathies. In: Calin A (Ed.): SPONDYLARTHROPATHIES, New York, Grune and Stratton 1984;323-37.
51. Khan MA, Kushner I. Diagnosis of ankylosing spondylitis. In Cohen AS (Ed.): PROGRESS IN CLINICAL RHEUMATOLOGY, VOL. I, New York, Grune and Stratton 1984;145-78.
52. van der Linden SM, Khan MA. The risk of ankylosing spondyltis in HLAB27 positive individuals: A reappraisal. (Editorial) J Rheumatol 1984;11:727-8.
53. Chung YM, Liao HT, Lin KC, et al. Prevalence of spondyloarthritis in 504 Chinese patients with HLA-B27-associated acute anterior uveitis. Scand J Rheumatol 2009; 38(2):84-90.
54. Huhtinen M, Karma A. HLA-B27 typing in the categorization of uveitis in a HLA-B27 rich population. Brit J Ophthalmol 2000; 84(4):413-6.
55. Fernandez-Melon J, Munoz-Fernandez S, Hidalgo V, et al. Uveitis as the initial clinical manifestation in patients with spondyloarthropathies. J Rheumatol. 2004; 31(3): 524-7.
56. Robinson J, Waller MJ, Fail SC, et al. The IMGT/HLA database. Nucleic Acids Research 2009; 37:(Database issue):D1013-7.
57. Akkoc N, Khan MA. Etiopathogenic role of HLA-B27 alleles in ankylosing spondylitis. APLAR J Rheumatol 2005; 8: 146-53.
58. Garcia-Fernandez S, Gonzalez S, Mina Blanco A, et al. New insights regarding HLA-B27 diversity in the Asian population. Tissue Antigens 2001; 58(4):259-62.
59. Khan MA. Prevalence of HLA-B27 in world populations. In Lopez-Larrea C (Ed.): HLA-B27 in the development of spondyloarthropathies. Austin, Texas, RG Landes Company 1997;95-112.
60. Wu Z, Lin Z, Wei Q, Gu J. Clinical features of ankylosing spondylitis may correlate with HLA-B27 polymorphism. Rheumatol Int 2009;29(4):389-92.
61. López-Larrea C, Sujirachato K, Mehra NK, et al. HLA-B27 subtypes in Asian patients with ankylosing spondylitis. Evidence for new associations. Tissue Antigens 1995;45(3):169-76.
62. Gonzalez-Roces S, Alvarez MV, Gonzalez S, et al. HLA-B27 polymorphism and worldwide susceptibility to ankylosing spondylitis. Tissue Antigens 1997; 49(2): 116 -23.
63. Madden DR, Gorga JC, Strominger JL, Wiley DC. The three-dimensional mage of HLA-B27 at 2.1 A resolution suggests a general mechanism for tight peptide binding to MHC. Cell. 1992 Sep 18;70(6):1035-48.
64. Khan MA. Spondyloarthropathies: Editorial review. Curr Opin Rheumatol 1994; 6:351-3.
65. Brown MA, Jepson A, Young A, Whittle HC, Greenwood BM, Wordsworth BP. Ankylosing spondylitis in West Africans—evidence for a non-HLA-B27 protective effect. Ann Rheum Dis. 1997 Jan;56(1):68-70.
66. Belachew DA, Sandu N, Schaller B, Guta Z. Ankylosing spondylitis in sub-Saharan Africa. Postgrad Med J 2009;85(1005):353-7.

67. Nasution AR, Mardjuadi A, Kunmartini S, et al. HLA-B27 subtypes positively and negatively associated with spondyloarthropathy. J Rheumatol 1997; 24(6):1111-4.
68. Sudarsono D, Hadi S, Mardjuadi A et al. Evidence that HLA-B*2706 is not protective against spondyloarthropathy. J Rheumatol 1999; 26(7):1534-6.
69. Cauli A, Vacca A, Mameli A, et al. A Sardinian patient with ankylosing spondylitis and HLA-B*2709 co-occurring with HLA-B*1403. Arthritis Rheum 2007; 56(8):2807-9.
70. Olivieri I, D'Angelo S, Scarano E, Santospirito V, Padula A. The HLA-B*2709 subtype in a woman with early ankylosing spondylitis. Arthritis Rheum 2007; 56(8): 2805-7.
71. Lopez de Castro J. HLA-B27 and the pathogenesis of spondyloarthropathies. Immunol Lett 2007;108(1):27-33.
72. Colbert RA, DeLay ML, Layh-Schmitt G, Sowders DP. HLA-B27 misfolding and spondyloarthropathies. Prion 2009;3(1):15-26.
73. Dazert E, Neumann-Haefelin C, Bressanelli S, et al. Loss of viral fitness and cross-recognition by CD8+ T cells limit HCV escape from a protective HLA-B27-restricted human immune response. J Clin Invest 2009; 119(2):376-86.
74. Marcilla M, López de Castro JA. Peptides: the cornerstone of HLA-B27 biology and pathogenetic role in spondyloarthritis. Tissue Antigens 2008;71(6):495-506.
75. Cragnolini JJ, Garcia-Medel N, Lopez de Castro J. Endogenous processing and presentation of T-cell epitopes from chlamydia trachomatis with relevance in HLA-B27-associated reactive arthritis. Mol Cell Proteomics. 2009;8(8):1850-9.
76. Taurog JD, Dorris ML, Satumtira N, et al. Spondylarthritis in HLA-B27/human beta(2)-microglobulin-transgenic rats is not prevented by lack of CD8. Arthritis Rheum 2009; 60(7):1977-84.
77. Hülsmeyer M, Welfle K, Pöhlmann T, et al. Thermodynamic and structural equivalence of two HLA-B27 subtypes complexed with a self-peptide. J Mol Biol 2005;346(5):1367-79.
78. Fiorillo MT, Rückert C, Hülsmeyer M, et al. Allele-dependent similarity between viral and self-peptide presentation by HLA-B27 subtypes. J Biol Chem 2005;280(4):2962-71.
79. Beltrami A, Rossmann M, Fiorillo MT, et al. Citrullination-dependent differential presentation of a self-peptide by HLA-B27 subtypes. J Biol Chem 2008;283(40):27189-99.
80. Kollnberger S, Chan A, Sun MY, et al. Interaction of HLA-B27 homodimers with KIR3DL1 and KIR3DL2, unlike HLA-B27 heterotrimers, is independent of the sequence of bound peptide. Eur J Immunol 2007;37(5):1313-22.
81. Boyle LH, Goodall JC, Gaston JS. Major histocompatibility complex class I-restricted alloreactive CD4+ T cells. Immunology 2004;112(1):54-63.
82. Robinson WP, van der Linden SM, Khan MA, et al. HLABw60 increases susceptibility to ankylosing spondylitis in HLAB27 positive individuals. Arthritis Rheum 1989;32:1135-41.
83. Brown MA, Pile KD, Kennedy LG, et al. HLA class I associations of ankylosing spondylitis in the white population in the United Kingdom. Ann Rheum Dis 1996;55(4):268-70.
84. Wei JC, Tsai WC, Lin HS, Tsai CY, Chou CT. HLA-B60 and B61 are strongly associated with ankylosing spondylitis in HLA-B27-negative Taiwan Chinese patients. Rheumatology (Oxford) 2004;43(7):839-42.
85. Martinez-Borra J, Gonzalez S, López-Vazquez A, et al. HLA-B27 alone rather than B27-related class I haplotypes contributes to ankylosing spondylitis susceptibility. Hum Immunol 2000;61(2):131-9.
86. Zinovieva E, Bourgain C, Kadi A, et al. Comprehensive linkage and association analyses identify haplotype, near to the TNFSF15 gene, significantly associated with spondyloarthritis. PLoS Genet 2009; 5(6): e1000528.
87. Brown MA. Breakthroughs in genetic studies of ankylosing spondylitis. Rheumatology (Oxford) 2008;47(2):132-37.
88. Wellcome Trust Case Control Consortium, et al. Association scan of 14,500 nonsynonymous SNPs in four diseases identifies autoimmunity variants. Nat Genet 2007;39(11):1329-37.
89. Rahman P, Inman RD, Gladman DD, Reeve JP, Peddle L, Maksymowych WP. Association of interleukin-23 receptor variants with ankylosing spondylitis. Arthritis Rheum 2008;58(4):1020-5.
90. Papp KA, Langley RG, Lebwohl M, et al. Efficacy and safety of ustekinumab, a human interleukin-12/23 monoclonal antibody, in patients with psoriasis: 52-week results from a randomised, double-blind, placebo-controlled trial (PHOENIX 2). Lancet 2008;371(9625): 1675-84.
91. Sandborn WJ, Feagan BG, Fedorak RN, et al. A Randomized Trial of Ustekinumab, a human Interleukin-12/23 monoclonal antibody, in patients with moderate to severe Crohn's disease. Gastroenterology 2008; 135(4):1130-41.
92. Maksymowych WP, Inman RD, Gladman DD, Reeve JP, Pope A, Rahman P. Association of a specific ERAP1/ARTS1 haplotype with disease susceptibility in ankylosing spondylitis. Arthritis Rheum 2009;60(5): 1317-23.
93. Sims AM, Timms AE, Bruges-Armas J, et al. Prospective meta-analysis of IL-1 gene complex polymorphisms confirms associations with ankylosing spondylitis. Ann Rheum Dis 2008;67(9):1305-9.
94. Martin TM, Zhang G, Luo J, et al. A locus on chromosome 9p predisposes to a specific disease manifestation, acute anterior uveitis, in ankylosing spondylitis, a genetically complex, multisystem, inflammatory disease. Arthritis Rheum 2005; 52:269-74.
95. Reynolds TL, Khan MA, van der Linden S, Cleveland RP. Differences in HLAB27 positive and negative patients with ankylosing spondylitis: Study of clinical disease activity and levels of serum IgA, Creactive protein, and haptoglobin. Ann Rheum Dis 1991;50:154-7.

96. Khan MA, Kushner I, Braun WE. Genetic heterogeneity in primary ankylosing spondylitis. J Rheumatol 1980;7:383-6.
97. Belachew DA, Sandu N, Schaller B, Guta Z. Postgrad Med J 2009;85(1005):353-7.
98. Thjodleifsson B, Geirsson AJ, Björnsson S, Bjarnason I. A common genetic background for inflammatory bowel disease and ankylosing spondylitis: A genealogic study in Iceland. Arthritis Rheum 2007;56(8):2633–9.
99. Khan MA. Heterogeneity and a wider spectrum of ankylosing spondylitis and related disorders. In Lipsky PE and Taurog JD (Eds.): HLAB27+ Spondyloarthropathies, New York, Elsevier 1991;133-43.
100. Végvári A, Szabó Z, Szántó S, Glant TT, Mikecz K, Szekanecz Z. The genetic background of ankylosing spondylitis. Joint Bone Spine. 2009 Jun 19. [Epub ahead of print]

Chapter

17

Immunogenetics of Rheumatoid Arthritis

Veena Taneja

INTRODUCTION

Rheumatoid arthritis (RA) is a chronic disease characterized by inflammation of the synovial joints leading to joint damage and disability. It has a worldwide distribution affecting approximately 1 percent of the population. It occurs two to three times more often in women than in men with about 70 percent of patients being women. It is denoted as an autoimmune disease, largely based on the presence of autoantibodies like rheumatoid factor (RF) and anti-cyclic citrullinated antibodies (ACPAs). Even though a lot of research has been done, pathogenesis of RA has not been fully elucidated. There is no known causative antigen that can lead to development of arthritis. It is considered a multifactorial disease that involves both genetic and environmental factors in predisposition. Genetic studies have estimated that 50 percent of risk of developing arthritis is due to genetic factors while the remaining is contributed by environmental factors. A strong genetic component is suggested by familial aggregation of disease and presence of autoantibodies in relatives of patients. The role of genetics in susceptibility to RA is strengthened by studies in twins. The MZ concordance rate for RA is four times greater than the dizygotic twin concordance rate, indicating a heritability of 40-60 percent.[1-3] Overall, the concordance rate for MZ twins is 12-15 percent suggesting a role of genetic and non-genetic factors.[4] Defining role of the genetic factors might explain pathogenesis of disease.

Population studies have shown that predisposition to autoimmune diseases is associated with few haplotypes only. However, these haplotypes are prevalent in general population suggesting that these haplotypes have been selected during evolution as they provide an advantage for clearing infections. Unfortunately these HLA class II alleles can positively select autoreactive T cells that can initiate autoimmunity.

MHC AND RHEUMATOID ARTHRITIS

Among genetic factors, major histocompatibility complex (MHC) is the region of the genome that has been consistently shown to be associated with disease. The MHC in humans is located on the short arm of chromosome 6, 6p21.3. The classical MHC genes are categorized as class I, class II and class III. Full details on MHC have been described in this book. The classical class I products include Human Leukocyte Antigen (HLA) – A, –B and –C molecules while classical class II includes HLA-DR and DQ molecules. The MHC gene complex is associated with most, if not all, of the common autoimmune conditions. The hallmark of MHC molecules is its remarkable polymorphism, which dictates the immune response to specific antigens. Education of the immune system in thymus teaches discrimination between self and non-self to ensure that an immune response is mounted against foreign antigen and not self. In the thymus, T cells are selected on the basis of their affinity and interaction with self-MHC molecules expressed in the thymus. Thus HLA molecules play a critical role in shaping T cell repertoire in the thymus by presenting self-peptides. However, not all self-antigens are expressed in the thymus, thus T cells specific for some self antigens can escape negative selection.

Population studies have shown that predisposition to almost all human autoimmune diseases is linked to HLA genes, primarily the class II genes. Despite a number of studies demonstrating an association of class II molecules with various autoimmune diseases, the mechanisms to explain these associations remains obscure. Since autoimmune diseases are generally heterogeneous, different mechanisms have been hypothesized to explain association with diseases; that implicate HLA molecule itself by virtue of its role in generation of immune response or as secondary molecule.[5] Other mechanisms by which HLA molecules could facilitate the development of some diseases is by influencing the T cell repertoire[6] or forming the basis for selection of T cell repertoire in the thymus.[7] The major problem has been the linkage disequilibrium of HLA class II alleles, DR and DQ, which makes it difficult to interpret the association of a disease with an allele. In humans it is difficult to dissect the mechanism due to following reasons (1) autoantigens are not defined, (2) frequency of autoreactive cells may be small, and (3) genetic variability makes it difficult to interpret the results.

HLA-DR Association with Rheumatoid Arthritis

Predisposition to Rheumatoid Arthritis has been linked to the major histocompatibility complex (MHC) class II HLA-DRB1 locus. Stastny in 1978 first reported an association of predisposition to RA with an HLA antigens, then called HLA-DW4.[8] HLA-DR4 has many alleles but only a few are associated with RA and some are protective (Fig. 17.1). Among the HLA-DR4 genes, DRB1*0401 (Dw4), DRB1*0404/0408 (Dw14), and DRB1*0405 (Dw15) alleles confer genetic predisposition to RA while DRB1*0402 (Dw10) does not.[9,10] Further, studies in certain ethnic populations showed that alleles other than DR4, notably DRB1*0101, *0102, *1402 and *1001, are associated with predisposition to RA.[11-13] The RA association with HLA alleles varies greatly in different ethnic groups. For example, while the Caucasians show a predominant association of *0401 and *0404 with RA, it is DRB1*0405 that shows the strongest association in Japanese and other Asian populations.[2] In the Indian population, all of these alleles, *0401, *0404, *0405 as well as *1001 have been found to be associated with susceptibility to develop RA;[13-15] however the relative risk of association with arthritis differs for all alleles (Fig. 17.2). As DR4 molecules mainly differ in the third hypervariable region (HV3), Gregerson and colleagues[16] proposed in their 'shared epitope' (SE) hypothesis that the amino acid motif Leu/Gly/Arg/Lys/Ala (L/Q/R or K/A) at position 67, 70, 71, and 74 of the

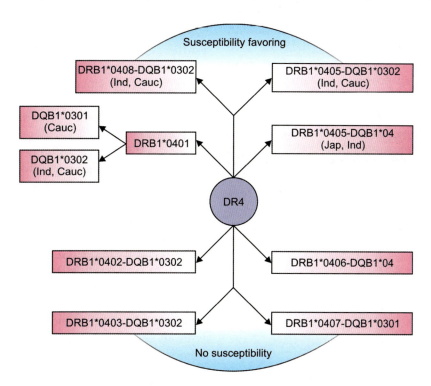

Fig. 17.1: DRB1*04 haplotypes predispose to develop rheumatoid arthritis in various populations. Not all of the known DRB1*04 subtypes favor susceptibility. Some of DRB1*04/DQB1 haplotypes have been associated with resistance to develop rheumatoid arthritis. Ind-Indian, Cau-Caucasian, Jap-Japanese

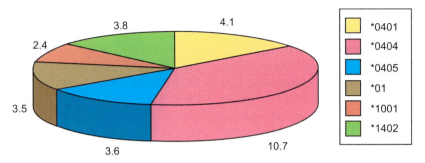

Fig. 17.2: Relative risk (RR) of developing rheumatoid arthritis in the presence of certain DRB1 alleles in multiple different groups including Caucasians, Asian Indians, Japanese, Chinese and Tlingit. Numbers indicate RR values

(hyper variable region) HVR3 of RA associated DRB1 alleles is the molecular basis for RA predisposition. According to their hypothesis, the 3rd hypervariable region comprising residues 67-74 is shared among susceptibility alleles and is a critical region for the selection of RA relevant autoreactive T cells. Importantly, the sequence motif of I/D/E/A expressed at positions[67,70,71,74] (as expressed in DRB1*0402, *0103, *0803, *1102, *1302, *1502) confers resistance to RA (Table 17.1). Although the mechanisms by which alleles affect RA susceptibility is not understood, it is thought that since these residues constitute the antigen binding site, antigen presentation may be a likely scenario by which the DRB1 alleles confer susceptibility or resistance to arthritis development. However, since not all individuals carrying the SE develop arthritis, it argues against the presentation of an arthritogenic peptide as a possible mechanism. Recent studies have suggested that individuals carrying DRB1 alleles expressing the "DERRA" sequence are less likely to develop arthritis and have less severe disease compared to those with 'DERRA' negative DRB1 alleles.[17,18] Although the mechanism is unknown, it has been proposed that the DERRA motif is naturally processed by DQ molecules leading to a possible deletion of T cells in the thymus.[19] An alternative explanation could be due to an association with one or more MHC genes, as well as contribution of non-MHC genes in influencing susceptibility to develop arthritis.

The shared epitope hypothesis, however, may not account for all DR alleles being linked to RA. For example, association of RA patients with DRB1*0301 in the Arab populations and with DRB1*09 in the Chilean population, are exceptions to the shared epitope hypothesis.[20,21] Further, even though association with DRB1 alleles is significant in most populations, penetrance of the genotype is low since the frequency of DRB1*0401 is around 30 percent in the normal Caucasian population. Further, 30-40 percent of the RA patients do not carry SE-encoding HLA-DR alleles, thus suggesting that the presence of SE is not absolutely necessary for the disease to occur, even though it provides a higher relative risk of developing arthritis. Thus, another susceptibility gene or environmental factor may be involved. These requirements are further highlighted by a hierarchy in the strength of association of various DRB1 alleles. Heterozygosity of certain alleles provides much greater risk than homozygosity. For example, presence of DRB1*0401/*0404 in an individual provided a relative risk (RR) of 31 compared to RR = 18 for *0401 homozygosity. Further, the former genotype is associated with an earlier onset and severe disease compared to homozygosity for either of the alleles.[22, 23] Similarly, *0401/*0101 has been reported to occur with the highest frequency in the Indian population.[24] These studies led some researchers to investigate haplotypic (rather than allelic) associations with RA.

Table 17.1: Amino acid differences among HLA alleles and H2E alleles associated with susceptibility to arthritis

Alleles	Amino acid at position						RA/CIA Susceptibility
	67	70	71	72	73	74	
DRB1*							
0101	L	Q	R	R	A	A	Yes
0401	L	Q	K	R	A	A	Yes
0402	I	D	E	R	A	A	No
0404	L	Q	R	R	A	A	Yes
0803	I	D	L	R	A	L	No
1102	I	D	E	R	A	A	No
1302	I	D	E	R	A	A	No
1502	I	Q	A	R	A	A	?
Eβ							
Eβk	F	Q	K	R	A	E	Yes
Eβd	I	D	A	R	A	S	No
Eβs	F	Q	R	R	A	A	Yes

RA- rheumatoid arthritis, CIA- Collagen-induced arthritis

Shared Epitope and Autoantibodies

Recent studies have shown that the presence of anti-cyclic citrullinated peptide antibodies (ACPAs) is a sensitive diagnostic criterion with 95 percent specificity for RA.[25] The peptidyl arginine deiminase-dependent conversion of positively charged arginine to neutral charge citrulline is known to occur in every individual. The post-translational modification like citrullination helps to generate efficient immune response to clear the infection. However, presentation of citrullinated self-peptides can generate T and B cell response. The demonstration that the presence of ACPAs precede the onset of symptoms of RA and predict disease severity implies a pathogenic role for these autoantibodies.[26,27] The observed association between SE and the occurrence of ACPAs may be explained by the fact that *0401 can bind citrullinated peptides with higher affinity than the native peptides. Further, environmental factors like smoking have been associated with an increase in citrullination and presence of ACPAs in the SE positive patients.[28] Smoking and SE interaction increases the risk, which is multiplicative rather than additive when combined with other known factors like the presence of PTPN22 alleles.[3] It may be mentioned that ACPA-negative RA patients do not show these associations. These observations point towards a possible heterogeneity in RA and suggest that ACPA negative and positive patients may represent two different subtypes that otherwise satisfy the American College of Rheumatology (ACR) criteria for arthritis.

Haplotype Association in RA

HLA class II molecules have been shown to play a role in shaping the T cell repertoire in the thymus by providing self-peptides.[29] This is supported by the findings that naturally processed peptides presented by class II molecules are derived from endogenous class II molecules.[19,30] Binding studies have shown that RA associated DR alleles bind limited numbers of human CII peptides compared to HLA-DQ8 which binds multiple peptides.[31,32] This has generated an interest in the role of DQ molecules in predisposition to develop arthritis. HLA-DQ occurs in linkage disequilibrium with DR genes and thus is inherited enbloc as a haplotype.[33] The DQB1*0301 (DQ7) and DQB1*0302 (DQ8) genes are in linkage disequilibrium with DRB1*0401 (DR4) alleles. RA patients in India have been shown to carry predominantly the DQ8/DR4 haplotype, and not DQ7/DR4[24] in which occurs primarily in the Caucasian population and shown to be associated with disease severity.[34] These data support a role for HLA-DQ alleles in genetic predisposition to RA. While the shared epitope hypothesis suggests that RA associated DRB1 molecules may bind similar arthritogenic peptides, it does not explain the differences in disease severity between these subtypes[35] or the increased severity of RA manifestations in patients homozygous for the shared epitope.[36] On the other hand, if we consider a potential role of haplotype in the predisposition to rheumatoid arthritis, most of the above inconsistencies can be explained. Thus, the HLA class II contribution to RA predisposition may be the result of an interaction between HLA-DQ and HLA-DR molecules on both haplotypes carried by the same individual. Support for this hypothesis comes from studies with animal models using transgenic mice expressing DR and DQ molecules (discussed below).

Interaction between HLA class II molecules is required for predisposition to develop rheumatoid arthritis and final outcome of the extent of severity of arthritis.

Non-inherited Maternal Antigen in RA

Recently, it has become clear that rheumatoid arthritis patients who are negative for the HLA-DRB1 shared epitope have a very high probability of their mothers being positive for the shared epitope compared to controls.[18] During pregnancy, cells of the mother migrate to the fetus and induce life-long microchimerism in the offspring.[37] Similar maternal microchimerism has been demonstrated in mice for inducing neonatal B and T cell tolerance.[38,39] Thus, a HLA-DRB1*0401+ve mother can predispose a *0401 negative child to rheumatoid arthritis through the process of microchimerism. Similarly, a mother who carries the protective DRB1*0402 gene can also protect a DRB1*0401+ve offspring from developing arthritis via non-inherited maternal antigens (NIMA).[40] Large scale family studies in the Netherlands and England have confirmed these two observations. Indeed a beneficial NIMA affect has already been demonstrated in organ and bone marrow transplantation. Maternal cells have been known to survive in the offspring for upto 50 years, and exert their effect through a change in the T cell repertoire of the child. As opposed to this, the non-inherited paternal antigens (NIPA) have not been shown to have a role in influencing susceptibility to RA disease. However, due to heterogeneity of the observations, further studies are required to delineate this possibility.

NON-HLA GENETIC ASSOCIATIONS

The contribution of HLA genes towards RA susceptibility is estimated to be ~33 percent only[41] suggesting a possible role of other genes within or outside the HLA complex. Association studies in families have shown that a parent with 2 SE haplotypes transmits one of the haplotype preferentially than the other, suggesting susceptibility allele on the over-transmitted haplotype. However, the role of MHC genes other than the HLA genes is difficult to interpret due to their strong linkage with the DRB1 locus and this can certainly skew their distribution. Using microsattellite markers, several regions have been implicated in susceptibility to arthritis,[2,42] the most significant being a region telomeric to the tumor necrosis factor (TNF) locus. The other candidate gene PTPN22, located on chromosome 1 has been extensively studied and validated. Genome wide association studies (GWAS) using genotyping for single nucleotide polymorphisms (SNPs) of RA patients have confirmed an association of both DRB1 and PTPN22 with RA.[43] In some populations, genes at several other loci have been shown to have an association of RA.[44] These include TNF-α-induced protein3 (TNFAIp3), tumor necrosis factor associated factor 1 (TRAF-1), CTLA-4 gene and PADI4 gene that encodes for peptidyl arginine deiminase isotype 4.[45-47] Environmental factors have also been shown to play an important role along with genetic susceptibility. The most notable of them is smoking which is known to increase citrullination and in association with SE haplotype increases the relative risk of developing RA.

> The most significant association of HLA and PTPN22 with RA probably makes up a combined effect of approximately half of the genetic contribution. The other minor associations as described above, along with gene-environmental interactions, are part of the other half that needs investigation and may explain the disease susceptibility factors.

EXPERIMENTAL MODEL OF ARTHRITIS

In humans most of the genetic associations with rheumatoid arthritis are based on epidemiological data. Even though many candidate genes are known to predispose, it is difficult to delineate mechanism(s) by which these genes are associated with the disease. Experimental models provide an important tool to design studies towards defining the mechanisms of disease pathogenesis and delineate effects made by specific genes. The advantage of using animal models is that most of the factors like environment and genes can be manipulated and experiments can be done in controlled conditions.

In RA, several experimental models have been studied including induced models like Collagen-induced arthritis (CIA), Proteoglycan induced arthritis (PGIA), streptococcal induced arthritis and spontaneous models like DBA/1 and SKG (mice with a point mutation in zeta-associated protein of 70 kD) mice. Of these, the mouse model of Collagen induced arthritis has been studied in greater details. This review will focus on CIA as a model of autoimmune/inflammatory arthritis.

Collagen-induced Arthritis as Model of Rheumatoid Arthritis

Experimental arthritis that shares a number of clinical, hematological, serological, and radiographic features with RA in humans can be induced in rats,[48,49] mice[50,51] and non-human primates[52] with type II collagen (CII). Collagen induced arthritis appears to represent an experimental autoimmune disease dependent upon the immune response to a tissue restricted, sequestered, organ protein where the immune and autoimmune responses are under immunogenetic regulation. David and coworkers were the first to show that susceptibility to CIA is mapped to the H2-A loci.[51] Their studies further showed that MHC class II polymorphism in H2A loci (H2A^q and H2A^r) determined susceptibility to CIA suggesting an important role of MHC-restricted T cells in development of disease.[53] H2A of mouse is homologous to HLA-DQ while H2E is homologous to HLA-DR in humans. H2E polymorphism modulates arthritis in mice and these molecules share HVR3 sequences at the peptide binding region of SE DRB1 molecules (Fig. 17.3). These studies led to the thought that in humans HLA-DRB1 polymorphism might play a similar role.

The role of class II molecules in CIA was further confirmed when Dr David and his associates showed significant reduction in the incidence, and severity of arthritis by pretreatment with specific anti-class II antibodies (54). Similar to RA, CIA is a T and B cell dependent disease. CII specific CD4+ T cells have been reported to be fundamental in initiation and perpetuation of the disease[55,56] and are essential for transferring arthritis into SCID mice.[57] Further evidence is provided by the observations that treatment of CIA mice with either anti-TCR antibody[58] or anti-CD4 antibodies[59] abrogates disease. On the other hand, CII-reactive CD4+ T cells have been reported in some circumstances to protect against CIA.[60]

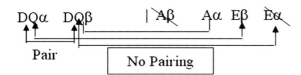

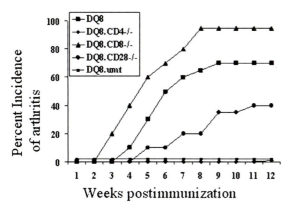

Fig. 17.3: Generation of HLA-DQ8. Aβo mice is described in reference 68. HLA-DQ8. Aβo mice express only DQ8 molecule on cell surface. The endogenous mouse class II chains do not pair with human DQalpha and DQbeta chains. Collagen induced arthritis in DQ8 mice and DQ8 mice deficient in CD4, CD8, CD28 and B cells (DQ8.umt) mice. All mice were immunized with type II collagen and monitored for onset and progression of arthritis. The graph shows the percent incidence and onset of arthritis in all strains suggesting role of CD4 and B cells in initiation and CD8 in regulation of arthritis

An extensive analysis of selective usage of T cell receptor Vβ genes has been done in CIA, thus implicating selective usage of T cell receptors in the susceptibility to an autoimmune disease similar to that shown in humans.[61] The findings of oligoclonal activated CD4+ T cells in the synovial fluid of affected joints suggests the involvement of CD4+ alpha/beta T cell receptor bearing class II restricted T cells in rheumatoid arthritis. This view is supported by the finding that partial elimination or inhibition of T cells by a variety of techniques can lead to amelioration of disease in certain patients. Using mouse strains with deletions in the T cell receptor Vβ genes, it was shown that specific T cell receptor Vβ genes may be involved in collagen induced arthritis[62] and the deletion of certain T cell receptor Vβ chains by mammary tumor virus (Mtv) antigens could also reduce the incidence of collagen induced arthritis.[63] Injection of monoclonal antibodies directed against the TCR alpha/beta framework in vivo prevented the onset of CIA.[64] The specificity of individual Vβ chains was confirmed by showing the prevention of CIA by treatment with anti-Vβ antibodies.

HLA Transgenic Mice as Model of RA

The CIA model has been extremely valuable in providing an insight into the immunobiology of autoimmune arthritis. However, since the immune response to an antigen in mouse model is restricted by the mouse major histocompatibility system, it is not applicable to human disease. The advent of transgenic mice expressing HLA genes has been greatly beneficial and their use in RA research has significantly advanced our understanding of the mechanism of association of MHC with disease. However, when only the alpha or beta chains from the human HLA-DR or DQ were introduced as transgenes in various strains of mice, no antigen-specific response could be generated. Soon it became clear that endogenous class II molecules were the major hurdle in deciphering the role of HLA in these animals. Consequently, mice with disrupted Aβ gene (Aβo) were successfully generated by Diane Mathis and Christophe Benoist.[65] The Aβo mice lacked expression of any functional endogenous class II molecules and had less than 2 percent of CD4+ T cells. Introduction of HLA transgenes in Aβo mice led to the expression of HLA molecules that could generate an antigen-specific response, suggesting that they were functional. The advantage of using HLA transgenic mice is that the T cell repertoire is selected by HLA transgenes in the thymus and hence the peripheral response to the antigen is restricted by HLA transgenes. In a comparison study, DR3. Aβo mice recognized only one epitope comprising of aa 1-20 for heat shock protein (hsp) 65 of mycobacterium tuberculosis which is similar to the epitope recognized by human DR3-restricted T cells.[66] T cells from HSP65 immunized HLA. DQ8. Aβo mice also responded to HSP65, but did not recognize the DR3-restricted peptide.[67] These results suggest that the MHC class II antigen processing pathways and peptide loading systems in transgenic mice can cooperate efficiently across the species barrier with human HLA molecules.

HLA transgenic mice can be used to define naturally processed epitopes for human T cells making them a useful model system to delineate relevant antigen and their presentation by MHC in disease. Knowledge of the pathogenic antigen is a crucial step towards finding a cure for arthritis.

HLA- DQ Transgenic Mice and CIA

Even though most studies have shown an association of shared epitope with RA, an association of HLA-DQ8 in the North Indian population suggested that DQ8 may play an important role in disease pathogenesis.[24] In order to understand the role of HLA-DQ molecules in RA, Aβo mice expressing RA susceptible HLA-DQ8 (DQB1*0302/DQA1*0301) and RA resistant HLA-DQ6 (DQB1*0601/DQA1*0103) were generated. The only class II molecules expressed in these mice is HLA-DQ molecules (Fig. 17.3). The HLA-DQ molecules were expressed on all antigen presenting cells. The CD4 T cells were restored in these mice and T cells expressing various T cell receptor Vβ's were either positively or negatively selected, similar to endogenous class II molecules, but unique for human HLA. The HLA-DQ8 and DQ6 transgenic mice were tested in the CIA model. Immunization with bovine type II collagen showed a moderate T cell response and antibody response in both strains. However, only DQ8 transgenic mice generated autoantibodies to mouse type II collagen and a pathogenic autoimmune CD4 mediated response leading to severe arthritis. About 75 percent of the HLA-DQ8 transgenic mice developed severe arthritis while about 15 percent of DQ6 transgenic mice developed mild arthritis.[68,69] The arthritic mice developed severe inflammation, swelling and joint deformity. Histologic examination of the arthritic hind limbs showed cellular infiltration, marked synovitis consisting of synovial cell hyperplasia and erosion of articular cartilage and subchondral bone. Thus, disease in these HLA-DQ mice was similar to the human linkage studies in RA. Double transgenic DQ8/DQ6 mice showed same incidence but a lower severity of the disease, similar to human patients who are heterozygous for the susceptible and resistant haplotype.[70] These experiments demonstrated that polymorphism in the DQB1 genes determines incidence, onset, and severity of collagen induced arthritis.

Development of arthritis in DQ8 mice requires the presence of both T as well as B cells (Fig. 17.3). Studies using DQ8 mice deficient in CD4, CD28 and CD8 suggested that CIA was mediated by CD4+T cells while CD8+ cells may be regulatory.[71] Interestingly, the DQ8 mice deficient in CD8 molecules developed much more severe disease than DQ8 mice and also produced rheumatoid factor and anti-nuclear antibodies (ANAs). Further, it was clear that costimulatory molecule CD28 is necessary for generating an optimal immune response as arthritis with late onset and milder disease was observed in DQ8 mice knocked out for CD28 compared to the parent DQ8 mice.[72] This was the first animal model in which the HLA transgenic mice were found to produce rheumatoid factor. These studies suggested that in humans, seropositive and seronegative RA could be related to the functional status of CD8 cells. In RA and CIA, B cells have generally been considered to be important for the production of autoantibodies. Our group generated DQ8. μ mt mice that lacked mature B cells due to disruption of the μ heavy chain transmembrane exon. Such mice were found to be resistant to develop arthritis.[73] Adoptive transfer of cells from parent mice to the B cell deficient mice and antigen presentation studies in these animals suggested that B cells are critical for antigen presentation and autoantibody production in CIA. A critical role of B cells is suggested in RA by the success of B cell depletion therapy. Thus, HLA transgenic mice have proved out to be an extremely valuable model system for providing important insights into the mechanism of RA pathogenesis.

> Even though most of the studies in humans have shown an association of HLA-DR4 with arthritis, studies using HLA-DQ transgenic mice suggest that DQ molecules play an important role in the predisposition to develop arthritis.

Structural studies have shown that DQ8 is an open molecule that can bind many peptides in various confirmations and probably can generate a high immune response. *In vitro* studies in DQ8 molecules showed that it can present multiple epitopes of type II collagen while CIA resistant DQ6 mice presented fewer epitopes.[74] On the other hand, DRB1*0401 can present one immunodominant peptide of CII. These studies suggest that DQ8 may actually predispose towards susceptibility to develop arthritis.

HLA-DR Transgenic Mice and Arthritis

As association of SE and RA is well established, we generated mice transgenic for RA associated DR alleles to determine the mechanism of such association. The first RA associated DR transgenic mice expressed a chimeric (human/mouse) DR1 molecule in the B10.M mouse.[75] This was followed by human/mouse chimeric molecule DRB1*0401/IE.B10M mice.[76] Inflammatory arthritis resembling rheumatoid arthritis can be induced in these DR1 and DR4 transgenic mice following immunization with CII.[75,76] An immunodominant epitope from human type II collagen was identified that was DR1 and DR4-restricted.[77] However, it was difficult to decipher the immune response in these mice because endogenous mouse class II molecules (IA^f) were also present, and those could shape the T cell repertoire. To overcome the problem of interaction of human DR molecules with mouse CD4 T cells, transgenic mice expressing DRB1*0401 and human CD4 were generated.[78] The major problem with these mice was the expression of hCD4 on all cell types. These mice developed arthritis only in a DBA/1 background.

We generated HLA-DR transgenic mice to determine the role of DRB1 polymorphism in RA. Mice lacking endogenous class II molecules, Aβo, but expressing, i) DR2 (DRB1*1502) a resistant gene in RA, ii) DR3 (DRB1*0301) a neutral gene in RA, or iii) DR4 (DRB1*0401) a susceptibility gene in RA were generated. Further, DRB1*1502 and DRB1*0401 mice were generated with both the DRB1 chain and E alpha chain as transgenes, which paired to form a DR molecule on the cell surface. The *0401 mice did not generate antigen specific response suggesting that they did not interact with the mouse CD4 molecules optimally. We also made an attempt to generate a functional HLA-DR4 transgenic mouse. For this the DR4 gene was altered at residues 110 and 139 by substituting asn for glycine and thr for lysine in order to resemble the mouse Eα gene for optimal interaction with the mouse CD4 molecule.[79] All mice expressed the transgene on the cell surface, and could positively select various Vβ T cell repertoire and thus generate an antigen-specific response. All mice were tested for CIA with the expectation that *0401 mice will develop arthritis. Surprisingly, none of the transgenic mice including Aβo.0401 mice developed arthritis. While it was expected for DR2 and DR3 transgenic mice, this was puzzling for those with a *0401 transgene. This lack of disease incidence in *0401 mice could be explained on the basis of two factors: (i) either the human DR4 molecule is not able to present many epitopes of CII as suggested by binding studies[31] or (ii) the Aβo.DR4 expresses the endogenous E alpha chain that could also pair with endogenous Eβ chain leading to expression of an H2E molecule. Indeed studies in mice have shown that H2E polymorphism is associated with protection from arthritis.[80] Thus the presence of endogenous chains made it difficult to interpret the results.

In their subsequent studies, Diane Mathis and Christophe Benoist generated knockout mice lacking all four of the classical murine MHC-II genes via a 80-kb deletion of the entire region.[81] To solve the problem of endogenous class II molecules, DRB1*0401 transgenic mice were generated in mice lacking all endogenous class II molecules (DR4.AEo). The only class II molecules expressed in these transgenic mice is HLA-DR4. The DR4.AE° mice developed normally and had no gross phenotypic abnormalities. The expression of DR4 in AEo mice was much higher than in Aβo mice. The CD4 to CD8 ratio was also comparable to other strains of mice together with the diverse T cell Vβ repertoire. Further, the expression of DR4 was normal in distribution. A major difference between the human class II molecules and mouse class II molecules is the expression of the former on T cells, especially activated T cells, while the mouse T cells do not express class II. The most significant observation in the DR4.AEo mice is the expression of DR molecules on 5-10 percent of CD3 cells, similar to that known in humans (Figs 17.4A to C). The level of expression is increased in activated T cells suggesting a role of class II positive T cells during inflammation.

HLA-DR4 Renders Sex-bias in Arthritis

Most of the current CIA models only reproduce a small segment of phenotype seen in human rheumatoid arthritis. Rheumatoid factors (RF) and anti-citrullinated peptide antibodies (ACPAs) are major manifestations in human RA, the mouse CIA models do not produce these autoantibodies. In addition, RA occurs predominantly in females while CIA occurs with similar incidence in both sexes. Induction of arthritis in DR4.AEo mice led to development of arthritis with female to male ratio of 3:1, similar to that reported for RA.[82] This sex-bias in arthritis was not observed in DQ8.AEo mice suggesting that HLA-DR4 renders sex-bias in arthritis (Fig. 17.4). Further, the arthritic mice produced ACPAs and RFs, IgG and IgM. Since a subset of CD4+ T cells is positive for the HLA transgene in AEo mice, we investigated if these CD4+ T cells are able to present the antigen. CD4+ T cells sorted from *0401 mice immunized with type II collagen or CII-derived peptide can present peptides but not the whole protein, suggesting that these T cells can not process the protein. The response was restricted by the DR molecule. These studies suggest that CD4+ T cells infiltrating the joint are able to present antigen locally, causing inflammation.

> DRB1*0401.AEo mice provide a better animal model to study arthritis as they mimic the major features of the human disease (a) in expressing class II molecules on CD4 T cells, (b) the activated CD4+ T cells can present peptides, and (c) develop autoimmunity in sex-biased manner (approximately 3F: 1M ratio) and produce autoantibodies, rheumatoid factor and ACPAs similar to RA.

Role of Shared Epitope in Arthritis

While, HLA-DRB1*0401 renders a person susceptible to develop arthritis, DRB1*0402 which differs by 3 amino acids in the 'P4 pocket' of the antigen binding groove is associated with resistance. To determine the mechanism by which *0402 gene provides protection against arthritis, our group generated transgenic mice lacking endogenous class II molecules but expressing DRB1*0402 gene, *0402.AEo mice. These mice do not develop CIA.[83] We decided to determine if a difference in antigen presentation was the reason for susceptibility/protection provided by the two subtypes of DR4. For the purpose, presentation of DR4-restricted CII-derived immunodominant peptide by *0401 and *0402 mice was investigated. While both molecules were found to bind the peptide, *0402 mice showed a very low response as compared to their *0401 counterparts. Further, *in vivo* and *in vitro* studies in *0402.AEo mice showed that the protection from arthritis in *0402 mice could be due to (i) negative selection of autoreactive cells in thymus, (ii)

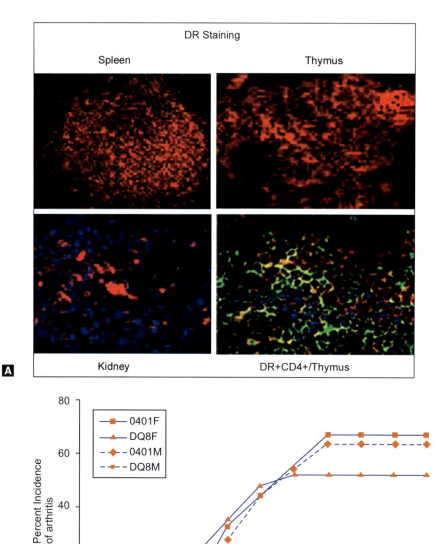

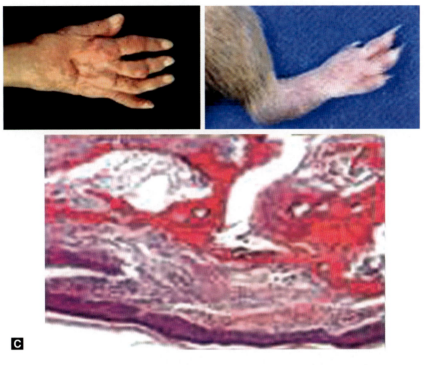

Figs 17.4A to C: (A) Expression of DR4 in various organs. Spleen, thymus, and kidney of DRB1*0401.AEo mice were studied by immunostaining with PE-conjugated anti-DR antibody and with DAPI. Thymus was also stained for CD4-PE and DR-FITC. Overlap of CD4 and DR staining showed some CD4+ cells positive for DR. (B) Incidence and onset of arthritis in male and female DRB1*0401.AEo mice show increased susceptibility and earlier onset in female DR4.AEo mice compared to males. DQ8.AEo mice do not show any sex-bias in CIA. (C) The phenotype and histopathology of arthritis in human and mouse show similarities. Right panel shows an arthritic paw, Hematoxylin and eosin staining of the section of paw of an arthritic DR4.AEo mouse shows infiltration of cells in the synovium and erosive arthritis in the digital joint. Left panel shows an arthritic hand

positive selection of T regulatory cells in thymus, (iii) generation of higher numbers of regulatory cells in the periphery that can suppress antigen-specific proliferation and lead to the production of anti-inflammatory cytokines like TGFβ and IL-10 and (iv) increased activation induced cell death. Indeed all of these factors together could be important for resistance to disease development.

The data with the DR transgenic mice demonstrating that genetic polymorphism of DR molecules modulates CIA, are similar to the studies conducted in the mouse CIA model. Based on these findings, a new hypothesis was proposed, suggesting that the 'shared epitope' shaped the T cell repertoire by serving as a self peptide for DQ molecules.[29] Thus high affinity DR-derived peptides binding to DQ molecules would negatively select an autoreactive T cell, while a low affinity DR-derived peptide would positively select the T cell. This hypothesis was tested *in vitro* by T cell proliferation to peptide 65-79 derived from RA-associated molecules, *0401 and *0404 and RA resistant *0402 molecule in the DQ8 mice. Observations from these studies suggested that HV3 peptides comprising of aa 65-79 derived from the non RA associated DRB1 molecules are highly immunogenic, while those derived from the RA associated DRB1 alleles fail to induce a DQ8 restricted T cell response (84). Intersetingly, *0401/DQ8 mice generated milder response to HVR3 peptide of *0401and a higher response to *0402 peptide. On the other hand, *0402/DQ8 mice did not generate an appreciate response to any peptide suggesting a possible deletion of self-reactive cells in the thymus (Fig. 17.5). This data suggested that presentation of self-derived peptide by the DQ molecule in thymus may delete self-reactive T cells in individuals with RA resistant haplotypes while RA susceptible haplotypes may select autoreactive cells due to low binding affinity. From these studies one can extrapolate that DRB1 polymorphism can modulate HLA-DQ mediated disease. Indirect support for this hypothesis comes from binding studies which show that DQ molecules bind multiple CII peptides compared to DR molecules.[31]

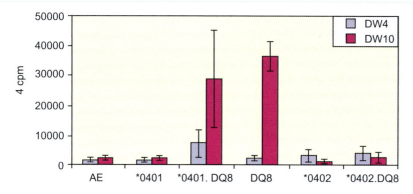

Fig. 17.5: T cell proliferation to self-peptides spanning 65-79 of *0401(DW4) and *0402 (DW10) in transgenic and control mice. The data shows that *0402 delete self-peptide reactive T cells in *0402/DQ8 mice while *0401 does not delete all cells generating response to DW4 peptide in *0401/DQ8 mice

This study shows that the protection from arthritis in *0402 mice could be due to (1) negative selection of autoreactive cells in thymus, (2) higher number of regulatory cells, (3) increased AICD and (4) low T cell proliferation and production of Th1 cytokines and TNF-α.

Interaction of Class II Molecules in Arthritis

In humans, the DR and DQ alleles occur as a haplotype and both may contribute to disease. Based on the *in vitro* results of presentation of DR-derived peptides by DQ8 molecule, we hypothesized that DQB1 polymorphism contributes to predisposition to arthritis while DRB1 polymorphism modulates disease. Thus interaction between DQ and DR may determine susceptibility/ protection to arthritis. To test this hypothesis, we introduced DR4 (DRB1*0401) gene into B10.RQB3 (H2-Aq) mice. The DR4/Aq mice were tested for susceptibility to CIA with porcine type II collagen since Aq are resistant to porcine induced CIA.[85] The *0401/H2Aq mice developed severe CIA with 65 percent incidence. This showed that the DR4 molecule can present porcine type II collagen to initiate the onset of the arthritis. These studies suggest that certain DR molecules can cause mild arthritis, but require H2-A or HLA-DQ for severe arthritis.

Since in humans two alleles of each loci are present, we proceeded to determine the epistatic modification by a protective allele. For the purpose, we generated mice expressing both DRB1*0401 and DRB1*0402 genes in H2Aq mice. Presence of *0402 delayed not only the onset but also caused reduced incidence of arthritis in *0401/ H2Aq mice, suggesting that protection is dominant. These studies are similar to humans where the presence of a susceptible and protective allele is generally low in patients. We further determined if DRB1 polymorphism could modulate DQ8-restricted arthritis by generating double transgenic DQ8/DR2 and DQ8/DR3 mice.[86] DQ8/ DR2 transgenic mice were resistant to CIA, suggesting that the DR2 molecule may actually function as a protective molecule, confirming some linkage data in the human RA. The incidence of arthritis in the DQ8/DR3 double transgenic mice was similar to that of DQ8 transgenic mice, suggesting the DR3 gene may be neutral and thus the presence of other factors may determine the final outcome.

These data clearly suggested that DRB1 polymorphism can modulate disease. In humans *0401 occurs in linkage with DQ8 and has been shown to occur with increased frequency in RA patients in certain ethnic groups. On the other hand, *0402/DQ8 is associated with resistance to arthritis. To simulate the human haplotype and understand interaction between DR and DQ molecules without the endogenous class II molecules of mouse, we generated DRB1*0401/DQ8.AEo and *0402/DQ8.AEo mice.[83] Our results showed that DRB1*0402 protects DQ8 mice from developing arthritis while *0401 is permissive (Fig. 17.6). Decreased incidence of arthritis in *0402.DQ8 mice is reminiscent of the model proposed for diabetes,[87] according to which MHC molecules provide dominant resistance to a given autoimmune disease by deleting the most pathogenic autoreactive T cells rather than all autoreactive T cells. Thus the reason that RA patients carrying *0402 are rare might be explained by the fact that most of the pathogenic autoreactive cells have been deleted in these individuals. Our observations showed that resistant mice have a higher number of regulatory T cells in the periphery as well as in the thymus compared to the susceptible mice. This suggests that MHC molecules are associated with protection by positively selecting T regulatory cells in thymus and deleting autoreactive T cells, while MHC susceptible alleles select lower number of regulatory cells. The regulatory cells in *0402/DQ8 resistant mice produced higher levels of anti-inflammatory

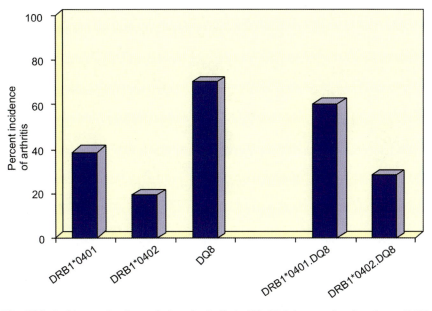

Fig. 17.6: Incidence of collagen-induced arthritis in AEo HLA transgenic mice shows *0402 is protective while *0401 is permissive for development of arthritis

cytokines like IL-10 and TGF and lower IL-23 and also suppressed antigen specific immune response as compared to the *0401/DQ8 mice.

Our studies suggest that both DR and DQ are involved in determining susceptibility/protection to disease. The transgenic mice expressing *0401 and DQ8 molecules and lacking complete endogenous molecules simulate the human haplotype and are a good model to study the mechanism of pathogenesis of RA. Further studies in these transgenic mice may help delineate the mechanism of HLA association with arthritis.

CONCLUDING REMARKS

Various *in vivo* and *in vitro* studies have shown that MHC and non-MHC genetic components are involved in influencing susceptibility/protection to rheumatoid arthritis and experimental arthritis. Thus polymorphism in MHC is an advantage for human survival. Evolutionarily only those HLA genes that can mount a strong immune response to infections, are selected. The constant mutations observed might lead to the generation of new subtypes of an allele to overcome autoimmunity. It is apparent that haplotypes, rather than single class II genes, function in the selection of T cell repertoire and expression of disease.

From studies with the HLA-DQ and DR transgenic mice, one can extrapolate that susceptibility to rheumatoid arthritis in humans is probably mediated by an additive effect, gene complementation, or interaction between DQ and DR molecules. Thus, self peptides derived from HLA molecules could potentially generate either tolerance or autoimmunity depending on their binding with the HLA molecule and affinity of interaction with T cell receptor. HLA molecules positively/negatively select T cells in thymus. RA susceptible alleles select autoreactive T cells while RA resistant alleles select T regulatory cells and delete autoreactive cells. An injury or constant infection can release self-antigens which when presented by RA susceptible haplotype can lead to the generation production of proinflammatory immune response, activation of NfkB pathway, increased survival of cells and pathogenesis. On the other hand, a RA resistant haplotype leads to an anti-inflammatory response to the same antigens, as most of the autoreactive cells are deleted in thymus, thus providing protection (Fig. 17.7). Transgenic mice expressing both DR and DQ molecule are an important tool to explore the mechanism of disease pathogenesis and successful treatment.

FUTURE DIRECTIONS

Rheumatoid arthritis is an autoimmune disorder with unknown etiology. The biggest challenge in finding a cure for arthritis is the identification of the initiating autoantigen(s). MHC class II association is the strongest genetic component in rheumatoid arthritis implying that autoantigen-specific T cells are important in pathogenesis

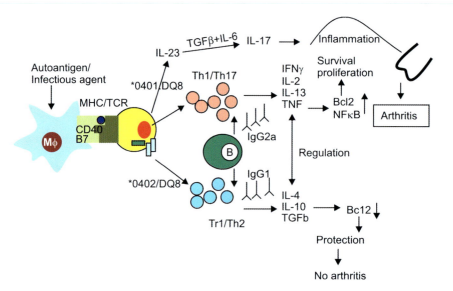

Fig. 17.7: A Scenario of HLA association with arthritis. In thymus *0401/DQ8 molecules positively select autoreactive positive cells while *0402/DQ8 molecules positively select T regulatory cells or delete autoreactive T cells. In the periphery, molecular mimicry or bystander effect after an infection or an injury can lead to the presentation of a self-peptide. In individuals carrying RA-susceptible alleles, it can lead to expansion of autoreactive T cells producing Th1 and Th17 cytokines and inflammation. The proinflammatory cytokines can activate NFkB pathway and BCl2 protein leading to hyperproliferation and increased survival of activated T cells. The autoreactive T cells and the inflammatory cytokines in the joint can lead to migration of other activated cells. HLA class II + CD4 T cells can also present peptides in the joint increasing the local immune response causing damage. In individuals with RA resistant HLA alleles, there is an increased selection of T regulatory cells that can control the autoreactive immune response leading to protection from disease

although the exact role of the MHC class II molecules is unknown. Transgenic mice expressing RA-associated HLA genes provide a biologically relevant situation to identify the autoantigens that could be involved in pathogenesis. No animal model can perfectly mimic the human disease but experimental animal models provide an opportunity to study the role of individual genes for genetic, environmental and pathogenic aspects of disease. Most of the studies are carried out to understand the mechanism of association for pathogenesis. Studies in CIA resistant *0402 and *0402/DQ8 mice can provide reasonably pertinent answers to the question as to how individuals carrying this haplotype are protected from arthritis. This will ultimately help to define the immunological pathway or identify cells that should be targeted for amelioration of RA disease.

RA is clinically heterogeneous disease. Understanding various predisposing factors in RA will help in prognosis and therapeutic strategies.

Despite considerable recent advances in the field, insight into pathogenesis of RA remains elusive. The transgenic mice that develop arthritis with clinical and histopathology features similar to RA may provide an insight into the mechanism of predisposition.

REFERENCES

1. Lawrence JS. The epidemiology and genetics of rheumatoid arthritis. Rheumatology 1969;2:1-36.
2. Newton JL, Harney SM, Wordsworth BP, Brown MA. A review of the MHC genetics of rheumatoid arthritis. Genes Immun 2004;5(3):151-7.
3. Pratt AG, Isaacs JD, Mattey DL. Current concepts in the pathogenesis of early rheumatoid arthritis. Best Pract Res Clin Rheumatol 2009;23(1):37-48.
4. Silman AJ, MacGregor AJ, Thomson W, Holligan S, Carthy D, Farhan A, et al. Twin concordance rates for rheumatoid arthritis: results from a nationwide study. Br J Rheumatol 1993;32(10):903-7.
5. Nelson JL, Hansen JA. Autoimmune diseases and HLA. Crit Rev Immunol 1990;10(4):307-28.
6. Mitchison NA. Specialization, tolerance, memory, competition, latency, and strife among T cells. Annu Rev Immunol 1992;10:1-12.
7. Moller E, Bohme J, Valugerdi MA, Ridderstad A, Olerup O. Speculations on mechanisms of HLA associations with autoimmune diseases and the specificity of "autoreactive" T lymphocytes. Immunol Rev 1990;118:5-19.
8. Stastny P. Association of the B-cell alloantigen DRw4 with rheumatoid arthritis. N Engl J Med 1978;298(16):869-71.
9. Wordsworth BP, Lanchbury JS, Sakkas LI, Welsh KI, Panayi GS, Bell JI. HLA-DR4 subtype frequencies in rheumatoid arthritis indicate that DRB1 is the major susceptibility locus within the HLA class II region. Proc Natl Acad Sci U S A 1989;86(24):10049-53.

10. Goldstein R, Arnett FC. The genetics of rheumatic disease in man. Rheum Dis Clin North Am 1987;13(3):487-510.
11. Willkens RF, Nepom GT, Marks CR, Nettles JW, Nepom BS. Association of HLA-Dw16 with rheumatoid arthritis in Yakima Indians. Further evidence for the "shared epitope" hypothesis. Arthritis Rheum 1991;34(1):43-7.
12. Yelamos J, Garcia-Lozano JR, Moreno I, Aguilera I, Gonzalez MF, Garcia A, et al. Association of HLA-DR4-Dw15 (DRB1*0405) and DR10 with rheumatoid arthritis in a Spanish population. Arthritis Rheum 1993;36(6):811-4.
13. Taneja V, Giphart MJ, Verduijn W, Naipal A, Malaviya AN, Mehra NK. Polymorphism of HLA-DRB, -DQA1, and -DQB1 in rheumatoid arthritis in Asian Indians: Association with DRB1*0405 and DRB1*1001. Hum Immunol 1996;46(1):35-41.
14. Taneja V, Mehra NK, Anand C, Malaviya AN. HLA-linked susceptibility to rheumatoid arthritis. A study of forty-one multicase families from northern India. Arthritis Rheum 1993;36(10):1380-6.
15. Taneja V, Mehra NK, Kailash S, Anand C, Malaviya AN. Protective & risk DR phenotypes in Asian Indian patients with rheumatoid arthritis. Indian J Med Res 1992;96:16-23.
16. Gregersen PK, Silver J, Winchester RJ. The shared epitope hypothesis. An approach to understanding the molecular genetics of susceptibility to rheumatoid arthritis. Arthritis Rheum 1987;30(11):1205-13.
17. Wagner U, Kaltenhauser S, Pierer M, Seidel W, Troltzsch M, Hantzschel H, et al. Prospective analysis of the impact of HLA-DR and -DQ on joint destruction in recent-onset rheumatoid arthritis. Rheumatology (Oxford) 2003;42(4):553-62.
18. Feitsma AL, van der Helm-van Mil AH, Huizinga TW, de Vries RR, Toes RE. Protection against rheumatoid arthritis by HLA: Nature and nurture. Ann Rheum Dis 2008;67 Suppl 3:iii61-3.
19. Snijders A, Elferink DG, Geluk A, van Der Zanden AL, Vos K, Schreuder GM, et al. An HLA-DRB1-derived peptide associated with protection against rheumatoid arthritis is naturally processed by human APCs. J Immunol 2001;166(8):4987-93.
20. Sattar MA, al-Saffar M, Guindi RT, Sugathan TN, Behbehani K. Association between HLA-DR antigens and rheumatoid arthritis in Arabs. Ann Rheum Dis 1990;49(3):147-9.
21. Massardo L, Jacobelli S, Rodriguez L, Rivero S, Gonzalez A, Marchetti R. Weak association between HLA-DR4 and rheumatoid arthritis in Chilean patients. Ann Rheum Dis 1990;49(5):290-2.
22. Wordsworth P, Pile KD, Buckely JD, Lanchbury JS, Ollier B, Lathrop M, et al. HLA heterozygosity contributes to susceptibility to rheumatoid arthritis. Am J Hum Genet 1992;51(3):585-91.
23. Hall FC, Weeks DE, Camilleri JP, Williams LA, Amos N, Darke C, et al. Influence of the HLA-DRB1 locus on susceptibility and severity in rheumatoid arthritis. Qjm 1996;89(11):821-9.
24. Taneja V, Mehra NK, Chandershekaran AN, Ahuja RK, Singh YN, Malaviya AN. HLA-DR4-DQw8, but not DR4-DQw7 haplotypes occur in Indian patients with rheumatoid arthritis. Rheumatol Int 1992;11(6):251-5.
25. Nishimura K, Sugiyama D, Kogata Y, Tsuji G, Nakazawa T, Kawano S, et al. Meta-analysis: Diagnostic accuracy of anti-cyclic citrullinated peptide antibody and rheumatoid factor for rheumatoid arthritis. Ann Intern Med 2007;146(11):797-808.
26. Nielen MM, van Schaardenburg D, Reesink HW, van de Stadt RJ, van der Horst-Bruinsma IE, de Koning MH, et al. Specific autoantibodies precede the symptoms of rheumatoid arthritis: A study of serial measurements in blood donors. Arthritis Rheum 2004;50(2):380-6.
27. Meyer O, Nicaise-Roland P, Santos MD, Labarre C, Dougados M, Goupille P, et al. Serial determination of cyclic citrullinated peptide autoantibodies predicted five-year radiological outcomes in a prospective cohort of patients with early rheumatoid arthritis. Arthritis Res Ther 2006;8(2):R40.
28. Klareskog L, Padyukov L, Lorentzen J, Alfredsson L. Mechanisms of disease: Genetic susceptibility and environmental triggers in the development of rheumatoid arthritis. Nat Clin Pract Rheumatol 2006;2(8):425-33.
29. Zanelli E, Gonzalez-Gay MA, David CS. Could HLA-DRB1 be the protective locus in rheumatoid arthritis? Immunol Today 1995;16(6):274-8.
30. Kirschmann DA, Duffin KL, Smith CE, Welply JK, Howard SC, Schwartz BD, et al. Naturally processed peptides from rheumatoid arthritis associated and non-associated HLA-DR alleles. J Immunol 1995;155(12):5655-62.
31. Matsushita S, Nishi T, Oiso M, Yamaoka K, Yone K, Kanai T, et al. HLA-DQ-binding peptide motifs. 1. Comparative binding analysis of type II collagen-derived peptides to DR and DQ molecules of rheumatoid arthritis-susceptible and non-susceptible haplotypes. Int Immunol 1996;8(5):757-64.
32. Krco CJ, Pawelski J, Harders J, McCormick D, Griffiths M, Luthra HS, et al. Characterization of the antigenic structure of human type II collagen. J Immunol 1996;156(8):2761-8.
33. Begovich AB, McClure GR, Suraj VC, Helmuth RC, Fildes N, Bugawan TL, et al. Polymorphism, recombination, and linkage disequilibrium within the HLA class II region. J Immunol 1992;148(1):249-58.
34. Lanchbury JS, Jaeger EE, Sansom DM, Hall MA, Wordsworth P, Stedeford J, et al. Strong primary selection for the Dw4 subtype of DR4 accounts for the HLA-DQw7 association with Felty's syndrome. Hum Immunol 1991;32(1):56-64.
35. Ploski R, Mellbye OJ, Ronningen KS, Forre O, Thorsby E. Seronegative and weakly seropositive rheumatoid arthritis differ from clearly seropositive rheumatoid

arthritis in HLA class II associations. J Rheumatol 1994; 21(8):1397-402.
36. Weyand CM, Hicok KC, Conn DL, Goronzy JJ. The influence of HLA-DRB1 genes on disease severity in rheumatoid arthritis. Ann Intern Med 1992;117(10): 801-6.
37. Lo YM, Lau TK, Chan LY, Leung TN, Chang AM. Quantitative analysis of the bidirectional fetomaternal transfer of nucleated cells and plasma DNA. Clin Chem 2000;46(9):1301-9.
38. Vernochet C, Caucheteux SM, Gendron MC, Wantyghem J, Kanellopoulos-Langevin C. Affinity-dependent alterations of mouse B cell development by noninherited maternal antigen. Biol Reprod 2005;72(2):460-9.
39. Andrassy J, Kusaka S, Jankowska-Gan E, Torrealba JR, Haynes LD, Marthaler BR, et al. Tolerance to noninherited maternal MHC antigens in mice. J Immunol 2003; 171(10):5554-61.
40. Feitsma AL, Worthington J, van der Helm-van Mil AH, Plant D, Thomson W, Ursum J, et al. Protective effect of noninherited maternal HLA-DR antigens on rheumatoid arthritis development. Proc Natl Acad Sci USA 2007; 104(50):19966-70.
41. Deighton CM, Walker DJ, Griffiths ID, Roberts DF. The contribution of HLA to rheumatoid arthritis. Clin Genet 1989;36(3):178-82.
42. Jawaheer D, Li W, Graham RR, Chen W, Damle A, Xiao X, et al. Dissecting the genetic complexity of the association between human leukocyte antigens and rheumatoid arthritis. Am J Hum Genet 2002;71(3):585-94.
43. Genome-wide association study of 14,000 cases of seven common diseases and 3,000 shared controls. Nature 2007;447(7145):661-78.
44. Kochi Y, Suzuki A, Yamada R, Yamamoto K. Genetics of rheumatoid arthritis: Underlying evidence of ethnic differences. J Autoimmun 2009;32(3-4):158-62.
45. Plenge RM, Cotsapas C, Davies L, Price AL, de Bakker PI, Maller J, et al. Two independent alleles at 6q23 associated with risk of rheumatoid arthritis. Nat Genet 2007;39(12):1477-82.
46. Han S, Li Y, Mao Y, Xie Y. Meta-analysis of the association of CTLA-4 exon-1 +49A/G polymorphism with rheumatoid arthritis. Hum Genet 2005;118(1):123-32.
47. Suzuki A, Yamada R, Chang X, Tokuhiro S, Sawada T, Suzuki M, et al. Functional haplotypes of PADI4, encoding citrullinating enzyme peptidylarginine deiminase 4, are associated with rheumatoid arthritis. Nat Genet 2003; 34(4):395-402.
48. Trentham DE, Townes AS, Kang AH. Autoimmunity to type II collagen an experimental model of arthritis. J Exp Med 1977;146(3):857-68.
49. Stuart JM, Cremer MA, Kang AH, Townes AS. Collagen-induced arthritis in rats. Evaluation of early immunologic events. Arthritis Rheum 1979;22(12):1344-51.
50. Courtenay JS, Dallman MJ, Dayan AD, Martin A, Mosedale B. Immunisation against heterologous type II collagen induces arthritis in mice. Nature 1980;283(5748): 666-8.

51. Wooley PH, Luthra HS, Stuart JM, David CS. Type II collagen-induced arthritis in mice. I. Major histocompatibility complex (I region) linkage and antibody correlates. J Exp Med 1981;154(3):688-700.
52. Gonnerman W, Cathcart E, Hayes K, Angello V, Lazzari A, Franzblau C. Anticollagen antibody specificity in arthritic nonhuman primates. Arthritis Rheum 1984; 27S:581.
53. Gonzalez-Gay MA, Zanelli E, Krco CJ, Nabozny GH, Hanson J, Griffiths MM, et al. Polymorphism of the MHC class II Eb gene determines the protection against collagen-induced arthritis. Immunogenetics 1995;42(1): 35-40.
54. Wooley PH, Luthra HS, Lafuse WP, Huse A, Stuart JM, David CS. Type II collagen-induced arthritis in mice. III. Suppression of arthritis by using monoclonal and polyclonal anti-Ia antisera. J Immunol 1985;134(4): 2366-74.
55. Mauri C, Chu CQ, Woodrow D, Mori L, Londei M. Treatment of a newly established transgenic model of chronic arthritis with nondepleting anti-CD4 monoclonal antibody. J Immunol 1997;159(10):5032-41.
56. Doncarli A, Stasiuk LM, Fournier C, Abehsira-Amar O. Conversion in vivo from an early dominant Th0/Th1 response to a Th2 phenotype during the development of collagen-induced arthritis. Eur J Immunol 1997;27(6): 1451-8.
57. Kadowaki KM, Matsuno H, Tsuji H, Tunru I. CD4+ T cells from collagen-induced arthritic mice are essential to transfer arthritis into severe combined immunodeficient mice. Clin Exp Immunol 1994;97(2):212-8.
58. Yoshino S, Cleland LG. Depletion of alpha/beta T cells by a monoclonal antibody against the alpha/beta T cell receptor suppresses established adjuvant arthritis, but not established collagen-induced arthritis in rats. J Exp Med 1992;175(4):907-15.
59. Chu CQ, Londei M. Induction of Th2 cytokines and control of collagen-induced arthritis by nondepleting anti-CD4 Abs. J Immunol 1996;157(6):2685-9.
60. Kakimoto K, Katsuki M, Hirofuji T, Iwata H, Koga T. Isolation of T cell line capable of protecting mice against collagen-induced arthritis. J Immunol 1988;140(1):78-83.
61. Banerjee S, Haqqi TM, Luthra HS, Stuart JM, David CS. Possible role of V beta T cell receptor genes in susceptibility to collagen-induced arthritis in mice. J Exp Med 1988;167(3):832-9.
62. Haqqi TM, Banerjee S, Jones WL, Anderson G, Behlke MA, Loh DY, et al. Identification of T-cell receptor V beta deletion mutant mouse strain AU/ssJ (H-2q) which is resistant to collagen-induced arthritis. Immunogenetics 1989;29(3):180-5.
63. Anderson GD, Banerjee S, Luthra HS, David CS. Role of Mls-1 locus and clonal deletion of T cells in susceptibility to collagen-induced arthritis in mice. J Immunol 1991; 147(4):1189-93.
64. Moder KG, Luthra HS, Kubo R, Griffiths M, David CS. Prevention of collagen induced arthritis in mice by treatment with an antibody directed against the T cell

receptor alpha beta framework. Autoimmunity 1992;11(4):219-24.
65. Cosgrove D, Gray D, Dierich A, Kaufman J, Lemeur M, Benoist C, et al. Mice lacking MHC class II molecules. Cell 1991;66(5):1051-66.
66. Geluk A, Taneja V, van Meijgaarden KE, Zanelli E, Abou-Zeid C, Thole JE, et al. Identification of HLA class II-restricted determinants of Mycobacterium tuberculosis-derived proteins by using HLA-transgenic, class II-deficient mice. Proc Natl Acad Sci U S A 1998;95(18):10797-802.
67. Geluk A, Taneja V, van Meijgaarden KE, de Vries RR, David CS, Ottenhoff TH. HLA-DR/DQ transgenic, class II deficient mice as a novel model to select for HSP T cell epitopes with immunotherapeutic or preventative vaccine potential. Biotherapy 1998;10(3):191-6.
68. Nabozny GH, Baisch JM, Cheng S, Cosgrove D, Griffiths MM, Luthra HS, et al. HLA-DQ8 transgenic mice are highly susceptible to collagen-induced arthritis: A novel model for human polyarthritis. J Exp Med 1996;183(1):27-37.
69. Bradley DS, Nabozny GH, Cheng S, Zhou P, Griffiths MM, Luthra HS, et al. HLA-DQB1 polymorphism determines incidence, onset, and severity of collagen-induced arthritis in transgenic mice. Implications in human rheumatoid arthritis. J Clin Invest 1997;100(9):2227-34.
70. Bradley DS, Das P, Griffiths MM, Luthra HS, David CS. HLA-DQ6/8 double transgenic mice develop auricular chondritis following type II collagen immunization: A model for human relapsing polychondritis. J Immunol 1998;161(9):5046-53.
71. Taneja V, Taneja N, Paisansinsup T, Behrens M, Griffiths M, Luthra H, et al. CD4 and CD8 T cells in susceptibility/protection to collagen-induced arthritis in HLA-DQ8-transgenic mice: Implications for rheumatoid arthritis. J Immunol 2002;168(11):5867-75.
72. Taneja V, Taneja N, Behrens M, Griffiths MM, Luthra HS, David CS. Requirement for CD28 may not be absolute for collagen-induced arthritis: Study with HLA-DQ8 transgenic mice. J Immunol 2005;174(2):1118-25.
73. Taneja V, Krco CJ, Behrens MD, Luthra HS, Griffiths MM, David CS. B cells are important as antigen presenting cells for induction of MHC-restricted arthritis in transgenic mice. Mol Immunol 2007;44(11):2988-96.
74. Krco CJ, Watanabe S, Harders J, Griffths MM, Luthra H, David CS. Identification of T cell determinants on human type II collagen recognized by HLA-DQ8 and HLA-DQ6 transgenic mice. J Immunol 1999;163(3):1661-5.
75. Rosloniec EF, Brand DD, Myers LK, Whittington KB, Gumanovskaya M, Zaller DM, et al. An HLA-DR1 transgene confers susceptibility to collagen-induced arthritis elicited with human type II collagen. J Exp Med 1997;185(6):1113-22.

76. Rosloniec EF, Brand DD, Myers LK, Esaki Y, Whittington KB, Zaller DM, et al. Induction of autoimmune arthritis in HLA-DR4 (DRB1*0401) transgenic mice by immunization with human and bovine type II collagen. J Immunol 1998;160(6):2573-8.
77. Rosloniec EF, Whittington KB, He X, Stuart JM, Kang AH. Collagen-induced arthritis mediated by HLA-DR1 (*0101) and HLA-DR4 (*0401). Am J Med Sci 2004;327(4):169-79.
78. Andersson EC, Hansen BE, Jacobsen H, Madsen LS, Andersen CB, Engberg J, et al. Definition of MHC and T cell receptor contacts in the HLA-DR4restricted immunodominant epitope in type II collagen and characterization of collagen-induced arthritis in HLA-DR4 and human CD4 transgenic mice. Proc Natl Acad Sci U S A 1998;95(13):7574-9.
79. Pan S, Trejo T, Hansen J, Smart M, David CS. HLA-DR4 (DRB1*0401) transgenic mice expressing an altered CD4-binding site: Specificity and magnitude of DR4-restricted T cell response. J Immunol 1998;161(6):2925-9.
80. Gonzalez-Gay MA, Nabozny GH, Bull MJ, Zanelli E, Douhan J, 3rd, Griffiths MM, et al. Protective role of major histocompatibility complex class II Ebd transgene on collagen-induced arthritis. J Exp Med 1994;180(4):1559-64.
81. Madsen L, Labrecque N, Engberg J, Dierich A, Svejgaard A, Benoist C, et al. Mice lacking all conventional MHC class II genes. Proc Natl Acad Sci USA 1999;96(18):10338-43.
82. Taneja V, Behrens M, Mangalam A, Griffiths MM, Luthra HS, David CS. New humanized HLA-DR4-transgenic mice that mimic the sex bias of rheumatoid arthritis. Arthritis Rheum 2007;56(1):69-78.
83. Taneja V, Behrens M, Basal E, Sparks J, Griffiths MM, Luthra H, et al. Delineating the role of the HLA-DR4 "shared epitope" in susceptibility versus resistance to develop arthritis. J Immunol 2008;181(4):2869-77.
84. Gonzalez-Gay MA, Zanelli E, Khare SD, Krco CJ, Zhou P, Inoko H, et al. Human leukocyte antigen-DRB1*1502 (DR2Dw12) transgene reduces incidence and severity of arthritis in mice. Hum Immunol 1996;50(1):54-60.
85. Pan S, Taneja V, Griffiths MM, Luthra H, David CS. Complementation between HLA-DR4 (DRB1*0401) and specific H2-A molecule in transgenic mice leads to collagen-induced arthritis. Hum Immunol 1999;60(9):816-25.
86. Taneja V, Griffiths MM, Luthra H, David CS. Modulation of HLA-DQ-restricted collagen-induced arthritis by HLA-DRB1 polymorphism. Int Immunol 1998;10(10):1449-57.
87. Schmidt D, Verdaguer J, Averill N, Santamaria P. A mechanism for the major histocompatibility complex-linked resistance to autoimmunity. J Exp Med 1997;186(7):1059-75.

Chapter 18

HLA Architecture of HIV Disease Pathogenesis

Xiaojiang Gao, Maureen P Martin, Mary Carrington

INTRODUCTION

Host genetic factors are believed to contribute to the remarkable inter-individual variation in response to human immunodeficiency virus (HIV) infection. Genetic variation, especially variation in genes encoding immunological components, is linked with the level of resistance to HIV infection among exposed individuals, as well as the rate of disease progression and the proficiency of viral transmission among HIV-infected individuals. Out of a dozen or so AIDS restriction genes that affect the natural history of HIV infection, *HLA* class I genes show the strongest association with HIV disease progression.[1,2] Genome wide association studies for genetic differences that influence individual variation in response to HIV-1 infection also point to *HLA* as the region most significantly associated with HIV-1 viral load control and AIDS progression.[3-5] *HLA* genes located on the short arm of chromosome 6 are the most polymorphic genes in the human genome. In the immune response against HIV infection, HLA proteins play important roles both in T-cell mediated adaptive immunity by presenting immunodominant HIV epitopes to cytotoxic T lymphocytes (CTL) and in natural killer (NK) cell mediated innate immunity by interacting with killer cell immunoglobulin-like receptors (KIR).[6] Interaction between HLA and HIV has led to the adaptation of HIV genes to the host *HLA* polymorphism, which may eventually change the established *HLA* associations at the population level.[7]

HLA polymorphism may impact many aspects of HIV/AIDS including HIV infection and transmission, selection pressure on HIV mutation, and HIV replication affecting the rate of progression to CD4+ T cell depletion (CD4 < 200) and AIDS-defining illnesses. This chapter will focus on *HLA* associations with AIDS progression that have been consistently confirmed in multiple cohort studies. We will consider *HLA* associations from several perspectives including the effects of *HLA* zygosity, individual *HLA* alleles, and HLA interactions with non-HLA factors, in particular, KIR. The *HLA* zygosity effect reflects the overall influence of *HLA* genotypes on AIDS pathogenesis and the fulfillment of the concept of overdominant selection believed to have driven *HLA* polymorphism in human populations.[8] Distinct HLA allotypes may mediate differential responses to HIV infection and have varied capacities to contain HIV replication. Detection of individual allele effects helps to specify critical peptide binding properties for specific HIV epitopes. Finally, class I *HLA* also regulates innate immunity through ligand binding with *KIR*. The effect of *HLA* and *KIR* compound genotypes provides an additional perspective of the influence of *HLA* on the host response to HIV infection.

Genetic associations with diseases are often complicated by statistical noise. A true disease association typically shows a consistent effect across cohort studies with adequate sample sizes and well-defined clinical information. Cohorts from the same ethnic group should exhibit the same allelic associations and cohorts from different ethnic groups are often associated with similar if not the same *HLA* alleles that share common features in peptide binding or other immunological functions. Therefore, *HLA* disease associations need to be replicated in distinct disease cohorts and validated in different populations. In this chapter we review the *HLA* associations with AIDS detected in multiple large cohorts of different racial origins.

HLA Heterozygote Advantage and Homozygote Disadvantage in AIDS Progression

It is generally believed that the extraordinary allelic diversity of *HLA* genes is driven and maintained by infectious pathogens interacting with the host *MHC*.[9,10] In this context the number of distinct HLA allotypes expressed on the cell surface is directly related to the capacity of the host to present a variety of antigens. An individual who is heterozygous at all three class I *HLA* loci expresses the maximum HLA diversity and is able to present a greater variety of viral peptides than an individual who is partially or fully homozygous. Theoretically, it may also take the virus a longer time to accumulate mutations to escape HLA surveillance in *HLA* heterozygous individuals than in homozygous individuals. If this model is correct, *HLA* homozygous individuals would be expected to progress more rapidly to AIDS than *HLA* heterozygous individuals after HIV infection.

We tested this hypothesis in a 1999, study of a cohort of 498 seroconverters (HIV-positive individuals with known dates of seroconversion) of different ethnic backgrounds (mainly European Americans and African Americans)[11] and updated the analysis recently with an enlarged cohort of 1,089 seroconverters. Survival and genetic association analyses showed a highly significant association of class I *HLA* zygosity with rate of progression to AIDS outcomes (CD4 < 200, onset of AIDS defining illness and AIDS related death). Individuals who are homozygous at any two or all three class I *HLA* loci progressed to AIDS significantly faster than individuals who are heterozygous at all three loci (Fig. 18.1). Individuals homozygous at only one locus showed an intermediate rate of progression compared to the other two groups. These results demonstrate that (a) All three class I loci, *HLA-A*, *-B* and *-C*, contribute separately to the zygosity effect since, homozygosity at any of the three loci showed more rapid progression to AIDS; (b) The homozygosity effect of any single class I *HLA* locus is enhanced when a second or third locus is also homozygous; (c) The *HLA* zygosity effect on AIDS progression is not confined to particular populations as it was detected in both European and African American cohorts. Similar results were also observed in a study of Dutch homosexual men infected with HIV-1 where *HLA-B* homozygosity showed a stronger association with an accelerated AIDS progression.[12] The same authors also reported a stronger homozygosity effect of *HLA-A* in a cohort of Rwandan heterosexual women infected with HIV-1.[12,13] In both the Dutch and the Rwandan cohorts,

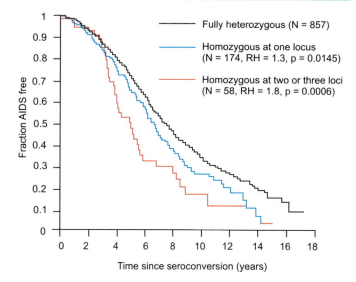

Fig. 18.1: Kaplan Meier survival analysis for class I HLA zygosity effect on progression to AIDS 1987 (the 1987 CDC definition of AIDS: HIV-positive and AIDS-defining illness or AIDS-related death) in 1,089 seroconverters that include multiple ethnic groups but mainly European and African Americans

however, *HLA-C* homozygosity did not show a significant effect on AIDS progression.

The *HLA* zygosity effect on AIDS progression is readily explained by its function of presenting antigenic peptides to modulate specific CTL responses against infection. A broader spectrum of viral epitopes that are recognized by HLA translates to a more efficient immune response against HIV infection. The observed heterozygote advantage in AIDS progression testifies to the notion that *HLA* polymorphism is maintained and driven by infectious diseases through balancing selection. Moreover, given the extremely rapid mutation rate of HIV-1,[14,15] it is more likely that the virus will escape recognition by common *HLA* alleles.[16,17] A study of the association of discrete *HLA* super types with HIV disease progression indicated that HIV adapts to the most frequent alleles in the population, providing a selective advantage for those individuals who express rare alleles.[7,18] Therefore, frequency-dependent selection favoring rare alleles may enhance the heterozygote advantage since rare alleles are more likely to be found in heterozygotes than in homozygotes.

Effect of Individual *HLA* Alleles on AIDS Progression

HLA genes encode allotypes with distinct peptide binding characteristics, which may result in varied immune responses and clinical consequences following

HIV infection. Therefore, a more direct approach to evaluate the influence of *HLA* on HIV/AIDS is to test individual *HLA* alleles. While the zygosity effect reflects the overall influence of *HLA* polymorphism, the effects of individual alleles correlate with specific immunogenetic traits interacting with different HIV epitopes. Several groups including our own have studied large cohorts for the effect of *HLA* allelic variation on HIV disease progression. Figure 18.2 illustrates a summary of the *HLA-B* alleles ranked from the most protective on the top to most susceptible at the bottom. Based on the effect on AIDS progression *HLA* alleles can be categorized into three groups: those associated with slower disease progression; those associated with more rapid progression and the majority of alleles showing no significant association. Three *HLA-B* alleles, *B*27*, *B*57* and *B*35*, have been repeatedly detected in independent studies as the alleles most significantly associated with AIDS progression. *B*27* and *B*57* show robust protection against AIDS progression whereas *B*35* (or *B*53* in Africans) confers a higher risk for more rapid disease progression. HLA-Bw4, a public epitope shared by members of HLA-B and -A molecules, was also found protective against AIDS progression even though it is not considered an independent allele.[19] These major *HLA* influences form the core of the *HLA* association with AIDS and have given impetus to numerous functional studies in an effort to explain the observed genetic associations. Other *HLA* associations are generally weak or inconsistent among different studies and there is very little known about the molecular basis of these 'minor' associations. However, those 'major' associations detected in survival analyses by no means represent the complete story of the *HLA* association with AIDS because some 'minor' *HLA* associations may only need a larger sample to boost their statistical significance; different analytical methods and cohort structures may also detect *HLA* associations that could not be seen by survival analyses with seroconverters.

HLA-B*27 Associated Protection against AIDS Progression

HLA-B*27 is well known for its high-risk association with autoimmune diseases. In HIV/AIDS, however, B*27 is protective and associates with slower progression to AIDS.[21-24] B*27 positive patients exhibit delayed progression to both CD4 < 200 and onset of an AIDS defining illness. Functional studies indicate that the protective effect of B*27 results from its recognition

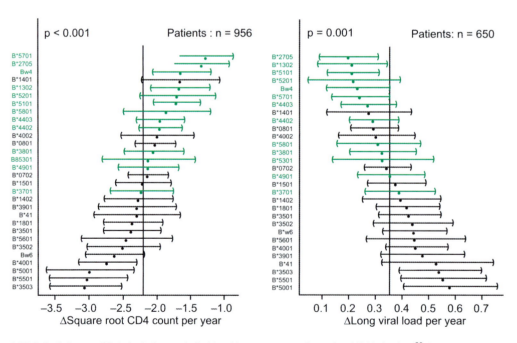

Fig. 18.2: Effect of *HLA-B* alleles on CD4 depletion and viral load increase over time after HIV infection.[20] Average change in the square root CD4 counts (left side) and log viral load measurements (right side) per year and 95 percent confidence intervals were determined using a linear mixed effects regression (LMER). *HLA-B* alleles that are most to least protective are listed from top to bottom, respectively. The vertical line in the middle of each plot represents the sample average and confidence intervals for alleles deviating significantly from this value do not cross the line. Alleles shown in green are *HLA-B Bw4+*, while those in black are *HLA-B Bw6+*

of an immunodominant HIV-1 Gag epitope KK10 (KRWIILGLNK p24$_{263-272}$).[25] Restriction of KK10 efficiently suppresses HIV replication and therefore delays disease progression. In fact most HLA class I molecules bind specific HIV epitopes and are able to contain the virus to an extent. What separates B*27 from most other HLA allotypes are some unique features in the B*27/KK10 interaction. The KK10 epitope in p24 Gag of HIV-1 is highly conserved and can tolerate very little variation. Mutation in the anchoring R$_{264}$ position of KK10 causes a severe defect in the ability of the virus to replicate.[26,27] A typical escape from B*27 surveillance is the result of clustered mutations of specific amino acids in specific positions both within the KK10 epitope and in adjacent locations. First, L$_{268}$ of KK10 needs to be replaced with a methionine (M), which serves as a prerequisite for the substitution of the anchoring R$_{264}$ for lysine (K). Mutations of the anchoring R$_{264}$ including the predominant R$_{264}$K dramatically compromises *in vitro* HIV replication[27] but the replication defect can be largely restored with an upstream S$_{173}$A mutation. Positions 173 and 264 are on the same planar surface of the folded p24 molecule even though they are quite far apart in the linear peptide sequence. The R$_{264}$K mutation of KK10 normally occurs rather late in the disease course, which explains the late but more lasting B*27 effect on resistance against AIDS progression. In our European American cohort, B*27 is predominantly the B*2705 subtype, whereas in African Americans, B*27 (B*2705) is only sporadically detected. There has been no clear evidence showing that the protective effect of B*27 is confined to particular B*27 subtypes.

Interestingly, HLA-B*27 shows a protective effect in other viral diseases as well. In hepatitis C it is associated with spontaneous viral clearance following acute HCV infection.[28] In Epstein-Barr virus related nasopharyngeal carcinoma (NPC) B*27 is associated with low risk for disease development.[29] The immunological basis of the B*27 protection in hepatitis C and NPC remains unknown but the apparently opposite clinical consequences in viral infections and autoimmune diseases may actually result from the same or similar mechanisms, in which the B*27-mediated response that contains viral replication in infectious diseases leads to tissue damage in autoimmune diseases.

HLA-B*57 Associated Protection against AIDS Progression

HLA-B*57 has been consistently associated with delayed progression to AIDS following HIV-1 infection. Large cohort studies have shown that B*57 confers the strongest and most consistent protection for AIDS progression among all HLA variants.[21,23,30-34] Genome-wide association studies also identified a B*5701-linked SNP in the HLA complex P5 (HCP5) gene as the strongest variant to associate with low HIV-1 viral load set point.[3] Survival analysis of seroconvertors detected a delayed progression to both CD4 <200 and the onset of AIDS-defining illness for individuals with B*5701.[22] In Caucasian HIV controllers B*5701 is the allele that is most consistently associated with long-term nonprogression.[35-37] In a small subset of HIV-infected individuals known as elite controllers (individuals who manage to contain HIV levels to less than 50 copies of the virus per ml plasma without treatment) 40 percent are positive for B*57 compared to 9 percent in non-controllers, which is about the same frequency as in the general population.[37]

Intensive efforts have been attempted to search for a functional explanation for the B*57-associated AIDS protection. It has been shown that the B*57 molecule is able to bind three immunodominant Gag epitopes: TW10 (TSTLQEQIAWp24$_{240-249}$), KF11 (KAFSPEVIPME p24$_{30-40}$), and ISW9 (ISPRTLNAW p24$_{147-155}$).[38,39] CTL responses to these highly conserved HIV epitopes can sufficiently maintain a low viral load. Viral escape mutations in these epitopes cause enormous viral constraints and compromise viral replication. Further, when HIV-1 escapes B*57 recognition and is transmitted to a B*57-negative individual, the B*57-imprinted TW10 mutants tend to revert to the wild type and the reversion is typically accompanied by a large increase in viral load.[39] There are two major B*57 subtypes: B*5701 in Europeans and B*5703 in Africans, which differ by two amino acids. They both bind the same Gag epitopes and can both efficiently contain viral load from the early stage of HIV infection even though they select mutually exclusive T-cell receptor (TCR) repertoires.[40]

In addition to its role in regulating the acquired immune response against HIV infection, B*57 also functions as a ligand for KIR and is therefore involved in NK-cell mediated innate immunity, which may enhance its protective effect on AIDS progression. Later in this chapter the HLA interaction with KIR and its influence on AIDS progression will be discussed.

HLA-B*35Px Associated Susceptibility to AIDS Progression

HLA-B*35 is among the first recognized HLA alleles that was found to be associated with AIDS[11, 32, 41-43] and so far it is the only HLA allele showing a consistent association with more rapid AIDS progression among a large number of other conflicting or unconfirmed associations. Our African American cohorts, however, did not show a B*35 susceptible effect as was shown in European Americans.[11] In a subsequent analysis of B*35 subtypes, we were able to solve the inconsistency and established the following: (1) The B*35 effect in Caucasians is subtype-dependent and can be entirely attributed to the less common subtypes of B*3502 and B*3503, but not the most common B*3501 (Fig.18.3). (2) Europeans and Africans have very different B*35 subtype distributions.[32] In Europeans, the neutral B*3501 accounts for about 55 percent of the B*35 gene frequency and the AIDS-related B*3502 and B*3503 account for ~45 percent. In African cohorts B*3501 is the predominant B*35 subtype found. B*3502 and B*3503 are only sporadically detected, which explains the lack of B*35 association with AIDS progression in this population. (3) Based on their peptide binding properties B*35 alleles can be divided into two groups, namely B*35Px and B*35PY, as shown in Table 18.1. All B*35 allotypes bind peptides with proline at the P2 anchor position but have different preferences for the carboxy-terminal P9 anchor[44, 45]. B*35PY (named for binding peptides with P at P2 and Y at P9), mainly composed of the common B*3501, prefers peptides with tyrosine (Y) at the P9 anchor whereas B*35Px (named for binding peptides with P at P2 and variable amino acids (x) at P9), mainly composed of B*3502, B*3503 and B*5301, a closely related African allotype, only accommodates small hydrophobic amino acids at the P9 position (B*3502, B*3503) or has no clear P9 preference (B*5301). In our AIDS cohorts B*35Px shows a consistent association with accelerated AIDS progression across races whereas B*35PY is neutral. (4) Minor variations in the class I MHC molecule can have a substantial impact on AIDS pathogenesis as exemplified by the single amino acid difference in position 116 between the AIDS-associated B*3503 (phenylalanine) and the neutral B*3501 (serine).[32] (5) The previously detected HLA-Cw*04 association with rapid AIDS progression[11]

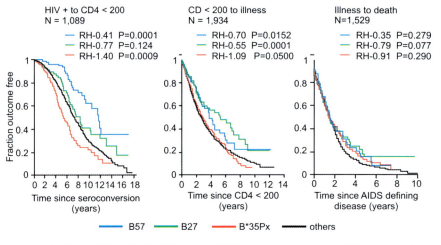

Fig. 18.3: Effect of HLA-B*27, B*35Px and B*57 on different stages of AIDS progression

Table 18.1: Variations of the peptide binding sites and peptide binding preferences of B*35 subtypes								
HLA Allele			Peptide binding site				Anchor residue	
	77	80	81	114	116	156	P2	P9
B*35Px								
B*3502	S	N	L	N	Y	L	P	L/V
B*3503	-	-	-	D	F	-	P	M/L
B*3504	-	-	-	-	-	-	P	L/V
B*5301	N	I	A	D	S	-	P	None
B*35PY								
B*3501	-	-	-	D	S	-	P	Y
B*3508	-	-	-	D	S	-	P	Y

can now be readily explained by its LD with both $B*35$ and $B*53$ since the $Cw*04$ effect is absent in patients positive for $Cw*04$ but negative for $B*35Px$.

Peptide binding assays have shown that amino acid substitutions $D_{114}N$ and Ser_{116} Tyr of $B*3502$ and Ser_{116}Phe of $B*3503$ abolished the ability of the P9 pocket of $B*3501$ to accommodate tyrosine. The resulting inability of $B*35Px$ to present $P_{P2}Y_{P9}$ peptides may be the critical distinction between $B*35Px$ and $B*35PY$ molecules, which affects their efficiency of presenting specific HIV-1 epitopes to CTLs. However, $B*35Px$ does not seem to behave simply as a null allele since its effect on AIDS progression is much stronger than that seen in individuals who are homozygous at HLA-B suggesting that $B*35Px$ may mediate an actively negative effect in AIDS pathogenesis. Though the specific HIV epitopes that discriminate $B*35Px$ from $B*35PY$ are yet to be identified, functional assays have shown that the level of the Gag-specific CTL is inversely correlated with HIV viral loads in $B*35PY$ but not $B*35Px$ individuals indicating a difference in the quality, if not the quantity, of HIV-specific CTL activity between $B*35Px$ and $B*35PY$ positive individuals.[46]

HLA-Bw4 Associated Protection against AIDS Progression and Lower Risk for HIV Transmission

The HLA-Bw4 epitope shared by members of HLA-B and –A molecules has been correlated with AIDS protection in a number of studies.[19,47] When treated as an independent allele, the $Bw4$ protection is typically weaker and less consistent compared to $B*27$ or $B*57$ both of which are Bw4 alleles. However, there is a clear trend in RH-ranked HLA class I alleles where the $Bw4$-positive B alleles cluster on the protective side (Fig. 18.2). Similar analyses of CD4+ T-cell depletion and viral load set point also showed a consistent protective effect of Bw4-positive HLA-B alleles.[20] In a separate study of HIV controllers, $Bw4$ homozygosity was found to be associated with profound suppression of HIV-1 viremia.[19] Our study of HIV-1 transmission in serodiscordant heterosexual couples also demonstrated that the presence of $Bw4$ is associated with a decreased risk of male-to-female HIV-1 transmission.[47] The exact mechanism of the $Bw4$-associated protection against AIDS is not clear but the highly heterogeneous peptide binding profiles among Bw4-carrying HLA-B molecules preclude HLA restriction of HIV epitopes as being the explanation. Recent studies of the immunogenetic partnership between KIR and HLA have shed more light on the nature of the $Bw4$ effect on AIDS and will be discussed later in this Chapter.

HLA Class II Polymorphism and AIDS Progression

Several genetic studies for the involvement of HLA class II alleles in AIDS progression detect some contradictory effects of certain DR, DQ haplotypes on AIDS progression.[21, 48-52] A study of a small cohort of early treated HIV-positive patients also showed an association of the DRB1*13-DQB1*06 haplotype with HIV suppression.[52] However, the reported class II HLA associations are often inconsistent, which might have been contributed by small sample sizes. Our survival analysis using large cohorts of seroconverters as well as analysis of odds ratios (OR) in high-risk seronegative men vs low-risk seroconverters both failed to find any significant class II HLA association with AIDS progression or HIV-1 infection.[53] It is possible that HLA association with AIDS is essentially a class I effect suggesting that in HIV immunopathogenesis, cell-mediated immunity may be more effective than humoral immunity. On the other hand, a thorough examination of all class II loci in larger cohorts with more detailed clinical outcomes is necessary before a convincing conclusion can be drawn regarding the role played by class II HLA polymorphisms in AIDS pathogenesis.

AIDS-associated HLA Alleles Target Distinct Intervals of the Disease Course

HLA-$B*27$, $B*57$ and $B*35Px$ consistently associate with altered rates of AIDS progression following HIV-1 infection but their influence appears to be in different clinical stages. The disease course of AIDS can be divided into three stages: (i) From seroconversion to CD4 < 200, (ii) From CD4 < 200 to the occurrence of an AIDS-defining illness; and (iii) From AIDS-defining illness to death. Our survival analysis of 2,627 HIV-1 infected individuals including 1,089 seroconverters[22] showed that none of the detected HLA associations lasts throughout the disease course, rather each of the three AIDS-associated HLA alleles targets a distinct interval of AIDS progression (Fig. 18.3). $B*35Px$ confers an early and short-lived susceptibility effect detectable only in the early stage of CD4 decline. After CD4 < 200 $B*35Px$ becomes neutral. The $B*57$-mediated protection also takes effect early and significantly delays CD4 decline. After CD4 < 200 the protective effect of $B*57$ begins to subside. In contrast, $B*27$ shows no clear protection against progression to

CD4 < 200 but significantly delays progression to AIDS-defining illness after CD4 depletion. However, once AIDS becomes full blown, all *HLA*-associated genetic effects disappear.

Hypothetical Models of *HLA* Associations with AIDS

On the basis of clinical associations and multiple functional studies, hypothetical models have been proposed to explain the diversified clinical impact of *HLA* allotypes on AIDS progression as summarized in Figure 18.4. All three major *HLA* associations especially *B*27* and *B*57*, may share the similar mechanism of peptide presentation and viral escape but two factors in the HLA-viral interaction lead to distinct clinical manifestations: The timing and consequence of viral escape. Viral escape from B*35Px and B*57 occurs in the early stage after HIV-1 infection, which leads to the early clinical effects. B*27 escape, on the other hand, occurs rather late compared to most HLA alleles, which leads to the late but longer lasting B*27 effect. Escape from both B*27 and B*57 results in compromised HIV fitness thus allowing continued viral load control and consequently delayed disease progression. On the other hand, escape from B*35Px may result in an even more robust virus leading to ineffective control of viral load and accelerated disease progression. However, the failure to identify specific HIV epitopes that discriminate B*35Px and B*35PY indicates that the susceptible effect of *B*35Px* may involve some other unknown mechanisms.

Other *HLA* Associations

Apart from the major *HLA* associations described above that have been universally detected, there are other *HLA* associations that have been reported by more than one study. These associations include the protective *HLA* alleles of *B*13* (Fig. 18.2),[54, 55] *B*5101* (Fig. 18.2),[21] and *B*5801*,[18, 56] and the deleterious alleles of *B*5802*[56, 57] and *B*5001* (Fig. 18.2).[58] Some of these alleles have highly confined frequency distributions across populations, which may explain their somewhat inconsistent associations in different cohort studies. Of particular interest are the identification of the B*13 restricted p1 $Gag_{429-437}$ epitope RQANFLGKI[59] and the B*51-restricted $RT_{128-135}$ epitope TAFTIPSI.[60] The RI9 and TI8 escape mutants may reduce viral fitness and delay AIDS progression. Since, *B*13 and B*51* are commonly detected in most populations the *B*13 and B*51* associated AIDS protection may have a general interest in terms of vaccine development. A recent study of HIV sequences and *HLA* alleles from > 2,800 subjects[7] demonstrated that the *HLA* association with HIV diseases is a dynamic process that is changing over time due to mutual adaptation between the virus and the host. Escape mutants of HLA-restricted HIV epitopes, especially non-reverting epitopes, accumulate over time at the population level. There is a strong correlation between the frequencies of escape mutants and the restricting *HLA* alleles. Therefore, in the long-term, some of the immunodominant HIV epitopes may reduce their significance in the CTL control of HIV infection and some of the well established AIDS-

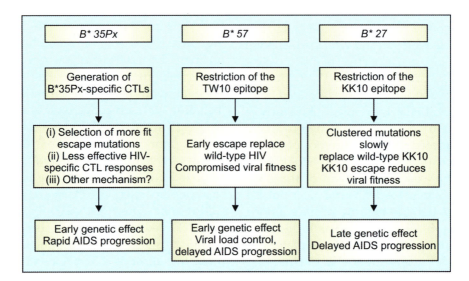

Fig. 18.4: Hypothetical models explaining distinct *HLA-B* effects on AIDS progression

restricting *HLA* alleles, especially those that are common, may lose their advantages and become neutral. These data would support the concept of frequency dependent selection.[18]

Effect of HLA Interaction with KIR on AIDS Progression

HLA plays a key role in both T-cell mediated adaptive immunity and natural killer (NK) cell mediated innate immunity. NK cells are central components of the innate immune system providing an early defense against intracellular infections before antigen-specific lymphocyte responses take effect. Class I HLA molecules serve as ligands for the killer cell immunoglobulin-like receptors (KIR), which are encoded by genes that map to chromosome 19q13.4.[61] Interaction between HLA ligands and KIRs regulates NK lysis of target cells. Inhibitory KIRs bind self HLA expressed in a normal context on cells and actively suppress NK lysis of these targets,[62] whereas activating KIRs are believed to recognize aberrantly expressed or altered class I HLA and actively stimulate NK cells to destroy virally infected or abnormal target cells.[63-65] Virally infected cells and tumor cells often downregulate class I HLA in an attempt to escape specific CTL responses,[66] but by doing so they become susceptible to NK cell cytotoxicity. The exact mechanism of maintaining the balance between KIR-mediated NK lysis and inhibition is not fully understood but it is likely that NK cell cytotoxicity is controlled by the equilibrium between activating and inhibitory signals mediated by corresponding NK cell receptors. *HLA* and *KIR* genes are both highly polymorphic encoding a variety of allotypes. It is therefore plausible that different combinations of *HLA/KIR* genotypes confer varied influences on NK cell activity and consequentially affect disease outcome. In light of recent developments in studies of KIR immunology and immunogenetics, we are now able to examine the functional interaction of these two genetically unlinked immunogenetic systems for their effect on a variety of diseases.

Synergism between *HLA-Bw4-80I* and *KIR3DS1* Protects against AIDS Progression

The inhibitory KIR3DL1 and activating KIR3DS1 are alleles encoded by the same *KIR* locus, an exception amongst the 15 known *KIR* loci. Ligand binding and lysis inhibition assays have shown that HLA-Bw4, especially a subtype of Bw4 with isoleucine at position 80 (referred to as HLA-B Bw4-80I) serves as the most efficient ligand for KIR3DL1.[67-69] The ligand for KIR3DS1 is unknown but given the ~97 percent amino acid similarity shared between KIR3DS1 and 3DL1 in their extracellular domains they may also share similar ligands. Indirect functional evidence supports the KIR3DS1/Bw4-80I partnership.[70,71] Our survival analyses of European and African seroconverters showed that the compound genotype of *KIR3DS1+ HLA-B Bw4-80I* is associated with delayed progression to AIDS.[72] HIV-1 positive patients possessing both *KIR3DS1* and *HLA-B Bw4-80I* showed a slower CD4+ T cell decline and disease development relative to patients without this genotype. Synergism between the two genes is implicated since having either *KIR3DS1* or *Bw4-80I* alone does not have any protective effect. In fact patients having *KIR3DS1* but not *Bw4-80I* showed the opposite effect with a more rapid CD4 decline. This is clearly demonstrated by the two groups of *KIR3DS1* homozygous individuals with or without *Bw4-80I* as shown in Figure 18.5. The protective effect of the *KIR3DS1 + HLA-B Bw4-80I* genotype is the strongest in delaying CD4 < 200 relative to other outcomes, suggesting that the synergistic interaction takes place

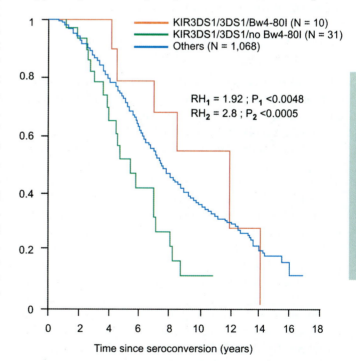

Fig. 18.5: Effect of *HLA-Bw4-80I* and *KIR3DS1* on progression to AIDS1993 (the 1993 CDC definition of AIDS: CD4 < 200 and/or AIDS defining illness or AIDS related death) in 1,109 seroconverters of mixed races. The survival analysis compares *Bw4-80I* homozygous genotypes with or without *KIR3DS1*. RH_1 and P_1 were estimated for the *Bw4-80I* homozygotes without *KIR3DS1* (the green curve) vs. all other samples (the red and blue curves). RH_2 and P_2 were estimated for the *Bw4-80I* homozygotes without *KIR3DS1* (the green curve) vs. the *Bw4-80I* homozygotes with *KIR3DS1* (the red curve)

soon after HIV-1 infection. The Bw4-80I motif is also carried by a number of HLA-A molecules including A*23, A*24, A*25 and A*32 but the *HLA-A* related *Bw4-80I* as a group, in combination with *KIR3DS1*, does not appear confer protection against AIDS progression, confirming that the concerted effect of *KIR3DS1* and *Bw4-80I* is apparently HLA-B-dependent. Other studies, however, arrived at somewhat contradictive results. One study of 191 individuals[73] showed that the *KIR3DS1/HLA-B Bw4-80I* genotype is actually associated with rapid progression to AIDS. Another study of 255 individuals[74] detected *KIR3DS1* and *HLA-B Bw4-80I* as independent protective factors, but not in a synergistic manner. While it would be interesting to further investigate the cause of the genetic inconsistency, recent functional studies are inclined to support the model of synergistic protection. In these experiments both the NK-cell mediated *in vitro* inhibition of HIV replication[70] and *in vivo* expansion of KIR3DS1+ NK cells[71] were found to be significantly enhanced in HIV-infected individuals possessing the compound genotype of *KIR3DS1 + Bw4-80I*, where both members of the compound genotype were necessary.

Innate Partnership of KIR and HLA Enhances HLA Protection against AIDS Progression

The HLA allotypes involved in both innate and adaptive immunological pathways are of particular interest when investigating the role of *HLA* in AIDS pathogenesis. This pleiotropic involvement is best exemplified by HLA-B*57, an allotype acting both as a presenter of critical HIV epitopes to CTLs in the adaptive immune response, and an efficient ligand (Bw4-80I) for KIR3DL1, and probably also KIR3DS1 in the innate immune response. *KIR3DL1* is one of the most polymorphic *KIR* loci with 52 alleles (46 being non-synonymous) identified thus far. Allotypes of KIR3DL1 are expressed at different levels on NK cells and the level of KIR3DL1 expression is closely related to the inhibitory capacity of NK cells.[75] Using a cohort of more than 1,500 HIV-1 infected individuals we demonstrated that among *HLA-B*57* positive patients those carrying the highly expressed 3DL1 allotypes (referred to as *KIR3DL1*h*) exhibit a higher level of protection against CD4 depletion and AIDS-defining illness compared to those carrying the low-expressing allotypes (referred to as *KIR3DL1*l*).[76] These observations suggest that the B*57 protection is due at least in part, to its interaction with KIR in addition to its well-characterized role in the adaptive immune system of presentation of HIV epitopes. Therefore, the epidemiological association of *HLA-B*57* with AIDS progression stems from at least three sources: (1) Restriction of critical HIV epitopes; (2) Epistatic interaction with KIR3DS1; and (3) Epistatic interaction with KIR3DL1, especially KIR3DL1*h. The other prominent protective HLA allotype B*27 (predominantly B*2705 in our cohorts) also carries Bw4 but mostly the Bw4-80T subtype. Individuals with *B*27-80T* showed borderline significant protection in the presence of *KIR3DL1*l* which suggests a role for *B*27* in the innate immune response to HIV.

The apparently contradictory *B*57* links with both the inhibitory KIR3DL1 and activating KIR3DS1 can be explained by a hypothetical model in which the activating KIR3DS1 directly stimulates NK cytotoxicity upon recognizing aberrantly expressed HLA ligands whereas the KIR3DL1 mediated NK inhibition functions as a necessary 'educational' process[77] during NK cell development and ultimately leads to more vigorous activation upon HIV infection. Other HLA allotypes that present immunodominant HIV epitopes and serve as a KIR ligand may also confer protection. One such allotype is HLA-A*11, a common allele in Asian populations but less common in Europeans and Africans. *A*11* has been implicated as a protective allele against HIV-1 infection in Asians[78,79] even though *A*11* is linked with the *B*35-Cw*04 –DRB1*01* haplotype which associates with faster progression to AIDS in Asian Indians.[80] In our European American cohorts *A*11* also showed a moderately delayed progression to AIDS (Fig. 18.2). A*11 also functions as a ligand for the inhibitory KIR3DL2[81] which happens to be one of the most polymorphic KIRs. It has been shown *in vitro* that the immunodominant Nef-derived peptide QVPLRPMTYK (position 73-82) can stimulate the A*1101-restricted CTL response[82] and A*1101 molecules loaded with viral peptides lead to weakened NK inhibition which potentiates NK lysis of target cells.[83] Therefore, the overall *A*11* protection is likely due to the combined effects of presenting critical HIV epitopes to CTLs, and possibly curtailing KIR3DL2 inhibition of NK lysis.

HLA-C Influences AIDS Progression through Interaction with KIR

HLA-C differs from other class I loci by some unique features including less diversity, lower surface expression and lack of HIV-1 Nef-mediated down-regulation.[84] Though HLA-C, as a classical class I HLA, can potentially present HIV epitopes to CTL, this potential may be limited by its lower cell surface expression compared to HLA-A and -B.[85] In fact, the *HLA-C* polymorphism has rarely been implicated as an independent AIDS restriction factor. The reported *HLA-C* associations with AIDS progression have been invariably attributed to its LD relationship with *HLA-B*.[56] HLA-C molecules also serve as KIR ligands and can be divided into two KIR binding groups determined by the amino acid at position 80.[86] Recent developments in KIR immunology and immunogenetics underscore *HLA-C* as a critical factor affecting NK cell mediated innate immunity and associate particular *HLA-C + KIR* compound genotypes with a variety of infectious, malignant and autoimmune diseases.[87-89] A recent GWAS also identified a SNP (rs9264942, -35C/T) located 35 kb upstream of the transcription initiation site of the *HLA-C* gene as the second most significant AIDS-related polymorphism.[3] The -35C allele of this SNP shows an independent protective effect on viral load set point and is also associated with higher HLA-C expression. These data strongly implicate high HLA-C expression levels in more effective control of HIV-1, potentially through better antigen presentation to CTLs and/or recognition and killing of infected cells by natural killer cells.

CONCLUSION

Host genetic factors play an important role in determining the level of resistance to HIV infection and AIDS progression. AIDS restriction genes are mainly those involved in HIV entry (chemokine receptors), intercellular signaling (cytokines) and acquired as well as innate immune responses (e.g. *HLA* and *KIR*). Diversity of these genes contributes to the varied responses to HIV infection. Recent GWAS estimated that the *B*57*-associated *HCP5* polymorphism alone explains 9.6 percent of the variation in viral load set point.[3] Both the candidate gene approach and GWAS point to *HLA* as the region harboring the most significant AIDS-restriction polymorphisms. Compared to chemokine receptors that affect HIV entry and therefore infection, *HLA* influence (especially *HLA-B*) on AIDS pathogenesis has post-infection involvement. In fact the AIDS restricting *HLA* factors that have been consistently confirmed in multiple cohort studies are essentially those associated with disease progression after HIV infection. Evaluation of the *HLA* influence on resistance to HIV infection has been difficult due to the lack of a precisely quantified measurement of HIV exposure. Our cohort studies have so far failed to detect any significant *HLA* association with HIV infection. However, there have been reports on *HLA* association with HIV susceptibility in exposed adults[90,91] and in infants of HIV seropositive mothers.[50,91] The most prominent AIDS-protective alleles, *B*27* and *B*57*, have never been associated with reduced risk of HIV infection. Therefore, if *HLA* polymorphism does indeed have an effect on HIV infection, the mechanism must be different from that in AIDS progression. Post-infection however, *HLA* may affect the infectivity of HIV transmitters through regulation of viral load in the blood as exemplified by the protective alleles *B*27* and *B*57* and the susceptible *B*35Px*. The strong and clear-cut *HLA* association with HIV diseases reflects the relatively short history of mutual adaptation between the host and virus. Given enough time *HLA* and HIV are likely to become more adapted to each other, which may change the landscape of the *HLA* associations.[7] However, viral adaptation to *HLA* is unlikely to lead to the fixation of escape mutations and thus the loss of CTL responses to HIV epitopes[92] because (i) A substantial proportion of escape mutations can rapidly revert to the wild type once the specific HLA pressure is lifted; and (ii) An escape mutation is still subject to renewed pressure when transmitted to a new HLA environment. *HLA* adaptation to HIV is also balanced by overdominant selection: A protective allele for AIDS can be a high-risk factor for other diseases and an AIDS-susceptible allele may need to be maintained in the population for its protective effect on other diseases. Further, given the involvement of *HLA* in both innate and adaptive immune responses the influence of *HLA* on AIDS needs to be appreciated from a multi-dimensional perspective. Genetic associations, especially those with disagreements, warrant functional studies to further investigate the molecular basis of the *HLA* impact on AIDS pathogenesis, which may hold the key to the development of better therapies and vaccines.

REFERENCES

1. Carrington M, SJ O'Brien. The influence of HLA genotype on AIDS. Annu Rev Med 2003;54:535-51.
2. O'Brien SJ, GW Nelson. Human genes that limit AIDS. Nat Genet 2004;36(6): 565-74.
3. Fellay J, et al. A whole-genome association study of major determinants for host control of HIV-1. Science 2007;317(5840):944-47.
4. Dalmasso C, et al. Distinct genetic loci control plasma HIV-RNA and cellular HIV-DNA levels in HIV-1 infection: The ANRS Genome Wide Association 01 study. PLoS One, 2008;3(12):e3907.
5. Limou S, et al. Genomewide association study of an AIDS-nonprogression cohort emphasizes the role played by HLA genes (ANRS Genomewide Association Study 02). J Infect Dis 2009;199(3):419-26.
6. Carrington M, MP Martin, J van Bergen. KIR-HLA intercourse in HIV disease. Trends Microbiol 2008;16(12): 620-27.

7. Kawashima Y, et al. Adaptation of HIV-1 to human leukocyte antigen class I. Nature 2009;458(7238):641-45.
8. Hughes AL, M Yeager. Natural selection at major histocompatibility complex loci of vertebrates. Annu Rev Genet 1998;32:415-35.
9. Parham P, T Ohta. Population biology of antigen presentation by MHC class I molecules. Science 1996;272(5258):67-74.
10. Hughes AL, M Yeager. Natural selection and the evolutionary history of major histocompatibility complex loci Front Biosci 1998;3:d509-16.
11. Carrington M, et al. HLA and HIV-1: Heterozygote advantage and B*35-Cw*04 disadvantage. Science 1999;283(5408):1748-52.
12. Tang J, et al. HLA class I homozygosity accelerates disease progression in human immunodeficiency virus type 1 infection. AIDS Res Hum Retroviruses, 1999;15(4):317-24.
13. Tang J, et al. Characteristics of HLA class I and class II polymorphisms in Rwandan women. Exp Clin Immunogenet 2000;17(4):185-98.
14. Roberts JD. K. Bebenek, TA Kunkel. The accuracy of reverse transcriptase from HIV-1. Science 1988;242(4882):1171-73.
15. Preston BD. Reverse transcriptase fidelity and HIV-1 variation. Science 1997; 275(5297):228-9; author reply 230-31.
16. McMichael A, P Klenerman. HIV/AIDS. HLA leaves its footprints on HIV. Science 2002;296(5572):1410-11.
17. Klenerman P, A McMichael. AIDS/HIV. Finding footprints among the trees. Science 2007;315(5818):1505-07.
18. Trachtenberg E, et al. Advantage of rare HLA supertype in HIV disease progression. Nat Med 2003;9(7):928-35.
19. Flores-Villanueva PO, et al. Control of HIV-1 viremia and protection from AIDS are associated with HLA-Bw4 homozygosity. Proc Natl Acad Sci USA 2001;98(9):5140-45.
20. Baker BM, et al. Elite control of HIV infection: Implications for vaccine design. Expert Opin Biol Ther 2009;9(1):55-69.
21. Kaslow RA, et al. Influence of combinations of human major histocompatibility complex genes on the course of HIV-1 infection. Nat Med 1996;2(4):405-11.
22. Gao X, et al. AIDS restriction HLA allotypes target distinct intervals of HIV-1 pathogenesis. Nat Med 2005;11(12):1290-92.
23. Hendel H, et al. New class I and II HLA alleles strongly associated with opposite patterns of progression to AIDS. J Immunol 1999;162(11):6942-46.
24. Magierowska M, et al. Combined genotypes of CCR5, CCR2, SDF1, and HLA genes can predict the long-term nonprogressor status in human immunodeficiency virus-1-infected individuals. Blood 1999;93(3):936-41.
25. Nixon DF, et al. HIV-1 Gag-specific cytotoxic T lymphocytes defined with recombinant vaccinia virus and synthetic peptides. Nature 1988;336(6198):484-87.
26. Kelleher AD, et al. Clustered mutations in HIV-1 Gag are consistently required for escape from HLA-B27-restricted cytotoxic T lymphocyte responses. J Exp Med 2001;193(3):375-86.
27. Schneidewind A, et al. Escape from the dominant HLA-B27-restricted cytotoxic T-lymphocyte response in Gag is associated with a dramatic reduction in human immunodeficiency virus type 1 replication. J Virol 2007;81(22):12382-93.
28. McKiernan SM, et al. Distinct MHC class I and II alleles are associated with hepatitis C viral clearance, originating from a single source. Hepatology 2004; 40(1):108-14.
29. Hildesheim A, et al. Association of HLA class I and II alleles and extended haplotypes with nasopharyngeal carcinoma in Taiwan. J Natl Cancer Inst 2002;94(23):1780-89.
30. Goulder P, et al. Coevolution of human immunodeficiency virus and cytotoxic T-lymphocyte responses. Immunol Rev 1997;159:17-29.
31. Salkowitz, JR, et al. Characterization of high-risk HIV-1 seronegative hemophiliacs. Clin Immunol 2001;98(2):200-11.
32. Gao X, et al. Effect of a single amino acid change in MHC class I molecules on the rate of progression to AIDS. N Engl J Med 2001;344(22):1668-75.
33. Klein MR, et al. Associations between HLA frequencies and pathogenic features of human immunodeficiency virus type 1 infection in seroconverters from the Amsterdam cohort of homosexual men. J Infect Dis 1994;169(6): 1244-49.
34. Costello C, et al. HLA-B*5703 independently associated with slower HIV-1 disease progression in Rwandan women. Aids 1999;13(14):1990-91.
35. Migueles SA, et al. HLA B*5701 is highly associated with restriction of virus replication in a subgroup of HIV-infected long-term nonprogressors. Proc Natl Acad Sci USA 2000;97(6):2709-14.
36. Lambotte O, et al. HIV controllers: A homogeneous group of HIV-1-infected patients with spontaneous control of viral replication. Clin Infect Dis 2005; 41(7):1053-56.
37. Emu B, et al. HLA class I-restricted T-cell responses may contribute to the control of human immunodeficiency virus infection, but such responses are not always necessary for long-term virus control. J Virol 2008;82(11):5398-407.
38. Altfeld M, et al. Influence of HLA-B57 on clinical presentation and viral control during acute HIV-1 infection. Aids 2003;17(18):2581-91.
39. Crawford H, et al. Evolution of HLA-B*5703 HIV-1 escape mutations in HLA-B*5703-positive individuals and their transmission recipients. J Exp Med 2009; 206(4):909-21.
40. Yu XG, et al. Mutually exclusive T-cell receptor induction and differential susceptibility to human immunodeficiency virus type 1 mutational escape associated with a two-amino acid difference between HLA class I subtypes. J Virol 2007;81(4):1619-31.

41. Scorza Smeraldi R, et al. HLA-associated susceptibility to AIDS: HLA B35 is a major risk factor for Italian HIV-infected intravenous drug addicts. Hum Immunol 1988;22(2):73-79.
42. Itescu S, et al. HLA-B35 is associated with accelerated progression to AIDS. J Acquir Immune Defic Syndr 1992; 5(1):37-45.
43. Sahmoud T, et al. Progression to AIDS in French haemophiliacs: Association with HLA-B35. Aids 1993; 7(4):497-500.
44. Hill AV, et al. Molecular analysis of the association of HLA-B53 and resistance to severe malaria. Nature 1992; 360(6403):434-39.
45. Falk K, et al. Peptide motifs of HLA-B35 and -B37 molecules. Immunogenetics, 1993;38(2):161-62.
46. Jin X, et al. Human immunodeficiency virus type 1 (HIV-1)-specific CD8+-T-cell responses for groups of HIV-1-infected individuals with different HLA-B*35 genotypes. J Virol 2002;76(24):12603-10.
47. Welzel TM, et al. HLA-B Bw4 alleles and HIV-1 transmission in heterosexual couples. Aids 2007;21(2): 225-29.
48. Just JJ. Genetic predisposition to HIV-1 infection and acquired immune deficiency virus syndrome: A review of the literature examining associations with HLA [corrected]. Hum Immunol 1995;44(3):156-69.
49. Keet IP, et al. The role of host genetics in the natural history of HIV-1 infection: The needles in the haystack. Aids 1996;10 Suppl A:S59-67.
50. Chen Y, et al. Influence of HLA alleles on the rate of progression of vertically transmitted HIV infection in children: Association of several HLA-DR13 alleles with long-term survivorship and the potential association of HLA-A*2301 with rapid progression to AIDS. Long-term Survivor Study. Hum Immunol 1997;55(2):154-62.
51. Kroner BL, et al. Concordance of human leukocyte antigen haplotype-sharing, CD4 decline and AIDS in hemophilic siblings. Multicenter Hemophilia Cohort and Hemophilia Growth and Development Studies. Aids 1995;9(3):275-80.
52. Malhotra U, et al. Role for HLA class II molecules in HIV-1 suppression and cellular immunity following antiretroviral treatment. J Clin Invest 2001;107(4):505-17.
53. Liu C, et al. Lack of associations between HLA class II alleles and resistance to HIV-1 infection among white, non-Hispanic homosexual men. J Acquir Immune Defic Syndr 2004;37(2):1313-17.
54. Harrer EG, et al. A conserved HLA B13-restricted cytotoxic T lymphocyte epitope in Nef is a dominant epitope in HLA B13-positive HIV-1-infected patients. Aids 2005;19(7):734-5 g of a CD8 T cell env epitope presented by HLA-B*5802 is associated with markers of HIV disease progression and lack of selection pressure. AIDS Res Hum Retroviruses 2008;24(1):72-82.
55. Honeyborne I, et al. Control of human immunodeficiency virus type 1 is associated with HLA-B*13 and targeting of multiple gag-specific CD8+ T-cell epitopes. J Virol 2007;81(7):3667-72.
56. Kiepiela P, et al. Dominant influence of HLA-B in mediating the potential co-evolution of HIV and HLA. Nature 2004;432(7018):769-75.
57. Ngumbela KC, et al. Targeting of a CD8 T cell env epitope presented by HLA-B*5802 is associated with markers of HIV disease progression and lack of selection pressure. AIDS Res Hum Retroviruses 2008;24(1):72-82.
58. Itescu S, et al. Grouping HLA-B locus serologic specificities according to shared structural motifs suggests that different peptide-anchoring pockets may have contrasting influences on the course of HIV-1 infection. Hum Immunol 1995; 42(1):81-89.
59. Prado JG, et al. Functional consequences of human immunodeficiency virus escape from an HLA-B*13-restricted CD8+ T-cell epitope in p1 Gag protein. J Virol 2009;83(2):1018-25.
60. Tomiyama H, et al. Identification of multiple HIV-1 CTL epitopes presented by HLA-B*5101 molecules. Hum Immunol 1999;60(3):177-86.
61. Lanier LL. NK cell recognition. Annu Rev Immunol 2005;23:225-74.
62. Storkus WJ, et al. Reversal of natural killing susceptibility in target cells expressing transfected class I HLA genes. Proc Natl Acad Sci USA 1989;86(7): 2361-64.
63. Hoglund P, et al. Recognition of β2 microglobulin-negative (β2 m) T-cell blasts by natural killer cells from normal but not from β2 m mice: Nonresponsiveness controlled by β2 m bone marrow in chimeric mice. Proc Natl Acad Sci USA 1991;88(22):10332-36.
64. Karre K, et al. Selective rejection of H-2-deficient lymphoma variants suggests alternative immune defence strategy 1986. J Immunol 2005;174(11):6566-69.
65. Wiertz E, et al. Cytomegaloviruses use multiple mechanisms to elude the host immune response. Immunol Lett 1997;57(1-3):213-16.
66. Collins KL, et al. HIV-1 Nef protein protects infected primary cells against killing by cytotoxic T lymphocytes. Nature 1998;391(6665):397-401.
67. Gumperz JE, et al. Conserved and variable residues within the Bw4 motif of HLA-B make separable contributions to recognition by the NKB1 killer cell-inhibitory receptor. J Immunol 1997;158(11):5237-41.
68. Carr WH, MJ Pando, P Parham. KIR3DL1 polymorphisms that affect NK cell inhibition by HLA-Bw4 ligand. J Immunol 2005;175(8):5222-29.
69. Cella M, et al. NK3-specific natural killer cells are selectively inhibited by Bw4-positive HLA alleles with isoleucine 80. J Exp Med 1994;180(4):1235-42.
70. Alter G, et al. Differential natural killer cell-mediated inhibition of HIV-1 replication based on distinct KIR/HLA subtypes. J Exp Med 2007;204(12): 3027-36.
71. Alter G, et al. HLA class I subtype-dependent expansion of KIR3DS1+ and KIR3DL1+ NK cells during acute human immunodeficiency virus type 1 infection. J Virol 2009;83(13):6798-805.
72. Martin MP, et al. Epistatic interaction between KIR3DS1 and HLA-B delays the progression to AIDS. Nat Genet 2002;31(4):429-34.

73. Gaudieri S, et al. Killer immunoglobulin-like receptors and HLA act both independently and synergistically to modify HIV disease progression. Genes Immun 2005; 6(8):683-90.
74. Barbour JD, et al. Synergy or independence? Deciphering the interaction of HLA Class I and NK cell KIR alleles in early HIV-1 disease progression. PLoS Pathog 2007; 3(4):e43.
75. Gardiner CM, et al. Different NK cell surface phenotypes defined by the DX9 antibody are due to KIR3DL1 gene polymorphism. J Immunol 2001;166(5): 2992-3001.
76. Martin MP, et al. Innate partnership of HLA-B and KIR3DL1 subtypes against HIV-1. Nat Genet 2007; 39(6):733-40.
77. Anfossi N, et al. Human NK cell education by inhibitory receptors for MHC class I. Immunity 2006;25(2):331-42.
78. Selvaraj P, et al. Association of human leukocyte antigen-A11 with resistance and B40 and DR2 with susceptibility to HIV-1 infection in south India. J Acquir Immune Defic Syndr 2006;43(4):497-99.
79. Stephens HA. HIV-1 diversity versus HLA class I polymorphism. Trends Immunol 2005;26(1):41-47.
80. Roger M. Influence of host genes on HIV-1 disease progression. Faseb J 1998; 12(9):625-32.
81. Hansasuta P, et al. Recognition of HLA-A3 and HLA-A11 by KIR3DL2 is peptide-specific. Eur J Immunol 2004;34(6): 1673-79.
82. Sriwanthana B, et al. HIV-specific cytotoxic T lymphocytes, HLA-A11, and chemokine-related factors may act synergistically to determine HIV resistance in CCR5 delta32-negative female sex workers in Chiang Rai, northern Thailand. AIDS Res Hum Retroviruses 2001; 17(8):719-34.
83. Gavioli R, QJ Zhang, MG Masucci. HLA-A11-mediated protection from NK cell-mediated lysis: Role of HLA-A11-presented peptides. Hum Immunol 1996; 49(1):1-12.
84. Cohen GB, et al. The selective downregulation of class I major histocompatibility complex proteins by HIV-1 protects HIV-infected cells from NK cells. Immunity 1999; 10(6): 661-71.
85. Snary D, et al. Molecular structure of human histocompatibility antigens: The HLA-C series. Eur J Immunol 1977;7(8): 580-85.
86. Boyington JC, PD Sun. A structural perspective on MHC class I recognition by killer cell immunoglobulin-like receptors. Mol Immunol 2002;38(14):1007-21.
87. Martin MP, et al. Cutting edge: Susceptibility to psoriatic arthritis: Influence of activating killer Ig-like receptor genes in the absence of specific HLA-C alleles. J Immunol 2002;169(6):2818-22.
88. Khakoo SI, et al. HLA and NK cell inhibitory receptor genes in resolving hepatitis C virus infection. Science 2004;305(5685):872-74.
89. Butsch Kovacic M, et al. Variation of the killer cell immunoglobulin-like receptors and HLA-C genes in nasopharyngeal carcinoma. Cancer Epidemiol Biomarkers Prev 2005;14(11 Pt 1): 2673-77.
90. Lockett SF, et al. Mismatched human leukocyte antigen alleles protect against heterosexual HIV transmission. J Acquir Immune Defic Syndr 2001;27(3):277-80.
91. MacDonald, KS, et al. The HLA A2/6802 supertype is associated with reduced risk of perinatal human immunodeficiency virus type 1 transmission. J Infect Dis 2001;183(3):503-06.
92. Brumme ZL, et al. Evidence of differential HLA class I-mediated viral evolution in functional and accessory/regulatory genes of HIV-1. PLoS Pathog 2007; 3(7):e94.

Chapter 19

Host Genetics of HIV-1/AIDS Infection

Gurvinder Kaur, Narinder K Mehra

BACKGROUND

The Acquired Immune Deficiency Syndrome (AIDS) caused by the human immunodeficiency virus (HIV-1) has already claimed nearly 21 million lives. More than 33.2 million people are currently living with this infection worldwide (http://data.unaids.org/pub/EPISlides/2007/2007epiupdate. en.pdf; http://www.nacoonline.org/NACO). The situation is particularly alarming in regions like the Sub-Saharan Africa where 22 million people are infected with HIV-1 and the adult prevalence rate is ~5%. Similarly, there are 4.2 million infected people living across South East Asia. According to the recent census published by the National AIDS control organization (NACO), there are ~2.5 million HIV infected people residing in the Indian sub-continent with the adult prevalence rate of ~ 0.36% (http://www.nacoonline.org/NACO). The menace of HIV-1/AIDS has emerged as one of the biggest health hazards of today and a matter of global priority for researchers, clinicians, policy makers, social workers and funding agencies alike. To this effect, a Joint United Nations Program on HIV/AIDS (UNAIDS) has been created by a constellation of important organizations like the UNHCR, UNICEF, WFP, UNDP, UNFPA, UNODC, ILO, UNESCO, WHO and world bank. The program has committed its '*Millenium development goal 6*' as "*To combat HIV/AIDS, malaria and other diseases*" and targets "*to have halted and begun to reverse the spread of HIV/AIDS*" by 2015.

Since the discovery of the virus in the early 1980s, important milestones in understanding the pathology, structural biology, clinical and immunological aspects of the infection have been achieved. The current focus is on defining the genetic and immunologic correlates of the host-pathogen interaction with a view to develop possible biomarkers for infection, transmission and disease progression. Further, despite impressive developments in anti-retroviral therapy and control of the disease, an universal anti HIV vaccine still eludes the researchers. Table 19.1 summarizes some of the important milestones achieved since the first instance of AIDS was documented in 1981.

It took more than four decades to develop a vaccine for polio or for chickenpox; similarly, it may take still a few more years to develop a successful vaccine against HIV-1. Lack of suitable animal model systems, inherent hypervariability of the virus and its extraordinary ability to adapt and evolve in the host are some of the major hurdles responsible for the delay in developing vaccine(s) against HIV (Table 19.2). The virus has devised its own mechanisms to escape immune recognition and surveillance through extensive glycosylation and surface masking. For example, the envelope glycoproteins gp120 and gp41 possess immunogenic epitopes but most of these are not exposed on the virus surface and therefore not available for eliciting an effector immune response. Likewise, the gp120 CD4-binding site is a recessed cavity in the virus and therefore inaccessible for the antibodies. Importantly, virus infection results in downregulation of HLA class I expression and perturbs antigen presentation. Antibodies to gp120 CD4-binding site have been reported to hinder antigen presentation and suppress gp120 specific CD4 T cell responses.[1] The CD4 T cells decline in number and their response gets compromised in HIV-1 infected patients although antigen stimulation in a fraction of Th cells can induce chemokine secretion and suppress HIV infection *in vitro*.[2]

Table 19.1: Important milestones in research in HIV/AIDS biology, diagnosis and genetics

\multicolumn{2}{c}{General}	\multicolumn{2}{c}{Diagnostics}	\multicolumn{2}{c}{Viral biology and therapeutics}	\multicolumn{2}{c}{Genetics}
Year	Event	Year	Event	Year	Event	Year	Event
1959	First case of AIDS confirmed retrospectively in Congo	1985	First ELISA test kit for screening of abs against HIV	1987	AZT (Zidovudine) approved as the first anti HIV drug	2004	First Meta analysis of AIDS restriction genes in multiple cohorts compiled [11]
1981	*Pneumocystis carinii* outbreak and Kaposi's sarcoma reported as Gay compromise syndrome or Gay-related immune deficiency (GRID)	1987	Western blot blood test kit for confirmation of infection	1995	Triple combination therapy approved as more effective ART	2007	First whole genome scan identified susceptibility loci in MHC at 6p21 [12]
1982	Syndrome renamed as Acquired Immunodeficiency syndrome (AIDS)	1996	Introduction of Amplicor HIV-1 monitor test for viral load	1998	First human trial of AIDS vaccine begins in the US	2008	Whole genome association identified susceptibility loci on 8q24.3 [13]
1983	Luc Montagnier isolated LAV (Lymphadenopathy-associated virus) – HIV-1	2001	Launch of TrueGene HIV-1 genotyping kit and Open Gene DNA sequencing	2007	Crystal structure of gp120 in complex with neutralizing ab b12	2008	Abacavir hypersensitivity syndrome HLA-B*5701 (F pocket residues 116 ser and 114 asp)[57]
1984	Identification of HIV-1 (HTLVIII) by Robert Gallo	2002	Versant HIV RNA 3.0 assay (bDNA) for viral load estimation	2008	Novel host derived factors for HIV-1 life cycle identified[8]	2009	International collaborative HIV controller consortium
1986	Global AIDS strategy launched by WHO	2002	Development of OraQuick Rapid HIV-1 ab test	2008	Nobel prize awarded to *Luc Montagnier, Francoise Barre-Sinoussi and Harald zur Hausen* for their discoveries of HIV and HPV		
1996	Launching of UNAIDS	2004	Introduction of OraSure rapid test for HIV-2				
1999	Source of origin of HIV traced to chimpanzee in West Central Africa	2004	Launching of Multispot HIV-1/HIV-2 rapid test				

[Adapted from (4)]

Table 19.2: Major obstacles encountered for the development of a successful vaccine against HIV-1

- Lack of suitable animal model systems
- Hyper-variability of the virus, particularly due to the extensive mutations in viral protein env and others
- Extensive glycosylation and surface masking of viral proteins (e.g., gp120 and gp41)
- Inaccessibility of antibody epitopes (e.g., CD4 binding site is a recessed cavity)
- Reduced antigen presentation (due to downregulation of HLA class I and development of antibodies against gp120 CD4-binding site)
- Decline in CD4 T cell numbers and dysfunction
- Inability to induce broadly neutralizing antibodies against the virus
- Rapid emergence of CTL escape mutants
- Population specific variability in host genetic and immunologic response factors
- Synergistic opportunistic infections and complications thereof

[Adapted from (4)]

HIV-1 infected T cells form a virological synapse with non-infected CD4+ T cells in order to efficiently transfer HIV-1 virions from cell to cell. The viral gp120 induces a transient stop signal and participates in the formation of a virological synapse that shares a similar supramolecular organization with that of an immunological synapse in uninfected CD4 T cells[3] and plausibly leads to further propagation of the virus.

Immune response against HIV-1 is modulated by multiple host genetic determinants, many of which are directly or indirectly implicated in recognition of the virus (includes chemokine receptors, HLA, T cell receptors-TCR, antibodies, Killer immunoglobulin like receptors - KIRs, Toll like receptors-TLRs), immune cell trafficking (includes Chemokines and receptors, adhesion molecules), and immune response amplification (includes molecules involved in signaling pathways, cytokine genes).[4,5]

HOST GENETICS: INDIVIDUAL VARIABILITY IN RESPONSE TO HIV/AIDS

Numerous studies have revealed that an extensive inter-individual variability exists in response to HIV infection. This includes susceptibility to virus, its transmission and course of disease progression, with phenotypes ranging from undetectable, asymptomatic state to fatal AIDS.[6,7] Individuals are not equally susceptible to infection and have differences in their viral set-points, rates of decline of CD4 T cells, levels of viremia, emergence of CTL escape mutants and development of opportunistic infections resulting in varying incubation periods of the AIDS virus. While a large majority of individuals infected with HIV-1 progress to AIDS, if untreated (called as 'Progressors'), most of them can, however, be turned aviremic by anti-retroviral therapy (Fig. 19.1). More importantly, ~ 5 to 10 percent of infected individuals do not develop AIDS for more than 7 years, remain naturally aviremic and are referred to as 'Long-term non-progressors' (LTNPs). This group of naturally resistant people represent 'spontaneous controllers' and include EUs partners of commercial sex workers as well as the discordant couples.[10]

Spontaneous Controllers

Spontaneous controllers possess a level of 'natural resistance' against HIV as they can combat infection after initial viral exposure and limit disease progression. Developing resistance against virus acquisition is one of the currently defined goals of the first generation vaccines.[8] Therefore, the underlying mechanisms that protect these people from HIV infection could hold the key to develop such an anticipated vaccine against the virus. The 'Elite' or 'Aviremic' controllers as they are often referred to, represent ~1 percent of total infected individuals and maintain viremia at almost undetectable levels of <75 copies of viral RNA/ml. The 'Intermediate' or 'Viremic' controllers manage to maintain their viremia at <2000 RNA copies/ml despite no treatment (Fig. 19.1) and do not allow consecutive episodes of viral blips of >200 copies (http://www2.massgeneral.org/aids/hiv_elite_controllers.asp). The progressors, on the other hand, permit virus propagation to > 10,000 RNA copies/ml but once on ART, their viral loads can be suppressed to undetectable levels.

An international collaborative HIV controller consortium has recently been established with the purpose of recruiting elite controllers from different ethnic groups.[8] This effort has already led to a collection of more than 300 elite controllers who are being checked through whole genome scans for their immune response to HIV and for the possible genetic mechanisms that may be responsible for spontaneous control of the virus (http://www2.massgeneral.org/aids/hiv_elite_controllers.asp, www.iasusa.org). The prime focus of the consortium is to understand host, viral and immunologic parameters that are associated with effective containment of HIV infection.

Recent studies have revealed specific immunologic and genetic features associated predominantly with Elite controllers that could be correlated to their ability to resist virus. For example, such persons have an over-representation of protective HLA-B*57 and B*27 alleles, high ratios of functional CD4:CD8 T cells, high generalized T activation levels (CD38 + DR +), high proportions of polyfunctional IL2 + γIFN + CD4 + T

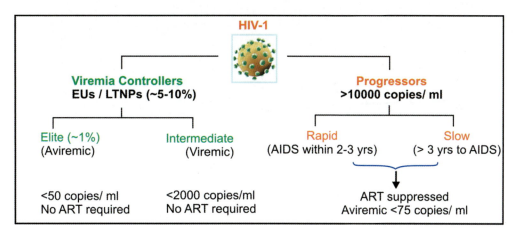

Fig. 19.1: Spontaneous controllers versus disease progressors following HIV-1 infection. The former include exposed uninfected (EUs) like the discordant couples, commercial sex workers (CSW) and Long-term non-progressors (LTNPs). The latter comprise of rapid and slow progressors as determined by their rates of disease progression [Adapted from (4)]

helpers, CD8 + CTL responses, preferential targeting of gag, env and high HIV specific antibody levels.[9] However, not all Elite controllers possess these resistance factors indicating an involvement of additional hitherto undetected restriction factors. For example, Brass and coworkers[10] have reported that HIV utilizes atleast 250 host derived HIV dependency factors (HDFs) for gaining entry into target cells and completing its life-cycle. Hence, multiple genetic factors are expected to be involved in disease pathogenesis and progression following HIV infection. A study carried out by O'Brien and colleagues[11] utilizing five different cohorts (MHCS, ALIVE, HGDS, MACS, SFCC) have revealed the existence of a number of 'AIDS restriction genes' (ARGs) that could determine the genetic propensity of an individual or a population and help predict survival kinetics following HIV infection.[6,7,11]

MULTIPLE GENES CONTROL HIV-1/AIDS

Structural genomic approaches aimed at defining chromosomal localization of a host of human genetic variants that regulate susceptibility to HIV infection, rate of CD4 decline, viral load, disease progression and response to therapy have revealed interesting results. More than 10 such set of genes that regulate expression of chemokines, cytokines, HIV-1 coreceptors, immune response following HIV-1 infection have been defined with their genetic loci located on variable chromosomes (Fig. 19.2).

Consortium approaches and their meta-analyses have revealed that only a fraction of the observed phenotypic differences can be explained by variability at such loci. Some of the genetic associations that have been established with HIV/AIDS conclusively involve (i) HLA polymorphic loci and their associated genes including HCP5, RNF39, ZNRD1 on the short arm of chromosome 6, (ii) chemokine receptors CCR2, CCR5 that act as HIV entry coreceptors and chemokine ligands like CCL3L1, CCL4L1, CCL5, (iii) anti-viral restriction factor TRIM5α on chromosome 11p15, (iv) APOBEC3 on chromosome 22q13, (v) DC-SIGN on chromosome 19p13, (vi) KIR3DS1 on chromosome 19q13, (vii) Interferon regulatory factor 1 (IRF1), (viii) LY6 family of G (GPI) -anchored proteins and others. Of these, two genetic regions namely, HLA-HCP5-RNF39-ZNRD1 region at 6p21[12] and the rs2572886-LY6 region at 8q24[13] have been established through genome wide association studies on a variety of population groups.

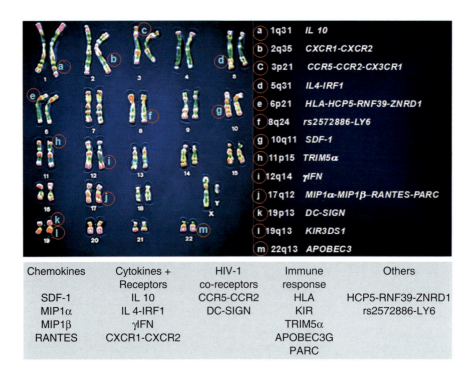

Fig. 19.2: Chromosomal localization of human genes involved in HIV/AIDS susceptibility, transmission, progression and response to therapy. For the sake of convenience, individual genes have been grouped according to their function at the bottom of the figure [Adapted from (4)]

Genes Influencing Viral Entry

Chemokines and their Receptors

Chemokines are low molecular weight potent chemoattractants produced by a variety of cell types that include T cells, macrophages, NK cells, B cells, fibroblasts and mast cells. These are involved in cell trafficking and immunomodulation of inflammation and immune responses. In certain instances, their receptors serve as entry portals for pathogens to gain entry into target cells and establish infection. For example, the Duffy Antigen Receptor for Chemokines (DARC) is utilized by *Plasmodium vivax*, while CCR5 and CXCR4 are preferentially opted by the HIV-1.

Vast majority of primary HIV-1 isolates are predominantly CCR5 tropic and gradually tend to become CXCR4 tropic during late infection. All non-syncitium inducing (NSI) strains of HIV-1 require chemokine receptor CCR5 to gain entry into target cells while the syncitium inducing (SI) virions utilize CXCR4 to enter (Fig. 19.3). The CCR5 expression is upregulated under the influence of IL 2 and IL 10 while IL 4 induces CXCR4 expression. The chemokines CCL3 (MIP1α), CCL4 (MIP1β) and CCL5 (RANTES) are natural ligands of CCR5 coreceptor that can block entry of nonsyncitium inducing virions. Similarly SDF-1 is a ligand for CXCR4 that is primarily used by syncitium inducing viruses.

Therefore, the availability of chemokine receptors expressed on cell surface and the levels of their ligands as well as cytokines are critical elements as they can enhance/suppress HIV entry. Functional genetic polymorphisms are known to occur in these proteins that affect their levels of expression and therefore might modulate their molecular interactions.

Of the known 50 genes for chemokines, 16 corresponding to the CC chemokine family are clustered together on chromosome 17q12. The primary HIV coreceptor CCR5 and CCR2 are located on chromosome 3p21 and constitute the extended CCR5 haplogroups.

CCR2: A valine to isoleucine substitution at position 64 (V64I or G190A) in the first transmembrane region of CCR2 has been associated with delayed progression to AIDS, by ~2 to 4 years than homozygous individuals carrying the wild-type allele.[14] The protective allele 'A' occurs at a population frequency of 8 to 10 percent among Caucasians, 15 to 17 percent in Chinese, ~ 12 percent in the North Indians[15] and 3 - 17 percent in the South Indian populations.[16] In an earlier study, Louisirirotchanakul and coworkers[17] reported that CCR264I homozygosity is associated with a reduced risk of acquiring infection among the HIV discordant couples in Thailand. However, in the Indian population, this polymorphism was not found to be protective against HIV-1.[15] Since the genetic loci for CCR2 and CCR5 are in strong linkage

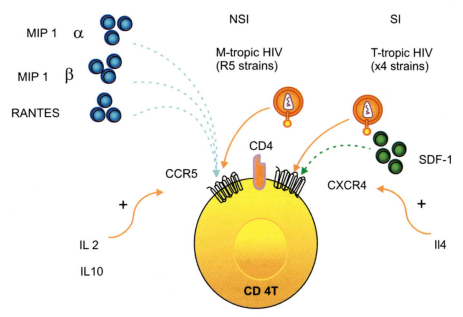

Fig. 19.3: Diagrammatic representation of binding of HIV to chemokine co-receptors CCR5 and CXCR4 expressed on the CD4 T cell. The level of expression of chemokine receptor CCR5, its ligands MIP1α, MIP1β, RANTES; and receptor CXCR4 and its ligand SDF-1 may enhance or suppress risk of HIV infection *[Adapted from (4)]*

disequilibrium, their combined analysis is greatly helpful to define CCR2-CCR5 extended haplotypes for disease association purposes.

CCR5: Multiple polymorphic variations have been described in the CCR5 gene.[18] Of these, a natural knockout deletion of 32 bases, i.e. CCR5 D32 introduces a premature stop codon resulting in truncated protein product.[19] In homozygous state, this deletion provides near complete protection in HIV infected individuals and upto 2-4 years delay in disease progression in the heterozygous state.[19,20] The CCR5D32 is found at a frequency of 10 to 16 percent in Northern Europe and this frequency decreases in a Southeast cline towards Mediterranean and gradually disappears in the African and Asian populations. It is extremely rare or almost absent in the Indian population.[21]

Based on a unique constellation of additional multisite polymorphisms in CCR5 regulatory 5' region, a number of CCR5 haplotypes have been identified[18,22] as illustrated in Figure 19.4. These have been designated based on the nucleotide position in the 5' UTR region and are referred to as haplogroups A to G. Of these, HHE has been associated with accelerated disease progression in Caucasians[18] and Thais[23] but not African Americans. In the latter, it is the HHD haplotype that shows positive association with fast progression to AIDS.[24] Similarly, HHC has been associated with fast disease progression in African Americans but with slow rate of progression in the Thai population. The HHG*2 and HHF*2 have been associated with slower progression among Caucasian and African American populations, respectively, plausibly because of the protective effects of D32 and CCR264I, respectively. In the Indian population, HHE has been implicated with susceptibility to infection and development of AIDS.[25] Whether this haplotype also influences disease progression is not clear since long term follow up is desirable to reach such a conclusion.

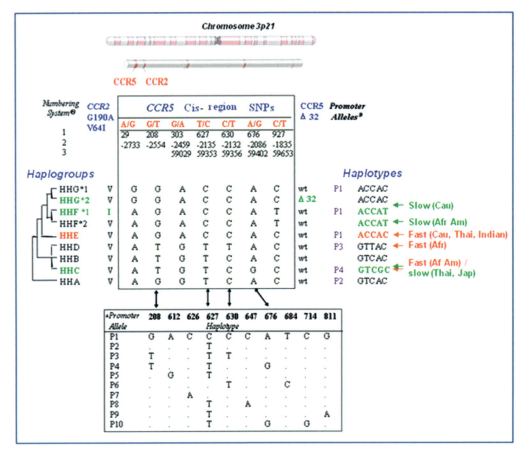

Fig. 19.4: Organization of CCR2 and CCR5 haplotypes on chromosome 3p21 and their association with HIV disease progression. There are seven haplogroups encompassing SNPs corresponding to CCR2 V64I, CCR5 cis region and the CCR5 deletion polymorphism. @Numbering system 1 is based on Genbank accession numbers AF031236, AF031237,[16] whereas 2 is relative to the translational site and 3 is based on accession number U95626. #The promoter alleles (P1 to P10) are numbered according to Martin et al[22] *[Adapted from (4)]*

CCL3-CCL4-CCL18 cluster: Genes coding for CCL3 (MIP1α), CCL4 (MIP1β) and CCL18 (PARC) are clustered together within a 47kb region on chromosome 17q12. These are potent chemokines produced by macrophages, NK cells, fibroblasts and T cells. Of these, CCL3 and CCL4 are natural ligands for the primary HIV co-receptor CCR5 and their genetic polymorphisms have been implicated in HIV-1 acquisition and disease progression[26] although these associations are complicated due to strong linkage disequilibrium between them.

Macrophage inflammatory protein-1 (MIP-1) is a monokine that is involved in the acute inflammatory state in the recruitment and activation of polymorphonuclear leukocytes. MIP1α (or the small inducible cytokine A3: SCYA3) and MIP1β (or the small inducible cytokine A4: SCYA4) are ~60 percent identical at protein level, their genes are separated by 14 kb, and are organized in a head-to-head fashion. The gene for CCL18, also referred to as the small inducible cytokine subfamily A member 18 (SCYA18) or the Pulmonary and activation-regulated chemokine (PARC) contains 3 exons and is 7.2 kb long. It is expressed at high levels in the lung, alveolar macrophages and in follicular dendritic cells of the germinal centers of lymph nodes. It is involved in the recruitment of Th2 cells and basophils in asthma allergic reactions and is upregulated by IL 4.

CCL3L1: Human CC chemokine ligand 3 like 1 gene (CCL3L1) also referred to as the macrophage inflammatory protein-1α (MIP-1αP) or the small inducible cytokine A3-like 1 (SCYA3L1) is a natural ligand of HIV co-receptor CCR5 and a potent HIV-1 suppressive chemokine that can physically block the entry of HIV-1. It is located on human chromosome 17q11.2 (Figs 19.5A and B) and shares 96 percent amino acid homology with CCL3. Although the CCL3 gene exists as a single copy per haploid genome, the copy number of the CCL3L1 gene varies among different individuals, and population groups.

The CCL3L1 and CCL4L1 genes harbor several SNPs and hotspots for duplication resulting in distinct haplotypes and copy number variations respectively in different individuals.[26] The copy numbers are the highest in Africans, followed by Asians, Amerindians, Central/South Asians, Middle East and Europeans.[27] It has been suggested that since CCL3L1 is a potent ligand of CCR5, variations in copy numbers and thus their expression might influence entry of the virus. Using real-time quantitative PCR, Townson et al[28] reported that CCL3L1 occurs as 2 copies per diploid genome in most Caucasians (49%), although 10 to 20 percent individuals could have 1, 3 or 4 copies.

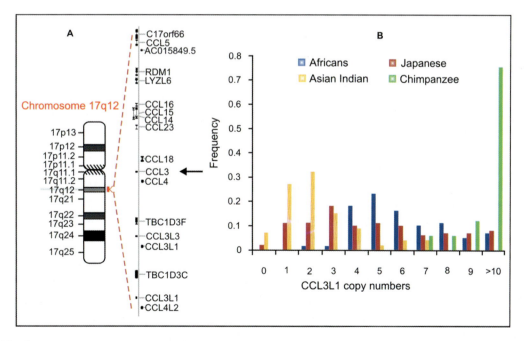

Figs 19.5A and B: Comparative genomic analysis of CCL3L1 copy numbers in different populations as compared to the Chimpanzee. (A) Gene map showing localization of CCL3L1 and other chemokines on chromosome 17q12, (B) Copy number variations in CCL3L1 in the Japanese, Asian Indian and African populations[27,30] *[Adapted from (4)]*

Copy number variations in CCL3L1 have been reported to be associated with susceptibility to HIV-1 infection.[27,29] However, such variations do not seem to have a significant effect on disease progression.[29] Further, subjects with 2 or less copies of CCL3L1 have significantly higher risk of acquiring HIV infection. A recent study carried out in the Japanese population[29] has shown that the average copy number of CCL3L1 in the HIV-1-infected subjects is significantly lower than in healthy controls (3.35±0.24 vs 5.00±0.22, p<0.001). On the contrary, studies on the North Indian population showed that the copy number variation in CCL3L1 has no effect on acquisition (2.13±0.15 in HIV infected individuals as compared to 2.34±0.17 in healthy controls).[30] It is worth mentioning that Chimpanzees who are naturally resistant to HIV-1 possess very high (~9-10) CCL3L1 copy numbers.[27,31]

Based on the combination of genotypes for CCL3L1 copy numbers and CCR5 deletion mutation, genetic risk groups can be defined that could help assess AIDS risk to HIV infection.[32,33] Individuals with CCL3L1 high copy numbers and CCR5 deletion point towards low risk as compared to those with CCL3L1 low copy numbers and CCR5 non-deletion genotypes. Further, these genotypes have been shown to influence CD4 recovery and immune reconstitution after HAART.[33] A recent study reported a correlation between higher CCL3L1 copy numbers and greater CD4+ and CD8+T cell responses to HIV-1 gag protein in the African population.[34]

RANTES: The chemokine 'Regulated upon Activation, Normally T-Expressed, and presumably Secreted' (RANTES), also referred to as small inducible cytokine A5 (SCYA5) is not only a mediator of inflammation, but also a significant regulator of differentiation in development. It is a natural ligand for CCR1, CCR3 and CCR5, and a potent inhibitor of infection by non-syncitium inducing CCR5 tropic HIV-1. It has been reported that a transversion of –28C to G in the promoter of RANTES increases its transcription and this polymorphism has been associated with delayed progression to AIDS in the Japanese population.[35] Another SNP, In1.1T/C (168923T/C) is found in a regulatory element in the first intron of RANTES. The 1n1.1C is associated with downregulated expression and has been implicated in accelerated progression to AIDS in African Americans and European Americans.[36] A recent study reported that the RANTES In1.1 T allele and haplotype II (ACT) may be a risk factor for HIV-1 transmission while RANTES In1.1 C allele may confer risk for disease progression among North Indians.[37] These data need to be replicated in larger cohorts, also in other population groups.

SDF-1: The **S**tromal cell **D**erived **F**actor 1 (SDF-1) or the CXCL12 is a highly potent α chemokine that binds CXCR4 (NPY3R), a co-receptor for syncitium inducing HIV-1 strains. It induces intracellular actin polymerization in lymphocytes and plays an important role in basal extravasation of lymphocytes and monocytes. It is therefore involved directly in regulating immune surveillance rather than in inflammation. SDF1-CXCR4 interactions are essential for the homing and retention of hematopoietic progenitor cells in the bone marrow and have been shown to control the navigation of progenitor cells between the bone marrow and blood. SDF1 is a ligand for CXCR4 and a potent entry inhibitor for syncitium inducing viruses that generally emerge during late stage HIV infection.

The gene for SDF-1 is ~ 10 kb long and located on human chromosome 10q11.1. It exists in two isoforms: alpha and beta obtained as a consequence of alternative splicing. The alpha form is derived from exons 1 to 3 while the beta form contains additional sequence from exon 4. A common polymorphism, i.e. presence of A at the SNP G801A in the 3' untranslated region of SDF-1β has been shown to have a recessive protective effect against HIV-1 and associated with delayed onset of AIDS.[38] The 801A allele is found at a frequency of 0.211 in Caucasians, 0.160 in Hispanics, 0.057 in African Americans, 0.257 in Asians and 0.24 in case of North Indians,[39,40] and 0.117 to 0.35 in South Indians.[16]

CXCR1-CXCR2: CXCR1 (IL 8RA) and CXCR2 (IL 8RB) are receptors for IL 8, a proinflammatory cytokine involved in chemoattraction and activation of neutrophils. Their genes are colocalized in a region spanning ~26 kb on chromosome 2q35 (Fig. 19.6) and have ~25 percent similarity in sequence to other neutrophil chemoattractants, fMet-Leu-Phe and C5a. Studies have indicated a dysregulated elevated IL-8 production and reduced expression of IL-8 receptors, CXCR1 and CXCR2 in HIV-1-infected patients. Reduced CXCR1 activity upon HIV-1 infection due to cross-receptor-mediated internalization with the major coreceptors CCR5 and CXCR4 has also been reported.[41] These observations suggest that CXCR1 and CXCR2 could affect AIDS-related conditions.

The CXCR1 and CXCR2 genes consist of several polymorphisms and depending on their linkage

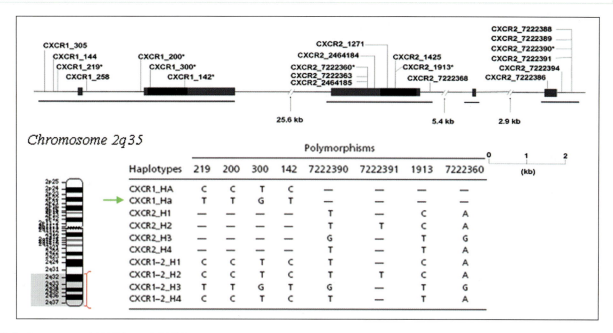

Fig. 19.6: Gene map of CXCR1 and CXCR2 on chromosome 2q35 with polymorphic positions and CXCR1 haplotypes indicated. Atleast 10 CXCR1 haplotypes are known.[42] Arrow indicates haplotype 'Ha' that has been associated with delayed progression in Caucasians [Adapted from (4)]

disequilibrium, have been classified into distinct haplotypes.[42] Two SNPs T92G (CXCR1 -300) and C1003T (CXCR1 -142), in particular, result in nonsynonymous substitutions M31R in the N terminal extracellular domain and R335C in the C terminal intracellular domain respectively. These two SNPs are an integral part of the CXCR1 haplotype 'Ha'. A recent genetic study on the French GRIV cohort comprising of 84 rapid and 253 slow progressors identified a strong association of CXCR1 haplotype 'Ha' with protection against rapid progression to AIDS.[42] It was suggested that the inhibitory effect of CXCR1 Ha could be mediated by suppressing CD4 and CXCR4 expression. This could be caused by either the direct involvement of palmitoylation of the cysteine introduced in the C terminus of CXCR1, or some other unknown CXCR1-mediated signaling, that regulate expression and intracellular trafficking of CD4 and CXCR4.

DARC

It has recently been shown that the **D**uffy **A**ntigen **R**eceptor for **c**hemokines (DARC), alternatively called as Glycoprotein D (GPD), conventionally used in the Duffy based blood grouping system and a known receptor for *P vivax*, can aid HIV-1 attachment to RBCs and its trans-infection to target cells.[43] The Duffy system is located on chromosome 1q21-22. The -46T-C SNP in particular, in the promoter of DARC is widely prevalent in populations of African descent, and its homozygous –46CC genotype results in selective loss of DARC expression on RBCs. This genotype has been shown to be associated not only with a high risk of HIV-1 infection but on the contrary, also with slower progression in terms of death or development of dementia. It has been suggested that there is interplay between DARC and chemokines that ultimately determine the amount of free virus bound to RBCs for eventual trans-infection.

DC-SIGN

Dendritic **C**ell-**S**pecific **I**ntracellular adhesion molecule-3-**G**rabbing **N**onintegrin (DC-SIGN, CD209) and its related protein DC-SIGNR are C-type lectins known to bind multiple pathogens such as HIV-1, HIV-2, *Mycobacterium tuberculosis, Helicobacter pylori, Klebsiella pneumoniae,* Dengue virus, Ebola virus, hepatitis C virus, CMV, measles, coronavirus, *Leishmania pifanoi, Shistosoma mansoni* and *Candida albicans*. The DC-SIGN and DC-SIGNR show 77 percent homology at amino acid sequence level; act as cell adhesion and pathogen recognition receptors and are involved in both innate as well as adaptive immunity. The two genes appear to have originated from a common ancestral gene by duplication and are therefore located in close proximity in head to head orientation on chromosome 19p13.

Polymorphisms in DC-SIGN and DC-SIGNR genes have recently been studied in Caucasian and African populations and several novel SNPs identified in 5′ and 3′ UTR regions.[44] These investigators have reported several significant differences in the prevalence of different alleles and haplotypes in the two population groups. In general, the African population shows greater genetic diversity in DC-SIGN than other populations. The DC-SIGN promoter variant -336C affects a Sp1 binding site and leads to decreased expression of DC-SIGN. This particular allele has been associated with susceptibility to parenteral HIV-1 infection in the European Americans.[45] This association has not been reported in patients known to be at risk for mucosally acquired infection.

A total of eight DC-SIGN haplotypes have been reported (Table 19.3). Of these, haplotype 4, that contains all of the high-risk SNPs, is associated with parenterally acquired infection (OR = 2.62, $P = 0.018$). On the other hand, the haplotype containing all of the protective SNPs (–139T, –336T, –939T, –1180T, and –1466T) is quite rare (frequency ≤ 0.001), making it difficult to test its influence on the actual risk following HIV-1 infection. Although this study did not find any significant association with HIV-1 disease progression, further evidence would be required to suggest that DCSIGN variants that bind the envelope glycoprotein of both R5 and X4 viruses more efficiently might also lead to enhanced virus infection.

The immune response generated by the host and the selection pressure exerted on the virus particularly at the time of early infection, directs the emergence of adaptive escape mutants. Accordingly, some mutations reduce the viral fitness and make it either revert to the wild type or gradually wane out, while others might rescue the virus from host surveillance. Thus viruses have the ability to adapt and evolve differentially at varying rates in different individuals depending on their host genetic architecture and concordance in the immunome. In general, greater the immune concordance between the virus donor and the recipient, easier it is for the virus to transcend and re-establish itself in the new host.

Genes Involved in Anti-HIV Immune Response

In addition to the genes that act at the level of viral entry, there are others that are critically involved in HIV restriction and influence the ensuing immune response. These include for example, the antiviral APOBEC3G gene family and the virus restriction factor TRIM5α that are described briefly in the following section.

APOBEC3G

Apolipoprotein B mRNA-editing enzyme, catalytic polypeptide-like 3G (APOBEC3G) is a host antiviral factor. It is a cytidine deaminase that induces G to A hypermutation in newly synthesized retroviral DNA resulting in instability of the nascent viral transcripts or lethal mutations.[46] However, this APOBEC3G mediated innate immune mechanism is counteracted by the HIV-1 vif thus allowing the virus to escape via mutations and even develop drug resistance to lamivudine (3TC).[47] It has been demonstrated that residues asp128 in APOBEC3G in humans and lys 128 in African green monkeys are involved in binding with viral vif resulting in its degradation. Further, an interchange of the asp128 with lys128 in human APOBEC3G switches its sensitivity from HIV vif to SIV vif.[48] APOBEC3G functions as a potent post-entry restriction factor for HIV-1 in naïve CD4 T cells but is not protective in activated CD4 T cells. In the latter, it is recruited into an enzymatically inactive high molecular mass ribonucleoprotein complex that depends on RNase for its conversion to its low molecular mass and active form. This inactivated form of APOBEC3G following T cell activation has been correlated with permissivity for HIV infection.[49] It has been suggested that creation of HIV vif resistant APOBEC3G mutations could provide an effective gene therapy approach against the virus.[50]

The gene for APOBEC3G exists as a tandem array of 7 APOBEC genes or pseudogenes on chromosome 22q12-q13.2. It has been reported that the antiviral activity of the APOBEC3H has been lost in the majority of human populations excluding Africans, via two polymorphisms and this may have important consequences for susceptibility to retroviral infections.[51]

Table 19.3: Major DC-SIGN haplotypes identified in the promoter region and investigated in HIV infection and disease progression studies (Adapted from: Martin)[45]

Haplotype	Nucleotide at position						
	–139	–336	–939	–1089	–1180	–1466	–1530
1	C	T	T	C	T	C	A
2	T	T	C	C	A	T	A
3	C	T	T	C	T	T	A
4	C	C	C	C	A	C	A
5	T	T	C	A	A	T	A
6	C	C	C	C	A	C	C
7	T	T	C	C	A	C	A
8	C	C	C	C	T	C	A

[Adapted from (4)]

TRIM5α

The antiviral factor, **T**ripartite **I**nteraction **M**otif 5α (TRIM5α) protects humans and other primates against a broad range of retroviruses in a species-specific manner. It targets the capsid molecules of the incoming retrovirus in the cytosol and disrupts its replication. Human TRIM5α can block N-tropic Murine leukemia virus (MLV) and equine anaemia virus, but is much less efficient in restricting HIV-1 replication, although TRIM5α escape mutants have been identified late in infection. Two SNPs (H43Y and R136Q) have been reported to affect the antiviral activity of this restriction factor. The 43Y allele is believed to impair the E3 ligase activity of TRIM and favors progression to AIDS. The other polymorphism 136Q is associated with greater anti-HIV activity and has earlier been reported to be more frequently observed in high risk seronegative African Americans as compared to HIV seropositive patients. Recently, Manen and coworkers[52] have analyzed the effect of polymorphisms in TRIM5α on the clinical course of HIV-1 infection in homosexual men enrolled in Amsterdam cohort studies (ACS). The study reported an accelerated disease progression in individuals homozygous for 43Y and established an *in vitro* protective effect of 136Q against the X4 viruses that infect naïve T cells. Further, these investigators reported that the 136Q allele along with -2GG genotype in the 5′UTR of TIM5α is associated with rapid progression to AIDS. In another recent study, TRIM5α sequence variants in exon 2 were investigated for association with susceptibility to HIV-1 infection in the Japanese and North Indian populations.[53] The study showed that the haplotypes carrying 43Tyr allele were significantly associated with reduced susceptibility in both these populations. Functional analyses revealed that the Gly110Arg substitution weakened the anti-HIV-1 and anti-HIV-2 activities of human TRIM5α, whereas the truncated G176del variant enhanced the anti-viral activity. It was concluded that the Gly110Arg and G176 del variants were associated with susceptibility and protection from HIV-1 infection respectively.

Among the various immunogenetic determinants that are known to influence HIV/AIDS, the HLA system which is the major histocompatibility complex (MHC) of man represents the central focal point because of its major biological function of presenting foreign peptides to the immune system. It is therefore the major driving force for shaping mutations in the virus. Further, specific HLA alleles are involved in hypersensitivity reactions to some of the antiretroviral drugs, for example abacavir therapy with HLA-B*5701 and nevirapine with DRB1*0101 allele.[54] The main focus of this review is to illustrate HLA allelic influences in governing immune response to HIV-1 infection and/or disease progression. In addition, the role of polymorphic gene determinants in pro- and anti-inflammatory cytokines in influencing HIV susceptibility has been discussed.

Major Histocompatibility Complex (MHC)

Human MHC is comprised of a set of highly polymorphic HLA (Human leukocyte antigen) class I and class II molecules (Fig. 19.7) whose main function is to regulate the development of an immune response. It is one of the important components of the human immunome whose gene products play a leading role in various stages of HIV-1 infection, disease progression and transmission. These include (i) selecting the repertoire of viral epitopes that are presented to T helper or CTLs, (ii) induction of NK cell mediated anti-viral cytotoxicity, and (iii) imprinting mutations in the virus thereby modulating kinetics of viral escape.

HLA Heterozygous Advantage

Since the major biological function of HLA class I and class II molecules is presentation of peptides (endogenous and exogenous respectively), the genetic polymorphism in these loci sets the stage for effective CD8+ and CD4+ T cell responses respectively against the virus. HLA system is, therefore, responsible for enforcing immune selection pressure on the virus and imprints viral mutations. Due to this, the virus continues to evolve into new mutants, albeit with varying degrees of fitness. An increased heterozygosity at HLA class I region is considered to be a selective advantage against AIDS as it empowers greater ability of the host to present a wide range of viral antigens and therefore evoke a broader T cell response. This results in delayed emergence of escape mutants and considerably prolongs the period before actual development of full blown AIDS. Carrington and coworkers (1999) have reported that 28 to 40 percent of HIV-1-infected Caucasian subjects who delayed AIDS for 10 or more years were fully heterozygous at HLA class I loci.[58]

HLA Sharing and Virus Transmission

An important observation that emerges from most HLA studies related to horizontal transmission of HIV

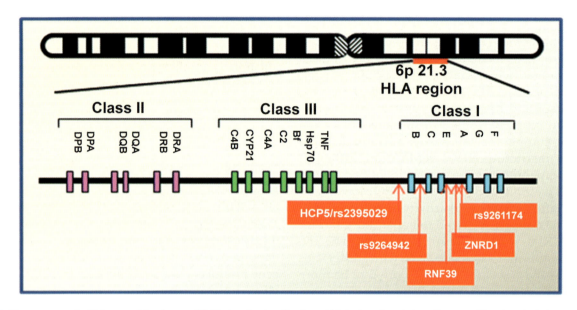

Fig. 19.7: Chromosome 6p21.3 map of the human MHC showing localization of HLA class I and class II genes. The classical HLA class I genes are located towards telomeric end and include HLA-A, B and C while class II are located towards the centromeric end and include genes like HLA-DR, DQ and DP. The HLA class III genes like TNF, Bf, Complement proteins are located in between class I and class II genes. Genes namely HCP5 (rs2395029), rs926494, RNF392 and ZNRD1 associated specifically with viremia control following HIV infection as suggested through genome scan and related studies[12,55] or linked with hypersensitivity to abacavir[56,57] also lie within the human MHC region and are indicated in red shaded boxes. *[Adapted from (5)]*

infection suggests that greater the MHC concordance between the virus donor and recipient, easier it is for the virus to passage itself to a new host.[59] The virus escape mechanisms are hence consistent among individuals with similar HLA class I alleles. A recent study carried out on Zambian discordant couples showed that HLA class I diversity influences heterosexual transmission. The study demonstrated that HLA-A*3601 on the A*36-Cw*04-B*53 haplotype was the most unfavorable marker of HIV-1 transmission by index partners, while Cw*1801 (primarily on the A*30-Cw*18-B*57 haplotype) was the most favorable.[60]

In the case of vertical transmission, (for example from mother to child), it is generally easier for the pre-adapted virus to re-establish itself in the progeny as the children are at least HLA haploidentical (sharing one haplotype) with their mothers. The virus therefore finds it convenient to continue to propagate unchecked, promote disease progression, and break through immune surveillance among such children, even if the shared HLA allele is apparently a 'protective' one like HLA-B27.[61] Walker and colleagues[61] reported that HLA-B27 +ve children born from mothers who were also B27+ve did not do well clinically despite their HLA-B27+ve status. This is in contrast to those who inherited B27 from their fathers instead and turned out to be slow/long-term non-progressors. Viral sequencing revealed that the former set of HLA-B27 positive children had in fact received the mutated virus from their mothers that had already learnt how to deal with the B27 molecules effectively, thus avoiding the protective immune cover conferred by the HLA molecule.

Similarly, a recent study by Schneidewind et al (2009)[62] investigated the role of maternal transmission of escape mutants against epitopes restricted by another 'protective' allele HLA-B57. The investigators found that the B57+ve infants born to B57+ve mothers could control the viremia and also possessed virions with attenuating mutations within TW10-Gag and other B57 restricted epitopes. On the other hand, the B57–ve infants born to B57 +ve mothers progressed rapidly to AIDS. The data suggested that B57 confers its advantage primarily by driving and maintaining a fitness-attenuating mutation in p24-Gag protein of the virus rather than depending solely on CD8 T cell recognition of B57 restricted epitopes.

It follows therefore that both the process of antigen presentation as well as the CTL escape are HLA class I restricted. These studies suggest that HLA class I footprints can be traced in the viral immune landscape in diverse populations and can be used to predict important possible sites of immune evasion in the virus.

Role of Rare HLA Alleles

Recently, investigations on the epitope mapping of HLA specific viral mutants have led to a conclusion that rare HLA alleles might drive additional viral evolution compared to the more common alleles particularly in relation to *env, nef* and *pol* HIV-1 genes.[63] Furthermore, individuals with rare HLA alleles are more likely to be heterozygous at HLA loci. Accordingly, HIV evades the immune pressure in individuals with common HLA alleles by emerging into escape variants that finally reach a point of fixation in the population (Fig. 19.8). On the contrary, when the virus encounters host(s) with rare HLA alleles, it is forced to evolve into additional variant forms albeit with low fitness. Several of such mutants therefore tend to revert to their more ancestral type suggesting that rare HLA alleles may confer selective advantage to such individuals. The pre-existing escape mutations transmitted among these people do not protect the virus against the immunity mediated by rare HLA alleles and leads to a reduced viral load. It is reasonable to believe that information on the epitope sequences in such reverting variants under the influence of rare HLA alleles would be highly advantageous and could be integrated in vaccine design against the HIV-1.

It is plausible that the population frequency of escape mutants correlates with the prevalence of restricting HLA alleles.[64] Since 25 years of HIV pandemic, the virus appears to be adapting to the restricting HLA alleles over time, particularly in populations where such alleles occur at high frequencies. For example, frequency of the viral mutant I135X [RT128-135] has been reported to correlate with the presence of HLA-B*51. This allele is highly prevalent amongst the Japanese (~20%) and a large majority of virus (>50%) in this population has gradually adapted the I135X mutation. Due to this, while B*51 was protective 25 years ago in Japan, this may not be the case at present.[64] Hence, there is apprehension among the HLA geneticists that the strong protection conferred by HLA alleles like the B*27, B*57 and B*51 may indeed decline with the passage of time. However, the brighter side of such an adaptive escape and loss of immunodominant epitopes is that subdominant CTL responses may be promoted, which may be more beneficial against circulating clade(s) of the virus in

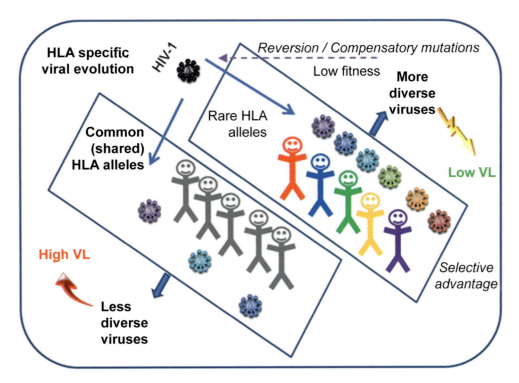

Fig. 19.8: Effect of HLA sharing between virus donor and recipient on the evolution of HLA specific HIV-1 escape mutants. Individuals with common HLA alleles (left panel) generally have limited virus diversification required to attain escape status and evade immunity leading to higher viral loads. On the other hand, in those with rare HLA class I alleles (right panel) there is possibly an unexpected encounter of the virus with HLA, leading to greater adaptive evolution albeit with low fitness/reversion. The emergence of latter results in low viral loads thereby suggesting that rare HLA alleles endow host with 'selective advantage' against the virus *[Adapted from (5)]*

various populations. These novel immune responses may turn out to be population specific due to differences in frequency of HLA alleles and the HLA mediated immune pressures on the virus. For example, B*1801 is associated with high viremia in C clade but not clade B, whilst the reverse is true for B*5301.[64]

HLA and Drug Hypersensitivity

A considerable inter-individual variability has been witnessed among HIV infected patients in terms of HAART hypersensitivity reactions. Abacavir (NRTI) is a commonly used drug against HIV-1 but can prove fatal if administered in patients who may have genetic predisposition to its toxic effects.[56] Approximately 2 to 8 percent of HIV infected Caucasian patients have been found to develop Abacavir Hypersensitivity syndrome (AHS) within 10 to 40 days after initiation of chemotherapy. Such patients show a strong association of AHS with an extended MHC Ancestral Haplotype 57.1 (AH57.1) carrying HLA-B*5701-DRB1*07.[65] Accordingly, presence of HLA-B*5701 is highly predictive of clinically diagnosed AHS and has been confirmed in several study cohorts.[66] Based on these studies, HIV treatment guidelines in the US and Europe have recommended mandatory screening of B*5701 before prescribing abacavir therapy. In European populations, B*5701 is found in strong linkage with the minor allele G corresponding to a SNP rs2395029 in the HCP5 gene in the MHC region.[56] These investigators have advocated HCP5 genotyping as an alternate marker for screening AHS particularly in low resource settings.[56] Recently, Chessman et al (2008) have explained the mechanism underlying abacavir induced AHS and reported that the drug induces specific HLA-B*5701 restricted CD8 + T cell responses through the conventional MHC class I antigen presentation pathway.[57] The specificity of abacavir recognition has been fine mapped particularly to residues 116 and 114 in the 'pocket F' of the peptide binding cleft of a B*5701 molecule.

Besides, a few other HAART formulations have shown specific genetic associations with drug efficacy and toxicities.[54] These include associations of i) HLA-DRB1*0101 and Cw8 with sensitivity to Nevirapine (NNRTI), ii) CYP2B6*6 with improved immunological recovery in response to NNRTIs; iii) CYP3A5*3 with faster PI (sequinavir and indinavir) oral clearance and others.[54]

HLA-KIR Interactions Modulate NK Cell Responses

It is known that HIV down-regulates expression of HLA-A and HLA-B, while sparing HLA-C. By doing so, the virus diminishes antigen presentation to T cells and also manages to evade an effective NK cell response. Killer cell Immunoglobulin like receptors (KIRs) are a set of polymorphic variants with their primary locus on chromosome 19 and control the activation or inhibition of NK cell response by recognition of specific HLA class I ligands. NK cell mediated target cell cytolysis occurs only when inhibitory signals are overcome by activating signals. The inhibitory and activating KIRs contain two or three external Ig-like domains (2D, 3D) with either long (2DL, 3DL) or short (2DS, 3DS) cytoplasmic tails, respectively. The inhibitory KIRs - KIR2DL2 and KIR2DL3 bind to HLA-Cw group 1 (HLA-C1), which have asparagine at position 80 whereas KIR2DL1 binds the mutually exclusive HLA-Cw group 2 (HLA-C2) with a lysine at this position. Group 1 comprises of the 2DL2, 2DL3, and 2DS2 binders, HLA-C*01, C*03, C*07 and C*08. In group 2 are the 2DL1 and 2DS1binders, namely HLA-C*02, C*04, C*05 and C*06.[67]

KIR3DL1 binds HLA-B molecules with the serologically defined Bw4 epitope, specified by five variable amino acids spanning positions 77–83. On the other hand, the alternative serotype, Bw6, is not known to bind any KIR. Despite high sequence similarity with inhibitory receptors, activating 2DS and 3DS KIRs show minimal binding to HLA class I. The KIR group A haplotypes contain two activating KIR genes KIR2DL4 and KIR2DS4, and five inhibitory KIR genes, KIR2DL1, KIR2DL3, KIR3DL1, KIR3DL2 and KIR3DL3. Whereas, group B haplotypes are defined by lack of KIR3DL1 and KIR2DS4 in the presence of inhibitory KIR2DL2 and KIR2DL5 and one or more of the activating KIR2DS1, KIR2DS2, KIR2DS3, KIR2DS5, and KIR3DS1.

Recently, Martin et al (2002)[68] showed that KIR3DS1, an activating receptor, is associated with rapid progression to AIDS but only in the absence of HLA-B alleles that encode Ile at position 40 (HLA-Bw4Ile). By contrast, when both KIR3DS1 and Bw4Ile were present, it resulted in an epistatic interaction with a synergistic protective effect. In the absence of KIR3DS1, the HLA-Bw4-80Ile allele was not associated with any effect on AIDS. Similarly, a study on seronegative female sex workers (FSWs) showed an increased occurrence of inhibitory KIRs in the absence of their specific ligands. For example, the inhibitory KIRs namely KIR2DL2/KIR2DL3 in heterozygous state and KIR3DL1 in homozygous state occur in the absence of their ligands HLA-C1 and HLA-Bw4 respectively.[69] On the contrary, seropositive FSWs had corresponding KIR and HLA ligands occurring together, for example, KIR2DL3 (homozygous) with HLA-C1 and KIR3DL1 in the presence of HLA alleles with Bw4 respectively. In agreement to this, the seronegative FSWs had a higher preponderance of AB haplotypes (containing higher number of activating KIRs) while seropositive FSWs had higher frequencies of the AA haplotypes (containing lower number of activating KIRs). Hence a lack of HLA ligands for inhibitory KIRs may lower the threshold for NK cell activation via activating KIRs, resulting in NK cytotoxicity and early elimination of HIV infected cells.

Non-classical HLA

The non-classical HLA class I molecules HLA-E and -G are ligands for the inhibitory NK cell receptors CD94/NKG2A and KIR2DL4, respectively. A recent study carried out on Zimbabwean women reported specific genetic variants of HLA-E (*0103) and HLA-G (*0105N) that are associated with a potentially lower affinity for their inhibitory NK cell receptors and decreased risk of HIV transmission.[70] It is now agreed that HLA-E and HLA-G polymorphisms can independently and synergistically influence susceptibility to heterosexual acquisition of HIV-1. These findings further support a role for NK cells in protection against HIV infection, its rate of progression and transmission and suggest that parallel inhibitory NK receptor/HLA ligand mechanisms may be involved.

HLA and HIV Mimicry

Chronic viral induced nonspecific immune stimulation is an important feature of progression to AIDS. It is often observed among the chronic progressors but is minimal in the LTNPs and the chimpanzees that are resistant to HIV-1. What induces this immunological hyperactivity is not clear although there are reports suggesting a strong sequence and structural similarity between C5 region of viral gp120 and the residues 67 to 80 of the hypervariable region 3 (HVR3) of the HLA-DRβ chain.[71] Such a mimicry may influence pathogenic immune activation through HLA/ TCR system[72] plausibly by binding similar peptides leading to allogeneic response similar to the one experienced during graft versus host disease (GvHD). HIV-1 may thus evade immune surveillance through peptide competition with HLA and result in loss of tolerance. Alternatively, this gp120-peptide complex may functionally mimic HLA-DR by binding with CD4[72] resulting in the presentation of sub-dominant cryptic self-epitopes and auto-activation. Molecular mimicry is well established between HIV-1 V3 loop sequences of gp120 and b strands in chemokines, and this might be a mechanism involved in directing selective coreceptor usage exploited by the virus.[73] It appears that targeting regions of mimic in the virus by antibodies even if non neutralizing, may promote therapeutic value of a vaccine designed to protect against progression.

HLA Class I Associations

Studies have shown that various viral proteins exhibit a hierarchy of immunogenicity (Nef> Gag> Pol> Env> Vif> Rev> Vpr> Tat> Vpu) and epitope recognition by CTLs.[74] It has been demonstrated that individual HLA class I alleles associated with delayed progression to AIDS contribute substantially to the total CD8 T cell response during primary infection in an immunodominant manner.[75] Different HLA class I alleles differ in their contribution to the total CD8 T cell response due to preferential recognition of a subset of HIV specific CTL epitopes. Recent data suggest that the 'protective' HLA class I alleles tend to present CTL epitopes derived mainly from the viral Gag capsid protein.

Several investigators have looked for an association of HLA class I alleles and their relative hazards with development and progression of HIV-1/AIDS in Caucasian and other populations. It has been demonstrated that HLA-B, in particular, plays a dominant role in selecting anti-viral CTL responses as compared to other class I molecules[76] and this difference can partially be explained by the greater diversity of HLA-B alleles compared to HLA-A and others. Figure 19.9 summarises various HLA alleles that have been associated with slow or fast disease progression following HIV infection. Of these, HLA- B*27[76] and B*57[77] show a particularly strong association with delayed progression to AIDS, while two other alleles, B*35[58,79] and B*53 are associated with rapid progression.[80] Further, HLA-B14, B44 and B51 have been associated with slow progression or viral control while A29 and B22 have been associated with rapid progression.

*HLA-B*27:* The HLA-B*27 allele that occurs with a frequency of ~ 4 to 6 percent among most human populations (http://www.allelefrequencies. net), is strongly associated with seronegative Spondyloarthropathies and Reiter's syndrome and is often used as a diagnostic aid worldwide. Of the 55 molecular subtypes of this allele, only four (*2702, *2704, *2705, *2707) have been reported to be associated with spondyloarthropathies, while others like *2706 and *2709 are not. HLA-B27 subtypes differ from the more common B*2705 'prototype' at one or more amino

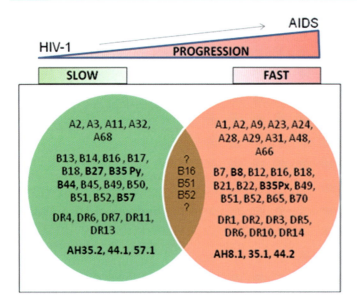

Fig. 19.9: HLA-A, B, DR alleles that have been reported to be associated with slow or fast progression following HIV infection. Allelic associations shown in bold have been found to be statistically significant in most studies [Adapted from (5)]

acid residues and show negative association with HIV infection. For example, presence of Glu^{2-} at position 45 contributes to an electronegative charge in the 'B pocket' of B*2705 and invites peptides with positively charged residues like Arg^{2+} at position P2 and thus contribute to slow pace of progression to AIDS. Most of the B*27 subtypes bind peptides with Arg at P2, but B*2701 also binds peptides with Gln^{2+}. Three major alleles, B*2705, *2703 and *2710 can present peptides with basic, aliphatic or aromatic C-terminal residues, whereas *2701, *2702, *2706, *2707 and *2709 present only peptides with C-terminal aliphatic or aromatic motifs. The crystal structure studies on B27 have demonstrated that a cysteine at position 67 alongwith glu at 45 and threonine at position 24 contribute to the specificity of 'pocket B' of the peptide binding site. It has been suggested that B*27 allotypes exert a moderate CTL mediated selection pressure on HIV-1. This leads to slow elimination of the virus and suppressed emergence of escape mutants.[81] The protective effect mediated by B*27 is therefore exerted at relatively late stages of the infection. However, HIV is in the process of adaptation and virus strains carrying CTL escape mutations against the main B27 epitope (Gag-p24 KK10, R264G) and additional compensatory mutation outside this epitope, like E260D, have been detected in circulation in the Netherlands.[82] Therefore, people carrying protective HLA alleles might not remain protected from HIV disease progression in the future.

*HLA-B*57:* Several studies have implicated an association of B*57 and related B*58, B*63 allelic family with low viremia and delayed onset of AIDS in various populations.[83] HLA-B*57 alleles bind peptides that carry large hydrophobic residues like tryptophan or phenylalanine at the carboxy terminus. Compared to B*27, the protective effect of B*57 is observed during early stages of infection. HLA-B*57 exerts a stronger selection pressure on virus forcing it to mutate rapidly. But this comes at the cost of its replicative fitness and the virus is finally eliminated.[80] Most patients carrying B*57 are relatively less symptomatic. Recent studies have shown that Elite controllers with B57 select rare Gag mutants with low fitness but strong CTL response[84] A particular Gag epitope KF11 can be presented by HLA-B*5701 and B*5703, subtypes that differ only by two amino acid residues at positions 114 and 116 near 'pocket F'.[85] This epitope undergoes limited escape variations in clade B virus under the influence of B*5701. However, it shows greater sequence variations in clade C among populations like those from Africa where *5703 is the major subtype. Hence even minor sequence differences in HLA may lead to totally divergent profiles of viral mutant forms.

*HLA-B*35:* Currently, 113 molecular subtypes of HLA-B*35 have become known and these can be categorized into two major groups based on their peptide binding abilities.[79] Of these, the B*35 'Py' group consists primarily of those alleles that bind epitopes with 'proline' at position 2 and 'tyrosine' at position 9, corresponding to 'pocket F' (Fig. 19.10). The B*35Px group of alleles, on the other hand, are more reactive and bind peptides with proline at P2 but several residues excluding tyrosine at P9. The HLA-B*35 Px and Py molecules differ primarily at position 116, which forms the floor of the peptide-anchoring 'F pocket' and determines the size of the peptide carboxy-terminal residues, and directly interacts with residues at P9 of the bound peptide. Variations at this position are critical not only in determining peptide preferences but also the peptide-loading machinery in the endoplasmic reticulum for optimizing the peptide repertoire.

The B*35Px molecules have been reported to favor rapid progression, i.e. accelerated transition from the time of seroconversion to a decline in CD4 counts to < 200.[80] However, the underlying mechanism(s) of such an association are not fully clear. A plausible hypothesis is that the HIV epitopes recognized by B*35Px act as 'immunological decoys' and induce CTLs that are

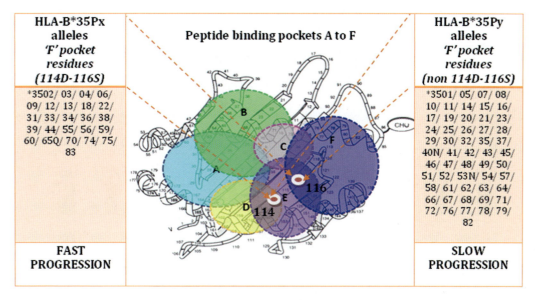

Fig. 19.10: Categorization of HLA-B*35'Px' and 'Py' alleles based on the peptide binding specificities of their F pockets for tyrosine towards the carboxy terminus of peptides. These two groups of alleles can be distinguished by the presence or absence of residues 114D and 116S that lie in and near the floor of the pocket F as shown in the middle panel of the figure *[Adapted from (5)]*

ineffective in destroying cells infected with HIV-1, thereby monopolizing CTL defense early during the infection.[80] In support of this possibility is the observation that carriers of HLA-B*35Py alleles reduce HIV-1 viral load far more effectively than those that have HLA-B*35Px alleles, despite having comparable quantitative CTL responses.[86] Preliminary studies on the Indian population have shown that population gene pool is 2 to 3 times more enriched with B*35Px alleles as compared to B*35Py, both in the healthy (58 percent Px versus 28 percent Py) and HIV infected individuals (70 percent Px versus 27 percent Py; RR = 1.17). However, these observations need to be further evaluated in terms of their effect on progression to AIDS in this and other populations.

An analysis of the data from various populations brings out a more holistic picture about the involvement of a 'trinity' of HLA alleles (B27, B57 and B35) that have been implicated in protection or susceptibility to HIV-1 infection and development of AIDS in different populations (Fig. 19.11). Interestingly, the susceptibility favoring HLA alleles and haplotypes are found as common constituents of gene pool in some populations (for example North Indians). Of these, the most common risk conferring classical HLA alleles appears to be B35. While further analyses is necessary to establish if B35 Px is more predominant than Py subtypes in different populations analogous to what has been observed in North Indians, the impact of such a profile at the population level with respect to HIV prevalence needs to be investigated. Furthermore, risk attributed by the MHC is only a fraction of the total genetic risk. Susceptibility to HIV/AIDS is under multigenic regulation and each host determinant contributes its own relative hazard towards the individuals' total genetic propensity to this infection. More importantly, the proportion of risk contributed by different factors may not necessarily be the same in different populations.

HLA Class II Associations

CD4 T cells play a central role in evoking an immune response against HIV as their help is critical for sustaining CTL and B cell responses. Immune prevalence of CD4 T cell epitopes depends on their capacity to bind to HLA class II molecules. As compared to CD8 T cells and their corresponding HLA class I associations, relatively little is known about the HLA class II molecules that could induce a protective CD4 T cell response and restrict viral infection.

A study carried out on acutely infected early treated HIV-1 positive patients suggested a significant association of HLA-DRB1*13 with suppressed viremia following treatment.[87] Another study on perinatal transmission reported a higher prevalence of DRB1*03 and DRB1*15 among infected and uninfected children

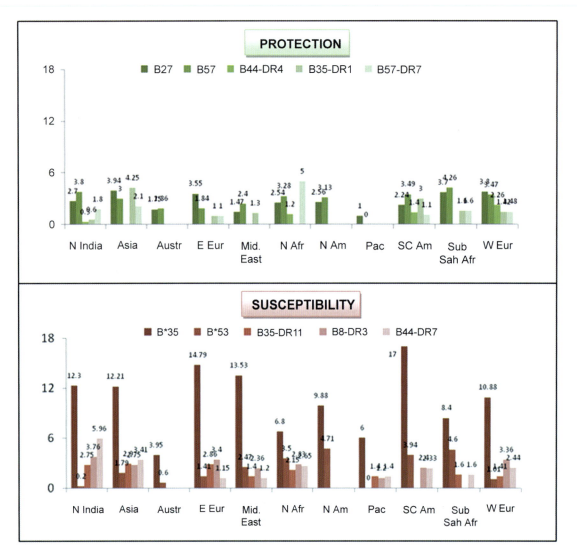

Fig. 19.11: Percent frequency distribution of HLA alleles and haplotypes associated with protection or susceptibility to HIV-1/AIDS in the healthy North Indian compared to other populations worldwide (*Adapted from: www.allelefrequencies.net*) [Adapted from (5)]

respectively born to infected mothers.[88] However, the HLA class II associations have not been reproducible and show variations in different populations.

Associations with HLA Supertypes

HLA supertypes represent a group of HLA alleles with overlapping peptide-binding properties. HLA class I supertype A*02/*6802 has been reported to protect Kenyan women from HIV-1 clade A infection and reduce mother to child transmission.[89] Similarly, HLA alleles A*0205/ *6802 belonging to the same supertype were observed more frequently among Highly Exposed Persistently Seronegative (HEPS) individuals in the 'Multi- center AIDS cohort study' (MACS) cohort which is an ongoing prospective study of HIV-1 infection in homosexual and bisexual men.[90] In case of HLA-B, B7 supertype which encompass alleles like B*0702-5, *1508, *3501-3, *5101, *5301, *5401, *5501-02, *5601, *5602, *6701, and *7801 (with specificities of proline at P2 and residues AILMVFWY at the C terminus) has been associated with high viremia, relatively poor CTL responses and accelerated progression to AIDS. This association was observed among Caucasians infected with the clade B virus but not in Africans who are infected predominantly with clade C.[58,81,91] The HLA supertypes A3 (*0301, *1101, *3101, *3301 and *6801) and B7 have been associated with susceptibility to HIV and development of AIDS in the North Indian HIV infected population.[92] The former, particularly the A*1101 has been found to restrict CTL epitopes derived from Nef protein of the virus in the HEPS and EUs among South East Asians.[93]

Associations with MHC Haplotypes

Extended MHC haplotypes that are conserved and inherited across generations due to strong linkage disequilibrium are referred to as 'Ancestral haplotypes' (AH). The classical Caucasian MHC haplotype, A1-B8-DR3-DQ2 (AH8.1) has been reported to be associated with faster progression to AIDS[91] although the underlying mechanism(s) are not clear. It is known that healthy people carrying this haplotype are immunologically hyper-responsive and have a significantly higher risk of developing autoimmune diseases. This haplotype is absent in the Indian population and is replaced by a totally different haplotype, designated as an AH8.1v where v refers to a 'variant form'.[94] Another related haplotype that occurs more commonly in this population is referred to as ancestral haplotype AH8.2 that is represented by A26-B8-DR3 with several genomic level differences from AH8.1.[94] Additionally, the Indian population is characterized by several other B8-DR3 haplotypes, which are unique and autoimmunogenic in the Indian population. However, there is no information on their role in HIV-1 infection and/or disease progression.

Another extended haplotype that shows positive association with rapid progression to AIDS among Caucasians is A11-Cw4-B35-DR1-DQ1,[91] apparently due to specific peptide binding motifs of B*35Px alleles. This study carried out on a French HIV infected cohort demonstrated that at least three haplotypes, namely AH35.1 [Ax-B35-DR11], 44.2 [A29-B44-DR7] and 8.1 [A1-B8-DR3] are associated with rapid progression and contribute an odds ratio (OR) of 5.7, 3.4 and 3 respectively. On the contrary, haplotypes like AH57.1 [A1-B57=DR7], 44.1 [A2-B44-DR4] and 35.2 [A11-B35-DR1] were associated with slow progression with OR of 5.8, 5.4 and 3.6 respectively. In the Zambian discordant couples, A*3601 on the A*36-Cw*04-B*53 haplotype has been reported to be the most unfavorable marker of HIV-1 transmission, while Cw*1801 (primarily on the A*30-Cw*18-B*57 haplotype) is the most favorable.[60] It is possible that B*53 and B*57 on these two haplotypes might also be involved in enhancement of infection or protection respectively.

Although there are no data available on the role of these key haplotypes associated with susceptibility or protection in HIV/AIDS in the Asian Indian population, baseline data available on the frequency distribution of these presumptive and related haplotypes carrying B8, B27, B44, B35 and B57 alleles in the North Indian population provides important leads (Fig. 19.12). For example, the germline gene pool of this population appears to be enriched particularly in the AH44.2 related haplotype, A33-B44-DR7 (as compared to A29-B44-DR7 that occurs in Caucasians). In fact this haplotype occurs predominantly in the North Indian population (3.4%) followed by A26-B8-DR3 (1.92%), A24-B52-DR15 (1.37%), A24-B40-DR15 (1.37%), A33-B58-DR3 (1.28%), A1-B57-DR7 (1.19%), A24-B8-DR3 (1.01%) and others. Further studies are needed to establish if such haplotype(s) are associated with HIV-1 disease pathogenesis in the Indian population where the virus background is predominantly of clade C type. It will be interesting to determine how haplotypes (such as AH8.2 or the A33-B44-DR7) that are unique to the Indian population would interact with the virus in this population and result in selection of perhaps different viral mutations. Information gained in this direction in diverse populations could help unravel target CTL epitopes for incorporation into future vaccine design against the HIV-1.

Genetic Polymorphisms in Pro- and Anti-inflammatory Cytokines

In addition to the genetic determinants belonging to MHC as described above and chemokine receptors along with their ligands, cytokine genes provide an additional set of host determined functional polymorphisms with a hitherto significant influence on HIV/AIDS pathogenesis. The role of cytokine gene polymorphisms (CGPs) in host defense against HIV-1 along with recent studies pertaining to whole genome scans for HIV-1/AIDS has been discussed here.

Cytokines are pleiotropic immunomodulators with functional genetic polymorphisms that affect their transcription levels. Ethnic differences in patterns of cytokine gene polymorphisms correlate well with population-based variations in the ability to mount an immune response. Accordingly, SNPs in relations to CGPs have been identified with differential association(s) with autoimmune and infectious diseases as well as graft function following organ and hematopoietic stem cell transplantation. Although the exact basis for the existence of variable cytokine genotypes in different ethnic groups is not clear, geographically localized natural selection imposed by invading microbes and host–pathogen interactions appears to be the most plausible explanation.

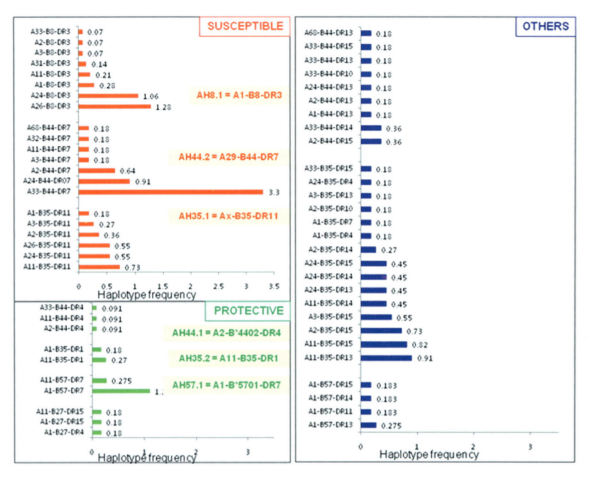

Fig. 19.12: A comparison of the haplotype frequencies of presumptive protective or susceptible haplotypes against HIV-1/AIDS and other haplotypes carrying HLA-B8, B27, B35, B44 and B57 alleles in the healthy North Indian population. The classical ancestral haplotypes (AH) that occur exclusively in the Caucasoids (AH8.1, 44.2, 35.1, 35.2 and 57.1) are shown in shaded background [Adapted from (5)]

Figures 19.13A to C summarizes the population distribution of various cytokine gene polymorphisms in the healthy North Indian population[95] along with a comparison with other major population groups.[96] The analyses reveals interesting results: (i) the low secretion IL 2 genotype (-330TT) is found predominantly in the Blacks, while the North Indians and Caucasians possess intermediate/high secretion genotypes, (ii) The high secretor genotype for IL 6 (-174 GG) occurs with the highest frequency in Blacks followed by Caucasians and North Indians, (iii) High IL 10 secretor haplotypes (-1082/-819/-592: GCC/GCC, GCC/ACC, GCC/ATA) are more predominant in the Black and Caucasian populations while Asians including North Indians are characterized by the low IL 10 secretor haplotypes (ATA/ATA, ATA/ACC, ACC/ACC),[29] (iv) The TNFα-308 low secretion genotype (GG) and TGFβ high secretion genotypes (codon 10/25: TT/GG, TC/GG) occur more frequently in all of the above populations.

That cytokines control HIV replication is now increasingly accepted.[97] The proinflammatory cytokines TNFα, TNFβ, IL1 and IL6 are found at elevated levels in HIV infected individuals and these have been reported to enhance viral replication. In contrast, IFNα, IFNβ and IL16 suppress HIV replication. The role of other cytokines like IL2, IL4, IL10, TGFβ and IFNγ is not very clear. However, these could either induce or suppress HIV expression depending on the cellular milieu. Interestingly, IL2 has been shown to upregulate expression of CCR1, CCR2 and CCR3. Further, cytokines are reported to have regulatory interactions as observed during HIV infection, for example, IL10 inhibits HIV replication by blocking secretion of TNFα and IL6.[98] In addition, opportunistic infections that are commonly observed during development of AIDS may lead to a burst of HIV inducing cytokines, particularly TNFα, IL6 and IL1 leading to increased viremia.

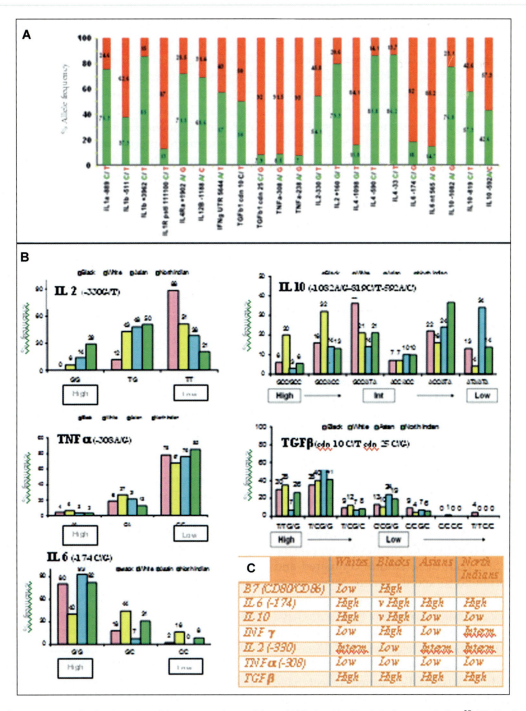

Figs 19.13A to C: Frequency distribution of cytokine gene polymorphisms (A) in healthy North Indian population,[95] (B) distribution of cytokine alleles/haplotypes associated with the high/ intermediate or low expressor phenotypes in major populations (Blacks, Whites, Asians and North Indians), (C) Levels of expressor phenotypes in different populations derived from information on their allelic and haplotype frequency distributions [Adapted from (5)]

As the HIV-1 infection progresses from nonsyncitium inducing (R5) to syncitium inducing (X4) viruses, it is accompanied simultaneously by a shift from Th1 to Th2 cytokine milieu. The anti-inflammatory cytokine, IL 4 induces expression of CXCR4 which favors the entry of X4 viruses. Further, increased levels of IL 10 are correlated with faster progression to AIDS. Amongst the pro-inflammatory cytokines, IL 1a has been found to be elevated in AIDS patients and it can enhance viremia through NF-kB mediated transactivation of viral LTRs. Similarly, TNFα which also occurs at increased levels in AIDS patients, is a potent inducer of HIV replication. The gene for TNFα is located within the MHC region and displays strong linkage disequilibrium with some of the conserved/ancestral haplotypes. As a result, the associations observed with TNFα may actually be secondary to haplotype associations. Again, polymorphism in cytokine genes has been reported to influence the development of immune restoration diseases (IRD) which occur frequently following ART.[99]

In a recent study on the North Indian HIV-1 infected individuals, we reported an overrepresentation of IL 4 -590 T, IL 10 -1082 G, TNFα -308A, IL1α -889T and γIFN UTR 5644T alleles, all of which are high secretor alleles except for γIFN.[92] These observations are consistent with those of others and support the suggestion of a dominant role of Th2 cytokines in HIV-1/AIDS.

Whole Genome Analysis for HIV Susceptibility Loci

With the advent of advanced molecular technologies and novel approaches of whole genome scans and gene expression profiling, it is now possible to identify novel susceptibility loci for various diseases as a virtue of their physical location and gene function. The first genome wide association study was carried out by Fellay et al (2007)[12] with the main purpose of defining the control of HIV infection by host determinant genes. This was quickly followed by another recent *in vitro* analysis of genetic determinants of susceptibility using multi-generation families from CEPH (Centre d'Etude du Polymorphisme Humain) resource.[13] Both these studies compared and estimated the contribution of specific genetic determinants that play a central role in HIV-1 pathogenesis against the total genomic background. The results of these scans have opened up new perspectives in our understanding of the host-pathogen interaction with respect to HIV. Details of these studies are discussed below.

In the first study,[12] ~30,000 HIV infected subjects have been screened in a consortium project (Euro-CHAVI) led by the Center for HIV-AIDS Vaccine Immunology (CHAVI) involving nine cohorts representing 8 European and 1 Australian study. Of this, 486 patients with consistent and accurate viral load measurements were finally selected for testing 555,352 SNPs loaded on Illumina's Human Hap 550 Bead chip. Nearly half of the top 50 SNPs associated with viremia control belonged to the MHC 6p21.3 region. The scan highlighted two independent polymorphisms, HCP5 (rs2395029) near HLA-B and rs9264942 near HLA-C locus (Fig. 19.7). The study showed that atleast 9.6 percent and 6.5 percent of the total variation in viral set-points observed across HIV-1 infected individuals could be attributed to these two polymorphisms respectively. The investigators suggested that HCP5 being a human endogenous retroviral element (HERV) with homology to retroviral *pol* gene might interact with HIV through an antisense mechanism. In this study, the associated HCP5 variant 'G' occurred in high linkage disequilibrium with HLA-B*5701, although it could not be established whether the associated viral control is an independent outcome or an effect of the presence of HLA-B*5701. Interestingly, the HCP5 protective allele G occurred with a relatively low frequency of 5 percent as compared to the rs9264942 protective allele C, which was found at a frequency of 41 percent. The latter variant is associated with increased expression of HLA-C suggesting an important role of HLA-C in the regulation of viral control. In addition to HCP5 and rs 9264942, a third group of seven genetic determinants nested near ring finger protein 39 (RNF39) and zinc ribbon domain-containing 1 (ZNRD1) genes may also be involved. Although the RNF39 gene is not yet fully characterized, the ZNRD1 gene encodes an RNA polymerase I subunit. This might interfere with the processing of HIV transcripts by the viral regulatory protein rev and thus explain the subtle differences in provirus transcription efficiency observed among individuals. The investigators reported that ~15 percent of the variation observed among individuals in viral load particularly during the asymptomatic set-point phase can be attributed to the above polymorphisms.

In a recent follow-up study on African Americans, the CC genotype at rs9264942 was found to be associated with decreased viremia.[100] On the other hand, no association of the G allele of rs2395029 (HCP5) gene could be established with reduced viremia. Incidentally, the G allele is linked to B*5701 in European populations, and with B*5703 in African populations suggesting that rs9264942 and B*57 (rather than HCP5) are actually associated with low viral loads atleast in European Americans. A similar study by Catano et al[55] reported that ZNRD-C was associated with disease retarding effects in AIDS at least in the European Americans, but not in African Americans. However, the protective effect of ZNRD1-C was evident only when it occurred on a haplotype carrying HLA-A10 (particularly A26). Similarly, the protective impact of rs9264942 (HLA-C5') C allele was greater in European Americans than African Americans and this may in part be due to its strong linkage with B*57 in the former. These results highlight the potential need to generate similar data in other populations so that consensus strategies towards control of viral load and disease progression may be formulated.

In the second whole genome scan study,[13] linkage analysis was performed on EBV transformed B cell lines of four generation families derived from CEPH. The B cell lines and purified CD4+T cells were transduced with VSV-G pseudotyped HIV-1 based vector (HIV.GFP) and checked for lentiviral infection. A quantitative genome-wide linkage analysis was performed using a panel of 2600 SNPs with an effective resolution of 3.9 cM and the candidate markers associated with in vitro susceptibility were identified. Differences in cellular susceptibility to infection were mapped to a region HSA8q24 (marker rs1398296) on chromosome 8, suggesting a role of LY6 family of GPI-anchored proteins in HIV-1 infection. Further, association analysis involving 521 tag SNPs in unrelated individuals from the Swiss HIV cohort study revealed that allele A of rs2572886 was associated with increased susceptibility to infection in both B and CD4+ T cells. This variant occurs with an allele frequency of 7 percent in Caucasians, 19 percent in Africans and 23 percent in Asians.[13] Presence of this variant explains an estimated 0.8 percent of variation in CD4 counts and 1 percent of variations in the viral load in HIV infected subjects.

Available data from case-control studies as well as genome wide scans thus point towards an important role of immune response associated host determined factors in HIV infection. Functional studies are required to decipher the relative contribution of these genes in disease susceptibility, transmission and progression. Information on these lines will help to understand the underlying mechanisms associated with disease expression in variable population groups.

CONCLUSION

A preventive vaccine against HIV/AIDS still eludes researchers but would possibly involve both cellular and humoral immune responses against the virus. It is expected that a first generation vaccine against HIV would be able to reduce viremia to <2000 copies RNA/ml and/or prevent disease progression thereby resulting in practically improved disease outcome and reduced transmission.

Genetic studies aimed at identifying host factors associated with natural resistance against the retrovirus would be helpful in developing screening tests that could identify people who have a greater or lower predisposition to HIV infection and who could progress at fast/slow pace to AIDS. Further, genetic testing could help in clinical diagnosis of drug hypersensitivity reactions prior to treatment and could possibly be translated in avoiding dug toxicities at an individual level. Since genetic variability is involved at several steps of the cascade of anti-viral immune surveillance, these could help in predicting vaccine responsiveness in population specific manner and help in our understanding of disease pathogenesis.

The genetic determinants that influence susceptibility to HIV-1 and limit AIDS vary in different populations and among individuals. Meta-analyses of large cohort studies have identified several genetic variants that regulate HIV cell entry (particularly chemokine co-receptors and their ligands with copy number variations), acquired and innate immunity (MHC, KIRs, cytokines) and others (TRIM5α, APOBEC3G) that influence outcome of HIV infection (reviewed in (1)). Of the various genes that contribute towards host genetic propensity, MHC turns out to be the major contributor as it is responsible both for restriction of CTL epitopes on one hand and the emergence of CTL escape mutants on the other. Atleast a trinity of HLA alleles, namely B27, B57 and B35 has already been shown to be associated with rate of disease progression. Others have been shown to be involved in ART drug toxicities, for example, B*5701 with abacavir and DRB1*0101 with nevirapine. Screening of such predictive biomarkers to avoid hypersensitivity reactions before actual administration of ART drugs is now a routine practice in several centers.

An important lesson learnt out of the genetic studies in HIV is that once a virus adapts to the commonly prevalent HLA molecules and succeeds in interrupting the immune competence of the host, it reaches a level of fixation and continues to circulate in the population. On the other hand, the viral replication is significantly hampered if it is passed on to an immune-competent host, who possesses less common or even rare HLA alleles, because of the need for it to undergo faster adaptive evolution and/or reversion to its original state. It is now becoming apparent that the protection rendered by 'protective alleles' may not remain effective in future since the virus is continuously evolving in a manner so as to mutate its immunodominant epitopes. However, the advantage of this process is that the virus may also expose novel dominant epitopes that were earlier cryptic and inaccessible for immune attack. Studies focused on the HLA-HIV interaction can thus predict immunodominant epitopes that may be protective and become potential candidate CTL epitopes that could be incorporated in future therapeutic or prophylactic vaccine approaches.

Nevertheless, several key issues have recently emerged through multidisciplinary approaches involving intensive international collaborations. It is clear that HIV-1/AIDS pathogenesis involves complex counter-interactive responses mediated by both viral and host derived factors. These are manifested differently in different individuals depending on host genomic and immunomic architecture. A number of host derived factors have been identified through case-control studies and multi-cohort meta-analyses. Whole genome scans, functional genomics and other experimental approaches have provided new insights into our understanding of the host-pathogen interactions. Future studies focused primarily on the mechanisms of protection from the virus in naturally resistant people especially the elite controllers could unravel the enigmatic approaches that could be utilized in favorable prognosis, vaccine design, therapy and clinical practice.

ACKNOWLEDGMENTS

The authors wish to thank the Department of Biotechnology (DBT), the Department of Science and Technology (DST) and the Indian Council of Medical Research (ICMR), Government of India for their financial support. The training obtained by GK through the Fogarty's AITRP fellowship program at the New York School of Medicine is gratefully acknowledged.

REFERENCES

1. Visciano ML, Tuen M, Chen PD, Hioe CE. Antibodies to the CD4-binding site of HIV-1 gp120 suppress gp120-specific CD4 T cell response while enhancing antibody response. Infect Agent Cancer 2008;18:11.
2. G Kaur, M Tuen, D Virland, S Cohen, NK Mehra, C Münz, S Abdelwahab, A Garzino-Demo, CE. Hioe. Antigen stimulation induces HIV envelope gp120-specific CD4+ T cells to secrete CCR5 ligands and suppress HIV infection. Virology 2007;369:214-25.
3. G Vasiliver-Shamis, M Tuen, T Wu, T Starr, TO Cameron, R Thompson, G Kaur, J Liu, ML Visciano, H Li, R Kumar, MW Cho, ML Dustin, CE Hioe. HIV-1 envelope gp120 induces a stop signal and virological synapse formation in non-infected CD4 T cells. J Virology 2008;82:9445-57.
4. Kaur G, Mehra N. Genetic determinants of HIV-1 infection and progression to AIDS: Susceptibility to HIV infection. Tissue Antigens 2009;73:289-301.
5. Kaur G, Mehra N. Genetic determinants of HIV-1 infection and progression to AIDS: Immune response genes. Tissue Antigens 2009;74:373-85.
6. Telenti A, Goldstein DB. Genomics meets HIV. Nat Rev Microbiol 2006;4:9-18.
7. Winkler C, An P, Brien SJO. Patterns of ethnic diversity among the genes that influence AIDS. Hum Mol Genet 2004;13:R9-R19.
8. Deeks SG, Walker BD. Human immunodeficiency virus controllers: Mechanisms of durable virus control in the absence of antiretroviral therapy. Immunity 2007;27: 406-16.
9. Baker BM, Block BL, Rothchild AC, Walker BD. Elite control of HIV infection: Implications for vaccines and treatments. Expert Opin Biol Ther. 2009;9:55-69.
10. Brass AL, Dykxhoorn DM, Benita Y, Yan N, Engleman A, Xavier RJ, Lieberman J, Elledge SJ. Identification of host proteins required for HIV infection through a functional genomic screen. Science 2008;319:921-26.
11. O'Brien SJ, Nelson GW. Human genes that limit AIDS. Nat Genet 2004;36:565-74.
12. Fellay J, Shianna KV, Ge D, Colombo S, Ledergerber B, Weale M, et al. A whole-genome association study of major determinants for host control of HIV-1. Science 2007;317:944-47.
13. Loeuillet C, Deutsch S, Cluffi A, Robyr D, Taffe P, Muñoz M, et al. In vitro whole-genome analysis identifies a susceptibility locus for HIV-1. PLoS Biol 2008;6(2): e32.doi:10.1371/journal.pbio.0060032.
14. Smith MW, Dean M, Carrington M, Winkler C, Huttley GA, Lomb DA, et al. Contrasting genetic influence of CCR2 and CCR5 variants on HIV-1 infection and disease progression. Hemophilia Growth and Development Study (HGDS), Multicenter AIDS Cohort Study (MACS), Multicenter Hemophilia Cohort Study (MHCS), San Francisco City Cohort (SFCC), ALIVE Study. Science 1997;277:959-65.
15. G Kaur, Singh P, Kumar N, Rapthap CC, Sharma G, Vajpayee M, Wig N, Sharma SK, Mehra NK. Distribution of CCR2 polymorphism in HIV-1 infected and healthy subjects in North India. Int J Immunogenetics 2007;34: 153-56.
16. Ramana GV, Vasanthi A, Khaja M, Su B, Govindaiah V, Jin L, Singh L, Chakraborty R. Distribution of HIV-1 resistance-conferring polymorphic alleles SDF-1-3'A, CCR2-64I and CCR5-Delta32 in diverse populations of Andhra Pradesh, South India. J Genet 2001;80:137-40.
17. Louisirirotchanakul S, Liu H, Roongpisuthipong A, Nakayama EE, et al. Genetic analysis of HIV-1 discordant couples in Thailand: Association of CCR2 64I homozygosity with HIV-1 negative status. J Acquir Immune Defic Syndr. 2002;29:314-15.
18. Gonzalez E, Bamshad M, Sato N, Mummidi S, Dhanda R, Catano G, Cabrera S, McBride M, Cao XH, Merrill G, et al. Race- specific HIV-1 disease-modifying effects associated with CCR5 haplotypes. Proc Nat Acad Sci 1999;96:12004-9.
19. Liu R, Paxton WA, Choe S, et al. Homozygous defects in HIV-1 coreceptor accounts for resistance of some multiply-exposed individuals to HIV-1 infection. Cell 1996;86: 367-77.

20. Dean M, Carrington M, Winkler C, Huttley GA, Smith MW, Allikmets R, Goedert JJ, Buchbinder SP, Vittinghoff E, Gomperts E, et al. Genetic restriction of HIV-1 infection and progression to AIDS by a deletion allele of the CKR5 structural gene. Science 1996;273:1856-62.
21. P Singh, G Kaur, G Sharma, NK Mehra. Immunogenetic basis of HIV-1 infection, transmission and disease progression. Vaccine 2008;26:2966-80.
22. Martin MP, Dean M, Smith MW, Winkler C, Gerrard B, Michael NL, et al. Genetic acceleration of AIDS progression by a promoter variant of CCR5. Science 1998;282:1907-11.
23. Nguyen L, Li M, Chaowanachan T, Hu DJ, Vanichseni S, Mock PA, van Griensven F, et al. CCR5 promoter haplogroups associated with HIV-1 discordant progression in Thai injection drug users. AIDS 2004; 18:1327-33.
24. Kostrikis LG, Neumann AU, Thomson B, Korber BT, et al. A polymorphism in the regulatory region of the CC chemokine receptor 5 gene influences perinatal transmission of HIV 1 to African American infants. J Virol 1999;73:10264-1071.
25. G Kaur, Singh P, Rapthap CC, Kumar N, Vajpayee M, Sharma SK, Wanchu A, NK Mehra. Polymorphism in the CCR5 gene promoter and HIV-1 infection in North Indians. Hum Immunol 2007;68:454-61.
26. Modi WS, Lautenberger J, An P, Scott K, Goedert JJ, Kirk GD, et al. Genetic variation in the CCL18-CCL3-CCL4 chemokine gene cluster influences HIV type 1 transmission and AIDS disease progression. Am. J. Hum. Genet. 2006;79:120-28.
27. Gonzalez E, Kulkarni H, Bolivar H, Mangano A, Sanchez R, Catano G, et al. The influence of CCL3L1 gene-containing segmental duplications on HIV-1/AIDS susceptibility. Science 2005;307:1434-40.
28. Towson JR, Barcellos LF, Nibbs RJB. Gene copy number regulates the production of the human chemokine CCL3-L1 J Immunol 2002;32:3016-26.
29. Nakajima T, Ohtani H, Naruse T, Shibata H, Mimaya J, Terunuma H, Kimura A. Copy number variations of CCL3L1 and long-term prognosis of HIV-1 infection in asymptomatic HIV-infected Japanese with hemophilia. Immunogen 2007;59:793-98.
30. Nakajima T, Kaur G, Mehra N, Kimura A. HIV-1/AIDS susceptibility and copy number variation in CCL3L1, a gene encoding a natural ligand for HIV-1 co-receptor CCR5. Themed Issue of Cytogenetics and Genome Research (in press).
31. Shao W, Tang J, Song W, Wang C, Li Y, Wilson CM, Kaslow RA. CCL3L1 and CCL4L1: Variable gene copy number in adolescents with and without HIV-1 infection. Genes Immun 2007;8:224-31.
32. Kulkarni H, Marconi VC, Agan BK, McArthur C, Crawford G, Clark RA, Dolan MJ, Ahuja SK. Role of CCL3L1-CCR5 genotypes in the epidemic spread of HIV-1 and evaluation of vaccine efficacy. PLoS ONE 2008;3(11):e3671. doi:10.1371/journal.pone.0003671.
33. Ahuja SK, Kulkarni H, Catano G, Agan BK, Camargo JF, He W, O'Connell RJ, Marconi VC, Delmar J, et al. CCL3L1-CCR5 genotype influences durability of immune recovery during antiretroviral therapy of HIV-1 infected individuals. Nat Med 2008;14:413-420.
34. Shalekoff S, Meddows-Taylor S, Schramm DB, Donninger SL, Gray GE, et al. Host CCL3L1 gene copy number in relation to HIV-1 specific CD4+ and CD8+ T cell responses and viral load in South African women. J Acquir Immune Defic Syndr 2008;48:245-54.
35. Liu H, Chao D, Nakayama EE, Taguchi H, Goto M, Xin X, Takamatsu J, Saito H, Ishikawa Y, Akaza T, Juji T, Takebe Y, et al. Polymorphism in RANTES chemokine promoter affects HIV-1 disease progression. Proc Nat Acad Sci 1999;96:4581-85.
36. An P, Nelson GW, Wang L, Donfield S, Goedert JJ, Phair, J et al. Modulating influence on HIV/AIDS by interacting RANTES gene variants. Proc Nat Acad Sci 2002;99: 10002-07.
37. Rathore A, Chatterjee A, Sivarama P, Yamamoto N, Singhal PK, Dhole TN. Association of RANTES –403 G/A, -28 C/G and In1.1 T/C polymorphism with HIV-1 transmission and progression among North Indians. J Med Virol 2008;80:1133-41.
38. Winkler C, Modi W, Smith MW, Nelson GW, Wu X, Carrington M, et al. Genetic restriction of AIDS pathogenesis by an SDF-1 chemokine gene variant. Science 1998;279:389-93.
39. Ramamoorti N, Kumarvelu J, Shanmugasundaram GK, Rani K, Banerjea AC. 2001 High frequency of G to A transition mutation in the stromal cell derived factor-1 gene in India, a chemokine that blocks HIV-1 (X4) infection: Multiple proteins bind to 3'-untranslated region of SDF-1 RNA Genes Immun. 2001;2:408-10.
40. Suresh P, Wanchu A, Sachdeva RK, Bhatnagar A. Gene polymorphisms in CCR5, CCR2, CX3CR1, SDF-1 and RANTES in exposed but uninfected partners of HIV-1 infected individuals in North India. J Clin Immunol 2006;26:476-84.
41. Richardson RM, Tokunaga K, Marjoram R, Sata T, Snyderman R. Interleukin-8-mediated heterologous receptor internalization provides resistance to HIV-1 infectivity. Role of signal strength and receptor desensitization. J Biol Chem 2003;278:15867-73.
42. Vasilescu A, Terashima Y, Enomoto M, Heath S, Poonpiriya V, Gatanaga H, et al. A haplotype of the human CXCR1 gene protective against rapid disease progression in HIV-1+ patients. Proc. Nat. Acad. Sci. 2007; 104:3354-59.
43. He W, Neil S, Kulkarni H, Wright E, Agan BK, Marconi VC, Dolan MJ, Weiss RA, Ahuja S K. Duffy antigen receptor for chemokines mediates trans-infection of HIV-1 from red blood cells to target cells and affects HIV-AIDS susceptibility. Cell Host Microbe 2008;4:52-62.
44. Boily-Larouche G, Zijenah LS, Mbizvo M, Ward BJ, Roger M. DC-SIGN and DC-SIGNR genetic diversity among different ethnic populations: Potential implications for

pathogen recognition and disease susceptibility. Hum Immunol 2007;68:523-30.
45. Martin MP, Lederman MM, Hutcheson HB, Goedert JJ, Nelson GW, van Kooyk Y, et al. Association of DC-SIGN promoter polymorphism with increased risk for parenteral, but not mucosal, acquisition of human immunodeficiency virus type 1 infection. J Virol 2004;78:14053-56.
46. Zhang J, Webb DM. Rapid evolution of primate antiviral enzyme APOBEC3G. Hum Molec Genet 2004;13:1785-91.
47. Mulder LC, Harari A, Simon V. Cytidine deamination induced HIV-1 drug resistance. Proc Natl Acad Sci 2008;105:5501-06.
48. Schrofelbauer B, Chen D, Landau NR. A single amino acid of APOBEC3G controls its species-specific interaction with virion infectivity factor (Vif). Proc Nat Acad Sci 2004;101:3927-32.
49. Chiu YL, Soros VB, Kreisberg JF, Stopak K, Yonemoto W, Greene WC. Cellular APOBEC3G restricts HIV-1 infection in resting CD4+ T cells. Nature 2005;435:108-14.
50. Xu H, Svarovskaia ES, Barr R, Zhang Y, Khan MA, Strebel K, Pathak VK. A single amino acid substitution in human APOBEC3G antiretroviral enzyme confers resistance to HIV-1 virion infectivity factor-induced depletion. Proc Nat Acad Sci 2004;101:5652-57.
51. OhAinle M, Kerns JA, Li MM, Malik HS, Emerman M. Antiretroelement activity of APOBEC3H was lost twice in recent human evolution. Cell Host Microbe 2008;4:249-59.
52. van Manen D, Rits MA, Beugeling C, van Dort K, Schuitemaker H, Kootstra NA. The effect of Trim5 polymorphisms on the clinical course of HIV-1 infection. PLoS Pathog 2008;4:e18.
53. Nakajima T, Nakayama EE, Kaur G, Terunuma H, Mimaya JI, Ohtani H, Mehra N, Shioda T, Kimura A. Impact of novel TRIM5alpha variants Gly110Arg and G176del on the anti-HIV-1 activity and the susceptibility to HIV-1 infection. AIDS 2009;23:2091-100.
54. Mahungu TW, Johnson MA, Owen A, Back DJ. The impact of pharmacogenetics on HIV therapy. Int J STD AIDS 2009;20:145-51.
55. Catano G, Kulkarni H, He W, et al. HIV-1 disease-influencing effects associated with ZNRD1, HCP5 and HLA-C alleles are attributable mainly to either HLA-A10 or HLA-B*57 alleles. PLoS One. 2008;3:e3636.
56. Colombo S, Rauch A, Rotger M, et al. The HCP5 single-nucleotide polymorphism: a simple screening tool for prediction of hypersensitivity reaction to abacavir. J Infect Dis 2008;198:864-67.
57. Chessman D, Kostenko L, Lethborg T, et al. Human leukocyte antigen class I-restricted activation of CD8+ T cells provides the immunogenetic basis of a systemic drug hypersensitivity. Immunity 2008;28:822-32.
58. Carrington M, Nelson GW, Martin MP, et al. HLA and HIV-1: Heterozygote advantage and B*35-Cw*04 disadvantage. Science 1999;283:1748-52.
59. Dalmau J, Puertas MC, Azuara M, et al. Contribution of immunological and virological factors to extremely severe primary HIV type 1 infection. Clin Infect Dis 2009;48:229-38.
60. Tang J, Shao W, Yoo YJ, et al. Human leukocyte antigen class I genotypes in relation to heterosexual HIV type 1 transmission within discordant couples. J Immunol 2008;181:2626-35.
61. Goulder PJ, Brander C, Tang Y, et al. Evolution and transmission of stable CTL escape mutations in HIV infection. Nature 2001;412:334-38.
62. Schneidewind A, Tang Y, Brockman MA, et al. Maternal transmission of HIV escape mutations subverts HLA-B57 immunodominance but facilitates viral control in the haploidentical infant. J Virol. 2009.
63. Rousseau CM, Lockhart DW, Listgarten J, et al. Rare HLA drive additional HIV evolution compared to more frequent alleles. AIDS Res Hum Retroviruses 2009;25:297-303.
64. Kawashima Y, Pfafferott K, Frater J, et al. Adaptation of HIV-1 to human leukocyte antigen class I. Nature 2009;458:641-45.
65. Mallal S, Nolan D, Witt C, et al. Association between presence of HLA-B*5701, HLA-DR7, and HLA-DQ3 and hypersensitivity to HIV-1 reverse-transcriptase inhibitor abacavir. Lancet. 2002;359:727-32.
66. Rauch A, Nolan D, Thurnheer C, et al. Refining abacavir hypersensitivity diagnoses using a structured clinical assessment and genetic testing in the Swiss HIV Cohort Study. Antivir Ther 2008;13:1019-28.
67. Boyton RJ, Altmann DM. Natural killer cells, killer immunoglobulin-like receptors and human leucocyte antigen class I in disease. Clin Exp Immunol. 2007;149:1-8.
68. Martin MP, Gao X, Lee JH, et al. Epistatic interaction between KIR3DS1 and HLA-B delays the progression to AIDS. Nat Genet 2002;31:429-34.
69. Jennes W, Verheyden S, Demanet C, et al. Cutting edge: Resistance to HIV-1 infection among African female sex workers is associated with inhibitory KIR in the absence of their HLA ligands. J Immunol 2006;177:6588-92.
70. Lajoie J, Hargrove J, Zijenah LS, Humphrey JH, Ward BJ, Roger M. Genetic variants in nonclassical major histocompatibility complex class I human leukocyte antigen (HLA)-E and HLA-G molecules are associated with susceptibility to heterosexual acquisition of HIV-1. J Infect Dis. 2006;193:298-301.
71. Habeshaw JA, Wilson SE, Hounsell EF, Oxford JS. How HIV-1 lentivirus causes immune deficiency disease. Med Hypotheses 1999;52:59-67.
72. Cadogan M, Austen B, Heeney JL, Dalgleish AG. HLA homology within the C5 domain promotes peptide binding by HIV type 1 gp120. AIDS Res Hum Retroviruses 2008;24:845-55.
73. de Parseval A, Bobardt MD, Chatterji A, et al. A highly conserved arginine in gp120 governs HIV-1 binding to

both syndecans and CCR5 via sulfated motifs. J Biol Chem 2005;280:39493-504.
74. Masemola A, Mashishi T, Khoury G, et al. Hierarchical targeting of subtype C human immunodeficiency virus type 1 proteins by CD8+ T cells: Correlation with viral load. J Virol. 2004;78:3233-43.
75. Altfeld M, Kalife ET, Qi Y, et al. HLA Alleles Associated with Delayed Progression to AIDS Contribute Strongly to the Initial CD8(+) T Cell Response against HIV-1. PLoS Med 2006;3:e403.
76. Kiepiela P, Leslie AJ, Honeyborne I, et al. Dominant influence of HLA-B in mediating the potential co-evolution of HIV and HLA. Nature 2004;432:769-75.
77. Goulder PJ, Phillips RE, Colbert RA, et al. Late escape from an immunodominant cytotoxic T-lymphocyte response associated with progression to AIDS. Nat Med 1997;3:212-17.
78. Migueles SA, Sabbaghian MS, Shupert WL, et al. HLA B*5701 is highly associated with restriction of virus replication in a subgroup of HIV-infected long term nonprogressors. Proc Natl Acad Sci USA 2000;97:2709-14.
79. Gao X, Nelson GW, Karacki P, et al. Effect of a single amino acid change in MHC class I molecules on the rate of progression to AIDS N Engl J Med 2001;344:1668-75.
80. Gao X, Bashirova A, Iversen AK, et al. AIDS restriction HLA allotypes target distinct intervals of HIV-1 pathogenesis. Nat Med 2005;11:1290-92.
81. Kaslow RA, Dorak T, Tang JJ. Influence of host genetic variation on susceptibility to HIV type 1 infection. J Infect Dis 2005;191 Suppl 1:S68-77.
82. Cornelissen M, Hoogland FM, Back NK, et al. Multiple transmissions of a stable human leucocyte antigen-B27 cytotoxic T-cell-escape strain of HIV-1 in The Netherlands. AIDS 2009.
83. Gillespie GM, Kaul R, Dong T, et al. Cross-reactive cytotoxic T lymphocytes against a HIV-1 p24 epitope in slow progressors with B*57. AIDS 2002;16:961-72.
84. Miura T, Brockman MA, Schneidewind A, et al. HLA-B57/B*5801 human immunodeficiency virus type 1 elite controllers select for rare gag variants associated with reduced viral replication capacity and strong cytotoxic T-lymphocyte [corrected] recognition. J Virol 2009;83:2743-55.
85. Yu XG, Lichterfeld M, Chetty S, et al. Mutually exclusive T-cell receptor induction and differential susceptibility to human immunodeficiency virus type 1 mutational escape associated with a two-amino-acid difference between HLA class I subtypes. J Virol. 2007;81:1619-31.
86. O'Brien SJ, Nelson GW. Human genes that limit AIDS. Nat Genet 2004;36:565-74.
87. Malhotra U, Holte S, Dutta S, et al. Role for HLA class II molecules in HIV-1 suppression and cellular immunity following antiretroviral treatment. J Clin Invest 2001;107:505-17.
88. Winchester R, Chen Y, Rose S, Selby J, Borkowsky W. Major histocompatibility complex class II DR alleles DRB1*1501 and those encoding HLA-DR13 are preferentially associated with a diminution in maternally transmitted human immunodeficiency virus 1 infection in different ethnic groups: Determination by an automated sequence-based typing method. Proc Natl Acad Sci USA 1995;92:12374-78.
89. MacDonald KS, Fowke KR, Kimani J, et al. Influence of HLA supertypes on susceptibility and resistance to human immunodeficiency virus type 1 infection. J Infect Dis 2000;181:1581-89.
90. Liu C, Carrington M, Kaslow RA, et al. Association of polymorphisms in human leukocyte antigen class I and transporter associated with antigen processing genes with resistance to human immunodeficiency virus type 1 infection. J Infect Dis 2003;187:1404-10.
91. Flores-Villanueva PO, Hendel H, Caillat-Zucman S, et al. Associations of MHC ancestral haplotypes with resistance/susceptibility to AIDS disease development. J Immunol 2003;170:1925-29.
92. Singh P, Kaur G, Sharma G, Mehra NK. Immunogenetic basis of HIV-1 infection, transmission and disease progression. Vaccine 2008;26:2966-80.
93. Stephens HA. HIV-1 diversity versus HLA class I polymorphism. Trends Immunol 2005;26:41-47.
94. Kaur G, Kumar N, Szilagyi A, et al. Autoimmune-associated HLA-B8-DR3 haplotypes in Asian Indians are unique in C4 complement gene copy numbers and HSP-2 1267A/G. Hum Immunol 2008;69:580-7.
95. Kaur G, Rapthap CC, Kumar N, Kumar S, Neolia S, Mehra NK. Frequency distribution of cytokine gene polymorphisms in the healthy North Indian population. Tissue Antigens 2007;69:113-20.
96. Hoffmann SC, Stanley EM, Cox ED, et al. Ethnicity greatly influences cytokine gene polymorphism distribution. Am J Transplant 2002;2:560-67.
97. Hogan CM, Hammer SM. Host determinants in HIV infection and disease. Part 2: Genetic factors and implications for antiretroviral therapeutics. Ann Intern Med 2001;134:978-96.
98. Weissman D, Poli G, Fauci AS. Interleukin 10 blocks HIV replication in macrophages by inhibiting the autocrine loop of tumor necrosis factor alpha and interleukin 6 induction of virus. AIDS Res Hum Retroviruses. 1994;10:1199-206.
99. Price P, Morahan G, Huang D, et al. Polymorphisms in cytokine genes define subpopulations of HIV-1 patients who experienced immune restoration diseases. AIDS 2002;16:2043-47.
100. Shrestha S, Aissani B, Song W, Wilson CM, Kaslow RA, Tang J. Host genetics and HIV-1 viral load set-point in African-Americans. AIDS 2009;23:673-77

Chapter 20

HLA and Drug Reactions

Elizabeth J Phillips, Simon Alexander Mallal

INTRODUCTION

Adverse drug reactions represent a significant burden from a hospital, healthcare and societal perspective comprising the 4th to 6th most common cause of death in some series.[1] Clinically, adverse drug reactions have been classified according to those that are predictable and dose-dependent on the basis of their pharmacological actions ("Type A") versus those that are believed to be immunogenetically mediated and not predictable based on traditional clinical and pharmacological properties of the drug ("Type B") (Table 20.1).[2,3] A major breakthrough has been the association between HLA class I and II alleles and Type B adverse drug reactions. Examples include the striking association between HLA-B*5701 and abacavir hypersensitivity syndrome (ABC HSR), HLA-B*1502 and Stevens-Johnson syndrome/Toxic epidermal necrolysis (SJS/TEN) associated with carbamazepine, and HLA-B*5801 and drug-induced hypersensitivity syndrome (DIHS) and SJS/TEN associated with allopurinol.[4-7] These associations have been facilitated by the introduction of molecular methods improving the accuracy and resolution of HLA typing and improved phenotyping of specific drug toxicities. Furthermore, the discovery of associations between specific HLA and these drug toxicities such as DIHS and SJS/TEN have fuelled our understanding of the immunopathogenesis of these syndromes. The associations between HLA and drug toxicity are hence important from both a clinical and scientific point of view. Drugs may be viewed as an experiment of man acting as a probe to provoke potentially vigorous and life-threatening HLA-restricted immune responses. From a clinical standpoint the association between HLA and drug toxicity represents an important opportunity to increase drug safety and prevent the traditionally unpredictable Type B reactions by excluding high-risk patients from the drug in question. The widespread uptake of HLA-B*5701 screening for ABC HSR provides a roadmap for the translation of HLA-based pharmacogenetics from discovery to clinical implementation.[8,9]

SYNDROMES OF DRUG TOXICITY AND HLA

Although almost all drugs have been associated with "Type B" adverse drug reactions certain classes of drugs such as antiretrovirals, allopurinol, anticonvulsants, and non-steroidal anti-inflammatory agents have been more commonly associated (Table 20.2). Although few HLA associations have been delineated to-date, the likely immunogenetic basis of these reactions identifies this as a fertile area of research. Type B reactions that have been associated with various class I and II HLA alleles include DIHS, TEN/SJS, single organ involvement (e.g. hepatitis, pancreatitis), drug exanthema, fixed drug eruption, and drug-induced lupus (Table 20.3).[4-40]

Drug Hypersensitivity Syndromes

Drug hypersensitivity syndromes include combinations of fever, rash, and internal organ involvement. Symptoms typically present greater than 1 week after the drug has been initiated. The rash can range from mild to severe. Organ involvement can be diverse and include lympadenopathy, hepatitis, pancreatitis, interstitial nephritis, interstitial lung disease, and hematological abnormalities (atypical lymphocytosis, eosinophilia). A more specific drug hypersensitivity syndrome has been termed DRESS or drug-induced hypersensitivity syndrome (DIHS).[41] Various definitions and criteria for

Table 20.1: Classification of adverse drug reactions into those that are predictable on the basis of the pharmacological actions of the drug (Type A) versus those that are believed to have an immunogenetic basis and are not predictable based on the known clinical and pharmacological properties of the drug (Type B)

Properties	Type A = Pharmacological	Type B = Bizarre
Predictable	Yes	No
Dose dependent	+++	+
Host dependent (Genetic factors)	+	+++
Immunologic basis	-	+++
Examples	Gastrointestinal intolerance, seizures with penicillin, etc.	Allergic and idiosyncratic syndromes, hypersensitivity syndromes

Table 20.2: Drugs most commonly associated with Type B adverse drug reactions

- Anticonvulsants
  - Phenytoin, phenobarbital, carbamazepine
  - Lamotrigine
- Antimicrobials
  - Sulfonamides (sulfa antimicrobials), penicillins, dapsone
  - Nitrofurantoin, minocycline, metronidazole
- Allopurinol
- Anti-inflammatories (e.g. oxicam-NSAIDS, Valdecoxib)
- Antiretrovirals
- Alternative medicines
  - Chinese herbals, etc.
- Antineoplastics
- Monoclonal antibodies
  - "Ximab" (infliximab, rituximab) > "Zumab" (omalizumab) > "Mumab" (adalimumab)

DIHS have been proposed that include at a minimum fever, rash, hepatitis and leukocyte abnormalities, with symptoms typically being delayed 3 weeks after starting drug.[41] Symptoms can recur in the third week or even later after the drug has been discontinued and have been attributed to human herpes virus 6 reactivation.[42-44] Reactivation of cytomegalovirus has also been described during the course of this syndrome.[43,45] Autoimmune phenomenon have been described in some patients months following the resolution of DIHS and have included autoimmune thyroiditis and less commonly systemic lupus erythematosis.[46,47] The pathogenesis of DIHS is hypothesized to be driven by a combination of immune, infectious, metabolic and genetic factors and several models which are not mutually exclusive of each other have been proposed. The danger hypothesis suggest that traditional antigenic responses often require that the immune system is first triggered by stressor or a "danger signal".[48,49] In a clinical context this could be any event that contributes to oxidative stress such as surgery, infection, or another pro-inflammatory process. The hapten hypothesis is based on the premise that small molecule drugs cannot independently stimulated an immune response and that the immune response is driven by a host protein which has been modified by reactive metabolite of the drug in question.[50] Another hypothesis, known as the pharmacological interaction theory proposed that under some circumstance drugs can directly interact with the MCH and/or T-cell receptor to activate T-cells.[51]

Common drugs associated with drug hypersensitivity syndromes have included antiretroviral agents (abacavir, nevirapine, fosamprenavir, amprenavir), sulfa antimicrobials, non-steroidal anti-inflammatory agents, aromatic amine anticonvulsants (carbamazepine, phenytoin, phenobarbital), lamotrigine, and allopurinol. Abacavir differs syndromically from other hypersensitivity syndromes in that it typically occurs in the second week of therapy, rash is a late manifestation of disease and rechallenge can result in severe hypotension and risk for severe morbidity or mortality.[52,53] For most drug hypersensitivity reactions a clear association between a specific HLA has either not been defined or has been defined but does not appear to be generalizable across different ethnicities. One hypothesis is that because the majority of drugs that cause drug hypersensitivity syndromes are oxidatively metabolized by cytochrome p450 enzymes, genetic variation in drug metabolism may underlie qualitative and quantitative differences in the generation of specific reactive metabolites in different populations. Another problem may be the inaccurate retrospective attribution of causality when it comes to defining a drug hypersensitivity related to a specific drug. Abacavir hypersensitivity is a notable exception where there is (1) 100 percent negative predictive value of HLA-B*5701 for abacavir hypersensitivity syndrome

Table 20.3: HLA-drug toxicity syndrome associations. +Odds ratio > 50 and reproduced in more than 1 study

Drug toxicity syndrome/Drug	HLA association	Ref
Toxic Epidermal Necrolysis/Stevens-Johnson Syndrome		
Allopurinol+	B*5801	7,10
Carbamazepine+	B*1502	6,11,12
Lamotrigine	B38	13
Oxicam	B73; B12; A2	13, 14
Phenytoin	B*1502	11, 12
Sulfonamides	A29, B12, DR7	14
Sulfamethoxazole	B38	13
Drug Hypersensitivity/DIHS		
Abacavir+	B*5701	4,5
Allopurinol	B*5801	7
Nevirapine		
- Rash associated hepatitis with CD4+ ≥ 25%	DRB1*0101	15
- DIHS in Italian population	Cw8-B14 haplotype	16
- DIHS in Japanese population	Cw8	17
- DIHS in Thai population	B*3505	18
Carbamazepine	promotor motlin gene (rs2894342)	19,20
Delayed Rash		
Aminopenicillins	A2, DRw52	21
Carbamazepine	A*3101	19
Efavirenz	DRB1*01	22
Nevirapine	DRB1*01	22
Drug-Induced Liver Disease		
Amoxicillin-clavulanate	DRB1*1501	23,24
Flucloxacillin	B*5701	25
Ximelagatran	DRB1*07, DQA1*02	26
Fixed-Drug Eruption		
Febrazone	B22	27,28
Sulfamethoxazole	A30-B13-Cw6 haplotype	29
Agranulocytosis		
Clozapine	B38, DR4, DQw3	30
Levamisole	B27	31
Drug-induced lupus erythematosis		
Hydralazine, procainamide, isoniazid, methyldopa, quinidine + others	DR4	32,32
Other Drug Reactions		
Aspirin (urticaria/angioedema)	DRB1*1302-DQB1*0609-DPB1*0201 haplotype	34
Aspirin (asthma)	DPB1*0301	35
Gold sodium thiomalate (proteinuria, thrombocytopenia, cutaneous reactions)	B8, DR3, DR5, DQ2	36,37
Nonsteroidal anti-inflammatory agents (anaphylactoid reaction)	DR11	38
D-penicillamine (myasthenia gravis)	DR1	39
D-penicillamine (proteinuria)	B8, DR3	40

which is generalizable across racial groups (2) A skin patch test exists to increase the specificity of diagnosis and overcome the common problem of false-positive clinical diagnosis.[56,57]

Abacavir

Abacavir is a nucleoside analogue effectively used as part of combination therapy in the treatment of HIV. Abacavir hypersensitivity was described in the pre-marketing development of the drug, being clinically diagnosed in approximately 8 percent of those initiating abacavir. Symptoms of abacavir hypersensitivity typically occur in the second week of therapy at a median of 9 days after initiating the drug. The syndrome differs phenotypically from other hypersensitivity syndromes in that intial symptoms such as fever, malaise and gastrointestinal and respiratory symptoms are common but nonspecific and difficult to differentiate from side effects of other HIV drugs, other infectious diseases or immune restoration disease. In addition, rash which is a consistent and early component of other drug hypersensitivity syndromes is only present in 70 percent of those with abacavir hypersensitivity, and if it does occur, often presents later in the course of disease. Upon discontinuation of abacavir symptoms disappear within 72 hours in most patients. Rechallenge after hypersensitivity reaction, however, can be associated with hypotension and morbidity or mortality.[58]

Early clues to a potential genetic association with abacavir hypersensitivity included lower frequency of the syndrome in those of African and Asian descent and a report of the syndrome in a father and daughter.[59,60] In 2002, two independent research groups reported an association between HLA-B*5701 and abacavir hypersensitivity.[4,5] Subsequent experimental work, demonstrated that abacavir hypersensitivity is HLA-B*5701 restricted and mediated by CD8+ T-lymphocytes.[57,61-64] It is likely that abacavir is metabolized by type 1 alcohol dehydrogenases to an aldehyde-reactive metabolite which can modify an endogenous peptide or protein which then undergoes classical MHC class 1 antigen processing.[65] The proposed mechanisms is illustrated (Fig. 20.1A). Further ex vivo research has

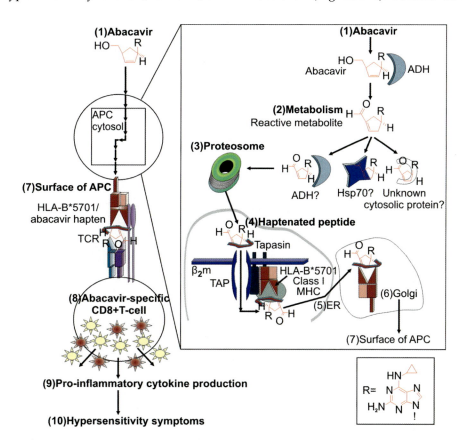

Fig. 20.1A: Model of the immunopathogenesis of the abacavir hypersensitivity syndrome as an example of how HLA-restricted antigen-presentation of a drug-haptened peptide can induce a T-Cell mediated drug hypersensitivity reaction. Abacavir hypersensitivity syndrome is strictly *HLA-B*5701*-restricted. Abacavir is postulated to diffuse freely into the cytosol (1), where it is metabolized by type 1 alcohol dehydrogenases to a reactive aldehyde metabolite (2) that can then haptenate an as of yet unidentified, endogenous protein or peptide. The peptide-HLA complex is then processed via the classical class I processing pathway [(3) to (7)] and presented to abacavir-specific CD8+ T-cells (8), culminating in the release of cytokines (9) and, finally, clinical manifestation of abacavir hypersensitivity (10). Concepts adapted from references Martin et al[61] and Chessman et al.[64] Reproduced with permission from Cell Press

β_2m β-2 microglobulin, ADH alcohol dehydrogenase, APC antigen-presenting cell, ER endoplasmic reticulum, TAP transporter-associated with antigen processing, TCR T-cell receptor

convincingly supported the specificity of HLA-B*5701 in this process as a single amino acid change within the peptide-binding domain of the HLA-B*5701 is enough to abrogate the predisposition to abacavir hypersensitivity.[64]

Following the discovery of the association between HLA-B*5701 and abacavir hypersensitivity hurdles to the clinical application of this tests were created by the apparent lack of sensitivity HLA-B*5701 for abacavir hypersensitivity in Blacks and other patients of non-White origin.[66] It was later determined that this apparent low negative predictive value of HLA-B*5701 for abacavir hypersensitivity was due to false-positive clinical diagnosis which particularly overshadowed true abacavir hypersensitivity in patients of non-White origin who have a low-carriage rate of HLA-B*5701 (Fig. 20.2). The high rate of false-positive clinical diagnosis has been supported by randomized, double-blind clinical trials showing 2 to 7 percent of patients not receiving abacavir were clinically diagnosed with abacavir hypersensitivity.[67-70]

This problem of false-positive clinical diagnosis was overcome by the development of an abacavir skin patch test which is highly specific for the diagnosis of abacavir hypersensitivity in patients who have been immunologically primed through previous ingestion of and therefore systemic exposure to, abacavir (Fig. 20.1B). It is likely that patch testing reproduces the systemic reaction of ABC HSR in the skin by alcohol dehydrogenase mediated metabolism of abacavir to a reactive metabolite that conjugates a host protein or peptide. Since alcohol dehydrogenase is abundant in the skin this may also explain why abacavir patch testing has a high diagnostic sensitivity for ABC HSR. Other drugs causing DIHS rely on metabolism to a reactive metabolite by CYP450, certain isoforms of which are inconsistently present in skin.[71] Studies have supported that 100 percent of abacavir patch test positive patients carry HLA-B*5701. The histopathology of the positive patch test shows an abundance of CD8+ and CD4+ T-cells consistent with histopathology of the rash in acute disease and the immunopathogenesis of abacavir hypersensitivity. Patch testing was used in the study design of two studies that support the clinical effectiveness of HLA-B*5701 screening, the Prospective, Randomized Evaluation of DNA Screening in a Clinical Trial (PREDICT-1) and the Study of Hypersensitivity to Abacavir and Pharmacogenetic Evaluation (SHAPE) studies.[54,55] The PREDICT-1 study was a seminal randomized, double-blind, controlled study specifically designed to examine the clinical effectiveness of HLA-B*5701 screening in the prevention of abacavir hypersensitivity.[54] Patients were randomized either to

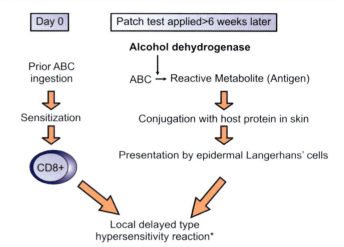

Fig. 20.1B: Proposed mechanism for the generation of a positive-patch test in a genetically predisposed HLA-B*5701 positive patient who has been previously immunologically primed to abacavir (ABC) and developed abacavir-specific CD8+ T-cells as a result of prior ingestion and systemic exposure to the drug. On re-exposure to abacavir in petrolatum applied to the skin at a later time, abacavir is metabolized via alcohol dehydrogenase to a reactive metabolite that can conjugate to a host protein or peptide in the skin and result in a local delayed hypersensitivity reaction via the same mechanisms shown in Figure 20.1A that underlie a systemic hypersensitivity reaction. * The local delayed type hypersensitivity response is read 24 to 48 hours after the abacavir patch test has been applied to the skin. Adapted from Phillips et al reference[8] with permission from Adis International

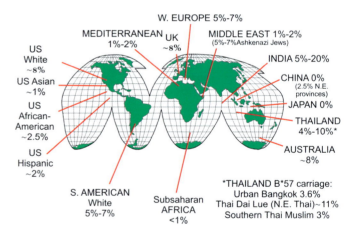

Fig. 20.2: HLA-B*5701 is predominantly a Caucasian allele: Carriage rate of HLA-B*5701 in different populations (Adapted from Phillips et al.[124] © 2006 by University of Chicago Press)

receive real-time HLA-B*5701 screening and exclusion of abacavir in those that were HLA-B*5701 positive or initiation of abacavir and clinical monitoring alone. The study, which enrolled a total of 1956 predominantly (84%) Caucasian patients from Europe and Australia, showed that patch test positive abacavir hypersensitivity did not occur in those who had a negative screening test for HLA-

B*5701 (Figs 20.3A and B). This confirmed a 100 percent negative predictive of HLA-B*5701 and hence its clinical utility as a screening test for prevention of abacavir hypersensitivity. The positive predictive value of HLA-B*5701 derived from the study was 55 percent supporting that HLA-B*5701 is necessary but not sufficient for the development of abacavir hypersensitivity. The study also showed that the diagnostic sensitivity of patch testing was approximately 87 percent and that the true rate of immunologically mediated ABC HSR in a PREDICT-1 predominantly Caucasian population will be approximately 3 percent (Fig. 20.3B). The SHAPE study was a case-control study conducted in both White and Black patients in the United States and designed to address the sensitivity and specificity of HLA-B*5701 for abacavir hypersensitivity in non-White populations.[55] This study showed that 100 percent of both White and Black patch-test positive patients carried HLA-B*5701 and suggested 100 percent negative predictive value of HLA-B*5701 for abacavir hypersensitivity generalizable across Black and White race. From combined data on 95 patch test positive patients from PREDICT-1, SHAPE and a multinational study, all patients have carried HLA-B*5701, adding further support to the strong association between HLA-B*5701 and ABC HSR.[72] However, it should be emphasized that these studies do not eliminate the possibility that a second rare HLA allele may yet be found to be associated with abacavir hypersensitivity.

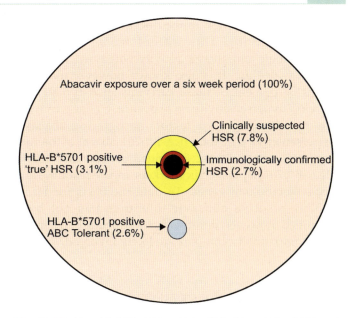

Fig. 20.3B: How HLA-B*5701 positivity (light blue circle, 2.6% and red black circle, 3.1%; total 5.7%) relates to clinical abacavir hypersensitivity (larger yellow circle, 7.8%) and immunologically confirmed (patch test positive, inner filled black circle, 2.7%) in a PREDICT-1, population. For every 100 patients started on abacavir in a typical Caucasian population, it can be predicted that 7.8 percent will be labelled with clinical abacavir hypersensitivity. Given the 100 percent sensitivity of the clinical outcome and the 100% specificity of the immunologically confirmed outcome it can be calculated the 3.1% of participants in the PREDICT-1 study had true hypersensitivity (red circle). Therefore with screening approximately 5.7 percent of the population would test positive (red/black and light blue circles) for HLA-B*5701, but only 3.1 percent would have developed true HSR (red/black circle) if they had been exposed to the drug and the other 2.6% (light blue circle) would have been abacavir tolerant despite being HLA-B*5701 positive (55% positive predictive value). Adapted from Phillips et al[9] with permission from Future Medicine Ltd.

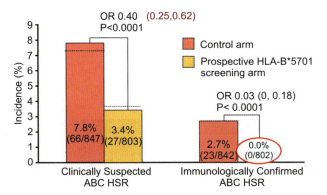

Fig. 20.3A: Results of the PREDICT-1 Study, a randomized, prospective, double-blind study of HLA-B*5701 screening for the prevention of abacavir hypersensitivity (yellow) versus no screening (orange). Co-primary endpoints were used: Clinically suspected abacavir hypersensitivity (right panel) which was a 100 percent sensitive but non-specific endpoint (the dotted lines show the anticipated outcome used in the power calculations for the study given the expected 3.6 percent false-positive clinical diagnosis rate observed in earlier studies) and abacavir hypersensitivity confirmed by a positive abacavir skin patch test (Immunologically confirmed hypersensitivity, right panel) which was a 100 percent specific but only 87 percent sensitive endpoint. Prospective screening for HLA-B*5701 and avoidance of abacavir in those positive for the allele eliminated immunologically confirmed hypersensitivity and reduced clinically diagnosed hypersensitivity to the extent expected given the expected 3.6 percent rate of false-positive clinical diagnoses

Observational studies have also supported the utility of HLA-B*5701 screening in clinical practice and numerous groups have shown that open screening significantly and substantially reduces false-positive clinical diagnoses in addition to reducing true ABC HSR.[73-78] It should be emphasized that false-positive clinical diagnoses could not be influenced by screening for HLA-B*5701 in the PREDICT-1 study as both clinicians and patients were blinded to whether screening had been undertaken or not.

Strong evidence exists to support that the carriage of HLA-B*5701 is necessary for, and is associated with a lifelong predisposition to the development of abacavir hypersensitivity. This differs from some other immunologic and allergic activity where reactivity can be lost over time. It is also known however that only about 55 percent of those carrying HLA-B*5701 will develop hypersensitivity on exposure to abacavir. In an attempt to explain the factors abrograting abacavir hypersensitivity in the HLA-B*5701 abacavir tolerant population studies have examined genetic variation in HLA-B*5701 haplospecific markers, innate response and drug metabolism genes. To-date the basis for HLA-B*5701 positive abacavir tolerance has not been identified, however, multiple factors outside of the major histocompatibility complex are likely involved.[79]

Nevirapine

Nevirapine is a non-nucleoside reverse transcriptase inhibitor (NNRTI) that is used in combination with other antiretroviral agents for the treatment of HIV. Nevirapine has been associated with the full spectrum of cutaneous side effects from isolated rash, drug-induced hypersensitivity syndrome comprising rash in combination with fever and internal organ involvement to SJS/TEN.[52] Rash, fever and hepatitis occur in approximately 5 percent or less of those initiating nevirapine and rash-related events are the major treatment limiting toxicities associated with nevirapine treatment.[52] Strategies to reduce nevirapine rash-related events have included initiating therapy with half the dose for 2 weeks with subsequent escalation to take into effect the auto-induction of metabolism that occurs at this time. Like many other drugs causing DIHS nevirapine is oxidatively metabolized by cytochrome p450, predominately the 3A4, but also the 2B6 isoform.[80] One CYP3A4 metabolite, 12-hydroxynevirapine has successfully reproduced cutaneous hypersensitivity in a Brown Norway rat model. These animal models have also supported the CD4+ T-cell dependence of nevirapine hypersensitivity and find that upregulation of MHC expression on antigen presenting cells in the skin leads to CD4+ T-cell activation mediated by nevirapine or its reactive metabolite.[81] Earlier clinical data which suggested that low CD4+ counts abbrogated clinical nevirapine hypersensitivity also adds support from animal models that the reaction is MHC Class II mediated. Severe nevirapine reactions, including DIHS and hepatitis have been reported in non-HIV infected patients taking nevirapine as post-exposure prophylaxis. More recent studies suggest that virologic as well as immunologic factors may be important in the pathophysiology of nevirapine rash and DIHS in that that patients with high CD4+ T-cell counts but suppressed HIV replication have been successfully switched to nevirapine therapy.[83,84]

Both Class I and Class II HLA associations have been described with nevirapine rash and DIHS and these may be related to genetic differences in both HLA and drug metabolism in the populations involved.[15-18,22] The generation of different reactive metabolites based on genetic differences in CYP enzymes may drive different HLA association with nevirapine rash (Fig. 20.4). The first reported study was from Western Australia demonstrating an HLA association between the class II allele HLA-DRB1*0101 and rash-associated hepatitis but not isolated skin rash.[15] This occurred in patients with CD4+ T-cell > 25 percent, again supporting the abrogating effect of low CD4+ T-cell count.[15] A French study differed from the Western Australian study in showing an association between HLA-DRB1*01 and isolated rash with both nevirapine and efavirenz, another NNRTI.[22] The small number of patients and lack of high resolution four digit HLA typing may hamper the interpretation of this study. Other studies have associated nevirapine rash and DIHS with Class I HLA alleles. HLA-B*1402 and HLA-Cw8 were

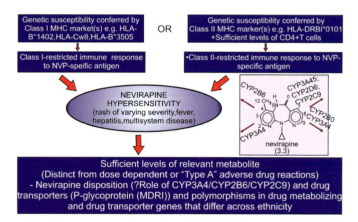

Fig. 20.4: A model for the immunopathogenesis of MHC class I- or class II-restricted responses to drug haptenated peptide using nevirapine hypersensitivity as an example. This model accounts for how pharmacological and immunological factors interact to produce ethnic-specific *HLA*-drug toxicity associations. It illustrates the potential contribution of immune response, and pharmacokinetic and pharmacodynamic factors that could potentially explain *HLA* associations that differ across race and phenotype. For example, genetic polymorphisms in drug-metabolizing and drug-transporter genes (in the case of nevirapine, cytochrome P450 (CYP)3A4, CYP2B6 and CYP2C9, and p-glycoprotein, respectively) may vary in different ethnic groups resulting in the generation of sufficient quantities of distinct reactive metabolites. These different metabolites may trigger specific MHC class I- or class II-restricted immune responses if the relevant *MHC* susceptibility alleles are present. Adapted from Phillips et al. Current Opinion in Molecular Therapeutics 2009;11:231-42, figure 1 with permission from Thomson Reuters

associated with nevirapine hypersensitivity in a Sardinian population, whereas HLA-Cw8 alone was associated with nevirapine hypersensitivity in Japanese.[16,17] A further recently published case-control study associated HLA-B*3505 with nevirapine rash or hypersensitivity with HLA-B*3505 occurring in 17.5 percent of HIV patients with nevirapine rash or hypersensitivity versus 1.1 percent of nevirapine tolerant controls and <1 percent of the general Thai population.[18] Currently no data exists as to HLA alleles that may be associated with nevirapine SJS/TEN although genetic factors are suggested by reports of the disease in first-degree family members.[85]

Stevens-Johnson Syndrome and Toxic Epidermal Necrolysis

SJS and TEN are rare but severe reactions which are largely drug-induced in adults. The mortality ranges from 1 to 5 percent for SJS but as high as 50 percent for TEN. Erythema multiforme which is often classified as being on the milder side of the SJS/TEN spectrum is a distinct syndrome characterized by classic targetoid lesions and can have mucous membrane involvement, but is typically related to reactivation of herpes simplex virus (HSV) rather than drug. Two studies suggested a possible association between HSV associated erythema multiforme and HLA-B15[86,87] and HLA-DQw3.[87] SJS was named after two American physicians who described a syndrome in two children of fever, stomatitis, disseminated skin rash with "purplish cutaneous macules and necrotic centres".[88] Complete blindness in one child and corneal scarring in the other. The term TEN or Lyell's syndrome was first described in 1956 to describe a severe and rapidly evolving syndrome with epidermal erythema, detachment and necrosis.[89] Since these early description of SJS/TEN the diseases have been defined in consensus papers.[90,91] A common classification defines TEN as being present when there is skin separation and > 30 percent of total body surface involved, SJS when there is <10 percent body surface area involved and SJS/TEN overlap when 10-30 percent of body surface area is involved.[90,91] For TEN, a severity of illness scale (SCORTEN) has been validated to predict mortality.[92]

SJS/TEN are extremely uncommon syndromes occurring at a rate of less than 10 cases per million per year in the general populations, but are 100-fold more common in HIV infected individuals, likely both as a consequence of their underlying immune state and the drugs that they are exposed to.[52]

Although SJS/TEN are extremely rare syndromes there are a smaller number of drugs that have been more commonly implicated such as aromatic amine anticonvulsants (Phenobarbital, carbamazepine), allopurinol, nonsteroidal anti-inflammatory drugs, antiretrovirals (nevirapine, amprenavir) and sulfa antimicrobials.[93-97]

The clinical syndrome of SJS/TEN typically has an onset of symptoms 1-3 weeks following first exposure to the drug in questions. Almost all patients present within 8 weeks of first exposure.[98] Early symptoms can include fever, malaise, myalgias followed by the development of atypical targetoid lesions with a dark red center and blistering. Epidermal separation can be elicited in early lesions by local pressure but typically progresses rapidly. Mucosal and ocular involvement are common as is internal organ involvement. Patients with full-blown TEN require aggressive clinical and supportive management, typically in the setting of a burn unit.[98,99] Sepsis is the most frequent cause of morbidity or mortality. Treatment is largely supportive with some evidence to support treatment with immunosuppressives such as cyclosporine.[99] Intravenous immunoglobulin has been used widely in treatment and may decrease morbidity and mortality.[99,100] The mechanism of action of intravenous immunoglobulin is not known but the immunoglobulin is postulated to block the CD95 cell surface receptor (Fas ligand) that triggers apoptosis of keratinocytes.[101] Anecdotal reports of success with TNF-alpha receptor antagonists such as infliximab have also been reported.[102,103]

It is postulated that TEN represents a state of an extreme immune response where exposure to the drug leads to widespread death of keratinocytes and mucosal cells and the clinical phenotype of TEN.[104,105] The process is likely triggered by pathway mediated by Fas and Fas ligand, granzyme B, TNF-alpha and TRAIL.[104,105] The immunopathology of TEN is believed to be mediated by CD8+ T cell class I HLA restricted process.[106,107] Analysis from blisters showed a predominance of IL2 soluble receptor and CD8+ T cells.[106,107] CD8+ T cells also predominate along the dermo-epidermal junction and epidermis.

Early clues that SJS/TEN could be genetically mediated came from reports of cases occurring in members of the same family and the increased prevalence of SJS/TEN amongst specific racial groups. More recently HLA associations between certain drug-induced SJS/TEN syndromes have been elucidated (Table 20.3).[6,7,10-14] These associations have been most significant for the aromatic amine anti-convulsant carbamazepine and allopurinol and HLA-B*1502 and HLA-B*5801 respectively (Table 20.2).[6,7,10-12]

Carbamazepine and Aromatic Amine Anticonvulsants

In 2004 a strong association was reported between HLA-B*1502 and carbamazepine SJS/TEN in Han Chinese.[6] This original study was a case control study showing that 100 percent of 44 Han Chinese patients with SJS/TEN carried HLA-B*1502 compared with 3 percent of 101 tolerant patients and 9 percent in an unexposed population. This suggested a 100 percent negative predictive value for HLA-B*1502 for carbamazepine associated SJS/TEN in Han Chinese. Subsequent case-control studies in Chinese and Thai populations confirmed these results, further supporting that carbamazepine SJS/TEN is a class I, HLA-B*1502 restricted process.[11,12] Further studies have suggested that this association is specific for SJS/TEN as an association between HLA-B*1502 and carbamazepine DIHS or exanthema could not be shown.[19] In addition an association between HLA-B*1502 and SJS/TEN has not been replicated in Caucasian or Japanese populations where the carriage rate of this allele is < 0.1 percent.[108-110] In Chinese and South-East Asian populations the carriage rate of HLA-B*1502 is estimated to be 10-15 percent and hence HLA-B*1502 is a marker for Chinese and South-East Asian ethnicity (Fig. 20.5). Carriage rates of HLA-B*1502 mirror those areas that have a high prevalence of carbamazepine induced SJS/TEN.[111]

In addition to carbamazepine, some data exists to support an association between HLA-B*1502 and SJS/TEN associated with another aromatic amine anticonvulsant, phenytoin.[11,12] Anticonvulsants such as carbamazepine, phenobarbital, and phenytoin share an aromatic benzene ring which is oxidized by cytochrome p450 to a toxic and reactive arene oxide metabolite which is normally detoxified by epoxide hydroxylase. Clinical cross-reactivity to a related aromatic amine anticonvulsants, after SJS/TEN or DIHS had been induced by one drug in the class, are thought to be between 70 and 80 percent.[112] In a case-control study in Thai patients 100 percent of 4 patients with phenytoin-associated SJS carried HLA-B*1502 compared with 8/45 (18%) phenytoin tolerant patients.[12] Data is currently being reviewed by the United States Food and Drug Administration and other regulatory agencies with regards to a label change on phenytoin similar to that for carbamazepine which warns against use in patients of Asian origin or known HLA-B*1502 status.[113] Data is currently not available on HLA-B*1502 and phenobarbital, another aromatic amine anticonvulsant. Although combined data on HLA and clinical cross-reactivity amongst aromatic amine anticonvulsants is lacking, available data suggests that a cautious approach may be to avoid all aromatic amine anticonvulsants in individuals known to be HLA-B*1502 positive. Furthermore in view of the availability of anticonvulsants that are not structurally related to aromatic amines; it seems prudent to avoid other aromatic amine convulsants when suspected SJS/TEN has occurred in association with any member of this class.

Allopurinol

Allopurinol is one of the few drugs available to prevent gout and hyperuricemia and it works by curbing production of uric acid through inhibition of xanthine oxidase. In 2005 a case-control study in Taiwanese Han Chinese was published demonstrating a strong association between HLA-B*5801 and allopurinol associated DIHS or SJS/TEN.[7] In this study 51/51(100%) of patients with allopurinol DIHS or SJS/TEN carried HLA-B*5801 versus 20/135 (15%) of tolerant patients and 19/93(20%) of population controls (p<0.00001, odds ratio = 580). A recent case-control study in Thai patients also supports a strong association between HLA-B*5801 and allopurinol SJS/TEN in other South-East Asian populations.[10] Although more prevalent in Han Chinese (9-11%), HLA-B*5801 is more broadly distributed across populations and is carried in 1-6 percent Caucasians, 2-4 percent Africans and < 0.4 percent Japanese.[111] A recent Japanese study reported four patients with allopurinol SJS/TEN that carried HLA-B*5801.[109] There is less data with regards to HLA-B*5801 and allopurinol associated DIHS/SJS/TEN in Caucasian populations. A recent study showed that 55 percent of patients of European ancestry and allopurinol associated SJS/TEN carried HLA-B*5801.[13]

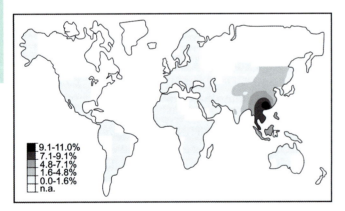

Fig. 20.5: Global carriage frequency of HLA-B*1502 showing concentration in individuals of Han Chinese ancestry across South East Asia and China. *Adapted from:* Franciotta et al. Current Opinion in Neurology 2009;22:144-49 with permission from Lippincott Williams & Wilkins

Drug-induced Liver Disease

Drug-induced liver disease (DILI) is still a major reason why drugs are withdrawn in the clinical and pre-clinical phase of drug development.[114] The causes of DILI are similar to the causes of type B reactions and most commonly include non-steroidal anti-inflammatory agents, analgesics, antimicrobials and statins.[114] Although liver disease can occur as part of a drug hypersensitivity or severe skin syndrome, DILI most commonly occurs without other signs such as fever, rash or extrahepatic internal organ involvement. As with DIHS, it is postulated that for some drugs the pathogenesis of DILI is driven by a combination of metabolic and immune factors and may involve any of the same theories of pathogenesis that apply to DIHS. The hapten hypothesis invokes that reactive metabolites are produced that covalently bind with hepatocytes or carrier proteins in the liver. There may be an interaction of multiple metabolic pathways including both production of reactive metabolites as well as disturbances in detoxification triggering hepatic or hepatobiliary aptosis and/or necrosis. Systemic inflammation, infection or the toxic metabolites themselves are likely to provide the danger signals that trigger the innate and cellular immune responses and cytokine production that facilitate liver injury. The association between both Class I and Class II HLA and DILI has been described and is outlined in (Table 20.3).[23-26,115]

Flucloxacillin

Flucloxacillin is an antibacterial agent used for the treatment of *Staphylococcus aureus* infections in Europe and Australia. Approximately 8.5/100,000 will develop a hepatitis with a cholestatic pattern in the first 6 weeks after initiating flucloxacillin. The exact mechanism of this is not known although flucloxacillin is metabolized by CYP3A4 to 5'hydroxymethylflucloxacillin that is selectively toxic to human biliary epithelial cells. A recent genome wide case-control study including 51 patients with flucloxacillin DILI, 282 matched controls and 64 flucloxacillin tolerant controls showed a very strong association between HCP5 (rs2395029[G]) (in strong linkage disequilibrium with HLA-B*5701 in Europeans) and HLA-B*5701 (OR = 80.6 p< 0.0001).[25] Cases with flucloxacillin DILI more commonly had the same HLA-B*5701 haplotype (HLA-DRB1*0701-DQB1*0303) observed in ABC HSR.[4,25] Another SNP (rs10937275) located on chromosome 3, which is an intronic SNP in the ST6GALI gene which encodes a sialic acid transfer enzyme was also found to be significantly associated with flucloxacillin DILI (OR; = 4.1; p<0.0001).[25]

Ximelagatran

Ximelagatran is a direct thrombin inhibitor developed for the prevention and treatment of thromboembolism that was never marketed due to elevated liver transaminases that occurred in approximately 8 percent of patients when treated for more than 5 weeks. Clinical studies had shown that there appeared to be a higher incidence of elevated alanine aminotransferase in Caucasian patients from Northern Europe. A retrospective case-control genome wide analysis was therefore carried out on 74 cases and 130 controls.[26] A strong association with the class II MHC alleles DRB1*07 and DQA1*02 was found supporting an immunogenetic basis for this syndrome and the findings were in keeping with the higher propensity for ximelagatran to occur in Northern Europe where HLA-DRB1*0701 has a carriage frequency of 11 percent.

USING HLA SCREENING TO PREVENT DRUG TOXICITY: CLINICAL AND LABORATORY IMPLICATIONS

The successful translation of HLA screening into clinical practice is contingent on a number of post-discovery steps whose execution is crucial to the widespread uptake of any pharmacogenetic test (Fig. 20.6). Abacavir acts as an example of a drug where each of these steps from (1) discovery of the initial HLA association, through (2) development of generalizable high-level clinical evidence supporting the clinical utility and 100 percent negative predictive value of HLA-B*5701 for immunologically-mediated ABC HSR, (3) development of efficient and cost-effective laboratory testing, reporting and quality assurance, and (4) evaluation of testing in real clinical practice have been accomplished. As a result HLA-B*5701 screening prior to abacavir prescription to prevent abacavir hypersensitivity has been widely incorporated into routine HIV clinical practice in much of the developed world and is now recommended as the standard of practice in international HIV treatment guidelines.[116,117] Particularly key to the success of HLA-B*5701 in clinical practice was the development of accurate, inexpensive and short- turn-around-time HLA-B*5701 PCR based tests such as sequence specific amplification and real-time PCR melting curve analysis that could provide cost-effective alternatives to high resolution HLA typing.[118,119] The development of internationally directed HLA-B*5701 specific quality assurance program now administered through the Australasian and South-East Asian Tissue Typing Association (ASEATTA) (MDiviney@arcbs.redcross.org.au), has also been critically important.[120] Ongoing

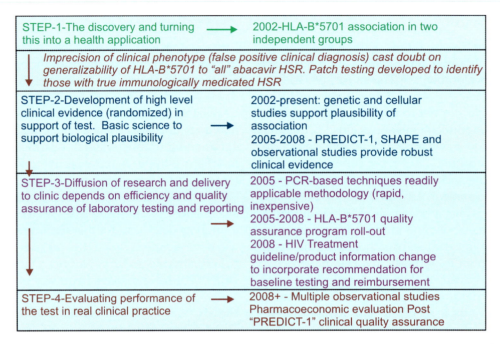

Fig. 20.6: Steps required to translate discovery of an HLA-drug toxicity association into primary clinical care use globally using *HLA-B*5701 and abacavir hypersensitivity as an example. Adapted from Phillips et al figure 2, ref [9] with permission from Future Medicine Ltd

laboratory participation in allele specific quality assurance has also been critically important in the prevention of potentially life-threatening hypersensitivity as the safety issues have now moved from the clinic to the laboratory. A recent report suggested that a taqman assay to detect an HCP5 SNP (rs2395029) within an endogenous retrovirus may be used as a surrogate marker for HLA-B*5701 as HCP5 was reported to be in complete linkage disequilibrium with HLA-B*5701 in European populations.[121] This may not apply to all populations, however, and genetic sub-studies of the PREDICT-1 and other studies have shown that patch test confirmed ABC HSR can occur in the setting of HCP5 negativity.[79] This example illustrates that no linked genetic surrogate of HLA-B*5701 can be safely implemented as a screening test. Other emerging technologies for HLA-B*57 detection include an HLA-B57/58(B17) flow cytometric technique which would offer a lower-cost option that could be incorporated onto the baseline CD4+/CD8+ testing in HIV patients.[122-23] The disadvantage of this technique is the need for confirmation of all B17 positives which would be a particular issue in non-Caucasian populations where HLA-B*58 and HLA-B*5703 are more prevalent. No matter what type of test is used, ongoing clinical vigilance will always be essential as the strong association between HLA-B*5701 and ABC HSR does not eliminate the possibility of a second rare, as of yet undiscovered, allele that may be associated with ABC HSR or that a laboratory error has occurred. It is, therefore, important for any reaction clinically compatible with ABC HSR that occurs despite negative HLA-B*5701 screening be carefully documented and investigated with independent high resolution HLA typing, abacavir patch testing and appropriate *ex vivo* cellular assays.

The successful and widespread incorporation of HLA-B*5701 as a screening test for abacavir hypersensitivity is illustrative and can now act as a roadmap for future implementation of a pharmacogenetic test. Other factors that made this both feasible and accomplishable that may not apply readily to other drugs however include (1) the high carriage rate of HLA-B*5701 in the Caucasian population and (2) the high prevalence of ABC HSR. This means that taking into account prevention of both true immunologically mediated ABC HSR and false positive clinically diagnosed cases, only should be 13 rather than 14 people in a predominantly Caucasian population need to be screened to prevent one case of ABC HSR. In addition the PREDICT-1 study suggested a 55 percent positive predictive value of HLA-B*5701 for ABC HSR meaning that for every 100 patients screened approximately 2 would be excluded that would have tolerated abacavir. From a cost-effectiveness standpoint, open screening significantly impacts on reducing false-positive clinical

diagnosis would largely cancel out the effect caused by excluding patients who would have tolerated abacavir (Fig. 20.7). The significant reduction in false-positive diagnosis with screening also suggests that testing will be cost-effective across different ethnicities.[124,125] Significantly higher hurdles exist for the development of HLA-B*5801 for allopurinol and HLA-B*1502 for carbamazepine as approximately 250 and 1000 for allopurinol patients respectively would need to be screened to prevent one case of disease even in the Han Chinese population of highest prevalence and allele carriage. Comparisons between abacavir, nevirapine, carbamazepine and allopurinol with regards to the prerequisites they satisfy for incorporating an HLA test into clinic practice are shown (Table 20.4). Similar considerations exist for a drug such as flucloxacillin where the positive predictive value of HLA-B*5701 for flucloxacillin DILI is less than 0.2 percent and over 13,000 patients would need to be screened to prevent a single case.

Regardless of the immediate clinical implications and hurdles to translation to the clinic, the lessons learned from HLA and drug-specific toxicity associations have been numerous and invaluable. Ultimately the greatest utility may be in the application of HLA pharmacogenomics in the premarketing phase of drug development to screen out the development of drugs likely to cause immunologically mediated drug reactions. In silico models may also serve as useful predictors as to drugs likely to elicit strong immune responses by identifying candidate peptides that would produce a haptenated peptide and bind a particular HLA allele.[126]

SUMMARY OF KEY ISSUES/CONCLUSIONS

- Associations between HLA and drug toxicities have been facilitated by the improvement in molecular methods that have improved the accuracy and resolution of HLA typing and improved phenotyping of specific drug toxicity syndromes.
- The discovery of a strong association between HLA-B*5701 and abacavir hypersensitivity and its translation as a widespread screening test used in clinical practice has acted as a roadmap identifying the essential components necessary to get a pharmacogenetic test to clinic.
- The strong association between HLA-B*1502 and carbamazepine SJS/TEN in Han Chinese and other Southeast Asian populations is illustrative of a class I restricted, CD8+ mediated reaction that may extend to other structurally related aromatic amine anticonvulsants such as phenytoin.
- The clinical application of HLA-B*1502 (carbamazepine), HLA-B*5801 (allopurinol) or HLA-B*5701 (flucloxacillin) will be mainly limited by their low positive predictive values (related to the low incidence of the relevant drug toxicity syndrome),

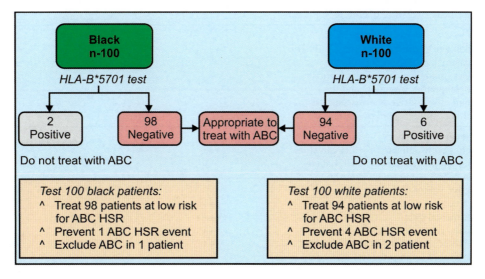

Fig. 20.7: Implications of HLA-B*5701 screening to prevent abacavir hypersensitivity in a black or white patient population. The main benefit of screening, regardless of race, is that it identifies the majority of the population to whom it is safe to administer abacavir. Although screening necessarily excludes some patients from abacavir therapy who would have tolerated the drug, this is compensated by the fall in false-positive clinical diagnoses achieved in an open screening program. The numbers shown are based upon the positive predictive values and prevalence of HLA-B*5701 in whites and blacks derived from PREDICT-1 and SHAPE studies respectively. Adapted from Phillips et al "Abacavir hypersensitivity" in "Uptodate" added October 2008

Table 20.4: A number of prerequisites must all be fulfilled for successful widespread integration of HLA pharmacogenetic testing into routine clinical care. Many of the necessary attributes of the test, drug, toxicity and environment are not modifiable (indicated by *) while other critical elements such as a sufficient levels and types of evidence, laboratory and clinical systems can be developed with sufficient time and resources. (Legend: ABC = abacavir/HLA-B*5701 association, CBZ = carbamazepine/HLA-B*1502, ALL = allopurinol/HLA-B*5801, NEV=nevirapine/HLA-DRB1*0101, FLUC= flucloxacillin/HLA-B*5701, +++ prerequisite present and very strongly influential, ++ prerequisite present and strongly influential , + prerequisite present and moderately influential, +/– prerequisite inconsistently present and dependent on external factors, – prerequisite absent)

Prerequisites	ABC	CBZ	ALL	NEV	FLUC
Test					
• HLA allele is strongly associated with the toxicity and the negative predictive value of the test is high*	+++	+	+	++	+
• Test validated across different populations	+++	–	–	–	–
• The number of patients needed for testing to prevent a case of toxicity is low*	+++	–	–	++	–
• HLA allele prevalent in a large, non-disenfranchised population*	++	+	+	++	++
• Recommendation for testing incorporated into national and international treatment guidelines	+++	–	–	–	–
• Recommendation for test incorporated into product monograph of drug	+++	+++	–	–	–
Drug					
• Drug exhibits favorable attributes, such as good efficacy, convenience, tolerability and pill burden*	++	+	++	+	++
• Alternative drug(s) with equal efficacy that do not need pharmacogenetic testing are either absent or have negative attributes*	++	+	+++	+	++
Drug toxicity					
• Toxicity can be severe and persistent* (i.e. not isolated mild rash)	++	++	++	++	++
• Toxicity is readily and accurately clinically phenotyped*	+/–	++	++	+/–	++
• An adjunctive diagnostic test, such as skin patch testing, can improve phenotypic precision and specificity of clinical diagnosis	+++	–	–	–	–
Environment					
• Champions available (e.g. clinical academics, industry [if drug not off patent*], professional bodies, regulatory agencies, guideline committees, patient advocacy groups, laboratory providers and the media), willing and able to drive pharmacogenetic test development and implementation	+++	–	–	–	–
Generation of high level of evidence					
• Case-control studies with estimated predictive values based on the assumed prevalence of the HLA allele	+++	++	++	–	+
• Population-based cohort studies with directly calculated predictive values of the test	++	–	–	++	–
• Open screening studies	+++	–	–	–	–
• Supportive experimental data	+++	–	–	–	–
• Blinded randomized controlled trials	+++	–	–	–	–
• Evidence across ethnic groups and geographic areas to determine the clinical settings the test may be applied to	+++	–	–	–	–
• Cost-effectiveness data	++	–	–	–	–
Development and availability of appropriate laboratory support					
• No patent restriction on use of the test	++	++	++	++	++
• Development of simple, inexpensive, robust unambiguous allele specific laboratory tests	+++	+	–	–	+++

Contd...

Contd...

Prerequisites	ABC	CBZ	ALL	NEV	FLUC
• Rapid and simple report and interpretation	++	–	–	–	++
• Development of reagents (e.g. mAbs, PCR-based kits)	++	–	–	–	++
• Global distribution and commercialization of allele-specific test	+	–	–	–	+
• Allele-specific quality assurance targeted to avoid false negative results and consequent morbidity or mortality	+	–	–	–	+
• Reimbursement of test in much of the developed world	+	–	–	–	–
Design and implementation of appropriate clinical systems					
• Education of clinicians, nurses, pharmacists, phlebotomists, patients	++	–	–	–	–
• Systems to ensure appropriate and routine triggering of ordering of the test	+	–	–	–	–
• Systems in clinic to ensure correct blood samples are sent to the correct laboratory for analysis	+	–	–	–	–
• Systems to ensure test results and correct interpretation is rapidly transmitted to, retained by and acted on by the healthcare team and patient	+	–	–	–	–

difficulty accruing the appropriate levels of evidence to support their use, and the availability of alternative drugs.

- After clinical evidence has been obtained to support the clinical utility of a specific HLA pharmacogenetic test the key feasibility and safety issues move to the laboratory and include the development of cost-effective tests with short turn-around times and the availability of an ongoing allele-specific quality assurance program.
- Future directions of HLA pharmacogenetics will likely focus on the insights it provides into the immunopathogenesis of type B reactions as well as the potential to help the development of drugs likely to cause immunologically mediated adverse drug reactions during the premarketing phase.

ACKNOWLEDGMENTS

The authors would like to thank the Australian National Health and Medical Research Council for funding support. The authors would also like to acknowledge Associate Professor David Nolan, Professor James McCluskey, Annalise Martin, Coral-Anne Almeida, Tessa Lethborg, Diana Chessman, Lyudmila Kostenko, and Mandvi Bharadwaj for their contributions.

REFERENCES

1. Lazarou J, Pomeranz BH, Corey PN. Incidence of adverse drug reactions in hospitalized patients: A meta-analysis of prospective studies. JAMA 1998;279:1200-5.
2. Gomes ER, Demoly P. Epidemiology of hypersensitivity drug reactions. Curr Opin Allergy Clin Immunol 2005;5:309-16.
3. Edwards JR, Aronson JK. Adverse drug reactions: Definitions, diagnosis and management. Lancet 2000;356:1255-9.
4. Mallal S, Nolan D, Witt C, et al. Association between presence of HLA-B*5701, HLA-DR7 and HLA-DQ3 and hypersensitivity to HIV-1 reverse transcriptase inhibitor abacavir. Lancet 2002;359;727-32.
5. Hetherington S, Hughes AR, Mosteller M, et al. Genetic variation in HLA-B region and hypersensitivity reactions to abacavir. Lancet 2002;359;1121-2.
6. Chung WH, Hung SI, Hong HS, et al. Medical genetics: A marker for Stevens-Johnson syndrome. Nature 2004;428:486.
7. Hung SI, Chung WH, Liou LB, et al. HLA-B*5801 allele as a genetic marker for severe cutaneous adverse reactions caused by allopurinol. Proc Natl Acad Sci USA 2005;102:4134-9.
8. Phillips E, Mallal S. Successful translation of pharmacogenetics into the clinic: the abacavir example. Mol Diagn Ther 2009;13:1-9.
9. Phillips E, Mallal S. Personalizing antiretroviral therapy: Is it a reality? Personalized Medicine 2009;6:393-408.
10. Tassaneeyakul W, Jantararoungtong T, Chen P, et al. Strong association between HLA-B*5801 and allopurinol-induced Stevens-Johnson syndrome and toxic epidermal necrolysis in a Thai population. Pharmacogenet Genomics 2009;19;704-9.
11. Man CB, Kwan P, Baum L, et al. Association between HLA-B*1502 and antiepileptic drug-induced cutaneous reactions in Han Chinese. Epilepsia 2007;48:1015-8.
12. Locharenkul C, Loplumlert J, Limotai C, et al. Carbamazepine and phenytoin induced Stevens-Johnson

syndrome is associated with HLA-B*1502 allele in Thai population. Epilepsia 2008;49:2087-91.
13. Lonjou C, Borot N, Sekula P, et al. A European study of HLA-B in Stevens-Johnson syndrome and toxic epidermal necrolysis related to five high-risk drugs. Pharmacogenet Genomics 2008;18:99-107.
14. Roujeau JC, Huynh TN, Bracq C, et al. Genetic susceptibility to toxic epidermal necrolysis. Arch Dermatol 1987;123:1171-3.
15. Martin AM, Nolan D, James I, et al. Predisposition to nevirapine hypersensitivity associated with HLA-DRB1*0101 and abrogated by low CD4 T cell count. AIDS 2005;19:97-9.
16. Littera R, Carcassi C, Masala A, et al. HLA- dependent hypersensitivity to nevirapine in Sardinian HIV patients. AIDS 2006;20:1621-6.
17. Gatanaga H, Yazaki H, Tanuma J, et al. HLA-Cw8 primarily associated with hypersensitivity to nevirapine. AIDS 2007;21;264-5.
18. Chantarangsu S, Mushiroda T, Maharasirimongkol S, et al. HLA-B*3505 allele is a strong predictor for nevirapine-induced skin adverse drug reactions in HIV-infected Thai patients. Pharmacogenet Genomics 2009;9:139-46.
19. Hung SI, Chung WH, Jee SH, et al. Genetic susceptibility to carbamazepine-induced cutaneous adverse drug reactions. Pharmcgenetic Genomics 2006;7:297-306.
20. Lonjou C, Thomas L, Borot N, et al. A marker for Stevens-Johnson syndrome: Ethnicity matters. Pharmacogenomics J 2006;6:265-8.
21. Romano A, De Santis A, Romito A, et al. Delayed hypersensitivity to aminopenicillins is related to major histocompatibility complex genes. Ann Allergy Asthma Immunol 1998;80:433-7.
22. Vitezica ZG, Milpied B, Lonjou C, et al. HLA-DRB1*01 associated with cutaneous hypersensitivity induced by nevirapine and efavirenz. AIDS 2008;22:540-1.
23. O'Donohue J, Oien KA, Donaldson P, et al. Co-amoxiclav jaundice : clinical and histological features and HLA class II association. Gut 2000;47:717-20.
24. Hautekeete ML, Horsmans Y, Van Waeyenberge C, et al. HLA association of amoxicilllin-clavulanate-induced hepatitis. Gastroenterology 1999;117:1181-6.
25. Daly A, Donaldson P, Bhatnagar P, et al. HLA-B*5701 genotype is a major determinant of drug-induced liver injury due to flucloxacillin. Nat Genet 2009;41:816-9.
26. Kindmark A, Jawaid A, Harbron CG, et al. Genome-wide pharmacogenetic investigation of a hepatic adverse event without clinical signs of immunopathology suggests an underlying immune pathogenesis. Pharmacogenomics J 2008;8:186-95.
27. Pellicano R, Lomuto M, Ciavarella G, et al. Fixed drug eruptions with feprazone are linked to HLA-B22 J Am Acad Dermatol 1997;36:782-4.
28. Pellicano R, Ciavarella G, Lomuto M, Di Giorgio G. Genetic susceptibility to fixed drug eruption: Evidence for a link with HLA-B22. J Am Acad Dermatol 1994;30: 52-4.
29. Ozkaya-Bayazit E, Akar U. Fixed drug eruption induced by trimethoprim-sulfamethoxazole: Evidence for a link to HLA-A30 B13 Cw6 haplotype. J Am Acad Dermatol 2001;45:712-7.
30. Lieberman JA, Yunis J, Egea E, et al. HLA-B38, DR4, DQw3 and clozapine induced agranulocytosis in Jewish patients with schizophrenia. Arch Gen Psychiatry 1990;47:945-8.
31. Diez RA. HLA-B27 and agranulocytosis by levamisole. Immunol Today 1990;11:270.
32. Batchelor JR, Welsh KI, Tinoco RM, et al. Hydralazine-induced systemic lupus erythematosis: Influence of HLA-DR and sex on susceptibility. Lancet 1980;1:1107-9.
33. Dalle Vedove C, Del Giglio M, Schena D, Girolomoni G, et al. Drug-induced lupus erythematosus. Arch Dermatol Res 2009;301:99-105.
34. Kim SH, Choi JH, Lee KW, et al. The human leucocyte antigen DRB1*1302-DQB1*0609-DPB1*0201 haplotype may be a strong genetic marker for aspirin induced urticaria. Clin Exp Allergy 2005;35:339-44.
35. Kim SH, Hur GY, Choi JH, Park HS. Pharmacogenetics of aspirin-intolerant asthma. Pharmacogenomics 2008;9:85-91.
36. Rodriguez-Perez M, Gonzalez-Dominguez J, Mataran L, et al. Association of HLA-DR5 with mucocutaneous lesions in patients with rheumatoid arthritis receiving gold sodium thiomalate. J Rheumatol 1994;21:41-3.
37. Speerstra F, Reekers P, Van de Putte LB, Vandenbroucke JP. HLA associations in aurothioglucose- and D-penicillamine-induced haematotoxic reactions in rheumatoid arthritis. Tissue Antigens 1985;26:35-40.
38. Quiralte J, Sanchez-Garcia F, Torres MJ, et al. Association of HLA-DR11 with the anaphylactoid reaction caused by nonsteroidal anti-inflammatory drugs. J Allergy Clin Immunol 1999;103;685-9.
39. Garlepp MJ, Dawkins RL, Christiansen FT. HLA antigens and acetylcholine receptor antibodies in penicillamine induced myasthenia gravis. Br Med J (Clin Res Ed) 1983;286:338-40.
40. Pachoula-Papasteriades C, Boki K, Varla-Leftheriotic M, et al. HLA-A-B- and –DR antigens in relation to gold and D-penicillamine toxicity in Greek patients with RA. Dis Markers 1986;4(1-2):35-41.
41. Shiohara T, Inaoka M, Kano Y. Drug induced hypersensitivity syndrome (DIHS) : A reaction induced by a complex interplay among herpesvirus and antiviral and antidrug immune responses. Allergol Int 2006;55: 1-8.
42. Tohyama M, Hasmimoto K, Yasukawa M, et al. Association of human herpesvirus 6 reactivation with the flaring and severity of drug-induced hypersensitivity syndrome. Br J Dermatol 2007;157:934-40.
43. Komura K, Hasegawa M, Hamaguchi Y, et al. Drug-induced hypersensitivity syndrome associated with human herpesvirus 6 and cytomegalovirus reactivation. J Dermatol 2005;32:976-81.
44. Sieishima M, Yamanaka S, Fujisawa T, et al. Reactivation of human herpesvirus(HHV) family members other than

HHV-6 in drug-induced hypersensitivity syndrome. Br J Dermatol 2006;155:344-9.
45. Asano Y, Kagawa H, Kano Y, Shiohara T. Cytomegalovirus disease during severe drug eruptions: Report of 2 cases and retrospective study of 18 patients with drug-induced hypersensitivity syndrome. Arch Dermatol 2009;145:1030-6.
46. Gupta A, Eggo MC, Uetrecht JP, et al. Drug-induced hypothyroidism: The thyroid as a target organ in hypersensitivity reactions to anticonvulsants and sulphonamides. Clin Pharmacol Ther 1992;51:56-67.
47. Aota N, Shiohara T. Viral connection between drug rashes and autoimmune diseases: how autoimmune responses are generated after resolution of drug rashes. Autoimmunity reviews. Epublished ahead of print 2009 Feb 23.
48. Matzinger P. The danger model: A renewed sense of self. Science 2002;296:301-5.
49. Seguin B, Uetrect J. The danger hypothesis applied to idiosyncratic drug reactions. Curr Opin Allergy Clin Immunol 2003;3:235-42.
50. Park BK, Naisbitt DJ, Gordon SF, et al. Metabolic activation in drug allergies. Toxicology 2001;158:11-23.
51. Pichler WJ, Beeler A, Keller M, et al. Pharmacological interaction of drugs with immune receptors: the p-i concept> Allergol Int 2006;55:17-25.
52. Phillips E, Mallal S. Drug hypersensitivity in HIV. Cur Opin Allergy Clin Immunol 2007;7:324-30.
53. Hetherington S, McGuirk S, Powell G, et al. Hypersensitivity reactions during therapy with the nucleoside reverse transcriptase inhibitor abacavir. Clin Ther 2001;23:1603-14.
54. Mallal S, Phillips E, Carosi G, et al. HLA-B*5701 screening for hypersensitivity to abacavir. N Eng J Med 2008;358:568-79.
55. Saag M, Balu R, Phillips E, et al. High sensitivity of human leucocyte antigen-B*5701 as a marker for immunologically confirmed abacavir hypersensitivity in white and black patients. Clin Infect Dis 2008;46:1111-8.
56. Phillips EJ, Sullivan JR, Knowles SR, Shear NH. Utility of patch testing in patients with hypersensitivity reactions associated with abacavir. AIDS 2002;16:2223-5.
57. Phillips EJ, Wong GA, Kaul R, et al. Clinical and immunogenetic correlates of abacavir hypersensitivity. AIDS 2005;19:979-81.
58. Shapiro M, Ward KM, Stern JJ. A near fatal hypersensitivity reaction to abacavir: Case report and literature review. AIDS Read 2001;11:222-6.
59. Symonds W, Cutrell A, Edwards M, et al. Risk factor analysis of hypersensitivity reactions to abacavir. Clin Ther 2002;24;565-73.
60. Peyriere H, Nicolas J, Siffert M, et al. Hypersensitivity related to abacavir in two members of a family. Ann Pharmacother 2001;35:1291-2.
61. Martin AM, Nolan D, Gaudieri S, et al. Predisposition to abacavir hypersensitivity conferred by HLA-B*5701 and a haplotypic Hsp70-Hom variant. Proc Natl Acad Sci USA 2004;101:4180-5.
62. Almeida CA, Martin AM, Nolan D, et al. Cytokine profiling in abacavir hypersensitivity patients. Antivir Ther 2008;13:281-8.
63. Martin AM, Almeida CA, Cameron P, et al. Immune responses to abacavir in antigen-presenting cells from hypersensitive patients. AIDS 2007;21:1233-44.
64. Chessman D, Kostenko L, Lethborg T, et al. Human leucocyte antigen class I restricted activation of CD8+ T cells provides the immunogenetic basis of a systemic drug hypersensitivity. Immunity 2008;28:822-32.
65. Walsh JS, Reese MH, Thurmond LM. The metabolic activation of abacavir by human liver cytosol and expressed human alcohol dehydrogenase isozymes. Chem Biol Interact 2002;142:135-54.
66. Hughes AR, Mosteller M, Bansal AT, et al. Association of genetic variations in HLA-B region wtih hypersensitivity to abacavir in some, but not all, populations. Pharmacogenomics 2004;5:203-11.
67. Dart Trial Team: Twenty-four week safety and tolerability of nevirapine vs. abacavir in combination with zidovudine/lamivudine as first-line antiretroviral therapy: A randomized double-blind trial (NORA) Trop Med Int Health 2008;13:6-16.
68. Guilick RM, Ribaudo H, Shikuma CM, et al. Three versus four-drug antiretroviral regimens for the initial treatment of HIV-1 infection: A randomized controlled trial. J Am Med Assoc 2006;296:769-81.
69. Dejesus E, Herrera G, Teofilo E, et al. Abacavir versus zidovudine combined with lamivudine and efavirenz for the treatment of antirretroviral naive HIV infected adults. Clin Infect Dis 2004;39:1038-46.
70. Hernandez J, Cutrell A, Bonny T, et al. Diagnosis of abacavir hypersensitivity reactions among patients not receiving abacavir in two blinded studies. Antivir Ther 2003;8:L88.
71. Merk HF. Drug skin metabolites and allergic drug reactions. Curr Opin All Clin Immunol 2009;9:311-5.
72. Shear NH, Milpied B, Bruynzeel DP, Phillips EJ. A review of drug patch testing and implications for HIV clinicians. AIDS 2008;22;999-1007.
73. Rauch A, Nolan D, Martin A, et al. Prospective genetic screening decreases the incidence of abacavir hypersensitivity reactions in the Western Australian HIV cohort study. Clin Inf Dis 2006;43:99-102.
74. Zucman D, Truchis P, Majerholc S, et al. Prospective screening for human leucocyte antigen B*5701 avoid abacavir hypersensitivity in the ethnically mixed French HIV population. J Acquir Immune Defic Syndr 2007;45:1-3.
75. Reeves I, Churchill D, Fisher M. Screening for HLA-B*5701 reduces the frequencies of abacavir hypersensitivity reactions. Antiviral Ther 2006;11(suppl 3):14.
76. Trottier B, Thomas R, Nguyen VK, Machouf N. How effectively HLA screening can reduce the early

discontinuation of abacavir in real life. Abstract IAS Sydney, Australia July 22-25, abstract MOPEB002 (2007).
77. Waters LJ, Mandalia S, Gazzard B, et al. Prospective HLA-B*5701 screening and abacavir hypersensitivity: A single centre experience. AIDS 2007;21:2533-4.
78. Young B, Squires K, Patel P, et al. First large multicenter open-label study utilizing HLA-B*5701 screening for abacavir hypersensitivity in North America. AIDS 2008;22:1673-5.
79. Phillips E, Nolan D, Thorborn D, et al. Genetic factors predicting abacavir hypersensitivity and tolerance in HLA-B*5701 positive individuals. Eur J Dermatol 2008;18:Abs 247.
80. Erickson DA, Mather G, Trager WF, et al. Characterization of the in vitro biotransformation of the HIV-1 reverse transcriptase inhibitor nevirapine by human hepatic cytochromes P-450. Drug Metab Dispos 1999;27:1488-95.
81. Shenton JM, Popovic M, Uetrect JP. Nevirapine hypersensitivity. In Drug Hypersensitivity. Pichler WJ (Ed), Karger AG, Basel Switzerland 2007;115-28.
82. Johnson S, Baraboutis JG, Sha BE, et al. Adverse effects associated with use of nevirapine in HIV post-exposure prophylaxis for 2 health care workers. JAMA 2000; 284:2722-3.
83. Wit FW, Kesselring AM, Gras L, et al. Discontinuation of nevirapine because of hypersensitivity reactions in patients with prior treatment experience, compared with treatment-naive patients: the ATHENA cohort study. Clin Infect Dis 2008;46;933-40.
84. Kesselring AM, Wit FW, Sabin CA, et al. Risk factors for treatment-limiting toxicities in patients starting nevirapine containing therapy. AIDS 2009; 23:1689-99.
85. Liechty CA, Solberg P, Mwima G, et al. Nevirapine-induced Stevens-Johnson syndrome in a mother and son. AIDS 2005;19:993-4.
86. Duvic M, Reisner EG, Dawson DV, Ciftan E. HLA-B15 association with erythema multiforme. J Am Acad Dermatol 1983;8:493-6.
87. Kampgen E, Brug G, Wank R. Association of herpes simplex-virus induced erythema multiforme with the human leukocyte antigen DQw3. Arch Dermatol 1988;124;1372-5.
88. Stevens AM, Johnson FC. A new eruptive fever associated with stomatitis and ophthalmia: Report of two cases in children. Am J Dis Child 1922;24:526-33.
89. Lyell A. Toxic epidermal necroylsis: An eruption resembling scalding of the skin. Br J Dermatol 1956;68: 355-61.
90. Bastuji-Garin S, Rzany B, Stern RS, et al. Clinical classification of cases of toxic epidermal necrolysis. Arch Dermatol 1993;129:92-6.
91. Stern RS, Albengres E, Carlson J, et al. An international comparison of case definition of severe adverse cutaneous reactions to medicines. Drug Saf 1993;8;69-77.
92. Bastuji-Garin N, Fouchard M, Bertocchi, et al. SCORTEN: A severity-of-illness score for toxic epidermal necrolysis. J Invest Dermatol 2000;115:149-53.
93. Roujeau JC, Kelly JP, Naldi L, et al. Medication use and the risk of Stevens-Johnson syndrome or toxic epidermal necrolysis. N Engl J Med 1995;333:1600-7.
94. Strom BL, Carson AC, Halpern R, et al. A population-based study of Stevens-Johnson syndrome. Incidence and antecedent drug exposures. Arch Dermatol 1991;127: 831-8.
95. Roujeau JC, Guillaume JC, Fabre JP, et al. Toxic epidermal necrolysis (Lyell syndrome). Incidence and antecedent drug exposures. Arch Dermatol 1990;126:37-42.
96. Mockenhaupt M, Viboud C, Dunant A, et al. Stevens-Johnson syndrome and toxic epidermal necrolysis: Assessment of medication risks with emphasis on recently marketed drugs. The EuroSCAR-study. J Invest Dermaol 2008;128:35-44.
97. Fagot JP, Mockenhaupt M, Bouwes-Bavinck JN, et al. Nevirapine and the risk of Stevens-Johnson syndrome or toxic epidermal necrolysis. AIDS 2001;15:1843-8.
98. Chia FL, Leon KP. Severe cutaneous adverse reactions to drugs. Curr Opin Allergy Clin Immunology 2007;7: 304-9.
99. Knowles S, Shear NH. Clinical risk management of Stevens-Johnson syndrome/toxic epidermal necrolysis spectrum. Dermatol Ther 2009;22:441-51.
100. Mittmann N, Chan B, Knowles S et al. Intravenous immunoglobulin in patients with toxic epidermal necrolysis and Stevens-Johnson syndrome. Am J Clin Dermatol 2006;7:359-68.
101. Viard I, Wehrli P, Bullani R, et al. Inhibition of toxic epidermal necrolysis by blockade of CD95 with human intravenous immunoglobulin. Science 1998;282;490-3.
102. Fisher M, Fiedler E, Marsh WC, Wohlrab J. Antitumour necrosis factor-alpha antibodies (infliximab) in the treatment of a patient with toxic epidermal necrolysis. Br J Deramtol 2002;146:707-9.
103. Gubinelli E, Canzona F, Tonanzi T, et al. Toxic epidermal necrolysis successfully treated with etanercept. J Dermatol 2009;36:150-3.
104. Verneuil L, Ratajczak P, Allabert C, et al. Endothelial cell apoptosis in severe drug-induced bullous eruptions. British J Derm 2009; Epub ahead of print [Jul 3 2009].
105. Abe R, Shimizu T, Shibaki A, et al. Toxic epidermal necrolysis and Stevens-Johnson syndrome are induced by soluble Fas ligand. Am J Pathol 2003;162:1515-20.
106. Le Cleach L, Delaire S, Boumsell L, et al. Blister fluid T lymphocytes during toxic epidermal necrolysis are functional cytotoxic cells which express human natural killer (NK) inhibitory receptors. Clin Exp Immunol 2000;119;225-30.
107. Nassif A, Bensussan A, Dorethee G, et al. Drug specific cytotoxic T-cells in the skin lesions of a patient with toxic epidermal necrolysis. J Invest Dermatol 2002;118:728-33.
108. Alfirevic A, Jorgensen AL, Williamson PR, et al. HLA-B locus in Caucasian patients with carbamazepine hypersensitivity. Pharmacogenomics 2006;7:813-8.
109. Kaniwa N, Saito Y Aihara M, et al. HLA-B locus in Japanese patients with anti-epileptics and allopurinol-

110. Ikeda H, Takahashi Y, Yamazaki E, et al. HLA Class I markers in Japanese patients with carbamazepine-induced cutaneous adverse reactions. Epilepsia 2009; epub ahead of print [August 19].
111. Hung SI, Chung WH, Chen YT. Genetics of severe drug hypersensitivity reactions in Han Chinese In: Drug Hypersensitivity Pichler WJ (Ed), Karger AG, Basel, Switzerland 2007;55-64.
112. Knowles SR, Shapiro LE, Shear NH. Anticonvulsant hypersensitivity syndrome: Incidence prevention and management. Drug Safety 1999;21:489-501.
113. FDA Alert: Phenytoin and Fosphenytoin: http://www.fda.gov/Drugs/DrugSafety/PostmarketDrugSafetyInformationforPatientsandProviders/ucm124788.htm.
114. Kaplowitz N. Idiosyncratic drug hepatotoxicity. Nat Rev Drug Discov 2005;4:489-99.
115. Daly A, Day C. Genetic association studies in drug-induced liver injury. Semin Liver Dis 2009;29:400-11.
116. Hammer SM, Eron JJ Jr, Reiss P, et al. Antiretroviral treatment of adult HIV infection: 2008 recommendations of the international AIDS Society-USA panel. J Am Med Assoc 2008;300:555-70.
117. Panel on antiretroviral guidelines for adults and adolescents: Guidelines for the use of antiretroviral agents in HIV-1 infected adults and adolesecents: Department of health and human services. Washington DC, USA 2008. http://www.aidsinfo.nih.gov/ContentFiles/AdultandAdolescentGL.pdf.
118. Martin AM, Nolan D, Mallal S: HLA-B*5701 typing by sequence specific amplification: Validation and comparison with sequence-based typing. Tissue Antigens 2005;65:571-4.
119. Hammond E, Mamotte C, Nolan D, et al. HLA-B*5701 typing: Evaluation of an allele-specific polymerase chain reaction melting assay. Tissue Antigens 2007;70:58-61.
120. Hammond E, Almeida CA, Mamotte C, et al. External quality assessment of HLA-B*5701 reporting: An International multicentre survey. Antivir Ther 2007;12:1027-32.
121. Colombo S, Rauch A, Rotger M, et al. The HCP5 single-nucleotide polymorphism: a simple screening tool for prediction of hypersensitivity reaction to abacavir. J Inf Dis 2008;198:864-7.
122. Martin AM, Krueger R, Almeida CA, et al. A sensitive and rapid alternative to HLA typing as a genetic screening test for abacavir hypersensitivity syndrome. Pharmacogenet Genomics 2006;16:353-7.
123. Kostenko L, Lucas A, Kjer-Neilsen, et al. A rapid and sensitive flow-based screening test for detection of HLA-B57 to avoid abacavir hypersensitivity. International AIDS Society Meeting Sydney July 22-25, 2007. Abstract WEPEB113LB.
124. Phillips EJ. Genetic screening to prevent abacavir hypersensitivity reaction: Are we there yet? Clin Infect Dis 2006;43:103-5.
125. Schackman BR, Scott CA, Walensky RP, et al. The cost effectiveness of HLA-B*5701 genotyping to guide initial antiretroviral therapy for HIV. AIDS 2008; 22:2025-33.
126. Yang L, Chen J, He L. Harvesting candidate genes responsible for serious adverse drug reactions from a chemical-protein interactome. Plos Computational Biology 2009;5:e1000441.

Chapter 21

Comparative Genomics: Insight into Human Health and Disease

Toshiaki Nakajima, Akinori Kimura

INTRODUCTION

Comparative genomics is an approach of extraordinary promise for studying the biological significance of the genome from the evolutionary points of view, because genome sequence is a record of the evolutionary history of organisms. It also has a crucial role in furthering our understanding of the pathophysiological mechanisms operated by human disease genes. The functional analyses of a homologue of disease gene in model organisms can provide important information in understanding the biochemical function of the human disease gene.

The comparative genomic analysis consists of 4 main processes, including the following steps. Step1: Generation of sequence data; Step 2: Identification of homologue sequences among related genomes; Step 3: Multiple-sequence alignment; and step 4: Analyses to determine the biological significance of the homologue sequences (Fig. 21.1).[1] The number of species available for genomic comparison has been rapidly increasing. The human genome project, which was started in the late 1980s and ostensibly "completed" in 2003, has actively stimulated the development of genome projects for model organisms, such as C. elegans, fruit fly, and mouse. Furthermore, the rapid progress in sequence technology, such as massive parallel sequencing technology,[2] has further accelerated the increase in the number of complete or semi-complete genome sequences of other organisms. These sequences serve as the material for large-scale analysis of comparative genomics. Moreover, rapid progress in the field of bioinformatics, which provides useful tools to reconstruct homologous sequences among related species and to generate base-pair alignment, has advanced studies of comparative genomics. There are several data-bases that are available for large-scale comparative sequence analyses (Table 21.1).[1]

In this chapter we will focus on the methods used to evaluate the biological significance of homologous sequences (step 4 in Fig. 21.1). In particular, we focus on the methods based on the theory of natural selection, but we will not touch on other steps of comparative genomics (Fig. 21.1). The underlying principle behind the identification of the biological significance is that the genomic regions, which have been evolving more rapidly (positive selection) or more slowly (negative selection) than the local rate of neutral evolution, are tightly linked to biological significance. Human diseases are occasionally linked to human evolutionary process and population history, so that comparative genomics will also provide insight into human health and disease.

HUMAN DISEASE AND EVOLUTION

The molecular evidence that the human evolutionary process is tightly linked to human disease has been steadily accumulating during the last decades. For example, the evolutionary processes, especially natural selection, affect the frequency of disease-related mutations in the general population. Disease-related mutations, which had been introduced through errors in DNA replication, are believed to be rapidly removed by natural negative selection triggered by the deleterious consequences induced by the mutations. However, certain environments may result in a special selective advantage for a disease mutation. For example, sickle-cell anemia provides a conspicuous example.[3] Sickle-cell mutations are relatively prevalent in Africa, where

Chapter 21 ■ Comparative Genomics: Insight into Human Health and Disease

Table 21.1: Main features of the data bases available for large-scale comparative genomics		
Data base	Web site	Main feature
Ensembl Genome Browser[63]	http://www.ensembl.org/index.html	Joint project between EMBL-EBI and the Sanger Center to develop a software system which produces and maintains automatic annotation on eukaryotic genomes.
Galaxy[64]	http://g2.bx.psu.edu.	Interactive system that combines the power of existing genome annotation databases with a simple Web portal to enable users to search remote resources, combine data from independent queries, and visualize the results.
UCSC Genome Browser[65]	http://genome.ucsc.edu/	The UCSC Genome Browser was created by the Genome Bioinformatics Group of UC Santa Cruz. The UCSC Genome Browser website contains the reference sequence and working draft assemblies for a large collection of genomes. It also provides a portal to the ENCODE project.
VISTA[49]	http://genome.lbl.gov/vista/index.shtml	The VISTA site includes computational tools for comparative genomics and provides whole-genome alignments of large vertebrate genomes

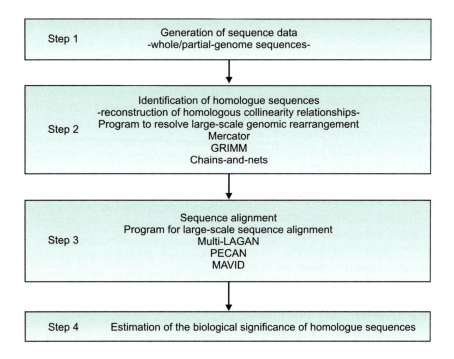

Fig. 21.1: Four main steps of the comparative genomic analyses
Step1: Generation of sequence data. **Step 2:** Identification of homologue sequences among related genomes. Mercator,[66] GRIMM,[67] and Chains-and-nets[68] are programs to resolve large-scale genomic rearrangement in genome-wide scale comparative genomics. **Step 3:** Multiple-sequence alignment. Multi-LAGAN,[69] PECAN,[70,71] and MAVID[72] are programs for large-scale sequence alignment. **Step 4:** Analyses to determine the biological significance of homologue sequences.[1]

Plasmodium falciparum malaria is common, because the individuals heterozygous for the sickle-cell mutation, who are resistant to malaria infection conferred by the mutation, have a distinct survival advantage. This example illustrates how disease mutations have arisen and maintained under the pressure of natural selection operating differently in different environments.

It has been reported that among primates humans and chimpanzees are sensitive to HIV infection, but chimpanzees are naturally resistant to the development of AIDS. Interestingly, the nucleotide diversity in the MHC class I genes in chimpanzees is much lower than that in humans, although nucleotide diversity in the chimpanzee genome in general is much higher than that in the human genome.[4, 5] Furthermore, common Patr-B alleles observed in chimpanzees have certain functional relationships to the HLA-B alleles, HLA-B27 and HLA-B57, which are known to be associated with the resistance and/or protection to HIV infection or development of AIDS.[5] The amino acid sequences of HIV-1 epitopes recognized by CTL in the context of these Patr-B alleles are more or less similar to those of the HIV-1 resistant human alleles, HLA-B27 and HLA-B57. Such evidence suggests that HIV-induced selective sweeps had occurred, and that only the descendants of chimpanzees that were resistant to HIV/AIDS have survived in the course of chimpanzee evolution. This is an example of disease susceptibility genes under the control of natural selection in the course of primate evolution.

The "thrifty genotype" hypothesis advanced by James V. Neel[6] is also an intriguing evolutionary scenario to account for the emergence of common human diseases. The genotypes predisposing to human common diseases (diabetes in Neel's original hypothesis) had previously been advantageous in the course of human evolution, but became deleterious in the changed context of the modern world. A change in the environment or life style factor, especially a dietary factor, may be responsible for the rapid increase in the prevalence of certain human diseases, such as diabetes mellitus and essential hypertension. Certain "thrifty" genotypes had thrived in scarce food environment. In our previous study,[7] genetic diversity in the human angiotensinogen gene, which is a susceptibility gene for essential hypertension,[8] was shown to be in support of this hypothesis.

Alternatively, it has been reported that the genes under the pressure of natural selection are occasionally associated with human diseases. HLA genes, which have the highest nucleotide diversity and the highest nonsynonymous substitution rate in the human genome, are a conspicuous example. The patterns of sequence variations in the HLA genes have been shaped by positive natural selection.[9] It is widely accepted that several human diseases are tightly linked to sequence variations in the HLA genes.[10]

These lines of evidence support a tight association between the evolution of human genome and certain human diseases, so that an improved understanding of the human genome from the evolutionary point of view might provide us with the critically important insight into human health and disease. In particular, understanding the effect of natural selection on the human genes might be helpful to understand the evolutionary aspects of human health and disease. Thus, in this chapter we will describe how to identify the genomic segments under the control of natural selection by comparative genomics.

COMPARATIVE GENOMICS AND NATURAL SELECTION

Assuming that all comparable organisms in a given lineage originate from a common ancestor and that the evolutionary process can be traced by means of genomic sequences, comparative genomics is a useful approach to study the evolution.[1, 11-13] The combined actions of mutation and selection are believed to be powerful driving forces of evolution. Mutations randomly occur in the genome, and their traits are then exposed to intense selective pressure. The fates of genetic mutations are tightly linked to their functional impacts on the phenotypic traits of organisms in the population.

Mutations are categorized into three types, advantageous, deleterious, or neutral mutations.[14] When a mutation confers a functional advantage on its carrier, it would increase the fitness of its carrier and eventually increase the chance of survival in the population (positive natural selection), resulting in a fixed difference between species. More frequently, a new mutation, which reduces the fitness of its carrier due to its deleterious impact on gene function, will be removed from the population (negative or purifying selection). Most new mutants arising in a population have no impact on gene function. Such mutations are selectively neutral and the fate in the population is determined by chance effect (neutral selection). Comparative genomics make it possible to trace all of these processes of natural selection in comparable organisms.

Evaluation of Selective Pressure on the Coding Regions: Synonymous and Nonsynonymous Nucleotide Substitution Rates

When comparing orthologous coding sequences from related species, the nucleotide differences among the orthologues are classified into two types, synonymous and nonsynonymous substitutions. Nucleotide substitutions which occur without affecting the amino acid sequence are called synonymous (silent) nucleotide substitutions, while those with amino acid replacements are called nonsynonymous nucleotide substitutions. As described in the following sections, estimates of synonymous (Ks) and nonsynonymous (Ka) substitution rates have provided important information for evaluating the selective pressure on the target genomic region in the evolutionary process. Ka and Ks are defined as the number of nonsynonymous substitutions (N_d) per nonsynonymous site (N), and the number of synonymous substitutions (S_d) per synonymous site (S) for any pair of sequences, respectively.[14]

Synonymous and nonsynonymous sites in coding sequence are the sites in a codon, where nucleotide changes would result in synonymous and nonsynonymous substitutions, respectively. One way to calculate them is based on the patterns of nucleotide substitutions in the genetic code and amino acid substitutions (degeneracy in the genetic code).[14] As shown in Table 21.2, nucleotide sites are classified into nondegenerate, twofold-degenerate, and fourfold-degenerate sites. A site is nondegenerate (denoted by G, A, T or C) when all possible changes at this site are nonsynonymous, twofold-degenerate (denoted by Y or R) when one of the three possible changes is synonymous, and fourfold-degenerate (denoted by N) when all possible changes at the site are synonymous. For simplicity, the third position in each of the three codons for Ile (denoted by H) is treated as a twofold-degenerate site, although the degeneracy at this position is actually threefold. When each of the average number of non-degenerate, twofold-degenerate, and fourfold-degenerate sites in the two compared sequences is denoted by L_0 (non-degenerate), L_2 (twofold-degenerate), and L_4 (fourfold-degenerate), respectively, the number of synonymous and nonsynonymous are given by the formula,

$$S = L_2 / 3 + L_4 \text{ and } N = 2L_2 / 3 + L_0$$

Table 21.2: Degeneracy in the mammalian genetic code

1st base	2nd base			
	T	C	A	G
T	TTY (Phe) TTR (Leu)	TCN (Ser)	TAY (Tyr) TAR (Stop)	TGY (Cys) TGA (Stop) TGG (Trp)
C	CTN (Leu)	CCN (Pro)	CAY (His) CAR (Gln)	CGN (Arg)
A	ATH (Ile) ATG (Met)	ACN (Thr)	AAY (Asn) AAR (Lys)	AGY (Ser) AGR (Arg)
G	GTN (Val)	GCN (Ala)	GAY (Asp) GAR (Glu)	GGN (Gly)

Non-degenerate sites are denoted by G, A, T, or C.
Twofold-degenerate sites are denoted by Y or R.
Threefold-degenerate sites are denoted by H.
Fourfold-degenerate sites are denoted by N.

For example, here are two coding sequences for three codons to estimate the value of Ks and Ka,

Sequence 1: GTC-TTT-GAT (Val-Phe-Asp)

Sequence 2: GTT-GTT-GCG (Val-Val-Ala)

The numbers of the three degenerate types of sites in each of the two sequences are as follows:

	Non-degenerate	Twofold-degenerate	Fourfold-degenerate
Sequence 1	6	2	1
Sequence 2	6	0	3
Average	6	1	2

Hence, $S = 1 \times 1/3 + 2 \cong 2.33$ and $N = 1 \times 2/3 + 6 \cong 6.67$

Next, to estimate the Ks and Ka, we need to compare codon by codon the two sequences and infer the nucleotide substitutions in each pair of codons. When comparing the two first codons, GTC (Val) and GTT (Val), a C to A synonymous nucleotide substitution at the four-degenerate site is easily inferred. Similarly, a T to G nonsynonymous nucleotide substitutions at the nondegenerate site is inferred in the comparison of the two second codons, TTT (Phe) and GTT (Val). For two codons with one nucleotide difference, the number of synonymous or nonsynonymous substitutions is easily inferred. However, the case of the two third codons is more complicated. For the two third codons, GAT (Asp) and GCG (Ala), there are two possible minimum evolutionary pathways;

Pathway 1: GAT (Asp) ↔ GCT (Ala) ↔ GCG (Ala)
Pathway 2: GAT (Asp) ↔ GAG (Glu) ↔ GCG (Ala)

In pathway 1, one nonsynonymous nucleotide substitution and one synonymous nucleotide substitutions are estimated, whereas the pathway 2 involves two nonsynonymous substitutions. For the estimation of the number of synonymous and nonsynonymous substitutions, we may apply the weight for the probability of each possible pathway, because synonymous substitutions have occurred more often than nonsynonymous substitutions in the course of evolution. There are several methods to estimate the weight for all possible codon pairs.[15-17] When estimated by Nei-Gojobori method,[16] which considers all pathways with equal probability, but which excludes those pathways that go through stop codons, the numbers of synonymous and nonsynonymous substitutions for sequence 1 and 2 are 1.50 and 2.50, leading the Ks and Ka for them to be 1.46 (1.50/2.33) and 0.52 (2.50/6.67), respectively.

As shown above, inferring the number of synonymous and nonsynonymous substitution is not simple or straightforward. Furthermore, the maximum-likelihood approach taking advantage of the probability theory has been developed.[18] It is necessary to pay attention to the differences in the estimated values of Ka and Ks by several different methods to obtain an accurate picture.

Natural Selection and Synonymous and Nonsynonymous Nucleotide Substitution Rates

In the comparisons of coding sequences from several species, estimates of synonymous (Ks) and non-synonymous (Ka) substitution rates between two given sequences are extremely useful in evaluating the selective pressure on the target genomic region in the evolutionary process. Because the value of Ks is proposed to be almost equal to the nucleotide substitution rate under the neutral selection, the Ka/Ks ratio is a good parameter for identifying genomic segments under the pressure of natural selection. In the absence of selective pressure, the values of Ks and Ka should be more or less the same (Ka/Ks $\cong$ 1). When the genomic segment has been under the pressure of negative (purifying) selection, the value of Ka is expected to be much lower than Ks (Ka/Ks<1), because selection would occur at the amino acid level. Amino acid sequences under the pressure of negative selection have been strictly conserved in the course of evolution. The functional significance of a target for the negative selection is considered as such that certain amino acid sequences have not been altered in the course of primate evolution. In clear contrast, if there has been a pressure of positive Darwinian selection, the value of Ka would be expected to be higher than Ks (Ka/Ks>1). In this scenario, rapid changes in amino acid sequences, which confer novel or gain in function, would have been advantageous in the course of evolution.

Genes under the Pressure of Natural Selection Derived from Whole-genome Comparative Analysis in Primates

Recently, large-scale genome sequences of chimpanzees[19] and rhesus macaque monkeys[20] have been available, and the whole genome sequencings of gorilla, orangutan, and marmoset are under way. Comparative genomic analyses among primates are definitely useful to address the issue of which genetic changes have made us uniquely human. Furthermore, they are also useful to identify the susceptibility genes for human diseases, and to understand the pathophysiological mechanisms of human disease genes, because biological differences among primates, such as differences in the susceptibility to several different diseases, have been reported.[21]

To resolve these issues, identification of the genes that have come under the pressure of natural selection in the course of primate evolution is of critical importance. Actually, comparisons between human and chimpanzee and between human and rhesus genome have already suggested that dozens of genes have been under the pressure of natural selection in the course of primate evolution, in particular those involved in host-pathogen interactions, reproduction, sensory system, and more.[19,20,22] However, it is difficult to establish the functional significance of the genes under the natural selection, because of the limitations on the functional experiments required by the ethical reasons. We cannot practically apply, for example, the knockout experiment in primates to reveal the functional differences induced by the genetic difference in the genes under the control of natural selection. Thus, further studies for comparative analyses of the genomes and phenotypes among primates should be undertaken.

Comparative Genomics in Coding Regions: Lesson from TLR Sequence Comparisons among Primates

In this section, we demonstrate an example of comparative genomic analysis. That is the analyses for Toll-like receptor (TLR)-related genes, which might be helpful in understanding how to study the biological significance of orthologous genes based on comparative genomics. TLRs recognize molecules derived from pathogens and play crucial roles in the innate immune system.[23,24] To investigate whether the TLR-related genes have come under the natural selection pressure in the course of primate evolution, we compared the nucleotide sequences of sixteen TLR-related genes, including ten *TLRs* (*TLR1-10*), four genes linked to signal transduction (*MYD88*, *TILAP*, *TICAM1*, and *TICAM2*), and 2 genes linked to *TLR4* (*MD2* and *CD14*), among seven primates, including human, chimpanzee, bonobo, gorilla, orangutan, crab-eating macaque, and rhesus macaque.[25] MD2 and CD14 are key molecules in the LPS signaling through TLR4.[26-28]

To evaluate the nonsynonymous/synonymous substitution ratio, we applied the Bn-Bs program.[29] This program uses a modified Nei-Gojobori method[16] to estimate pairwise synonymous and nonsynonymous distances among the sequences, and then estimates the branch lengths in terms of synonymous (bs) and nonsynonymous substitutions (bn) per site by using the ordinary least-squares method, while the tree topology is given. Σbn and Σbs indicate the value summing up the bn and bs scores, respectively, in the lineages. The values of bs and bn are almost identical to those of Ka and Ks, respectively, which were described in the previous section. When the value of Σbn and Σbs and the ratio of Σbn/Σbs were evaluated for the entire coding sequences from each gene, all values of the Σbn/Σbs ratio from the analyzed genes were much lower than 1.0, suggesting that these genes have been under the pressure of negative selection (Table 21.3).

Next, we performed a sliding window plot analysis (600 bp-window with 30 bp-steps) throughout these genes to identify the genomic segments that might have undergone the natural selection. Analysis of the Σbn/Σbs ratio revealed the presence of both the strictly conserved and rapidly evolving regions among the TLR-related genes. Three candidate segments, where the pressure of the negative or positive natural selection might have operated, were identified in *TLR7*, *MYD88*, and *TLR4* (Fig. 21.2A).

Two target segments showed little nonsynonymous nucleotide differences (Σbn/Σb<<1) among seven primates (Fig. 21.2B). One segment was located at the coding segment for the C-terminal of TLR7 and the other segment was that for the C-terminal of MYD88, both of which encode the intracellular Toll/interleukin 1 receptor (TIR) domain (Fig. 21.2B), implying that the genomic regions corresponding to the TIR domains were the targets of negative natural selection. We then evaluated the Σbn/Σbs ratios for the TIR domains for fourteen genes carrying the TIR domains. The sizes of the genomic segments encoding TIR domains were between 249 and 426 base pairs (bp) (average 393 bp) that were smaller than the window size (600 bp) used in our analysis, implicating that the window analysis would underestimate the Σbn/Σbs ratios for the TIR domains. The values of Σbn and Σbn/Σbs ratio for TIR domains displayed lower values when compared with those of the non-TIR coding sequences, except for the Σbn/Σbs ratio from *TLR10* (Fig. 21.3). In particular, *TLR7*, *TLR8*, *TLR9*, *MYD88*, and *TICAM2* have much lower values for Σbn in the TIR domains. Taken together, these observations suggest that the TIR domains were under the control of negative/purifying selection. The TIR domains are key components in the TLR signal transduction. In particular, the adaptor protein MYD88 is tightly linked to all the TLR signaling pathways except for TLR3.[23,24] This may be the reason for that the amino acid sequences have not been altered in the course of primate evolution. Most of the mutations arising at the TIR domains would in all likelihood were deleterious, and thus reduced the fitness of primates which had harbored such changes.

Table 21.3: The nonsynonymous and synonymous substitution ratio, GC content and CBI for 16 TLR-related genes among 7 primates

Gene	Chromosome (Human)	Σbn	Σbs	Σbn/Σbs	G + C 2nd	G + C 3rd	G + C all	CBI
TLR1	4p14	0.041	0.095	0.429	0.319	0.433	0.394	0.188
TLR2	4q32	0.025	0.086	0.290	0.344	0.452	0.417	0.213
TLR3	4q35	0.032	0.121	0.267	0.314	0.419	0.399	0.193
TLR4	9q32-33	0.038	0.085	0.447	0.323	0.472	0.428	0.214
TLR5	1q41-42	0.030	0.108	0.282	0.33	0.487	0.438	0.189
TLR6	4p14	0.030	0.120	0.240	0.307	0.408	0.384	0.195
TLR7	Xp22.3-p22.2	0.014	0.069	0.202	0.317	0.442	0.409	0.193
TLR8	Xp22.3-p22.2	0.020	0.095	0.209	0.321	0.41	0.394	0.144
TLR9	3p21.3	0.029	0.153	0.187	0.418	0.804	0.619	0.631
TLR10	4p14	0.024	0.106	0.228	0.311	0.368	0.378	0.262
MYD88	3p22-p21.3	0.009	0.096	0.094	0.435	0.712	0.588	0.484
TIRAP	11q23-q24	0.035	0.164	0.216	0.531	0.691	0.608	0.497
TICAM1*	19p13.3	0.039	0.171	0.227	0.523	0.732	0.64	0.486
TICAM2	5q23.1	0.020	0.119	0.167	0.383	0.383	0.427	0.318
MD2	8q21.11	0.015	0.054	0.269	0.353	0.361	0.361	0.408
CD14	5q31.1	0.013	0.040	0.332	0.488	0.704	0.63	0.422

* TICAM1 has a CCT (Pro)-repeat variation.

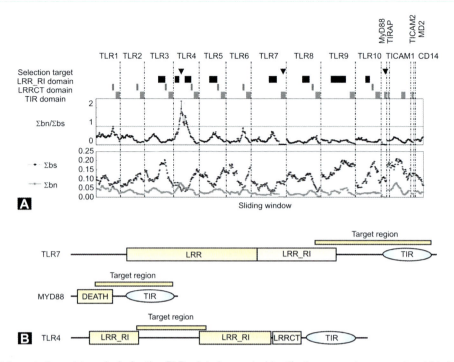

Figs 21.2A and B: Sliding window plot analysis for the TLR-related gene to identify the genomic segments which have undergone natural selection. (A) The values of $\Sigma bn/\Sigma bs$, $\acute{O}bn$, and $\acute{O}bs$ based on the sliding window plot analysis for the TLR-related gene (600 bp-window with 30 bp-steps). The arrow heads indicate the candidate segments for the pressure of positive or negative natural selection. Three conserved domain structures, LRR_RI (Leucine-rich repeats, ribonuclease inhibitor-like subfamily), LRRCT (Leucine rich repeat C-terminal domain), and TIR (Toll/interleukin-1 receptor homology domain), were referred from CD-search.[73] (B) Natural selection target in *TLR7* (negative selection), *MYD88* (negative selection), and *TLR4* (positive selection)

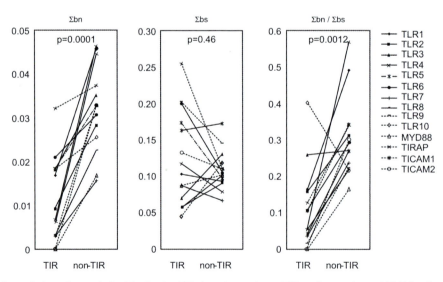

Fig. 21.3: The values of Σbn, Σbs, and $\Sigma bn/\Sigma bs$ for the TIR domains and non-TIR coding regions of TLR family and related genes. Data for fourteen genes, including *TLRs (TLR1-10)*, *MYD88*, *TILAP*, *TICAM1*, and *TICAM2*, are presented

On the other hand, sequence comparisons among the primates support positive Darwinian selection at the extracellular domain of TLR4, for which the $\Sigma bn/\Sigma bs$ ratios were much higher than 1.0 and the highest value in the 600 bp-window was 2.37 that was significant on Z-test[29,30] with Z-score 2.16 (p-value < 0.01) (Fig. 21.2). The TLR4 target region encoding the extracellular domain next to the domain with Leucine-rich repeats (Fig. 21.2B) has been reported to be hypervariable and contribute to the species-specific recognition of several molecules, such as taxol, lipid IVa, and LPS.[31-33] This target region also was reported to be linked to LPS susceptibility in humans.[34] The missense mutation D299G, where an aspartic acid was replaced by a glycine at the 299 amino acid position of human TLR4, was associated with a blunted response to LPS and increased susceptibility to Gram-negative bacterial infections. An aspartic acid corresponding to the 299 amino acid position of human TLR4 has been highly conserved among great apes and gibbons, whereas it was replaced by a glycine in the lineage of Old World Monkeys. These results indicate that the sensitivity to a certain type of LPS might differ between the lineage of great apes and that of the Old World Monkeys.

Given that TLR4 recognizes a wide variety of ligands such as LPS and viral envelope proteins, the differences in the species-specific susceptibility to infectious disease might be linked to the natural selection pressure. As shown in the case of TLR-related genes, comparative sequence analyses provide us with the useful information to evaluate the functional significance of genes from an evolutionary point of view.

OTHER FACTORS AFFECT SYNONYMOUS NUCLEOTIDE SUBSTITUTION RATE IN CODING REGIONS

In previous sections, the ratio of Ka/Ks was used as a parameter to estimate the selective pressure on the genomic segment. Since the synonymous substitutions do not cause any changes in amino acid sequences, they were proposed to be equal to the nucleotide substitution rate under the neutral selection. However, several lines of evidence suggest that the synonymous changes have not, in fact, been selectively neutral in the course evolution.[35] It has been reported that the following several factors would affect the synonymous nucleotide substitution rates. Although many synonymous mutations are no doubt free from the selection, the assumption that they are all neutral no longer appears tenable. It is important to keep in mind these effects when evaluating the selective pressure.

Base Composition and the Nucleotide Substitution Rate

The correlation between the synonymous substitution rate (Ks) and the GC content of the genome has been the subject of debate.[36, 37] It is likely that the GC content would affect the nucleotide substitution rates, because the GC content might affect the DNA structure. Therefore, we evaluated the correlation of the GC content with the synonymous and nonsynonymous nucleotide substitution rates by using sixteen TLR-related genes. As shown in Figures 21.4A to D, the synonymous substitution rate, but not the nonsynonymous substitution rate, weakly correlates with the GC content. The genes with higher levels of GC content

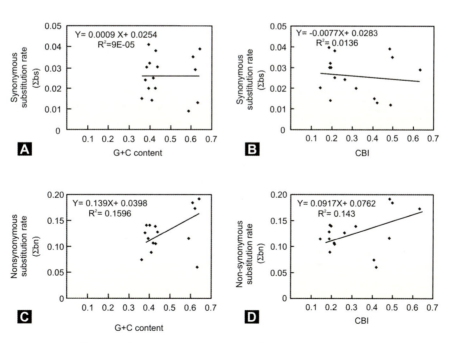

Figs 21.4A to D: Correlation analyses of comparative genomics parameters. Correlations between Σbs and the GC comtent (A), Σbs and CBI (B), Σbn and the GC comtent (C), and Σbn and CBI (D) in sixteen TLR-related genes are shown. All values of Σbs, Σbn, the GC content, and CBI were evaluated for the entire coding sequences for the TLR-related gene

appeared to be linked to the higher levels of synonymous substitution rates.

Nonrandom Codon Usage and the Nucleotide Substitution Rate

Table 21.4 shows the frequencies of codon usage in human genes, based on 40, 662, 582 codons from 93, 487 coding sequences (Codon usage data base. See http://www.kazusa.or.jp/codon/). If the synonymous changes were completely neutral in the course of evolution, the synonymous codons for an amino acid should have equal frequencies. However, the pattern of codon usage for synonymous codon was apparently nonrandom in the human genome. For example, in the comparisons of the frequencies of six codon usages for leucine, a large bias was observed in their usage (The amino acid, leucine, was most frequently coded by CUG and less often by CUA), suggesting that the pattern of synonymous codons was distinctly nonrandom.

There are several methods to evaluate the nonrandom usage of synonymous codons. We applied the codon bias index (CBI) as a measure of the deviation from the equal use of synonymous codons to investigate the TLR-related genes. Bennetzen and Hall[38] arbitrarily chose twenty-two codons encoding for seventeen amino acids as preferred codons for species of interest. Based on these preferred codons, the value of CBI was defined as:

$$CBI = (N_{pfr} - N_{ran}) / (N_{tot} - N_{ran})$$

where N_{pfr} is the total number of occurrences of the preferred codons, N_{ran} is the expected number of the preferred codons if all synonymous codons were used equally, and N_{tot} is the total number of the seventeen amino acids encoded by the preferred codons. The CBI values range from 0 (uniform use of synonymous codons) to 1 (maximum codon bias).

Figure 21.4 shows the correlation of nucleotide substitution rates using the CBI for sixteen TLR-related genes, that is, a correlation of CBI with the synonymous substitution rates, but not the nonsynonymous substitution rates. The departure of codon usage from random should be associated with the higher levels of synonymous substitution rates. We do not know the exact reason why the CBI was linked to the synonymous substitution rate in TLR-related genes. Since the degree of nonrandom codon usage has been reported to be linked to the levels of gene expression,[39-41] expression levels of the TLR-related genes might be linked to the synonymous substitution rates. An alternative possible

Table 21.4: The frequencies of codon usage in human genes based on 40,662,582 codons from 93,487 coding sequences

1st base	2nd base U		2nd base C		2nd base A		2nd base G	
U	UUU (Phe)	17.6	UCU (Ser)	15.2	UAU (Tyr)	12.2	UGU (Cys)	10.6
	UUC (Phe)	20.3	UCC (Ser)	17.7	UAC (Tyr)	15.3	UGC (Cys)	12.6
	UUA (Leu)	7.7	UCA (Ser)	12.2	UAA (Stop)	1	UGA (Stop)	1.6
	UUG (Leu)	12.9	UCG (Ser)	4.4	UAG (Stop)	0.8	UGG (Trp)	13.2
C	CUU (Leu)	13.2	CCU (Pro)	17.5	CAU (His)	10.9	CGU (Arg)	4.5
	CUC (Leu)	19.6	CCC (Pro)	19.8	CAC (His)	15.1	CGC (Arg)	10.4
	CUA (Leu)	7.2	CCA (Pro)	16.9	CAA (Gln)	12.3	CGA (Arg)	6.2
	CUG (Leu)	39.6	CCG (Pro)	6.9	CAG (Gln)	34.2	CGG (Arg)	11.4
A	AUU (Ile)	16	ACU (Thr)	13.1	AAU (Asn)	17	AGU (Ser)	12.1
	AUC (Ile)	20.8	ACC (Thr)	18.9	AAC (Asn)	19.1	AGC (Ser)	19.5
	AUA (Ile)	7.5	ACA (Thr)	15.1	AAA (Lys)	24.4	AGA (Arg)	12.2
	AUG (Met)	22	ACG (Thr)	6.1	AAG (Lys)	31.9	AGG (Arg)	12
G	GUU (Val)	11	GCU (Ala)	18.4	GAU (Asp)	21.8	GGU (Gly)	10.8
	GUC (Val)	14.5	GCC (Ala)	27.7	GAC (Asp)	25.1	GGC (Gly)	22.2
	GUA (Val)	7.1	GCA (Ala)	15.8	GAA (Glu)	29	GGA (Gly)	16.5
	GUG (Val)	28.1	GCG (Ala)	7.4	GAG (Glu)	39.6	GGG (Gly)	16.5

The frequencies are shown per thousand.

explanation is that the GC content might affect the synonymous substitution rate, because the CBI has a positive correlation with the GC content in the TLR-related genes (data not shown).

Synonymous Nucleotide Substitutions Having Functional Impact

It is widely accepted that a part of synonymous substitutions would have a functional impact on the genome through their effects on the mRNA stability, translational efficiency, and/or splicing control. It is easily supposed that the synonymous substitutions with these functional affects have not taken place under the control of neutral evolution.

It was reported that some synonymous substitutions could affect the mRNA secondary structure and mRNA stability,[42] which were occasionally associated with the disease susceptibility. Human dopamine receptor D2 gene (*DRD2*) is a well known example of how a synonymous mutation can affect the mRNA stability.[43] Among six synonymous variants in *DRD2*, only the mutation that decreased the mRNA half-life and induced a conspicuous change in the predicted secondary structure was linked to the disease. For another example, synonymous variants in the gene for Catechol-O-methyltransferase (*COMT*), an enzyme responsible for degrading catecholamines, are associated with the enzymatic activity.[44] *COMT* is a key regulator of pain perception, cognitive function, and affective mood. Several haplotypes divergent in synonymous changes exhibited the largest difference in COMT enzymatic activity, due to a reduced amount of translated protein. These synonymous variants affect the mRNA stability due to the resulting difference in the local stem-loop structures of mRNA. The most stable structure was associated with the lowest protein level and enzymatic activity.

Synonymous substitutions could also affect the translational efficiency through the use of codons with rare tRNA.[39-41] Alternative codons specifying particular amino acids can differ in translational efficiency, in part due to the relative abundance of tRNA and the use of codons that are specified by rare tRNA might be linked to slow translation. For example, *MDR1* encodes an ATP-binding cassette transporter, P-gp, which contributes the pharmacokinetics of drugs with altered transport. A synonymous variant in exon 26 was found to be associated with the P-gp activity.[45] This synonymous variant in *MDR1* affected the timing of co-translational folding due to a slow translation resulting form rare codon usage, which might result in the altered function of P-gp.

The evidence for the synonymous mutations leading to human disease by disrupting the splicing process is abundant.[35] These synonymous mutations might create new cryptic splice sites or change splicing-control elements, such as exonic splicing enhancers (ESEs) and silencers (ESSs), which are oligomeric motifs that recruit splicesomal proteins to facilitate splice-site recognition. Alternatively, splicing-control elements were reported to have come under the control of negative selection, because the disruption of splicing-control elements induced by nucleotide substitutions would be deleterious for the gene function.

COMPARATIVE GENOMICS IN NON-CODING REGIONS

The comparison of non-coding genomic sequences is also useful for identifying the genomic regions for regulatory elements, such as components of promoters and enhancers.[1, 11-13] We briefly touch on such comparisons in this section. This approach is based on the idea that functionally important regions should be conserved in the course of evolution. In fact, it has been reported that putative-transcription factor binding sites are enriched in the evolutionary conserved non-coding genomic sequences.[46-48] Furthermore, experimentally determined regulatory elements are indeed enriched in the evolutionary conserved genomic segments. For the prediction of regulatory-regions, comparisons among relatively distant species appears to be more effective than those among closely related species, because the higher similarity in the non-coding sequences can be found among the closely related species, but presumably hard to be observed in the distantly related ones if there were no evolutionary pressures to maintain the sequences.

Two main approaches have been broadly available in the discovery of regulatory regions in the non-coding regions. The first approach is based on the global alignment of orthologous sequences, followed by the identification of conserved regions. Figure 21.5 shows the comparisons of 20-kb genomic sequences encoding human TLR4 gene with its orthologues from six vertebrate species, including mouse, rat, chicken, dog, rhesus, and horse, which were aligned with the computational tool, VISTA.[49] Highly conserved non-coding genomic segments observed between two distant

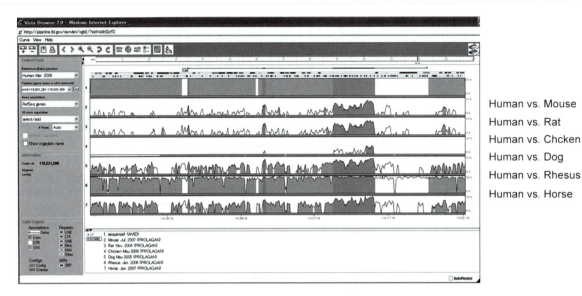

Fig. 21.5: Comparative genomic analysis using a computational tool, VISTA.[49] The 20-kb genomic sequences encoding TLR4 gene among seven vertebrate species including human, mouse, rat, chicken, dog, rhesus, and horse were analyzed

species, such as the human and mouse, are potential candidate regions for regulatory elements.

The second approach endeavors to find multiple orthologous sequences from related species, followed by the evaluation of their functional significance. For instance, we tried to identify and compare orthologous sequences of the human microRNA (miRNA), miR759, from other vertebrate species. miRNA is a class of short, non-coding RNAs that post-transcriptionally regulate gene expression by interaction with partially complementary target sites on mRNAs. It has been reported that mammalian miRNAs may regulate the expression of ~30 percent of the protein-coding genes.[50] We identified homologous sequences of miR759 from eight vertebral species. Figure 21.6 shows the sequence alignment among human, rhesus, mouse, rabbit, rat, cattle, and dog. miR759 sequences was found to be strictly conserved in the course of vertebrate evolution, suggesting the biological significance of miR759 in the control of gene expression. The human miRNA miR759 regulates the expression level of human fibrinogen-alpha gene through its binding to the 5'-untransrated region of the human fibrinogen-alpha gene (Chen et al unpublished data).

APPLICATION OF COMPARATIVE GENOMICS TO AN IDENTIFICATION OF HUMAN DISEASE GENES

As discussed in the previous sections, comparative genomics is a promising approach for identifying the genes that may control the susceptibility to human diseases, especially in combination with comparative analyses of phenotype, such as differences in disease susceptibility, among primates. It has been reported that the susceptibility to various diseases differs among primates.[21] For example, Asian Old World monkeys are highly susceptible to infection with *M. tuberculosis bacilli*, while New World monkeys are reported to be more resistant.[51] Furthermore, as described previously, the species-specific restrictions operating on HIV-1 infection are well-known (4; 52; 5). Humans, as well as chimpanzees, but not New and Old World monkeys, are susceptible to HIV-1 infection. Such differences in the species-specific susceptibility to infectious disease might be associated with the differences in gene functions linked to the defense against infectious diseases, which would lead the differences in defense mechanisms mounted against invading pathogens. Natural selection pressure has advanced the species-specific evolution in the susceptibility genes for infectious diseases. In fact, dozens of genes under the control of natural selection in the course of primate evolution have been identified to date. Taking all things into consideration, these genes are candidates for determining the susceptibility to human diseases. In the following sections, we describe the examples.

Comparative Genomics Might Uncover Susceptibility Genes for Human Diseases

TRIM5α plays crucial roles in the intracellular defense against HIV-1,[52] and sequence differences in the SPRY domain of TRIM5α contribute to the differences in anti-HIV-1 activity among primate species.[52] Comparative

```
                       ***..*****************************************************
Mature miR-759    1:                                            GCAGAGUGCAAACAAUUUUGAC  22
human             1: TTATGGAAAGGATTATAATAAATTAAATGCCTAAACTGGCAGAGTGCAAACAATTTTGAC  60
rhesus            1: TTATAGAAAGGATTATAATAAATTAAATGCCTAAACTGGCAGAGTGCAAACAATTTTGAC  60
mouse             1: TTATGGGCAGGATTATAATAAATTAAATGCCTAAACTGGCAGAGTGCAAACAATTTTGAC  60
rat               1: TTATGGGAAGGATTATAATAAATTAAATGCCTAAACTGGCAGAGTGCAAACAATTTTGAC  60
rabbit            1: TTATGTAAAGGATTATAATAAATTAAATGCCTAAACTGGCAGAGTGCAAACAATTTTGAC  60
cattle            1: TTACGGGAAGGATTATAATAAATTAAATGCCTAAACTGGCAGAGTGCAAACAATTTTGAC  60
dog               1: TTATGGGAAGGATTATAATAAATTAAATGCCTAAACTGGCAGAGTGCAAACAATTTTGAC  60

                     **************************************************.******.**....
human            61: TCAGATCTAAATGTTTGCACTGGCTGTTTAAACATTTAATTTGTTAGAATGGAAGTAGCG 120
rhesus           61: TCAGATCTAAATGTTTGCACTGGCTGTTTAAACATTTAATTTGTTAGAATGGAAGTAGCG 120
mouse            61: TCAGATCTAAATGTTTGCACTGGCTGTTTAAACATTTAATTTGTTCCAATGGAGGTAGCA 120
rat              61: TCAGATCTAAATGTTTGCACTGGCTGTTTAAACATTTAATTTGTTCGAATGGAGGTAGAG 120
rabbit           61: TCAGATCTAAATGTTTGCACTGGCTGTTTAAACATTTAATTTGTTAGAATGGAAGTAGCA 120
cattle           61: TCAGATCTAAATGTTTGCACTGGCTGTTTAAACATTTAATTTGTTAGAATGGAGGTTCCA 120
dog              61: TCAGATCTAAATGTTTGCACTGGCTGTTTAAACATTTAATTTGTTAGAATGGAGGTAGCA 120
```

Fig. 21.6: Sequence alignment of miR-759-like sequences in human, rhesus, mouse, rabbit, rat, cattle, and dog. The pri-miR-759 sequences are underlined. The mature miR-759 sequence is 22 bp long, as indicated on the top

genomics for TRIM5α shows that this gene has rapidly evolved in the course of primate evolution, and that natural selection has shaped the sequence difference in the SPRY domain. Sequence variations in TRIM5 have been reported to be associated with the susceptibility to HIV-1/AIDS in humans. For another example, APOBEC3G, that also plays an important role in the defense against HIV-1, has been under positive Darwinian selection.[53] A comparison of APOBEC3G sequences among primates suggests a rapid evolution of APOBEC3G in the course of primate evolution.

Given that TRIM5α and APOBEC3G are the genes associated with the susceptibility to HIV/AIDS in humans, comparative genomics can be a useful tool for both identifying the candidate genes for controlling the HIV/AIDS susceptibility and evaluating the pathophysiological roles of the genes from an evolutionary point of view. These examples suggest that comparative genomics is a promising approach to identify the susceptibility genes for infectious diseases. Since susceptibilities differ among primates to not only infectious, but also other common diseases, such as Alzheimer's disease and cardiovascular diseases, comparative genomics may be a crucial tool in providing candidate genes to determine the susceptibility for the other diseases as well.

Bioinformatics Tool to Evaluate Functional Impact of Nonsynonymous Variations based on Comparative Genomics

It is estimated that there are 67,000-200,000 common nonsynonymous single nucleotide polymorphisms (SNPs) in the human genome, and that each individual is heterozygous for 24,000-40,000 nonsynonymous SNPs.[54] Because nonsynonymous SNPs would affect the protein function, some of them might be associated with human health and disease. Recently, various computational approaches to assessing the functional significance of nonsynonymous SNPs have been developed.[55-61] They predict whether an amino acid substitution induced by nonsynonymous SNPs affects protein function based on the comparative genomics, physical properties of amino acids, and/or three-dimensional (3D) structures of proteins. The main features of the representative methods are summarized in Table 21.5. These programs are also useful to estimate the significance of functional impact induced by nonsynonymous mutations in the genes for single-gene disorders.

Some of the programs are sequence-based amino acid substitution prediction method based on the comparative genomics, which are founded on the concept that the amino acid substitutions affecting protein function tend to occur at conserved evolutionary sites. Such conserved sites, as described in the previous sections, have come under the control of negative (purifying) selection, and are considered to be important for protein function. A multiple sequence alignment among the homologous sequences indicates the conserved sites throughout the course of evolution. The sequence-based amino acid substitution prediction method scores the levels of amino acid substitution based on the amino acids appearing in the multiple alignments, and the severity of the amino acid change based on the physical properties. It has been reported that 25-35 percent of nonsynonymous SNPs are predicted to affect the protein function by the most

Table 21.5: The main features of representative prediction methods used to evaluate the impact of nonsynonymous SNPs on protein function

Method	Web site	
SIFT [55]	http://sift.jcvi.org/	Sequence-based prediction method using position-specific scoring matrices with Dirichlet priors
PolyPhen[56]	http://coot.embl.de/PolyPhen/	Structure/sequence-based prediction method
SNPs3D[57]	http://www.snps3d.org/	Structure/sequence-based prediction method
PANTHER PSEC[58]	http://www.pantherdb.org/tools/csnpScoreForm.jsp	Sequence-based prediction method using PANTHER Hidden Markov Model families
PMUT [59]	http://mmb2.pcb.ub.es:8080/PMut/	Structure/sequence-based prediction method
TopoSNP[60]	http://gila.bioengr.uic.edu/snp/toposnp/	Structure/sequence-based prediction method. A database of topographic mapping of SNPs
MAPP[61]	http://mendel.stanford.edu/SidowLab/downloads/MAPP/index.html	Sequence-based prediction method

widely used prediction methods. Currently, automated prediction methods are being applied on a genome-wide scale, which might accelerate the findings of human disease susceptibility genes in the near future. However, it has been pointed out that there are limitations to the current prediction methods. For example, Thomas et al[62] have reported that the current method may not be useful for identifying certain nonsynonymous SNPs involved in human common diseases. In any events, however, it is reasonable to expect further progress in the field of bioinformatics using these and related methods.

CONCLUSION

In this chapter, we introduced concepts and methods for evaluating the biological significance of homologues sequences, especially focusing on the methods that are based on the theory of natural selection. Although the comparative genomics are not definitive in determining the biological significance of conserved sequences, this approach is nonetheless highly useful as the first step for identifying and characterizing functional regions in the genome. We have introduced here only a small part of comparative genomics. We recommend referring to a number of reviews to cover the wide variety of the features of comparative genomics.[1, 11-13]

Recent rapid progress in the field of bioinformatics and sequencing technology has brought about a breakthrough in the comparative genomic analysis. It is therefore expected that further progress in the comparative genomics will provide a stream of novel insight into health and disease in humans.

ACKNOWLEDGMENTS

This work was supported in part research grants from the Ministry of Health, Labor and Welfare, Japan, the Japan Health Science Foundation, the program of Founding Research Centers for Emerging and Reemerging Infection Disease, the Japan Health Science Foundation, the program of Research on Publicly Essential Drugs and Medical Devices, Grant-in-Aids for Scientific research from the Ministry of Education, Culture, Sports, Science, and Technology (MEXT), Japan, grants for Indo-Japan collaboration research from DST and JSPS, and a grant from Heiwa Nakajima Foundation.

REFERENCES

1. Margulies EH, Birney E. Approaches to comparative sequence analysis: Towards a functional view of vertebrate genomes. Nat Rev Genet 2008;9:303-13.
2. Shendure J, Mitra RD, Varma C, Church GM. Advanced sequencing technologies: Methods and goals. Nat Rev Genet 2004;5:335-44.
3. Vogel F, Motulsky AG. Human Genetics problems and approaches 3rd ed. Springer 1996.
4. de Groot NG, Otting N, Doxiadis GG, et al. Evidence for an ancient selective sweep in the MHC class I gene repertoire of chimpanzees. Proc Natl Acad Sci USA 2002;99:11748-53.
5. Bontrop RE, Watkins DI. MHC polymorphism: AIDS susceptibility in non-human primates. Trends Immunol 2005;26:227-33.
6. Neel JV. Diabetes mellitus: A "thrifty" genotype rendered detrimental by "progress"? Am J Hum Genet 1962;14:353-62.

7. Nakajima T, Wooding S, Sakagami T, et al. Natural selection and population history in the human angiotensinogen gene (AGT): 736 complete AGT sequences in chromosomes from around the world. Am J Hum Genet 2004; 74:898-916.
8. Inoue I, Nakajima T, Williams CS, et al. A nucleotide substitution in the promoter of human angiotensinogen is associated with essential hypertension and affects basal transcription in vitro. J Clin Invest 1997;99:1786-97.
9. Hughes AL, Nei M. Pattern of nucleotide substitution at major histocompatibility complex class I loci reveals overdominant selection. Nature 1988;335: 167-70.
10. Horton R, Wilming L, Rand V, et al. Gene map of the extended human MHC. Nat Rev Genet 2004;5:889-99.
11. Pennacchio LA, Rubin EM. Genomic strategies to identify mammalian regulatory sequences. Nat Rev Genet 2001;2:100-9.
12. Ureta-Vidal A, Ettwiller L, Birney E. Comparative genomics: Genome-wide analysis in metazoan eukaryotes. Nat Rev Genet 2003;4:251-62.
13. Boffelli D, Nobrega MA, Rubin EM. Comparative genomics at the vertebrate extremes. Nat Rev Genet 2004; 5:456-65.
14. Li WH. Molecular Evolution. Sinauer Associates, Inc 1997.
15. Miyata T, Yasunaga T. Molecular evolution of mRNA: A method for estimating evolutionary rates of synonymous and amino acid substitutions from homologous nucleotide sequences and its application. J Mol Evol 1980;16:23-36.
16. Nei M, Gojobori T. Simple methods for estimating the numbers of synonymous and nonsynonymous nucleotide substitutions. Mol Biol Evol 1986;3:418-26.
17. Li WH, Wu CI, Luo CC. A new method for estimating synonymous and nonsynonymous rates of nucleotide substitution considering the relative likelihood of nucleotide and codon changes. Mol Biol Evol 1985;2: 150-74.
18. Yang Z. PAML 4: Phylogenetic analysis by maximum likelihood. Mol Biol Evol 2007;24:1586-91.
19. Chimpanzee Sequencing and Analysis Consortium. Initial sequence of the chimpanzee genome and comparison with the human genome. Nature 2005; 437:69-87.
20. Rhesus Macaque Genome Sequencing and Analysis Consortium, Gibbs RA, Rogers J, Katze MG, et al. Evolutionary and biomedical insights from the rhesus macaque genome. Science 2007;316:222-34.
21. Olson MV, Varki A. Sequencing the chimpanzee genome: Insights into human evolution and disease. Nat Rev Genet 2003;4:20-8.
22. Nielsen R, Bustamante C, Clark AG, et al. A scan for positively selected genes in the genomes of humans and chimpanzees. PLoS Biol 2005;3:e170.
23. Akira S, Uematsu S, Takeuchi O. Pathogen recognition and innate immunity. Cell 2006: 124: 783-801.
24. Bowie A, O'Neill LA. The interleukin-1 receptor/Toll-like receptor superfamily: Signal generators for pro-inflammatory interleukins and microbial products. J Leukoc Biol 2000;67:508-14.
25. Nakajima T, Ohtani H, Satta Y, et al. Natural selection in the TLR-related genes in the course of primate evolution. Immunogenetics 2008;60:727-35.
26. Poltorak A, He X, Smirnova I, et al. Defective LPS signaling in C3H/HeJ and C57BL/10ScCr mice: Mutations in Tlr4 gene. Science 1998;282:2085-8.
27. Shimazu R, Akashi S, Ogata H, et al. MD-2, a molecule that confers lipopolysaccharide responsiveness on Toll-like receptor 4. J Exp Med 1999; 189:1777-82.
28. Nagai Y, Akashi S, Nagafuku M, et al. Essential role of MD-2 in LPS responsiveness and TLR4 distribution. Nat Immunol 2002;3:667-72.
29. Zhang J, Rosenberg HF, Nei M. Positive Darwinian selection after gene duplication in primate ribonuclease genes. Proc Natl Acad Sci USA 1998;95:3708-13.
30. Tamura K, Dudley J, Nei M, Kumar S. MEGA4: Molecular Evolutionary Genetics Analysis (MEGA) Software Version 4.0. Mol Biol Evol 2007;24:1596-9.
31. Smirnova I, Poltorak A, Chan EK, McBride C, Beutler B. Phylogenetic variation and polymorphism at the toll-like receptor 4 locus (TLR4). Genome Biol 2000; 1: research002.1-002.10.
32. Hajjar AM, Ernst RK, Tsai JH, Wilson CB, Miller SI. Human Toll-like receptor 4 recognizes host-specific LPS modifications. Nat Immunol 2002;3:354-9.
33. Lien E, Means TK, Heine H, et al. Toll-like receptor 4 imparts ligand-specific recognition of bacterial lipopolysaccharide. J Clin Invest 2000;105:497-504.
34. Arbour NC, Lorenz E, Schutte BC, et al. TLR4 mutations are associated with endotoxin hyporesponsiveness in humans. Nat Genet 2000;25:187-91.
35. Chamary JV, Parmley JL, Hurst LD. Hearing silence: Non-neutral evolution at synonymous sites in mammals. Nat Rev Genet 2006;7:98-108.
36. Bielawski JP, Dunn KA, Yang Z. Rates of nucleotide substitution and mammalian nuclear gene evolution. Approximate and maximum-likelihood methods lead to different conclusions. Genetics 2000;156:1299-1308.
37. Hurst LD, Williams EJ. Covariation of GC content and the silent site substitution rate in rodents: Implications for methodology and for the evolution of isochores. Gene 2000;261:107-14.
38. Bennetzen JL, Hall BD. Codon selection in yeast. J Biol Chem 1982;257:3026-31.
39. Urrutia AO, Hurst LD. The signature of selection mediated by expression on human genes. Genome Res 2003;13:2260-4.
40. Lavner Y, Kotlar D. Codon bias as a factor in regulating expression via translation rate in the human genome. Gene 2005;345:127-38.
41. Comeron JM. Selective and mutational patterns associated with gene expression in humans: Influences on synonymous composition and intron presence. Genetics 2004;167:1293-304.
42. Shen LX, Basilion JP, Stanton VP Jr. Singlenucleotide polymorphisms can cause different structural folds of mRNA. Proc Natl Acad Sci USA 1999;96:7871-6.

43. Duan J, Wainwright MS, Comeron JM, et al. Synonymous mutations in the human dopamine receptor D2 (DRD2) affect mRNA stability and synthesis of the receptor. Hum Mol Genet 2003;12:205-16.
44. Nackley AG, Shabalina SA, Tchivileva IE, et al. Human catechol-O-methyltransferase haplotypes modulate protein expression by altering mRNA secondary structure. Science 2006;314:1930-3.
45. Kimchi-Sarfaty C, Oh JM, Kim IW, et al. A "silent" polymorphism in the MDR1 gene changes substrate specificity. Science 2007;315:525-8.
46. Wasserman WW, Palumbo M, Thompson W, Fickett JW, Lawrence CE. Human-mouse genome comparisons to locate regulatory sites. Nat Genet 2000; 26:225-8.
47. Levy S, Hannenhalli S, Workman C. Enrichment of regulatory signals in conserved non-coding genomic sequence. Bioinformatics 2001;17:871-7.
48. Fickett JW, Wasserman WW. Discovery and modeling of transcriptional regulatory regions. Curr Opin Biotechnol 2000;11:19-24.
49. Frazer KA, Pachter L, Poliakov A, Rubin EM, Dubchak I. VISTA: Computational tools for comparative genomics. Nucleic Acids Res 2004:32(Web Server issue): W273-9.
50. Filipowicz W, Bhattacharyya SN, Sonenberg N. Mechanisms of post-transcriptional regulation by microRNAs: Are the answers in sight? Nat Rev Genet 2008;9:102-14.
51. Isaza R. Tuberculosis in all taxa. In Fowler ME and Miller RE, (eds.) Zoo and Wild Animal Medicine. 5th ed. Elsevier, St Louis, MO, 2003;689-96.
52. Stremlau M, Owens CM, Perron MJ, Kiessling M, Autissier P, Sodroski J. The cytoplasmic body component TRIM5a restricts HIV-1 infection in Old World monkeys. Nature 2004;427:848-53.
53. Sheehy AM, Gaddis NC, Choi JD, Malim MH. Isolation of a human gene that inhibits HIV-1 infection and is suppressed by the viral Vif protein. Nature 2002;418:646-50.
54. Rebbeck TR, Spitz M, Wu X. Assessing the function of genetic variants in candidate gene association studies. Nat Rev Genet 2004;5:589-97.
55. Ng PC, Henikoff S. SIFT: Predicting amino acid changes that affect protein function. Nucleic Acids Res 2003;31:3812-4.
56. Ramensky V, Bork P, Sunyaev S. Human non-synonymous SNPs: Server and survey. Nucleic Acids Res 2002;30:3894-900.
57. Yue P, Melamud E, Moult J. SNPs3D: Candidate gene and SNP selection for association studies. BMC Bioinformatics 2006;7:166.
58. Mi H, Guo N, Kejariwal A, Thomas PD. PANTHER version 6: Protein sequence and function evolution data with expanded representation of biological pathways. Nucleic Acids Res 2007;35(Database issue):D247-52.
59. Ferrer-Costa C, Gelpí JL, Zamakola L, Parraga I, de la Cruz X, Orozco M. PMUT: A web-based tool for the annotation of pathological mutations on proteins. Bioinformatics 2005;21:3176-8.
60. Stitziel NO, Binkowski TA, Tseng YY, Kasif S, Liang J. topoSNP: A topographic database of non-synonymous single nucleotide polymorphisms with and without known disease association. Nucleic Acids Res 2004: 32(Database issue): D520-2.
61. Stone EA, Sidow A. Physicochemical constraint violation by missense substitutions mediates impairment of protein function and disease severity. Genome Res 2005;15: 978-86.
62. Thomas PD, Kejariwal A. Coding single-nucleotide polymorphisms associated with complex vs. Mendelian disease: Evolutionary evidence for differences in molecular effects. Proc Natl Acad Sci USA 2004;101: 15398-403.
63. Hubbard TJ, Aken BL, Ayling S, et al. Ensembl 2009. Nucleic Acids Res 2009: 37(Database issue):D690-7.
64. Giardine B, Riemer C, Hardison RC, et al. Galaxy: A platform for interactive large-scale genome analysis. Genome Res 2005;15:1451-5.
65. Kuhn RM, Karolchik D, Zweig AS, et al. The UCSC Genome Browser Database: Update 2009. Nucleic Acids Res 2009;37(Database issue):D755-61.
66. Dewey CN. Aligning multiple whole genomes with Mercator and MAVID. Methods Mol Biol. 2007;395: 221-36.
67. Tesler G. GRIMM: Genome rearrangements web server. Bioinformatics. 2002; 18:492-3.
68. Kent WJ, Baertsch R, Hinrichs A, Miller W, Haussler D. Evolution's cauldron: Duplication, deletion, and rearrangement in the mouse and human genomes. Proc Natl Acad Sci USA 2003;100:11484-9.
69. Brudno M, Do CB, Cooper GM, et al. LAGAN and Multi-LAGAN: Efficient tools for large-scale multiple alignment of genomic DNA. Genome Res 2003; 13:721-31.
70. Notredame C, Higgins DG, Heringa J T-Coffee: A novel method for fast and accurate multiple sequence alignment. J Mol Biol 2000;302:205-17.
71. Do CB, Mahabhashyam MS, Brudno M, Batzoglou S. ProbCons: Probabilistic consistency-based multiple sequence alignment. Genome Res 2005:15:330-40.
72. Bray N, Pachter L. MAVID: Constrained ancestral alignment of multiple sequences. Genome Res 2004;14: 693-9.
73. Marchler-Bauer A, Bryant SH. CD-Search: Protein domain annotations on the fly. Nucleic Acids Res 2004;32(W): 327-31.

Chapter 22

Genetic Architecture of Mycobacterial Diseases

Marianna Orlova, Erwin Schurr

MYCOBACTERIAL PATHOGENS AND THEIR HUMAN DISEASES

The genus *Mycobacterium* represents gram-positive bacteria that are characterized by the presence of mycolic acids in their cell walls resulting in their characteristic acid- and alcohol-fast stain in histological preparations. Since the description of *Mycobacterium leprae* as first human mycobacterial pathogen in 1873 over 135 species and subspecies of mycobacteria have been identified (http://www.bacterio.cict.fr). The vast majority of mycobacterial species are environmental free-living saprophytes that rarely cause disease in humans.[1] An important exception is the saprophyte *Mycobacterium ulcerans,* the cause of Buruli ulcer. Nevertheless, a small but important subset of mycobacerial species causes a wide spectrum of human diseases with distinct epidemiological, clinical and pathological features. Most notably, *Mycobacterim tuberculosis*, and to a lesser extent *Mycobacterium bovis* and *Mycobacterium africanum,* are the cause of clinical tuberculosis,[2,3] a disease that claims close to 2 million lives annually.[4] A second medically important species is *Mycobaterium leprae* which is the cause of leprosy. Leprosy is a chronic granulomatous disease of skin and peripheral nerves that affects over 250,000 new subjects each year.[5] The disease is rarely life threatening but in the absence of treatment leaves patients with severe disfigurations and deformities due to irreversible nerve damage. The third most common mycobacterial disease globally is Buruli ulcer[6] which is caused by the environmental *M. ulcerans*. The number of patients with Buruli ulcer has dramatically increased during recent years, especially in West Africa.[7] Unlike other pathogenic mycobacteria, *M. ulcerans* is captured by host phagocytes only in the early stage of infection, but later resides in the subcutaneous fat tissue.[8] If left untreated, *M. ulcerans* infection can result in tissue destruction and severe necrotizing ulcers due to secretion of the necrotizing toxin mycolactone.[9]

Occasionally, mildly virulent mycobacteria can cause clinical disease in humans. For example, the majority of the global population (85% of all children) are inoculated with live vaccine strains of Bacille Calmette-Guérin (BCG), an attenuated form of *M. bovis*. In rare instances BCG vaccination may result in local adenitis (BCG-itis) or systemic disease (BCG-osis).[10] Humans constantly come in contact with water- and air-borne environmental mycobacteria (EM) through skin, digestive and respiratory epithelia. Under certain host conditions, including immune deficiencies, immune impairment and related genetic disorders, EM can cause a wide variety of clinical symptoms in humans. The lung is the most commonly affected organ by EM disease, e.g. pneumonitis caused by *M. avium, M. malmoense, M. intracellulare* and others.[11] In addition, EM species may be the cause of skin granulomas (*M. marinum*[1]), cervical adenitis (*M. avium*), and disseminated mycobacterial disease may be caused by *M. smegmatis*,[12] *M. avium*,[13] *M. chelonae*,[14] or *M. flavescens*.[15] However, compared to the three major mycobacterial diseases, the number of patients suffering from EM disease is relatively small.

Host Genetics Underlies Disease Susceptibility

A complex interplay of microbial and nonmicrobial environmental factors (e.g. mycobacterial virulence, cell tropism, crowding, sanitation) and genetic and nongenetic host factors (e.g. hygiene, nutrition, inherited defects of the immune system, acquired immunodeficiencies) governs to what extent exposure to infectious agents will result in infection and subsequent clinical disease (Fig. 22.1). This complex system of host, pathogen and environment underlies the large inter-individual and inter-population differences in susceptibility to both infection and development of clinical disease for all mycobacterial pathogens. In practical terms this implies that not all persons exposed to pathogenic mycobacteria will become infected and only a minority of persistently infected individuals will develop clinical disease. This holds true not only for weakly virulent BCG and EM, but also for human pathogenic *M. leprae*,[16] *M. tuberculosis*[17] and *M. ulcerans*.[9] If and to what extent host genetic factors contribute to this large variability in susceptibility to both infection and development of clinical disease has been one of the key questions of infectious diseases research ever since Charles Nicole described the occurrence of non-diseased carriers of infectious pathogens.

One of the classical examples of genetic control of resistance/susceptibility to tuberculosis was an accident that occurred in the city of Lübeck in northern Germany. During the BCG vaccination campaign between December 1929 and May 1930, 251 newborns were accidentally infected with a virulent strain of *M. tuberculosis* by three repetitive *per os* administration within their first 10 days of life. Within the next 12 months 72 children died from tuberculosis and 5 from non-tuberculosis causes, while 173 children displayed variable signs of tuberculosis but recovered from the infection. Of these 173 children, 61 displayed symptoms of severe tuberculosis disease, 95 displayed mild clinical symptoms of tuberculosis disease and 17 showed a positive tuberculin reaction but no clinical signs. On the contrary, none of 164 unvaccinated infants born during the same period died of tuberculosis within the next three years.[18]

During the investigation of this accident it became quickly evident that the BCG vaccine strain had been contaminated with a virulent *M. tuberculosis* strain. This contamination was not uniform and 4 different "virulence" levels of the vaccine preparation could be distinguished according to when the vaccine had been prepared. For example, virulence level 4, the most virulent vaccine preparation, was given to 74 children. Of these, 53 (72%) died while 18 (24%) showed severe illness and only 3 (4%) showed mild signs of tuberculosis. By contrast, virulence level 2 was given to 93 children.

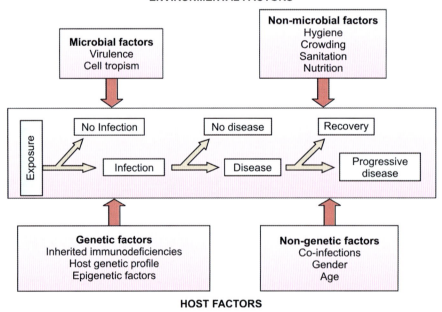

Fig. 22.1: Schematic representation of the interplay of environmental- and host-factors in the pathogenesis of infectious diseases. A complex interaction of various factors (microbial and non-microbial, genetic and non-genetic) influence how exposure of humans to pathogens leads to infection and clinical disease. There are multiple decision points on the path from exposure to clinical disease when the combination of this multitude of factors may influence the progress of pathogenesis. Thus, to detect the action of genetic factors it is of pivotal importance to keep non-genetic factors constant across the sample enrolled in a genetic study. Therefore, a clear understanding of the epidemiology and the clinical presentations of a given infectious disease is a critical necessity for the successful identification of host genetic susceptibility factors

Of these 6 died, 9 displayed severe illness and 78 displayed only mild forms of tuberculosis. Moreover, the virulence level 3 vaccine preparation approximately evenly split children into deceased, severe and mild forms of tuberculosis disease. It was shown that the socioeconomic status of the infants had no impact on clinical picture or prognosis.[18] Given that the preparation was given to newborns, the results of the accident provide strong evidence for an important role of innate (genetic) resistance/susceptibility factors to tuberculosis. These factors are not absolute since increased exposure (higher virulence level) was able to overcome innate resistance in a large proportion of vaccinees directly demonstrating the crucial interplay between exposure intensity and genetically controlled tuberculosis susceptibility factors.

In addition, numerous epidemiological and experimental studies supported the hypothesis of a strong host genetic contribution to mycobacterial diseases. For example, incidence of tuberculosis is often particularly high in populations with no or low ancestral experience of *M. tuberculosis* infection. In such ethnic groups the disease often takes a more fulminant course suggesting absence of selection for tuberculosis resistance during the natural history of the disease in these populations.[19] Strong support of host genetic predisposition to leprosy and tuberculosis was obtained from twin studies where monozygotic twins displayed substantially higher disease concordance rates compared to dizygotic pairs.[20-22] Yet, perhaps the most elegant and convincing work for a pivotal role of host genetics was provided by the classic work of Max Lurie who demonstrated that strains of rabbits resistant and susceptible to *M. tuberculosis* disease could be obtained by selective breeding. This result formally established the key role of host genetic factors in tuberculosis disease.

Observations made by Lurie on survival time, histopathology and bacillary load in the lungs of animals were particularly informative since the natural respiratory route of infection was used for the studies. Aerosol infection of diverse rabbit families was done by continuous exposure of uninfected rabbits to sick animals suffering from cavitary disease,[23,24] which is an excellent approximation to natural infection. Lurie observed that resistant rabbits developed well defined cavities, whereas rabbits from the susceptible strain demonstrated disseminated disease. Also, animals from the resistant strain lived twice as long as susceptible rabbits, and required 6-15 fold higher infectious dose to demonstrate the same number of primary pulmonary foci.[25] From Lurie's studies we know that about 20-40 percent of all exposed animals, regardless of susceptibility group, did not develop disease by the end of the experiment, and the majority of them did not demonstrate tuberculin positivity even after 11 months of continuous exposure to *M. tuberculosis*.[26] Although Lurie considered these tuberculin-negative animals a result of limitations in the infection procedure, an alternative interpretation was given by Werneck-Barroso.[26] Based on experimental exposure pattern, the latter author argued that the group of tuberculin negative animals represented innately resistant animals that were able to eliminate the bacilli from alveoli prior to stimulation of adaptive immunity, thus avoiding a positive tuberculin response. In this view, Lurie's rabbits showed two distinct phases of genetic resistance, innate resistance/susceptibility to infection and innate resistance/susceptibility to progression from infection to tuberculosis disease.

Experimental Approaches in Genetic Studies

While epidemiological and animal studies made a strong case for an important role of host genetic factors in susceptibility to mycobacterial diseases, the nature and molecular identity of the corresponding susceptibility genes remained unknown. However, over the last decade the field of genetic epidemiology has developed an array of experimental and analytical approaches to identify the genes that influence susceptibility to complex traits, including mycobacterial diseases. In broad outline, two strategies are used to investigate the genetic component of complex traits, including susceptibility to *M. tuberculosis* and *M. leprae*: Linkage analyses, which aim to identify chromosomal regions that co-segregate with the phenotype of interest within families, and association studies, which aim to identify alleles that are non-randomly associated with the disease trait.[27,28]

Linkage-based Strategies

Linkage analysis can be used to test existing hypotheses by studying candidate genes, or to perform unbiased genome-wide screens. Based on the initial understanding of the genetic model of the susceptibility trait two methods of linkage analysis can be used: Model-based and model-free. Model-based linkage analysis, performed by the lod-score method,[29] necessitates a model which specifies the relationship between the phenotype, genetic factors that influence the expression of the phenotype and co-variates, for example age, gender, or exposure intensity. It is assumed that all the parameters (allele frequency, penetrance, degree of dominance etc.) are known for each locus. The information on the genetic model is often provided by segregation analysis, which ascertains the mode of inheritance of the phenotype. Parametric linkage analysis is a very powerful approach if the assumed genetic model reflects the real model. However, misspecification of genetic parameters may lead to significant loss of power to detect linkage and false-negative results.[30-32] To avoid the problem of misspecification, a number of hypothetical genetic models can be tested systematically. In this case it is critically important to introduce appropriate corrections for multiple testing by adjusting the level of significance for significant linkage.[31,32]

Model-free linkage methods are used when little is known about the genetic model. Just like model-based linkage studies, model-free approaches also require multi-case families. Most non-parametric linkage studies enroll a large number of sib-pair families. The basic approach is then to study the extent of alleles identical-by-decent (IBD) that shared among affected sib-pairs. An excess of alleles shared IBD among affected sib-pairs indicates linkage of the genetic markers with a gene impacting on the phenotype. For the analysis of sib-pair data two powerful maximum likelihood methods were developed: The maximum likelihood score (MLS)[33] method, and the maximum likelihood binomial approach (MLB),[34] which offers a natural extension of allele sharing methods to sib-ships with more than two affected children. If used in the context of whole genome scans, both parametric and model-free linkage approaches will only be able to identify an approximate location for susceptibility loci. These approximate locations are defined as so-called linkage peak intervals and usually span 10-20 million base pairs (Mbp). For the final identification of disease causing genes association-based method are required.

Overview of Genotype-phenotype Association Studies

The focal point of efforts aimed at the identification of genetic disease risk factors (i.e. susceptibility genes) is the testing of alleles in candidate genes for association with the disease susceptibility trait. The designs employed in such association studies can be either population-based (e.g. the classic epidemiology case-control design) or family-based (e.g. transmission disequilibrium testing in families with one affected offspring). The genetic markers that are being used for present association studies are so called single nucleotide polymorphisms (SNPs). SNPs represent a very common type of genetic variation in which at identical points on the human DNA two alternative nucleotides can be found in a given population. These alternative nucleotides are also referred to as SNP alleles. With the development of new techniques, high-throughput SNP genotyping is now a widely used and powerful approach to correlate genetic variation to disease phenotype. Analysis of fully sequenced individual genomes[35-38] suggests that the average human genome contains at least 11 million SNPs that can be used in genetic studies.

How do we identify suitable candidate genes for detailed association studies? One approach is to use genome wide linkage analysis to identify chromosomal regions that segregate non-randomly with the phenotype under study in families with multiple affected offspring. The genes of the identified chromosomal segment can then be considered candidate genes and subjected to more detailed association studies (see above). Candidate genes can also be obtained by genome wide association studies (GWAS) and then fine mapped in more dedicated follow-up experiments. Analysis of differential gene expressions in various tissues of patients and healthy individuals is another approach to identify mycobacterial candidate susceptibility genes. While in the above approaches candidate genes are identified based on experimental evidence, candidate genes can also be selected based on the known biology of the trait or on results obtained from suitable animal models. However, irrespective of the way a candidate gene was selected or the strength of association with the tested disease phenotype that is being detected, association studies cannot provide formal evidence for causality with disease susceptibility. Functional studies are necessary to confirm association results and to formally implicate the associated gene variant in the pathogenesis of disease.

A typical population-based candidate gene-disease association study tests for differences in the frequencies of selected marker alleles in groups of unrelated patients and unrelated healthy controls. This is an epidemiological design where genotypes are considered "exposure factors" and the risk for disease of such genotypic exposure is statistically evaluated. Since cases and controls can be enrolled in a straightforward way, this is a popular study design to evaluate genotype-phenotype associations that is also usually employed in GWAS. Several GWAS are in progress for tuberculosis and leprosy but the results are currently unknown. From a genetic point of view the case-control design has the disadvantage of providing only an approximate estimate of haplotype-specific effects. In a family-based design, a disease-associated variant is analyzed for under- or over-transmission from heterozygous parents to affected offspring (transmission disequilibrium test, TDT). In this approach, parental alleles that are not transmitted to affected children are used as control alleles. Moreover, family-based samples are protected from the problem of population stratification, which can lead to false significant associations between genotype and phenotype in case-control studies, especially if small samples are employed in the testing of a small number of candidate alleles.

LINKAGE DISEQUILIBRIUM

In the rare case where the disease causing genetic effect (e.g. a particular SNP allele resulting in premature termination of the translated protein) is known such a SNP can be used in association studies. This situation is referred to as direct association. More commonly, the disease causing molecular lesion is not known. In this situation, one will aim to use SNPs that are tightly correlated with the unknown disease causing variant. The fact that alleles at two loci are correlated is called linkage disequilibrium (LD). Technically speaking, LD is the difference between the observed genotypic combinations of the alleles at two loci and the genotype frequency expected by random allele combination. For pair-wise LD (two bi-allelic loci, with alleles A, a at locus 1, and alleles B, b at locus 2) there are four haplotype probabilities: pAB, pAb, paB and pab. Under complete linkage equilibrium two alleles A and B, with frequencies pA and pB, respectively, are completely randomly associated with each other, i.e. observed and expected genotypes are identical: pAB=pApB. When this condition is not met, the alleles are said to be in linkage disequilibrium. The extent of LD, i.e. the deviation of observed genotypic frequency from expected, is measured by D =pAB-pApB. A popular measure of pair-wise LD is Lewontin's $|D'|$, which is: $|D'|=D/D_{max}$, where D_{max} is the maximum possible LD, given the allelic frequencies, and D_{max} = min[pApb,papB], if D>0; or D_{min}=max[-pApB,-papb], if D<0. D' takes the value of 1 if one of the haplotypes is not present in the population. Another popular measure of LD is r^2 which describes the level of correlation between alleles at the two SNPs. The r^2 measure is particularly useful for indirect association studies. If two SNPs are correlated at the level of 80 percent (r^2=0.8), then the genotype of SNP1 will reflect the genotype of SNP2 80 percent of the time. Similar to D', r^2 is normalized to the allele frequencies:

r^2=D^2/pApBpapb. The correlation coefficient r^2 is a more strict measure of LD and for r^2 to take a value of 1, only two haplotypes can be present.

Regions of high LD display low haplotype diversity. Such regions are called haplotype blocks and represent segments of adjacent SNPs that are inherited in blocks. Common haplotypes can be efficiently tagged with only a subset of all common variants, knows as "haplotype tagging SNPs". Unless the tag SNPs is highly correlated with the other LD block SNPs (which is usually not the case), the use of such tag SNPs results in loss of power of detection of all SNPs on the same block in association studies. For this reason the procedure of tag SNP selection is commonly based on pair-wise r^2.[39] Such r^2-defined tag SNPs simply represent a group of highly correlated (usually $r^2 \geq 0.8$) not necessarily adjacent SNPs that are commonly referred to as a "SNP bin" (Fig. 22.2).

GENETIC SPECTRUM OF HUMAN INFECTIOUS DISEASES

Clinical, epidemiological and genetic data led to the concept of a continuous genetic spectrum of infectious diseases.[40,41] In this view, conventional primary immunodeficiencies (PIDs) and common diseases with polygenic control reside at the opposite ends of the spectrum and are joined by new PIDs and major gene effects on susceptibility. Conventional PIDs render patients susceptible to multiple infectious diseases, which vary in nature and number, depending on the affected gene.[42] Hence, they follow the paradigm of one gene – multiple infections. The mutations that give rise to PIDs have a strong effect on protein function and allow an easy link to the phenotypes observed. New PIDs, or pathogen-specific PIDs, confer monogenic susceptibility to a single type of infection. These conditions, e.g. Mendelian Susceptibility to Mycobacterial Diseases (MSMD), largely follow the rule of one gene-one infection. As for conventional PIDs there is a relatively strong genotype-phenotype correlation. Due to the rarity of the causative mutations, conventional and known new PIDs contribute only marginal to the burden of disease at the population level. Compared to PIDs, major genes have significantly weaker correlation between a disease predisposing mutation and expression of the phenotype at the level of the individual person. However, due to the often high frequency of the susceptibility allele major genes can explain a large proportion of disease on the population level. Major genes have been traditionally identified as linkage peaks in genome-wide linkage scans.

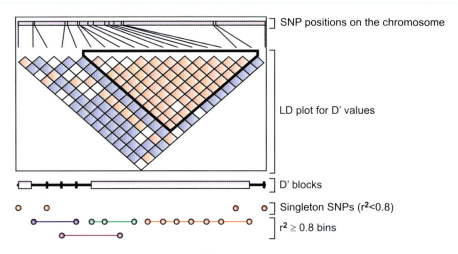

Fig. 22.2: Linkage disequilibrium (LD) between SNPs based on r^2 and D'. A schematic representation of a 12.7 kb fragment on chromosome region 19q13 which corresponds to the 3' region of the *NALP12* gene is shown for SNP data obtained from the Chinese HapMap population (CHB). SNPs with minor allele frequency (MAF) ≥ 5% are shown according to their chromosomal position. D' and r^2 are two commonly used measures of LD. D' highlights the extent of haplotypic diversity within the region, identifying the haplotype blocks. r^2 describes the correlation between the SNP alleles. The plot shown is based on pair-wise D' values between the SNP markers. The extent of LD as measured by D' is depicted by the box colour: red indicates high linkage (D'=1), white represents linkage equilibrium (D' = 0), and intermediate values are represented by colour diamonds. The LD block, shown on the plot with the black border, is identified using a confidence interval algorithm (Haploview software). Below the LD plot, the corresponding D'-based haplotype blocks are shown by rectangles. Below the haplotypes, the LD organization based on the r^2 measure is shown. Uncorrelated SNPs, so called singletons ($r^2 < 0.8$), are shown as independent red circles. The bins (multiple SNPs with $r^2 \geq 0.8$) are represented by coloured circles (indicating a SNP) that are connected by solid bars. Of note, the D' blocks contain adjacent SNPs and do not overlap with other blocks, whereas r^2 bins may overlap each other, as well as contain SNPs that may be located outside the gene boundaries (not shown)

Polygenic contribution to infectious diseases refers to the presence of a relatively large number of susceptibility genes, each with a small impact on disease susceptibility. One of the widely accepted hypothesis of polygenic susceptibility is the common disease-common variant hypothesis, which proposes that common polymorphisms (with minor allele frequency [MAF] above 1%) contribute to susceptibility to common human diseases.[43,44] Under this assumption the identification of such alleles can be done by GWAS,[45,46] or by candidate gene association studies. While this hypothesis underlies the vast majority of candidate gene studies in mycobacterial diseases, it is important to realize that polygenic susceptibility may also involve alleles with MAF <1 percent. Collectively, such rare and mild susceptibility variants may still explain a substantial proportion of genetic susceptibility to disease.[47,48] The main difference to PIDs is that the genotype-phenotype correlation would be substantially weaker and the recognition of disease causing variants would pose enormous analytical difficulties. To what extent these different genetic susceptibility models explain the overall disease burden is a hotly disputed area of current research.

MENDELIAN SUSCEPTIBILITY TO MYCOBACTERIAL DISEASES

MSMD was probably clinically first described in 1951 and became the subject for thorough genetic studies in the mid-1990s.[49,50] Clinically, MSMD represents disseminated or localized but recurrent disease, which is mostly caused by mildly virulent mycobacterial species such as BCG vaccine and environmental mycobacteria.[51] Unlike other conventional PIDs which result in susceptibility to multiple infectious agents, MSMD confers susceptibility almost exclusively to *Mycobacteria* and *Salmonella*, and is now considered as the prototypic example of a "pathogen-specific" PID.[41] So far, five autosomal genes: *IFNGR1*,[50,52] *IFNGR2*,[53] *IL12B*,[54] *IL12RB1*,[54] *STAT1*,[55] and one X-linked gene, *NEMO*,[56] have been implicated in MSMD. Mutations in *IFNGR1*, encoding the IFNγ receptor ligand-binding chain, *IFNGR2*, coding for a complementary chain for IFNγ receptor, and *STAT1*, coding for the signal transducer and activator of transcription 1, result in impaired cellular responses to IFNγ. In contrast, defects in *IL12B*, encoding the p40 subunit of IL12 and IL23, *IL12RB1*, encoding the β1 chain of the IL12 and IL23 receptor, and *NEMO*, encoding the NF-B essential modulator, are associated with impaired IL12/IL23-dependant IFNγ production. *IFNGR1* and *IL12RB1* mutations are the most common MSMD-predisposing defects, each responsible for approximately 40 percent of all cases, whereas deficiencies in *IL12B*, *STAT1*, *IFNGR2* and *NEMO*, respectively, account for 9 percent, 5 percent, 4 percent and 3 percent of MSMD-affected patients. The high degree of allelic heterogeneity of the six MSMD-causing genes, including variable modes of inheritance, the presence of hypomorphic and null alleles, and different alleles affecting various functional domains of the same protein, give rise to 13 distinct genetic disorders associated with different degrees of mycobacterial infection. There are still numerous cases with clinical MSMD but unknown genetic etiology. Consequently, additional genes are likely to be identified in future studies.[57]

The first described genetic etiology for mycobacterial susceptibility was a mutation in *IFNGR1* leading to complete deficiency of the IFNγ receptor ligand-binding chain.[50,52] Since this initial discovery, 30 different mutations in *IFNGR1* have been described. The majority of *IFNGR1* mutations are nonsense or frameshift mutations that result in premature termination of translation with either no IFNGR1 expression on the cell surface,[12,50,52,58,59] or the plasma membrane expression of dysfunctional forms of IFNGR1 that are unable to recognize IFNγ.[60,61] Such INFGR1 deficiencies show a recessive mode of inheritance and are therefore referred to as "recessive complete INFGR1 deficiencies." Due to their complete clinical penetrance, these INFGR1 deficiencies manifest themselves in early childhood as severe and often fatal infections caused by BCG (in BCG-vaccinated cases)[62] or by EM such as *M. fortuitum*,[61,63] *M. chelonae*,[52,64] or *M. smegmatis*.[12,58] The prognosis for such cases is poor since antibiotic treatment does not provide a sustained clinical remission and recombinant IFNγ does not have a beneficial effect in the absence of a functional IFNγ receptor.

A specific 187T mutation of *IFNGR1* is the only known defect that causes a partial recessive IFNγ-R1 deficiency. *In vitro* studies demonstrated that patients with this mutation possess partially functional receptor for IFNγ, as STAT1 DNA-binding and induction of HLA-II were detected in response to high concentrations of IFNγ.[65,66] Although patients with this defect are still susceptible to BCG and EM infections, the disease is much less severe than with complete IFNGR1 deficiency. Prognosis is good as patients can be treated with antibiotics and recombinant IFNγ. Partial recessive IFNGR1 deficiency was the first MSMD-causing mutation to be associated with clinical tuberculosis,[65] highlighting the critical role of IFNγ-mediated immunity in susceptibility to *M. tuberculosis* infection and the possible contribution of Mendelian effects to complex diseases. A different type of partial deficiency of IFNγ receptor is caused by defects in *IFNGR1* demonstrating a dominant mode of inheritance. In such cases mutant IFNGR1 molecules lack a recycling motif and accumulate on the cell surface, but cannot transmit a signal due to the absence of JAK1 and STAT1 binding domains. Patients with dominant partial IFNGR1 deficiency have a weak, but not entirely abrogated IFNγ-mediated response.[67,68]

Autosomal recessive deficiency of the gene encoding the accessory chain of the IFNγ receptor, *IFNGR2*, is a much rarer cause for mycobacterial susceptibility than *IFNGR1* mutations.[56] Like *INFGR1*, genetic defects in *IFNGR2* can lead to complete or partial inhibition of ligand recognition function. Mutations identified in patients with complete IFNGR2 deficiency can result in abrogation of expression of receptor on the cell surface,[53] or result in expression of a dysfunctional receptor unable to respond to IFNγ. Interestingly, studies of *INFGR2* detected a novel mechanism of genetic susceptibility, i.e. the creation of new N-glycosylation sites. An in-frame non-synonymous mutation in *INFGR2* generated a new N-glycosylation site that led to the formation of a new polysaccharide chain and abolished receptor function.[69] Clinically, complete IFNGR2 deficiency resembles mycobacterial disease in IFNGR1-deficient patients. The infection, usually triggered by BCG, *M. avium* or *M. fortuitum*, starts in early childhood and rapidly develops into severe and often fatal disease.[53,69,70]

STAT1 encodes the signal transducer and activator of transcription-1, which is critical for cellular responses during viral infection via the IFNα/β signaling pathway and for mycobacterial infection due to its involvement in the IFNγ signaling cascade. Depending on the position of the mutation in *STAT1* the resulting STAT1 protein can have more severe effects on susceptibility to mycobacterial,[55,71] or viral disease[72] or may impact both types of infections equally.[73] Patients with complete *STAT1* deficiency display disseminated mycobacterial disease, but may succumb to severe viral infections. Again, patients with partial loss of STAT1 function display a milder clinical phenotype with good prognosis. This further supports a strict genotype-phenotype correlation between the level of IFNγ responsiveness and the severity of mycobacterial disease.[66]

An uncommon (approx. 10% of all cases) MSMD-causing gene, *IL12B*, encodes the IL-12 p40 subunit shared by the IL-12 and IL-23 cytokines. Currently, all genetic defects identified in this gene result in recessive complete IL-12 p40 deficiency leading to a low level of IFNγ production *in vitro* and predisposing to mycobacterial infections *in vivo*.[54,74] Patients with *IL12B* deficiency typically develop disseminated BCG infection after BCG vaccination, or disseminated EM infection.[74] Since INFγ can be used therapeutically prognosis for such patients is good. Interestingly, approximately half of the patients with IL12 p40 deficiency are also infected with *Salmonella*, in contrast to a much smaller number (~6%) of *Salmonella* infections in MSMD-affected patients with defective IFNγ signaling. These observations suggest an important IFNγ-independent role of the IL12/IL23 signaling cascade in effective anti-*Salmonella* immunity.

Mutations in *IL12RB1* are the most common genetic etiology of MSMD. All known *IL12RB1* mutants are recessive and result in loss-of-function of the IL12β1 receptor (reviewed in detail by Ref 56). Patients with IL12Rβ1 deficiency display mycobacterial disease and salmonellosis.[75,76] Similar to patients with IFNGR1 and IFNGR2 complete deficiencies, infections start before age of 12 in symptomatic patients. However, the outcome of infection is fairly good as the majority of patients survive into adulthood. The penetrance of IL12RB1 mutations is low as most genetically affected siblings of known cases remain free of symptoms.[76] Environmental factors have been demonstrated to play a role in the inter-individual variability in mycobacterial susceptibility, as BCG vaccination confers resistance to EM.[76] Clinical observations suggest the critical role of IL12/IL23 signaling for primary, rather than secondary immunity to mycobacterial infections. Alternatively, it seems to be equally important for primary and secondary immunity to *Salmonella*.

Of interest was the discovery of IL12β1 deficiency as an etiology for Mendelian susceptibility to childhood tuberculosis. The majority of young IL12RB1 deficient patients with primary tuberculosis did not demonstrate other mycobacteria-triggered disease, despite documented BCG vaccination and exposure to environmental mycobacteria, providing the proof of concept that tuberculosis in children can present a *bona fide* Mendelian predisposition. Based on these observations there is a possibility that a substantial portion of childhood tuberculosis cases occur due to a Mendelian predisposition.[77,78] Although the sample size of these studies is rather small, the importance of rare molecular defects in understanding the mechanisms of tuberculosis pathogenesis, as well as other mycobacterial diseases, is evident.

The identification of MSMD-causing genes provided a better understanding of the mechanisms that confer resistance/susceptibility to mycobacterial diseases. Similarly, studies of patients with various pathogen-specific PIDs allowed the dissection of the machinery of protective immunity to several infectious agents. While being exposed to the same microbial environment, patients with deficiencies in IL12-IL23-IFNγ circuit are susceptible to mycobacterial infection and salmonellosis,[56,75] patients with defects in their IFNα/β response acquire susceptibility to viral infections[79] while dysfunction of TIR/IRAK signaling pathway results in susceptibility to *Staphylococcus* and *Streptococcus* infections.[80] Interestingly the study of MSDM has so far failed to provide evidence for a role of TLRs, IL-1 and IL-18 in mycobacterial susceptibility although these molecules are widely thought to be critical players of innate immunity.[81,82]

A mutation in the *IL23R* gene, has been identified as a risk factor for Crohn's disease.[83] Since IL12B is also a risk of Crohn's disease this suggests a contribution of the IL12/IL23 signaling pathway in the etiology of IBD. As defects in the IL12/IL23 signaling axis grant susceptibility to a narrow spectrum of infectious agents, i.e. *Mycobacteria* and *Salmonella*, this raises the question to what extent mycobacteria are part of the pathogenesis of Crohn's disease. The hypothesis of mycobacteria, especially *M. paratuberculosis*, as causative agents for Crohn's disease has been actively pursued in recent years, however, unambiguous results are still outstanding.[84,85]

Identification of Chromosomal Regions Carrying Major Susceptibility Genes by Genome wide Linkage Studies

The concept of "major genes" was initially derived in the context of complex segregation analysis. Indeed, for a number of infectious diseases major genes have been identified by segregation analysis.[86-89] At the same time, advances in genotyping technologies as well as in parametric and non-parametric linkage analysis made it possible to conduct genome wide linkage (GWL) scans. It became customary to refer to significant linkage peaks in GWL scans as "major loci." On the level of the genetic effect size, it is now common to refer to alleles that predispose to susceptibility with a relative risk of approximately 5 as major genetic effects.

In mycobacterial diseases, first evidence for the presence of a major gene in leprosy susceptibility was obtained by segregation analysis of leprosy families on Desirade Island in 1988.[86] More recently, three genome-wide linkage studies were carried out and reported three different major leprosy susceptibility loci. One major locus was mapped to chromosome region 10p13 in South-Indian patients with paucibacillary leprosy.[90] A second independent locus was identified on chromosome region 20p13 in the same population.[90] Interestingly, a GWL scan in Brazilian families identified strong evidence for a leprosy susceptibility locus on the same chromosomal interval.[91] However, the molecular identity of the gene(s) underlying the chromosome 20p13 locus remains unknown. The Brazilian study also detected suggestive evidence for a linkage hit with HLA-DQA (lod score of 3.28) and weaker evidence for linkage to chromosome region 17q11.[91] A follow-up study of the chromosome 17 region identified a cluster of genes that impact on leprosy susceptibility.[92] A third major locus for susceptibility to leprosy *per se* was identified on chromosome region 6q25-q26 in Vietnamese patients.[93] Systematic linkage disequilibrium mapping of this region resulted in the identification of polymorphic risk factors in the promoter region shared by two genes: *PARK2*, coding for an E3-ubiquitin ligase designated Parkin, and *PACRG*, the Parkin coregulated gene.[94] This study was the first successful positional cloning of a major gene in a common infectious disease, which also revealed a new ubiquitin-dependent pathway of immunity to infection with *M. leprae*.[95]

The GWL scan, involving multi-case leprosy families from Vietnam, provided additional evidence for suggestive linkage between chromosome region 6p21, including the HLA region, and leprosy *per se*.[93] This region was subjected to high resolution linkage disequilibrium mapping in a sample of 197 simplex, i.e. one affected child and both parents, Vietnamese families. From the 103 genes underlying the targeted region, the most significantly associated SNP was rs2071590 (*LTA-293*; p<0.001) which is located in the promoter region of *LTA*.[96] Subsequent high-resolution association mapping allowed the identification of *LTA+80* as strongest susceptibility factor candidate. This SNP had previously been shown to impact on *LTA* transcription in an allele specific manner.[97] Interestingly, the leprosy risk "A" allele was shown to promote reduced *LTA* transcription due to its preferential binding of the ABF1 transcriptional repressor.

For validation of the association of *LTA+80A* with leprosy two additional case-control cohorts from India and Brazil were used. While it was possible to replicate association of *LTA+80A* with leprosy *per se* in the Indian population (p = 0.01; OR = 1.60 (95% CI 1.10–2.33), similar attempts in the Brazilian sample failed. Careful consideration of the Vietnamese and Brazilian samples revealed the age at diagnosis as major difference. Indeed, when individuals were stratified by age at diagnosis a much stronger effect was detected in Vietnamese patients less than 16 years at diagnosis (P=0.00004, OR=5.76 (95% CI 2.25–14.78) and India (p = 0.006, OR=2.95 (95% CI 1.32–6.58). Similarly, a clear enrichment of the *LTA+80*A allele was observed in the youngest Brazilian age group (16–25 years) (p = 0.07). These results indicated the association of *LTA+80A* with early-onset leprosy. To test the predominant age dependency of the *LTA+80A* allele, an additional independent sample of 104 simplex leprosy families from Vietnam was recruited. Again, a significant association of *LTA+80A* with leprosy risk in the overall sample was observed (p=0.003, OR=2.34, 95% CI 1.27–4.31), and the strongest association was reported for group of patients < 16 years of age (OR=5.31, 95% CI 1.19–23.60). When the two Vietnamese samples were combined the evidence for association of *LTA+80A* with leprosy diagnosis before 16 years became very strong (p = 0.0000004, OR=5.63, 95% CI 2.54–12.49).

The results of the genetic analysis are further supported by data obtained in the mouse. Construction of bone marrow chimeric mice, unable to secrete LTA and lymphotoxin-beta (LTB), resulted in extreme susceptibility to *M. tuberculosis* infection.[98] The essential role of LTA in immune response to infection with *M. leprae* was confirmed in a recent study.[99] In this study, the critical importance of LTA for the development of a disease protective granulomatous response and effective T-cell recruitment to the site of infection was clearly demonstrated. Therefore, the association of the *LTA+80* suppressive A allele with increased risk of leprosy could be explained by inadequate recruitment of lymphocytes to sites of infection.

GWL scans have been also applied to tuberculosis but have not yet resulted in the positional cloning of susceptibility genes. The strongest evidence for a major susceptibility gene has been obtained in a sample of Moroccan families.[100] Here a region on chromosome 8q12-q13 next to anonymous marker D8S1723 was significantly linked to tuberculosis (LOD score = 3.49; P = 3 × 10⁻⁵). A closer look at the linkage peak revealed 26 known genes, which met the criteria of candidates for tuberculosis susceptibility genes.[100] Experiments on identification of a true susceptibility variant are ongoing. Interestingly, analysis of a subsample of 39 families with at least one tuberculosis affected parent demonstrated very strong evidence of linkage to the same region linkage (LOD score = 3.94; P = 10^{-5}). This finding strongly supported a dominant mode of inheritance of the major susceptibility locus. The presence of a dominant acting tuberculosis susceptibility locus was unexpected. However, if genetic control of susceptibility generally followed a dominant model this would open the possibility of strong evolutionary selection against such loci.

A number of other studies found evidence for suggestive linkage of diverse chromosomal regions with tuberculosis disease. One study was performed in 92 sib-pairs with TB from Gambia and South Africa. Suggestive evidence for linkage was detected on chromosome regions 15q and Xq.[101] Subsequently, the UBE3A locus was identified as candidate susceptibility locus on chromosome 15.[102] A genome scan for TB in a Brazilian population found three regions with suggestive evidence for linkage: 10q26, 11q12, and 20p12.[91] A linkage study of TB affected sibling-pairs from South Africa and Malawi identified two loci with suggestive linkage on chromosomes 6p21-q23 and 20q13.[103] Association testing was done in an independent population from West Africa and positive association was detected with two genes on chromosome 20q13: The Melanocortin 3 Receptor (MC3R), a member of a family of proteins involved in obesity and weight control, and Cathepsin Z (CTSZ), a member of the cathepsin protease family.[103] Linkage at 20q13, although not attaining significance, was also detected in a scan of TB patients from Uganda.[104] Finally, a genome-scan in a Thai population of multiplex families detected evidence of suggestive linkage with TB on chromosome 5q23.2-31.3. Interestingly, in an ordered subset analysis using minimum age at onset of TB as the covariate, this study identified two other suggestive linkages on chromosome regions 17p13 and 20p20, implying different disease mechanisms in young versus older patients.[105]

Candidate Gene Studies

Polygenic control of disease susceptibility is best demonstrated by numerous candidate gene studies that can be found in the literature. In these studies, the genetic effect size is usually modest (OR <2) and the identified risk alleles have usually high allele frequencies.

Unfortunately, many of the results obtained in candidate gene studies have not been replicated and it is often difficult to decide which represent a true genetic effect. Indeed, independent replication was obtained for only few genes. For example, consistent results were obtained with some HLA class II genes,[106-109] and the Natural Resistance-Associated Macrophage Protein 1 (NRAMP1) gene.[110]

HLA

The association between major histocompatibility complex (MHC) genes (human leukocyte antigen [HLA] system) and their alleles with mycobacterial diseases has been extensively studied for the past twenty years.[106,111-113] Earlier studies might have suffered from methodological problems or genetic heterogeneity of the studied populations.[106-108,112,114-116] Indeed, it has been suggested that studies based on serologic techniques, due to high cross-reactivity and low-grade specificity, might have produced wrong HLA class II designations in about 25 percent of samples.[117] The history of HLA typing and the development of highly sensitive DNA-based techniques throughout past 25 years are reviewed by Middleton and will not be repeated here.[118]

Class I

The critical role of MHC class II-restricted CD4+ lymphocytes in immune defense against tuberculosis has long been established,[119] however the role of CD8+ cells remains largely undefined. Mouse studies provided evidence for the important role of this cell type in the control of tuberculous infection by creating mouse strains with a dysfunctional β_2–microglobulin gene,[120] as well as CD4 and CD8 knock-out strains.[121] Additionally, several studies demonstrated the presence of CD8+ cells specific to mycobacterial antigen in patients with active tuberculosis as well as healthy contacts who tested positive for purified protein derivative (PPD).[122-125] These observations indicate a possible function of class I molecules in tuberculosis and related phenotypes.

Based on the functional similarities of MHC-peptide interactions during antigen presentation "supermotifs" of HLA-A and HLA-B molecules are subdivided into nine supertypes.[126] A case-control study, performed in an Indian sample demonstrated significantly decreased frequencies of A1-like supertypes and increased frequencies of A3-like supertypes in tuberculosis patients compared to control subjects. These two allele groups share a similar peptide-binding motif with the exception of the residues in the pocket F of the HLA class I molecules.[127] The same study also reported the B-44 supertype as being protective against infection with tuberculosis, as this allelic group was more frequently identified in healthy controls compared to patients. This finding is in agreement with a previous report of lower frequencies of the B-44 supertype in Indonesian tuberculosis patients.[128] Similarly, based on a meta-analysis of 22 studies the presence of the B13 supertype was found to be associated with lower risk of developing pulmonary tuberculosis.[129]

HLA-C molecules are the main ligands for killer inhibitory receptors (KIRs) of natural killer (NK) cells. It has been demonstrated that the degree of targeted cell lysis by NK cells is inversely related to the expression of class I molecules by the target cell.[130,131] HLA-Cw alleles can be classified on the basis of KIR binding according to a dimorphism at position 80 in their alpha helix: Group 1 allotypes (e.g. Cw1, Cw3 and Cw7) specifically bind KIR2DL2 receptors, whereas group 2 allotypes (e.g. Cw2, Cw4 and Cw6) bind KIR2DL1 receptors.[132] A study of Indian tuberculosis patients revealed higher frequencies of HLA-Cw alleles of both allotype groups in patients, including those with disseminated tuberculosis, compared to healthy controls, but also a significant over-representation of the HLA-Cw allotype 1 among patients with pulmonary tuberculosis (p<0.001). These results suggest inhibition of NK cell activity against *M tuberculosis* infected cells as possible susceptibility mechanism.[127,133]

Association of HLA alleles with multibacillary (MB) leprosy was tested in an Indian case control sample.[134] In this study both, serological and DNA-based methods of HLA genotyping were used. A significant increase in HLA A2, A11, B40 and Cw7 alleles was demonstrated by micro-lymphotoxicity assays, while a decrease of A28, B12, B15 and Cw3 molecules was observed among MB leprosy patients compared to controls. Molecular subtyping of leprosy patients revealed a significant increase in frequency of HLA A*0203, A*0206, A*1102, B*1801, B*4016, B*5110, Cw*0407 and Cw*0703 alleles, while the frequency of HLA A*0101, A*0211, B*4006, Cw*03031, Cw*04011 and Cw*0602 alleles was significantly decreased in leprosy patients as compared to healthy controls. Furthermore, haplotypes A*1102-B*4006-Cw*1502; A*0203-B*4016-Cw*0703 and A*11-B*40 were significantly associated with increased susceptibility to multibacillary leprosy.[134]

A recent study evaluated the association between HLA alleles and lung disease caused by environmental mycobacteria (*M. avium, M. intracellulare* and *M. abscessus*) in Korean patients.[135] Genotyping of HLA-A, -B, and –DRB1 alleles was done by the polymerase chain reaction method. Among eleven identified HLA-A alleles none was over- or underrepresented in the group of patients. In the group of 26 HLA-B alleles only one, B*46, was borderline significantly overrepresented in the group of patients with *M. avium/M. intracellulare* infection (P_{corr}=0.044, OR=2.23, 95% CI = 1.05-4.73). Similarly, only HLA-DRB1*11 showed borderline significant higher frequency in the overall group of patients, as compared to healthy subjects (P_{corr}=0.045, OR=1.91, 95% CI=1.01-3.64). Earlier studies in Japanese patients with *M. avium/M. intracellulare* lung infections described elevated frequencies of HLA-A33 and HLA-DR6 antigens in patients, and an association of HLA-A26 antigen with the deterioration of such pulmonary infection.[136,137]

Class II

A number of serological studies from the early 1980s, reported associations between HLA class II alleles and risk of mycobacterial diseases. Increased frequency of HLA-DR2 was reported in Indonesian[106] and Indian patients affected by pulmonary tuberculosis (PTB),[107,108] with particularly strong evidence in patients non-responding to drug treatment (p=0.0001, OR=3.7). Additional support for the role of HLA-DR2 in PTB susceptibility came from family-based studies that demonstrated over-transmission of DR2 to affected offspring from heterozygous parents in Indian multicase families.[114] However, due to low resolution of HLA techniques, ethnic heterogeneity, discrepancies in definition of phenotype and occasionally low power, some case-control studies failed to confirm HLA-DR2 association with tuberculosis in Chinese,[115] Mexican[116] and Indian[112] populations. With the development of DNA-based genotyping techniques more accurate analysis of underlying HLA alleles became possible. As an example, identification of two alleles, DRB1*1501 and DRB1*1502, which belong to the HLA-DR2 serotype, shed new light on the role of HLA-DRB1 molecules in tuberculosis susceptibility. Increased frequency of the DRB1*1501 allele (with a very strong OR range of 2.7-8.0) was demonstrated in Indian and Mexican PTB patients,[138-140] respectively. In addition, the DQB1*0501 and DQB1*0503 alleles were found associated with PTB but each in a different population: DQB1*0501 in Mexico[140] and DQB1*0503 in Cambodia.[141] For the latter, a substitution of alanin at position 57 by aspartic acid (Asp57) was shown to play a critical role. Independently, it had been shown previously that the amino acid polymorphism Ala57Asp in binding pocket P9 of the DQ β chain (DQ β57) influences charge of the pocket and spatial limitations of the peptide binding groove.[142,143] A significant enrichment of alleles encoding Asp57, compared to non-Asp57 alleles, was observed among patients with pulmonary tuberculosis.[144] Particularly, individuals homozygous for the Asp57 allele were at higher risk for developing pulmonary tuberculosis (p=0.001, OR=3.05, 95% CI 1.53-6.07). Additionally, presence of DQ β57-Asp leads to a 5-fold decrease of binding to *M. tuberculosis* peptide ESAT6, and as a result to significantly lower induction of protective IFNγ secretion by CD4+ T cells.[144]

The role of HLA class II alleles has been studied extensively for leprosy. For review of early work see Ref. 145. While HLA-DR3 was identified as risk factor for tuberculoid leprosy,[146] the majority of studies reported on associations between HLA-DR2 and leprosy subtypes.[109] Two family-based association studies performed in India and Egypt demonstrated overtransmission of the DR2 serotype to offspring affected with tuberculoid leprosy.[147,148] Similarly, HLA-DR2 alleles *DRB1*1501* and *DRB1*1502* were associated with tuberculoid leprosy in Northern Indians.[149] Detailed molecular analysis of the DR2 alleles most commonly associated with tuberculoid leprosy revealed that 87 percent of tuberculoid leprosy patients carried alleles containing arginin at positions 13 or 70-71. The cumulative relative risk of arginine at these positions was estimated at a very high OR=8.8 (p=0.000005). This strong effect on leprosy susceptibility was attributed to resulting polarity changes in the peptide binding groove leading to altered profiles of antigen presentation and T-cell activation.[150]

Strong evidence for the involvement of the HLA region in leprosy susceptibility was provided by multiple sib-pair studies. Over-transmission of parental HLA haplotypes to offspring affected by tuberculoid leprosy was demonstrated in populations from Surinam,[151] Central India,[147] South India,[152] Venezuela[146] and Egypt.[148] HLA class II alleles were also associated with lepromatous leprosy in multicase families from Venezuela and China.[146,153] Interestingly, attempts to detect an effect of HLA alleles on susceptibility to leprosy *per se* failed consistently arguing against a role of HLA-linked susceptibility factors in leprosy *per se*.[146,152] This led to the conclusion that HLA genes play a role at later stages of leprosy by stimulating the polarization of immune response towards the lepromatous or tuberculoid form. However, at least one study of multiplex families found association and linkage of leprosy *per se* with a number of MHC genes,[154] hence indicating some degree of HLA genetic heterogeneity of leprosy *per se* genetic control.

Class III Genes: TAP, MICA and MICB, TNF, LTA

The major histocompatibility complex (MHC) contains numerous genes coding non-class I/II genes involved in the innate immune response (for a recently updated MHC gene map see.[155] Many of these genes have been studied for their role in susceptibility to mycobacterial infection.[96,156-158]

The *TAP1* and *TAP2* genes, for transporter associated with antigen processing, are located in the class II HLA subregion between *HLA-DR* and *HLA-DP*. The products of *TAP1/TAP2* form a heterodimer that transports antigenic peptides from the cytoplasm to the endoplasmic reticulum for binding to HLA class I molecules and subsequent presentation to CD8+ cytotoxic T cells.[159] The contribution of polymorphisms in these genes to susceptibility to pulmonary tuberculosis and tuberculoid leprosy was studied in a Northern Indian case-control sample.[156] No association was found between *TAP1* alleles and tuberculosis or leprosy. However, two *TAP2* variants were observed more frequently in the group of affected patients compared to controls. The *TAP2-A/F* allele was enriched among patients with pulmonary tuberculosis as compared to controls (p_{corr}<0.01, OR=4.3) while the *TAP2-B* allele was enriched among the group of tuberculoid leprosy patients (P_{corr}<0.003, OR=3.5). These results suggested a role of TAP2 variants in preferential transport of mycobacterial antigens leading to increased susceptibility to disease most likely via CD8 T-cells mediated mechanism.

The MHC class I chain-related genes, *MICA* and *MICB* encode stress-inducible proteins expressed on the cell surface and recognized by γδ T cells, CD8+ αβ T cells and NK cells via the NKG2D receptor.[160,161] These genes were analyzed in a family-based association study of paucibacillary leprosy in Southern India.[157] The study reported strong association of the *MICA*5A5.1* allele with paucibacillary leprosy. The latter allele encodes a truncated transmembrane domain of MICA and presumably impacts negative on MICA function. These results are opposite to findings reported for Southern Chinese leprosy patients where the *MICA*5A5.1* allele showed a protective effect against multibacillary leprosy.[162] Although there are no genetic studies on the role of *MICA* and *MICB* polymorphisms in susceptibility to tuberculosis, a functional study demonstrated that infection with *M. tuberculosis* led to increased MICA expression and activation of cytotoxic γδ T cells.[161]

The tumor necrosis factor-alpha and lymphotoxin-alpha cytokines, encoded by the genes *TNF* and *LTA* play a crucial role in the protective host response against mycobacterial infection (for example reviewed in Ref. 163,164 and 98,165-167). The role of the promoter variant at position –308 of *TNF-α* has been assessed in several case-control studies. The –308 G → A substitution was designated TNF2 to identify the "A" allele. The effect of TNF2 on risk of mycobacterial disease susceptibility has been inconsistent. No association between TNF2 and risk of developing leprosy was reported in Brazil[168-170] and Cambodia,[141] whereas higher frequencies of TNF2 were observed in lepromatous leprosy patients in India[171,172] and lepromatous and tuberculoid leprosy patients in an independent study in Brazil.[154] Yet another study in Brazilian leprosy patients reported a significant overrepresentation of TNF2 in the control group compared to leprosy patients ($p<0.05$), suggesting a protective effect of the TNF2 polymorphism.[173] The role of TNF2 in tuberculosis susceptibility is equally unclear: A positive association between TNF2 and risk of tuberculosis was reported in Southern Russia,[174] whereas lack of association was found in Thailand[175] and Colombia.[176]

Selected non-HLA Candidate Gene Studies

Numerous non-HLA genes have been implicated as candidate tuberculosis or leprosy susceptibility loci. The implications and limitations of such studies have been described in several reviews and will not be re-iterated here (reviewed in Ref. 177-180). Instead, we will only discuss some selected examples of such candidate susceptibility genes. One of the most common candidate genes is *NRAMP1*, also referred to as *SLC11A1* in the systematic nomenclature. The mouse orthologue gene was first identified as a susceptibility locus to mycobacterial diseases and termed *Bcg*.[181,182] *Nramp1* was identified as the molecular equivalent of the *Bcg* locus by positional cloning.[183] *Nramp1* encodes an integral membrane transporter of divalent metal cations which is recruited to the membrane of the phagosome.[184] It has been shown that *Nramp1* affects mycobacterial growth via the regulation of the intraphagosomal concentration of cationic iron.[185] The function of the human NRAMP1 protein is unknown but thought to be identical to the one described for the mouse protein. Indeed, a recent study showing that NRAMP1 impacts on phagosome maturation in human macrophages provided direct experimental support for the conservation of NRAMP1/Nramp1 function.[186] Based on the results in the mouse model, *NRAMP1* was selected for a case-control study in a Gambian tuberculosis population. Two independent *NRAMP1* variants located in intron 4 and the 3'UTR region were significantly associated with pulmonary tuberculosis. Moreover, combined heterozygosity for these two polymorphisms was associated with a very strong risk of tuberculosis (OR=4.1; $p<0.001$).[187] These initial positive results prompted a large number of follow-up studies in numerous population groups that largely replicated and validated *NRAMP1* as a prime tuberculosis susceptibility gene.[110]

The above results were obtained in adult tuberculosis populations with reactivational patients representing the majority of cases. By contrast, a study of a tuberculosis outbreak in a North Canadian aboriginal community allowed timing of infection and focused on primary tuberculosis. This family-based study demonstrated strong linkage of *NRAMP1* to tuberculosis susceptibility (RR=10; $p<10^{-5}$). This study also highlighted the importance of taking into account the exposure history of a person. Indeed, neglecting information about past mycobacterial exposure resulted in loss of the linkage signal.[188,189] This surprising effect was confirmed in an independent study of primary tuberculosis in Houston, TX. The *NRAMP1* effect was the highest in the families with low exposure to *M. tuberculosis*.[190]

The role of the *NRAMP1* gene was also studied in leprosy and related phenotypes. In Vietnamese leprosy families significant linkage ($p<0.005$) was observed between *NRAMP1* haplotypes and leprosy *per se*.[191] In a study in Malawi, *NRAMP1* polymorphisms were implicated in leprosy subtype control.[192] Perhaps the most interesting results were obtained by studying the genetic control of Mitsuda reactivity. The *in vivo* Mitsuda reaction measures the infectious granuloma forming capacity in response to intradermally injected lepromin. Despite the use of lepromin, Mitsuda reactivity is independent of exposure to *M. leprae*. In two studies, highly significant linkage of the *NRAMP1* gene to extent of Mitsuda reactivity was observed.[193,194] Hence, it is tempting to hypothesize that NRAMP1 is involved in early protective immunity against *M. leprae*, consistent with previous results in the mouse model.[182,184] Interestingly, the D543N *NRAMP1* polymorphisms was demonstrated to be associated with susceptibility to Buruli ulcers (OR=2.89; 1.41-5.91 95% confidence interval),[9] suggesting a role of *NRAMP1* in the early, still intracellular stage of *M. ulcerans*. To our knowledge, this is the only study showing a role of genetic factors in development of *M. ulcerans* infection.

An involvement of the *VDR* gene in tuberculosis and leprosy susceptibility has been suggested in a number of studies. The active form of vitamin D, 1α, 25 (OH)$_2$D$_3$, modulates the differentiation, growth and function of a broad range of cells, including antigen-presenting cells. A number of studies have analyzed vitamin D levels among tuberculosis patients and matched controls. Generally, vitamin D levels are lower in patients. However, the absolute levels vary substantially from study-to-study so that patients in one study have higher levels than controls in another study. To better establish the role of vitamin D levels in tuberculosis the results of prospective studies are needed.

Nevertheless, the immune-modulatory potency of vitamin D especially on macrophages and dendritic cells is well established.[195,196] The effect of vitamin D is transduced through its receptor molecule, VDR. Recent data point to a connection of TLR-signalling with vitamin D metabolism and microbial activity.[197] A number of allelic variants have been described for the *VDR* gene.[198,199] In a Gambian case-control study, the *tt* genotype of a *TaqI* polymorphism was underrepresented among patients with PTB (OR=0.5; p<0.02).[200] Similarly, polymorphisms in the 5' promoter and 3' UTR were identified as risk factors for tuberculosis in independent population samples from West Africa,[201,202] and South India[203-205] and South Americans.[206] Interesting evidence for a possible interaction of *VDR* polymorphisms, vitamin D levels and risk of tuberculosis was described in a case control study among Gujarati Indiana residing in England. While, VDR polymorphism *per se* were not associated with risk of PTB, in persons with low serum vitamin D levels *VDR* polymorphism were highly significant PTB risk factors.[207] A case control study of *VDR* polymorphisms and leprosy patients in India found the *TaqI* polymorphism with a higher frequency of tt genotypes among tuberculoid leprosy patients (OR=3.2, p<0.001) whereas the *TT* genotype was overrepresented in lepromatous patients (OR=1.7, p<0.04).[208] Under the hypothesis that the homozygous *tt* genotype impairs the function of VDR these data are consistent with an immunosuppressive effects of 1α, 25 (OH)$_2$D$_3$.

MCP1. Linkage studies in a large collection of Brazilian multiplex tuberculosis and leprosy families reported a suggestive linkage peak on chromosomal fragment 17q11-q21, which was subsequently narrowed down to the 17q11.2 region.[92,169] The linkage signal overlaps a chemokine gene cluster and the Nitric Oxide Synthase 2A (*NOS2A*) gene. Flores-Villanueva et al,[209] performed a positional candidate gene study in the Mexican PTB patients and analyzed the association of *NOS2A*, *RANTES*, *MIP-1α*, and Monocyte Chemo-attractant Protein-1 (*MCP1*) with PTB. Only a regulatory polymorphism at position -2581 relative to the ATG start codon of *MCP1* was associated with PTB. The carriers of *AG* and *GG* genotypes at position -2581 were 2.3 and 5.8 times more likely to develop tuberculosis. Since, all subjects of the control group were positive for latent infection with *M. tuberculosis* as measured by TST, this result implicated *MCP1* as very strong tuberculosis progression susceptibility gene. The genetic association was further supported by functional data which showed that carriers of the *GG* genotype demonstrated the highest levels of MCP1 and the lowest level of IL12p40 in plasma, thus increasing the likelihood of progression of *M. tuberculosis* infection to active pulmonary disease. These finding were replicated in an independent population of South Korean patients with PTB. Surprisingly, in this validation study the odds of developing tuberculosis were even higher than in the initial study (OR = 2.8 and 6.9 for *AG* and *GG* genotypes vs *AA* genotype).

On the other hand, a number of results are not consistent with this very strong effect of the *MCP1* -2581 SNP on tuberculosis susceptibility. First, this polymorphism did not show significant evidence of association with tuberculosis susceptibility in the initial Brazilian study.[92] Secondly, a very large study of *MCP1* polymorphisms in West Africa observed an inverse association with the "G" MCP-1 -2581 allele being a resistance factor for PTB in cases versus controls [odds ratio (OR) 0.81, corrected P-value (P$_{corr}$ = 0.0012].[210] Moreover, an independent large case-control sample from Russia failed to provide significant evidence for association of PTB with *MCP1-2581*.[210] Clearly, the effect of MCP1 levels and the role of polymorphism within *MCP1* in tuberculosis pathogenesis require additional careful investigation.

CONCLUSION

Stimulated by powerful new genotyping techniques, the access to complete sequence data of human genomes, and the availability of high density SNP arrays, linkage disequilibrium maps and improved methods for the analysis of genetic epidemiological data, the genetic analysis of mycobacterial disease has experienced tremendous advances in the past decade. Further progress is expected due to the emerging possibility to perform whole genome resequencing. The analysis of mycobacterial diseases, however, is lagging in adjusting the phenotypic description of patient samples with the same level of accuracy that is provided by the laboratory. There is a need to analyze different phenotypes which take into account various stages of the disease, particularly different steps of immune response, starting from the exposure to the pathogen to the eventual progression to clinical disease. Another area that is in need of improvement is the integration of genetic findings into ongoing studies of the human immune response to mycobacterial diseases. Without considering the critical contribution of host genetics in susceptibility to mycobacterial diseases, the success of these studies is an unlikely event. The ultimate approach to the study of mycobacterial pathogenesis must be to combine the expertise of different disciplines to benefit the shared effort of combating the spread of mycobacterial diseases.

REFERENCES

1. Falkinham JO, III. Epidemiology of infection by nontuberculous mycobacteria. Clin. Microbiol Rev 1996;9:177-215.
2. Bloom BR. Tuberculosis: Pathogenesis, Protection, and Control. AMS Press, Washingoton, DC 637, 1994.
3. Collins CH. The bovine tubercle bacillus. Br J Biomed Sci 2000;57:234-40.
4. WHO. WHO Report 2008. Global Tuberculosis Control. 1-1-2008.
5. WHO. WHO. 2007. The leprosy burden at the end of 2006. Wkly Epidemiol Rec 25, 225-232. 1-1-2006.
6. van der Werf TS, van der Graaf WT, Tappero JW, et al. Mycobacterium ulcerans infection. Lancet 1999;354: 1013-18.
7. Debacker M, Aguiar J, Steunou C, et al. Mycobacterium ulcerans disease (Buruli ulcer) in rural hospital, Southern Benin, 1997-2001. Emerg Infect Dis 2004;10:1391-98.
8. Coutanceau E, Marsollier L, Brosch R, et al. Modulation of the host immune response by a transient intracellular stage of Mycobacterium ulcerans: The contribution of endogenous mycolactone toxin. Cell Microbiol 2005;7:1187-96.
9. Stienstra Y, van der Werf TS, Oosterom E, et al. Susceptibility to Buruli ulcer is associated with the SLC11A1 (NRAMP1) D543N polymorphism. Genes Immun 2006;7:185-89.
10. Lotte A, Wasz-Hockert O, Poisson N, et al. A bibliography of the complications of BCG vaccination. A comprehensive list of the world literature since the introduction of BCG up to July 1982, supplemented by over 100 personal communications. Adv Tuberc Res 1984;21:194-245.
11. Holland SM. Nontuberculous mycobacteria. Am J Med Sci 2001;321:49-55.
12. Pierre-Audigier C, Jouanguy E, Lamhamedi S, et al. Fatal disseminated Mycobacterium smegmatis infection in a child with inherited interferon gamma receptor deficiency. Clin Infect Dis 1997;24:982-84.
13. Doffinger R, Smahi A, Bessia C, et al. X-linked anhidrotic ectodermal dysplasia with immunodeficiency is caused by impaired NF-kappaB signaling. Nat Genet 2001;27: 277-85.
14. Brooks EG, Klimpel GR, Vaidya SE, et al. Thymic hypoplasia and T-cell deficiency in ectodermal dysplasia: Case report and review of the literature. Clin Immunol Immunopathol 1994;71:44-52.
15. Allen DMChng HH. Disseminated Mycobacterium flavescens in a probable case of chronic granulomatous disease. J Infect 1993;26:83-86.
16. Jacobson RRKrahenbuhl JL. Leprosy. Lancet 1999;353: 655-60.
17. Bloom BR Small PM. The evolving relation between humans and Mycobacterium tuberculosis. N Engl J Med 1998;338:677-78.
18. Moegling A. Die Epidemiologie der Lûbecker Säuglingstuberkulose. Arbeiten a.d.Reichsges.-Amt 1935;69:1-24.
19. Stead WW. Genetics and resistance to tuberculosis. Could resistance be enhanced by genetic engineering? Ann Intern Med 1992;116:937-41.
20. Comstock GW. Tuberculosis in twins: A re-analysis of the Prophit survey. Am Rev Respir Dis 1978;117:621-24.
21. Kallmann FJ, Reisner D. Twin studies on the significance of genetic factors in tuberculosis. Am Rev Tuber 1943;74:549-74.
22. Chakravartti MR, Vogel FA Twin study on Leprosy. Topics in Human Genetics. Stuttgart, Georg Thieme Publishers 1973;1:1-124.
23. Lurie MB. Mechanisms of immunity in tuberculosis. J Exp Med 1936;63:923-60.
24. Lurie MB. Heredity, constitution and tuberculosis. An experimental study. Am Rev Tuber 1941;44(Suppl):1-125.
25. Lurie MB, Heppleston AG, Bramson S, et al. Evaluation of the method of quantitative airborne infection and its use in the study of the pathogenesis of tuberculosis. Am Rev Tuberc 1950;61:765-97.
26. Werneck-Barroso E. Innate resistance to tuberculosis: Revisiting Max Lurie genetic experiments in rabbits. Int J Tuberc Lung Dis 1999;3:166-68.
27. Lander ES, Schork NJ. Genetic dissection of complex traits. Science 1994;265:2037-48.
28. Abel LDessein AJ. The impact of host genetics on susceptibility to human infectious diseases. Curr Opin Immunol 1997;9:509-16.
29. Morton NE. Sequential tests for the detection of linkage. Am J Hum. Genet 1955;7:277-318.
30. Clerget-Darpoux F, Bonaiti-Pellie C,Hochez J. Effects of mis-specifying genetic parameters in lod score analysis. Biometrics 1986;42:393-99.

31. Lander EKruglyak L. Genetic dissection of complex traits: Guidelines for interpreting and reporting linkage results. Nat Genet 1995;11:241-47.
32. MacLean CJ, Bishop DT, Sherman SL, et al. Distribution of lod scores under uncertain mode of inheritance. Am J Hum. Genet 1993;52:354-61.
33. Risch N. Linkage strategies for genetically complex traits. III. The effect of marker polymorphism on analysis of affected relative pairs. Am J Hum Genet 1990;46:242-53.
34. Abel LMuller-Myhsok B. Robustness and power of the maximum-likelihood-binomial and maximum-likelihood-score methods, in multipoint linkage analysis of affected-sibship data. Am J Hum. Genet 1998;63:638-47.
35. Levy S, Sutton G, Ng PC, et al. The diploid genome sequence of an individual human. PLoS Biol 2007;5:e254.
36. Wheeler DA, Srinivasan M, Egholm M, et al. The complete genome of an individual by massively parallel DNA sequencing. Nature 2008;452:872-76.
37. Wang J, Wang W, Li R, et al. The diploid genome sequence of an Asian individual. Nature 2008;456:60-65.
38. Bentley DR, Balasubramanian S, Swerdlow HP, et al. Accurate whole human genome sequencing using reversible terminator chemistry. Nature 2008;456:53-59.
39. Ke X, Miretti MM, Broxholme J, et al. A comparison of tagging methods and their tagging space. Hum Mol Genet 2005;14:2757-67.
40. Abel LCasanova JL. Genetic predisposition to clinical tuberculosis: Bridging the gap between simple and complex inheritance. Am J Hum Genet 2000;67:274-77.
41. Casanova JLAbel L. Human genetics of infectious diseases: A unified theory. EMBO J 2007;26:915-22.
42. Notarangelo L, Casanova JL, Conley ME, et al. Primary immunodeficiency diseases: An update from the International Union of Immunological Societies Primary Immunodeficiency Diseases Classification Committee Meeting in Budapest 2005. J Allergy Clin Immunol 2006;117:883-96.
43. Lander ES. The new genomics: Global views of biology. Science 1996;274:536-39.
44. Lohmueller KE, Pearce CL, Pike M, et al. Meta-analysis of genetic association studies supports a contribution of common variants to susceptibility to common disease. Nat Genet 2003;33:177-82.
45. Hirschhorn JNDaly MJ. Genome-wide association studies for common diseases and complex traits. Nat Rev Genet 2005;6:95-108.
46. McCarthy MI, Abecasis GR, Cardon LR, et al. Genome-wide association studies for complex traits: Consensus, uncertainty and challenges. Nat Rev Genet 2008;9:356-69.
47. Pritchard JK. Are rare variants responsible for susceptibility to complex diseases? Am J Hum Genet 2001;69:124-37.
48. Pritchard JKCox NJ. The allelic architecture of human disease genes: Common disease-common variant...or not? Hum Mol Genet 2002;11:2417-23.
49. Mimouni J. Our experiences in three years of BCG vaccination at the center of the OPHS at Constantine; study of observed cases (25 cases of complications from BCG vaccination). Alger Medicale 1951;55:1138-47.
50. Jouanguy E, Altare F, Lamhamedi S, et al. Interferon-gamma-receptor deficiency in an infant with fatal bacille Calmette-Guerin infection. N Engl J Med 1996;335:1956-61.
51. Casanova JL, Jouanguy E, Lamhamedi S, et al. Immunological conditions of children with BCG disseminated infection. Lancet 1995;346:581.
52. Newport MJ, Huxley CM, Huston S, et al. A mutation in the interferon-gamma-receptor gene and susceptibility to mycobacterial infection. N Engl J Med 1996;335:1941-49.
53. Dorman SE, Holland SM. Mutation in the signal-transducing chain of the interferon-gamma receptor and susceptibility to mycobacterial infection. J Clin Invest 1998;101:2364-69.
54. Altare F, Lammas D, Revy P, et al. Inherited interleukin-12 deficiency in a child with bacille Calmette-Guerin and Salmonella enteritidis disseminated infection. J Clin Invest 1998;102:2035-40.
55. Dupuis S, Dargemont C, Fieschi C, et al. Impairment of mycobacterial but not viral immunity by a germline human STAT1 mutation. Science 2001;293:300-03.
56. Filipe-Santos O, Bustamante J, Chapgier A, et al. Inborn errors of IL-12/23- and IFN-gamma-mediated immunity: Molecular, cellular, and clinical features. Semin Immunol 2006;18:347-61.
57. Al-Muhsen SCasanova JL. The genetic heterogeneity of mendelian susceptibility to mycobacterial diseases. J Allergy Clin Immunol 2008;122: 1043-51.
58. Altare F, Jouanguy E, Lamhamedi-Cherradi S, et al. A causative relationship between mutant IFNgR1 alleles and impaired cellular response to IFNgamma in a compound heterozygous child. Am J Hum Genet 1998;62:723-26.
59. Roesler J, Kofink B, Wendisch J, et al. Listeria monocytogenes and recurrent mycobacterial infections in a child with complete interferon-gamma-receptor (IFNgammaR1) deficiency: Mutational analysis and evaluation of therapeutic options. Exp Hematol 1999;27:1368-74.
60. Allende LM, Lopez-Goyanes A, Paz-Artal E, et al. A point mutation in a domain of gamma interferon receptor 1 provokes severe immunodeficiency. Clin Diagn Lab Immunol 2001;8:133-37.
61. Jouanguy E, Dupuis S, Pallier A, et al. In a novel form of IFN-gamma receptor 1 deficiency, cell surface receptors fail to bind IFN-gamma. J Clin Invest 2000;105:1429-36.
62. Jouanguy E, Altare F, Lamhamedi-Cherradi S, et al. Infections in IFNGR-1-deficient children. J Interferon Cytokine Res 1997;17:583-87.
63. Dorman SE, Picard C, Lammas D, et al. Clinical features of dominant and recessive interferon-gamma receptor 1 deficiencies. Lancet 2004;364:2113-21.
64. Levin M, Newport MJ, D'Souza S, et al. Familial disseminated atypical mycobacterial infection in childhood: A human mycobacterial susceptibility gene? Lancet 1995;345:79-83.

65. Jouanguy E, Lamhamedi-Cherradi S, Altare F, et al. Partial interferon-gamma receptor 1 deficiency in a child with tuberculoid bacillus Calmette-Guerin infection and a sibling with clinical tuberculosis. J Clin Invest 1997;100:2658-64.
66. Dupuis S, Doffinger R, Picard C, et al. Human interferon-gamma-mediated immunity is a genetically controlled continuous trait that determines the outcome of mycobacterial invasion. Immunol Rev 2000;178:129-37.
67. Jouanguy E, Lamhamedi-Cherradi S, Lammas D, et al. A human IFNGR1 small deletion hotspot associated with dominant susceptibility to mycobacterial infection. Nat Genet 1999;21:370-78.
68. Villella A, Picard C, Jouanguy E, et al. Recurrent Mycobacterium avium osteomyelitis associated with a novel dominant interferon-gamma receptor mutation. Pediatrics 2001;107:E47.
69. Vogt G, Chapgier A, Yang K, et al. Gains of glycosylation comprise an unexpectedly large group of pathogenic mutations. Nat Genet 2005;37:692-700.
70. Vogt G, Bustamante J, Chapgier A, et al. Complementation of a pathogenic IFNGR2 misfolding mutation with modifiers of N-glycosylation. J Exp Med 2008;205:1729-37.
71. Chapgier A, Boisson-Dupuis S, Jouanguy E, et al. Novel STAT1 alleles in otherwise healthy patients with mycobacterial disease. PLoS Genet 2006;2:e131.
72. Dupuis S, Jouanguy E, Al-Hajjar S, et al. Impaired response to interferon-alpha/beta and lethal viral disease in human STAT1 deficiency. Nat Genet 2003;33:388-91.
73. Chapgier A, Wynn RF, Jouanguy E, et al. Human complete STAT-1 deficiency is associated with defective type I and II IFN responses in vitro but immunity to some low virulence viruses in vivo. J Immunol 2006;176:5078-83.
74. Picard C, Fieschi C, Altare F, et al. Inherited interleukin-12 deficiency: IL12B genotype and clinical phenotype of 13 patients from six kindreds. Am J Hum Genet 2002;70:336-48.
75. MacLennan C, Fieschi C, Lammas DA, et al. Interleukin (IL)-12 and IL-23 are key cytokines for immunity against Salmonella in humans. J Infect Dis 2004;190:1755-57.
76. Fieschi C, Dupuis S, Catherinot E, et al. Low penetrance, broad resistance, and favorable outcome of interleukin-12 receptor beta1 deficiency: Medical and immunological implications. J Exp Med 2003;197:527-35.
77. Alcais A, Fieschi C, Abel L, et al. Tuberculosis in children and adults: Two distinct genetic diseases. J Exp Med 2005;202:1617-21.
78. Casanova JL Abel L. Inborn errors of immunity to infection: The rule rather than the exception. J Exp Med 2005;202:197-201.
79. Zhang SY, Boisson-Dupuis S, Chapgier A, et al. Inborn errors of interferon (IFN)-mediated immunity in humans: Insights into the respective roles of IFN-alpha/beta, IFN-gamma, and IFN-lambda in host defense. Immunol Rev 2008;226:29-40.
80. Picard C, Puel A, Bonnet M, et al. Pyogenic bacterial infections in humans with IRAK-4 deficiency. Science 2003;299:2076-79.
81. O'Neill LA. Signal transduction pathways activated by the IL-1 receptor/toll-like receptor superfamily. Curr Top Microbiol Immunol 2002;270:47-61.
82. Nakanishi K, Yoshimoto T, Tsutsui H, et al. Interleukin-18 regulates both Th1 and Th2 responses. Annu Rev Immunol 2001;19:423-74.
83. Duerr RH, Taylor KD, Brant SR, et al. A genome-wide association study identifies IL23R as an inflammatory bowel disease gene. Science 2006;314:1461-63.
84. Behr MA, Schurr E. Mycobacteria in Crohn's disease: A persistent hypothesis. Inflamm Bowel Dis 2006;12:1000-04.
85. Feller M, Huwiler K, Stephan R, et al. Mycobacterium avium subspecies paratuberculosis and Crohn's disease: A systematic review and meta-analysis. Lancet Infect Dis 2007;7:607-13.
86. Abel L, Demenais F. Detection of major genes for susceptibility to leprosy and its subtypes in a Caribbean island: Desirade island. Am J Hum Genet 1988;42:256-66.
87. Abel L, Cot M, Mulder L, et al. Segregation analysis detects a major gene controlling blood infection levels in human malaria. Am J Hum Genet 1992;50:1308-17.
88. Abel L, Vu DL, Oberti J, et al. Complex segregation analysis of leprosy in southern Vietnam. Genet Epidemiol 1995;12:63-82.
89. Alcais A, Abel L, David C, et al. Evidence for a major gene controlling susceptibility to tegumentary leishmaniasis in a recently exposed Bolivian population. Am J Hum Genet 1997;61:968-79.
90. Siddiqui MR, Meisner S, Tosh K, et al. A major susceptibility locus for leprosy in India maps to chromosome 10p13. Nat Genet 2001;27:439-41.
91. Miller EN, Jamieson SE, Joberty C, et al. Genome-wide scans for leprosy and tuberculosis susceptibility genes in Brazilians. Genes Immun 2004;5:63-67.
92. Jamieson SE, Miller EN, Black GF, et al. Evidence for a cluster of genes on chromosome 17q11-q21 controlling susceptibility to tuberculosis and leprosy in Brazilians. Genes Immun 2004;5:46-57.
93. Mira MT, Alcais A, Van TN, et al. Chromosome 6q25 is linked to susceptibility to leprosy in a Vietnamese population. Nat Genet 2003;33:412-15.
94. Mira MT, Alcais A, Nguyen VT, et al. Susceptibility to leprosy is associated with PARK2 and PACRG. Nature 2004;427:636-40.
95. Schurr E, Alcais A, de LL, et al. Genetic predisposition to leprosy: A major gene reveals novel pathways of immunity to Mycobacterium leprae. Semin Immunol 2006;18:404-10.
96. Alcais A, Alter A, Antoni G, et al. Stepwise replication identifies a low-producing lymphotoxin-alpha allele as a major risk factor for early-onset leprosy. Nat Genet 2007;39:517-22.

97. Knight JC, Keating BJ, Kwiatkowski DP. Allele-specific repression of lymphotoxin-alpha by activated B cell factor-1. Nat Genet 2004;36:394-99.
98. Roach DR, Briscoe H, Saunders B, et al. Secreted lymphotoxin-alpha is essential for the control of an intracellular bacterial infection. J Exp Med 2001;193: 239-46.
99. Hagge DA, Saunders BM, Ebenezer GJ, et al. Lymphotoxin-{alpha} and TNF Have Essential but Independent Roles in the Evolution of the Granulomatous Response in Experimental Leprosy. Am J Pathol 2009.
100. Baghdadi JE, Orlova M, Alter A, et al. An autosomal dominant major gene confers predisposition to pulmonary tuberculosis in adults. J Exp Med 2006;203:1679-84.
101. Bellamy R, Beyers N, McAdam KP, et al. Genetic susceptibility to tuberculosis in Africans; A genome-wide scan. Proc Natl Acad Sci US A 2000;97:8005-09.
102. Cervino AC, Lakiss S, Sow O, et al. Fine mapping of a putative tuberculosis-susceptibility locus on chromosome 15q11-13 in African families. Hum Mol Genet 2002;11:1599-1603.
103. Cooke GS, Campbell SJ, Bennett S, et al. Mapping of a novel susceptibility locus suggests a role for MC3R and CTSZ in human tuberculosis. Am J Respir Crit Care Med 2008;178:203-07.
104. Stein CM, Zalwango S, Malone LL, et al. Genome scan of M tuberculosis infection and disease in Ugandans. PLoS. ONE 2008;3:e4094.
105. Mahasirimongkol S, Yanai H, Nishida N, et al. Genome-wide SNP-based linkage analysis of tuberculosis in Thais Genes Immun 2009;10:77-83.
106. Bothamley GH, Beck JS, Schreuder GM, et al. Association of tuberculosis and M. tuberculosis-specific antibody levels with HLA. J Infect Dis 1989;159:549-55.
107. Brahmajothi V, Pitchappan RM, Kakkanaiah VN, et al. Association of pulmonary tuberculosis and HLA in south India. Tubercle 1991;72:123-32.
108. Rajalingam R, Mehra NK, Jain RC, et al. Polymerase chain reaction—based sequence-specific oligonucleotide hybridization analysis of HLA class II antigens in pulmonary tuberculosis: Relevance to chemotherapy and disease severity. J Infect Dis 1996;173:669-76.
109. Meyer CG, May J, Stark K. Human leukocyte antigens in tuberculosis and leprosy. Trends Microbiol 1998;6:148-54.
110. Li HT, Zhang TT, Zhou YQ, et al. SLC11A1 (formerly NRAMP1) gene polymorphisms and tuberculosis susceptibility: A meta-analysis. Int J Tuberc Lung Dis 2006;10:3-12.
111. Khomenko AG, Litvinov VI, Chukanova VP, et al. Tuberculosis in patients with various HLA phenotypes. Tubercle 1990;71:187-92.
112. Sanjeevi CB, Narayanan PR, Prabakar R, et al. No association or linkage with HLA-DR or -DQ genes in south Indians with pulmonary tuberculosis. Tuber Lung Dis 1992;73:280-84.
113. Pospelov LE, Matrakshin AG, Chernousova LN, et al. Association of various genetic markers with tuberculosis and other lung diseases in Tuvinian children. Tuber Lung Dis 1996;77:77-80.
114. Singh SP, Mehra NK, Dingley HB, et al. Human leukocyte antigen (HLA)-linked control of susceptibility to pulmonary tuberculosis and association with HLA-DR types. J Infect Dis 1983;148:676-81.
115. Hawkins BR, Higgins DA, Chan SL, et al. HLA typing in the Hong Kong Chest Service/British Medical Research Council study of factors associated with the breakdown to active tuberculosis of inactive pulmonary lesions. Am Rev Respir Dis 1988;138:1616-21.
116. Cox RA, Downs M, Neimes RE, et al. Immunogenetic analysis of human tuberculosis. J Infect Dis 1988;158: 1302-08.
117. Opelz G, Mytilineos J, Scherer S, et al. Survival of DNA HLA-DR typed and matched cadaver kidney transplants. The Collaborative Transplant Study. Lancet 1991;338: 461-63.
118. Middleton D. HLA Typing from Serology to Sequencing Era. Iran J Allergy Asthma Immunol 2005:4:53-66.
119. Cooper AMFlynn JL. The protective immune response to Mycobacterium tuberculosis. Curr Opin Immunol 1995;7:512-16.
120. Flynn JL, Goldstein MM, Triebold KJ, et al. Major histocompatibility complex class I-restricted T cells are required for resistance to Mycobacterium tuberculosis infection. Proc Natl Acad Sci U SA 1992;89:12013-017.
121. Mogues T, Goodrich ME, Ryan L, et al. The relative importance of T cell subsets in immunity and immunopathology of airborne Mycobacterium tuberculosis infection in mice. J Exp Med 2001;193: 271-80.
122. Lalvani A, Brookes R, Wilkinson RJ, et al. Human cytolytic and interferon gamma-secreting CD8+ T lymphocytes specific for Mycobacterium tuberculosis. Proc Natl Acad Sci USA 1998;95:270-75.
123. Smith SM, Klein MR, Malin AS, et al. Human CD8(+) T cells specific for Mycobacterium tuberculosis secreted antigens in tuberculosis patients and healthy BCG-vaccinated controls in The Gambia. Infect Immun 2000;68:7144-48.
124. Mohagheghpour N, Gammon D, Kawamura LM, et al. CTL response to Mycobacterium tuberculosis: Identification of an immunogenic epitope in the 19-kDa lipoprotein. J Immunol 1998;161:2400-06.
125. Lewinsohn DM, Zhu L, Madison VJ, et al. Classically restricted human CD8+ T lymphocytes derived from Mycobacterium tuberculosis-infected cells: Definition of antigenic specificity. J Immunol 2001;166:439-46.
126. Sette A, Sidney J. Nine major HLA class I supertypes account for the vast preponderance of HLA-A and -B polymorphism. Immunogenetics 1999;50:201-12.
127. Balamurugan A, Sharma SK, Mehra NK. Human leukocyte antigen class I supertypes influence susceptibility and severity of tuberculosis. J Infect Dis 2004;189:805-11.
128. Bothamley GH. Differences between HLA-B44 and HLA-B60 in patients with smear-positive pulmonary

tuberculosis and exposed controls. J Infect Dis 1999;179: 1051-52.
129. Kettaneh A, Seng L, Tiev KP, et al. Human leukocyte antigens and susceptibility to tuberculosis: A meta-analysis of case-control studies. Int J Tuberc Lung Dis 2006;10:717-25.
130. Harel-Bellan A, Quillet A, Marchiol C, et al. Natural killer susceptibility of human cells may be regulated by genes in the HLA region on chromosome 6. Proc Natl Acad Sci USA 1986;83:5688-92.
131. Storkus WJ, Howell DN, Salter RD, et al. NK susceptibility varies inversely with target cell class I HLA antigen expression. J Immunol 1987;138:1657-59.
132. Colonna M, Spies T, Strominger JL, et al. Alloantigen recognition by two human natural killer cell clones is associated with HLA-C or a closely linked gene Proc Natl Acad Sci USA 1992;89:7983-85.
133. Fernando SL, Britton WJ. Genetic susceptibility to mycobacterial disease in humans. Immunol Cell Biol 2006;84:125-37.
134. Shankarkumar U. HLA associations in leprosy patients from Mumbai, India. Lepr Rev 2004;75:79-85.
135. Um SW, Ki CS, Kwon OJ, et al. HLA Antigens and Nontuberculous Mycobacterial Lung Disease in Korean Patients. Lung 2009.
136. Takahashi M, Ishizaka A, Nakamura H, et al. Specific HLA in pulmonary MAC infection in a Japanese population. Am J Respir Crit Care Med 2000;162:316-18.
137. Kubo K, Yamazaki Y, Hanaoka M, et al. Analysis of HLA antigens in Mycobacterium avium-intracellular pulmonary infection. Am J Respir Crit Care Med 2000;161: 1368-71.
138. Mehra NK, Rajalingam R, Mitra DK, et al. Variants of HLA-DR2/DR51 group haplotypes and susceptibility to tuberculoid leprosy and pulmonary tuberculosis in Asian Indians Int J Lepr Other Mycobact Dis 1995;63:241-48.
139. Ravikumar M, Dheenadhayalan V, Rajaram K, et al. Associations of HLA-DRB1, DQB1 and DPB1 alleles with pulmonary tuberculosis in south India. Tuber Lung Dis 1999;79:309-17.
140. Teran-Escandon D, Teran-Ortiz L, Camarena-Olvera A, et al. Human leukocyte antigen-associated susceptibility to pulmonary tuberculosis: Molecular analysis of class II alleles by DNA amplification and oligonucleotide hybridization in Mexican patients. Chest 1999;115:428-33.
141. Goldfeld AE, Delgado JC, Thim S, et al. Association of an HLA-DQ allele with clinical tuberculosis. JAMA 1998;279:226-28.
142. Nepom BS, Nepom GT, Coleman M, et al. Critical contribution of beta chain residue 57 in peptide binding ability of both HLA-DR and -DQ molecules. Proc Natl Acad Sci USA 1996;93:7202-06.
143. Kwok WW, Domeier ME, Johnson ML, et al. HLA-DQB1 codon 57 is critical for peptide binding and recognition. J Exp Med 1996;183:1253-58.
144. Delgado JC, Baena A, Thim S, et al. Aspartic acid homozygosity at codon 57 of HLA-DQ beta is associated with susceptibility to pulmonary tuberculosis in Cambodia. J Immunol 2006;176:1090-97.
145. Ottenhoff TH, de Vries RR. HLA class II immune response and suppression genes in leprosy. Int J Lepr Other Mycobact Dis 1987;55:521-34.
146. van EW, Gonzalez NM, de Vries RR, et al. HLA-linked control of predisposition to lepromatous leprosy. J Infect Dis 1985;151:9-14.
147. de Vries RR, Mehra NK, Vaidya MC, et al. HLA-linked control of susceptibility to tuberculoid leprosy and association with HLA-DR types. Tissue Antigens 1980;16:294-304.
148. Dessoukey MW, el-Shiemy S, Sallam T. HLA and leprosy: Segregation and linkage study. Int J Dermatol 1996;35: 257-64.
149. Rani R, Fernandez-Vina MA, Zaheer SA, et al. Study of HLA class II alleles by PCR oligotyping in leprosy patients from North India. Tissue Antigens 1993;42:133-37.
150. Zerva L, Cizman B, Mehra NK, et al. Arginine at positions 13 or 70-71 in pocket 4 of HLA-DRB1 alleles is associated with susceptibility to tuberculoid leprosy. J Exp Med 1996;183:829-36.
151. de Vries RR, Fat RF, Nijenhuis LE, et al. HLA-linked genetic control of host response to Mycobacterium leprae. Lancet 1976;2:1328-30.
152. Fine PE, Wolf E, Pritchard J, et al. HLA-linked genes and leprosy: A family study in Karigiri, South India. J Infect Dis 1979;140:152-61.
153. Xu KY, de Vries RR, Fei HM, et al. HLA-linked control of predisposition to lepromatous leprosy. Int J Lepr Other Mycobact Dis 1985;53:56-63.
154. Shaw MA, Donaldson IJ, Collins A, et al. Association and linkage of leprosy phenotypes with HLA class II and tumour necrosis factor genes. Genes Immun 2001;2: 196-204.
155. Shiina T, Hosomichi K, Inoko H, et al. The HLA genomic loci map: Expression, interaction, diversity and disease. J Hum Genet 2009;54:15-39.
156. Rajalingam R, Singal DP, Mehra NK. Transporter associated with antigen-processing (TAP) genes and susceptibility to tuberculoid leprosy and pulmonary tuberculosis. Tissue Antigens 1997;49:168-72.
157. Tosh K, Ravikumar M, Bell JT, et al. Variation in MICA and MICB genes and enhanced susceptibility to paucibacillary leprosy in South India. Hum Mol Genet 2006;15:2880-87.
158. Sadek M, Yue FY, Lee EY, et al. Clinical and immunologic features of an atypical intracranial mycobacterium avium complex (MAC) infection compared with those of pulmonary MAC infections. Clin Vaccine Immunol 2008;15:1580-89.
159. Spies T, Bresnahan M, Bahram S, et al. A gene in the human major histocompatibility complex class II region controlling the class I antigen presentation pathway. Nature 1990;348:744-47.
160. Steinle A, Li P, Morris DL, et al. Interactions of human NKG2D with its ligands MICA, MICB, and homologs of

160. the mouse RAE-1 protein family. Immunogenetics 2001;53:279-87.
161. Das H, Groh V, Kuijl C, et al. MICA engagement by human Vgamma2Vdelta2 T cells enhances their antigen-dependent effector function. Immunity 2001;15:83-93.
162. Wang LM, Kimura A, Satoh M, et al. HLA linked with leprosy in Southern China: HLA-linked resistance alleles to leprosy. Int J Lepr. Other Mycobact Dis 1999;67:403-08.
163. Mootoo A, Stylianou E, Arias MA, et al. TNF-alpha in tuberculosis: A cytokine with a split personality. Inflamm. Allergy Drug Targets 2009;8:53-62.
164. Lin PL, Plessner HL, Voitenok NN, et al. Tumor necrosis factor and tuberculosis. J Investig Dermatol Symp Proc 2007;12:22-25.
165. Knight JC, Kwiatkowski D. Inherited variability of tumor necrosis factor production and susceptibility to infectious disease. Proc Assoc Am Physicians 1999;111:290-98.
166. Bopst M, Garcia I, Guler R, et al. Differential effects of TNF and LT-alpha in the host defense against M. bovis BCG. Eur J Immunol 2001;31:1935-43.
167. Jacobs M, Brown N, Allie N, et al. Fatal Mycobacterium bovis BCG infection in TNF-LT-alpha-deficient mice. Clin Immunol 2000;94:192-99.
168. Sarno EN, Santos AR, Jardim MR, et al. Pathogenesis of nerve damage in leprosy: Genetic polymorphism regulates the production of TNF alpha Lepr Rev 2000;71 Suppl:S154-S158.
169. Blackwell JM, Black GF, Peacock CS, et al. Immunogenetics of leishmanial and mycobacterial infections; The Belem Family Study. Philos Trans R Soc Lond B Biol Sci 1997;352:1331-45.
170. Franceschi DS, Mazini PS, Rudnick CC, et al. Influence of TNF and IL10 gene polymorphisms in the immunopathogenesis of leprosy in the South of Brazil. Int J Infect Dis 2008.
171. Roy S, McGuire W, Mascie-Taylor CG, et al. Tumor necrosis factor promoter polymorphism and susceptibility to lepromatous leprosy. J Infect Dis 1997;176:530-32.
172. Vejbaesya S, Mahaisavariya P, Luangtrakool P, et al. TNF alpha and NRAMP1 polymorphisms in leprosy. J Med Assoc Thai 2007;90:1188-92.
173. Santos AR, Suffys PN, Vanderborght PR, et al. Role of tumor necrosis factor-alpha and interleukin-10 promoter gene polymorphisms in leprosy. J Infect Dis 2002;186:1687-91.
174. Bikmaeva AR, Sibiriak SV, Valiakhmetova DK, et al. [Polymorphism of the tumor necrosis factor alpha gene in patients with infiltrative tuberculosis and from the Bashkorstan populations]. Mol Biol (Mosk) 2002;36:784-87.
175. Vejbaesya S, Chierakul N, Luangtrakool P, et al. NRAMP1 and TNF-alpha polymorphisms and susceptibility to tuberculosis in Thais. Respirology 2007;12:202-06.
176. Correa PA, Gomez LM, Anaya JM. [Polymorphism of TNF-alpha in autoimmunity and tuberculosis]. Biomedica 2004;24 Suppl 1:43-51.
177. Schurr E, I Kramnik. Genetic control of host-susceptibility to tuberculosis. In Handbook of Tuberculosis. Kaufmann SHE, WJ Britton, editors. Wiley-VCH, Weinheim 2008; 305-46.
178. Casanova JL, Abel L. Genetic dissection of immunity to mycobacteria: The human model. Annu Rev Immunol 2002;20:581-620.
179. Quintana-Murci L, Alcais A, Abel L, et al. Immunology in natura: Clinical, epidemiological and evolutionary genetics of infectious diseases. Nat Immunol 2007;8:1165-71.
180. Alcais A, Mira M, Casanova JL, et al. Genetic dissection of immunity in leprosy. Curr Opin Immunol 2005;17:44-48.
181. Skamene E, Gros P, Forget A, et al. Genetic regulation of resistance to intracellular pathogens. Nature 1982;297:506-09.
182. Buu N, Sanchez F, Schurr E. The Bcg host-resistance gene. Clin Infect Dis 2000;31 Suppl 3:S81-S85.
183. Vidal SM, Malo D, Vogan K, et al. Natural resistance to infection with intracellular parasites: Isolation of a candidate for Bcg. Cell 1993;73:469-85.
184. Gruenheid S, Gros P. Genetic susceptibility to intracellular infections: Nramp1, macrophage function and divalent cations transport Curr Opin Microbiol 2000; 3:43-48.
185. Jabado N, Jankowski A, Dougaparsad S, et al. Natural resistance to intracellular infections: Natural resistance-associated macrophage protein 1 (Nramp1) functions as a pH-dependent manganese transporter at the phagosomal membrane. J Exp Med 2000;192:1237-48.
186. Gallant CJ, Malik S, Jabado N, et al. Reduced in vitro functional activity of human NRAMP1 (SLC11A1) allele that predisposes to increased risk of pediatric tuberculosis disease. Genes Immun 2007;8:691-98.
187. Bellamy R, Ruwende C, Corrah T, et al. Variations in the NRAMP1 gene and susceptibility to tuberculosis in West Africans. N Engl J Med 1998;338:640-44.
188. Greenwood CM, Fujiwara TM, Boothroyd LJ, et al. Linkage of tuberculosis to chromosome 2q35 loci, including NRAMP1, in a large aboriginal Canadian family. Am J Hum Genet 2000;67:405-16.
189. Schurr E. Is susceptibility to tuberculosis acquired or inherited? J Intern Med 2007;261:106-11.
190. Malik S, Abel L, Tooker H, et al. Alleles of the NRAMP1 gene are risk factors for pediatric tuberculosis disease. Proc Natl Acad Sci USA 2005;102:12183-188.
191. Abel L, Sanchez FO, Oberti J, et al. Susceptibility to leprosy is linked to the human NRAMP1 gene. J Infect Dis 1998;177:133-45.
192. Meisner SJ, Mucklow S, Warner G, et al. Association of NRAMP1 polymorphism with leprosy type but not susceptibility to leprosy per se in west Africans. Am J Trop Med Hyg 2001;65:733-35.
193. Alcais A, Sanchez FO, Thuc NV, et al. Granulomatous reaction to intradermal injection of lepromin (Mitsuda reaction) is linked to the human NRAMP1 gene in Vietnamese leprosy sibships. J Infect Dis 2000;181:302-08.

194. Ranque B, Alter A, Mira M, et al. Genomewide linkage analysis of the granulomatous Mitsuda reaction implicates chromosomal regions 2q35 and 17q21. J Infect Dis 2007; 196:1248-52.
195. Piemonti L, Monti P, Sironi M, et al. Vitamin D3 affects differentiation, maturation, and function of human monocyte-derived dendritic cells. J Immunol 2000;164: 4443-51.
196. D'Ambrosio D, Cippitelli M, Cocciolo MG, et al. Inhibition of IL-12 production by 1,25-dihydroxyvitamin D3. Involvement of NF-kappaB downregulation in transcriptional repression of the p40 gene. J Clin Invest 1998;101:252-62.
197. Liu PT, Stenger S, Li H, et al. Toll-like receptor triggering of a vitamin D-mediated human antimicrobial response. Science 2006;311:1770-73.
198. Uitterlinden AG, Fang Y, van Meurs JB, et al. Genetics and biology of vitamin D receptor polymorphisms. Gene 2004;338:143-56.
199. Selvaraj P, Chandra G, Jawahar MS, et al. Regulatory role of vitamin D receptor gene variants of Bsm I, Apa I, Taq I, and Fok I polymorphisms on macrophage phagocytosis and lymphoproliferative response to mycobacterium tuberculosis antigen in pulmonary tuberculosis. J Clin Immunol 2004;24:523-32.
200. Bellamy R, Ruwende C, Corrah T, et al. Tuberculosis and chronic hepatitis B virus infection in Africans and variation in the vitamin D receptor gene. J Infect Dis 1999;179:721-24.
201. Bornman L, Campbell SJ, Fielding K, et al. Vitamin D receptor polymorphisms and susceptibility to tuberculosis in West Africa: A case-control and family study. J Infect Dis 2004;190:1631-41.
202. Olesen R, Wejse C, Velez DR, et al. DC-SIGN (CD209), pentraxin 3 and vitamin D receptor gene variants associate with pulmonary tuberculosis risk in West Africans. Genes Immun 2007;8:456-67.
203. Alagarasu K, Selvaraj P, Swaminathan S, et al. 5' regulatory and 3' untranslated region polymorphisms of vitamin D receptor gene in south Indian HIV and HIV-TB patients. J Clin Immunol 2009;29:196-204.
204. Selvaraj P, Chandra G, Sunil Mathan, Kurian Reetha AM, Narayanan PR. Association of vitamin D receptor gene variants of BsmI, and FokI polymorphism with susceptibility or resistance to pulmonary tuberculosis. Current Science 2003;8:1564-68.
205. Selvaraj P, Alagarasu K, Harishankar M, et al. Regulatory region polymorphisms of vitamin D receptor gene in pulmonary tuberculosis patients and normal healthy subjects of south India. Int J Immunogenet 2008;35: 251-54.
206. Wilbur AK, Kubatko LS, Hurtado AM, et al. Vitamin D receptor gene polymorphisms and susceptibility M tuberculosis in native Paraguayans. Tuberculosis 2007;87:329-37.
207. Wilkinson RJ, Llewelyn M, Toossi Z, et al. Influence of vitamin D deficiency and vitamin D receptor polymorphisms on tuberculosis among Gujarati Asians in West London: A case control study. Lancet 2000;355: 618-21.
208. Roy S, Frodsham A, Saha B, et al. Association of vitamin D receptor genotype with leprosy type. J Infect Dis 1999;179:187-91.
209. Flores-Villanueva PO, Ruiz-Morales JA, Song CH, et al. A functional promoter polymorphism in monocyte chemoattractant protein-1 is associated with increased susceptibility to pulmonary tuberculosis. J Exp Med 2005;202:1649-58.
210. Thye T, Nejentsev S, Intemann CD, et al. MCP-1 promoter variant -362C associated with protection from pulmonary tuberculosis in Ghana, West Africa. Hum Mol Genet 2009;18:381-88.

Chapter 23

MHC and Non-MHC Genes in Tuberculosis and Leprosy

Narinder K Mehra, Paras Singh, Prashant Sood, Gurvinder Kaur

INTRODUCTION

Infectious diseases represent a major health problem worldwide, both in terms of morbidity and mortality. Rapid advances in genomics and a growing appreciation of the potential of biomarkers in medicine and molecular targets of intervention have necessitated the need to further delineate genetic susceptibility parameters in defined mycobacterial infections like leprosy and tuberculosis. The two mycobacterial diseases have been the scourge of humanity since antiquity and continue to be major public health problem even in the 21st century. Although evolutionary selection pressure has equipped our immune system to defend and eradicate the innumerable pathogens constantly attempting to invade the human body, a few like the mycobacteria have evolved to achieve greater genetic fitness, evade the host immune system and circumvent intracellular destruction. In >90% of infected individuals the host-mycobacterial interaction results in containment of disease whereby the pathogen is rendered metabolically quiescent and is prevented from propagation and dissemination. The remaining individuals however develop progressive and even fulminant disease. This inter-individual variability in susceptibility to infection and clinical disease spectrum is believed to be a consequence of variations in the host immune response genes.

New information emerging from genomics and high-throughput sequencing has generated unprecedented opportunities for defining the genetic basis of susceptibility to complex diseases. This is of particular relevance to mycobacterial infections, permitting genetic dissection of the anti-mycobacterial immunity leading to new vistas of preventive and therapeutic measures. It is known that only a subset of individuals exposed to the mycobacterial pathogens ultimately go on to develop clinical disease and even among them there is a great variability of disease expression across a broad clinical spectrum. Accordingly, the outcome of infection is controlled to a large extent by the host determined factors that influence the initial infection and the type of immune response that develops subsequently. A clear understanding of the genetic determinants that may influence host susceptibility/resistance is desirable for deciphering the mechanisms underlying disease pathogenesis. While important major genes have been identified through genome scan of multi-case affected families; mouse genetics has also contributed significantly in mapping and identification of several other genes. Similarly, a large majority of known susceptibility loci has emerged from screening of likely candidate genes. The emerging picture is of highly polygenic diseases, with a few major genes, along with significant inter-population heterogeneity. This complex genetic architecture reflects the role that evolutionary selection has played in generating and maintaining a diverse repertoire of susceptibility/resistance loci, most with individually small effects. Genome-wide association studies with large sample sizes could help unravel other relevant genes and the interaction among them. This chapter presents a comprehensive review of the genetic aspects of *M. leprae* as well as *M. tuberculosis* infection, the role of immune response genes linked with the major histocompatibility complex (MHC) as well as other candidate genes including non-MHC and positional genes identified through genome wide studies.

DISEASE BURDEN

Tuberculosis (TB) also referred to as the "captain of death" affects more than 9.2 million people globally every year, and exacts a toll of nearly 1.3 million annually.[1] The WHO Global Tuberculosis Control report 2009 reveals that India, China, Indonesia, Nigeria and South Africa shoulder the highest incidence of TB worldwide. The epidemic of HIV has added fuel to fire and has created new populations of individuals highly susceptible to TB. Of the 9.2 million persons affected by TB in 2007, nearly 1.4 million (14.8%) were HIV-positive and this resulted in 456,000 deaths from TB among HIV-positive individuals. The growing menace of multi-drug resistant tuberculosis also contributes to the escalating death toll due to this disease. Current surveillance data from the WHO reports 511,000 cases of MDR-TB from 113 countries, with the highest burden in India, China, South Africa and the Russian Federation.

The prevalence of leprosy on the other hand stands at 212,802 cases, spread over 118 countries and territories, with 254,525 new cases detected in 2007 alone. The number of new cases detected globally has fallen by 11,100 cases (a 4% decrease) during 2007 compared with 2006 but it continues to remain a public health problem in at least 24 countries and a cause of severe disability in many parts of the world.[2] In 1981, India recorded a prevalence of 57.6 cases per 10,000 population, with a total burden of 2.91 million cases, and a dismal leprosy elimination area-population of only 12.92 million. Since the inception of National Leprosy Eradication Program (NLEP) in the year 1983, spectacular success has been achieved in reducing the disease burden. The goal of leprosy elimination as a public health problem was achieved at the National level by December 2005, and the prevalence of leprosy in India has come down to 0.72 cases per 10,000 population with a total burden of 83,000 cases. The leprosy elimination area-population has increased to a landmark 897.03 million. Nevertheless, this must be viewed with caution because during 2006-07, of the nearly 139,000 new leprosy cases detected, 45% were of the multibacillary type.[3]

HOST GENETIC DETERMINANTS

Evidence that host genetic factors contribute to susceptibility to leprosy and TB comes from epidemiological data, family segregation analysis and twin studies.[4-6] The goal of identification of host genetic factors that underlie susceptibility to leprosy can be approached in at least two ways: *firstly*, candidate gene studies on genes of known function that have a possible biological role in the control of infection or disease. A *second* approach utilizes a non-targeted genome-wide linkage analysis, in which increased sharing of chromosomal regions by affected individuals leads to identification of positional candidates. Although mechanisms underlying *M. leprae* targeting of Schwann cells, and killing of the bacteria in macrophages have not been fully elucidated, several hypotheses have been put forward. It is possible that host genes influence these processes and thus the outcome of infection. In this context, a battery of genes including those that may modulate innate immunity (Killer immunoglobulin like receptors or KIRs), cell-mediated immune response (MHC genes, cytokines/chemokines and their receptors) as well as other candidate genes (TLRs, NRAMP1, PACRG, PARK2) have been investigated. In addition, there are a host of others that have been reported to govern susceptibility to leprosy *per se*. Table 23.1 summarizes the current status of genes implicated in leprosy and tuberculosis suggesting them to be multigenic diseases.

PATHOGENESIS OF MYCOBACTERIAL INFECTIONS

The generic name *Mycobacterium* was introduced by Lehmann and Neumann in 1896.[38] The organisms were named so because of the mold like (*myco*: fungus; *bacterium*: bacteria) pellicular growth of these organisms in liquid medium. The true bacterial nature of these organisms was, however soon established. The genus *Mycobacterium* is the only genus in the family Mycobacteriaceae and order Actinomycetales. The guanine + cytosine (G+C) ratio in the deoxyribonucleic acid (DNA) of mycobacteria is 62 to 70 mol percent. Mycobacteria have been classified in a variety of ways but a more practical, clinical classification is given in Table 23.2.

The genus *Mycobacterium* consists of a diverse group of acid-fast, alcohol-fast, aerobic bacilli that are characterized by a high lipid content and slow growth. The genus contains >50 well-defined species, most of which are non-pathogenic saprophytes. Species can be differentiated using various microbiological, biochemical and molecular genetic techniques. The major pathogenic mycobacterial species include *M. tuberculosis*, which causes tuberculosis (TB) and is directly responsible for more deaths worldwide than any other pathogen, and *M. leprae*, which causes leprosy.

Table 23.1: Leprosy and tuberculosis are multigenic diseases: Gene loci implicated in mycobacterial susceptibility have been grouped into (i) Those that control immune responsiveness (ii) Candidate genes that control susceptibility per se and (iii) Genome wide scan suggesting involvement of other genes

Genes/locus	Chromosome location	Main function of protein encoded/ immune function of gene product(s)	Disease	References
Gene controlling immune response				
MHC class II (DR2)	6p21.3	Immune response genes	TB, leprosy	7-15
Cytokine genes	On different chromosomes	Immune response genes	TB, leprosy	16
SLC11A1	2q35	Acquired antibacterial immunity (Divalent cation transporter)	TB and leprosy	17, 18
C4B	6p21.3	Opsonization and immune complex clearance	Leprosy	19
CTL4A	2q31-33	Negative regulator of T cell activation	Leprosy	20
Col3A	2q31-33	Extracellular matrix structural constituent	Leprosy	20
Candidate genes/marker Controlling Susceptibility				
HSPA1A	6p21.3	Heat shock protein	Leprosy	21
MICA	6p21.3	Augment T cell activation	Leprosy	22
CCL2	17q11.2-q12	Monocyte chemoattractant protein-1 chemokine	TB	23
P2X7	12q24	ATP receptor	TB	24
DC-SIGN	19p13.3	C-type lectin receptor on dendritic cells	TB	25
TAP2	6p21.3	Peptide translocation	TB, Leprosy	26
TNFα	6p21.3	Pleiotropic both innate and acquired immunity	Leprosy	18, 27
VDR	12q12-14	Suppression of inflammation	TB, Leprosy	15, 28
TLR2	4q32	Role in pathogen recognition and activation of innate immunity	TB, Leprosy	15, 29, 30
PARK2, PACRG	6q25	E3 polyubiquitin ligase	Leprosy	31, 32
Genome wide scan				
	10p13	-	Susceptibility to Leprosy	33
	20p12	-	Susceptibility to leprosy	34
	6q25, 10p13	-	Susceptibility and severity of leprosy	35
	17q11	-	Paucibacillary leprosy	36, 37

Table 23.2: Classification of mycobacteria based on their function and species specificity

Group 1: Obligate pathogens	*Mycobacterium tuberculosis* *Mycobacterium leprae* *Mycobacterium bovis*
Group 2: Skin pathogens	*Mycobacterium marium* *Mycobacterium ulcerans*
Group 3: Opportunistic pathogens	*Mycobacterium kansasii* *Mycobacterium avium intracellulare* (MAIC)
Group 4: Non- or rarely pathogenic	*Mycobacterium gordonae* *Mycobacterium smegmatis*
Group 5: Animal pathogens	*Mycobacterium paratuberculosis* *Mycobacterium lepraemurium*

The Etiological Agents: *M. leprae* versus *M. tuberculosis*

Several remarkable characteristics distinguish *M. leprae* from most other human bacterial pathogens, such as an unusually long generation time, an optimal growth temperature between 27-30°C and a notorious resistance to grow in artificial media. The unique characteristics of *M. leprae* can be better understood in light of the finding that the bacterium displays remarkable reductive evolution. The recently published complete genome sequence of *M. leprae* has provided evidence for extensive genomic downsizing and rearrangement, making it a highly specialized obligate intracellular parasite. Importantly, the loss of genes involved in crucial metabolic pathways provides an appealing explanation for the difficulties encountered to cultivate the bacterium, as well as its slow duplication. A comparison of the *M. leprae* genome with that of its close relative *M. tuberculosis* suggests that it has undergone an extreme reductive evolution, which is reflected by its smaller genome (~3.3 Mb vs. 4.4 Mb) and a major reduction in G+C content (58% vs. 66%). Further, *M. leprae* annotated genome contains only 1,614 open reading frames potentially encoding functional proteins, compared to 3,993 open reading frames predicted in *M. tuberculosis*. One of the most striking features of *M. leprae* genome is that it possesses 1,133 inactivated genes (genes lost through mutation, or pseudogenes), compared to only six pseudogenes in *M. tuberculosis*. In addition, a large number of genes apparently have been entirely deleted from the genome. The result of this massive gene loss leaves *M. leprae* with < 50% of its genome encoding functional genes, compared to *M. tuberculosis*, in which 90% of the genome encodes functional genes. Interestingly, 34% of *M. leprae* proteins identified in silico appear to be the products of gene duplication events or share common domains.[39]

A detailed study of *M. leprae* provides important comparative lessons for tuberculosis. Although *M. tuberculosis* isolates are strikingly homogenous at the level of primary nucleotide sequence, insertion and deletion events provide evidence of significant genome plasticity. There is considerable interest in the possibility that these changes impact on clinical and epidemiological manifestations of tuberculosis, with the number of deletions in a particular isolate seen to correlate with ability to cause cavitary disease. Viewing these events in the context of the more extreme genetic changes in *M. leprae* will help in understanding their mechanisms and biological relevance in *M. tuberculosis*. Leprosy represents a classical example of the way in which the host response influences the course of infection and provides an exciting challenge to understanding the genetics of disease susceptibility. Studies to date suggest that different disease phenotypes result from variations at multiple genetic loci, each making some small contribution to susceptibility, rather than any single dominant determinant.[39]

Clinical Spectrum and Disease Progression

M. leprae Infection

The pathogenesis of leprosy can be described as a two stage process (Figs 23.1A and B). In the first stage, individuals who are intrinsically susceptible to leprosy are infected by *M. leprae*. Such infection may develop into a single skin lesion (*indeterminate leprosy*) that often remains undetected and in most individuals may heal by itself. Those individuals who do not self heal and are not treated, progress to the second stage: A spectrum of clinical forms of leprosy that ranges from localized to severe, systemic disease. Collectively, these individuals are described as susceptible to leprosy *per se*, i.e. leprosy regardless of the type of clinical manifestation. The variability of the clinical presentation of the disease relates to the type of immune response presented by the host, with the localized forms being associated with a stronger cell-mediated, Th1 immune response, and the systemic forms being associated with a predominantly humoral, Th2 immune response. A classic classification system proposed in 1966 by Ridley and Jopling, states five groups of leprosy spanning the entire disease spectrum: Tuberculoid (TT), borderline tuberculoid (BT), mid borderline (BB), borderline lepromatous (BL) and lepromatous (LL) leprosy. More recently, a treatment-oriented system suggested by the WHO classifies leprosy patients into two groups: I) those presenting with a single skin lesion with scanty or no bacilli are classified as single-lesion *paucibacillary* (PB) cases. A subtype in PB leprosy includes all cases presenting five or fewer skin lesions and; II) patients presenting six or more skin lesions with detectable *M. leprae* are classified as multibacillary leprosy (MB). When comparing the two systems, the single and multi-lesion PB patients are generally equivalent to the TT + BT, while MB patients represent BB + BL +LL disease of the Ridley Jopling system.

Clinical manifestations of leprosy occur mainly in the skin and most importantly, peripheral nerves, with sensorial loss, physical deformities and permanent nerve damage being common findings.[40] The hallmark of the disease is the presence of one or more macular, often dry,

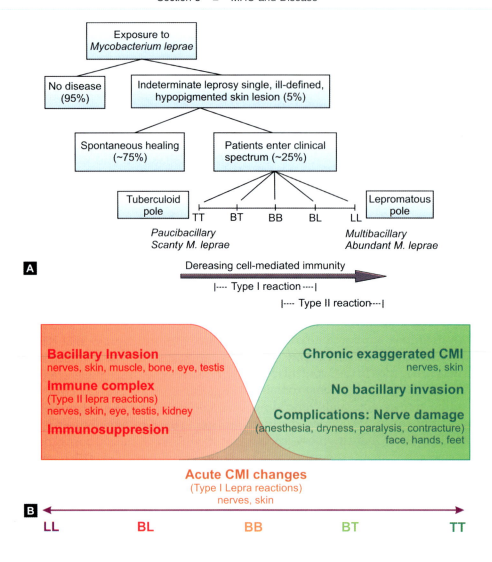

Figs 23.1A and B: Clinico-immunological spectrum of leprosy. A: Flowchart depicts the progression of leprosy from initial exposure to full blown disease which is further subdivided into various clinical types depending on the host immune response. B: Elaborates the interplay of host immune response to *M. leprae* and the consequent disease manifestations, emphasizing the importance of host immunity in determining the fate of *M. leprae* infection

hypopigmented or erythematous anaesthetic skin lesions with sharp, well defined margins. While TT/ BT patients present few skin lesions with no detectable bacilli and often neural affection detectable near the lesions, BB patients present lesions intermediate in number and size between TT and LL forms. BL/LL cases are characterized by numerous small skin lesions and widespread nerve damage. Deformities of hands and feet are common, and if untreated, lepromatous leprosy may slowly progress to bacteremia. Death due directly to leprosy is uncommon, and is usually a result of a complication such as laryngeal obstruction.

M. tuberculosis Infection

Epidemiological evidence suggests that protective immunity against *M. tuberculosis* exists in most exposed humans. The proportion of non-immunocompromised individuals who undergo primary infection or reactivation disease following *M. tuberculosis* infection is low. Only 5-10% of *M. tuberculosis*–infected individuals develop tuberculosis during their lifetime. The study of human immunity to *M. tuberculosis* infection is critical to the understanding of the mechanisms that contain the initial tuberculous focus and maintain clinical latency.

Tubercle bacilli are transmitted from person to person by aerosol infection. The percentage of individuals becoming infected varies, mainly depending on environmental conditions, frequency of exposure and concentration of mycobacteria in the air, but is in general considered very low. Of the infected individuals, >90% successfully contain the infection by virtue of an efficient immune response. Replication and dissemination of the pathogen are restricted by mononuclear phagocytes, while T cells recruited to the site of primary infection help to contain the bacilli. In an attempt to avoid direct confrontation with the host immune defense, M. tuberculosis successively retards its replication rate and transforms into a dormant state (dormant M. tuberculosis is defined as being in a state of low replication and strongly reduced metabolic activity). Thus, approximately one third of the world's population, i.e. 2 billion people, is latently infected with the pathogen. Latent tuberculosis is used here to describe mycobacterial infection that does not present any clinical symptoms and is restricted to a contained primary site of infection harboring intact but dormant mycobacteria. The immune system is not able to clear the mycobacteria from the host. The bacilli remain dormant until the balance between mycobacterial persistence and the immune response gets disturbed and leads to reactivation and disease.[41]

Disease Progression

Progression to clinical disease shows great inter-individual variation following infection with the two most common mycobacteria. A dramatic illustration of this variable response was provided by the accidental immunization of children with a virulent strain of M. tuberculosis in 1926 in Lübeck, Germany. Of the 251 children who received the same dose of mycobacteria, 72 died within 1 yr, 175 developed radiological signs of the disease, while the remaining four showed no detectable disease. In natural conditions of infection, it is generally estimated that only 10% of individuals infected by M. tuberculosis actually develop clinical tuberculosis[42] while the proportion of subjects infected by M. leprae who will develop symptomatic leprosy is likely to be lower. Although the most common expression of tuberculosis is pulmonary, which can be more or less severe, the disease can involve numerous extra-pulmonary sites and thus have lymphatic, pleural, meningeal, bone, peritoneal, and other localization. Leprosy patients also display a wide spectrum of disease that is correlated with their immunological response.[40]

At one extreme of this spectrum, patients with specific tuberculoid leprosy show well-developed specific cellular responses with low M. leprae antibody levels and lesions that are paucibacillary, whereas, at the other extreme, lepromatous patients have poorly developed specific cellular responses, high antibody levels and multibacillary lesions.

HOST IMMUNE RESPONSE TO MYCOBACTERIAL INFECTIONS

Effective control of TB requires the generation of antigen-specific T-cell responses, activation of infected macrophages and formation of granulomatous lesions to wall off infected macrophages and prevent dissemination of the bacilli.[43] Macrophages play multiple roles during mycobacterial infection since they are not only the key antigen presenting cells (APCs) but also act as the inadvertent principal hosts for intracellular replication of mycobacteria. Mycobacterial phagocytosis by macrophages is mediated through the mannose (MR) and complement receptors of later these and other dendritic cells (DC) are activated through the toll-like receptors (TLR) borne by them. The latter comprise a family of mammalian cell-surface proteins that stimulate pro-inflammatory cytokine gene transcription and DC maturation on binding to pathogen-associated molecules. Of the 11 known TLR genes, TLR2 is involved in the recognition of the mycobacterial lipoproteins, lipoarabinomannan and phosphatidylinositolmannan. Mycobacteria have evolved efficient mechanisms to enhance their survival within macrophages. These include maturation arrest of mycobacteria-containing phagosomes, prevention of phagosome acidification[44] and inhibition of phagolysosomal fusion.[45]

The immunological control of M. tuberculosis infection is dependent on the activity of CD4+ T cells. Differentiation of these cells into Th1 cells is promoted by MHC class II-restricted mycobacterial antigen presentation as well as the early cytokine milieu, which includes IL-12, IL-18 and IL-23.[46] This milieu is partially induced through the activation of TLR2.[47, 48] The Th1 response results in the production of IFN-γ, which promotes phagosomal maturation and the production of antimycobacterial molecules, such as reactive oxygen and nitrate intermediates.[49] Other cytokines, particularly the tumor necrosis factor (TNF) are also important in the formation and maintenance of granulomas.[50] By cross-priming, mycobacterial antigens can also access the MHC class I pathway and activate CD8+ T cells. These cells can kill mycobacteria through the action of granulysin and perforin.[51] CD8+ T cells can also lyse infected macrophages and facilitate the translocation of mycobacteria from incapacitated cells to the more proficient effector cells.[52]

Mycobacterium leprae has the unique property of tropism for macrophages, particularly the Schwann cells. Once inside the Schwann cell, the leprosy bacilli replicate slowly over a period of years, although the exact mechanism of this persistence remains largely unclear. Specific T cells recognize the presence of mycobacterial antigens within the nerve and initiate a chronic inflammatory reaction. Schwann cells express HLA class II molecules and are able to present mycobacterial peptides to HLA class II restricted CD4+ T cells.

Genetic Contribution to the Immune Response

Twin studies strongly suggest that genetic factors play a significant role in modulating the immune response to infectious agents.[53, 54] This is in contrast to many autoimmune diseases, where concordance among monozygotic twins is almost always <50% suggesting a more significant role of environmental factors in autoimmune disease pathogenesis. For this reason, much interest has been generated on the possible contribution of host genetic factors to the often diverse clinical manifestations seen in infectious diseases. Besides the intrinsic virulence of a mycobacterial species and socioeconomic factors, the large inter-individual variability of clinical outcome observed among exposed individuals is thought to result, to a large extent, from variability in the genes that control host defense. This was first shown in animal models in the context of experimental infections by different mycobacteria species.[55] More recently, this was also demonstrated in humans with the identification of the syndrome of *Mendelian susceptibility to mycobacterial disease* (MSMD) owing to infection by poorly virulent mycobacteria. All humans are exposed to water- or air-borne environmental mycobacteria (EM) and approx 85% of children in the world are inoculated with the live BCG vaccine. Generally, these species do not cause any disease, but in some rare individuals localized or disseminated disease has been diagnosed. So far, different types of mutations in five genes involved in interferon-γ (IFN-γ)-mediated immunity (*IFNGR1*, *IFNGR2*, *STAT1*, *IL12B*, and *IL12RB1*) have been identified (Discussed in detail in Chapter 22), leading to the first demonstration that genetic defects could cause severe mycobacterial infections in humans. It is worthwhile to note that some mutations in the genes *IFNGR1* and *IFNGR2* leading to incomplete defects of corresponding IFN-γ receptors are responsible for much less severe clinical phenotypes, consistent with the view that IFN-γ mediated immunity is a continuous trait. This may regulate, at least in part, the outcome of host-mycobacterial interactions.[56]

In contrast, the genetic control of common mycobacterial infections is expected to be more complex, and the genes involved are expected to exert a less deleterious effect than in MSMD. Several studies have demonstrated that a person's resistance level to *M. tuberculosis* infection correlates with the region of his/her ancestry. For example, the incidence of tuberculosis has been shown to be particularly high during outbreaks in populations with no ancestral experience of the infection, such as Native Americans. Further, Black populations have greater susceptibility to tuberculosis than their white counterparts, probably because the disease has been endemic in Europe for a much longer period and survivors are likely to be more resistant individuals.[57] Other convincing sources of evidence came from familial aggregation studies and those conducted on twins. The latter reported much higher concordance rates among monozygotic than dizygotic pairs for both clinical tuberculosis[54] as well as leprosy.[4] Finally, several segregation analyses have provided convincing evidence that susceptibility to leprosy must have a significant genetic component. In particular, a study conducted on Desirade Island in the French West Indies showed that a major recessive major gene controlled susceptibility to leprosy *per se* regardless of the clinical subtype.[58]

Two Stage Model of Leprosy Immunopathogenesis

It is clear that only a small fraction of persons exposed to *M. leprae* ultimately develop leprosy. Molecular nature of the genetic component has consistently identified HLA region genes as the major susceptibility factor. In addition, genome-wide scan has identified a susceptibility locus on chromosome region 10p13 in Indian families[33] and another one conducted in Brazil suggesting an important role of 6p21[35] and 17q22 regions.[36, 37] *M. leprae* specific immune reactions, histopathology of lesions and response to treatment are strikingly different between pauci- and multibacillary patients. A critical, unknown question is whether pauci- and multibacillary leprosy develop as two entirely different pathologies from the onset of infection or develop as subtypes as the infection progresses. This question has direct bearing on the enrolment of patients and the design of any leprosy genetics study.

Following close contact with a leprosy patient, the contact person may be infected with *M. leprae*, most likely via the respiratory route, leading to clinical manifestation of the disease, either multibacillary or paucibacillary. By definition, all forms of leprosy are categorized as "*leprosy per se.*" Assuming that all patients share a common initial non-symptomatic stage of pathogenesis, this stage can be considered as the manifestation of the leprosy per se phenotype. The two-stage model of leprosy pathogenesis is supported by the genetic findings that have identified genes that act only on leprosy per se and a second set of genes that influence and control immune response and hence act as risk factors for the development of specific clinical forms. For example, PARK2/PACRG variants are risk factors for leprosy per se while a locus on chromosome 10p13 is a risk factor for paucibacillary leprosy (Fig. 23.2). Allelic variants within the MHC which in humans is the HLA system can be risk factors for pauci- or multibacillary forms of leprosy. It is not known if this so defined "leprosy per se" stage imposes a commitment on the patient to advance to one of the clinical forms of leprosy, or if it represents a distinct stage of disease arrest that by necessity needs additional stimuli to trigger and advance to clinical disease. The prevalence of non-symptomatic *leprosy per se* patients is not known but may be substantial and we propose that such patients may contribute to leprosy transmission.

A two-stage process of disease has direct implications for the design of genetic studies aiming to identify genes that are risk factors for leprosy per se. Assuming that clinically defined leprosy patients represent only a subgroup of leprosy per se patients – those who received a necessary second hit – traditional (clinical) case control studies will suffer from a lack of power since a sizeable proportion of apparently unaffected controls may indeed be non-symptomatic leprosy per se cases. In such a scenario, family-based association designs are expected to be substantially more powerful.

METHODS TO STUDY INFLUENCE OF GENES ON HUMAN DISEASE

Two study designs have traditionally been used to identify human susceptibility genes for complex traits including TB, according to the groups studied. Firstly, population-based association studies search for genetic differences between individuals who have the disease (cases) compared to those who do not (controls). The second approach involves family-based 'linkage' studies that aim to detect genetic similarities in affected family members. Each approach has its benefits and drawbacks. In association studies, large number of cases and controls are recruited, and this approach has the power to detect relatively small gene effects. However, it is important

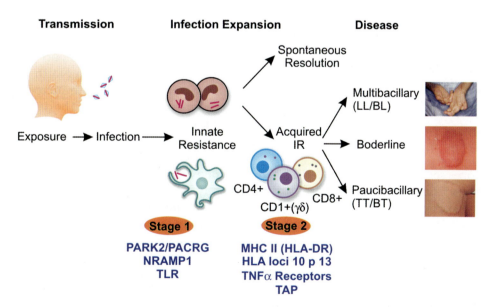

Fig. 23.2: Two stage model of genetic influence on human immunity to *M. leprae*. Following exposure to the infectious agent a set of genes, (e.g. PARK2/PACRG) influence development of leprosy *per se*. However, a second set of genes (represented by HLA loci and other genes) influence the host immune response, and hence the clinical staging of the disease [Adapted from Ref. 59)

that cases and controls are properly matched for their ethnicity and socio-economic status. Linkage analysis requires a reasonably good cohort of families in order to obtain a significant result. Such families should have more than one affected sib, at least one healthy sib and both parents available for haplotype analysis. More often than not, such families are uncommon and hence vast majority of studies involving genetics of infectious diseases have been the association studies.

Essentially, two methodological approaches have been employed to investigate the involvement of specific genes in a disease. These include the candidate gene approach and the genome wide scanning. The former targets specific gene(s), implicated in disease pathogenesis, and this could be studied for defining linkage in families or an association at the population level. Genome wide scan, on the other hand, is currently limited to family-based linkage studies. Polymorphic markers across the whole genome are studied on family members and when co-inheritance of markers with the trait occurs, the marker is said to be *linked* to the disease. This approach has the capacity to identify new genes that are important in disease pathogenesis but so far undiscovered.[60]

Infectious diseases pose an additional problem of poor reproducibility of results across populations. This could be due to the relatively small sample size for analysis in most studies, inadequate information on the ethnic status, methodology and technology issues and faulty statistical procedures. Involvement of environmental factors in addition to the host factors in mycobacterial diseases suggests that unless bigger cohorts are included for analysis, the observed genetic associations could only be modest. Clinical heterogeneity of patients in various studies is a further confounding factor which may explain differences in the observed associations.

HLA ASSOCIATION STUDIES IN MYCOBACTERIAL DISEASES

Table 23.3 summarizes some of the prominent HLA and disease associations. The MHC is considered to be associated with any particular disease, if one or more alleles are increased or decreased significantly in patients when compared with ethnically matched healthy controls. However, the underlying mechanisms for most disease associations are still poorly understood. Accumulating evidence suggests a direct disease related role for polymorphic HLA proteins, whereby they recognize peptide motif signatures and allow/prohibit their binding to antigen-binding groove. An increasing number of HLA-binding motifs are being discovered for several autoimmune and infectious agents. One main limitation in identifying primary determinants within the MHC, however, is the linkage disequilibrium that keeps several genes linked together on a haplotype. Generally, it is more difficult to demonstrate a negative association of MHC with a disease. These associations vary greatly among populations and defined ethnic groups.

Several investigators have searched for an association of mycobacterial diseases with either HLA class I (HLA-A, -B,-C)[61,62] or class II (HLA-DR,-DQ) antigens.[13,14] Particularly in Asian Indians, strong association of HLA-DR2 and its two most common molecular subtypes, both (DRB*1501 and DRB*1502) has been reported in leprosy.[8,10,14,63-65] The first report in tuberculosis came from a study conducted in North India by our group demonstrating a moderate increase of HLA-DR2 in sporadic patients with PTB. The data was also confirmed in multiplex family studies suggesting a DR2 linked control of susceptibility to the disease.[66] Almost all published studies on HLA and tuberculosis have involved patients with pulmonary tuberculosis and only scantly information is available regarding other clinical forms of the disease including extrapulmonary disease. Our group investigated HLA association across various clinical subgroups including pulmonary TB, multi-drug resistant TB (MDR-TB), miliary/disseminated TB and lymph node TB. Molecular subtyping of polymorphic DRB1 alleles revealed that in addition to the increased occurrence of DR2 subtypes, a positive association of specific DR6 subtype was noticed in different clinical forms of tuberculosis, particularly DRB1*1301 in patients

Table 23.3: Prominent HLA and disease associations observed in most populations

Disease	HLA association
Type 1 diabetes	Susceptibility: DQB1*0201, *0302; DRB1*0301; *0401, *0404. Protection: DQB1*06, some DRB1*04 (e.g. *0403)
Ankylosing spondylitis	B*27 (most alleles except *2706)
Rheumatoid arthritis	Specific alleles of DRB1*04 (*0401, *0404, *0405), *0101
HIV	HLA-B*35, HLA-B*27, HLA-B*57
Narcolepsy	DRB1*1501-DQA1*0102-DQB1*0602 haplotype
Celiac disease	DQA1*0501-DQB1*02, to a lesser extent DQB1*0302
Mycobacterial infections (leprosy and TB)	DRB1*1501/02, *1404

with pulmonary TB (PTB and MDR-TB) and DRB1*1302 in extrapulmonary TB (M/DTB and LNTB). A detailed clinical and immunogenetic analysis repeated that in addition to the poor past compliance to treatment and presence of higher number of cavities in the chest radiographs, presence of HLA-DRB1*14 allele in patients with pulmonary TB acts as an independent predictor for the development of MDR-TB.[67]

The population frequency of HLA alleles in the North Indian population has revealed that two alleles, namely DRB1*1501 and DRB1*1502 constitute >90% of the DR2 alleles in this population. Other alleles such as DRB1*1506 and DRB1*1602 are represented at much decreased frequencies. DRB1*1601 occurred in only 4% of DR2+ healthy controls. Studies carried out both in North as well as South India have indicated a population association of DRB1*1501(rather than other subtypes of DR2) with patients of tuberculosis.[68] Sequence analysis of the DRB1 first domain residues has disclosed that only one amino acid variation can discriminate the products of DRB1*1501 from DRB1*1502 and DRB1*1601 from DRB1*1602. Particularly DRB1*1501 carries *valine* at aminoacid position 86 while it is substituted with *glycine* in DRB1*1502. Similarly, DRB1*1601 subtype has the aromatic amino acid phenylalanine at position 67 which is substituted by aliphatic leucine in DRB1*1602. Studies on pulmonary tuberculosis did not favor a preferential involvement of any of these common subtypes of DR2 suggesting that the whole DR2 molecule or its closely linked gene(s) may be involved in governing susceptibility to pulmonary tuberculosis and the expression of its various clinical forms. However, analysis of DR2 subtypes and the differences in radiographic severity based on the extent of lung lesions (UL, UE, BL and BE) revealed an increased trend in the frequency of DRB1*1501 as the pulmonary severity increased from the unilateral limited disease (49% in UL vs 55% in controls) to bilateral extensive (82% in BE vs. 55% in controls) lung lesions. Similar trends have been observed in leprosy suggesting inverse relationship of V^{86}/G^{86} as the disease severity progressed from paucibacillary to the BL/LL multibacillary leprosy type.[69]

Knowledge on the three dimensional crystallography structure of the human class II HLA molecule has revealed that residues at position 67 and 86 of the α-helix of the β-chain are actively involved in the binding of a foreign peptide. Accordingly, the peptide binding and subsequent immune triggering capability of the host depends critically on these single amino acid variants. It is possible that DRB1*1501 and 1502 alleles may be selectively implicated in the presentation of pathogenic mycobacterial peptides leading to the development of pulmonary tuberculosis.

In depth sequence analysis of the HLA associated alleles has been carried out on Indian patients with leprosy as well TB patients by our group. These studies have yielded crucial information on critical sites in the peptide-binding groove of the DR molecule that affects peptide binding and/or T cell interaction in immune response against mycobacteria.[70] A large majority of leprosy patients (87%) carry specific alleles of DRB1 characterized by *positive* charged residues Arg^{13} or Arg^{70} or Arg^{71} as compared to 43 percent controls conferring a relative risk of 8.8. Thus, susceptibility to tuberculoid leprosy involves three critical amino acid positions of the β-chain, the side chains of which when modeled on the DR1 crystal structure, line a pocket (Pocket 4) accommodating the side chain of a bound peptide. Characteristically, pocket 4 is formed by the side chains of aminoacids $α^9$, $β^{13}$, $β^{70}$, $β^{71}$, $β^{74}$ and $β^{78}$. Substitutions of any of these can affect the local charge. For example, presence of positive charged Arg at position ^{13} or Arg at position ^{70} or ^{71} will probably accommodate the binding of a negatively charged residue of the same foreign peptide (Fig. 23.3).

On the basis of physicochemical properties, particularly on the amino acid charges in these positions, the HLA class II molecules can be further grouped into four different DR-restricted supertypes. Each of these supertypes includes a group of alleles with the similar anchor residues during MHC-peptide interaction. In support to this hypothesis, presence of promiscuous T cell epitopes recognized by several different HLA-DR molecules has been well established.[71] Thus, based on the polymorphism in charged residues at positions 70, 71 and 74, we classified HLA-DRB1 alleles into four major supertypes namely i) positively charged (with Q70, K/R71, A74) ii) negatively charged with (D70, E71, A74) iii) di –charged (positive/negative) (with D/R70, R71, A/L/E/Q74) and iv) no charged/neutral charged (with Q70, A71, A74) allele groups.[72] Based on this classification, an analysis of the DRB1 alleles revealed that "pocket 4" motifs with positive charge (Q70, K/R71, A74) or neutral charge (Q70, A71, A74) residues at position 70, 71 and 74 of DR β chain play an important role in influencing susceptibility to *M. leprae* infection and disease manifestation to various clinical forms. This is in contrast to the situation in tuberculosis where negative charge (D70, E71, A74) or neutral charge (Q70, A71, A74) in "pocket 4' increase the risk to acquire the infection.

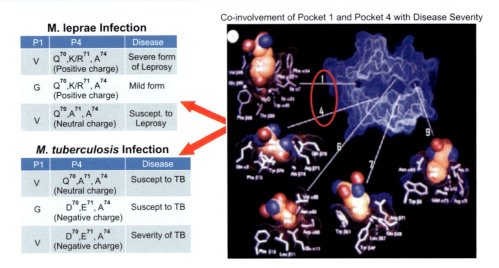

Fig. 23.3: Crystallographic representation of MHC Class II molecule showing peptide binding motifs and involvement of 'pocket 4' and 'pocket 1' residues in controlling disease susceptibility and severity. Note difference in 'pocket 4' net charge in tuberculosis and leprosy whereas 'pocket 1' residues affect disease severity similarly in both diseases

Further, the result of our study analyzed by including the supertypes based on the pocket 1 region suggest that patients with V86 in the DR β chain along with negatively or no charged (neutral) pocket 4 motifs are at higher risk to develop more severe tuberculosis disease by either inducing anergy or insufficient immune response to *M. tuberculosis* infection. From the results, it implies that the negatively charged or neutral charged pocket-4 binding motifs of DRB1 alleles may be responsible for the initial infection with *M. tuberculosis* and subsequent development of localized pulmonary disease. On the other hand, presence of valine at codon 86 of DRβ chain in association with these pocket 4 binding motifs may increase the complexity or severity of the disease by causing poor binding of the DRB1 alleles with *M. tuberculosis* antigens.

According to the leprosy model, it is likely that peptides originating from *M. leprae* bind preferentially to HLA allelic forms characterized by *arginine* at positions 13 or 70-71 and stimulate particular T cell-clones that result in detrimental immune response as seen in tuberculoid leprosy. Identification of peptide motifs that bind different allelic forms associated with disease would contribute significantly to the search for mycobacterial antigenic determinants that initiate this response.

It is hypothesized that net positive or neutral charges in binding 'pocket 4' cause poor binding of the DRB1 molecule to *M. leprae* antigens. As HLA molecules with the highest affinity to peptides produce the greatest T-cell proliferation and IFN-γ response,[73] peptide presentation by low affinity class II molecules may result in muted cell-mediated immunity.[74] Alternatively, peptide presentation by specific class II molecules may result in activation of suppressor/regulatory T cells that might be correlated with disease severity.

NON-HLA GENES IN MYCOBACTERIAL INFECTIONS

Most HLA associations with diseases and relative risk conferred by a particular HLA antigen/allele differ among various populations and this can be attributed to the assumption that in polygenic diseases, there can be more than one-pathway and involvement of other candidate genes. The combination of such genes and their polymorphic forms favor investigations into a possible role of non-HLA/MHC polymorphic gene variants. These include transporter associated with antigen processing (TAP), tumor necrosis factor α and β (TNF α and β), mannose binding lectin (MBL), vitamin D receptor (VDR), natural resistance associated macrophage protein (NRAMP1) genes and interleukin-1 receptor antagonists (IL-1RA). Further, a genome wide scan of various genes in mycobacterial diseases could provide crucial information on the involvement of non-HLA genes in governing susceptibility to these diseases. Beside MHC, a number of non-HLA genes have been implicated in leprosy susceptibility. Studies carried out in various ethnic groups on this set of genes are summarized in Table 23.4. Further, relevant studies for each non-HLA gene have been discussed, except those on NRAMP 1 (SLC11A1), which has been dealt with in Chapter 22.

Table 23.4: Non–HLA candidate gene variants associated with susceptibility/ resistance to tuberculosis and leprosy

Gene	Population	SNP/Haplotype	Phenotype	Reference
VDR	Indian	Codon 352 (TT)	Susceptibility to LL	28
		Codon 352 (CC)	Susceptibility to TT	
	Malawi	Codon 352 (CT)	Protection from leprosy & TB	78
		Codon 352 (CC)	Susceptibility to Leprosy & TB	
CR1	Malawi	K1590E (GG)	Protection or susceptibility to lepromatous	78
TNF	Indian	-308A	Susceptibility to lepromatous form, TB	27
	Brazilian	-308A	Protection to leprosy per se Multibacillary forms	79, 80
	Malawi	-238/-308/-376/-863	No association	78
	Brazil	-819T	Susceptibility	80
	Brazil	-3575A/-2849G/-2763C	Protection against Leprosy per se and Multibacillary forms	81
IL10	Indian	-3575T/-2849A/-2763C	Susceptibility	16
		-3575T/-2849G/ -2763C/-1082A/ -819C/-592C5	Protection	
	Malawi	-592/-819/-1082	No association	78
IL12RB2	Japan	-1035G/-1023G/-464G	Susceptibility	82
COL3A1	India	250bp	Susceptibility	20
CTLA4	India	CTLA4 size allomorphs	Protection from MB	20
HSPA1A	India	HSPA1A	PB	21
TAP2	North India	TAP1 I333V, N637G,TAP2: V379L, A565T, A665T	PB(TAP-2B)	26
C4B	Brazil	C4B, C2, BF, C4A, C4B*Q0	ENL	19
TLR2	Korea	R677W	MB	29
SLC11A1	India	Promoter microsatellite, Exon 2, 469+14G/C, (TGTG)n	No association (Leprosy and TB)	28
SLC11A1	Mali	Promoter microsatellite, 469+14G/C, (TGTG)n	TGTG het.	17

Amongst the non-HLA genes, combined occurrence of TAP2 along with HLA-DR2 and their association with susceptibility to pulmonary tuberculosis has been reported.[26] Similarly, an association with haptoglobin 2-2 phenotype has been shown in Russian patients,[75] although, this could not be corroborated in Indonesians[76] and Indian patients.[77] Genome-wide linkage studies on sib-pairs of families affected with the tuberculosis has led to the identification of several candidate genes, some of which show association with the susceptibility to tuberculosis.

Tumor Necrosis Factor (TNF-α)

TNF-α is a cytokine that plays multiple roles in immune responses against TB. Mice deficient in TNF have been observed to have severe susceptibility to tuberculosis and are unable to form protective granulomas.[83] M. tuberculosis induces TNF secretion by macrophages, DC and T cells.[84] TNF along with IFN-γ induces nitric oxide synthetase-2 expression in macrophages and studies have also noted disseminated TB as a complication of TNF neutralizing therapy in rheumatoid arthritis.[85] Many of the described polymorphisms in the TNF promoter may be involved in the regulation of TNF expression. The -308 TNF promoter polymorphism (a G/A transition known as TNF2) was associated with increased TNF levels in some studies[86] but not in others.[87] The TNF2 allele was associated with MB leprosy in Bengali Indians,[27] whereas in Brazil this allele was found to be protective against MB leprosy.[88] No association has been found between pulmonary TB and TNF2 in populations from Cambodia and Brazil.[89]

Interferon-gamma (IFN-γ)

IFN-γ is crucial for host defense against mycobacteria. An SNP in intron 1 (1874A/T) lies within a binding site for the transcription factor NFkB. The 1874T and the 1874A alleles correlate with high and low IFN-γ expression, respectively. In a South African colored population, the1874A allele was associated with an increased risk of TB (OR 1.64).[90] Another study from Spain corroborated the above findings and reported an increased susceptibility to TB in individuals homozygous for the 1874A polymorphism over wild-type individuals (OR 3.75).[91] Interestingly although no Mendelian mutations predisposing to severe mycobacterial infections have yet been found in IFN-γ, an SNP has been defined which predisposes to TB in the general population. On the other hand null mutations in IFN-γR1 have been described, that predispose to mycobacterial infections, but no association has been noted with the common polymorphisms in the gene and mycobacterial diseases.[92]

Heat Shock (70 kDa) Protein 1A

The heat shock (70 kDa) protein 1A (HSPA1A) gene is located in the class III region of the MHC, between the genes for TNF and C2. One of three 70 kDa heat shock proteins encoded in this region, HSPA1A is expressed constitutively at a low-level and its expression is increased in response to thermal stress. Antigenic peptides can associate with heat shock proteins, leading to their uptake and presentation by APC. Furthermore, HSP70 activates macrophages by induction of pro-inflammatory cytokine production by the Myd88/NFkB pathway.[93] An allele in the HSPA1A gene was found to be associated with PB leprosy in a small North Indian study.[21] Further studies are warranted to explore the precise role played by this gene in susceptibility to mycobacterial infections.

Interleukin-1Rα (IL-1Rα)

Experiments in mice models have highlighted the importance of IL-1 signaling in the control of pulmonary TB. Studies have also noted a significant elevation of IL-1b levels in the bronchoalveolar lavage fluid of TB patients, suggesting its contribution to lung inflammation. The antagonist IL-1 receptor-a (IL-1Ra) competes for the IL-1 receptor and down regulates the pro-inflammatory response to Il-1b. Analysis of an 86 bp variable nontandem repeat (VNTR) in intron 2 of IL-1Rá showed that allele 2, which consists of two 86 bp repeats, was associated with a 1.9-fold higher level of IL-1Rα production than in nonallele-2 carriers.[94] The allele 2 of IL-1Rα was found to be significantly less frequent in TB patients from Gambia (OR 0.45; P 0.09).[95] But on the other hand no association was evident when IL-1Rα polymorphisms were assessed in Gujarati Indian patients suffering from TB.

IL-12 and IL-12 Receptor

Remus and co-workers,[96] in their study on Moroccan TB patients found a strong linkage disequilibrium between two IL-12RB1 promoter polymorphisms pulmonary tuberculosis. Further, Tso et al[97] noted that Chinese individuals resident in Hong Kong have a significantly increased risk of TB when they are homozygous for an IL-12p40 intron 2 repeat marker. Certain diplotypes of IL-12p40 in this population rendered them susceptible to TB, whereas others conferred protection against TB. Hence, it appears that there is a gradation of genetic defects in the IL-12/IFN-γ axis that ranges from rare Mendelian null mutations predisposing to severe overwhelming infections with less virulent mycobacteria to more common polymorphisms that exert detectable, but less pronounced, effects on the genetic control of TB in the general population.

Pulmonary Surfactant Proteins

Pasula and co-workers demonstrated that the pulmonary surfactant protein SP-A aids *M. tuberculosis* to latch onto murine alveolar macrophages,[98] whereas Ferguson et al found that SP-D agglutinates mycobacteria and reduces their phagocytosis by the macrophages.[99] Such observations have prompted investigation into the genes encoding these pulmonary surfactant proteins. The SP-A locus consists of two genes, SP-A1 and SP-A2. In a small case-control study of Mexican subjects, allele 1A of the SP-A2 gene, 6A allele of the SP-A1 gene and the DA11_C of the SP-D gene were found to be overrepresented in TB patients (OR 9.28, 2.71, and 1.57, respectively).[100]

P2X7 Receptor

The P2X7 receptor (P2X7), a member of the purinergic family of receptors, is a ligand-gated cation channel with two transmembrane domains and a trimeric structure in the plasma membrane. Treatment of mycobacteria-infected macrophages with ATP activates P2X7, resulting in an influx of calcium, which leads to the death of both the host cell and the internalized bacilli.[101] This mycobacterial killing occurs through the activation of phospholipase-D2 and the subsequent promotion of phagolysosomal fusion.[102] Heterogeneity of ATP-induced killing of BCG was shown in a small number of patients, suggesting possible genetic differences in P2X7. A Gambian study showed a weakly protective effect against pulmonary TB for a polymorphism in the putative promoter (OR 0.70).[103] Subjects with loss-of-function SNP in P2X7 show reduced ATP-mediated apoptosis and mycobacterial killing[104] and more extensive studies are required to determine if these SNP predispose to TB.

The PARK2/PACRG Genes

Studies by Erwin Schurr's group from Montreal, Canada have shown conclusively that *PARK2/PACRG* genes, originally shown to be linked to Parkinson's disease and expressed on chromosome 6q25, could also be strong leprosy *per se* susceptibility markers. These proteins are an integral component of the cellular proteasome ubiquitination system that is involved in protein degradation. In addition, PARK2, an E3-ubiquitin ligase is known to have an important role in intracellular signaling including induction of apoptosis. The PARK2/PACRG variability provides an instructive example for the power of unbiased genome-wide forward genetics approaches in the study of complex traits like mycobacterial infections.

A recent genome-wide scan has resulted in the first successful positional cloning of genetic variants that may play a major role in controlling susceptibility to leprosy. Genome-wide, non-parametric linkage analysis was performed on 86 multiplex leprosy families from South Vietnam presenting similar proportion of MB and PB cases. Strong evidence for linkage was obtained for chromosomal region 6q25-q27, with a maximum multipoint LOD score of 4.31 (P= 2.5×10^{-4}).[35] In their subsequent study, an independent population of 197 Vietnamese simplex families was recruited and investigated in order to construct a high resolution association map of the 6q25-q27 candidate region. Detailed association mapping led to the identification of 17 SNPs associated with leprosy per se susceptibility in the Vietnamese population. Linkage disequilibrium (LD) analysis of the candidate region showed that 15 of the 17 associated SNPs were located on a single LD block of 80 kb spanning a regulatory region shared by two genes, an autosomal recessive juvenile Parkinsonism (AR-JP) gene (Parkin/PARK2) and the Parkin co-regulated gene (PACRG).[31] Similar results were obtained on Indian leprosy subjects.

GENOME SCREENS

Development of high throughput genotyping technologies and identification of thousands of polymorphic microsatellite markers have made genome-wide linkage studies an attractive proposition for defining the relevant region of interest. This approach has the advantage that no disease model or prior knowledge of the structure, function or location of the disease gene is required. The chromosomal region identified by this approach is initially much larger than that utilized for an association study (several megabases compared to a few hundred kilobases) nevertheless, fine mapping and subsequent identification of the relevant genes is greatly aided greatly by the release of the draft human genome sequence. The genome-wide approach has the additional advantage that genes of unknown function and those not previously suspected as possible candidates can also be identified.

The two genome screens performed in tuberculosis and leprosy have been based on affected sib-pair linkage studies. The first study was conducted on pulmonary tuberculosis (PTB) in families originating from Gambia (85 sibpairs) and South Africa (88 sib-pairs).[105] Most affected subjects had smear-positive pulmonary disease and the remaining patients were diagnosed using clinical and X-ray criteria. No region of the genome showed significant evidence for linkage, ruling out the presence of a gene with a strong effect on tuberculosis in these families. In particular, no linkage was found with the regions containing the *NRAMP1* and *VDR* genes for which associations were previously reported in the Gambian population,[106, 107] indicating that those genes did not have a major effect on PTB in this population. Two other regions located on chromosome 15q ($P < 0.001$) and Xq ($P < 0.005$) provided only suggestive evidence for linkage.

The use of genomic scans in leprosy has the ability to uncover a region/gene not apparently associated with disease to be tested as candidate genes. This is a great advantage in the study of complex diseases, especially leprosy in which low mortality rates enable the collection of samples from several generations, which is necessary in this kind of a test. Table 23.5 summarizes various studies performed that define genetic linkage and chromosomal location of relevant genes in leprosy through genome wide scan approach.

The second genome screen involved 245 leprosy affected sib-pairs from South India.[33] Patients were

Table 23.5: Genetic linkage studies in leprosy using genomic wide scan approach

Gene/ Region	Population	Phenotype Observed	Reference
10p13	Indian	Susceptibility	33
20p12	Indian	Susceptibility	34
6q25, 10p13	Vietnamese	Susceptibility, severity (paucibacillary form)	35
17q11	Brazilian	Susceptibility	36, 3

diagnosed using WHO guidelines and all siblings except four were affected by paucibacillary leprosy. Significant evidence for linkage ($P < 2 \times 10^{-5}$) was found with chromosome 10p13 indicating that a gene located within this region can have a substantial influence in paucibacillary leprosy. Surprisingly, no linkage was observed with the HLA region, whereas several previous sibpair studies, including those in South India, provided some evidence for HLA-linked genes playing a role in paucibacillary/tuberculoid leprosy.

Chromosomal Regions 10p13 and 20p12

The first genome wide scan of leprosy susceptibility was performed in a collection of paucibacillary families obtained from the endemic regions of the states of Tamil Nadu and Andhra Pradesh, in India. In a two-step approach the authors first genotyped 103 sib pairs and their parents for 388 microsatellite markers covering the entire genome. Non-parametric sib pair linkage analysis identified 21 chromosomal regions showing weak evidence for linkage with leprosy susceptibility (LOD score> and equal 1.0). Next, 37 additional markers covering these 21 regions were genotyped in an independent sample of 142 sib pairs. Significant evidence for linkage was obtained only for the chromosomal region 10p13, with a multipoint maximum LOD score of 3.52. Finally, eight additional markers on chromosome 10p13 were investigated bringing the maximum LOD score to 4.09 ($P < 2 \times 10^{-5}$).[33] The finding of strong linkage between the 10p13 region and paucibacillary leprosy (but not leprosy per se or other forms of clinical disease), was confirmed by a second genome scan performed in a Vietnamese population.[35] In a follow up study, further analysis of the 185 sib pairs of the Tamil Nadu sub-set of the Indian population identified significant linkage between leprosy and chromosomal region 20p12, with a single point maximum LOD score of 3.48 (P =0.00003).[34] Curiously, multipoint analyses resulted in a lower maximum LOD score of 3.16. In addition, no significant linkage was observed after multipoint analysis when the families from Andhra Pradesh were included. Although encouraging, these findings should be interpreted carefully since paucibacillary leprosy cannot be taken as representative of all clinical forms of the disease.

Chromosomal Region 6q25-q27

Recent positional cloning of the PARK2/PARCG polymorphisms, points to variants shared by these two genes as major contributors for the linkage effect observed between leprosy per se and the 6q25-q27 region.[31] However, positive association between leprosy and alleles of both a microsatellite and SNP markers located upstream of the PARK2/PACRG regulatory locus suggests the presence of additional candidate genes for leprosy susceptibility in this chromosomal location. Further fine mapping of the genomic sequence underlying linkage peak is necessary for complete elucidation of the impact of genes located in the 6q25-q27 chromosomal region on leprosy susceptibility.

Chromosomal Region 17q11-q21

The most recent genome-wide scan for leprosy genes was conducted on a collection of 71 extended, multiplex Brazilian leprosy families. The authors report suggestive evidence for linkage between the 17q11-q21 region and leprosy susceptibility. The linkage signal was distributed in two peaks, with a maximum LOD score of 2.67 (P =0.004). Families presenting the LL phenotype contributed most to one of the peaks. Unfortunately, the number of leprosy trios was insufficient for family based association analysis. The same paper reports weak evidence for linkage between the 20p13 region and leprosy (LOD score 1.51, P = 0.004), a region located 3.5 Mb distal to that reported in the Indian study.[36]

INNATE IMMUNITY TO MYCOBACTERIAL INFECTIONS

During the innate immune response, pathogen-associated molecular patterns displayed on many microorganisms are recognized by *pattern recognition receptors* expressed on immune cells at the sites of initial exposure. One class of pattern recognition receptors contains the calcium-dependent or C-type lectins, which bind specific carbohydrate moieties on pathogens and facilitates internalization for antigen processing and presentation. A second category of pattern recognition receptors is comprised of Toll like receptors. Engagement of these receptors can trigger release of antimicrobial products which can exert preliminary assault on the pathogen as well as signal expression of co-stimulatory molecules and production of cytokines which induce the adaptive immune system. Yet another class of receptors important for mycobacterial uptake relates to the complement receptors. The exact influence of these receptors is not fully elucidated as yet.

Role of Toll-like Receptors

Toll-like receptors (TLRs) are important polypeptides involved in the regulation of innate immune response regulation. Of the ten TLRs, TLR2 is able to respond to many microbial components, including mycobacterial lipoproteins and lipoarabinomannan[108, 109] and is thus important in generating a pro-inflammatory, protective immune response against mycobacteria.[110] In both mice and humans, TLR2 activation by *M. tuberculosis* lipoprotein leads to killing of the intracellular pathogen. While this process is nitric oxide (NO) dependent in mice, it is NO independent in humans.[111] Recent evidence suggests that genetic variations of TLRs could be involved in increased susceptibility to leprosy also. For example, a coding non-synonymous base pair substitution at nucleotide 2029 (Arg677Trp) of the TLR2 gene occurs in 10 out of 45 LL leprosy patients as compared to its complete absence in patients with TT leprosy or healthy controls.[29] Functional studies have suggested a possible role for TLR2 in controlling disease susceptibility and clinical progression of leprosy.[112, 113] It is noteworthy that despite attempts, Arg677Trp polymorphism favoring leprosy susceptibility has not been reported in leprosy. In fact, screening of an Indian population for the Arg677Trp variation led to the conclusion that the supposed functional mutation is actually located 23 kb upstream of TLR2, in a duplicated sequence sharing 93% homology with the exon 3 of the TLR2 gene.[114] Recently, 86 Korean leprosy patients were screened for polymorphisms in a highly conserved part of the TLR2 intracellular domain. No other polymorphisms were found in the region and it was hypothesized that the substitution may affect the intracellular signaling of TLR2. Another polymorphism of a conserved C-terminal arginine in TLR2 reduces NF kappa B activation in response to Gram-positive bacterial peptides and may be associated with susceptibility to staphylococcal infection.[115] Besides TLR2, no other TLRs have shown an association with leprosy susceptibility and/or resistance.

In pulmonary tuberculosis on the other hand, TLR4 polymorphism shows a positive association, particularly in patients who develop more severe disease as assessed by bacteriological and radiological criteria. In a study carried out by us at the AIIMS, SNP analysis of TLR promoter polymorphism revealed a positive correlation of TLR4 896 A/G (Asp 299 Gly) and 1196 C/T (Thr 399 Ile) gene variants with susceptibility, contributing to disease manifestation and modulating disease severity.[116]

PERSPECTIVES

Understanding the evolutionary impact of infectious diseases on the human genome and vice versa may shed light on the origin of recent or other common diseases. An important task is to develop vaccines and improved treatment strategies for major infectious diseases like leprosy, tuberculosis, HIV infection and AIDS, and malaria. It is now possible to screen the whole genome for genetic determinants that control susceptibility to such diseases and identify critical pathways of host defense and thus generate novel strategies for disease prevention. There are three important facets of research into a MHC based vaccine design: (i) Understanding of peptide-MHC molecular interactions, (ii) Identification of immunodominant T cell epitopes that can be presented by HLA molecules on the basis of maximum population coverage and (iii) Use of adjuvants that can selectively modulate MHC class I or class II mediated Th1 or Th2 responses, which is very important for protection against infectious diseases. MHC class I tetramers are being used extensively to track the responsive CD8+ T cytotoxic cells in autoimmune and infectious diseases. Likewise, the class II tetramers have been developed successfully to stain responsive CD4+ T cells in different immuno-pathological conditions. A number of transformed B cell lines expressing HLA molecules of interest have been created. Information on all of these could lead to a better understanding of the MHC-peptide interactions and for devising novel therapeutic strategies.

Thus far, genes suggested to have a role in influencing susceptibility to leprosy have been shown to act either by directly modulating of the adaptive immune response (HLA, MICA, TAP2, CTLA4, VDR), or may bridge the innate and adaptive responses (NRAMP1, TLR2, HSP70, TNFα, MRC1). Lack of correlation in results in other populations should not necessarily be regarded as a negation of initial associations but may instead reflect heterogeneity in the genetic susceptibility to this enigmatic disease. High throughput techniques to genotype large number of SNPs and statistical tools to organize and test this information are now available. The recruitment of large samples and correct choice of controls and patients is critical to better design and reliable results. The replication in different populations is also expected and the ultimate validation will only be achieved when the functional significance of epidemiologically associated SNPs/genes are discovered, which is essential to understanding leprosy immunopathogenesis and finally control the disease. It is quite possible that in the near future, these genetic tools will be used to better diagnose and treat patients as well as to help eradicate leprosy and TB.

REFERENCES

1. Global tuberculosis control: Epidemiology, strategy, financing, WHO report 2009. Report No: ISBN 978 92 4 156380 2.
2. WHO Weekly epidemiological record. 2008;83(33): 293-300.
3. National Leprosy Eradication Programme (NLEP) [homepage on the internet]. Annual report 2007; Available from http://nlep.nic.in/annual.html
4. Chakravartti MR, Vogel F. A twin study on leprosy. Top Hum Genet 1973;1: 1-123.
5. Haile RW, Iselius L, Fine PE, et al. Segregation and linkage analyses of 72 leprosy pedigrees. Hum Hered 1985;35: 43-52.
6. Feitosa MF, Borecki I, Krieger H, et al. The genetic epidemiology of leprosy in a Brazilian population. Am J Hum Genet 1995; 56:1179-85.
7. Kikuchi I, Zawa T, Hirayama K, Sasasuki T. An HLA-linked gene controls susceptibility to lepromatous leprosy through T-cell regulation. Lepr Rev 1986; 57(Suppl 2): 139-42.
8. de Vries RR, Fat RF, Nijenhuis LE, et al. HLA-linked genetic control of host response to *Mycobacterium leprae*. Lancet 1976;2:1328-30.
9. de Vries RR, van Eden W, Ottenhoff TH. HLA class-II immune response genes and products in leprosy. Prog Allergy 1985;36:95-113.
10. van Eden W, de Vries RR, Mehra NK, et al. HLA segregation of tuberculoid leprosy: Confirmation of the DR2 marker. J Infect Dis 1980;141(6):693-701.
11. van Eden W, de Vries RR, D'Amaro J, et al. HLA-DR-associated genetic control of the type of leprosy in a population from Surinam. Hum Immunol 1982;4: 343-50.
12. Gorodezky C, Alaez C, Munguia A, et al. Molecular mechanisms of MHC linked susceptibility in leprosy: Towards the development of synthetic vaccines. Tuberculosis 2004;84:82-92.
13. Mehra, NK. Role of HLA linked factors in governing susceptibility to leprosy and tuberculosis. Trop Med Parasitol 1990;41:352-54.
14. Mehra NK, Rajalingam R, Mitra DK, et al. Variants of HLA-DR2/DR51 group haplotypes and susceptibility to tuberculoid leprosy and pulmonary tuberculosis in Asian Indians. Int J Leprosy 1995;63(2):241-48.
15. Hill AV. Aspects of genetic susceptibility to human infectious diseases. Annu Rev Genet 2006;40:469-86.
16. Malhotra D, Darvishi K, Sood S, et al. IL-10 promoter single nucleotide polymorphisms are significantly associated with resistance to leprosy. Hum Genet 2005;118:295-300.
17. Meisner SJ, Mucklow S, Warner G, et al. Association of NRAMP1 polymorphism with leprosy type but not susceptibility to leprosy per se in west africans. Am J Trop Med Hyg 2001;65:733-35.
18. Hill AV. The genomics and genetics of human infectious disease susceptibility. Ann Rev Genomics Hum Genet 2001;2:373-400.
19. de Messias IJ, Santamaria J, Brenden M, et al. Association of C4B deficiency (C4B*Q0) with erythema nodosum in leprosy. Clin Exp Immunol 1993;92: 284-87.
20. Kaur G, Sachdeva G, Bhutani LK, Bamezai R. Association of polymorphism at COL3A and CTLA4 loci on chromosome 2q31–33 with the clinical phenotype and in-vitro CMI status in healthy and leprosy subjects: A preliminary study. Hum Genet 1997;100:43-50.
21. Rajalingam R, Mehra NK, Singal DP. Polymorphism in heatshock protein 70-1 (HSP70-1) gene promoter region and susceptibility to tuberculoid leprosy and pulmonary tuberculosis in Asian Indians. Indian J Exp Biol 2000; 38:658-62.
22. Tosh K, Ravikumar M, Bell JT, Meisner S, Hill AVS, Pitchappan R. Variation in MICA and MICB genes and enhanced susceptibility to paucibacillary leprosy in South India. Hum Mol Genetics 2006;15(19):2880-87.
23. Buijtels PCAM, van de Sande WWJ, Parkinson S, et al. Polymorphism in CC-chemokine ligand 2 associated with tuberculosis in Zambia. Int J Tuberc Lung Dis. 2008;12(12):1485-88.
24. Li CM, Campbell SJ, Kumararatne DS, et al. Association of a polymorphism in the P2X7 gene with tuberculosis in a Gambian population. J Infect Dis 2002; 186:1458-62.
25. Barreiro LB, Neyrolles O, Babb CL, et al. Promoter Variation in the DC-SIGN–Encoding Gene CD209 Is Associated with Tuberculosis. PLoS Med 2006 February;3(2):e20.
26. Rajalingam R, Singal DP, Mehra NK. Transporter associated with antigen-processing (TAP) genes and susceptibility to tuberculoid leprosy and pulmonary tuberculosis. Tissue Antigens 1997;49(2):168-72.
27. Roy S, McGuire W, Mascie-Taylor CG, et al. Tumor necrosis factor promoter polymorphism and susceptibility to lepromatous leprosy. J Infect Dis 1997; 176: 530-32.
28. Roy S, Frodsham A, Saha B, et al. Association of vitamin D receptor genotype with leprosy type. J Infect Dis 1999;179:187-91.
29. Kang TJ, Chae GT, et al. Detection of Toll-like receptor 2 (TLR2) mutation in the lepromatous leprosy patients. FEMS Immunol Med Microbiol 2001; 31(1):53-58.
30. Schroder, M. and Bowie, A.G, TLR3 in antiviral immunity: Key player or bystander? Trends Immunol 2005;26: 462-68.

31. Mira MT, Alcais A, VanThuc N, et al. Susceptibility to leprosy is associated with PARK2 - PACRG. Nature 2004;427:636-40.
32. Malhotra D, Darvishi K, Lohra M, et al. Association study of major risk single nucleotide polymorphisms in the common regulatory region of PARK2 and PACRG genes with leprosy in an Indian population. Eur J Hum Genet 2006;14(4):438-42.
33. Siddiqui MR, Meisner S, Tosh K, et al. A major susceptibility locus for leprosy on chromosome 10p13. Nat Genet 2001;27:439-41.
34. Tosh K, Meisner S, Siddiqui MR, et al. A region of chromosome 20 is linked to leprosy susceptibility in a South Indian population. J Infect Dis 2002;186:1190-93.
35. Mira MT, Alcais A, Van Thuc N, et al. Chromosome 6q25 is linked to susceptibility to leprosy in a Vietnamese population. Nat Genet 2003;33:412-15.
36. Miller EN, Jamieson SE, Joberty C, et al. Genome-wide scans for leprosy and tuberculosis susceptibility genes in Brazilians. Genes Immun 2004;5:63-67.
37. Jamieson SE, Miller EN, Black GF, et al. Evidence for a cluster of genes on chromosome 17q11-q21 controlling susceptibility to tuberculosis and leprosy in Brazilians. Genes Immun 2004;5:46-57.
38. Grange JM. Mycobacterial disease-a challenge to biotechnology. MIRCEN Journal 1985;1:1-21.
39. Cole ST, Eiglmeier K, Parkhill J, et al. Massive gene decay in the leprosy bacillus, Nature 2001;409(6823):1007-11.
40. Jacobson RR, Krahenbuhl JL. Leprosy. Lancet 1999; 353(9153):655-60.
41. Kaufmann SHE, Hanh H. Mycobacteria and TB. Issues in Infectious Diseases, Vol. 2. Basel (Switzerland): S Karger AG; 2003.
42. Bloom BR, Small PM. The evolving relation between humans and *Mycobacterium tuberculosis*. N Engl J Med 1998;338:677-78.
43. Saunders BM, Cooper AM. Restraining mycobacteria: Role of granulomas in mycobacterial infections. Immunol. Cell Biol 2000;78:334-41.
44. Sturgill-Koszycki S, Schlesinger PH, Chakraborty P, et al. Lack of acidification in Mycobacterium phagosomes produced by exclusion of the vesicular proton-ATPase. Science 1994;263:678-81.
45. Armstrong JA, Hart PD. Phagosome-lysosome interactions in cultured macrophages infected with virulent tubercle bacilli. Reversal of the usual nonfusion pattern and observations on bacterial survival. J Exp Med 1975;142:1-16.
46. Flynn JL, Chan J. Immunology of tuberculosis. Annu Rev Immunol 2001;19: 93-129.
47. Means TK, Wang S, Lien E, Yoshimura A, Golenbock DT, Fenton MJ. Human toll-like receptors mediate cellular activation by *Mycobacterium tuberculosis*. J Immunol 1999;163:3920-27.
48. Ladel CH, Szalay G, Riedel D, Kaufmann SH. Interleukin-12 secretion by *Mycobacterium tuberculosis*-infected macrophages. Infect Immun 1997;65:1936-38.
49. Schaible UE, Sturgill-Koszycki S, Schlesinger PH, Russell DG. Cytokine activation leads to acidification and increases maturation of Mycobacterium avium-containing phagosomes in murine macrophages. J Immunol 1998; 160: 1290-96.
50. Bean AG, Roach DR, Briscoe H, et al. Structural deficiencies in granuloma formation in TNF gene-targeted mice underlie the heightened susceptibility to aerosol *Mycobacterium tuberculosis* infection, which is not compensated for by lymphotoxin. J Immunol 1999; 162:3504-511.
51. Stenger S, Hanson DA, Teitelbaum R, et al. An antimicrobial activity of cytolytic T cells mediated by granulysin. Science 1998;282:121-5.
52. Kaufmann SHE. Immunity to infectious agents. In: Paul W (ed.) Fundamental Immunology, 4th edn. New York: Lippincott-Raven 1999:1335-71.
53. Kallmann FJ, Reisner D. Twin studies on the significance of genetic factors in tuberculosis. Am Rev Tuberc 1942; 47:549-74.
54. Comstock G. Tuberculosis in twins: A re-analysis of the Prophit study. Am Rev Respir Dis 1978;117:621-24.
55. Buu N, Sanchez F, Schurr E: The Bcg host-resistance gene. Clin Infect Dis 2000;31 Suppl 3:S81-S85.
56. Casanova JL, Abel L. Genetic dissection of immunity to mycobacteria: The Human Model. Annu Rev Immunol 2002;20:581-620.
57. Stead WW. Genetics and resistance to tuberculosis. Could resistance be enhanced by genetic engineering? Ann Intern Med 1992;116:937-41.
58. Abel L, Demenais F. Detection of major genes for susceptibility to leprosy and its subtypes in a Caribbean island: Desirade island. Am J Hum Genet 1988;42: 256-66.
59. Schurr E, Alcäis A, de Leseleuc L, Abel L. Genetic predisposition to leprosy: A major gene reveals novel pathways of immunity to *Mycobacterium leprae*. Sem Immunol 2006;18:404-10.
60. Bellamy R. Susceptibility to mycobacterial infections: the importance of host genetics. Genes Immun 2003; 4: 4-11.
61. Rajalingam R, Mehra NK, Mehra RD, et al HLA class I profile in Asian Indian patients with pulmonary tuberculosis. Indian J Exp Biol 1997;35:1055-59.
62. Balamurugan A, Sharma SK, Mehra NK. Human leukocyte antigen class I supertypes influence susceptibility and severity of tuberculosis. J Infect Dis 2004;189(5):805-11.
63. de Vries RR, Mehra NK, Vaidya MC, et al. HLA-linked control of susceptibility to tuberculoid leprosy and association with HLA-DR types. Tissue Antigens 1980;16:294-304.
64. Rani R, Fernandez-Vina MA, Zaheer SA, et al. Study of HLA class II alleles by PCR oligotyping in leprosy patients from north India. Tissue Antigens 1993;42(3):133-37.
65. van Eden W, Gonzalez NM, de Vries RR, et al. HLA-linked control of predisposition to lepromatous leprosy. J Infect Dis 1985;151(1):9-14.

66. Singh SP, Mehra NK, Dingley HB, Pande JN, Vaidya MC. Human leukocyte antigen (HLA)-linked control of susceptibility to pulmonary tuberculosis and association with HLA-DR types. J Infect Dis 1983;148(4):676-81.
67. Sharma SK, Turagaa KK, Balamurugan A, et al. Clinical and genetic risk factors for the development of multi-drug resistant tuberculosis in non-HIV infected patients at a tertiary care center in India: A case-control study. Inf Genetics and Evolution 2003;3(3):183-88.
68. Pitchappan RM. Castes, Migration, Immunogenetics and infectious diseases in South India. Community Genetics 2002;5:157-61.
69. Singh M, Balamurugan A, Katoch K, Sharma SK, Mehra NK. Immunogenetics of mycobacterial infections in the North Indian population. Tissue Antigens 2007;69(s1):228-30.
70. Zerva L, Cizman B, Mehra NK, et al. Arginine at positions 13 or 70-71 in pocket 4 of HLA-DRB1 alleles is associated with susceptibility to tuberculoid leprosy. J Exp Med 1996;183(3):829-36.
71. Ou D, Mitchell LA, Tingle AJ. HLA-DR restrictive supertypes dominate promiscuous T cell recognition: Association of multiple HLA-DR molecules with susceptibility to autoimmune diseases. J Rheumatol 1997;24(2):253-61.
72. Singh M. PhD thesis, All India Institute of Medical Sciences, New Delhi, India.
73. Agrewala JN, Wilkinson RJ. Influence of HLA-DR on the phenotype of CD4+ T lymphocytes specific for an epitope of the 16-kDa alpha-crystallin antigen of *Mycobacterium tuberculosis*. Eur J Immunol 1999 Jun; 29(6):1753-61.
74. Uko GP, Lu LY, Asuquo MA, et al. HLA-DRB1 leprogenic motifs in Nigerian population groups. Clin Exp Immunol 1999;118(1):56-62.
75. Kharakter ZZ, Mazhak KD, Pavlenko AV. The role of genetically determined haptoglobin phenotypes in patients with destructive pulmonary tuberculosis. Probl Tuberk 1990;7:50.
76. Grange JM, Kardjito T, Beck JS, Ebeid O, Kohler W, Prokop O. Haptoglobin: An immunoregulatory role in tuberculosis? Tubercle 1985;66:41.
77. Papiha SS, Singh BN, Lanchbury JSS, et al. Association of HLA and other genetic markers in south Indian patients with pulmonry tuberculosis. Tubercle 1987;68:159.
78. Fitness J, Floyd S, Warndorff DK, et al. Large-scale candidate gene study of leprosy susceptibility in the Karonga district of Northern Malawi. Am J Trop Med Hyg 2004;71:330-40.
79. Santos AR, Almeida AS, Suffys PN, et al. Tumor necrosis factor promoter polymorphism (TNF2) seems to protect against development of severe forms of leprosy in a pilot study in Brazilian patients. Int J Lepr Other Mycobact Dis 2000;68:325-27.
80. Santos AR, Suffys PN, Vanderborght PR, et al. Role of tumor necrosis factor-a and interleukin-10 promoter gene polymorphisms in leprosy. J Infect Dis 2002;186:1687-91.
81. Moraes MO, Pacheco AG, Schonkeren JJ, et al. Interleukin-10 promoter single-nucleotide polymorphisms as markers for disease susceptibility and disease severity in leprosy. Genes Immun 2004;5:592-95.
82. Ohyama H, Ogata K, Takeuchi K, et al. Polymorphism of the 50 flanking region of the IL-12 receptor beta2 gene partially determines the clinical types of leprosy through impaired transcriptional activity. J Clin Pathol 2005;58:740-43.
83. Bean AG, Roach DR, Briscoe H, et al. Structural deficiencies in granuloma formation in TNF gene-targeted mice underlie the heightened susceptibility to aerosol *Mycobacterium tuberculosis* infection, which is not compensated for by lymphotoxin. J Immunol 1999;162:3504-11.
84. Henderson RA, Watkins SC, Flynn JL. Activation of human dendritic cells following infection with *Mycobacterium tuberculosis*. J Immunol 1997;159:635-43.
85. Maini R, St Clair EW, Breedveld F, et al. Infliximab (chimeric anti-tumour necrosis factor alpha monoclonal antibody) versus placebo in rheumatoid arthritis patients receiving concomitant methotrexate: A randomised phase III trial. ATTRACT Study Group. Lancet 1999;354:1932-39.
86. Wilson AG, Symons JA, McDowell TL, McDevitt HO, Duff GW. Effects of a polymorphism in the human tumor necrosis factor alpha promoter on transcriptional activation. Proc Natl Acad Sci. USA 1997;94:3195-99.
87. Somoskovi A, Zissel G, Seitzer U, Gerdes J, Schlaak M, Muller Quernheim J. Polymorphisms at position -308 in the promoter region of the TNF-alpha and in the first intron of the TNF-beta genes and spontaneous and lipopolysaccharide-induced TNFalpha release in sarcoidosis. Cytokine 1999;11:882-7.
88. Santos AR, Suffys PN, Vanderborght PR, et al. Role of tumor necrosis factor-alpha and interleukin-10 promoter gene polymorphisms in leprosy. J Infect Dis 2002;186:1687-91.
89. Blackwell JM, Black GF, Peacock CS, et al. Immuno-genetics of leishmanial and mycobacterial infections: The Belem Family Study. Philos Trans R Soc Lond B Biol Sci 1997;352:1331-45.
90. Rossouw M, Nel HJ, Cooke GS, van Helden PD, Hoal EG. Association between tuberculosis and a polymorphic NFkappaB binding site in the interferon gamma gene. Lancet 2003;361:1871-72.
91. Lopez-Maderuelo D, Arnalich F, Serantes R, et al. Interferon-gamma and interleukin-10 gene polymor-phisms in pulmonary tuberculosis. Am J Respir Crit Care Med 2003;167:970-75.
92. Awomoyi AA, Nejentsev S, Richardson A, et al. No association between interferon-gamma receptor-1 gene polymorphism and pulmonary tuberculosis in a Gambian population sample. Thorax 2004;59:291-94.
93. Vabulas RM, Ahmad-Nejad P, Ghose S, Kirschning CJ, Issels RD, Wagner H. HSP70 as endogenous stimulus of the Toll/interleukin-1 receptor signal pathway. J Biol Chem 2002; 277:15 107-12.

94. Wilkinson RJ, Patel P, Llewelyn M, et al. Influence of polymorphism in the genes for the interleukin (IL)-1 receptor antagonist and IL-1beta on tuberculosis. J Exp Med. 1999;189:1863-74.
95. Bellamy R, Ruwende C, Corrah T, McAdam KP, Whittle HC, Hill AV. Assessment of the interleukin 1 gene cluster and other candidate gene polymorphisms in host susceptibility to tuberculosis. Tuber Lung Dis 1998;79: 83-89.
96. Remus N, El Baghdadi J, Fieschi C, et al. Association of IL12RB1 polymorphisms with pulmonary tuberculosis in adults in Morocco. J Infect Dis 2004;190:580-87.
97. Tso HW, Lau YL, Tam CM, Wong HS, Chiang AK. Associations between IL12B polymorphisms and tuberculosis in the Hong Kong Chinese population. J Infect Dis 2004;190:913-19.
98. Pasula R, Downing JF, Wright JR, Kachel DL, Davis TE Jr, Martin WJ 2nd. Surfactant protein A (SP-A) mediates attachment of *Mycobacterium tuberculosis* to murine alveolar macrophages. Am J Respir Cell Mol Biol 1997;17: 209-17.
99. Ferguson JS, Voelker DR, McCormack FX, Schlesinger LS. Surfactant protein D binds to *Mycobacterium tuberculosis* bacilli and lipoarabinomannan via carbohydrate-lectin interactions resulting in reduced phagocytosis of the bacteria by macrophages. J Immunol 1999;163:312-21.
100. Floros J, Lin HM, Garcia A, et al. Surfactant protein genetic marker alleles identify a subgroup of tuberculosis in a Mexican population. J Infect Dis 2000;182:1473-78.
101. Lammas DA, Stober C, Harvey CJ, Kendrick N, Panchalingam S, Kumararatne DS. ATP-induced killing of mycobacteria by human macrophages is mediated by purinergic P2Z(P2X7) receptors. Immunity 1997;7:433-44.
102. Kusner DJ, Barton JA. ATP stimulates human macrophages to kill intracellular virulent *Mycobacterium tuberculosis* via calcium-dependent phagosome-lysosome fusion. J Immunol 2001;167:3308-15.
103. Li CM, Campbell SJ, Kumararatne DS, et al. Association of a polymorphism in the P2X7 gene with tuberculosis in a Gambian population. J Infect Dis 2002;186:1458-62.
104. Saunders BM, Fernando SL, Sluyter R, Britton WJ, Wiley JS. A loss-of-function polymorphism in the human P2X7 receptor abolishes ATP-mediated killing of mycobacteria. J Immunol 2003;171:5442-46.
105. Bellamy R, Beyers N, McAdam KP, et al. Genetic susceptibility to tuberculosis in Africans: a genome-wide scan. Proc Natl Acad Sci. USA 2000;97:8005-09.
106. Bellamy R, Ruwende C, Corrah T, McAdam KP, Whittle HC, Hill AV. Variations in the NRAMP1 gene and susceptibility to tuberculosis in West Africans. N Engl J Med 1998;338:640-44.
107. Bellamy R, Ruwende C, Corrah T et al. Tuberculosis and chronic hepatitis B virus infection in Africans and variation in the vitamin D receptor gene. J Infect Dis 1999;179:721-24.
108. Means TK, Wang S, Lien E, et al. Human toll-like receptors mediate cellular activation by *Mycobacterium tuberculosis*. J Immunol 1999;163:3920-27.
109. Lien E, Sellati TJ, Yoshimura A, et al. Toll-like receptor 2 functions as a pattern recognition receptor for diverse bacterial products. J Biol Chem 1999; 274:33419-25.
110. Underhill DM, Ozinsky A, Smith KD, et al. Toll-like receptor-2 mediates mycobacteria-induced proinflammatory signaling in macrophages. Proc Natl Acad Sci. USA 1999;96:14459-63.
111. Thoma-Uszynski S, Stenger S, Takeuchi O, et al. Induction of direct antimicrobial activity through mammalian toll-like receptors. Science 2001;291:1544-47.
112. Krutzik SR, Ochoa MT, Sieling PA, et al. Activation and regulation of Toll-like receptors 2 and 1 in human leprosy. Nat Med 2003;9(5):525-32.
113. Krutzik SR, Tan B, Li H, et al. TLR activation triggers the rapid differentiation of monocytes into macrophages and dendritic cells. Nat Med 2005;11:653-60.
114. Malhotra D, Relhan V, Reddy BSN, et al. TLR2 Arg677Trp polymorphism in leprosy: Revisited. Hum Genet 2005;116: 413-15.
115. Lorenz E, Mira JP, Cornish KL, et al. A novel polymorphism in the toll-like receptor 2 gene and its potential association with staphylococcal infection. Infect Immun 2000;68:6398-401.
116. Najmi N. PhD thesis, All India Institute of Medical Sciences, New Delhi, India; 2009.

Chapter 24

Killer Cell Immunoglobulin-like Receptors in Health and Disease

Raja Rajalingam, Elham Ashouri

NATURAL KILLER CELLS

Natural killer (NK) cells are bone marrow derived large granular lymphocytes, and they mount early immune responses in an antigen independent manner by direct cytotoxicity.[1] NK cell deficiencies in humans results in overwhelming fatal infection during childhood.[2] NK cells produce granzymes and perforin, and their lytic response can be triggered within minutes, without requiring transcription, translation, or cell proliferation.[3] NK cells further secrete pro-inflammatory cytokines such as interferon-γ (IFN-γ), tumor necrosis factor-α (TNF-α), macrophage inflammatory protein-1β (MIP-1β) and granulocyte macrophage colony-stimulating factor (GM-CSF) upon activation. The IFN-γ is considered the prototypic NK cell cytokine, and its production by NK cells is known to shape the Th1 immune response,[4] activate antigen presenting cells to further up-regulate MHC class I expression,[5] activate macrophage killing of obligate intracellular pathogens,[6] and have antiproliferative effects on viral-infected and malignant-transformed cells.[7]

The traditional cell surface phenotype defining human NK cells within the lymphocyte gate on the flow cytometric analyzer shows an absence of CD3 (thereby excluding T cells) and expression of CD56, the 140-kDa isoform of neural cell adhesion molecule (NCAM) found on NK cells and a minority of T cells. Approximately 5–15 percent of the peripheral blood mononuclear cells are NK cells.[8] Two distinct subsets of human NK cells have been identified by cell surface density of CD56 and CD16 (FcγRIII).[9] Approximately 90 percent of circulating NK cells belongs to the $CD56^{dim}CD16^{pos}$ type and secrete large quantities of perforin and granzyme. These cells are effective killers, mediate antibody dependent cellular cytotoxicity (ADCC), natural cytotoxicity and produce low levels of pro-inflammatory cytokines. In contrast, approximately 10 percent of circulating NK cells belongs to the $CD56^{bright}CD16^{neg}$ NK cells. These cells secrete large amounts of pro-inflammatory cytokines upon activation. Interestingly, the distribution of these two subsets is reversed in healthy secondary lymphoid organs such as the lymph nodes, where 90 percent of the cells belong to the cytokine secreting $CD56^{bright}CD16^{neg}$ NK cell subset and only 10 percent of the cells belong to the $CD56^{dim}CD16^{pos}$ cytolytic compartment of NK cells.

NK CELLS SENSE 'MISSING-SELF', 'INDUCED-SELF', 'ALTERED-SELF', AND 'NON-SELF'

NK cells share several common features with cytotoxic T lymphocytes (CTL) in development, morphology, cell-surface phenotypes, and triggering effector function against infection and tumors.[10,11] Despite these similarities, NK cells and CTLs differ in their cell surface receptors used to recognize the infected/transformed cellular targets. The CTLs interact with the class I human leukocyte antigen (HLA) and its bound peptide complex expressed on target cells through specific T cell receptors (TCR), which initiates cytolytic activity if the peptide is derived from a pathogen. HLA class I expression is generally down-regulated in virally-infected or transformed cells, rendering the cells resistant to cytolysis by CTLs. The aberrant levels of class I expression can result in spontaneous destruction by NK cells, a concept originally termed the "missing-self" hypothesis.[12,13] In support of this concept, human NK cells kill Epstein-Barr virus-transformed B-lymphoblastoid cell lines lacking

HLA class I, whereas re-expression of class I in these lines inhibits cytolysis. Therefore, the normal healthy cells are protected from spontaneous NK cell killing when they express an appropriate ligand for an inhibitory receptor expressed by NK cells (Fig. 24.1). In contrast to the CTLs, the NK cells use a vast combinatorial array of germline-encoded non-arranging receptors that can trigger either inhibitory or activating signals.[14, 15] The inhibitory receptors recognize self-HLA class I molecules while the activating receptors recognize either 'induced-self' (such as, MHC class I-like chains A and B [MICA and MICB] and unique long binding proteins [ULBP]), 'altered-self' (HLA class I molecules loaded with foreign peptide) or pathogen encoded 'non-self' molecules associated with infection and tumor transformation. Therefore, the net signal integrated from the inhibitory and activating receptors determines the effector function of NK cells.[14]

NATURAL KILLER CELL RECEPTORS

There are many different receptors on NK cells that provide activating or inhibitory signals in response to target cells.[14, 16] Human NK cells utilize structurally two distinct families of receptors: killer cell immunoglobulin-like receptors (KIR) and killer cell lectin-like receptors (KLR).[16-18] The KIRs are the key receptors that human NK cells use to distinguish the unhealthy targets from the healthy-self.[19]

KLR receptors are expressed as heterodimers (CD94-NKG2A, CD94-NKG2C, CD94-NKG2E, and CD94-NKG2F) or homodimers (NKG2D-NKG2D) and are encoded by genes within the NK gene complex (NKC) located on chromosome 12p12.3-p13.1 (20-25). CD94-NKG2A is an inhibitory receptor while the remaining receptors display activating functions. Both inhibitory (CD94-NKG2A) and activating (CD94-NKG2C) receptors recognize the non-classical class I HLA-E complexed to peptides derived from the leader sequences of certain HLA-A, B, C, G, and H heavy chains.[26-28] The NKG2D receptor interacts with MICA, MICB, and ULBP proteins.[29-31] The ligands for CD94-NKG2E and CD94-NKG2F receptors are unknown.

KIR Receptor Nomenclature

Fourteen distinct KIR receptors have been identified in humans (Fig. 24.2). They contain either two or three C2-type immunoglobulin-like domains in the extra-cellular region and either a long or short cytoplasmic tail. Based on the protein structure, each KIR receptor and its encoding gene have been given the following specific name: KIR2DL1, 2DL2, 2DL3, 2DL4, 2DL5, 3DL1, 3DL2, 3DL3, 3DS1, 2DS1, 2DS2, 2DS3, 2DS4, and 2DS5.[32] The first digit following the KIR acronym corresponds to the number of Ig-like domains (2D or 3D) in the receptor (D denotes domain). The 'D' is followed by either an 'L' indicating a 'Long' cytoplasmic tail, or an 'S' indicating a 'Short' cytoplasmic tail or a 'P' for pseudogenes (KIR3DP1 and KIR2DP1). The final digit indicates the number of the gene encoding a protein with this

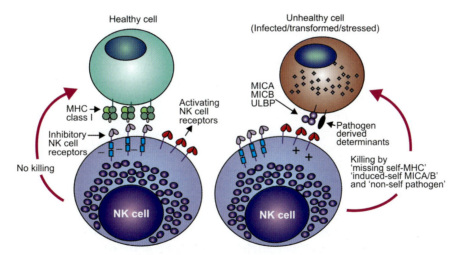

Fig. 24.1: Natural killer (NK) cell recognition. NK cells patrol for abnormal cells that lack self-HLA class molecules, over expression of 'induced-self' (MICA, MICB, ULBP), expression of 'altered-self' (HLA-class I loaded with foreign peptide), and/or pathogen encoded 'non-self' molecules associated with infection and tumor transformation. By expressing HLA-A, B, and C molecules, the healthy cells become resistant to NK surveillance. Downregulation of HLA class I expression due to tumor transformation or viral infection relieves the inhibitory influence on NK cells, permitting NK cells to lyse these unhealthy target cells, a phenomenon first described as the 'missing-self' hypothesis. The net signal integrated from the inhibitory and activating receptors determines the effector function of NK cells

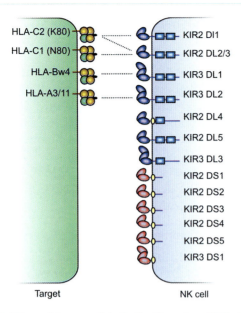

Fig. 24.2: Killer cell Immunoglobulin-like Receptors (KIR). Fourteen distinct KIR receptors have been characterized in humans that comprise either 2 or 3 (2D or 3D) extracellular Ig-like domains and either a long (L) or short (S) cytoplasmic tail. Six KIR receptors are activating types and the remaining KIR are inhibitory types. The ITIM motifs in the cytoplasmic tails of inhibitory KIRs are shown as blue boxes, and positively charged residues in the transmembrane regions of activating KIRs are shown as yellow circles. The inhibitory KIR receptors bind to distinct HLA class I allotypes (shown by dotted lines) and the ligands for the activating KIR receptors not known

structure. Thus KIR2DL1, 2DL2 and 2DL3 all encode receptors having two extracellular Ig-like domains and a long cytoplasmic tail. The long cytoplasmic tails include one or two copies of immunereceptor tyrosine-based inhibitory motifs (ITIM) that recruit and activate SHP-1 and SHP-2 phosphatases for inhibitory signal transduction. The short cytoplasmic tails do not carry any signaling motifs. The short-tailed KIRs carry a charged amino acid residue in their transmembrane region, which allow these receptors to bind to the adapter molecule, DAP12 (DNAX activation protein of 12 kDa).[33] The DAP12 adapter chain contains immunereceptor tyrosine-based activation motifs (ITAM), which trigger activating signals upon the short-tailed KIR receptor bound to a relevant ligand.

KIR allele sequences are named in an analogous fashion to HLA alleles.[32] After the gene name, an asterisk (*) is used as a separator before a numerical allele designation. The first three digits of the numerical designation are used to indicate alleles that differ in the sequences of their encoded proteins (e.g., 2DL1*001 and 2DL1*003). The next two digits is used to distinguish alleles that only differ by synonymous (non-coding) differences within the coding sequence (e.g., 2DL1*00301 and 2DL1*00302). The final two digits are used to distinguish alleles that only differ by substitutions in an intron, promoter, or other non-coding region of the sequence (e.g., 2DL1*0030201 and 2DL1*0030202). A complete listing of all KIR allele sequences assigned official names can be found at the IPD-KIR database that serves as a central depository for KIR sequences (http://www.ebi.ac.uk/ipd/kir/index.html). Since the KIR3DL1 and 3DS1 behave as alleles of the same loci, the alleles of these genes are combined under one gene name. To avoid confusion, the alleles of both genes are named in a single numerical series, thus 3DL1*001–3DL1*009 are followed by 3DS1*010–3DS1*014. Likewise the alleles of the 2DL5A and 2DL5B genes have also been named in a single series, because of the similarity of these sequences. Like other cell surface molecules of the immune system, the KIR molecules have also been given a CD designation and are recognized as members of the CD158 series.[34]

KIR Genomic Organization

The KIR receptors are encoded by a family of polymorphic and highly homologous genes located in the leukocyte receptor complex (LRC) that maps to chromosome 19q13.4.[35-37] LRC is a highly polymorphic region containing at least 30 members encoding Ig-like receptors other than KIRs, as well as additional receptors, e.g. the leukocyte Ig-like receptor family (LILR), leukocyte-associated inhibitory receptor (LAIR-1 and LAIR-2), Fcα receptor, collagen-binding receptors, and natural cytotoxicity receptor (NCR1). The number and type of KIR genes arranged differ substantially between haplotypes (Fig. 24.3). Nearly 30 distinct KIR haplotypes have been characterized that differ in gene content.[38-43] Only four KIR genes (3DL3, 3DP1, 2DL4, and 3DL2) present on all haplotypes, are referred to as 'framework' genes. KIR3DL3 and 3DL2 mark the centeromeric and telomeric boundaries of the KIR gene complex respectively, while 3DP1 and 2DL4 are located in the middle of the KIR gene complex. KIR3DP1 and 2DL4 genes are separated by a 14 kb sequence enriched with L1 repeats, while the distance between other KIR genes is only a 2 kb homogeneous sequence. The 14 kb DNA sequence between 3DP1 and 2DL4 divides the KIR haplotypes into two halves.[36] KIR3DL3 at the 5'-end and 3DP1 at the 3'-end mark the centromeric half, while 2DL4 at the 5'-end and 3DL2 at the 3'-end mark the telomeric half. Values of linkage disequilibrium are higher between the genes of the same half as compared to those between genes of the different halves.[44]

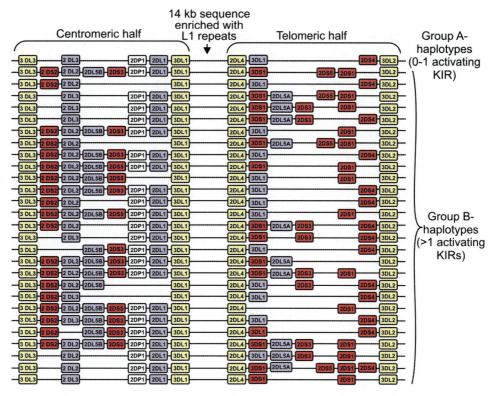

Fig. 24.3: KIR haplotypes have variable gene content. Map of KIR haplotypes as determined by family segregation analyses. The first haplotype on the top represents the group-A KIR haplotype and the remainder group-B haplotypes. The framework genes, present in all haplotypes are shown in yellow; genes encoding activating KIR are in orange; and those for inhibitory receptors are in blue

On the basis of gene content, KIR haplotypes are broadly classified into two groups.[45] Group A haplotypes have a fixed gene content comprising KIR3DL3-2DL3-2DP1-2DL1-3DP1-2DL4-3DL1-2DS4-3DL2, but are diversified through allelic polymorphism of the individual genes (Fig. 24.3). In contrast, group B haplotypes have variable gene content comprising several genes and alleles that are not part of the A haplotype. Particularly, KIR2DS1, 2DS2, 2DS3, 2DS5, 2DL2, 2DL5 and 3DS1 are associated only with group B haplotypes, and thus B haplotypes generally encode more activating KIR receptors than the A haplotype that encodes a single activating receptor, KIR2DS4. The gene content varies dramatically between group-B haplotypes.[36, 38, 39, 43] Even more complicated haplotypes have been identified with two copies of KIR2DL5 (2DL5A and 2DL5B) and/or KIR2DS3 on the same haplotype, and thus individuals homozygous for these haplotypes may carry four copies of KIR2DL5 and four copies of KIR2DS3 sequences.[39, 40, 46-50] Furthermore, several KIR haplotypes with unusual KIR gene content due to reciprocal recombinations have been described.[50] Inheritance of paternal and maternal haplotypes comprising different KIR gene contents generates human diversity in KIR genotypes. For example, homozygotes for group-A haplotypes have only seven functional KIR genes, while the heterozygotes for group-A and group-B haplotypes may have all 14 functional KIR genes.

All human populations have both group A and B haplotypes, but their frequencies vary considerably.[40,42,43,51-71] A website developed by Professor Derek Middleton (http://www.allelefrequencies.net) compiles the frequency of KIR genes and genotypes of different populations.[72] A panel of 242 KIR genotypes that vary in the gene content have been published in about 4638 individuals studied to date in 51 populations.[71] However, only 38 (15.7%) of them occurred greater than 5 percent in at least one population study (Fig. 24.4). In Africans and Caucasians, the A and B haplotypes are equally distributed suggestive of a balancing selection. Conversely, the A haplotype is overrepresented in Northeast Asians (Chinese, Japanese and Koreans), while the B haplotype occurred most frequently in the natives of India, Australia and America. NK cells of group-B haplotypic individuals express more activating NK receptors and respond more vigorously to pathogens. It

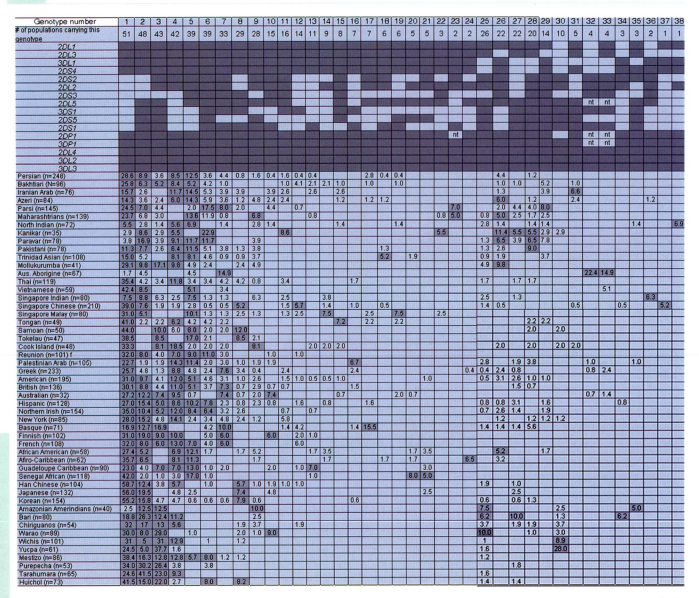

Fig. 24.4: Diverse KIR genotypes in ethnic populations. Genotyping studies reveal a significant ethnic difference in the distribution of KIR genotypes. A total of 242 distinct KIR genotypes in the combined pool of 4638 unrelated individuals were observed, which differ from each other by the presence (shaded box) or absence (white box) of 16 *KIR* genes. Only the frequencies of selected KIR genotypes that occur ≥ 5 percent in at least one population (highlighted with gray shade) are listed, and are compared with the frequencies in other populations. "nt" indicates not tested for the given *KIR* gene, and "n" indicates the number of individuals studied in each population. The frequency of each genotype is expressed as a percentage and defined as the number of individuals having the genotype divided by the number of individuals studied in the population group

is likely that group-B haplotypes were positively selected by nature over time in natives of India, Australia and America to survive in an ever changing environment during their prehistoric migrations from Africa.[65]

Exon-intron Organization of KIR Genes

Organization of the exon-intron structure of the various KIR genes is fairly consistent with the following basic arrangement: the signal sequence is encoded by the first two exons, each Ig domain (D0, D1, and D2, starting from the N-terminus) corresponds to a single exon (exons 3–5, respectively), the stem and transmembrane regions are each encoded by a single exon (exons 6 and 7), and the cytoplasmic domain is encoded by two final exons (Fig. 24.5).[73] KIR2DL1, 2DL2/3, and all 2DS genes have an identical genomic organization to that encoding KIR molecules with three Ig domains. However, exon 3 is a pseudoexon in these two-domain KIR genes, which often remains in-frame but is eventually spliced out. The protein products of these two-domain KIR are therefore missing the D0 domain. KIR2DL4 and 2DL5 are characterized by the complete absence of exon 4,[74,75] and therefore their protein product has no D1 domain. The KIR3DL3 gene closely resembles the other 3D genes, except that it is missing exon 6.

Nucleotide Polymorphism of KIR Genes

In addition to haplotypic diversity, each KIR gene exhibits considerable sequence polymorphism.[43,76-80] A total of 224 KIR sequences that differ in predicted protein sequence have been deposited to date into the GenBank (http://www.ncbi.nlm.nih.gov/Genbank/genomesubmit.html) and IPD-KIR databases (Fig. 24.6) (http://www.ebi.ac.uk/ipd/kir/index.html). The most abundant allelic polymorphism was reported for KIR3DL1 comprising 46 variants.[80] The framework genes KIR3DL2 and 3DL3 are relatively more polymorphic, while the activating KIR genes are generally conserved. The amino acid substitutions that distinguish allelic diversity of KIR3DL1 is rich in the region where the receptor contacts the polymorphic HLA-Bw4 ligands.[80,81] The sequence polymorphism of KIR3DL1 is shown to influence their expression, ligand binding and cytolytic and cytokine secretion functions.[41,81-85] Some nucleotide mutations affect the cell-surface expression of KIR receptors. For example, some of the frequently occurring KIR2DS4 sequences have a 22 bp deletion in exon-5, which shifts the reading-frame and results in a premature stop codon causing 2DS4 to be non-expressed at the cell surface.[40,86] Furthermore, chain-terminating frame-shift

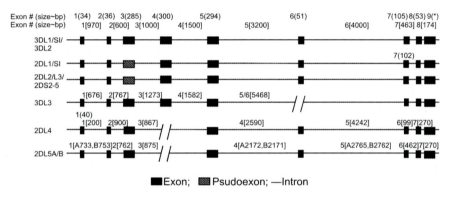

Fig. 24.5: The intron-exon organization of KIR genes. KIR genes sharing similar structural organization have been grouped accordingly, while KIR genes with structural peculiarities are shown on their own

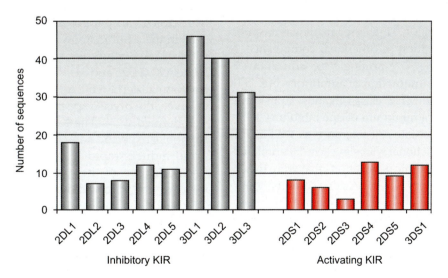

Fig. 24.6: Allelic polymorphism of KIR genes. The number of sequences identified for each KIR gene that can encode distinct proteins are shown. These statistics were obtained from the IPD-KIR database, release 2.1.0, January 2008 (http://www.ebi.ac.uk/ipd/kir/stats.html)

deletions were reported for KIR2DL4.[87-89] Similarly, sequence variation in the promoter region is associated with the lack of KIR2DL5 expression[90] and amino acid polymorphism is largely responsible for the intracellular retention of 3DL1*004[91] and 2DL2*004.[83] The synergistic combination of allelic polymorphism and variable gene content individualize KIR genotypes to an extent where unrelated individuals almost always have different KIR types.[76] This level of diversity likely reflects a strong pressure from pathogens on the human NK cell response.

Clonal Expression of KIR Receptors and 'NK Cell Licensing'

KIR receptors are clonally expressed on NK cells, so that each NK cell clone expresses only a portion of the genes within the gene profile.[92] Stochastic expression of different combinations of receptors by NK cells results in this repertoire of NK clones with a variety of ligand specificities. Once a given KIR receptor is expressed on an NK cell clone or T cell, it is stably maintained in the progeny of the clone. This pattern of expression appears to be regulated by methylation of the silent KIR loci.[93]

The majority of NK cells in peripheral blood express at least one inhibitory receptor for self-MHC class I and is functionally competent to recognize and eliminate target cells that have down-regulated the respective MHC class I ligands.[15,92] Additionally, a subpopulation of developmentally immature NK cells exists that lack inhibitory receptors for self-MHC class I and are generally hyporesponsive to target cells that are deficient in MHC class I expression.[94-96] Furthermore, NK cells from MHC class I deficient mice and humans were shown to be defective in target killing.[97,98] In this regard, it was recently shown that the acquisition of functional competence, a process called 'licensing',[95,99] 'arming'[100] or 'education',[94] is mediated through interaction of inhibitory NK cell receptors with cognate MHC class I ligands. Consistent with the need to have a minimum of one inhibitory KIR-HLA interaction to mediate self-tolerance as well as for the development of functional NK cells, each 759 unrelated individuals from four ethnic populations that were tested had at least one inhibitory KIR-HLA gene combination.[59] Expression of progressively higher numbers of inhibitory KIRs for self-HLA-B and HLA-C molecules have been correlated with an increased effector capacity.[101] In summary, interactions of KIR to HLA class I ligands set the threshold of NK cell capacity as well as control the NK cell response.

LIGAND FOR KIR RECEPTORS

The inhibitory KIR receptors recognize a distinct motif on the COOH-terminal portion of polymorphic HLA class I molecules and trigger signals that stop NK cell action (Fig. 24.2). The HLA proteins are encoded by a fascinating genetic region located in the major histocompatibility complex (MHC) that comprises about 3.6 Mb DNA located on the short arm of chromosome 6 (6p21.3). The HLA genes in the human MHC encodes cell-surface glycoproteins displaying a remarkable degree of polymorphism.[102,103] The extensive allelic diversity at these loci is generated by point mutations, recombinations, and gene conversions. Rapidly evolving viruses and pathogens drive HLA polymorphism, and consequently the presence of KIR-binding HLA ligands are variable in individuals.[103-105]

Members of the KIR2D subfamily recognize a polymorphism in HLA-C proteins at amino acid position 80 on the α1 domain of the HLA-C heavy chain.[106] All known alleles of HLA-C have either Asparagine or Lysine at position 80, and these are recognized by different isoforms of KIR2DL. Specifically, KIR2DL1 recognizes HLA-C alleles characterized by a Lysine 80 residue located in the F-pocket of the peptide binding groove (Cw*02, Cw*0401, Cw*05, Cw*06 and Cw*15 - termed C2 group).[107-109] KIR2DL2 and KIR2DL3 recognize the remaining HLA-C allotypes (Cw*01, Cw*03, Cw*07 and Cw*08) with asparagine at position 80 (termed C1 group). The inhibitory signals triggered by the KIR2DL2/3+HLA-C1 interaction is relatively weaker as compared to those triggered by the KIR2DL1+HLA-C2 interaction.[82] KIR3DL1 binds to the Bw4 serological epitope, defined by amino acid residues 77-83 in the α1 domain, which is presents on 40 percent of the HLA-B allotypes and certain HLA-A allotypes (HLA-A23, 24, 25 and 32).[110-112] KIR3DL2 has been shown to recognize certain HLA-A ligands (HLA-A3 and A11); however, the precise specificity of this receptor has not been defined.[113,114] The KIR2DL4 receptor binds to the trophoblast-specific non-classical class I molecule HLA-G and induces rapid IFN-γ production that promotes vascularization of the maternal decidua during early pregnancy.[115-118] In addition to its activation function, the KIR2DL4 receptor carries a single ITIM motif in its cytoplasmic tail and exhibits inhibitory function.[119-121] Although the cell-surface expression of two other inhibitory receptors KIR3DL3 and 2DL5 was recently confirmed,[122,123] the ligands for these receptors have yet to be discovered.

Although the specificity of the inhibitory KIR have been extensively characterized, very little is known about the ligands for the activating KIRs. Certain activating KIRs are predicted to bind to the same HLA class I ligands as their structurally related inhibitory KIRs. For instance, 3DS1 that shares the highest sequence homologies with 3DL1 in their extracellular Ig-domain is believed to bind to HLA-Bw4.[124] Whereas KIR2DL1 and 2DS1 differ by only 7 amino acids in their extracellular domain, KIR2DL1 binds to HLA-C*0401 much more strongly than KIR2DS1.[82] Similarly, KIR2DL2 and 2DL3 bind to HLA-C*0304, but KIR2DS2, whose extracellular domain differs from KIR2DL2 and 2DL3 by only 3 or 4 amino acids, respectively, failed to bind any HLA class I molecule examined. Taken as a whole, an intact HLA class I trimer, composed of heavy chain, β2-microglobulin, and peptide, is required for KIR recognition. The strength of these specific KIR-HLA class I interactions are highly sensitive to the HLA class I bound peptide sequence.[82, 112, 125-129] Although KIR recognition is clearly both peptide dependent and peptide selective, these receptors do not distinguish self from nonself peptides; thus, the biological relevance is not obvious.

HUMAN DIVERSITY IN KIR-HLA COMPOUND GENOTYPES

Given that KIR genes at chromosome 19q13.4 and HLA genes at chromosome 6p21.3 are polymorphic and display significant variations, the independent segregation of these unlinked gene families produce diversity in the number and type of KIR-HLA pairs inherited in individuals.[59] Individuals carrying homozygous group-A KIR genotypes (AA genotypes) are frequent (30-58%) in most ethnic populations (Fig. 24.4, Genotype#1). The exceptions are the natives of America, Australia and India, in which the individuals carrying AB and BB genotypes are frequent. The NK cells from the AA homozygous individuals can express a maximum of four inhibitory KIR receptors (2DL1, 2DL3, 3DL1 and 3DL2) and one activating KIR2DS4 receptor. In contrast, the individuals carrying AB or BB KIR genotypes can express a maximum of five inhibitory KIR receptors (2DL1, 2DL2/3, 2DL5, 3DL1, and 3DL2) and 2 to 6 activating KIR receptors. The function of the inhibitory KIR receptors depends on the availability of their specific cognate HLA class I ligands. Only a few individuals carry cognate HLA class I ligands for all inhibitory KIR receptors, but most individuals carry ligand for 2 to 3 inhibitory KIR receptors.[59] Around 20 percent of most populations carried a single inhibitory KIR-HLA pair. Genotypes encoding a dominant inhibitory KIR receptor repertoire (inhibitory KIR+HLA>activating KIR) are likely protective against autoimmunity but susceptible for infection and tumor. Genotypes encoding a dominant activating KIR receptor repertoire (inhibitory KIR+HLA<activating KIR) are presumably susceptible to autoimmunity but instrumental in antiviral and anti-tumor immunity.

KIR RECEPTORS EXPRESSED ON CTL CAN CONTROL ADAPTIVE IMMUNITY

In addition to NK cells, KIR receptors are expressed on a subset of T lymphocytes, in particular on γδ T cells and memory/effector CD8+ T cells indicating that the KIRs can regulate the antigen-specific T cell immune response, affirming their role in adaptive immunity.[130, 131] Similar to NK cells, HLA class I-specific inhibitory receptors might subserve on T cells an important negative control that participates in the prevention of autologous damage. Furthermore, recognition of HLA class I molecules by inhibitory KIR receptors on T cells down-regulates the activation-induced cell death, and promotes the survival of CD8+ memory T cells.[132] The majority of CD4+ T cells constitutively expresses the CD28 molecule, a key player in providing co-stimulatory signals to induce T cell activation and to prevent T cell apoptosis.[133] CD4+ T cells lacking the CD28 molecule are distinctly infrequent in most normal individuals (comprising 0.1–2.5 percent of T cells).[134] However, CD4+CD28^{null} cells are expanded in RA patients expressing variable KIR receptors.[135] Particularly, a preponderance of activating KIR receptors on CD4+CD28^{null} T cells and their co-stimulatory function on CD28 negative T cells prompted the hypothesis that the activating KIR receptors may predispose a person to autoimmune manifestation.[136-138]

KIR GENES ORIGINATED RECENTLY AND ARE RAPIDLY EVOLVING

NK cells of humans and mice perform analogous tasks in mediating early immune response against infected and tumor transformed cellular targets. However, they use a distinct family of NK cell receptors (Fig. 24.7). Mice do not have KIR genes, but use only NKC encoded receptors. Both human and mice NK cells use KLR receptors (CD94:NKG2 family), and these genes are highly conserved between mice and men showing 60-80 percent nucleotide sequence homologies.[26, 139] In addition to KLR encoding genes, the mouse NKC cluster at chromosome 6 includes 15-20 polymorphic LY49 receptor genes.[140, 141] In

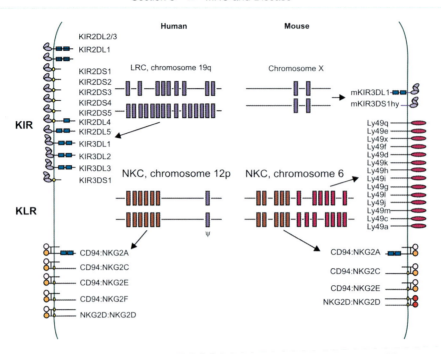

Fig. 24.7: Human and mouse NK cells use distinct families of MHC class I-specific receptors. The CD94:NKG2 family of NK receptors are used by both human and mouse NK cells. Ly49 receptors are exclusively used by mouse NK cells, which are reduced to a single pseudogene in humans. The humans use KIR receptors as major class I specific NK cell receptors, which are under developed in the mouse

humans, the Ly49 family has been reduced to a single unexpressed pseudogene.[142, 143]

Despite their structural differences, the KIR gene family in the LRC in man and the functional equivalents in mice, the Ly49 genes of the NKC share many common features: (a) Both are small gene families (10–15 closely linked genes) that arose by gene duplication and have diversified by gene conversion; (b) both demonstrate substantial genetic polymorphism; (c) both are expressed on subsets of NK cells and memory type CD8+ T cells by a stochastic process, with the receptor repertoire in the individual being shaped by subtle influences of the host MHC class I molecules; (d) both families contain genes that encode inhibitory receptors with ITIMs in their cytoplasmic domains and activating receptors that associate with the ITAM-bearing DAP12 adapter protein; and (e) both recognize polymorphic determinants on MHC class I ligands.

Humans use KIR receptors as the major class I specific NK cell receptors. In mice, only two KIR-like genes have been identified on the X-chromosome.[144] However, the expression and function of these molecules is not defined. Comparison between human and mice revealed that the KIR system originated recently after the divergence of human and mouse lineages, which occurred around 65 million years ago.[145, 146] Further comparison between humans and higher primates indicates that KIR genes are rapidly evolving. The chimpanzee and gorilla are the closest living relatives to man. Their common ancestor is estimated to have existed around 5-8 million years ago.[147] The chimpanzees and gorillas share >98 percent homology with humans in their genome. Further, the MHC class I genes in these apes are the direct counterparts (orthologs) to human HLA-A, B and C genes.[148] However, only three KIR genes are conserved among humans, chimpanzees and gorillas.[149-151] Most chimpanzee and gorilla KIR genes have diverged to the point where the orthologous relationships with human KIRs are lost. These findings suggest that the KIR genes are a rapidly evolving system, and the driving force of this dynamic evolution is not limited to the polymorphic MHC class I genes. The nature of rapid evolution could potentially contribute to KIR diversity within and between species.

CLINICAL IMPLICATIONS OF VARIABLE KIR-HLA INTERACTIONS

Since the MHC class I and KIR loci are both highly polymorphic yet their products interact and are inherited independently, one could imagine that certain combinations of HLA class I and KIR alleles could result in beneficial or deleterious interactions.[152, 153] Efforts to modulate NK cell trafficking into inflamed tissues and/or lymph nodes, and to counteract NK cell suppressors, might prove fruitful clinically.[154] Some of the promising clinical implications of KIR-HLA interactions are summarized here.

Hematopoietic Stem Cell Transplantation (HCT)

Allogeneic (genetically different) HCT is an effective therapy for an increasing number of life-threatening hematological, oncological, hereditary and immunological diseases.[155-157] Patients undergoing matched unrelated donors (MUD) HCT, compared to those receiving sibling HCT, display a higher incidence of graft-versus-host disease (GVHD), suggesting the role of non-T cell-mediated mechanism(s) involved in GVHD and graft-versus-tumor effect (GVT). Studies with mice suggest the role of NK alloreactivity in bone marrow transplant rejection.[158-160] Recent studies with HLA-haploidentical transplantation revealed a potential role of NK cells in mediating enhanced anti-leukemic effect, decreased GVHD, and survival advantage of allogeneic HCT.[161,162]

Following allogeneic HCT, the recipient reconstitutes NK cells from the donor stem cell graft, and thereby the donor NK receptor and recipient HLA class I ligand determines the alloreactivity of the reconstituted NK cells. The central hypothesis is that patients reconstituted with more inhibitory 'receptor-ligand' combinations develop a lower degree of GVHD, and patients reconstituted with more activating receptors show a high GVT effect. The donor graft from group-A homozygotes develops NK cells expressing four inhibitory KIRs and one or no activating KIR. The alloreactivity of the donor NK cells depends on the recipient's HLA type. If the recipient expresses most of the HLA class I ligands (HLA-C1, C2, Bw4, and A3/11), the donor NK cells are likely inhibited and become tolerant to recipient tissue, so that less or no GVHD will result. In contrast, recipients lacking these HLA ligands (missing-self model) fail to inhibit all donor NK cells and result in NK mediated GVHD. Since the group-A homozygotes express just one or no activating KIR, these NK cells may poorly recognize tumors, and thus low GVT effect is expected. The grafts from AB or BB haplotypic donors develop NK cells expressing more than one activating KIR in addition to 4 to 6 inhibitory KIRs. The inhibitory KIRs will recognize relevant HLA ligands on recipient tissues and stop NK alloreactivity. The activating KIRs will presumably recognize and kill recipient tumors leading to an increased GVT effect. If the recipient does not have ligands for all inhibitory KIRs, the GVHD effect is increased. In summary, the degree of KIR-HLA interactions may determine the success rate of hematopoietic cell replacement therapy for certain leukemias.

Solid Organ Transplantation

Human NK cells are not affected by the currently used clinical regimen of immunosuppressive agents such as Cyclosporine,[163] FK506,[164] mycophenolate mofetil,[165] azathioprine[166] and rapamycin,[167] and thus NK cells may play an important role in the outcome of solid organ transplants. Infiltration of recipient NK cells into the renal,[168] as well as cardiac,[169] lung[170] and liver[171] allografts shortly after clinical transplantation have been observed indicating human NK cell's capacity to recognize and respond to solid organ grafts. Two studies compared kidney transplant outcome with the recipient's KIR genotypes. Kunert et al[172] found an association between a higher number of inhibitory receptors in the recipient's genotype and patients with stable renal function. Vampa et al[173] found recipients carrying more activating KIR genes triggered more NK cytotoxicity against their donors than recipients carrying fewer activating KIR genes. The most direct and compelling evidence of NK cell mediated rejection was observed with the cardiac allograft missing self-MHC class I in CD28$^{-/-}$ recipient mice.[174]

The recipient NK cells can recognize and react to the allograft by three possible mechanisms: 1. missing-self recognition, 2. induced-self recognition, and 3. antibody-dependent cell-mediated cytotoxicity (ADCC).[175] If the allograft does not express relevant HLA class I ligands for the recipient's inhibitory KIR receptors, the NK cells of the recipient will release cytolytic granules that will damage the allograft—a phenomenon of the 'missing-self' hypothesis.[13] The allograft may express stress-induced proteins that could serve as ligands for the activating receptors and enhance NK response – 'induced-self' killing. The expression of CD16 (Fc-γ R III), an Fc receptor for IgG, allows NK cells to trigger ADCC against specific targets. If the recipient carries donor-specific HLA antibodies, the recipient NK cells can elicit specific cytolysis against the allograft through the antibody-mediated NK cell recognition.

KIR-HLA in Infection

NK cells play a critical role in successful resolution of viral infections in both mice and humans.[176-178] In acute HIV infection, there is an expansion of the CD56^{dim}CD16^{pos} subset of NK cells, which are cytotoxic and express KIRs.[179] The genetic association between HIV disease progression and number of HLA-B alleles containing Bw4 serological motif was the first line of evidence to suggest the involvement of KIR in protection against the virus, since Bw4 allotypes have the potential to interact with KIR3DL1 and possibly KIR3DS1.[180] Consistent with these data, the presence of homozygosity for HLA-Bw4 was associated with a slower decline in CD4+ T-cell count, a marker for disease progression in HIV infection, among a group of HIV-infected patients.[181] Analysis of KIR and MHC class I in a cohort of over 1000 HIV-infected individuals demonstrated that those with the compound genotype KIR3DS1 and a subset of HLA-Bw4 alleles that encode for an isoleucine at position 80 of the MHC class I heavy chain progress more slowly to AIDS than those without this activating KIR–HLA combination.[124, 182]

Individuals exposed to HCV either resolve acute infection or progress to chronic infection. The 80 percent of individuals who become chronically infected have a substantial risk of developing end-stage liver disease, including liver cirrhosis and hepatocellular carcinoma.[183] A role for KIR and HLA genotypes in clearance versus persistence of HCV infection has been indicated by a multicenter study.[184] Particularly, protection against chronic hepatitis C virus was shown to be conferred by homozygosity of the genes for the inhibitory NK receptor KIR2DL3 and its ligand HLA-C^{Asn80}, particularly in cases of low inoculum of virus.[184]

Tumor Immunotherapy

Elimination of NK cells in mice results in a higher incidence of spontaneous tumors, impaired clearance of inoculated tumor cells, and an increased rate of tumor metastasis.[185] A large body of evidence argues that enhancement of NK cell numbers and function in human cancer patients is associated with increases in tumor clearance and duration of clinical remission.[186] This observation is largely based on clinical trials with interleukin-2 (IL-2).[187] IL-2 was shown to promote proliferation, cytokine production, and cytolytic activity by human NK cells *in vitro*. When IL-2 was infused at moderately high doses in patients with melanoma, a dramatic increase in peripheral blood CD56^{bright} CD16^{neg} cells was observed with some partial and complete responses.[188, 189] In addition, peripheral blood leukocytes from these patients demonstrated increased killing of tumor cells *in vitro*. KIR receptors seem to influence malignancies, specifically those associated with viral infections. Women developing cervical carcinoma are more likely to express KIR and HLA genotypes associated with activation,[190] whereas reduced susceptibility to hepatocellular carcinoma is associated with activating KIR and HLA allotypes.[191]

Autoimmune Disease

Psoriasis vulgaris is a common inflammatory skin disorder associated with HLA-Cw6, which is further associated with the activating KIR rich group B haplotypes.[192] Particularly, KIR2DS1 is significantly overrepresented in the affected population, and there is also a non-significant lower frequency of KIR2DL1. KIR2DS1, either alone[193] or in combination with HLA-Cw6,[194] is also associated with the presence of psoriasis. A weak association of the activating receptor–ligand pair KIR2DS2:HLA-C^{Asn80} is observed in diabetes mellitus.[195] Additionally, the unusual genotype of KIR2DS2 in the absence of its inhibitory counterpart KIR2DL2 is found at high frequency in patients with scleroderma (12%) as compared with controls (2%).[196] Overall, autoimmune and inflammatory conditions appear associated with a surplus of activating genotypes.

CONCLUSIONS

NK cells are more than simple killers and have been implicated in control and clearance of malignant and virally infected cells, regulation of adaptive immune responses, rejection of bone marrow transplants, autoimmunity and the maintenance of pregnancy. Human NK cells use a variable number and type of inhibitory and activating KIR receptors to discriminate healthy and unhealthy cells. The inhibitory KIRs recognize distinct HLA class I molecules and trigger signals that stop NK killing. The activating KIRs recognize determinants associated with infections and tumors, and trigger signals that activate NK killing. The effector function of a given NK cell depends upon the number and type of receptors it expresses and ligands it recognizes on the targets. Genes encoding KIRs and HLA ligands are located on different chromosomes, and feature variation in the number and type of genes. The independent segregation of KIR and HLA genes results in variable KIR-HLA combinations in individuals, which may determine the individual's immunity and susceptibility to diseases as diverse as autoimmunity, viral infections, and cancer.

ACKNOWLEDGMENTS

This work was supported by start-up funds from the UCLA Department of Pathology and Laboratory

Medicine. Elham Ashouri was supported by a fellowship from the Ministry of Health and Medical Education, The Islamic Republic of Iran.

REFERENCES

1. Trinchieri G. Biology of natural killer cells. Adv Immunol 1989;47:187-376.
2. Orange JS. Human natural killer cell deficiencies. Curr Opin Allergy Clin Immunol 2006;6:399-409.
3. Stetson DB, Mohrs M, Reinhardt RL, et al. Constitutive cytokine mRNAs mark natural killer (NK) and NK T cells poised for rapid effector function. J Exp Med 2003;198:1069-76.
4. Mocikat R, Braumuller H, Gumy A, et al. Natural killer cells activated by MHC class I(low) targets prime dendritic cells to induce protective CD8 T cell responses. Immunity 2003;19:561-9.
5. Wallach D, Fellous M, Revel M. Preferential effect of gamma interferon on the synthesis of HLA antigens and their mRNAs in human cells. Nature 1982;299:833-6.
6. Filipe-Santos O, Bustamante J, Chapgier A, et al. Inborn errors of IL-12/23- and IFN-gamma-mediated immunity: molecular, cellular, and clinical features. Semin Immunol 2006;18:347-61.
7. Maher SG, Romero-Weaver AL, Scarzello AJ, Gamero AM. Interferon: Cellular executioner or white knight? Curr Med Chem 2007;14:1279-89.
8. Blum KS, Pabst R. Lymphocyte numbers and subsets in the human blood. Do they mirror the situation in all organs? Immunol Lett 2007;108:45-51.
9. Cooper MA, Fehniger TA, Turner SC, et al. Human natural killer cells: A unique innate immunoregulatory role for the CD56(bright) subset. Blood 2001;97:3146-51.
10. Spits H, Blom B, Jaleco AC, et al. Early stages in the development of human T, natural killer and thymic dendritic cells. Immunol Rev 1998;165:75-86.
11. Colucci F, Caligiuri MA, Di Santo JP. What does it take to make a natural killer? Nat Rev Immunol 2003;3:413-25.
12. Karre K, Ljunggren HG, Piontek G, Kiessling R. Selective rejection of H-2-deficient lymphoma variants suggests alternative immune defence strategy. Nature 1986;319:675-8.
13. Ljunggren HG, Karre K. In search of the 'missing self': MHC molecules and NK cell recognition. Immunol Today 1990;11:237-44.
14. Lanier LL. NK cell recognition. Annu Rev Immunol 2005;23:225-74.
15. Raulet DH, Vance RE, McMahon CW. Regulation of the natural killer cell receptor repertoire. Annu Rev Immunol 2001;19:291-330.
16. McQueen KL, Parham P. Variable receptors controlling activation and inhibition of NK cells. Curr Opin Immunol 2002;14:615-21.
17. Long EO, Barber DF, Burshtyn DN, et al. Inhibition of natural killer cell activation signals by killer cell immunoglobulin-like receptors (CD158). Immunol Rev 2001;181:223-33.
18. Moretta A, Bottino C, Vitale M, et al. Activating receptors and coreceptors involved in human natural killer cell-mediated cytolysis. Annu Rev Immunol 2001;19:197-223.
19. Vilches C, Parham P. KIR: Diverse, rapidly evolving receptors of innate and adaptive immunity. Annu Rev Immunol 2002;20:217-51.
20. Renedo M, Arce I, Rodriguez A, et al. The human natural killer gene complex is located on chromosome 12p12-p13. Immunogenetics 1997;46:307-11.
21. Suto Y, Yabe T, Maenaka K, et al. The human natural killer gene complex (NKC) is located on chromosome 12p13.1-p13.2. Immunogenetics 1997;46:159-62.
22. Yabe T, McSherry C, Bach FH, et al. A multigene family on human chromosome 12 encodes natural killer-cell lectins. Immunogenetics 1993;37:455-60.
23. Plougastel B, Trowsdale J. Sequence analysis of a 62-kb region overlapping the human KLRC cluster of genes. Genomics 1998;49:193-9.
24. Lazetic S, Chang C, Houchins JP, Lanier LL, Phillips JH. Human natural killer cell receptors involved in MHC class I recognition are disulfide-linked heterodimers of CD94 and NKG2 subunits. J Immunol 1996;157:4741-5.
25. Carretero M, Cantoni C, Bellon T, et al. The CD94 and NKG2-A C-type lectins covalently assemble to form a natural killer cell inhibitory receptor for HLA class I molecules. Eur J Immunol 1997;27:563-7.
26. Braud VM, Allan DS, O'Callaghan CA, et al. HLA-E binds to natural killer cell receptors CD94/NKG2A, B and C. Nature 1998;391:795-9.
27. Lee N, Llano M, Carretero M, et al. HLA-E is a major ligand for the natural killer inhibitory receptor CD94/NKG2A. Proc Natl Acad Sci USA 1998;95: 5199-204.
28. Borrego F, Ulbrecht M, Weiss EH, Coligan JE, Brooks AG. Recognition of human histocompatibility leukocyte antigen (HLA)-E complexed with HLA class I signal sequence-derived peptides by CD94/NKG2 confers protection from natural killer cell-mediated lysis. J Exp Med 1998;187:813-8.
29. Groh V, Rhinehart R, Randolph-Habecker J, et al. Costimulation of CD8alphabeta T cells by NKG2D via engagement by MIC induced on virus-infected cells. Nat Immunol 2001;2:255-60.
30. Cosman D, Mullberg J, Sutherland CL, et al. ULBPs, novel MHC class I-related molecules, bind to CMV glycoprotein UL16 and stimulate NK cytotoxicity through the NKG2D receptor. Immunity 2001;14:123-33.
31. Bauer S, Groh V, Wu J, et al. Activation of NK cells and T cells by NKG2D, a receptor for stress-inducible MICA. Science 1999;285:727-9.
32. Marsh SG, Parham P, Dupont B, et al. Killer-cell immunoglobulin-like receptor (KIR) nomenclature report, 2002. Tissue Antigens 2003;62:79-86.

33. Lanier LL, Bakker AB. The ITAM-bearing transmembrane adaptor DAP12 in lymphoid and myeloid cell function. Immunol Today 2000;21:611-4.
34. Andre P, Biassoni R, Colonna M, et al. New nomenclature for MHC receptors. Nat Immunol 2001;2:661.
35. Steffens U, Vyas Y, Dupont B, Selvakumar A. Nucleotide and amino acid sequence alignment for human killer cell inhibitory receptors (KIR). Tissue Antigens 1998;51:398-413.
36. Wilson MJ, Torkar M, Haude A, et al. Plasticity in the organization and sequences of human KIR/ILT gene families. Proc Natl Acad Sci USA 2000;97:4778-83.
37. Trowsdale J. Genetic and functional relationships between MHC and NK receptor genes. Immunity 2001;15:363-74.
38. Uhrberg M, Parham P, Wernet P. Definition of gene content for nine common group B haplotypes of the Caucasoid population: KIR haplotypes contain between seven and eleven KIR genes. Immunogenetics 2002;54:221-9.
39. Hsu KC, Chida S, Geraghty DE, Dupont B. The killer cell immunoglobulin-like receptor (KIR) genomic region: Gene-order, haplotypes and allelic polymorphism. Immunol Rev 2002;190:40-52.
40. Hsu KC, Liu XR, Selvakumar A, et al. Killer Ig-like receptor haplotype analysis by gene content: Evidence for genomic diversity with a minimum of six basic framework haplotypes, each with multiple subsets. J Immunol 2002;169:5118-29.
41. Yawata M, Yawata N, Draghi M, et al. Roles for HLA and KIR polymorphisms in natural killer cell repertoire selection and modulation of effector function. J Exp Med 2006;203:633-45.
42. Whang DH, Park H, Yoon JA, Park MH. Haplotype analysis of killer cell immunoglobulin-like receptor genes in 77 Korean families. Hum Immunol 2005;66:146-54.
43. Middleton D, Meenagh A, Gourraud PA. KIR haplotype content at the allele level in 77 Northern Irish families. Immunogenetics 2007;59:145-58.
44. Yawata M, Yawata N, Abi-Rached L, Parham P. Variation within the human killer cell immunoglobulin-like receptor (KIR) gene family. Crit Rev Immunol 2002;22:463-82.
45. Uhrberg M, Valiante NM, Shum BP, et al. Human diversity in killer cell inhibitory receptor genes. Immunity 1997;7:753-63.
46. Gomez-Lozano N, Gardiner CM, Parham P, Vilches C. Some human KIR haplotypes contain two KIR2DL5 genes: KIR2DL5A and KIR2DL5B. Immunogenetics 2002;54:314-9.
47. Williams F, Maxwell LD, Halfpenny IA, et al. Multiple copies of KIR 3DL/S1 and KIR 2DL4 genes identified in a number of individuals. Hum Immunol 2003;64:729-32.
48. Vyas Y, Selvakumar A, Steffens U, Dupont B. Multiple transcripts of the killer cell immunoglobulin-like receptor family, KIR3DL1 (NKB1), are expressed by natural killer cells of a single individual. Tissue Antigens 1998;52:510-9.
49. Martin MP, Bashirova A, Traherne J, Trowsdale J, Carrington M. Cutting edge: Expansion of the KIR locus by unequal crossing over. J Immunol 2003;171:2192-5.
50. Ordonez D, Meenagh A, Gomez-Lozano N, et al. Duplication, mutation and recombination of the human orphan gene KIR2DS3 contribute to the diversity of KIR haplotypes. Genes Immun 2008;9:431-7.
51. Single RM, Martin MP, Gao X, et al. Global diversity and evidence for coevolution of KIR and HLA. Nat Genet 2007;39:1114-9.
52. Jiang K, Zhu FM, Lv QF, Yan LX. Distribution of killer cell immunoglobulin-like receptor genes in the Chinese Han population. Tissue Antigens 2005;65:556-63.
53. Yawata M, Yawata N, McQueen KL, et al. Predominance of group A KIR haplotypes in Japanese associated with diverse NK cell repertoires of KIR expression. Immunogenetics 2002;54:543-50.
54. Toneva M, Lepage V, Lafay G, et al. Genomic diversity of natural killer cell receptor genes in three populations. Tissue Antigens 2001;57:358-62.
55. Norman PJ, Stephens HA, Verity DH, Chandanayingyong D, Vaughan RW. Distribution of natural killer cell immunoglobulin-like receptor sequences in three ethnic groups. Immunogenetics 2001;52:195-205.
56. Gendzekhadze K, Norman PJ, Abi-Rached L, Layrisse Z, Parham P. High KIR diversity in Amerindians is maintained using few gene-content haplotypes. Immunogenetics 2006;58:474-80.
57. Witt CS, Dewing C, Sayer DC, et al. Population frequencies and putative haplotypes of the killer cell immunoglobulin-like receptor sequences and evidence for recombination. Transplantation 1999;68:1784-9.
58. Denis L, Sivula J, Gourraud PA, et al. Genetic diversity of KIR natural killer cell markers in populations from France, Guadeloupe, Finland, Senegal and Reunion. Tissue Antigens 2005;66:267-76.
59. Du Z, Gjertson DW, Reed EF, Rajalingam R. Receptor-ligand analyses define minimal killer cell Ig-like receptor (KIR) in humans. Immunogenetics 2007;59:1-15.
60. Niokou D, Spyropoulou-Vlachou M, Darlamitsou A, Stavropoulos-Giokas C. Distribution of killer cell immunoglobulin-like receptors in the Greek population. Hum Immunol 2003;64:1167-76.
61. Norman PJ, Carrington CV, Byng M, et al. Natural killer cell immunoglobulin-like receptor (KIR) locus profiles in African and South Asian populations. Genes Immun 2002;3:86-95.
62. Rajalingam R, Krausa P, Shilling HG, et al. Distinctive KIR and HLA diversity in a panel of north Indian Hindus. Immunogenetics 2002;53:1009-19.
63. Lee YC, Chan SH, Ren EC. Asian population frequencies and haplotype distribution of killer cell immunoglobulin-like receptor (KIR) genes among Chinese, Malay, and Indian in Singapore. Immunogenetics 2008;60:645-54.

64. Kulkarni S, Single RM, Martin MP, et al. Comparison of the rapidly evolving KIR locus in Parsis and natives of India. Immunogenetics 2008;60:121-9.
65. Rajalingam R, Du Z, Meenagh A, et al. Distinct diversity of KIR genes in three southern Indian populations: Comparison with world populations revealed a link between KIR gene content and pre-historic human migrations. Immunogenetics 2008;60:207-17.
66. Santin I, de Nanclares GP, Calvo B, et al. Killer cell immunoglobulin-like receptor (KIR) genes in the Basque population: Association study of KIR gene contents with type 1 diabetes mellitus. Hum Immunol 2006;67:118-24.
67. Velickovic M, Velickovic Z, Dunckley H. Diversity of killer cell immunoglobulin-like receptor genes in Pacific Islands populations. Immunogenetics 2006;58:523-32.
68. Gutierrez-Rodriguez ME, Sandoval-Ramirez L, Diaz-Flores M, et al. KIR gene in ethnic and Mestizo populations from Mexico. Hum Immunol 2006;67:85-93.
69. Flores AC, Marcos CY, Paladino N, et al. KIR genes polymorphism in Argentinean Caucasoid and Amerindian populations. Tissue Antigens 2007; 69:568-76.
70. Ewerton PD, Leite Mde M, Magalhaes M, Sena L, Melo dos Santos EJ. Amazonian Amerindians exhibit high variability of KIR profiles. Immunogenetics 2007;59: 625-30.
71. Ashouri E, Farjadian S, Reed EF, Ghaderi A, Rajalingam R. KIR gene content diversity in four Iranian populations. Immunogenetics 2009;(in press).
72. Middleton D, Menchaca L, Rood H, Komerofsky R. New allele frequency database: http://www.allelefrequencies.net. Tissue Antigens 2003;61:403-7.
73. Barten R, Torkar M, Haude A, Trowsdale J, Wilson MJ. Divergent and convergent evolution of NK-cell receptors. Trends Immunol 2001;22:52-7.
74. Selvakumar A, Steffens U, Dupont B. NK cell receptor gene of the KIR family with two IG domains but highest homology to KIR receptors with three IG domains. Tissue Antigens 1996;48:285-94.
75. Vilches C, Rajalingam R, Uhrberg M, et al. KIR2DL5, a novel killer-cell receptor with a D0-D2 configuration of Ig-like domains. J Immunol 2000;164:5797-804.
76. Shilling HG, Guethlein LA, Cheng NW, et al. Allelic polymorphism synergizes with variable gene content to individualize human KIR genotype. J Immunol 2002;168:2307-15.
77. Garcia CA, Robinson J, Guethlein LA, et al. Human KIR sequences 2003. Immunogenetics 2003;55:227-39.
78. Rajalingam R, Gardiner CM, Canavez F, Vilches C, Parham P. Identification of seventeen novel KIR variants: Fourteen of them from two non-Caucasian donors. Tissue Antigens 2001;57:22-31.
79. Du Z, Sharma SK, Spellman S, Reed EF, Rajalingam R. KIR2DL5 alleles mark certain combination of activating KIR genes. Genes Immun 2008;9:470-80.
80. Norman PJ, Abi-Rached L, Gendzekhadze K, et al. Unusual selection on the KIR3DL1/S1 natural killer cell receptor in Africans. Nat Genet 2007;39:1092-9.
81. Gardiner CM, Guethlein LA, Shilling HG, et al. Different NK cell surface phenotypes defined by the DX9 antibody are due to KIR3DL1 gene polymorphism. J Immunol 2001;166:2992-3001.
82. Winter CC, Gumperz JE, Parham P, Long EO, Wagtmann N. Direct binding and functional transfer of NK cell inhibitory receptors reveal novel patterns of HLA-C allotype recognition. J Immunol 1998;161:571-7.
83. VandenBussche CJ, Dakshanamurthy S, Posch PE, Hurley CK. A single polymorphism disrupts the killer Ig-like receptor 2DL2/2DL3 D1 domain. J Immunol 2006;177:5347-57.
84. O'Connor GM, Guinan KJ, Cunningham RT, et al. Functional polymorphism of the KIR3DL1/S1 receptor on human NK cells. J Immunol 2007;178:235-41.
85. Carr WH, Pando MJ, Parham P. KIR3DL1 polymorphisms that affect NK cell inhibition by HLA-Bw4 ligand. J Immunol 2005;175:5222-9.
86. Maxwell LD, Wallace A, Middleton D, Curran MD. A common KIR2DS4 deletion variant in the human that predicts a soluble KIR molecule analogous to the KIR1D molecule observed in the rhesus monkey. Tissue Antigens 2002;60:254-8.
87. Witt CS, Martin A, Christiansen FT. Detection of KIR2DL4 alleles by sequencing and SSCP reveals a common allele with a shortened cytoplasmic tail. Tissue Antigens 2000;56:248-57.
88. Goodridge JP, Lathbury LJ, Steiner NK, et al. Three common alleles of KIR2DL4 (CD158d) encode constitutively expressed, inducible and secreted receptors in NK cells. Eur J Immunol 2007;37:199-211.
89. Goodridge JP, Witt CS, Christiansen FT, Warren HS. KIR2DL4 (CD158d) genotype influences expression and function in NK cells. J Immunol 2003; 171:1768-74.
90. Vilches C, Gardiner CM, Parham P. Gene structure and promoter variation of expressed and nonexpressed variants of the KIR2DL5 gene. J Immunol 2000; 165: 6416-21.
91. Pando MJ, Gardiner CM, Gleimer M, McQueen KL, Parham P. The Protein Made from a Common Allele of KIR3DL1 (3DL1*004) Is Poorly Expressed at Cell Surfaces due to Substitution at Positions 86 in Ig Domain 0 and 182 in Ig Domain 1. J Immunol 2003;171:6640-9.
92. Valiante NM, Uhrberg M, Shilling HG, et al. Functionally and structurally distinct NK cell receptor repertoires in the peripheral blood of two human donors. Immunity 1997;7:739-51.
93. Santourlidis S, Trompeter HI, Weinhold S, et al. Crucial role of DNA methylation in determination of clonally distributed killer cell Ig-like receptor expression patterns in NK cells. J Immunol 2002;169:4253-61.
94. Anfossi N, Andre P, Guia S, et al. Human NK Cell Education by Inhibitory Receptors for MHC Class I. Immunity 2006.
95. Kim S, Poursine-Laurent J, Truscott SM, et al. Licensing of natural killer cells by host major histocompatibility complex class I molecules. Nature 2005; 436:709-13.

96. Cooley S, Xiao F, Pitt M, et al. A subpopulation of human peripheral blood NK cells that lacks inhibitory receptors for self MHC is developmentally immature. Blood 2007;110:578-86.
97. Bix M, Liao NS, Zijlstra M, et al. Rejection of class I MHC-deficient haemopoietic cells by irradiated MHC-matched mice. Nature 1991;349:329-31.
98. Furukawa H, Yabe T, Watanabe K, et al. Tolerance of NK and LAK activity for HLA class I-deficient targets in a TAP1-deficient patient (bare lymphocyte syndrome type I). Hum Immunol 1999;60:32-40.
99. Yokoyama WM, Kim S. How do natural killer cells find self to achieve tolerance? Immunity 2006;24:249-57.
100. Raulet DH, Vance RE. Self-tolerance of natural killer cells. Nat Rev Immunol 2006;6:520-31.
101. Yu J, Heller G, Chewning J, et al. Hierarchy of the Human Natural Killer Cell Response Is Determined by Class and Quantity of Inhibitory Receptors for Self-HLA-B and HLA-C Ligands. J Immunol 2007;179:5977-89.
102. Parham P, Adams EJ, Arnett KL. The origins of HLA-A,B,C polymorphism. Immunol Rev 1995;143:141-80.
103. Marsh SG, Albert ED, Bodmer WF, et al. Nomenclature for Factors of the HLA System, 2004. Hum Immunol 2005;66:571-636.
104. Prugnolle F, Manica A, Charpentier M, et al. Pathogen-driven selection and worldwide HLA class I diversity. Curr Biol 2005;15:1022-7.
105. Parham P, Ohta T. Population biology of antigen presentation by MHC class I molecules. Science 1996;272:67-74.
106. Colonna M, Spies T, Strominger JL, et al. Alloantigen recognition by two human natural killer cell clones is associated with HLA-C or a closely linked gene. Proc Natl Acad Sci USA 1992;89:7983-5.
107. Colonna M, Borsellino G, Falco M, Ferrara GB, Strominger JL. HLA-C is the inhibitory ligand that determines dominant resistance to lysis by NK1- and NK2-specific natural killer cells. Proc Natl Acad Sci USA 1993;90:12000-4.
108. Wagtmann N, Biassoni R, Cantoni C, et al. Molecular clones of the p58 NK cell receptor reveal immunoglobulin-related molecules with diversity in both the extra- and intracellular domains. Immunity 1995;2:439-49.
109. Winter CC, Long EO. A single amino acid in the p58 killer cell inhibitory receptor controls the ability of natural killer cells to discriminate between the two groups of HLA-C allotypes. J Immunol 1997;158:4026-8.
110. Gumperz JE, Litwin V, Phillips JH, Lanier LL, Parham P. The Bw4 public epitope of HLA-B molecules confers reactivity with natural killer cell clones that express NKB1, a putative HLA receptor. J Exp Med 1995;181:1133-44.
111. Cella M, Longo A, Ferrara GB, Strominger JL, Colonna M. NK3-specific natural killer cells are selectively inhibited by Bw4-positive HLA alleles with isoleucine 80. J Exp Med 1994;180:1235-42.
112. Thananchai H, Gillespie G, Martin MP, et al. Cutting Edge: Allele-specific and peptide-dependent interactions between KIR3DL1 and HLA-A and HLA-B. J Immunol 2007;178:33-7.
113. Pende D, Biassoni R, Cantoni C, et al. The natural killer cell receptor specific for HLA-A allotypes: A novel member of the p58/p70 family of inhibitory receptors that is characterized by three immunoglobulin-like domains and is expressed as a 140-kD disulphide-linked dimer. J Exp Med 1996;184:505-18.
114. Dohring C, Scheidegger D, Samaridis J, Cella M, Colonna M. A human killer inhibitory receptor specific for HLA-A1,2. J Immunol 1996;156:3098-101.
115. Rajagopalan S, Long EO. A human histocompatibility leukocyte antigen (HLA)-G-specific receptor expressed on all natural killer cells. J Exp Med 1999;189:1093-100.
116. Moffett-King A. Natural killer cells and pregnancy. Nat Rev Immunol 2002;2:656-63.
117. Rajagopalan S, Bryceson YT, Kuppusamy SP, et al. Activation of NK cells by an endocytosed receptor for soluble HLA-G. PLoS Biol 2006;4:e9.
118. Kikuchi-Maki A, Yusa S, Catina TL, Campbell KS. KIR2DL4 Is an IL-2-Regulated NK Cell Receptor That Exhibits Limited Expression in Humans but Triggers Strong IFN-gamma Production. J Immunol 2003;171:3415-25.
119. Faure M, Long EO. KIR2DL4 (CD158d), an NK cell-activating receptor with inhibitory potential. J Immunol 2002;168:6208-14.
120. Yusa S, Catina TL, Campbell KS. SHP-1- and phosphotyrosine-independent inhibitory signaling by a killer cell Ig-like receptor cytoplasmic domain in human NK cells. J Immunol 2002;168:5047-57.
121. Ponte M, Cantoni C, Biassoni R, et al. Inhibitory receptors sensing HLA-G1 molecules in pregnancy: Decidua-associated natural killer cells express LIR-1 and CD94/NKG2A and acquire p49, an HLA-G1-specific receptor. Proc Natl Acad Sci U S A 1999;96:5674-9.
122. Trundley AE, Hiby SE, Chang C, et al. Molecular characterization of KIR3DL3. Immunogenetics 2006;57:904-16.
123. Estefania E, Flores R, Gomez-Lozano N, et al. Human KIR2DL5 Is an Inhibitory Receptor Expressed on the Surface of NK and T Lymphocyte Subsets. J Immunol 2007;178:4402-10.
124. Martin MP, Gao X, Lee JH, et al. Epistatic interaction between KIR3DS1 and HLA-B delays the progression to AIDS. Nat Genet 2002;31:429-34.
125. Peruzzi M, Parker KC, Long EO, Malnati MS. Peptide sequence requirements for the recognition of HLA-B*2705 by specific natural killer cells. J Immunol 1996;157:3350-6.
126. Rajagopalan S, Long EO. The direct binding of a p58 killer cell inhibitory receptor to human histocompatibility leukocyte antigen (HLA)-Cw4 exhibits peptide selectivity. J Exp Med 1997;185:1523-8.

127. Maenaka K, Juji T, Nakayama T, et al. Killer cell immunoglobulin receptors and T cell receptors bind peptide-major histocompatibility complex class I with distinct thermodynamic and kinetic properties. J Biol Chem 1999; 274:28329-34.
128. Zappacosta F, Borrego F, Brooks AG, Parker KC, Coligan JE. Peptides isolated from HLA-Cw*0304 confer different degrees of protection from natural killer cell-mediated lysis. Proc Natl Acad Sci USA 1997;94:6313-8.
129. Boyington JC, Motyka SA, Schuck P, Brooks AG, Sun PD. Crystal structure of an NK cell immunoglobulin-like receptor in complex with its class I MHC ligand. Nature 2000;405:537-43.
130. Phillips JH, Gumperz JE, Parham P, Lanier LL. Superantigen-dependent, cell-mediated cytotoxicity inhibited by MHC class I receptors on T lymphocytes. Science 1995;268:403-5.
131. Uhrberg M, Valiante NM, Young NT, et al. The repertoire of killer cell Ig-like receptor and CD94:NKG2A receptors in T cells: Clones sharing identical alpha beta TCR rearrangement express highly diverse killer cell Ig-like receptor patterns. J Immunol 2001;166:3923-32.
132. Ugolini S, Arpin C, Anfossi N, et al. Involvement of inhibitory NKRs in the survival of a subset of memory-phenotype CD8+ T cells. Nat Immunol 2001;2:430-5.
133. Greenwald RJ, Freeman GJ, Sharpe AH. The B7 Family Revisited. Annu Rev Immunol 2005;23:515-48.
134. Martens PB, Goronzy JJ, Schaid D, Weyand CM. Expansion of unusual CD4+ T cells in severe rheumatoid arthritis. Arthritis Rheum 1997;40:1106-14.
135. Schmidt D, Goronzy JJ, Weyand CM. CD4+ CD7- CD28- T cells are expanded in rheumatoid arthritis and are characterized by autoreactivity. J Clin Invest 1996; 97:2027-37.
136. Namekawa T, Snyder MR, Yen JH, et al. Killer cell activating receptors function as costimulatory molecules on CD4+CD28null T cells clonally expanded in rheumatoid arthritis. J Immunol 2000;165:1138-45.
137. Groh V, Bruhl A, El-Gabalawy H, Nelson JL, Spies T. Stimulation of T cell autoreactivity by anomalous expression of NKG2D and its MIC ligands in rheumatoid arthritis. Proc Natl Acad Sci USA 2003;100:9452-7.
138. Snyder MR, Muegge LO, Offord C, et al. Formation of the killer Ig-like receptor repertoire on CD4+CD28null T cells. J Immunol 2002;168:3839-46.
139. Shum BP, Flodin LR, Muir DG, et al. Conservation and variation in human and common chimpanzee CD94 and NKG2 genes. J Immunol 2002;168:240-52.
140. Brown MG, Scalzo AA, Matsumoto K, Yokoyama WM. The natural killer gene complex: A genetic basis for understanding natural killer cell function and innate immunity. Immunol Rev 1997;155:53-65.
141. Karlhofer FM, Ribaudo RK, Yokoyama WM. MHC class I alloantigen specificity of Ly-49+ IL-2-activated natural killer cells. Nature 1992;358:66-70.
142. Barten R, Trowsdale J. The human Ly-49L gene. Immunogenetics 1999;49:731-4.
143. Westgaard IH, Berg SF, Orstavik S, Fossum S, Dissen E. Identification of a human member of the Ly-49 multigene family. Eur J Immunol 1998;28:1839-46.
144. Welch AY, Kasahara M, Spain LM. Identification of the mouse killer immunoglobulin-like receptor-like (Kirl) gene family mapping to Chromosome X. Immunogenetics 2003;54:782-90.
145. Glazko GV, Nei M. Estimation of divergence times for major lineages of primate species. Mol Biol Evol 2003;20: 424-34.
146. Abi-Rached L, Parham P. Natural selection drives recurrent formation of activating killer cell immunoglobulin-like receptor and Ly49 from inhibitory homologues. J Exp Med 2005;201:1319-32.
147. Horai S, Hayasaka K, Kondo R, Tsugane K, Takahata N. Recent African origin of modern humans revealed by complete sequences of hominoid mitochondrial DNAs. Proc Natl Acad Sci USA 1995;92:532-6.
148. Parham P, Adams EJ, Arnett KL. The origins of HLA-A,B,C polymorphism. Immunol Rev 1995;143:141-80.
149. Khakoo SI, Rajalingam R, Shum BP, et al. Rapid evolution of NK cell receptor systems demonstrated by comparison of chimpanzees and humans. Immunity 2000;12:687-98.
150. Rajalingam R, Hong M, Adams EJ, et al. Short KIR haplotypes in pygmy chimpanzee (Bonobo) resemble the conserved framework of diverse human KIR haplotypes. J Exp Med 2001;193:135-46.
151. Rajalingam R, Parham P, Abi-Rached L. Domain shuffling has been the main mechanism forming new hominoid killer cell Ig-like receptors. J Immunol 2004; 172:356-69.
152. Khakoo SI, Carrington M. KIR and disease: a model system or system of models? Immunol Rev 2006;214: 186-201.
153. Kulkarni S, Martin MP, Carrington M. The Yin and Yang of HLA and KIR in human disease. Semin Immunol 2008;20:343-52.
154. Terme M, Ullrich E, Delahaye NF, Chaput N, Zitvogel L. Natural killer cell-directed therapies: Moving from unexpected results to successful strategies. Nat Immunol 2008;9:486-94.
155. Appelbaum FR. The current status of hematopoietic cell transplantation. Annu Rev Med 2003;54:491-512.
156. Thomas ED. History, current results, and research in marrow transplantation. Perspect Biol Med 1995;38: 230-7.
157. Armitage JO. Bone marrow transplantation. N Engl J Med 1994;330:827-38.
158. Cudkowicz G, Bennett M. Peculiar immunobiology of bone marrow allografts. II. Rejection of parental grafts by resistant F 1 hybrid mice. J Exp Med 1971; 134:1513-28.
159. Cudkowicz G, Bennett M. Peculiar immunobiology of bone marrow allografts. I. Graft rejection by irradiated responder mice. J Exp Med 1971;134:83-102.

160. George T, Yu YY, Liu J, et al. Allorecognition by murine natural killer cells: Lysis of T-lymphoblasts and rejection of bone-marrow grafts. Immunol Rev 1997;155:29-40.
161. Ruggeri L, Capanni M, Urbani E, et al. Effectiveness of donor natural killer cell alloreactivity in mismatched hematopoietic transplants. Science 2002;295:2097-100.
162. Ruggeri L, Capanni M, Casucci M, et al. Role of natural killer cell alloreactivity in HLA-mismatched hematopoietic stem cell transplantation. Blood 1999;94:333-9.
163. Petersson E, Qi Z, Ekberg H, et al. Activation of alloreactive natural killer cells is resistant to cyclosporine. Transplantation 1997;63:1138-44.
164. Kageyama S, Matsui S, Hasegawa T, et al. Augmentation of natural killer cell activity induced by cytomegalovirus infection in mice treated with FK506. Acta Virol 1997;41:215-20.
165. Shapira MY, Hirshfeld E, Weiss L, et al. Mycophenolate mofetil does not suppress the graft-versus-leukemia effect or the activity of lymphokine-activated killer (LAK) cells in a murine model. Cancer Immunol Immunother 2005;54:383-8.
166. Pedersen BK, Beyer JM. A longitudinal study of the influence of azathioprine on natural killer cell activity. Allergy 1986;41:286-9.
167. Luo H, Chen H, Daloze P, Wu J. Effects of rapamycin on human HLA-unrestricted cell killing. Clin Immunol Immunopathol 1992;65:60-4.
168. Blancho G, Buzelin F, Dantal J, et al. Evidence that early acute renal failure may be mediated by CD3- CD16+ cells in a kidney graft recipient with large granular lymphocyte proliferation. Transplantation 1992;53:1242-7.
169. Petersson E, Ostraat O, Ekberg H, et al. Allogeneic heart transplantation activates alloreactive NK cells. Cell Immunol 1997;175:25-32.
170. Fildes JE, Yonan N, Tunstall K, et al. Natural killer cells in peripheral blood and lung tissue are associated with chronic rejection after lung transplantation. J Heart Lung Transplant 2008;27:203-7.
171. Navarro F, Portales P, Candon S, et al. Natural killer cell and alphabeta and gammadelta lymphocyte traffic into the liver graft immediately after liver transplantation. Transplantation 2000;69:633-9.
172. Kunert K, Seiler M, Mashreghi MF, et al. KIR/HLA ligand incompatibility in kidney transplantation. Transplantation 2007;84:1527-33.
173. Vampa ML, Norman PJ, Burnapp L, et al. Natural killer-cell activity after human renal transplantation in relation to killer immunoglobulin-like receptors and human leukocyte antigen mismatch. Transplantation 2003;76:1220-8.
174. Maier S, Tertilt C, Chambron N, et al. Inhibition of natural killer cells results in acceptance of cardiac allografts in CD28-/- mice. Nat Med 2001;7:557-62.
175. Rajalingam R. Variable interactions of recipient killer cell immunoglobulin-like receptors with self and allogenic human leukocyte antigen class I ligands may influence the outcome of solid organ transplants. Curr Opin Organ Transplant 2008;13:430-7.
176. Biron CA, Nguyen KB, Pien GC, Cousens LP, Salazar-Mather TP. Natural killer cells in antiviral defense: Function and regulation by innate cytokines. Annu Rev Immunol 1999;17:189-220.
177. French AR, Yokoyama WM. Natural killer cells and viral infections. Curr Opin Immunol 2003;15:45-51.
178. Orange JS, Ballas ZK. Natural killer cells in human health and disease. Clin Immunol 2006;118:1-10.
179. Alter G, Teigen N, Davis BT, et al. Sequential deregulation of NK cell subset distribution and function starting in acute HIV-1 infection. Blood 2005; 106: 3366-9.
180. Carrington M, O'Brien SJ. The influence of HLA genotype on AIDS. Annu Rev Med 2003;54:535-51.
181. Flores-Villanueva PO, Yunis EJ, Delgado JC, et al. Control of HIV-1 viremia and protection from AIDS are associated with HLA-Bw4 homozygosity. Proc Natl Acad Sci USA 2001;98:5140-5.
182. Lopez-Vazquez A, Mina-Blanco A, Martinez-Borra J, et al. Interaction between KIR3DL1 and HLA-B*57 supertype alleles influences the progression of HIV-1 infection in a Zambian population. Hum Immunol 2005;66:285-9.
183. Alter HJ, Seeff LB. Recovery, persistence, and sequelae in hepatitis C virus infection: A perspective on long-term outcome. Semin Liver Dis 2000;20:17-35.
184. Khakoo SI, Thio CL, Martin MP, et al. HLA and NK cell inhibitory receptor genes in resolving hepatitis C virus infection. Science 2004;305:872-4.
185. Waldhauer I, Steinle A. NK cells and cancer immunosurveillance. Oncogene 2008;27:5932-43.
186. Zamai L, Ponti C, Mirandola P, et al. NK cells and cancer. J Immunol 2007;178:4011-6.
187. Smyth MJ, Hayakawa Y, Takeda K, Yagita H. New aspects of natural-killer-cell surveillance and therapy of cancer. Nat Rev Cancer 2002;2:850-61.
188. Wu J, Lanier LL. Natural killer cells and cancer. Adv Cancer Res 2003;90:127-56.
189. Hayakawa Y, Smyth MJ. Innate immune recognition and suppression of tumors. Adv Cancer Res 2006;95:293-322.
190. Carrington M, Wang S, Martin MP, et al. Hierarchy of resistance to cervical neoplasia mediated by combinations of killer immunoglobulin-like receptor and human leukocyte antigen loci. J Exp Med 2005;201:1069-75.
191. Lopez-Vazquez A, Rodrigo L, Martinez-Borra J, et al. Protective effect of the HLA-Bw4I80 epitope and the killer cell immunoglobulin-like receptor 3DS1 gene against the development of hepatocellular carcinoma in patients with hepatitis C virus infection. J Infect Dis 2005;192:162-5.

192. Suzuki Y, Hamamoto Y, Ogasawara Y, et al. Genetic polymorphisms of killer cell immunoglobulin-like receptors are associated with susceptibility to psoriasis vulgaris. J Invest Dermatol 2004;122:1133-6.
193. Holm SJ, Sakuraba K, Mallbris L, et al. Distinct HLA-C/KIR genotype profile associates with guttate psoriasis. J Invest Dermatol 2005;125:721-30.
194. Luszczek W, Manczak M, Cislo M, et al. Gene for the activating natural killer cell receptor, KIR2DS1, is associated with susceptibility to psoriasis vulgaris. Hum Immunol 2004;65:758-66.
195. van der Slik AR, Koeleman BP, Verduijn W, et al. KIR in type 1 diabetes: disparate distribution of activating and inhibitory natural killer cell receptors in patients versus HLA-matched control subjects. Diabetes 2003;52:2639-42.
196. Momot T, Koch S, Hunzelmann N, et al. Association of killer cell immunoglobulin-like receptors with scleroderma. Arthritis Rheum 2004;50:1561-5.

Chapter 25

Role of Non-classical HLA Antigens in Pregnancy

Suraksha Agrawal, Prashant Sood, Narinder K Mehra

INTRODUCTION

Normal pregnancy is one of the most imposing immunological paradoxes of nature. Even after decades of scientific inquiry into this enigma, immunologists continue to grapple with the intricate orchestration of immunomodulatory pathways operating at the fetomaternal interface. The paradox of this successful symbiosis of an antigenically foreign fetus and placenta, growing in an immunologically foreign maternal environment with a region of potential histocompatibility at the maternal-fetal interface, was first presented by Sir Peter Medawar in the early 1950s.[1] Ever since, then several milestones have been achieved in understanding the immunological aspects of fetomaternal interface and disorders caused by the disruption of this exquisite natural immunomodulation.

Normal pregnancy refers to the maternal state of carrying a developing fetus *in utero* which culminates in successful live birth after 37 to 40 weeks' period of gestation, through a normal vaginal delivery. Aberrations leading to unsuccessful pregnancy can vary from simple miscarriages to baffling idiopathic recurrent spontaneous abortions. Simple *miscarriage* refers to the loss of a pregnancy before 24 weeks. It is a common complication, occurring in 12-30 percent of all clinical pregnancies. The World Health Organization defines *spontaneous abortion* as the "expulsion or extraction of a fetus weighing 500 grams or less (approximately equal to 20-22 weeks of gestation) or another product of gestation of any weight and specifically designated (e.g. hydatidiform mole) irrespective of gestational age and whether or not there is evidence of life".[2] *Recurrent spontaneous abortions* (RSA) on the other hand, are defined as three or more consecutive pregnancy losses prior to the 20th week of gestation, conceived with the same partner in the absence of uterine, genetic or autoimmune abnormalities.[3] RSA can be further subdivided into three subgroups: (i) Primary aborters – women who have had three or more consecutive abortions and no history of live births; (ii) Secondary aborters – women who have suffered three or more consecutive abortions after minimum one live birth, the risk of subsequent pregnancy loss being ~24 percent after two, 30 percent after three and 40 percent after four consecutive abortions; and (iii) Potential aborters – women who have suffered two consecutive abortions.[4-6] Hence, pregnancy is not a uniformly successful phenomenon. While ~70 percent of fertilized ova are lost prior to implantation,[7] 10-15 percent of clinically recognized pregnancies abort spontaneously in the first trimester. Most of these spontaneous abortions are sporadic and non-recurrent and only 0.5–2 percent of couples suffer from RSA. A cause is determined in only 50 percent of these cases. This translates to an unexplained RSA rate of approximately 1 in every 200 to 400 women who wish to have children.[4,8]

A successful pregnancy involves local immune-modulation and immune-suppression, without compromise to the systemic immune system of the mother. While the former helps in fetal survival and growth, the latter protects the growing fetus from infectious assaults. Disruption of this delicate immune balance results in implantation failures, spontaneous abortions and pregnancy complications like pre-eclampsia and abnormalities of placentation. In this chapter, we discuss the prevailing concepts in reproductive immunology with a specific emphasis on human leukocyte antigen (HLA) sharing, non-classical HLA antigens, non-major histocompatibility complex (MHC) genes, uterine natural killer (uNK) cells and their role in normal pregnancy and RSA. Further in an attempt to resolve the consensus pathways orchestrating immune tolerance at this critical cross-section, the role of various cytokine, cellular, MHC, non-MHC, and neuroendocrine players operating at the maternal-fetal interface has been discussed. The chapter also discusses the available immunotherapeutic modalities for the management of RSA, and highlights potential research directions in the area of reproductive immunology with a focus on translational solutions.

THE MAJOR HISTOCOMPATIBILITY COMPLEX AND PREGNANCY

The HLA System – Brief Overview

The MHC was discovered in the mid to late 1930s, through studies involving exchange of skin grafts in different strains of mice. The HLA region spans 4×10^6 nucleotides on chromosome 6p21.1 to p21.3, with class II, class III and class I genes located from the centromeric to the telomeric end (Fig. 25.1).

Most of the genes are in linkage disequilibrium and are therefore inherited as a combined block or a haplotype. Recombination occurs rarely, at a frequency of 1-3 percent, mostly at the HLA-A or HLA-DP ends. The HLA genes are codominantly expressed and follow the Mendelian pattern of inheritance. Detailed description on the human MHC has been given in Chapter 4 by Brian Tait. The classical HLA genes involved in immune regulation are located primarily in the class I and II regions. The latter spans approximately 1.1 Mb and contains the HLA-DP, DQ and DR loci, which are found as pairs encoding the α and β chains. These chains encode the heterodimeric class II antigens expressed on the cell surface of antigen-presenting cells (APCs) like macrophages, dendritic cell, Langerhans' cell, Kupffer cell, B cells and activated T cells. The class I region on the other hand lies at the telomeric end and contains the classical HLA-A, B, C (HLA class Ia); non-classical HLA-E, F, G (HLA class Ib); and other related loci, spread over a region of approximately 2 Mb. Class Ia molecules are highly polymorphic and are more ubiquitously expressed on all nucleated cells. They form heterodimers with the non-MHC encoded β2 microglobulin whose gene lies on chromosome 15. Class Ib molecules on the other hand exhibit a much more limited degree of polymorphism and have a more restricted tissue distribution than their class Ia counterparts. Class III region placed between class I and II regions consists of genes with immune functions such as C2, C4, Bf, properdin factor B, which are involved in the complement cascade and others such as tumor necrosis factor (TNF), LTA, LTB and heat shock proteins (HSP). The second set of genes within class III region with non-immune functions and not directly related to antigen presentation include G7a (valyl tRNA), OSG and others. The gene densities are very high with approximately one gene per 14.1 Kb in the class I, per 25 Kb in the class II and per 14.3 Kb in class III regions. Currently, a total of 3201 alleles in the HLA region have been defined according to the ImMunoGeneTics (IMGT)/HLA database statistics (http://www.ebi.ac.uk/imgt/hla), updated by the European Bioinformatics Institute. Of these: in the MHC

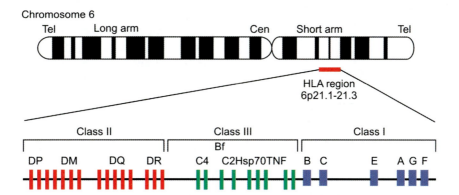

Fig. 25.1: Gene map of the human leukocyte antigen (HLA) region that spans 4×10^6 nucleotides on chromosome 6p21.1 to p21.3, with class II, class III and class I genes located from the centromeric (Cen) to the telomeric (Tel) end. HLA class I are further subdivided into class Ia (HLA-A, B, C) and class Ib (HLA-E, F, G) antigens. The latter unlike other HLA loci have restricted expression, show very little polymorphism and are bracketed under the non-classical HLA. HLA-G and E are the major antigens expressed on the fetal syncytiotrophoblast and are believed to play a key role in the normal immunological response during pregnancy and in the immunopathogenesis of complications like RSA

class I region, 673 alleles have been identified in HLA-A, 1077 in HLA-B and 360 in HLA-C; in the MHC class II region, 585 alleles have been identified in HLA-DRB1, 93 in HLA-DQB1, 34 in DQA1, 128 in DPB1 and 27 in DPB1.

Three cardinal features of the MHC include extraordinarily high polymorphism, tight linkage among various loci and its multipeptide binding ability. The sequence variation between alleles is predominantly localized within exons 2 and 3 for HLA-A, B and C, and within exon 2 for HLA-DRB, DQA, DQB, DPA and DPB loci. A large number of non-synonymous substitutions are concentrated in the peptide binding cleft that determines the specificity of peptides finally presented. The MHC class I and class II antigens are cell surface glycoproteins with a prime function of presenting antigens to effector cells and thereby regulating T cell mediated immune response. HLA molecules interact with the antigen-specific T cell receptor to condition the recognition of antigens by T cells, thereby bringing about T cell activation and resulting in an immune response. HLA class I-encoded molecules restrict CD8+ cytotoxic T-lymphocyte (CTL) function and mediate immune responses against 'endogenous' antigens and virally infected targets. On the other hand HLA class II molecules are involved in the presentation of 'exogenous' antigens to CD4+ T helper (Th) cells.[9,10]

Role of HLA in Normal Pregnancy

Trophoblast cells, including the syncytiotrophoblast and villous cytotrophoblast are one of the few physiological cellular populations in the human body that lack typical MHC class Ia (HLA-A and B) and MHC class II antigens. This renders these semiallogenic fetal cells 'invisible' to the maternal immune system. However, cells which do not express MHC/HLA antigens on their surface are prone to undergo NK cell mediated lysis. Hence, the invasive extravillous cytotrophoblast and endovascular trophoblast cell subsets, which come in direct contact with the uterine NK cells, express MHC class Ib antigens including HLA-G, E and F and also demonstrate expression of MHC class Ia HLA-C antigens.[11,12]

HLA Sharing and RSA

Interaction between MHC genes and the immune system in RSA is a subject of intense discussion. While several hypotheses have been put forward to explain the pathogenesis of RSA, no clear understanding of the precise mechanisms responsible for this complication has prevailed. In recent years, an immunogenetic basis of RSA has been advocated by several groups of investigators. Two schools of thought namely the "immunotrophic theory" and the "genetic hypothesis" attempt to summarize these immunogenetic mechanisms. The "genetic hypothesis" states that there is a high degree of sharing of HLA antigens in couples suffering from RSA.[13] Accordingly, the fetal loss in RSA results from homozygosity of recessive lethal or deleterious alleles in gametic disequilibrium with HLA antigens, in specific HLA haplotypes. The probability that a fetus would be unviable when the parents share HLA antigens at one to two loci, which are in absolute disequilibrium with a recessive lethal gene, is ¼ to ½. For some haplotypes when three antigens are shared at three loci, the probability of an unviable offspring is ¾.[14,15] Recent studies have localized the genetic defects involved to the HLA-B, DR and DQ region of the MHC. The shared HLA antigens can be potential markers for the sharing of closely linked susceptibility genes or genetic defects.[16]

Besides the genetic hypothesis the 'immunotrophic theory' put forward by Thomas Gill (1983) states that the presence of an immune response when the mother and fetus differ at the HLA loci is necessary for proper implantation and fetal growth. Conversely, sharing of HLA antigens in a parental couple, results in a fetus similar to the mother and consequently an immune response that is abnormal in some way by the mother to the fetus, thus preventing successful establishment of pregnancy.[17] This concept was further substantiated by Wegmann in 1987,[18] who showed that certain cytokines produced by maternal cells recognize fetal antigens and promote the proliferation of trophoblastic cells to sustain pregnancy. Inadequate immunological interactions between partners or between the mother and fetus are a potential cause of pregnancy failure.[19] Although the fetal syncytiotrophoblast does not express polymorphic MHC class I or II antigens, the fetus itself expresses HLA-DR antigens as early as the 9th week of gestation, which possibly elicits maternal immune responses. HLA-DR molecules, bind peptides derived from the degradation of proteins ingested by MHC class II expressing antigen presenting cells (APC), and display them at the cell surface for recognition by CD4+ T-lymphocytes. In the decidua, CD4+ T-lymphocytes expressing HLA-DR antigens are reported to be activated during early pregnancy. Thus, there is a possibility that significant compatibility of HLA-DR and -DQ alleles in couples with recurrent abortions might suppress the appropriate immune response of the mother against her fetus.[18,19]

The common thread between the genetic and immunotrophic hypothesis stands out to be the maternal-fetal or maternal-paternal HLA sharing. This sharing is the predecessor of possible downstream mechanisms causing RSA (Fig. 25.2). HLA sharing literally implies sharing of HLA antigens at one or more loci between the two parents. It is presumed that when the fetus expresses paternally derived HLA that is shared with maternal HLA, the initial maternal immune response to fetal antigens will be deficient.[20] Considerable evidence points to HLA compatibility or sharing being more prevalent in couples experiencing reproductive failure, especially RSA couples, compared to those having normal childbearing capabilities.[13] Therefore, HLA incompatibility between mother and fetus, rather than histocompatibility (as hypothesized in earlier studies), appears to confer a selective advantage in terms of fertility and reproductive success.[19-23]

HLA maternal-fetal sharing: Maternal recognition of paternally derived fetal antigens occurs at the time of mating and conception, as well as implantation and throughout pregnancy, and is believed to be beneficial for the establishment and maintenance of pregnancy. Sharing of HLA alleles between mother and fetus is the primary exposure of interest while couple sharing is merely a proxy measure. Studies have shown that while an increased incidence of RSA is noted in women who shared HLA-A, B or DR alleles with their offspring, there was no significant association between RSA and couple sharing of HLA alleles.[24] Table 25.1 summarizes some of the studies in this context.

HLA maternal-paternal/couple sharing: As against the above, increased HLA sharing among spouses has been reported with RSA by several investigators (Table 25.2). Most studies point out that HLA-DR and/or HLA-DQ sharing, specifically HLA-DQA1*0505 predispose to abortion when shared between partners,[26,27] although others have failed to confirm these findings.[28-30]

Studies that focused on couple HLA sharing as a proxy of fetal-maternal sharing have yielded inconsistent results, in terms of whether or not couple sharing is significantly related to RSA and which particular HLA genes may be responsible. Recently, Beydoun and co-workers[20] performed analysis on selected case control studies and found significantly increased risk of RSA among couples who shared at least one allele at the HLA-DR locus, but not at other HLA loci. The genes controlling virtually all immune responses in humans are situated

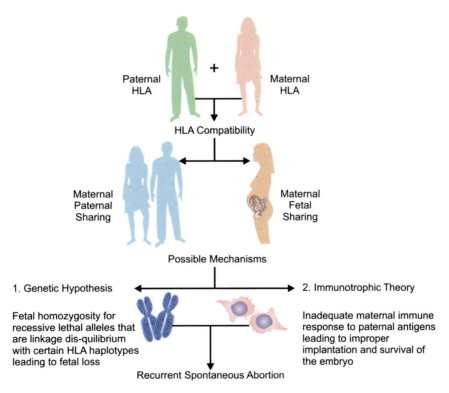

Fig. 25.2: The two main conceptual models of recurrent spontaneous abortion are based on the common observation of HLA compatibility (sharing) between the mother and fetus and/or the mother and father in couples suffering from recurrent spontaneous abortions

Table 25.1: Maternal-fetal HLA sharing and the risk[25] of recurrent spontaneous abortion

Ethnic group	Ref.	RSA triads	Fertile couples	HLA loci studied
Studies showing positive association				
British	24	36 RSA mother, father, baby triads	None	A, B, DR
Studies showing no difference				
Finnish	25	35 primary RSA triads, 15 secondary RSA triads	40 randomly selected Finnish families	DQ
North American	26	40 RSA abortus	31 live born children to RSA couples	DQA1, DQB1

Table 25.2: Maternal-paternal HLA sharing and the risk of recurrent spontaneous abortion

Ethnic group	Ref.	RSA couples	Fertile couples	HLA loci studied
Studies showing positive association				
Croatian	31	303	79	A, B
Swedish	32	8	General population	A, B, DR
French	33	20	132	DR
North American	15	344	84	A
Italian	34	18	23	A, B
Caucasian	13	21	568	B, DR
North American	35	161[a]	103	Overall HLA[d]
North American	28	59[a]	51	DR[d], DQ[e]
Taiwanese	36	123[a]	51	A, DQ1; ≥ 3 of A, B, DR, DQ[d&e]
Japanese	37	99	3070[b]	DR, DQ1
British	4	103	1772[b]	A, B, DR
Hutterite	38	111; (251 abortions)	None	B, C, C4 (entire 16 loci haplotype)
Danish	39	588	562	DRB1*03
Japanese	19	91	72	DRB1, DQB1
Studies showing no difference				
French	33	20	132	A, B
North American	15	344	84	B, DR
Caucasian	13	21	568	A
North American	35	161[a]	103	Overall HLA[e]
Australian	40	85[a]	Fertile couples	A, B, DR
Hutterite	23	111	None	A, B, DR
Italian	41	96	328	A, B, C, DR
Spaniards	29	57	57	A, B, DR
Danish	30	56	33	A, B, DR
Taiwanese	42	36	35	A, B, C, DR
Japanese	37	99	3070[b]	A, B, C
Japanese	43	22	20	DQB
British	24	36	None	A, B, DR
North American	26	40 RSA abortus	31[c]	DQA1, DQB1
Hutterite	38	111; (251 abortions)	None	A, DR, DQ
Caucasoid, Mongoloid	44	158	81	A, B, C, G, E, DR, DQ, DP

[a] Primary and secondary RSA subgroups, [b] MHC I and MHC II subgroups, [c] live borne children to RSA couples, [d] primary RSA group, [e] secondary RSA group.

in the HLA complex, that also contains many non-HLA 'passenger' genes. This raises the question whether the effect of HLA in the pathogenesis of RSA is indeed direct or due to linkage disequilibrium with neighboring genes (e.g. TNF α) embedded in the HLA haplotype. No definitive conclusions have been reached because of small study cohorts and application of serological techniques for determining HLA class II alleles in these studies.

HLA-G AND FETOMATERNAL INTERFACE IMMUNOMODULATION

HLA-G was the first HLA class I antigen to be identified on trophoblast cells by Ellis et al.[45] In the growing fetoplacental unit, it is mainly expressed on the invading extravillous cytotrophoblast but the villous cytotrophoblast and the syncytiotrophoblast also express certain isoforms of HLA-G.[12] Physiological HLA-G expression has also been noted in the thymus, eye and kidney. HLA-G belongs to the non-classical HLA class Ib antigens, which also include HLA-E and F. It differs from the classic class I genes by its unique promoter region, atypical splicing patterns, shortened cytoplasmic tail, minimal genetic variation, and restricted tissue distribution.[46,47] While a detailed description on HLA-G, E and F has been given in Chapter 9 by Antonio Arnaiz-Villena, only the most relevant aspects of these genes are discussed here.

HLA-G gene is located telomeric to HLA-A locus on chromosome 6. It consists of eight exons, seven introns and a 32 untranslated region (3'UTR) (Figs 25.3A to C).

Exon 1 codes for the signal peptide, exons 2-4 encode for the α1, α2, and α3 domains of the molecule, exons 5 encodes for the transmembrane domain and exons 6 and 7 carry the intracellular domain code. While α1 and α2 contribute to the peptide binding cleft; the candidate-binding site for leukocyte Ig-like receptor is borne by the α3 domain.[48-50] HLA-G antigen is nearly monomorphic owing to relatively little polymorphism in its coding region. Only 13 polymorphisms have been identified till date in the exons 1-4, and one 14 bp insertion/deletion

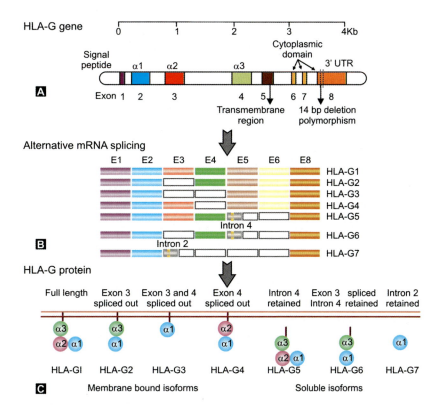

Figs 25.3A to C: (A) The HLA-G gene consists of 8 exons, of which exons 2, 3, and 4 encode the α1, α2, and α3 peptide chains of the HLA-G molecule respectively. The gene structure differs from HLA class Ia genes, in having a shorter cytoplasmic domain and very little polymorphism. The 3' untranslated region (3'UTR) contains a 14 bp insertion/deletion polymorphism associated with decreased HLA-G expression. (B and C) Alternative splicing of the mRNA transcript yield seven isoforms of HLA-G, including membranous and soluble forms. The intron 4 and 2 retained in the soluble isoforms (HLA-G5, -G6, -G7) contain stop codons (shown as thin yellow bar within the gray introns), which prevent the translation of the transmembrane anchor

polymorphism in exons 8 in the 3' untranslated region (UTR). The polymorphisms that alter the protein sequence define five alleles, called G*0101, G*0103, G*0104, G*0105N, and G*0106. Silent variation within these allelic classes defines subtypes, referred to as G*010101, G*010102, etc. HLA-G exists in 4 membrane bound isoforms (HLA-G1-G4) and 3 soluble isoforms (HLA-G5-G7). These are generated by alternative splicing of the HLA-G mRNA which yields 7 transcripts. The soluble forms (sHLA-G) are generated from transcripts that include sequences derived from intron 4 and 2, which contain premature stop codons that preclude the generation of the transmembrane and cytoplasmic domains of the antigen.

HLA-G alleles containing the 14 bp insertion/deletion polymorphism sequence in exons 8 are associated with lower HLA-G mRNA levels for most isoforms in heterozygous trophoblast samples. This polymorphism has been shown in recent studies to impact mRNA transcript size and stability. In addition to the four alleles that differ at the protein level, a polymorphic 1 bp deletion of a cytosine (C) residue at codon 130 in exons 3 results in a null allele (G*0105N), which does not encode functional HLA-G1 or -G5 protein isoforms. The mutation leads to loss of disulfide bridge between residues 101 and 164, rendering the HLA-G molecule unstable. This mutation, called 1597 ΔC, occurs in the homozygous form in apparently healthy individuals, indicating that HLA-G1 and -G5 isoforms are not essential for fetal survival. Interestingly HLA-G2/G6 expression has been noted in many of the same cells as HLA-G1, suggesting that in women carrying the null allele (G*0105N) that does not encode functional HLA-G1 or HLA-G5 protein isoforms yet have uneventful pregnancies, because in these situations HLA-G2/G6 may comprise an adequate substitute.[12,48]

HLA-G expression in the fetoplacental unit follows a distinct pattern. HLA-G1 and HLA-G2/G6 have been identified only at the leading edge of trophoblast columns and the chorion membrane cytotrophoblast cells immediately adjacent to the decidua. HLA-G5 on the other hand is ubiquitous in trophoblast subpopulations, including villous and extravillous cytotrophoblast and syncytiotrophoblast cells and in maternal blood.[12] HLA-G antigens play a major role in tolerance induction in immune cells. Broadly, their effects include downregulated NK cell killing, migration, and cell viability; regulation of IFNγ and cytokine production in blood mononuclear cells and cytotoxic T lymphocytes (CTLs); suppression of CTL killing and viability; inhibition of proliferation and induction of a suppressive phenotype in T-helper cells; and alteration of dendritic cell stimulatory capacity and maturation of this lineage.

HLA-G appears to be recognized mainly by immunoglobulin-like transcript (ILT) receptors, which are expressed by T and B lymphocytes, NK cells and mononuclear phagocytes, and abrogate activating signals received by these cells. Direct interaction of its α1 domain with ILT2 and ILT4 receptors and killer Ig-like receptors 2 DL4 (KIR2DL4) have been demonstrated in recent studies. Both membrane bound and soluble HLA-G (sHLA-G) have been noted to induce apoptosis of alloreactive (antipaternal) CD8+ T cell through the Fas/FasL pathway and also prevent CD4+ T cell proliferation while simultaneously shifting them towards an immunosuppressive phenotype.[12,47] Diminished or aberrant HLA-G expression seems to be associated with certain complications of pregnancy like implantation failure in IVF, pre-eclampsia, and RSA. Hunt et al[49] hypothesized mechanisms by which HLA-G contributes to maternal immune tolerance and maintenance of pregnancy. One possible explanation is that maternal cells programmed to recognize HLA class II associated peptides, bind the circulating sHLA-G2 and thus initiate a peptide-specific immune response. A second possibility is that lymphocytes bearing HLA-G specific T cell receptors recognize circulating sHLA-G2 and are induced to "commit suicide" through the Fas–Fas ligand apoptosis pathway. This is an attractive hypothesis that could account for the lack of circulating maternal antifetal T lymphocytes. Third, sHLA-G2 might interact with killer inhibitory receptors on NK cells at the maternal-fetal interface and prevent attack on the placenta. Further details of the interaction between HLA-G antigens with NK cells are deliberated in the section on uterine NK cells below.

Reduced sHLA-G serum levels have been observed in women experiencing early RSA as compared to those with intact pregnancies. Substantial part of sHLA-G detected in maternal circulation is produced by immunocompetent cells of the mother, and much of this expression has been found to be steady in the course of a normal pregnancy.[47,51] HLA-G*0103 and *0105 (null allele) mutations have been associated with decreased HLA-G levels. Immunostaining of extravillous and endovascular cytotrophoblast have shown decreased HLA-G expression in cases of recurrent miscarriage as compared to normal pregnancy.[47] Isoform specific HLA-G variations have been reported in RSA women in India.[46] In this study, while the G1 isoform was equally prevalent in both normal and RSA women, the G2 and G3 isoforms were decreased in controls (68-80 percent) as compared with RSA (88-100 percent). On the other hand the G4 isoform occurred with higher in the controls (56 percent) versus RSA women (47%). Although these differences are not significant, the study highlights a trend towards differential expression among the two cohorts and further suggests that a relatively lower transcription of the truncated isoforms of HLA-G may also contribute to RSA.

Studies on HLA-G gene polymorphism, expression and sharing in RSA have been performed in different ethnic groups with variable conclusions.[47,52] Owing to the small number of well controlled studies involving large cohorts, empirical evidence appears to be ambiguous as to whether one or several specific HLA-G alleles may be involved in the pathogenesis of RSA. It is also not clear whether these HLA alleles are themselves the susceptibility factors or represent other major linked genes within the HLA complex. Table 25.3 summarizes various studies evaluating the association of HLA-G expression and polymorphism with the risk of RSA.

EVOLVING ROLE OF HLA-E AND HLA-F

The extravillous cytotrophoblast cells express HLA-E and F in addition to HLA-G. While the former has two alleles, HLA-F has no allelic variants reported till date. Two non-synonymous (amino acid) substitutions of HLA-F reported in online databases (http://genome.ucsc.edu) are believed to be uncommon in the general population. The role of HLA-F in the immunomodulation of successful pregnancy remains to be elucidated.[12]

HLA-E on the other hand has been discovered to play a critical role in maternal-fetal immunology. It is the least polymorphic of all the MHC-I molecules, with only eight alleles encoding three different proteins described in the human population. Only two of these alleles, HLA-E*0101 and HLA-E*0103, exist with a reasonable frequency at the population level. Interestingly, surface expression of HLA-E requires it to bind leader sequence peptides (residues 3-11) derived from other HLA class I antigens. The loading of these peptides into HLA-E is dependent on the "transporter associated with antigen processing" (TAP) and cells deficient in TAP are unable to express HLA-E at the cell surface. The acquisition of these peptides by HLA-E is tightly controlled and dependent on the expression of other MHC-I molecules, which serve as a source of these peptides. In the extravillous cytotrophoblast cells which have markedly reduced expression of HLA class Ia antigens, HLA-E utilizes the leader sequence peptide

Table 25.3: HLA-G expression/polymorphism and the risk of recurrent spontaneous abortion				
Ethnic group	Ref.	RSA couples	Fertile couples	Allelic Associations
Studies showing positive association				
North American	53	113	None	G*0104, G*0105 N
German	54	78	52	G*01013, G*0105 N
Indian	55	120	120	G*010103
Danish	56	61	47	G*0106
Hutterite	57	42	None	Promoter region SNP
Danish	58	61	93	14 bp deletion/insertion in exons 8 of HLA-G
Dutch	59	9 RSA tissue sections	11 non-RSA tissue sections	Low HLA-G expression
Indian	60	300 ACLA/APL+ RSA women	120 RSA women	+14/+14 bp HLA-G genotype
Studies showing no difference				
Finnish	61	38	26	G
Hungarian	62	21	72	G*01011, G*01013
Japanese	63	20	54	G*01011, G*01012, G*01013, G*0104
Chinese (Han)	64	69	146	G*010101, G*010102, G*010103, G*010108, G*0103, G*010401, G*010402, G*010403, G*0105N

ACLA, anticardiolipin antibody; APL, antiphospholipid antibody

derived from HLA-G, that constitutes the predominant HLA antigen on these cells. Further, it has been shown that Phe at P8 in the HLA-G leader sequence (VMAPRTLFL) is preferentially recognized by both CD94-NKG2A and -NKG2C receptors of uNK cells.[65] These findings have helped evolve our understanding of HLA-E and HLA-G interaction with uterine NK cells (uNK) in the maternal decidua.

HLA-E is recognized by CD94-NKG2 receptors expressed largely but not exclusively by uNK cells. These receptors are members of the C-type lectin superfamily and consists of an invariant CD94 subunit disulfide-linked to a member of the NKG2 family. The NKG2 family comprises inhibitory (2A and 2B) and activating (2C, 2E and 2H) isoforms and when in complex with CD94 are capable of transducing opposing signals upon ligation with HLA-E. The inhibitory isoforms contain immunoreceptor tyrosine-based inhibitory motifs (ITIM) in their cytoplasmic tail, and their engagement leads to recruitment and activation of Src homology 2 domain-bearing tyrosine phosphatase 1 (SHP-1). In contrast, the activating isoforms contain a lysine residue in their transmembrane regions, which associate with the immunoreceptor tyrosine-based activating motif (ITAM) containing adaptor molecule DAP-12.[65] This molecular engagement further triggers appropriate inhibitory/stimulatory downstream signals resulting in corresponding immune effects, which have been further detailed under the section of uterine NK cells below. The role of HLA-E in conjunction with HLA-G is an intense area of research and a better elucidation of innate and adaptive immune mechanisms regulated by these antigens is anticipated in the near future.

THE UTERINE NK CELL–CONDUCTOR OF THE FETOMATERNAL ORCHESTRA

Natural killer (NK) cells are a vital component of the innate immune system and comprise of lymphocytes involved in the first line of immune surveillance. They are characterized by the expression of CD56 and absence of CD3 antigens. These cells are endowed by a broad array of activating receptors that ligate specific ligands on target cells and trigger cytotoxic activity and/or cytokine and chemokine production. As a counter measure to balance unwanted reactivity, NK cells also express various inhibitory receptors, most of which are HLA class I-dependent. These inhibitory receptors control activation signals mediated by the activating receptors. The downstream effect of NK cell activation is target cell lysis, expression of inflammatory cytokines, including TNF-α and IFN-γ, which aid in abrogating viral infection and spread of cancer cells. NK cells are found in the peripheral blood (10-15 percent of the lymphocytes) and in secondary lymphoid organs from which they migrate to infected or inflammatory sites.

Uterine NK cells are a unique subset constituting the predominant leukocyte population (70 percent of total immune cells), in the maternal decidua during the first and second trimesters. Subsequent to blastocyst implantation, massive recruitment of pre-NK cells to the decidua ensues. This dramatic change is brought about by the macrophage inflammatory protein (MIP-1α), a chemo-attractant secreted by the extravillous cytotrophoblast cells. Under the influence of neuro-hormonal stimuli of progesterone and progesterone induced blocking factor (PIBF) and cytokines like IL-15 and IL-18, these pre-NK cells undergo activation to uterine NK (uNK) cells in the decidua basalis. While the circulatory NK cells in the peripheral blood are CD56+ CD16+ CD160+, the hallmark of uNK cells is the CD56+ CD16- CD160- phenotype. Interestingly, CD16 is a low affinity receptor for FcRIII, responsible for antibody-dependent cellular cytotoxicity and CD160 renders the NK cell a high cytotoxic potential. Morphologically, peripheral blood CD56 bright NK cells are small and agranular, while CD56 bright uNK cells are large granular lymphocytes. These phenotypic dissimilarities suggest that uNK cells play a functionally different yet critical role in immunomodulation at the fetomaternal interface. As discussed previously, the fetal trophoblast does not express the polymorphic HLA-A and -B antigens and although this protects it from attack by maternal T cells, it renders it susceptible to lysis by uNK cells, present in abundance around the invading trophoblast. This is believed to be prevented by the expression of non-classical HLA-G, E, F antigens on the trophoblast cells.[66,67]

The possibility that uterine NK cells interact with the extravillous fetal trophoblast is suggested by the observations that these cells express a series of NK receptors (NKR) including the killer immunoglobulin-like-receptor (KIR) family, the C-type family CD94/NKG2 heterodimers, and Ig-like receptor ILT2/CD85j. HLA-C, E and G expressed on trophoblast are natural ligands to these receptors. However, it is intriguing whether the purpose of these class I ligands is to activate receptors on NK cells, thereby stimulating them to secrete cytokines like interferon-γ (IFN-γ) which regulate decidual spiral artery remodeling; or to interact with inhibitory receptors, thereby protecting the trophoblast from NK cell mediated lysis.[67,68] It is believed that a fine balance between the uNK cytotoxicity and cytokine production is important for the maintenance of fetal-maternal immunotolerance. Leftherioti and co-workers[44] have reported that an imbalance between inhibitory and activating KIR receptors, in favor of decidual NK cell activation, could damage the trophoblast and hence avert pregnancy.

The KIR receptors possess variable number of immunoglobulin domains (Fig. 25.4) and each member interacts with a specific HLA class I antigen HLA-C and/or HLA-G. Each receptor has an inhibitory or activating motif associated with its cytoplasmic domain, which renders the entire molecule an inhibitory or activating isoform respectively. Inhibitory KIRs have immunoreceptor tyrosine-based inhibitory (ITIM) motifs at their cytoplasmic domain which recruit and activate SHP-1 and/or SHP-2 phosphatases and prevent downstream activating signaling cascades. Activating KIRs on the other hand, have immunoreceptor tyrosine-based activating (ITAM) motifs which transmit signals to molecules like KARAP/DAP12 and activate specific downstream NK cell effector cascades. HLA-C is a natural ligand for KIR and by virtue of its dimorphism at position 80 of the α1 domain, defines two major epitopes. While HLA-C^{asn80} ligates with KIR2DL2/3 inhibitory and KIR2DS2 activating receptors; HLA-C^{lys80} is the ligand for inhibitory KIR2DL1 and activating KIR2DS1 counterparts.[69] HLA-G also ligates KIRs and is the specific natural ligand of the KIR2DL4/CD158d receptor on uNK cells, and depending on the two functionally different alleles of KIR2DL4 mediates either cytotoxic activation or mere cytokine expression by the uNK cells.[70] Interestingly, there is considerable genetically determined variation in the repertoire of KIR receptors between different individuals. Based on this observation, it has been hypothesized that a particular KIR repertoire might predispose to complications of pregnancy like RSA. Nevertheless, others failed to find an association between KIR repertoire especially of KIR2DL4 and RSA, suggesting that the HLA-G–KIR2DL4 interaction may have only a limited role in pregnancy.[71]

The Ig-like receptor ILT2/CD85j (Fig. 25.4) naturally binds HLA-G antigens expressed on the extravillous trophoblast. They have been noted on 20-25 percent uNK cells in normal pregnancy. The ILT2 receptor essentially possesses an ITIM motif in its cytoplasmic tail, but this receptor has the ability to exert dual inhibitory/activating functions.[72] The C-type lectin family of NK receptors are CD94/NKG2 heterodimers composed of covalently associated CD94 and C-type lectin-like inhibitory NKG2A/NKG2B, or activating NKG2C molecules (Fig. 25.4). The HLA-E antigen acts as a natural ligand for the NKG2 moiety. As described earlier, HLA-E is incapable of independent surface expression without the aid of a leader sequence peptide derived from other HLA class I

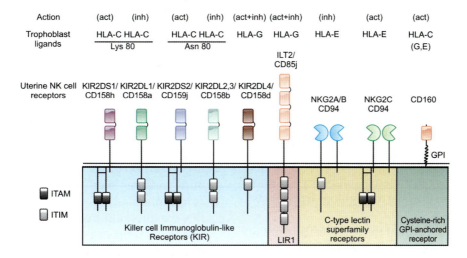

Fig. 25.4: Types of NK cell receptors—Killer cell immunoglobulin-like receptors (KIR) are inhibitory or activating depending on the presence of immunoreceptor tyrosine-based inhibitory motif (ITIM) or immunoreceptor tyrosine-based activating motif (ITAM) motif in their cytoplasmic domain. KIR2DL4 is an exception in possessing an ITIM motif but has both activating and inhibitory actions. Leukocyte immunoglobulin-like receptors (LIR) are characterized by the presence of 2 to 4 Ig-like extracellular domains. LIRs along with KIRs constitute the immunoglobulin-like receptor superfamily. Another group of receptors is the C-type lectin superfamily which consists of disulphide linked heterodimers of CD94 glycoprotein and one member of NKG2. The CD160 receptor is a cysteine-rich GPI-anchored receptor having an immunoglobulin external domain, and is expressed on a minor uNK cell subpopulation. (act – activating function; inh – inhibitory function)

antigens. Recent studies have indicated that in context of the extravillous cytotrophoblast, which is devoid of HLA-A, B antigens, only the HLA-G leader sequence peptide complexed with HLA-E binds CD94/NKG2 with an affinity that is great enough to trigger an NK cell response. Hence contrary to earlier belief, HLA-G has a facilitatory role rather than a direct impact on uNK cell suppression. It recruits HLA-E to the trophoblast cell surface by contributing its leader peptide. This HLA antigen complex further binds CD94/NKG2 receptor on uNK cells and the resultant trimeric complex undergoes conformational change triggering inhibitory signals and finally suppressing the uNK cell cytotoxic activity.[73,74]

From the above, it is apparent that uNK cells possess a heterocladic repertoire of receptors for the recognition of different HLA class I molecules. The co-expression of multiple NKR combinations with specificity for different HLA alleles ultimately determines the level of immune response at the maternal-fetal interface. The NKR repertoire has been shown to vary among individuals, and it is the expression on all mature uNK cells of at least one dominant inhibitory receptor recognizing self-HLA class I antigens that prevents autoreactivity in a normal pregnancy.[75] On the other hand, women who tend to abort have increased numbers of cytotoxic NK cells of the more conventional type (CD3–CD56+CD16+) in their decidua. However, the systemic and microenvironmental triggers that prompt the uNK cells to revert to cytotoxic phenotype and attack the trophoblast, remain largely unresolved. Hiby et al have reported that the maternal KIR of AA genotype lacks nearly all activating KIRs on their NK cells.[76] When such an NKR repertoire interacts with fetal trophoblast HLA-C^{lys80} ligands, women suffer from severe pre-eclampsia. Hence, excessive inhibitory uNK cell activity prevents proper trophoblast invasion and implantation. In the same vein, others have found that nearly 60 percent of women suffering from RSA lack the KIR2DL1 inhibitory receptor on their uNK cells.[77] Such selective lack of a specific KIR leads to improper epitope matching between maternal inhibitory KIRs and the HLA-Cw alleles on the fetal extravillous trophoblast, leading to miscarriage.

In conclusion, it is apparent that uNK cells maintain a delicate balance between their cytotoxic lytic versus secretory non-lytic phenotypic status in the decidua. These critical players of maternofetal immune tolerance, unlike their peripheral blood counterparts, express several cytokines including M-CSF, GM-CSF, TNF-α, IFN-γ, TGF-β, leukemia inhibitory factor (LIF) and angiogenic growth factor angiopoietin-2. It is believed that these cytokines aid in trophoblast invasion, implantation and spiral artery remodeling leading to placental augmentation and successful establishment of pregnancy. Nevertheless precise pathways and signaling cascades operating between these cells and the fetal trophoblast are not fully understood.

CONVERGENCE OF IMMUNOENDOCRINE PATHWAYS AT THE FETOMATERNAL INTERFACE

Possible mechanisms for induction of immune tolerance leading to a successful pregnancy have been a subject of intense debate. The fertilized egg initiates a cascade of events involving a complex orchestration of immuneendocrine signaling. The preimplantation blastocyst prior to hatching and endometrial invasion bathes in a progesterone-rich milieu which stimulates increased expression of Th2 cytokines (IL-4, IL-10) and leukemia inhibitory factor (LIF) by the CD4+ T cells and macrophages harbored in the cumulus oophorus.[78] Microenvironmental signals direct the homing-in and implantation of the blastocyst. Once, the blastocyst adhesion and invasion commences, a series of events ensue in tandem in the maternal decidua as shown in Figure 25.5 and discussed sequentially as under:

a. The resident decidual macrophages and endometrial stromal cells are stimulated by the progesterone surge and progesterone-induced blocking factor (PIBF) to liberate IL-15 and IL-18 cytokines. The former induces multiple uNK cell effector functions including their clonal proliferation, release of cytokines (IFN-γ, GM-CSF, MIP-1α, MIP-1β, TNF-α and IL-18), upregulation of cytolytic mediators (perforin and FasL) and NK receptor expression (activating: NKp44, NKp46 and inhibitory: CD94/NKG2-A).[79,80]

b. IL-18 on the other hand is not only produced by endometrial stromal cells and activated macrophages but also by giant extravillous trophoblast cells. It induces perforin expression on uNK cells; regulates trophoblast invasion through IL-18R constitutively expressed on uNK cells and syncytiotrophoblast; and induces Fas expression on extravillous cytotrophoblast.[81]

c. IFN-γ expression by uNK cells is induced by IL-15 and IL-18. It plays a key role in spiral artery vascular remodeling and apoptosis of T and B cells. It also enhances secretion of IL-18 binding protein (IL-18BP) which decreases proinflammatory activity of IL-18.

d. Further, chemoattractants MIP-1α and MIP-1β liberated by uNK cells aid in homing of pre-NK cells from the maternal circulation. A positive feedback loop thus attracts more pre-NK cells which undergo activation to mature uNK cells in the decidua. This

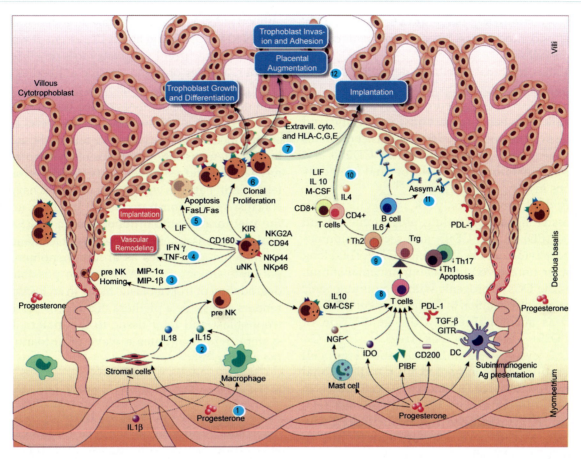

Fig. 25.5: A hypothetic model of immunological cross-talk at the maternal-fetal interface. (1) Progesterone acts as a neuroendocrine trigger activating decidual macrophages and endometrial stromal cells to secrete IL-15 and IL-18. (2) These cytokines activate resident pre-NK cells to uNK cells. (3) MIP-1α and MIP-1β attract more circulatory pre-NK cells, and the uNK cells become the predominant decidual immune cells. (4) IFN-γ, TNF-α and LIF expressed by uNK cells help regulate spiral artery remodeling, thereby increasing blood supply to the developing fetoplacental unit and facilitating implantation. (5) Cytolytic mediators, FasL and perforin delete antipaternal lytic uNK cell clones, which express a predominance of activating NKp44 and NKp46 receptors. (6) GM-CSF and M-CSF induce preferential clonal proliferation of uNK cells endowed with inhibitory KIR and NKG2A/CD94 receptors. (7) Interaction of these receptors with HLA-E, F, G ligands on the extravillous cytotrophoblast cells shifts the uNK cell phenotype from cytotoxic-lytic to secretory non-lytic state rendering them immune-tolerant. (8 and 9) Immunomodulators like IDO, NGF, CD200, PDL-1 and sub-immunogenic fetal antigen presentation by dendritic cells converge to tilt the Th1/Th2 balance at the maternal-fetal interface towards a pro-pregnancy Th2 profile. (10) Th2 cytokines IL-4, IL-10 along with M-CSF and LIF collaborate to aid placental augmentation and implantation. (11) Th2 cytokines upregulate synthesis of antipaternal IgG asymmetric blocking antibodies, which block paternal antigen induced activation of inflammatory cascades. (12) All of the above cellular and acellular mediators converge their downstream effects towards successful invasion, implantation, growth and development of the fetoplacental unit. (Assym. Ab.— Asymmetric blocking antibodies; DC—dendritic cell; GM-CSF—Granulocyte-macrophage colony stimulating factor; IDO—Indoleamine 2,3-dioxygenase; KIR—killer immunoglobulin-like receptors; LIF—leukemia inhibitory factor; M-CSF—Macrophage colony stimulating factor; MIP—macrophage inflammatory protein; NGF—nerve growth factor; PDL-1—programmed death ligand 1; PIBF—progesterone-induced blocking factor; Treg – T regulatory cells; uNK – uterine NK cell)

along with the clonal proliferation triggered by IL-15 shifts the dominance of cellular immune cells in the decidua basalis towards uNK cells. The positive feedback is kept in balance by release of cytokines like IL-1β, which provide a negative feedback.

e. The HLA class I antigens HLA-C, E, F, G expressed on invasive extravillous cytotrophoblast cells ligate to the heterocladic uNK cell receptors. This interaction shifts the uNK cell phenotype from cytotoxic-lytic to secretory non-lytic state rendering them tolerant towards the immunologically foreign fetus, thereby allowing normal placentation and fetal development.

f. Several immunomodulatory mediators trigger signaling cascades to tilt the Th1/Th2 balance at the maternal-fetal interface towards a Th2 profile. The key neuroendocrine trigger is progesterone, although other hormones like estrogen, prolactin, relaxin also influence the expression and function of these mediators. Progesterone directly or indirectly (through PIBF) directs the expression of indoleamine

2,3-dioxygenase (IDO), nerve growth factor (NGF), CD200, and modulates the activity of decidual dendritic cells.

g. IDO inhibits maternal T cells by depriving them of tryptophan and inducing apoptosis of activated Th1 and Th17 cells.[82] NGF, a neurotrophin mediates the cross-talk between the nervous, endocrine and immune system, and at moderate levels contributes to the local Th2 cytokine milieu.[83] CD200 is a glycoprotein immunomodulator that prevents abortions in very early pregnancy.[84]

h. The decidual dendritic cells (DC) upregulate their suppressive ligands including programmed death ligand 1 (PDL-1) and CD95, and secrete immunoregulatory cytokines like IL-10 and TGF-β. This along with other unresolved microenvironmental stimuli renders the DCs tolerogenic with subimmunogenic fetal antigen presentation to T cells. Consequent T cell anergy is accompanied by the generation of CD4+CD25+ T regulatory cells (Treg).

i. The Th2 cytokine dominance and Treg cell proliferation is accompanied by parallel clonal deletion (apoptosis) of Th1 and Th17 T cell subsets to prevent proinflammatory reactivity against fetal antigens. Th2 cytokines like IL-4 and IL-10 along with GM-CSF, M-CSF and LIF ultimately aid in implantation and trophoblast development.

j. The Th2 cytokines (IL-4, IL-6) also upregulate the proportion of asymmetrically glycosylated antipaternal IgG antibodies (asymmetric antibodies), which have an extra carbohydrate moiety in one of their Fab regions. This glycosylation affects their antigen interaction turning them into functionally univalent blocking antibodies, which are unable to fix complement or incite a proinflammatory reaction against paternal antigens.[85]

In summation all of these activities revolve around uNK, Th2 and Treg cells, and ultimately translate into successful trophoblast adhesion, invasion and implantation, followed by spiral artery remodeling, placental augmentation and trophoblast growth and development into a healthy fetus.

NON-MHC MEDIATORS OF RSA

Role of Autoantibodies

Recent evidence indicates that a small percentage of RSA cases are autoimmune in character. Indeed antiphospholipid antibodies (APL), lupus anticoagulant (LAC), anticardiolipin antibodies (ACL), antinuclear antibody (ANA) and anti-double-stranded antibodies (a-ds-DNA) are present in about 10 percent of women with a history of recurrent pregnancy loss or ≥ 1 fetal death. Further, a series of organ specific antibodies including antithyroid peroxidase antibodies (anti-TPO), antithyroglobulin antibodies (anti-Tg) have been reported to be increased in RSA. Notwithstanding several association studies incriminating a causative role for these antibodies in RSA, demonstration of plausible pathophysiological mechanisms and a significantly higher rate of subsequent fetal loss in patients with these antibodies have not been conclusively demonstrated.[86,87] It has been argued that the plethora of autoantibodies seen in RSA women could be a consequence of concurrent formation of non-pathogenic antibodies as an epiphenomenon to the pathophysiology of RSA. It is also possible that the degradation of trophoblastic tissue in an RSA pregnancy renders accessible a plethora of antigens present on the trophoblast and fetal tissue to the maternal immune system; which initiates a wave of autoantibodies in the mother.[86,88]

MTHFR Gene Polymorphism and Factor V Leiden

Substitution of cytosine to thymine mutation at nucleotide position 677 in the gene encoding for methylenetetrahydrofolate reductase (MTHFR) has been reported to be associated with repeated early fetal losses.[89] This observation suggests an important role for hypercoagulability, abnormal uteroplacental vasculature and impaired placental development and function in the causation of repeated pregnancy loss. The MTHFR mutation effect is mediated through hyperhomocysteinemia and its resulting procoagulant effect, endothelial injury and a low serum folate status contributing to the deleterious effect. Conversely, appropriately targeted folic acid supplements may, by catalyzing homocysteine remethylation into methionine, reduce plasma homocysteine levels and reduce RSA related pregnancy loss. Unexplained RSA has been associated with diverse prothrombotic states, such as the presence of APL or activated protein C resistance, and factor V Leiden mutation which is a known independent risk factor for unexplained RSA.[90] Based on these observations it is hypothesized that hyperhomocysteinemia and its resulting damaging effect plays an important role in RSA pathogenesis. Most studies on the possible involvement of MTHFR gene polymorphism in RSA have been inconclusive. Lissak and co-workers[89] reported an increased prevalence of the MTHFR C677T mutation among patients with unexplained RSA. However no significant association of homozygosity or heterozygosity of the mutation with prevalence of RSA was noted in this study. Further studies are needed to unravel the true significance of this mutation in RSA.

Mannan Binding Lectin

Mannan binding lectin (MBL) is a C-type serum lectin that participates in the innate immune defense by recognizing the mannose-rich oligosaccharides present on a wide range of bacteria, viruses, fungi, and parasites and by activating the MBL pathways of complement. The serum level of MBL in an individual is determined genetically by an interaction between polymorphism in exon 1 of the MBL gene and of the promoter region. Similarities of idiopathic RSA with autoimmune disorders and reports of MBL deficiency predisposing to a number of autoimmune diseases have prompted investigations of MBL levels in RSA. Most studies have reported significantly lower levels of MBL in RSA couples, as compared to fertile controls, and this is even more significant with the number of previous spontaneous abortions. Interestingly, while the fetal and paternal MBL genotype is not of much significance for the development of RSA, only the maternal MBL deficiency seems to be associated with RSA. It may be pointed out that, since most women with low MBL levels do not experience RSA, this is unlikely to be an independent factor mediating RSA. It is possible that low MBL levels increase the risk of fetal loss when prevalent in conjunction with abnormal cytokine profiles at the fetomaternal interface or increased NK cell activity. Hence, a proportion of the women with low MBL levels could be exposed to hypothetic microorganisms leading to spontaneous abortion.[91]

MANAGEMENT OF RSA

Recurrent spontaneous abortion presents a difficult and often frustrating circumstance for both the couple and the physician. Extensive and emotionally harrowing investigation protocols may throw up no results. Notwithstanding the complexity of the problem, and increased risk of subsequent pre-term deliveries in RSA women, it is important to bear in mind that the spontaneous salvage rate with a normal subsequent pregnancy resulting in a normal childbirth is 55-70 percent.[92] The treatment of recurrent miscarriage should be directed towards the underlying cause if defined. Several modes of therapy have been under trial with the primary aim of boosting the maternal immune system, so as to allow an optimal fetomaternal interface, essential for the successful continuation of pregnancy to term.

The concept of immunotherapy is based on the hypothesis that miscarriage occurs due to a failure of maternal 'immunological adaptation' to the developing semiallogenic conceptus resulting in a form of transplant rejection. Immunotherapy for RSA may be either active or passive. In the active mode, either paternal leukocyte injection or trophoblast membrane infusion is used with a view to boost the subsequent maternal immune recognition of a developing conceptus. In passive immunotherapy on the other hand, regular intravenous infusion of immunoglobulins is employed to produce beneficial immunomodulatory effects including neutralization of circulating autoantibodies, inhibition of complement mediated cytotoxicity, and modulation of cytokine release by the lymphocytes.[93] Despite variable results of immunotherapy in treating RSA, its use in induction of immune tolerance in the mother has been attempted by several investigators. The most commonly employed modes of immunotherapy alongwith their benefits and disadvantages are reviewed here briefly.[8,94]

Paternal Lymphocyte Alloimmunization Therapy (PLAT)

Taylor and Faulk (1981), were the first to report on the use of active immunization of RSA women with allogenic blood cells. Their rationale for this treatment was to create antipaternal cytotoxic or "blocking antibodies" believed to prevent miscarriage.[86] The first successful trial of immunotherapy in women suffering from RSA was done in 1985, where women were injected with purified lymphocytes from their husband's blood.[8,95] The following inclusion criteria have been advocated for PLAT by most trials: (i) Women sharing several HLA alleles with their spouse; (ii) Women negative for complement-dependent cytotoxic antibodies and (iii) Women negative for blocking antibodies. In majority of the studies, immunization was offered exclusively to those experiencing first trimester RSA, while in others only to those with primary RSA and/or cases negative for autoantibodies. Suitable RSA patients should be adequately informed of the fair prognosis of achieving a successful pregnancy without any treatment at all and the established and potential risks associated with the treatment. No immunization should be given to patients with significant titers of autoantibodies or to those who do not carry the HPA-1a thrombocyte allotype, which increases the risk thrombocyte antibody formation. The lymphocyte donor should, display negative tests for HIV, hepatitis B and hepatitis C. Immunization is usually performed using the husbands' lymphocytes separated and administered intradermally, s.c. or i.v., as reported by Mowbray et al.[96] Others have used buffy coat or leukocyte-rich erythrocyte concentrates. The protocol employed at Nippon Medical School, Japan is presented in Table 25.4. The rates of successful pregnancies in immunized women with this protocol have been reported to range from 50 to 88 percent.[97]

Immunological events leading to beneficial effects of allogenic lymphocyte immunization are unknown. Changes in the level of IL receptors, suppression of NK cell activity or alterations in the numbers of CD8+ T cells are hypothetical possibilities.[86] It has been argued that transfusion/immunization leads to stimulation of maternal allogeneic recognition leading to the formation of lymphocytotoxic and/or non-cytotoxic antibodies which inhibit Fc-rosette formation, immune phagocytosis or mixed lymphocyte reaction.[98] Pandey et al[99] have recently demonstrated that PLAT upregulates the synthesis of IgG_3 type mixed lymphocyte reaction blocking factors (MLR-Bf) in women with RSA and correlated the same with success of pregnancy.

Notwithstanding the potential advantages of a successful pregnancy, PLAT has associated disadvantages including the risk of infection with blood borne pathogens, hepatitis B virus and HIV, complications like local reaction at the injection site, blood group alloimmunization, transfusion reaction and graft-versus-host reaction. It can also cause adverse pregnancy outcomes including abruptio placenta, intrauterine growth restriction and in rare cases neonatal alloimmune thrombocytopenia and intracranial hemorrhage.[8,100]

Table 25.5 summarizes some of the important randomized controlled trials comparing the utility of PLAT in unexplained RSA patients. Although results from early trials appeared to suggest PLAT as a beneficial mode of therapy for RSA, Clarke and co-workers[95] critically analyzed these studies and highlighted improper selection of subjects in many trials and consequent misleading conclusions. A meta-analysis of all published and ongoing placebo-controlled trials of allogenic lymphocyte immunization was undertaken by the Recurrent Miscarriage Immunotherapy Trialists Group (RMITG) under the American Society for Reproductive Immunology in 1994. A total of 1753 cases from eight trials were analyzed. The results revealed significantly increased success rate in primary RSA patients with a therapeutic gain of 8 percent in the total patient group. This gain reached ~16 percent when patients with no previous pregnancy beyond the 20th gestational week, no HLA antibodies against the partner and any ANA or ACL were analyzed. Others have shown therapeutic gains of 23-38 percent in primary RSA group while no benefit was observed in women with secondary RSA.[86,95] Recently Cochrane reviews meta-analyzed 20 well designed randomized controlled trials evaluating leukocyte immunization, and concluded that the live birth outcome between the treatment (65%) and the non-treatment groups (60%) were not statistically different.[94,100] As of date, the value of PLAT remains unproven and hence, this therapy is recommended only within the context of a carefully designed randomized controlled trial.

Table 25.4: Protocol for paternal lymphocyte alloimmunization therapy followed at Nippon Medical School[97]

1. **Indications**
    a. Women with ≥ 3 consecutive spontaneous abortions with the same partner
    b. Women with 2 recurrent spontaneous abortions with documented genetically normal fetus
    c. Women with 2 recurrent spontaneous abortions with elevated peripheral blood NK cell activity
2. **Contraindications**
    a. Women with > 1 live birth with the same partner
    b. Women with malignant disease
    c. Women positive for APL, ANA
    d. Women with spouses who do not fit blood donor selection criteria
3. **Procedure protocol**
    a. Lymphocytes are prepared by Ficoll-Paque centrifugation from husbands or partners and then 3000 Gy irradiated. The cells are washed 3 times with sterile saline and resuspended in 1ml at a concentration of $4\text{-}7 \times 10^7$/ml. The cells are given intradermally 4 times at an interval of 2-3 wks
    b. The skin reaction at the injection site is measured
    c. If the skin reaction does not reduce after the 4th immunization, additional immunization is performed until it does.

APA = anti-phospholipid antibodies; ANA = anti-nuclear antibodies

Table 25.5: Summary of randomized controlled trials of allogenic leukocyte immunotherapy in unexplained RSA patients[101-110]

Population	No. of patients	Live birth rate Patients[a]	Live birth rate Controls[b]	Odds ratio	Conclusions	Ref
Maltese	20	65 percent	72.7 percent	0.70	Negative study	101
Danish	8	50 percent	57.1 percent	0.75	Negative study	102
Australian	19	68.4 percent	60 percent	1.43	Favors immunotherapy	103
Chinese	42	78.6 percent	65.3 percent	1.90	Favors immunotherapy	104
Italian	16	62.5 percent	78.6 percent	0.48	Negative study	105
British	12	66.7 percent	60 percent	1.32	Favors immunotherapy	106
British	37	67.6 percent	46.7 percent	2.33	Favors immunotherapy	96
North American	68	45.6 percent	65.1 percent	0.46	Negative study	107
French	26	65.4 percent	53.8 percent	1.60	Favors immunotherapy	108
North American	10	60 percent	41.7 percent	2.01	Favors immunotherapy	109
North American	25	84 percent	30 percent	9.03	Favors immunotherapy	110

[a]RSA patients immunized with paternal leukocytes; [b] RSA patients given placebo or no treatment

Intravenous Immunoglobulin Infusion (IVIG) Therapy

Several investigators have evaluated the potential utility of IVIG therapy in RSA patients. Mueller-Eckhardt (1986-89)[98] and Christiansen (1992)[111] were the first to report the beneficial effects of IVIG in a large series of RSA patients. They employed 30g IVIG infusions at 3 weekly intervals up to 24 weeks. Both groups found a success rate of > 80 percent in the treated group. Christiansen in a subsequent study[112] enrolled patients who displayed no benefit from paternal leukocyte infusions and gave them 380 to 550 g of IVIG over 17 infusions. The study reported a therapeutic gain of 24 percent. In another study Coulam[113] initiated IVIG therapy during the months before conception and continued if conception occurred, and demonstrated significant therapeutic gain of 28 percent, suggesting that the preconceptional treatment regimen may be effective in preventing some very early miscarriages.[86] Several other studies thereafter have shown success rates ranging from 60-82 percent. Nevertheless several inadequacies in methodology used have been noted, and authors have cautioned against the false belief that these 'therapies' are effective, especially because the results in these patients differed only marginally from those left untreated.[92,98] Cochrane review analysis of eight trials and 305 women showed that there was no significant effect of IVIG on pregnancy outcome, with 64 percent live births seen in the treatment group compared to 59 percent in the control group.[8,114] Overall, current evidence suggests that there is as yet no firm evidence to suggest IVIG might benefit women with unexplained RSA, but within this context, its use should only occur as part of a randomized controlled trial. IVIG could be more efficacious in women presenting with secondary RSA or those with repeated second trimester intrauterine fetal deaths.[114]

Although the exact therapeutic mechanism of IVIG in the treatment of RSA remains unclear, the immunomodulatory effects achieved may be attributed to several factors. These include blockade of Fc receptors, blockade of complement C3 fragment binding to target cells, action of anti-idiotypic antibodies, increase in the numbers of T suppressor cells, blockage of Th lymphocyte receptors, blockade of placental transport of maternal endogenous IgG, reduction of NK cell activity and feedback inhibition of autoantibody synthesis.[86,98] IVIG infusion has its risks, such as life-threatening anaphylaxis, fever, flushing, muscle pain, nausea, headache and viral transmission, in addition to its extremely high cost.[8,114]

Trophoblast Membrane Infusion

Trophoblast membrane infusion is an immunotherapeutic modality based on a single intravenous infusion with isolated placental trophoblast plasma membrane vesicle preparations, derived from early embryos. Ramsden and Johnson,[115] in a combined randomized double-blind and open study, reported that trophoblast membrane infusion did not confer any benefit in women with apparently unexplained RSA. Only one trial on trophoblast membrane immunization has been covered in Cochrane review. The live birth rates for the treatment and control groups in this analysis were 47 percent and 70 percent respectively. The results were again statistically insignificant.[100] Hence, the utility of this therapy remains questionable.

Third Party Donor Cell Immunization

Third party donor cell immunization involves infusion of leukocytes obtained from an unrelated donor. Cochrane review covered three trials on this therapy. The live birth rates for treatment and control groups were found to be 63 percent and 60 percent respectively and these were statistically insignificant. The review concluded that third party donor cell immunizations do not lower the risk of future miscarriages in women suffering from RSA.[8]

Finally, a word of caution has been sounded by several international organizations. The Royal College of Obstetricians and Gynaecologists (RCOG) maintain that none of the above-mentioned methods of immunotherapy improve the live birth rate. Similarly, the Sociedad Colombiana de Obstetricia y Ginecología (SCOG) recommends against the use of these methods of immunotherapy. The body of American College of Obstetricians and Gynecologists (ACOG) maintains that mononuclear cell (leukocyte) immunization and IVIG are not effective in preventing recurrent pregnancy loss. The Food and Drug Administration (FDA) does not approve these products for routine use and cautions that they can be administered only in the context of an approved clinical trial.[8,100]

Aspirin/Heparin Therapy

The concept of anticoagulation therapy for treatment of RSA is based on the observation that APL positive women suffer from an increased risk of thrombosis in placental endothelial cells. This modality is now a routine treatment for RSA women with antiphospholipid antibody syndrome and inherited thrombophilia. A meta-analysis of randomized controlled trials has revealed that combined therapy with unfractionated heparin and aspirin reduces the incidence of pregnancy loss by as much as 54 percent in women suffering with RSA.[114] However, Di Nisio et al[116] in their Chocrane meta-analysis contend that studies on the use of anticoagulants for the treatment of RSA in women without APS are too limited to recommend their routine use as yet. Corticosteroids including prednisone have also been investigated in combination with aspirin/heparin therapy. Owing to their equivocal results, further trails are warranted before, it can be recommended for routine treatment of RSA.

1α, 25-dihydroxy-vitamin-D3 (VD3) Therapy

1alpha, 25-dihydroxy-vitamin-D3 (VD3) and its analogs are known to be effective therapeutic immunomodulators for certain Th1 response immune disorders. Recently Bubanovic et al[117] used VD3 at a dose of 5-10 μg/kg of body weight with or without immunosuppressive/anticoagulant combinations to assess its utility in the treatment of RSA, and encouraging results have been reported. The mechanism of VD3 activity, however, is not yet fully understood. It is believed to downregulate the production of Th1 cytokines such as IL-1, IL-2 and IFN-γ while simultaneously augmenting the Th2 T cell response. The observed similarities in the effects of VD3 with those of IL-10 have encouraged investigators to try it as a local immunomodulatory drug for the treatment of RSA. However, extensive clinical trials are needed prior to incorporating it as a regular therapeutic modality for RSA.

PERSPECTIVES

Notwithstanding the key milestones achieved in reproductive immunology, several gaps in our knowledge remain, that prevent us from translating this wealth of information into bedside solutions for women suffering from reproductive failures and complications. Some of the issues that need an answer include: (a) There is a need to ascertain the precise microenvironmental signals and pathways which define and regulate functional uNK cell subsets. How and why do perivascular uNK cells vary from their counterparts in other parts of the maternal decidua, might contain the answers to what defines and fine tunes local immune modulation of these key immune cells. Simultaneously there is a need to understand what signals/factors trigger uNK cells (CD16- CD56+) to revert to lytic CD16+ CD56+ NK cells in RSA? (b) Precise mechanisms/signaling cascades which regulate the antigen presenting cells to present and handle fetal antigens in a tolerance inducing way also need to be understood. This arrest of APCs in an intermediate/immature state of antigenic stimulation suggests possibilities of hitherto unknown mechanisms which can render local immune suppression without effecting overall systemic immunity. (c) Little work has been done yet on the intracellular cascades including JAK-STAT and GATA3 pathways active at the maternal-fetal junction. Further investigation in this area would help complete the jig-saw puzzle as to how immune cells homing in from the circulation undergo such drastic functional immune tolerance when they arrive in the decidua. (d) Although a plethora of immunomodulatory agents operating at the maternal-fetal interface have been defined, translational solutions need to be developed to imitate peripheral tolerance at will for therapeutic and preventive use.

It is believed that future studies will not only help to forge solutions for problems like RSA, implantation failures, pre-eclampsia and other reproductive ailments; but also suggest common solutions for the field of transplant immunology, autoimmunity, allergies and infection immunology as well.

EXECUTIVE SUMMARY

Perhaps the greatest riddle in reproductive immunology is the quintessential query on what precisely regulates the peripheral maternal tolerance towards the antigenically foreign fetus, permitting a successful pregnancy. It is now becoming clear that non-classical HLA antigens including HLA-E, F and G along with uNK cells are the key immunomodulators operating at the maternal-fetal interface. The non-classical HLA antigens shift the uNK cell phenotype from cytotoxic-lytic to secretory non-lytic state rendering them tolerant towards the immunologically foreign fetus, thereby allowing normal placentation and fetal development. The evolving role of HLA-E is re-establishing several concepts, hitherto believed to be regulated solely by HLA-G. While a lot has been unraveled about the uNK cells, recent reports are redirecting the attention of researchers worldwide towards T regulatory cells and the critical links they bridge with uNK cells and individual immunomodulators in the maternal decidua. Extrapolation of regulatory pathways operating in normal pregnancy towards understanding of pathophysiology of RSA is yet another critical area of investigation. HLA sharing between mother and fetus and that between parents along with certain non-MHC factors like autoimmune antibodies, MBL and MTHFR gene polymorphism are believed to precipitate RSA. But our current understanding of RSA is far from complete and further investigation to unravel this baffling ailment is essential. Several immunotherapeutic modalities have been evolved to manage RSA, but so far equivocal results have prevented their routine clinical use. Future research promises to bring forth new translational solutions with far reaching ramifications not only in reproductive immunology but also in other fields of immunology as a whole.

REFERENCES

1. Medawar PB. Some immunological and endocrinological problems raised by the evolution of vivparity in vertebrates. Symp Soc Exp Biol 1953;44:320-38.
2. WHO Recommended definitions, terminology and format for statistical tables related to the perinatal period and use of a new certificate for cause of perinatal deaths (modifications recommended by FIGO as amended by October 14, 1976). Acta Obstet Gynecol Scand 1977;56: 247-53.
3. Casper RF. Abstracts of the First World Congress On: Controversies in Obstetrics, Gynecology and Infertility. Prague, Czech Republic – 1999. Definition and Etiology of Recurrent Spontaneous Abortion.
4. Purandare AS, Smith DS, Wilson PJ. HLA frequency, HLA sharing and immunotherapy in the management of recurrent miscarriage. Int J Fertil Menopausal Stud 1993;38:219-24.
5. Stirrat GM. Recurrent miscarriage I: Definition and epidemiology. Lancet 1990;336:673-75.
6. Bulletti C, Flamigni C, Giacomucci E. Reproductive failure due to spontaneous abortion and recurrent miscarriage. Hum Reprod Update 1996;2(2):118-36.
7. Meka A, Reddy BM. Recurrent spontaneous abortions: An overview of genetic and non-genetic backgrounds. Int J Hum Genet 2006;6:109-17.
8. Tien JC, Tan TYT. Non-surgical interventions for threatened and recurrent miscarriages. Singapore Med J 2007;48(12):1074.
9. McCluskey J, Peh CA. The human leukocyte antigens and clinical medicine: An overview. Rev Immunogenet 1999;1:3-20.
10. Shiina T, Tamiya G, Oka A, Takishima N, Inoko H. Genome sequencing analysis of the 1.8 Mb entire human MHC class I region. Immunol Rev 1999;167:193-99.
11. Colbern GT, Main EK. Immunology of the maternal-placental interface in normal pregnancy. Semin Perinatol 1991;15:196-205.
12. Hunt JS. Stranger in a strange land. Immunol Rev 2006;213:36-47.
13. Thomas L, Hargerd JH, Wageserb K, Rabin S, Gill TJ. HLA sharing and spontaneous abortion in humans. Am J Obstet Gynecol 1985;151:1053-58.
14. Hedrick PW. HLA-sharing, Recurrent Spontaneous Abortion, and the Genetic Hypothesis. Genetics. May 1988;119:199-204.
15. Schacter B, Weitkamp LR, Johnson WE. Parental HLA compatibility, fetal wastage and neural tube defects: Evidence for a T/t-like locus in humans. Am J Hum Genet 1984;36:1082-91.
16. Jin K, Ho HN, Speed TP, Gill III TJ. Reproductive Failure and the Major Histocompatibility Complex. Am J Hum Genet 1995;56:1456-67.
17. Gill TJ. Immunogenetics of spontaneous abortions in humans. Transplantation 1983;35:1-6.
18. Wegmann TG. Placental immunotrophism: Maternal T cell enhance placental growth and function. Am J Reprod Immunol Microbiol 1987;15:67-69.
19. Takakuwa K, Honda K, Yokoo T, Hataya I, Tamura M, Tanaka K. Molecular genetic studies on the compatibility of HLA class II alleles in patients with unexplained recurrent miscarriage in the Japanese population. Clin Immunol 2006;118:101-07.

20. Beydoun H, Saftlas AF. Association of human leukocyte antigen sharing with recurrent spontaneous abortions. Tissue Antigens 2005;65:123-35.
21. Lauritsen JG, Jorgensen J, Kissmeyer-Nielson F. Significance of HLA and blood-group incompatibility in spontaneous abortion. Clin Genet 1976;7:575-82.
22. Komlos L, Zamir R, Joshua H, Halbrecht I. Common HLA antigens in couples with repeated abortions. Clin Immunol Immunopathol 1977;7:330-35.
23. Ober C, Elias S, O'Brien E. HLA sharing and fertility in Hutterite couples: Evidence for prenatal selection against compatible fetuses. Am J Reprod Immunol Microbiol 1988;18:111-15.
24. Kilpatrick DC, Liston WA. Parental HLA sharing, fetomaternal compatibility and neonatal birthweight in families with a history of recurrent spontaneous abortion. Dis Markers 1993;11:125-30.
25. Laitinen T, Koskimies S, Westman P. Fetomaternal compatibility in HLA-DR, -DQ, and - DP loci in Finnish couples suffering from recurrent spontaneous abortions. Eur J Immunogenet 1993;20:249-58.
26. Ober C, Steck T, Van der Ven K. MHC class II compatibility in aborted fetuses and term infants of couples with recurrent spontaneous abortion. J Reprod Immunol 1993;25:195-207.
27. Ober CL, Hauck WW, Kostyu DD. Adverse effects of human leukocyte antigen-DR sharing on fertility: A cohort study in a human isolate. Fertil Steril 1985;44:227-32.
28. Coulam CB, Moore SB, O'Fallon WM. Association between major histocompatibility antigen and reproductive performance. Am J Reprod Immunol Microbiol 1987;14:54-58.
29. Balasch J, Coll O, Martorell J, Jove IC, Gaya A, Vanrell JA. Further data against HLA sharing in couples with recurrent RSAs. Gynecol Endicrinol 1989;3:63-69.
30. Christiansen OB, Riisom K, Lauritsen JG, Grunnet N. No increased histocompatibility antigen sharing in couples with idiopathic habitual abortion. Hum Reprod 1989;4:160-62.
31. Gerencer M, Drazancic A, Kuvacic I, Tomaskovic Z, Kastelan A. HLA antigen studies in women with recurrent gestational disorders. Fertil Steril 1979;31:401-04.
32. Unander AM, Olding LB. Habitual abortion: Parental sharing of HLA antigens, absence of maternal blocking antibody, and suppression of maternal lymphocytes. Am J Reprod Immunol 1983;4:171-78.
33. Reznikoff-Etievant MF, Edelman P, Muller JY, Pinon F, Sureau C. HLA-DR locus and maternal-fetal relation. Tissue Antigens 1984;24:30-34.
34. Casciani CU, Pasetto N, Forleo R, Adorno D, Valeri M, Piazza A. HLA sharing in couples with recurrent abortion. Exp Clin Immunogenet 1985;2:65-69.
35. McIntyre JA, Faulk WP, Nicholas-Johnson VR, Taylor CG. Immunologic testing and immunotherapy in recurrent spontaneous abortion. Obstet Gynecol 1986;67:169-74.
36. Ho HN, Gill TJ, Nsieh RP, Hsieh HJ, Lee TY. Sharing of human leukocyte antigens in primary and secondary recurrent spontaneous abortions. Am J Obstet Gynecol 1990;163:178-88.
37. Koyama M, Saji F, Takahashi S. Probabilistic assessment of the HLA sharing of recurrent spontaneous abortion couples in the Japanese population. Tissue Antigens 1991;37:211-17.
38. Ober C, Hyslop T, Elias S, Weitkamp LR, Hauck WW. Human leukocyte antigen matching and fetal loss: Results of a 10 years prospective study. Hum Reprod 1998;13:33-38.
39. Kruse C, Steffensen R, Varming K, Christiansen OB. A study of HLA-DR and -DQ alleles in 588 patients and 562 controls confirms that HLA-DRB1*03 is associated with recurrent miscarriage. Hum Reprod 2004;19:1215-21.
40. Cauchi MN, Tait B, Wilshire MI, et al. Histocompatibility antigens and habitual abortion. Am J Reprod Immunol 1988;18:28-31.
41. Sciorelli G, Bontempelli M, Carella G, et al. HLA sharing in Italian recurrent abortion couples. Acta Eur Fertil 1988;19:257-61.
42. Chang MY, Soong YK, Huang CC. Comparison of histocompatibility between couples with idiopathic recurrent spontaneous abortion and normal multipara. J Formos Med Assoc 1991;90:153-59.
43. Takakuwa K, Higashino M, Ueda H, et al. Significant compatibility does not exist at the HLA-DQB gene locus in couples with unexplained recurrent abortions. Am J Reprod Immunol 1992;28:12-16.
44. Leftherioti MV, Keramitsoglou T, Vlachou MS, et al. 14th International HLA and Immunogenetics Workshop: Report from the reproductive immunology component. Tissue Antigens 2007;69(Suppl 1):297-303.
45. Ellis SA, Palmer MS, McMichael AJ. Human trophoblast and the choriocarcinoma cell line BeWo express a truncated HLA Class I molecule. J Immunol 1990;144:731-35.
46. Abbas A, Javed S, Agrawal S. Transcriptional status of HLA-G at the maternal-fetal interface in recurrent spontaneous abortion. Int J Gynecol Obstet 2006;93:148-49.
47. Hviid TVF. HLA-G in human reproduction: Aspects of genetics, function and pregnancy complications. Hum Reprod Update 2006;12(3):209-32.
48. Hunt JS, Petroff MG, McIntire RH, Ober C. HLA-G and immune tolerance in pregnancy. FASEB J 2005;19:681-93.
49. Hunt JS, Jadhav L, Chu W, Geraghty DE, Ober C. Soluble HLA-G circulates in maternal blood during pregnancy. Am J Obstet Gynecol. September 2000; 183(3):682-88.
50. Ober C, Aldrich C. HLA-G polymorphisms: Neutral evolution or novel function? J Reprod Immunol 1997;36:1-21.
51. Laird SM, Tuckerman EM, Cork BA, Linjawi S, Blakemore AIF, Li TC. A review of immune cells and molecules in women with recurrent miscarriage. Hum Reprod Update 2003;9(2):163-74.
52. Yan WH, Lin A, Chen XJ, et al. Association of the maternal 14-bp insertion polymorphism in the HLA-G gene in

women with recurrent spontaneous abortions. Tissue Antigens 2006;68:521-23.
53. Aldrich CL, Stephenson MD, Karrison T, et al. HLA-G genotypes and pregnancy outcome in couples with unexplained recurrent miscarriage. Mol Hum Reprod 2001;7:1167-72.
54. Pfeiffer KA, Fimmers R, Engels G, van der Ven H, van der Van K. The HLA-G genotype is potentially associated with idiopathic recurrent spontaneous abortion. Mol Hum Reprod 2001;7(4):373-78.
55. Abbas A, Tripathi P, Naik S, Agrawal S. Analysis of human leukocyte antigen (HLA)-G polymorphism in normal women and in women with recurrent spontaneous abortions. Eur J Immunogen 2004;31:275-78.
56. Hviid TV, Hylenius S, Hoegh AM, Kruse C, Christiansen OB. HLA-G polymorphisms in couples with recurrent spontaneous abortions. Tissue Antigens 2002;60:122-32.
57. Ober C, Aldrich CL, Chervoneva I, et al. Variation in the HLA-G promoter region influences miscarriage rates. Am J Hum Genet 2003;72:1425-35.
58. Hviid TV, Hylenius S, Lindhard A, Christiansen OB. Association between human leukocyte antigen-G genotype and success of in vitro fertilization and pregnancy outcome. Tissue Antigens 2004;64:66-69.
59. Emmer PM, Steegers AP, Kerstens HMJ, et al. Altered phenotype of HLA-G expressing trophoblast and decidual natural killer cells in pathological pregnancies. Hum Reprod 2002;17:1072-80.
60. Tripathi P, Abbas A, Naik S, Agrawal S. Role of 14 bp deletion in the HLA-G gene in the maintenance of pregnancy. Tissue Antigens 2004;64:706-10.
61. Karhukorpi J, Laitinen R, Tiilikainen AS. HLA-G polymorphism in Finnish couples with recurrent spontaneous miscarriage. BJOG 1997;104:1212-14.
62. Penzes M, Rajczy K, Gyodi E, et al. HLA-G gene polymorphism in the normal population and in recurrent spontaneous abortion in Hungary. Transplant Proc 1999;31:1832-33.
63. Yamashita T, Fujii R, Tokunaga K, et al. Analysis of human leukocyte antigen-G polymorphism including intron-4 in Japanese couples with habitual abortion. Am J Reprod Immunol 1999;41:159-63.
64. Yan WH, Fan LA, Yang JQ, Xu LD, Ge Y, Yao FJ. HLA-G polymorphism in a Chinese Han population with recurrent spontaneous abortion. Int J Immunogen 2006;33:55-58.
65. Sullivan LC, Clements CS, Rossjohn J, Brooks AG. The major histocompatibility complex class Ib molecule HLA-E at the interface between innate and adaptive immunity. Tissue Antigens 2008; 72:415-24.
66. Dosiou C, Giudice LC. Natural Killer Cells in Pregnancy and Recurrent Pregnancy Loss: Endocrine and Immunologic Perspectives. Endocr Rev 2005;26:44-62.
67. Lanier L. Natural killer cell receptor signaling. Curr Opin Immunol 2003;15:308-14.
68. Rajagopalan S, Long EO. A Human Histocompatibility Leukocyte Antigen (HLA)-G–specific Receptor Expressed on All Natural Killer Cells. J Exp Med. April 1999;189(7): 1093-99.
69. Mandelboim O, Reyburn HT, Sheu EG, et al. The binding site of NK receptors on HLA-C molecules. Immunity 1997;6:341-50.
70. Rajagopalan S, Fu J, Long EO. Cutting edge: Induction of IFN-gamma production but not cytotoxicity by the killer cell Ig-like receptor KIR2DL4 (CD158d) in resting NK cells. J Immunol 2001;167:1877-81.
71. Witt CS, Goodridge J, Gerbase-DeLima MG, Daher S, Christiansen FT. Maternal KIR repertoire is not associated with recurrent spontaneous abortion. Hum Reprod 2004;19(11): 2653-57.
72. Saverino D, Merlo A, Bruno S, Pistoia V, Grossi CE, Ciccone E. Dual effect of CD85/leukocyte Ig-like receptor-1/Ig-like transcript 2 and CD152 (CTLA-4) on cytokine production by antigenstimulated human T cells. J Immunol 2002;168:207-15.
73. Braud VM, Allan DS, O'Callaghan CA, et al. HLA-E binds to natural killer cell receptors CD94/NKG2A, B and C. Nature 1998;391:795-99.
74. Vales-Gomez M, Reyburn HT, Erskine RA, Lopez-Botet M, Strominger JL. Kinetics and peptide dependency of the binding of the inhibitory NK receptor CD94/NKG2-A and the activating receptor CD94/NKG2-C to HLA-E. EMBO J 1999;18:4250-60.
75. Uhrberg M, Valiante NM, Shum BP, et al. Human diversity in killer cell inhibitory receptor genes. Immunity 1997;7:753-63.
76. Hiby SE, Walker JJ, O'Shaughnessy KM, et al. Combinations of maternal KIR and fetal HLA-C genes influence the risk of pre-eclampsia and reproductive success. J Exp Med 2004;200:957-65.
77. Varla-Leftherioti M, Spyropoulou-Vlachou M, Keramitsoglou T, et al. Lack of the appropriate natural killer cell inhibitory receptors in women with spontaneous abortion. Hum Immunol 2005;66:65-71.
78. Piccinni M-P, Scaletti C, Mavilia C, et al. Production of IL-4 and leukemia inhibitory factor by T cells of the cumulus oophorus: A favorable microenvironment for preimplantation embryo development. Eur J Immunol 2001;31:2431-37.
79. Fehniger TA, Shah MH, Turner MJ, et al. Differential cytokine and chemokine gene expression by human NK cells following activation with IL-18 or IL-15 in combination with IL-12: Implications for the innate immune response. J Immunol 1999;162:4511-20.
80. Cooper MA, Fehniger TA, Turner SC, et al. Human natural killer cells: A unique innate immunoregulatory role for the CD56 (bright) subset. Blood 2001;97:3146-51.
81. Rukavina D, Bogovic T, Sotosek V, et al. Physiological role(s) of IL-15 and IL-18 at the maternal-fetal (m-f) interface. 8th Congress of the AASIR, Weimar, Germany. Am J Reprod Immunol. 2002;48:139.
82. Mellor AL, Munn DH. IDO expression by dendritic cells: Tolerance and tryptophan catabolism. Nat Rev Immunol 2004;4:762-74.

83. Aloe L, Simone MD, Properzi F. Nerve growth factor: A neurotrophin with activity on cells of the immune system. Microsc Res Tech 1999;45:285-91.
84. Gorczynski RM, Chen Z, Clark DA, et al. Structural and functional heterogeneity in the CD200R family of immunoregulatory molecules and their expression at the fetomaternal interface. Am J Reprod Immunol. 2004;52:147-63.
85. Voisin G, Chaouat G. Demonstration, nature and properties of maternal antibodies fixed on placenta and directed against paternal alloantigens. J Reprod Fertil 1974;21:89-103.
86. Christiansen OB. A fresh look at the causes and treatments of recurrent miscarriage, especially its immunological aspects. Hum Reprod Update 1996;2(4):271-93.
87. Esplin MS, Branch DW, Silver R, Stagnaro-Green A. Thyroid autoantibodies are not associated with recurrent pregnancy loss. Am J Obstet Gynecol. December 1998; 179(6):1400-78.
88. Lee RM, Branch DW, Silver RM. Immunoglobulin A Anti β2-glycoprotein antibodies in women who experience unexplained recurrent spontaneous abortion and unexplained fetal death. Am J Obstet Gynecol. 2001; 185:748-53.
89. Lissak A, Sharon A, Fruchter O, Kassel A, Sanderovitz J, Abramovici H. Polymorphism for mutation of cytosine to thymine at location 677 in the methylenetetrahydrofolate reductase gene is associated with recurrent early fetal loss. Am J Obstet Gynecol 1999;181:126-30.
90. Wang X, Ma Z, Lin Q. Inherited thrombophilia in recurrent spontaneous abortion among Chinese women. Int J Gynecol Obstet. 2006;92:264-65.
91. Kruse C, Rosgaard A, Steffensen R, Varming K, Jensenius JC, Christiansen OB. Low serum level of mannan-binding lectin is a determinant for pregnancy outcome in women with recurrent spontaneous abortion. Am J Obstet Gynecol 2002;187:1313-20.
92. Hammoud AO, Merhi ZO, Diamond M, Baumann P. Recurrent pregnancy loss and obstetric outcome. Int J Gynecol Obstet 2007;96:28-53.
93. Li TC, Makris M, Tomsu M, Tuckerman E, Laird S. Recurrent miscarriage: Aetiology, management and prognosis. Hum Reprod Update 2002;8(5):463-81.
94. Scott JR. Immunotherapy for recurrent miscarriage. Cochrane Database Syst Rev. 2003;1:CD000112.
95. Clark DA, Coulam CB, Daya S, Chaouat G. Unexplained sporadic and recurrent miscarriage in the new millennium: A critical analysis of immune mechanisms and treatments. Hum Reprod Update. 2001;7(5):501-11.
96. Mowbray JF, Gibbings C, Liddell H, Reginald PW, Underwood JL, Beard RW. Controlled trial of treatment of recurrent spontaneous abortion by immunisation with paternal cells. Lancet 1985;1:941-43.
97. Takeshita T. Diagnosis and treatment of recurrent miscarriage associated with Immunological disorders: Is Paternal lymphocyte immunization a relic of the past? J Nippon Med Sch. 2004;71(5):308-13.
98. Heine O, Eckhardt GM. Intravenous immune globulin in recurrent abortion. Clin Exp Immunol. 1994;97 (Suppl 1):39-42.
99. Pandey MK, Agrawal S. Prevalence of anti-idiotypic antibodies in pregnancy v/s recurrent spontaneous (RSA) women. Obs and Gynae Today 2003;7:574-78.
100. Porter TF, LaCoursiere Y, Scott JR. Immunotherapy for recurrent miscarriage. Cochrane Database of Systematic Reviews 2006, Issue 2. Art. No.: CD000112. DOI: 10.1002/14651858.CD000112.pub2.
101. Cauchi MN. Abstracts of Contributors' Individual Data Submitted to the Worldwide Prospective Observation Study on Immunotherapy for Treatment of Recurrent Spontaneous Abortion. Am J Reprod Immunol 1994; 32:263.
102. Christiansen OB, Christiansen BS, Husth M, Mathiesen O, Lauritsen J, Grunnet N. Prospective study of anticardiolipin antibodies in immunized and untreated women with recurrent spontaneous abortions. Fertil Steril 1992;58:328-34.
103. Gatenby PA, Cameron K, Simes RJ, et al. Treatment of recurrent spontaneous abortion by immunization with paternal lymphocytes: Results of a controlled trial. Am J Reprod Immunol 1993;29:88-94.
104. Ho HN, Gill TJ, Hsieh HJ, Jiang JJ, Lee TY, Hsieh CY. Immunotherapy for recurrent spontaneous abortions in a Chinese population. Am J Reprod Immunol 1991;25:10-15.
105. Illeni MT, Marelli G, Parazzini F, et al. Immunotherapy and recurrent abortion: A randomized clinical trial. Hum Reprod 1994;9:1247-49.
106. Kilpatrick DC, Liston W. Abstracts of Contributors' Individual Data Submitted to the Worldwide Prospective Observation Study on Immunotherapy for Treatment of Recurrent Spontaneous Abortion. Am J Reprod Immunol 1994;32:264.
107. Ober C, Karrison T, Odem RB, Barnes RB, Branch DW, Stephenson MD. Mononuclear-cell immunisation in prevention of recurrent miscarriages: A randomized trial. Lancet 1999;354:365-69.
108. Reznikoff-Etievant MF. Abstracts of Contributors' Individual Data Submitted to the Worldwide Prospective Observation Study on Immunotherapy for Treatment of Recurrent Spontaneous Abortion. Am J Reprod Immunol 1994;32:266-67.
109. Scott JR, Branch WD, Dudley DJ, Hatasaka HH. Immunotherapy for recurrent pregnancy loss: The University of Utah perspective. In: DonderoF, JohnsonP editor(s). Reproductive immunology. Serono Symposium Publications, Raven Press 1997:255-57.
110. PandeyMK, Agrawal S. Induction of MLR-Bf and protection of fetal loss: A current double blind randomized trial of paternal lymphocyte immunization for women with recurrent spontaneous abortion. Int Immunopharmacol 2004;4:289-98.

111. Christiansen OB, Mathiesen O, Lauritsen JG, Grunnet N. Intravenous immunoglobulin treatment of women with multiple miscarriages. Hum Reprod 1992;7:718-22.
112. Christiansen OB, Mathiesen O, Husth M, et al. Placebo-controlled trial of treatment of unexplained secondary recurrent spontaneous abortions and recurrent late spontaneous abortions with intravenous immunoglobulin. Hum Reprod 1995;10:2690-95.
113. Coulam CB, Krysa L, Stern JJ, Bustillo M. Intravenous immunoglobulin for treatment of recurrent pregnancy loss. Am J Reprod Immunol 1995;34:333-37.
114. Jauniaux E, Farquharson RG, Christiansen OB, Exalto N. Evidence-based guidelines for the investigation and medical treatment of recurrent miscarriage. Hum Reprod 2006;21(9):2216-22.
115. Ramsden GH, Johnson PM. Unexplained recurrent miscarriage and the role of immunotherapy. Contemp Rev Obstet Gynaecol 1992;4:29-35.
116. Di Nisio M, Peters LW, Middeldorp S. Anticoagulants for the treatment of recurrent pregnancy loss in women without antiphospholipid syndrome. Cochrane Database Syst Rev 2005, Issue 2. Art. No.: CD004734.
117. Bubanovic I. 1alpha, 25-dihydroxy-vitamin-D3 as new immunotherapy in treatment of recurrent spontaneous abortion. Med Hypotheses 2004;63:250-53.

Section 4

MHC and Transplantation

Chapter 26

Donors Selection Strategies for Hematopoietic Stem Cell Transplantation

Uma Kanga, Narinder K Mehra

INTRODUCTION

Hematopoietic Stem Cell transplantation (HSCT) is a recognized curative therapy for a variety of malignant and non-malignant diseases, inherited blood disorders, acquired or congenital disorders of hematopoietic system or for patients with chemosensitive, radiosensitive or immunosensitive tumors. Additionally, HSCT has been proposed in an array of severe pathologic states including autoimmune diseases, HIV and AIDS. A major limitation in this procedure is the availability of a genetically matched donor particularly with respect to the immune response genes. In the same way as the blood transfusion needs to be matched for a particular blood group, stem cell transplants need to be matched for the genes at the Major Histocompatibility Complex (MHC). These genes in the humans are collectively referred to as Human Leukocyte Antigens (HLA).

An important landmark in biomedical research has been the discovery of the MHC in the late 40's and of the HLA system in mid 50's. The system consists of a cluster of genes on human chromosome 6 and is only about one thousandth of the total genome. The most influential genes are the class I genes namely, HLA-A, -B, -C and the HLA class II genes, HLA-DRB1,-DQB1,-DPB1.

According to the current International Immunogenetics HLA database (IMGT statistics), a total of 4124 HLA alleles (2968 HLA class I and 1156 class II alleles) are identified (Table 26.1). Indeed, there is no other genetic system so far known in man with as many closely linked polymorphic loci as the HLA system. Major advances in recent years have revealed that besides major barriers to transplantation, this cluster of few genes has additional functional relevance due to its vast genetic complexity.

During development, the immune system becomes tolerant to the normal components of the human body, which are recognized as self and develops tolerance for the self-MHC antigens expressed on the cell surface. This tolerance however does not develop for the thousands of other types of MHC molecules to which it has not been exposed during the stages of development. Preformed or newly generated antibodies in the recipient to donor HLA antigens lead to immediate destruction of the transplanted tissue in varying time periods. Therefore the best option is to transplant stem cells/bone marrow from a donor that is completely matched at the HLA allele level with the recipient so that it would be recognized as self and accepted by the host immune system. Hence, the success of transplantation can be achieved through

Table 26.1: Polymorphism of the HLA system – IMGT statistics (Oct 2009)

HLA loci	Numbers identified		HLA loci	Numbers identified	
	Antigens	Alleles*		Antigens	Alleles*
A	24	893	DR	20	814
B	49	1431	DQ	9	141
C	10	569	DP	6	164

*HLA antigens are serologically defined while alleles refer to those defined at the DNA level. In HSCT, donor-recipient pair matching at the allelic level is mandatory.

better understanding of the immunobiology of the HLA system and through precise and comprehensive matching of the recipient and the donor.

SOURCES OF HEMATOPOIETIC STEM CELLS

Past two decades have seen rapid strides in our understanding of the intricacies of the HSCT whereby it has evolved from an experimental procedure to the standard treatment algorithm for various diseases. The tremendous progress in preparative regimens, improved supportive care, HLA testing technologies, novel conditioning regimens have extended the use of HSCT for new disease indications and new patient categories. Transplantation of hematopoietic stem cells to any recipient who is not HLA identical presents an allogenic challenge similar to any other kind of allograft. In addition, cord blood transplantation using stem cells derived from the umbilical cord has been successfully used for reconstitution of bone marrow particularly in children with many disease conditions.[1-3] The approaches to transplantation are distinguished by the type of donors used in providing the stem cell component. The possible sources of stem cells are:

1. Peripheral blood stem cells and/or Bone marrow from a family member. These include: (i) Syngeneic, i.e. from an identical twin. The donor is perfectly matched with the recipient for HLA, non-HLA as well as other relevant unknown genes (ii) Allogeneic – This is the commonest form of HSCT/BMT and is dependent on the availability of an HLA -identical sibling (iii) Autologous – Stem cells or Bone marrow of the self with or without purging.
2. Cord blood: Stem cells obtained from the umbilical cord and placenta.
3. Marrow Donor Registries: Stem cells from an HLA-A, B, DR "full house" matched donor can be made available from the database of the unrelated donor marrow registries.

In addition to the above, stem cells can be obtained through laboratory manipulations involving embryonal stem cells and creation of HLA compatible homozygous stem cell lines. A few such options have recently been described and discussed here briefly.

HUMAN EMBRYONIC STEM CELLS (hESCs) HOMOZYGOUS AT HLA LOCI

A highly promising source of stem cell for replacement of diseased or damaged tissue is the undifferentiated products of the embryonic stem cells (hESCs) that retain their pluripotency. The HLA expression of these undifferentiated progeny would lead to graft rejection and therefore the need to develop a bank of HLA typed hESCs. A recent study is the UK population has estimated that nearly 150 hESCs might be sufficient to provide a beneficial match for a majority of recipients and extending beyond this number may not confer a great benefit for matching. The authors argued that having just 10 such lines homozygous for common HLA types in the population might be sufficient.[4] Nevertheless, extensive diversity of the HLA system poses a substantial challenge in identifying matched donors. Data from HLA typing of half the hESC lines eligible for US Federal support indicates none to be homozygous at all HLA loci and also these lines do not reflect the ethnic diversity and minority proportion of the US population.[5] Hence the necessary number of lines and the optimum range of HLA tissue types will vary between populations depending on the ethnic makeup. A recent study on the Japanese population indicates that if a bank of 170 hESC lines is established from selected donated embryos, 80 percent of patients will be able to find at least one beneficial HLA matched line. With 5000 spare embryos discarded annually by the fertility clinic, establishment of 200 hESC lines will be feasible with less bioethical and social concerns.[6] As parthenogenetic hESC have similar and sufficient ability of pluripotency and have no greater risks, less number of hESC could provide a full match. The hESC lines with uniparental disomy (UPD) have complete homozygosity at all genomic loci, their unique advantage in transplantation therapy is the possibility to be transplanted to both homozygous and heterozygous patients. Extrapolation in the Japanese study revealed that 80 percent of patients could be offered a UPD hESC line established from out of only 55 randomly selected donated oocytes. A potential concern is the epigenetic status of such lines, but studies have suggested that they retain the pluripotency to produce derivatives of all three germ layers. These are clearly important options to be evaluated in future.

DIRECT REPROGRAMMING OF ADULT CELLS

Human embryonic stem cells hold the promise of differentiating into a variety of cell types from all primitive germ layers. Expression of alpha fetoprotein (AFP) and human chorionic gonadotrophin (HCG) typically produced by trophoblast cells is observed on *in vitro* differentiation of human embryonic cells. Stage specific embryonic antigen (SSEA)-3, SSEA-4, tumor rejection antigen (TRA)-1-16, and TRA-1-81 surface antigens are expressed on human embryonic cells prior to differentiation.[7,8] Maintenance of pluripotency of human ESCs is supported by highly expressed transcription factors REX1 and a POU transcription factor (POU5F1).[9] Studies on mouse embryonic stem cells suggest that a network of transcription factors including Sox-2, Nanog and Oct-4 may be sufficient to establish self renewal and/or suppress lineage differentiation. A recent report by Silva, et al has revealed important role of Nanog in reprogramming and acquisition of both embryonic and induced pluripotency.[10]

During embryonal cell differentiation, there is a decrease in the expression of several candidate proteins like Zn-finger transcription factor, LIN28, a RNA binding protein, NPM1, a nucleolar protein on human embryonic cells. The REX-1, POU5F1, UTF-1 and SOX-2 are transcription factors with a defined role in maintenance of pluripotency and their expression is down regulated upon differentiation. A cocktail of these proteins are capable of converting adult human cells into embryonic stem cells that can grow and replace tissues.

Pluripotency can be imposed by fusion of embryonic cells with differentiated cell nuclei. A homodomain protein Nanog is a molecule that is capable of mediating this conversion. Increased levels of Nanog[11] stimulates pluripotent gene activation from the somatic cell genome and enables recovery of stem cell colonies, which show all the characteristics of embryonic stem cells. Depending on the differentiation status of the somatic cells, pluripotency can be infused with 100 percent efficiency when embryonic stem cells are fused with somatic cells in presence of elevated Nanog. The developments in field of cell therapy would enable using a set of proteins to reprogram patient's own cells to first transform them into embryonic stem cells and further differentiate into blood, pancreas or any other tissue that can replace/cure the damaged tissue/organ. The bottlenecks in generating inducible pluripotent stem cell (iPS) have been investigated and stochastic models for iPS generation are recently reported.[12] A discussion by four pioneering iPS researchers has expressed hope for improved understanding and treatment of human disease and proposes establishment of iPS cell banks.[13]

HLA MATCHED STEM CELL BANK

The diversity of the HLA system is the major challenge in our efforts to identify compatible donors for patients requiring HSCT. Currently more than 4000 HLA alleles have been identified and this number is still growing.

The distribution of these alleles displays ethnic variability among different population groups. For donor selection purposes, majority of patients requiring HSCT could be served through a stem cell bank with reasonable number of cell lines representing the 'common HLA alleles and haplotypes' observed in a given population. If cell lines homozygous at HLA haplotypes are developed, smaller stem cell banks could serve as an optimal donor pool. Immense heterogeneity at HLA class I and II loci has been observed in the Indian population. Studies from our group have revealed that the HLA gene pool of Indians resembles the Caucasians and also has appreciable oriental influence. In the Indian population ~90 percent of allelic diversity at the HLA class I region (Fig. 26.1) is represented by few alleles at locus A i.e HLA –A*02, A*11, A*24, A*01 and A*33 and HLA-B*05, B*35, B*40, B*44 and B*07 at the HLA-B locus.

Further analysis indicate that (i) A26-B8-DR3, (ii) A1-B57-DR15, (iii) A2-B44-DR15 and (iv) A2-B60-DR15 are the most common three locus HLA-A-B-DR haplotypes encountered in the Indian population with significant linkage disequilibrium. Additionally, the two locus HLA class I haplotypes, e.g. A11-B35, A24-B40 and two locus HLA class II haplotypes, e.g. DR3-DQ2, DR15-DQ6, DR4-DQ3 are observed with appreciable frequency. A large number of unique haplotypes are also encountered at significant frequencies in the Indian population, which have not been reported in other ethnic groups (Table 26.2). These include for example, the A2-B50-DR7, A24-B7-DR13, A24-B35-DR3 and others. Some of these are disease associated and encountered frequently in patients with autoimmune and/or infectious diseases.[14]

Depending on the ethnic group being evaluated, the probability of finding an individual with homozygous HLA haplotypes varies between 0.01 to 0.8 percent in the Indian population. It is therefore envisaged that a set of cryopreserved stem cells that are representative of the most commonly occurring HLA alleles and haplotypes of a population can serve as a ready source of donor pool for patients awaiting stem cell transplantation.

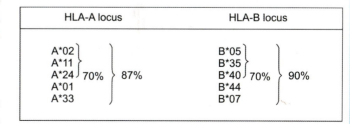

Fig. 26.1: The common HLA class I alleles in the Indian population covering the maximum population

Table 26.2: Commonly occurring HLA haplotypes representing >70 percent of the Indian population	
HLA class I haplotypes	HLA class II haplotypes
A*26-B*0801	DRB1*03-DQB1*0201-DQA1*0501
A*11-B*5801	DRB1*07-DQB1*DQB1*0201-DQA1*0201
A*3303-B*5801	DRB1*1502-DQA1*0103-DQB1*0601
A*01 B*5701	DRB1* 0403-DQB1*0302-DQA1*03
A*02-B*5001	DRB1*11-DQB1*0301-DQA1*0501
A*24-B*35	DRB1*14-DQB1*0503-DQA1*0104

SELECTION OF DONORS

The Ideal Donor: HLA Identical Sibling

HLA antigens being diploid in nature, each individual inherits two antigens of each of the locus A,B,C,DR,DQ and DP. A complete set of antigens on the same chromosome usually inherited en bloc (one unit) is referred to as a *haplotype*. All humans inherit half of their entire genetic make-up, and thus of their HLA phenotypes, from each parent, i.e. one haplotype from mother and the other from the father. Therefore the most likely place to find a match is within the patient's own family. Sibling donors that match for both maternal as well as the paternal HLA haplotypes are chosen as donors for HSCT. Because of the haplotypic inheritance pattern of the MHC, there is a 25 percent chance of finding an HLA identical sibling through family testing. Atypical HLA segregation patterns have been observed in leukemic families that includes a higher frequency of HLA-identical unaffected siblings, increased HLA homozygosity and increased maternal HLA-DR identity.[15] The overall chance of having an HLA-identical sibling is correlated with the family size (equal to [1-$(0.75)^n$] where n is the number of siblings) (http://www.ibmtindy.com/faq/hla-typing.htm). This probability may go up in cases where families are traditionally large. With the average family size of 2-3 children, only about 30-35 percent patients are able to find an HLA-identical sibling within the family and the remaining 70-75 percent of patients have to depend on other sources of donors.

Partially Matched Donor

For patients without an HLA matched sibling, extended family testing is done to include first cousins or near relatives. In offsprings of first cousin marriages and where consanguinity is practiced, there is a 1-8 percent probability of either the parent or another first degree relative in the family to be HLA phenotypically identical. All patients have a haploidentical parent, child, sibling or relative who can serve as a donor.[16] In some cases of consanguineous marriages, the parents have also been shown to be HLA matched with a patient. In children with non-malignant hematologic or metabolic diseases that are eventually fatal and which can be cured or ameliorated by allogeneic HSCT, CD34+selected stem cell transplants from mismatched or even haploidentical parents has been suggested if no other suitable donor is available.[17,18]

In AML patients with primary induction failure, BMT using partially mismatched related donors (PMRDs) showed timely engraftment and less GVHD (acute and chronic), where as disease relapse was the major cause of failure.[19,20] Thus transplants with PMRDs has been suggested as a viable option along with matched related or unrelated donors.

Antenatal HLA Testing

The technology of testing HLA genes with the DNA obtained from chorionic villous samples (ultrasound guided collection at 10 weeks of gestation) has helped in identifying potential sibling donors at the prenatal stage. Prenatal screening for thalassemia mutations are advised to parents with a thalassemic child and they can simultaneously benefit from this technology since there is a 25 percent chance of matching. Knowledge of fetal HLA types can be important since it might influence choice of treatment and timing of transplantation. This also helps in planning for storage of cord blood that can subsequently be used for transplantation purposes.

HLA 'Full House' Matched Unrelated Donor

Since HSCT/BMT is more sensitive to HLA differences than solid organ transplants, immunological compatibility between the prospective donor and the recipient is an absolute necessity for successful therapy. Patients requiring HSCT but without a family donor, have to depend on the availability of a perfectly matched unrelated donor. The diversity in the MHC has proved to be a major hindrance in selection of HLA matched donors, considering that the probability of any two unrelated individuals sharing the same genotype is less than 1 in 150 billion, which is very low. A unique feature of the HLA system, closely related to its biological significance is its extraordinary polymorphism that means that an exceptional inter-individual variability exists as far as HLA antigen profile of a population is considered. This extraordinary figure makes it virtually impossible to have a perfect match donor for transplants from amongst the general population. This is quite in contrast to the ABO blood groups where there is one locus with three alleles and a maximum of six different combinations. Probability of finding a full house HLA matched donor is possible only through a pool of several million potential donors, but problems arise when rare HLA genes or haplotypes occur in a patient. The more unique or unusual the HLA type, the more difficult it will be to find a sufficiently matched unrelated donor. Patients from mixed ethnic background may have very uncommon HLA types. However, since 1987, large registries have been developed in various countries and successful BMTs have been performed for patients without an HLA identical sibling, using allele matched unrelated donors.

INITIATION OF BONE MARROW REGISTRIES: INTERNATIONAL EFFORT

Establishment of 'bone marrow donor registries' having large groups of voluntary unrelated donors, has been of great help to patients requiring HSCT/BMT and who do not have an HLA identical sibling in the family. Pioneers in the field of BMT/HSCT have emphasized the need for such registries[21] and their structure and functioning has been discussed in Chapter 33. The rarity of finding two individuals with an identical HLA type emphasizes the necessity for very large pools of donors with representation from all major ethnic groups to increase probabilities of finding optimum donors from the registry. As expected, the probability of finding a well-matched donor in the registry varies with the HLA type of the patient and its frequency in the population represented in the registry. Thus patients with common HLA types would find many HLA matched donors whereas those with uncommon or novel alleles or combinations would find it hard to find even one.

The first successful bone marrow transplant using an unrelated donor was performed in 1973. Since bone marrow can be donated without any major inconvenience to the donor, large bone marrow registries have been set up to provide donors for unrelated patients. In 1974, the first registry of volunteer donors was initiated and named Anthony Nolan Bone Marrow Trust (ANBMT) in the UK now called as Anthony Nolan Trust (ANT). This registry has currently enrolled 402,373 volunteers. Subsequently, other independent registries were established in many countries. The largest registry in the world is the National Marrow Donor Program (NMDP) in the USA having nearly 7 million donors on the list. The NMDP currently facilitates more than 3600 recipients annually. Since its inception in 1986, the number of unrelated transplants facilitated by NMDP is increasing each year (Fig. 26.2) and untill 2007 the total number has already reached >29,000 transplants.[22]

Since the initiation of such registries in the late 1980's, 13.67 million volunteer donors are currently registered with various organizations in several countries. These include France Grafffe de Moelle (171,875 donors), Australian Bone Marrow Donor registry (181,443 donors), German Registry of Bone Marrow Donors (3,645,872 donors), Izrael Ezer Mizion (487,480) and Canada (248,193 donors). These national registries are linked with each other and facilitate international searches. To assist patients in finding an unrelated donor, an organization with an international network of donor exchanges was developed under the auspices of 'Europe Donor Foundation'.[23] The organization functions under the name, 'Bone Marrow Donors Worldwide (BMDW) and was initiated in 1989 with a total of 155,000 donors from 8 registries. Currently, BMDW has 63 stem cell registries from 44 countries as its members. In addition, 43 Cord blood registries from 26 countries have submitted data to BMDW (September 2009 update of BMDW, http://www.bmdw.org). Around 725 users from 450 organizations have an access to the BMDW database. This collaborative international effort has been able to overcome the problem of finding HLA matched unrelated donors to a large extent. Further, the quantitative effort has been paralleled by an improvement in the quality of registries and in the efficiency of their donor search procedures.

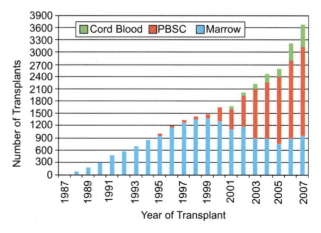

Fig. 26.2: Hematopoietic stem cell transplants using unrelated donors through the NMDP[17]

UNRELATED DONOR SEARCHES

The probability of finding a suitable unrelated donor depends on selection criteria and patients racial and ethnic background.[24] The World Marrow Donor Association (WMDA) has set standards for unrelated donor search (UDS) strategies.[25] The duration of unrelated searches are significantly shorter for patients with common HLA haplotypes and are longer and less successful for patients with uncommon HLA types. The median time and success of searches has improved over the last few years.[26,27] Newer donor recruitment activities, access to over 13 million donors, increased number of allele level typed donors have influenced donor searches.[28] However, stringent matching criteria influence the duration and success rates that are reported to be 60-80 percent.[29,30] The outcome of UDS is influenced by the registry size and studies have assessed the gene and haplotype frequencies in a population to estimate an optimal size of the registry.[31] These theoretical considerations are complemented by informatics challenges and search algorithms that are developed on the basis of changes in the HLA typing technology and resolution of HLA typing. The WMDA information technology working group has proposed a set of guidelines for use of HLA nomenclature for international exchanges and HLA information required for operation of search algorithms. The study recommends HLA data collection format including assignments and primary data for most HLA typing technologies.[32] A recent study that retrospectively evaluated 549 searches in Germany, indicates remarkably shortened overall UDS duration and better success rate when predicting on the basis of patients HLA DRB1 allele and DRB1-DQB1 haplotype frequencies.[33] Since this study was based on Caucasians, the information may not be reproducible while analysing patients belonging to other racial groups. These predictions are of clinical importance when therapeutic alternatives for patients (e.g. high risk AML patients in first complete remission) are discussed at the beginning of the treatment.

HLA TYPING—RESULT PRESENTATION AND DONOR SELECTION

Methods of HLA analysis and presentation of the results are important and crucial aspects of donor selection for HSCT. In recent years, various modifications of the DNA based HLA typing methods have been introduced. The most frequently used technologies for first time donor testing are sequence specific primer amplification, sequence specific oligo probe (Reverse line Strip/Luminex) hybridization based technologies while sequenced based typing (SBT) and high resolution (HR) Luminex SSO frequently employed for confirmatory typing. The presentation of results could be low/intermediate/high resolution based on the technology employed. The intermediate resolution result often display several ambiguous alleles belonging to one low resolution (LR) HLA group. The notation for an ambiguous result is often abbreviated by NMDP codes and this helps to resolve genotypes of most common alleles (http://bioinformatics.nmdp.org/HLA/Allele_Codes/DNA_Type_Lookup/dnatyp.pl?dna =). A study on large cohort of 25,000 patients has provided the definition of common and well documented alleles (CWD) which are used for representing the HR results.[34] Although ambiguous descriptions produced by nucleotide substitutions in the Antigen Recognition Site (ARS) domains are accepted for inclusion in the HR results, they seem to be not valid for HSCT outcome. The reasonable basis for clinical histocompatibility decision seems to be the combined criteria of the 'maximum one genotype with upto two CWD allele plus non-ARS substitution'.[35] These criteria have helped in achieving the HSCT donor matching rapidly at the high resolution level which is of clinical importance.[36]

These strategies help in identifying 10/10 HLA allele matched donors for 30-70 percent of patients requiring such donors. Remaining patients in need of allogeneic HSCT are dependent on alternative donors, meaning those with varying degrees of HLA incompatability. The subsets of such alternative donors are haploidentical family donors, partially matched unrelated donors and partially mismatched cord blood units. The transplant physicians are advised to accept such donors only with the 'permissive mismatches'. It is a permanent debate to define permissiveness. The adverse effect on HSCT outcome is dependent on the locus of mismatch, number of mismatched alleles and level of mismatches (antigen or allele) and could be influenced also by the amino acid substitutions in or out of the antigen recognition site of the HLA.[35] All these types of incompatabilities influence the HSCT outcome; hence, alternate methods of therapy need to be applied.

The alternative sources like the haploidentical related donor or umbilical cord blood (UCB) significantly expand the donor pool since all patients have a haploidentical parent, child, sibling or relative who can serve as a donor immediately.[37] Several centers have reported successful outcomes through use of haploidentical donors.[38,39] Such transplants require positive selection of CD34+ cells in the PBSC grafts to attain high CD34 recovery with effective T cell depletion. These regimens allow full donor engraftment in over 95 percent of adult patients.[40] Inclusion of ATG and OKT3 for T cell depletion *in vivo*, have helped reduce incidence of GVHD.[41] However, in such transplants delayed immune reconstitution leads to significantly high infection related mortality rates. Use of cytokines such as IL7 and keratinocyte growth factor enhance thymopoiesis[42,43] as well as graft manipulation by regulatory T Cells and T cells specific for tumor associated viral antigen[44] are few strategies being developed to improve immune reconstitution.

Cryopreserved UCB is a stem cell source used to circumvent the difficulties faced in locating a matched unrelated donor (MUD) donor. UCB transplants are becoming common in patients under 20 years of age as the small volume of blood yields fewer cells for transplantation.[2] The barriers to UCB success are the longer engraftment time and low cell dose of single unit.[45] The benefit however is that the UCB can be procured readily and requires less stringent matching[46] because mismatched UCB transplantation cause less severe GVHD than unrelated donor Bone Marrow (BM)/ Peripheral Blood (PB) transplantation.[3] Given the promising results of UCB transplantation, establishment of public cord blood banks are supported by many agencies expecting an increased likelihood of a transplant candidate matching to a UCB unit. A study on comparison of UCB verses BMT revealed that the 5 year disease free survival (DFS) was similar in transplantation either with 1-2 antigen mismatch UCB or 8/8 matched BM grafts and DFS was higher (60%) after transplantation of 6/6 matched UCB compared to 38 percent in 8/8 matched BM.[47] Several studies have estimated that a reasonable size of UCB bank is necessary to find acceptable matched donors for majority of the patients. For example, in a UK study, UCB bank with 50,000 units was sufficient for finding donors for 80 percent patients at 5/6 allele match.[48] Using data from NMDP (in a bank size of 38,108), a recent study revealed 70 fold relative value of a UCB unit versus each BM donor recruited, assuming the matched unit has sufficient cells. The 5/6 match probability of a UCB unit was approx 91.2 percent which was close to 87.3 percent chance of finding a 6/6 match donor from a 2.2 M bone marrow donor pool.[45] The cost effectiveness of maintaining UCB banks have also been evaluated and since smaller UCB inventories than bone marrow registries could allow similar match probabilities, developing public cord blood banks may be worth the effort. This would avoid donor retention issues, quick searches and early transplants with better outcome. A high uptake rate from a new UCB bank in Mexico supports the concept of UCB in parallel with the BM registries.[49]

WORLD MARROW DONOR ASSOCIATION

With the initiation of matched unrelated donor transplants in various countries, a need was felt for international cooperation in terms of exchanging donors across international borders. A worldwide forum for discussion and joint activities has led to the establishment of World Marrow Donor Association (WMDA) whose main goal is to facilitate efficient, timely and reliable exchange of marrow/stem cells and to promote interests of donors. The numerous other goals of WMDA include establishing guidelines on ethical, technical, medical and financial issues that concern the donor and the transfer of cells.[50,51] The WMDA has a strength of five working groups, i.e. Donor Registry Working Group, Quality Assurance Working Group, Ethics Working Group, Finance Group, and Clinical Working Group that help is assessing and defining the guidelines and international standards for setting up registries, unrelated donor searches,[52] stem cell donation and consenting at various stages of recruitment, donor evaluation and donor workup,[53] quality assurance,[25] donor commitment and patient needs.[54] The international guidelines are in correlation with the NMDP's guidelines and experience on advances in donor selection based on refinements in HLA typing.[55,56]

REGIONAL DIFFERENCES IN TRANSPLANTATION ACTIVITY

With the rapid expansion in HSCT activity, current data indicates that 25,000 patients are treated annually in Europe with HSCT and an estimated 100,000 patients worldwide.[57,58] The data from CIBMTR and EBMT indicates significant differences in the number of transplants performed in different countries.[59] Additionally there are differences in indications for transplants and in techniques which is mainly attributed to the differences in the prevalence of diseases and in the economic structure of the countries. These are evident from annual HSCT activity survey of organizations like EBMT. A recent such survey including more than 600 teams from more than 40 countries over a time span of 15 years have revealed interesting data. The survey included evaluation of disease indications, transplant numbers, retransplants, transplants rates, team density and distribution, economic factors, etc. The major factors having impact on the transplant activity were the gross national income per capita, number of transplant teams per 10 million inhabitants or per 10,000 km², team size and experience. More research in various geographic regions would help understand the mechanism of HSCT activity and that could enable health care agencies for providing the necessary infrastructure for HSCT in any part of the world.[60]

STEM CELL TRANSPLANTATION IN THE ASIAN REGION

Although the BMT/HSCT activity was initiated in late 80's in Europe and North America, other countries in rest of the world have also developed efficient stem cell transplant programs and have established unrelated marrow donor registries and cord blood banks (Table 26.3). These organizations help support the national transplant activity with international collaborations.

Japan: The Japanese Marrow Donor Program was initiated in 1991 and currently has 300,000 volunteers on the register. The annual number of stem cell transplants is nearly 3500 (1000 BM/HSCT from siblings, 900 MUDs, 600 CBT and 1000 autologous) performed by more than 300 transplant teams across the country. The JMDP has accepted >20,000 patients and has facilitated >8000 unrelated BMTs. Similarly, the Japanese cord blood bank network initiated in 1999, has already collected 20,000 units and facilitated nearly 4000 CBTs untill 2008.[61]

China: The first allogeneic BMT was performed in 1981 in China and the number gradually increased especially since 1991. In recent years, approximately 2000 SCTs are performed annually by >100 transplant centers in mainland China. These transplants are mainly from identical sibling (38.6%), related mismatched or haploidentical (19.4%), unrelated matched (17.2%) and autologous (24.5%). The Chinese Marrow Donor Program (CMDP) was initiated under the Red Cross Society of China in 1992 and has recruited 950,000 donors until 2008.[62-64] More than 1100 stem cell transplants have been performed from the CMDP of which 50 were overseas exchanges.

Taiwan: Since inception of Budhist Tzu Chi Marrow Donor registry (BTCMDR) in 1993, nearly 310,000 volunteer donors are recruited and currently offers on an average, one case of stem cell donation each day. The BTCMDR has facilitated >1800 cases of donation for patients in 27 countries till date. The Tzu Chi Cord Blood Bank (TCCBB) has an inventory of 12,000 CB units and 47 of these cryopreserved units have been employed in 37 transplants from both Pediatrics and Adult patients domestically and internationally.[65,66] The BTCMDR and TCCBB are Non- Governmental Organizations operating under the umbrella of Buddhist Tzu Chi Stem Cell Center.

Korea: The first HSCT in Korea happened in 1983 and during the past 25 years, 38 HSCT centers have been developed. As of Dec 2006, 9561 HSCT were carried out (5617 allogeneic and 3944 autologous).[67] There are two registries in Korea, the Korean Marrow Donor Program (KMDP) and the Catholic Hematopoietic Stem Cell Bank (CHSCB). The actual donation rate is 50-80 percent and of the 1477 unrelated HSCT cases, 250 (17%) found donors through international registries mainly JMDP, BTCSCC, NMDP and DKMS. Untill Dec 2007, the Korean Network of Organ Sharing registered 144, 970 donors.[68] The Korean Network for Cord Blood was established in 2001 and 14,302 CB units are preserved. 364 CBTs were done till 2007 and 223 cases facilitated by KMDP.

Singapore: The Bone Marrow Donors Program (BMDP) in Singapore was established in 1993 with a goal to recruit 5000 donors annually and has currently 47,500 registered donors. A total of 245 BMT/HSCT have been performed which include 82 bone marrow, 70 peripheral blood, 93 UCB donations of which 75 were using BMDP donors (personal communication).

Table 26.3: HSCT/CBT activity of Asian Registries and Transplant Centers

Country	Registry	Year of Establishment	No of donors	MUD transplantation
Japan	Japan Marrow Donor Program	1991	300,000	>8000
China	Chinese Marrow Donor Program	1992	950,000	>1117
Singapore	Bone Marrow Donor Program	1993	47,500	245
Taiwan	Budhist Tzu Chi Marrow Donor Registry	1993	319,000	>1800
Korea	Korea Marrow Donor Program	1994	144,970	>1477
Thailand	Thai Stem Cell Donor Registry	2002	50,000	60
India	Asian Indian Donor Marrow Registry	1994	5000	11

Thailand: The Thai Stem Cell Donor Registry was established under the Thai Red Cross Society in the year 2002 and currently has 50,000 donors on the register that has facilitated 60 transplants till date (personal communication).

India: The BMT/HSCT activity in India was initiated in 1983 at the Tata Memorial Hospital, Mumbai. Subsequently a number of other centers in India have developed the expertise for performing BMT/HSCT (Fig. 26.3). In the absence of any country specific organization/group to maintain the record of transplant activity it is difficult to state the exact numbers of transplants carried out and their long term outcome. Estimates indicate that ~2000 patients have undergone transplants at these centers. Published results from these centers,[69-72] indicate that achieving results comparable to international

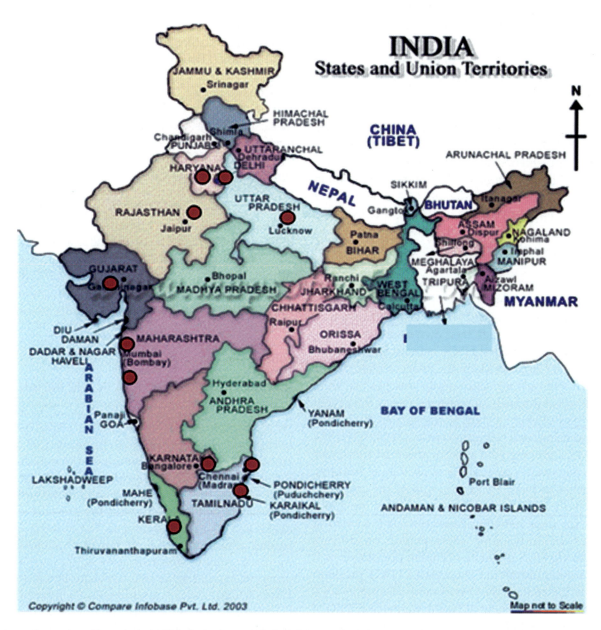

● denotes active centers. These include All India Institute of Medical Sciences (AIIMS)- New Delhi, Army Hospital Research and Referral-New Delhi, Christian Medical College-Vellore, Sahyadri Hospital, Pune, Tata Memorial Hospital-Mumbai, Sanjay Gandhi Post Graduate Institiute-Lucknow, Apollo Hospital-Chennai.

Fig. 26.3: Location of hematopoietic stem cell transplant centers in India

standards is possible. However, keeping in mind the number of patients requiring transplants, there is a need for more trained manpower, clinicians and nurses, more recognized centers for HLA typing, more transplant centers, financial resources for patients. With a population of over a billion, only about 5 percent are able to afford the very best treatment, 25 percent in the middle class with increasing income and 70 percent who cannot support a transplant without support from the state. Considering other health problems, support for transplants is not enough.[73]

The CMC Vellore, a center in India performing highest number of HSCTs offers transplants for a variety of diseases, of which the largest disease category is thalassemia major. With 20 Million thalassemia carriers and ~10,000 children being born with thalassemia major each year, if 30-35 percent find a suitable matched sibling donor for transplantation, there is a potential to offer HSCT cure to 3000 children each year.[74] Considering 6 per million as the incidence for Aplastic Anemia (AA), there would be 6000 new cases per year and if 10 percent of these are suitable for treatment by HSCT, there would be a need to perform 600 transplants per year for AA alone.[75] With increase in India's per capita GDP from $370 in 1999 to $3460 in 2006 (World population data sheet 1999/2006), it appears that many patients would not require resources from the insurance/state and would be able to afford a stem cell transplant through their own resources.

The matched unrelated HSCT activity was initiated in India at the Christian Medical College, Vellore in the year 2008. Of the few unrelated donor searches that were activated with international registries, nearly 50 percent were successful and till date 11 transplants have been performed using stem cells provided by the NMDP, USA and DKMS, Germany with a reasonable post-transplant outcome (personal communication, abstract at ASH 09). Other centers in India are keen to initiate the unrelated HSCT activity and are awaiting success with the donor searches for their patients. Expansion of the existing registries in India and recruitment of donors encompassing HLA diversity of Indian population will provide a major thrust to the unrelated HSCT program in India. In this context, the Department of Biotechnology (DBT) and the Department of Health Research (DHR) of the Government of India have recently undertaken a joint effort towards the expansion of Asian Indian Donor Marrow Registry (AIDMR) of voluntary donors representing various ethnic groups.

THE INDIAN POPULATION

The Indian population has time and again been described as a melting pot of various racial groups. Historically, the Indian peninsula has attracted travelers, historians, pilgrims and writers as it underwent an onslaught of invasions from foreigners mainly from the Northwest frontiers. The migration began by Aryans during 1750-1000 BC, followed by Buddhist's (around 500 BC) and by Mauryans in 324-200 BC. After the Indo-Aryan civilization settled, there were series of invasions to the subcontinent during 200-78 BC by the Greeks, Pahalavas and Kushanas. During the period 455-528 AD the Huns, Jews and Parsi's invaded the West coast and then Muslims (during 711-1000 AD), Turks (1192-1526 AD) and Mughals (1526-1585 AD) entered in from time to time. Infusions by the Dutch in 1609, European, Portuguese, French in 1674 and British in 1800 led to the development of an Indo-European community. The comparatively virgin side of the east of the country was home for invaders from South East Asia. From the above account, it is not difficult to appreciate that the Indian milieu consists of descendants of a large number of diverse populations who from time to time came to India and intermingled with the local population and each other. Several attempts have been made to anthropologically study the Indian population and classify it into distinct racial groups. A two-fold division of the population has led to classification into two basic races, the Aryans or North Indians and Non-Aryans or South Indian Dravidians races (Deniker).

UNIQUE DIVERSITY OF HLA IN THE INDIAN POPULATION

HLA studies in the North Indian population have confirmed the historical documentation of racial admixture. Although population studies indicate that the major HLA gene pool is much similar to that of Western Caucasoids, the DNA based studies have revealed appreciable heterogeneity with the presence of 'novel' alleles and 'unique' haplotypes. For example, diversity studies among the HLA-A2 family of alleles indicates the predominant occurrence of A*0211, an allele not observed in other major population groups. Remarkably, HLA-A*0201 which comprises 95 percent of the Caucasian HLA-A2 repertoire is found in very low frequency in the Indian population.[76,77] Similar studies in the HLA-A19 family of alleles reveals the presence of both Caucasian as well as Oriental genes[78] along with a novel gene A*3306 that occurs only in the North Indian population.[79] Further investigations on the polymorphism in HLA-B27 molecule among North Indians revealed the presence of B*2705, B*2702 (Caucasian alleles), B*2704 (oriental allele), B*2707 (only reported in Thai population) and B*2714 (rarely reported) alleles.[80] Similarly, among the class II alleles presence of a new allele DRB1*1506,[81] unique HLA-DR2 haplotypic combinations,[82-84] unique HLA-A,B,DR haplotypes[85] and some novel HLA-DRB1*04 haplotypes[86] have been reported in the North Indian population.

The data indicates the presence of both Caucasoid and Oriental HLA genes, as well as new recombinants amongst Indians. In addition, the population gene pool has a significant number of unique alleles and haplotypic combinations both in the MHC class I as well as class II region. Thus the Indian population appears to constitute a 'transition zone' between Caucasians and Negroids on one hand and Australoids and Mongoloids on the other (Fig. 26.4). The allelic diversity and uniqueness of HLA-A, B loci among North Indians is contributed by new allele sequences and immense heterozygosity in haplotypic combinations. The novel alleles and haplotypes may confer some selective survival advantage to the population as a whole. Immense racial admixture, influence of natural selection and potential genetic conversions over centuries in this subcontinent are thought to be probable causes for the observed allelic repertoire and generation of these ubiquitous and unique alleles.

Knowledge on the occurrence of the novel alleles and unique HLA haplotypes is of critical importance for donor selection during organ and bone marrow transplantation. Therefore developing a reasonable size Asian Indian registry would be of immense help to patients from India and also from around the world who are waiting to find an unrelated HLA-matched donor from such registries. Due to the large size of the population, with thousands of communities, endogamous groups and extended families, genetic diversity studies in the Indian population are of paramount importance not only in the transplantation context but also for vaccine development and disease associations especially with reference to the immune response genes.

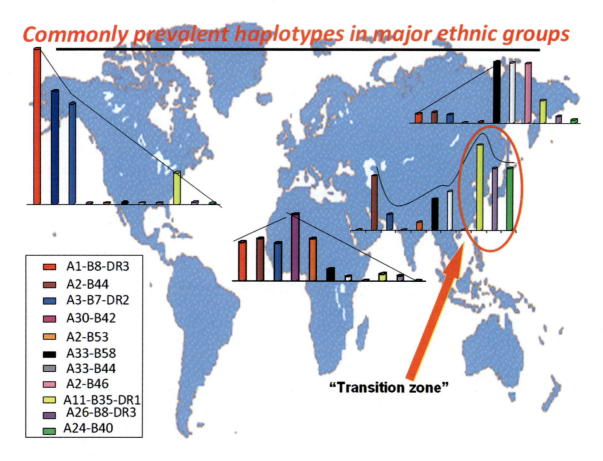

Fig. 26.4: Commonly prevalent HLA haplotypes in major ethnic groups around the world

INADEQUATE DONOR POOL IN BMDW

With the increase in volunteer donor registries as members in the Bone Marrow Donors Worldwide (BMDW), the number of available donors having different ethnic background has increased worldwide. Yet accurate definition of the HLA polymorphism within different ethnic groups poses a major challenge for donor selection. As noted above, ethnic groups differ in the representation and frequencies of their alleles and haplotypes. Therefore patients from minority ethnic groups often find it difficult to have optimally matched donors from the major registries that have an inherent biased composition of donors from a few select major ethnic groups.

The records of large registries indicate that very few Asians are registered as volunteer bone marrow donors in them. A search in the website of Anthony Nolan Trust (ANT) mentions that only approx 1.5-2 percent of the 402,373 donors are Asians and in the NMDP list, only 4-5 percent of the nearly 7 million registered donors are Asians/Pacific islanders of which only 0.05 percent are South Asians (http://www.marrow.org). The corresponding figures for Caucasians is significantly higher in both the ANT as well as the NMDP donor pool. Therefore while the chances of a Caucasian patient finding an HLA matched donor from this pool are much higher compared to one of an Asian Indian descent. Indeed searches for Asian patients with unique HLA profile are realistically limited to a small donor pool and are therefore often unsuccessful. Availability of matched donors is generally low for patients belonging to populations poorly represented in the registry in comparison to those from well represented populations. The NMDP records indicate that matched donors for Caucasians are more often identified. Of the 29,000 transplants facilitated by the NMDP till 2008, only a minor percentage of these patients were Asian/Pacific islanders. Indeed, search for a proper donor is dependent on the composition of the registry with respect to the number of donors, diversity of their ethnic background, representation of haplotypes (frequent vs rare vs unique), and the accuracy of HLA typing and therefore the quality control procedures used in HLA typing.[87]

ASIAN INDIAN DONOR MARROW REGISTRY

The *'Asian Indian Donor Marrow Registry'* (AIDMR) was established in 1994 at the All India Institute of Medical Sciences (AIIMS) with a view to recruit voluntary Indian donors. With the main objective of recruiting large donor pool, This modest effort has resulted in the enrolment of ~5000 donors, majority of which belong to the states from North India. These are already tested for HLA class I alleles by serological/molecular methods and approximately 50 percent of them are also tested for HLA class II alleles using molecular technologies.

The AIDMR is the only registry of voluntary donors in India and has developed collaborative arrangements with similar registries elsewhere, e.g. NMDP (USA), SAMAR (USA), BMDW (Holland). It is our endeavor to expand the registry appreciably in the near future for the benefit of those unfortunate patients who may not have an HLA identical sibling in the family. AIDMR receives 4-5 search requests per week from within and outside India. The registry also supports Indian patients living abroad for HLA testing and selecting donors from among their family members living in India. A computerized software developed by AIDMR, 'Soft HLA' is utilized for data maintenance of all voluntary donors and patient search requests. This enables efficient donor searches and identification of appropriate donors for all patients. Only restricted and authorized individuals, primarily the search coordinators and scientific supervisors have access to this software via a unique login and password.

Owing to the extensive polymorphism in the HLA system and the need for a large donor pool of Asian Indian volunteers, a regular structure of AIDMR has now been developed. Major objectives of the Indian Registry are: (i) recruitment of voluntary donors on regular basis and maintenance of a database on their HLA profile, (ii) Develop links with other HLA testing laboratories in India so as to increase representation of other Indian populations in the AIDMR, (iii) provide counseling to patients requiring stem cell transplantation and their family members on the availability of HLA matched donors, (iv) development of computer programs with matching algorithms that minimize the donor selection time, (v) increasing the donor pool tested for HLA-A,-B,-DR alleles by DNA based methods and (vi) provide confirmatory typing services.

As HLA antigens or the tissue types are inherited genetic characteristics, the probability of finding a suitable donor increases if the search is made from amongst the group of people who share similar genetic history to the patient, i.e. from same ethnic background. In practice, this means that an Indian with 'unique HLA alleles' has the greatest opportunity of finding a donor from within his or her own community, i.e. the Indian donor pool rather than the Caucasian population. Indeed, Indian population represents a pool of all HLA alleles which would be desirable in any unrelated donor registry. All patients, especially those of Indian origin would benefit immensely from an Asian Indian Donor Registry since the probability of finding a matched donor from this pool will be greatly enhanced. The ultimate goal is to provide an HLA matched donor to all patients who might benefit from a stem cell transplant.

REFERENCES

1. Gluckman E, Rocha V, Boyer-Chammard A, et al. Outcome of cord blood transplantation from unrelated and related donors. Eurocord Transplant Group and the European Blood and Marrow Transplantation Group. N Engl J Med 1997;337:373-81.
2. Urbano-Ispizua, A. Risk assessment in haematopoietic stem cell transplantation: stem cell source. Best Practice and Research Clinical Haematology 2007;20:265-80.
3. Gluckman E, Rocha V. Donor selection for unrelated cord blood transplants. Curr Opin Immunol 2006;18:565-70.
4. Taylor CJ, Bolton EM, Pocock S, et al. Banking on human embryonic stem cells: Estimating the number of donor cell lines needed for HLA matching. Lancet 2005; 366(9502):2019-25.
5. Rao MS, Auerbach JM. Estimating human embryonic stem-cell numbers. Lancet 2006;367(9511):650.
6. Nakajima F, Tokunaga K, Nakatsuji N. Human leukocyte antigen matching estimations in a hypothetical bank of human embryonic stem cell lines in the Japanese population for use in cell transplantation therapy. Stem Cells 2007;25(4):983-5.
7. Thompson JA, Itskoviz-Eldor J, Shapiro SS, et al. Embryonic stem cell lines derived from human blastocysts. Science 1998;282:1145-7.
8. Henderson JK, Draper JS, Baillie HS, et al. Preimplantation human embryos and embryonic stem cells show comparable expression of stage-specific embryonic antigens. Stem Cells 2002;20:329-37.
9. Nichols J, Zevnik B, Anastassiadis K, et al. Formation of pluripotent stem cells in the mammalian embryo depends on the POU transcription factor Oct.4. Cell 1998;95: 379-91.
10. Silva J, Nichols J, Theunissen TW, et al. Nanog is the gateway to the pluripotent ground state. Cell 2009;138(4): 722-37.
11. Mitsui K, Tokuzawa Y, Itoh H, et al. The homeoprotein Nanog is required for maintenance of pluripotency in mouse epiblast and ES cells. Cell 2003;113:631-42.
12. Belmonte JC, Ellis J, Hochedlinger K, Yamanaka S. Induced pluripotent stem cells and reprogramming: Seeing the science through the hype. Nat Rev Genet [Epub ahead of print], 2009.
13. Yamanaka S. Elite and stochastic models for induced pluripotent stem cell generation. Nature 2009;460(7251): 49-52.
14. Mehra NK, Kaur G, Kaur J, et al. Hematopoietic Stem Cell Transplantation: Strategies for expansion of HLA compatible donor pool. Proceedings of the Ranbaxy Science Foundation 2005;45-52.
15. Dorak MT, Burnett AK. Major histocompatibility complex, t-complex, and leukemia. Cancer Causes Control 1992;3:273-82.
16. Spitzer TR. Haploidentical stem cell transplantation: The always present but overlooked donor. Hematology Am Soc Hematol Educ Program 2005;390-5.
17. Kremens B, Basu O, Peceny R, et al. Allogeneic CD34+ - selected peripheral stem cell transplantation from parental donors in children with non-malignant diseases. Bone Marrow Transplant 2002;29:9-13.
18. Xiao-Jun H, Lan-Ping X, Kai-Yan L, et al. Partially matched related donor transplantation can achieve outcomes comparable with unrelated donor transplantation for patients with hematologic malignancies. Clin Cancer Res 2009;15(14):4777-83.
19. Chiang KY, Van Rhee F, Godder K, et al. Allogeneic bone marrow transplantation from partially mismatched related donors as therapy for primary induction failure acute myeloid leukemia. Bone Marrow Transplant 2001;5:507-10.
20. Godder KT, Metha J, Chiang KY, et al. Partially mismatched related donor bone marrow transplantation as salvage for patients with AML who failed autologous stem cell transplant. Bone Marrow Transplant 2001; 28:1031-6.
21. Hansen JA. Development of registries of HLA -typed volunteer marrow donors. Tissue Antigens 1996;47: 460-3.
22. Confer D, Robinett P. The US National Marrow Donor Program role in unrelated donor hematopoietic cell transplantation. Bone Marrow Transplant 2008;42 Suppl 1:S3-S5.
23. Oudshoorn M, van Leeuwen A, Zanden HGM, van Rood JJ. Bone Marrow donors worldwide: a successful exercise in international cooperation. Bone Marrow Transplantation 1994;14:3-8.
24. Johansen KA, Schneider JF, McCaffree MA, Woods GL. Council on Science and Public Health, American Medical Association. Efforts of the United States' National Marrow Donor Program and Registry to improve utilization and representation of minority donors. Transfus Med 2008; 18(4):250-9.
25. Wiegand T, Raffoux C, Hurley CK, et al. World Marrow Donor Association Quality Assurance Work Group; WMDA Donor Registries Working Group. A special report: Suggested procedures for international unrelated donor search from the donor registries and quality assurance working groups of the World Marrow Donor Association (WMDA). Bone Marrow Transplant 2004; 34(2):97-101.

26. Heemskerk MBA, van Walraven SM, Cornelissen JJ, et al. How to improve the search for an unrelated haematopoietic stem cell donor. Faster is better than more! Bone Marrow Transplant 2005;35:645-652.
27. Barker JN, Krepski TP, DeFor TE, et al. Searching for unrelated donor hematopoietic stem cells: Availability and speed of umbilical cord blood versus bone marrow. Biol Blood Marrow Transplant 2002;8:257-60.
28. van Rood JJ, Oudshoorn M. Eleven million donors in Bone Marrow Donors Worldwide! Time for reassessment? Bone Marrow Transplant 2008;41:1-9.
29. Hurley CK, Fernandez Vina M, Setterholm M. Maximizing optimal hematopoietic stem cell donor selection from registries of unrelated adult volunteers. Tissue Antigens 2003;61:415-24.
30. Tiercy JM, Nicoloso G, Passweg J, et al. The probability of identifying a 10/10 HLA-matched unrelated donor is highly predictable. Bone Marrow Transplant 2007;40:515-22.
31. C. K. Hurley, M. Maiers, S. G. E. Marsh & M. Oudshoorn. Overview of registries, HLA typing and diversity, and search algorithms. Tissue Antigens 2007;69 Suppl. 1(3-5).
32. Muller CR, Ehninger G, Goldmann SF. Gene and haplotype frequencies for the loci HLA-A, HLA-B, and HLA-DR based on over 13 000 German blood donors. Hum Immunol 2003;64:137-51.
33. K Hirv, K Bloch, M Fischer, et al. Prediction of duration and success rate of unrelated hematopoietic stem cell donor searches based on the patient's HLA-DRB1 allele and DRB1-DQB1 haplotype frequencies. Bone Marrow Transplantation 2009;44:433-40.
34. Cano P, Klitz W, Mack SJ, et al. Common and well-documented HLA alleles: Report of the Ad-Hoc committee of the american society for histocompatiblity and immunogenetics. Hum Immunol 2007;68(5):392-417.
35. Nowak J. Role of HLA in hematopoietic SCT. Bone Marrow Transplant. 2008;42 Suppl 2:S71-6.
36. Tiercy JM, Nicoloso G, Passweg J, et al. The probability of identifying a 10/10 HLA allele-matched unrelated donor is highly predictable. Bone Marrow Transplant 2007;40(6):515-22.
37. Spitzer TR. Haploidentical stem cell transplantation: The always present but overlooked donor. Hematology Am Soc Hematol Educ Program 2005;390-5.
38. Andolina M, Maximova N, Rabusin M, et al. Haploidentical bone marrow transplantation in leukemia and genetic diseases. Haematologica 2000;85:37-40.
39. Yoshihara T, Morimoto A, Nakauchi S, et al. Successful transplantation of haploidentical CD34+ selected bone marrow cells for an infantile case of severe combined immunodeficiency with aspergillus pneumonia. Pediatr Hematol Oncol 2002;19:439-43.
40. Aversa F. Hematopoietic stem cell transplantation from full-haplotype mismatched donors. Transfus Apher Sci 2002;27:175-81.
41. Handgretinger R, Klingebiel T, Lang P, et al. Megadose transplantation of highly purified haploidentical stem cells: current results and future prospects. Pediatr Transplant 2007;7 Suppl 3:51-5.
42. Fry TJ, Mackall CL. Interleukin-7: From bench to clinic. Blood 2002;99:3892-904.
43. Min D, Taylor PA, Panoskaltsis-Mortari A, et al. Protection from thymic epithelial cell injury by keratinocyte growth factor: A new approach to improve thymic and peripheral T-cell reconstitution after bone marrow transplantation. Blood 2002;99:4592-600.
44. Kennedy-Nasser AA, Brenner MK. T-cell therapy after hematopoietic stem cell transplantation. Curr Opin Hematol 2007;14:616-24.
45. William YK Hwang, Shin Y Ong. Allogeneic Haematopoietic Stem Cell Transplantation without a Matched Sibling Donor: Current Options and Future Potential. Ann Acad Med Singapore 2009;38:340-5.
46. Goldstein G, Toren A, Nagler A. Transplantation and other uses of human umbilical cord blood and stem cells. Curr Pharm Des 2007;13(13):1363-73.
47. Eapen M, Rubinstein P, Zhang MJ, et al. Outcomes of transplantation of unrelated donor umbilical cord blood and bone marrow in children with acute leukaemia: A comparison study. Lancet 2007;369:1947-54.
48. Querol S, Mufti GJ, Marsh SG, et al. Cord blood stem cells for hematopoietic stem cell transplantation in the UK: How big should the bank be? Haematologica 2009;94(4):536-41.
49. Novelo-Garza B, Limon-Flores A, Guerra-Marquez A, et al. Establishing a cord blood banking and transplantation program in Mexico: A single institution experience. Transfusion 2008;48:228-36.
50. Hurley CK, Wade JA, Oudshoorn M, et al. Histocompatibility testing guidelines for hematopoietic stem cell transplantation using volunteer donors: Report from The World Marrow Donor Association. Quality Assurance and Donor Registries Working Groups of the World Marrow Donor Association. Bone Marrow Transplant 1999;24:119-21.
51. Cleaver SA, Warren P, Kern M, et al. Donor work-up and transport of bone marrow—recommendations and requirements for a standardized practice throughout the world from the Donor Registries and Quality Assurance Working Groups of the World Marrow Donor Association (WMDA). Bone Marrow Transplant 1997;20:621-9.
52. Hurley CK, Setterholm M, Lau M, et al. Hematopoietic stem cell donor registry strategies for assigning search determinants and matching relationships. Bone Marrow Transplant 2004;33(4):443-50.
53. Rosenmayr A, Hartwell L, Egeland T. Ethics Working Group of the World Marrow Donor Association. Informed consent—suggested procedures for informed consent for unrelated haematopoietic stem cell donors at various

stages of recruitment, donor evaluation, and donor workup. Bone Marrow Transplant 2003;31(7):539-45.
54. Bakken R, van Walraven AM, Egeland T. Ethics Working Group of the World Marrow Donor Association. Donor commitment and patient needs. Bone Marrow Transplant 2004;33(2):225-30.
55. Bray RA, Hurley CK, Kamani NR, et al. National marrow donor program HLA matching guidelines for unrelated adult donor hematopoietic cell transplants. Biol Blood Marrow Transplant 2008;14(9 Suppl):45-53.
56. Spellman S, Setterholm M, Maiers M, et al. Advances in the selection of HLA-compatible donors: Refinements in HLA typing and matching over the first 20 years of the National Marrow Donor Program Registry. Biol Blood Marrow Transplant 2008;14(9 Suppl):37-44.
57. Copelan EA. Haematopoietic stem-cell transplantation. N Engl J Med 2006;354:1813-26.
58. Ljungman P, Urbano-Ispizua A, Cavazzana-Calvo M, et al. European Group for Blood and Marrow. Allogeneic and autologous transplantation for haematological diseases, solid tumours and immune disorders: Definitions and current practice in Europe. Bone Marrow Transplant 2006;37:439-49.
59. Gratwohl A, Baldomero H, Horisberger B, et al. Accreditation committee of the European group for blood and marrow transplantation (EBMT). Current trends in haematopoietic stem cell transplantation in Europe. Blood 2002;100:2374-86.
60. A Gratwohl, H Baldomero, K Frauendorfer and D Niederwieser, for the Joint Accreditation Committee of the International Society for Cellular Therapy ISCT and the European Group for Blood and Marrow Transplantation EBMT (JACIE)Why are there regional differences in stem cell transplantation activity? An EBMT analysis. Bone Marrow Transplantation 2008;42:S7-S10.
61. Kodera Y. The Japan Marrow Donor Program, the Japan Cord Blood Bank Network and the Asia Blood and Marrow Transplant Registry. Bone Marrow Transplant 2008;42 Suppl 1:S6.
62. Wu T, Lu DP. Blood and marrow transplantation in the People's Republic of China. Bone Marrow Transplant 2008;42 Suppl 1:S73-S75.
63. Hong JL. A brief introduction of the Chinese Marrow Donor Program. Hong Kong Med J 2009;3 Suppl 3:45-7.
64. Lu DP. Blood and marrow transplantation in mainland China. Hong Kong Med J 2009;3 Suppl 3:9-12.
65. Chen PM, Hsiao LT, Tang JL, et al. Haematopoietic stem cell transplantation in Taiwan: Past, present, and future. Hong Kong Med J 2009;3 Suppl 3:13-6.
66. Yang KL, Chang CY, Lin S, et al. Unrelated haematopoietic stem cell transplantation in Taiwan and beyond. Hong Kong Med J 2009;3 Suppl 3):48-51.
67. Lee JW, Kim CC. The activity of hematopoietic stem cell transplantation in Korea. Bone Marrow Transplant 2008;42 Suppl 1:S92-S95.
68. J Seo, E Choi, H Im, B Kim. Current status of the Korea marrow donor program (KMDP), and its international cooperative activities. Hematologica 2008;93(s1):138 Abs 0339.
69. Chandy M, Srivastava A, Dennison D, et al. Allogeneic bone marrow transplantation in the developing world: Experience from a center in India. Bone Marrow Transplant 2001;27:785-90.
70. Saikia TK, Parikh PM, Tawde S, et al. Allogeneic blood stem cell transplantation in chronic myeloid leukaemia-chronic phase following conditioning with busulphan and cyclophosphamide: a follow up report. Natl Med J India 2004;17(2):71-3.
71. Kumar L, Raju GM, Ganessan K, et al. High dose chemotherapy followed by autologous haemopoietic stem cell transplant in multiple myeloma. Natl Med J India 2003;16(1):16-21.
72. Kumar R, Prem S, Mahapatra M, et al. Fludarabine, cyclophosphamide and horse antithymocyte globulin conditioning regimen for allogeneic peripheral blood stem cell transplantation performed in non-HEPA filter rooms for multiply transfused patients with severe aplastic anemia. Bone Marrow Transplant 2006;37(8):745-9.
73. Chandy M. Childhood acute lymphoblastic leukaemia in India: an approach to management in a three-tier society. Med Paediatr Oncolo 1995;25:197-203.
74. Weatherall DJ, Clegg JB. Inherited haemoglobin disorders: an increasing global health problem. Bull World Health Organ 2001;79:704-12.
75. M Chandy. Stem cell transplantation in India. Bone Marrow Transplantation 2008;42:S81-S84.
76. Mehra N.K. Rajalingam R, Kanga U, et al. Genetic diversity of HLA In the population of India, Sri Lanka, and Iran. In: Genetic Diversity of HLA: Functional and Medical Implications, Vol.1. eds. Dominique Charron, EDK Publishers, Paris 1996;314-20.
77. Mehra NK, Jaini R, Rajalingam R, et al. Molecular diversity of HLA-*02 in Asian Indians Predominance of A*0211. Tissue Antigens 2001;57:502-7.
78. Jaini R, Naruse T, Kanga U, et al. Molecular diversity of HLA-A*19 group of alleles in North Indians: possible oriental influence. Tissue Antigens 2002;59:487-91.
79. Rozemuller EH, Mehra NK, van der Zwan A-W, et al. A*3306, a novel variant in the Indian population. Tissue Antigens 2002;59:421-3.
80. Mehra NK, Kanga U. Molecular diversity of the HLA-B27 gene and its association with disease. Modern Rheumatol 2002;11:275-85.
81. Rani R, Mukherjee R, Stastny P. Diversity of HLA-DR2 in North Indians: the changed scenario after the discovery of DRB1*1506. Tissue Antigens 1998;52:147-52.
82. Mehra NK, Bouwens AGM, Naipal A, et al. Asian Indian HLA-DR2, DR4 and DR5 related DR-DQ genotypes analysed by PCR based non-radioactive oligonucleotide

typing: unique haplotypes and a novel DR4 subtype. Hum Immunol 1994;39:202-10.
83. Mehra NK, Rajalingam R, Mitra DK, et al. Variants of HLA-DR2/DR51 group haplotyes and susceptibility to tuberculoid leprosy and pulmonary tuberculosis in Asian Indians. Internat. J. Leprosy 1995;63:241-8.
84. Mehra NK, Rajalingam R, Giphart MJ. Generation of DR51 associated DQA1, DQB1 haplotypes in Asian Indians. Tissue Antigens 1996;47:85-9.
85. Mehra NK, Kaur G, Kanga U, Tandon N. Immunogenetics of autoimmune diseases in Asian Indians. Ann. N.Y. Acad. Sciences 2002;958:333-6.
86. Jaini R, Kaur G, Mehra NK. Heterogeneity of HLA-DR*04 and its associated haplotypes in the North Indian population. Hum Immunol 2002;63:24-9.
87. Charron DJ. HLA matching in unrelated donor marrow transplantation. Curr Opinion in Hematology 1996;3:416-22.

Chapter 27

Allorecognition

Frans HJ Claas

INTRODUCTION

The HLA antigens are the most important transplantation antigens, which is the reason why the best transplant results are obtained with HLA identical donors. This holds true both for solid organ transplantation and hematopoietic stem cell transplantation. In solid organ transplantation HLA mismatches are associated with a higher incidence of graft rejection and graft loss. In bone marrow transplantation or hematopoietic stem cell transplantation the main complication associated with HLA mismatches is graft-versus-host disease. Although efforts are made to select a fully HLA matched donor for every recipient, this is not feasible due to the enormous polymorphism of the HLA system.

We have to accept that many patients will be transplanted with an HLA mismatched donor. Recent data suggest that not every HLA mismatch leads to the same detrimental alloimmune response. Based on population data it became clear that certain HLA mismatches should be avoided as they are associated with a very poor graft survival whereas other HLA mismatches have hardly any impact on graft survival or function.[1] The challenge is to find an optimal HLA mismatched donor for an individual patient, for whom no HLA identical donor is available. In order to be able to do so it is essential that one understands the alloimmune response leading to the different clinical complications. Different regulatory and effector cells are involved in the alloimmune response leading to graft rejection and/or graft-versus-host disease. In this chapter we will discuss the different aspects of the alloimmune response and the important cells involved (Fig. 27.1).

Allorecognition by B Lymphocytes

B lymphocytes are responsible for the humoral alloimmune response. Donor specific HLA antibodies have found to be associated with rejection of bone marrow grafts and hyperacute, acute and chronic rejection of solid organ allografts. Extensive analyses of the humoral alloimmune response after transplantation, blood transfusion or pregnancy show that only a proportion of the individuals will make antibodies to a particular HLA mismatch. The challenge is to predict whether an individual patient will indeed make antibodies against a foreign HLA antigen or whether the foreign HLA antigen will not be immunogenic for the patients B cell allorepertoire. The introduction of molecular HLA typing techniques has made it possible to determine the exact amino acid sequence of every HLA molecule and this knowledge is certainly helpful if one would like to determine the immunogenicity of a foreign HLA molecule for an individual patient. If one compares the different HLA alleles it becomes clear that every HLA molecule has many polymorphic sites; some of them are specific for a certain HLA allele but others are shared amongst HLA alleles (Fig. 27.2). This knowledge enables to analyze whether a certain HLA is likely to induce an antibody response or not. Very important in such an analysis is the assumption that a patient will make only antibodies against epitopes on foreign HLA molecules which are not present on the patients own HLA antigens. Therefore in order to determine the immunogenicity of a HLA mismatch one should always consider the immunogenicity of a HLA mismatch in the context of the self-HLA epitopes of the antibody producer. This is

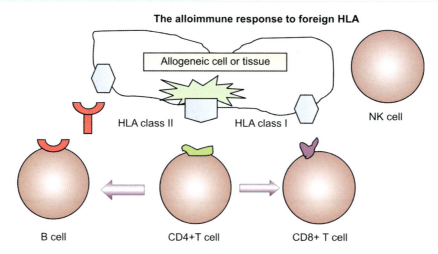

Fig. 27.1: The alloimmune response is very complicated and includes different types of immune cells. Foreign HLA class I molecules are recognized by HLA antibodies and CD8 positive T cells, foreign HLA class II molecules are recognized by antibodies and CD4 positive T cells whereas the lack of self-HLA class I may lead to the induction of NK reactivity

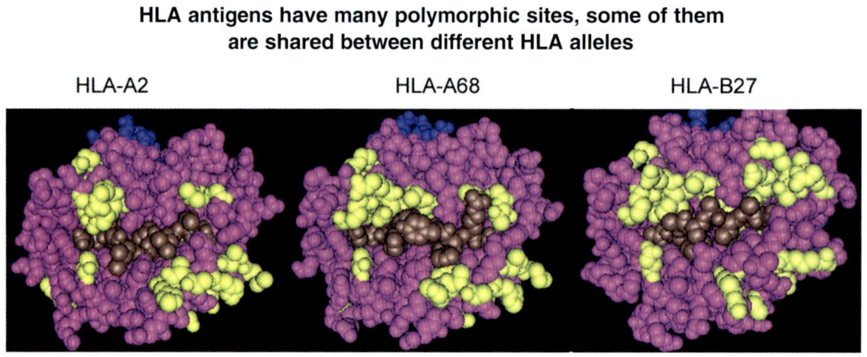

Fig. 27.2: HLA antigens have many polymorphic sites (indicated by the yellow amino acids). Some of these sites are specific for individual HLA antigens while others are shared between different HLA alleles

the principal of a computer algorithm, HLAMatchmaker, developed by Rene Duquesnoy.[2] In this algorithm the different HLA antigens are defined by a string of potential epitopes on antibody acceptable sites of the HLA molecules. If one would like to know the immunogenicity of a HLA mismatch, all epitopes of the mismatched HLA antigen should be compared with the epitopes present on the different self-HLA molecules of a patient. Several studies have shown that the number of foreign epitopes present on a HLA mismatch indeed predicts the chance that a patient will form antibodies against that particular mismatch.[3,4] Both after graft rejection and also after pregnancy an almost linear association was found between the number of epitopes mismatched on the foreign HLA molecule and the chance that a patient will form antibodies. In order to select the optimal HLA mismatch for the humoral alloimmune response one should select a foreign HLA antigen with as few as possible foreign epitopes. If there are no foreign epitopes present on a mismatch HLA molecule the chance is very low that the patient will develop a humoral immune response.

Allorecognition by CD8 Positive Cells

CD8 positive T cells are effector or cytotoxic T cells, which will recognize foreign HLA class I antigens. A HLA class I antigen can be foreign, if it is an allogeneic HLA antigen but, in case donor and recipient have the same HLA antigen class I antigen, a shared HLA antigen may also become foreign if this HLA class I molecule contains peptides derived from polymorphic proteins present in the donor but not in the recipient, the so called minor transplantation antigens (Fig. 27.3). So even in a fully HLA matched situation CD8 positive cells may become

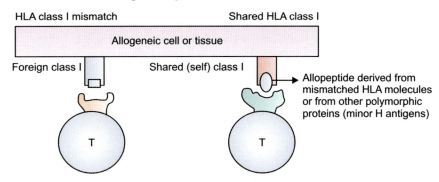

Fig. 27.3: CD8 positive T cells recognize foreign HLA class I molecules. The foreign HLA class I molecule may either be an allogeneic HLA molecule or a self-HLA molecule containing an allogeneic peptide

activated. However, the strongest alloimmune response by CD8 positive cells is directed against allogeneic HLA class I mismatches. In order to analyze whether the HLAMatchmaker program is also fruitful for the prediction of the alloimmune response of CD8 positive T cells, it was checked whether there was a direct association between the number of foreign epitopes on an allogeneic HLA molecule and the cytotoxic T cell response. However, no direct relationship was found. This is not surprising as HLAMatchmaker is mainly focusing on the antibody accessible sites of the HLA class I molecules whereas T cell recognition involves recognition of amino acids in and around the groove of the HLA class I molecules. Very recent analyses suggest that if one looks at the amino acid substitutions in and around the groove of the mismatched HLA molecule, a relationship exists between the number of amino acid differences and the chance that the patient makes a strong CTL response. However, the association is quite different than that observed with respect to the antibody response. When the immune system of the patient is confronted with a mismatched HLA antigen which is very different from the patient's own HLA antigens (many amino acid substitutions), often no cytotoxic T cell response is induced while HLA mismatches with only one amino acid substitution may already lead to a strong CTL response.[5] This differential immunogenicity is probably based on T cell education in the thymus where T cells are positively selected when they have a low affinity for self-HLA molecules. T cells with no affinity for self are deleted from the T cell repertoire. In case an allogeneic HLA molecule is very different from self we probably do not have a T cell repertoire for this foreign HLA molecule. In contrast to B cell allorecognition where the immunogenicity of a HLA molecule increases with the number of epitopes mismatches, the immunogenicity of a HLA molecule for a T cell alloimmune response seems to be higher in case of less amino acid differences.[6]

Allorecognition by CD4 Positive T Cells

B cells and CD8 positive T cells are involved in the effector phase of the alloimmune response. They are able to destruct the transplanted organ or cause the graft-versus-host disease. However, activation of both types of effector cells is dependent on triggers by CD4 positive regulatory T cells. CD4 positive T cells react against foreign HLA class II molecules which are mainly expressed on professional antigen presenting cells. We can distinguish two ways of allorecognition by CD4 positive T cells. In case of **direct allorecognition**, CD4 positive T cells recognize the mismatched donor MHC class II molecule directly on the antigen presenting cells of the donor. This type of allorecognition occurs in the first few months after organ transplantation because the transplanted organ contains antigen presenting cells from donor origin. However, later after the transplantation these antigen presenting cells, which are bone marrow derived, are replaced by recipient antigen presenting cells. These recipient antigen presenting cells are able to internalize MHC molecules from the donor and present these as peptides in the presence of the recipient's own HLA class II. Recognition of this complex is called **indirect allorecognition**. This type of allorecognition plays a very important role late after transplantation. Different populations of CD4 positive T cell using indirect allorecognition have been described (Fig. 27.4). Some of the CD4 positive cells may serve as helper cells for the alloimmune response by CD8 positive T cells whereas others provide help to B cells with respect to IgG antibody formation.[7] Recently a third population, called TH17, has

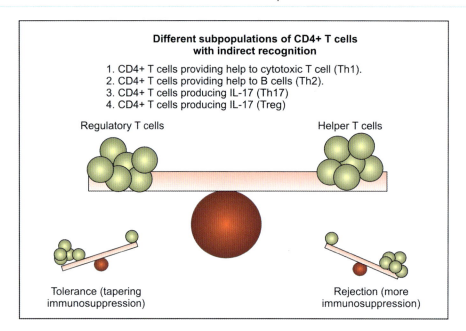

Fig. 27.4: Indirect allorecognition involves different types of CD4 positive T cells, which may up regulate or down regulate the immune response to the graft

been described which is also involved in inflammatory responses.

However, there are also CD4 positive T cells using indirect allorecognition which are involved in downregulation of the alloimmune response. The challenge is now to develop reliable tools to monitor the equilibrium between the different CD4 positive regulatory T cells in order to be able to fine-tune immunosuppression in transplantation recipients.

Allorecognition by NK Cells

Allorecognition of B cells and T cells involves active recognition of a foreign structure on the donor organ. However, allorecognition is still possible even in a situation where there is no recognition of a foreign HLA molecule by B cells and T cells. The cells involved in this type of allorecognition are the NK cells. There is a fundamental difference in allorecognition by NK cells versus T and B cells. Most NK cells do not react on basis of recognition of a foreign HLA molecule but they are triggered by an absence of self-HLA. If certain receptors or NK cells, the so called KIR receptors, are not able to associate with self-HLA molecules, they tend to kill that target cell. Different HLA class I molecules are ligands for KIR receptors on NK cells (Table 27.1). In the normal situation NK cells will be inhibited by the self-HLA molecules of an individual. In case of a bone marrow or kidney transplantation where the target cell, which is

Table 27.1: KIR receptors on NK cells bind epitopes on classical HLA class I molecules

Receptor	Ligand	Epitope
KIR2DL1	HLA-C (e.g. Cw2, 4, 5, 6)	N77/K80
KIR2DL 2, 3	HLA-C (e.g. Cw1, 3, 7, 8)	S77/N80
KIR3DL1	HLA-Bw4	77-80
KIR3DL2	HLA-A3/A11	Unknown

When inhibitory receptors on NK cells do not recognize their ligands, this will lead to activation of the NK cells. The indicated HLA class I alleles are targets for these receptors

fully compatible for and can not be recognized by the T cell and B cell repertoire, lacks a relevant self-HLA molecule, NK cells tend to attack this target cell (Fig. 27.5). This type of reactivity has shown to be relevant for complications after bone marrow transplantation[8] and recent studies suggest also that in very well matched kidney transplants, NK cells may also play a destructive immune response.

CONCLUSIONS ON THE DIFFERENTIAL IMMUNOGENICITY OF AN HLA MISMATCH

It is clear from the previous part that allorecognition is a very complex phenomenon and it is not surprising that it is very difficult to predict the immunogenicity of a particular HLA mismatch. If we consider the T cell and B cell alloimmune response, it is clear that an antigen which

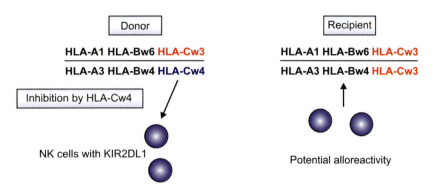

Fig. 27.5: NK cells with receptor KIR2DL1 in the donor are inhibited by the HLA-CW4 antigen present on the cells of the donor. After bone marrow transplantation to a CW4 negative recipient these NK are no longer inhibited by CW4 and will be activated

is very immunogenic with respect to the T cell repertoire can be non-immunogenic for the B cell repertoire and the other way around. It is therefore very important to define the clinical complication which one would like to avoid. For instance, in order to prevent HLA antibody formation late after kidney transplantation, which is associated with chronic rejection, one should select an HLA mismatch with almost no foreign epitopes. In contrast, in order to prevent a cytotoxic T cell response leading to graft-versus-host disease after a HLA mismatched bone marrow transplantation, it might be useful to select a donor with a HLA mismatch with many amino acid substitutions in and around the groove. Therefore, different clinical situations need different algorithms to find the optimal donor. In most of the cases, the different cell types are all involved in the alloimmune response and it is not clear which immune mechanism is dominant in the destructive alloimmune response, which makes it very difficult to select the optimal HLA mismatch. One of the options, one could explore in such a situation is to select donors on basis of the non-inherited maternal HLA antigens. Different studies have shown that confrontation with maternal HLA antigens during pregnancy and/or early in life by breastfeeding, may have an impact on both the alloreactive T and B cell repertoire of a child. Both in organ- and hematopoietic stem cell transplantation, mismatches for the non-inherited maternal HLA antigens have been associated with favorable outcome.

KEY ISSUES

The best transplant results are obtained with HLA matched donors but due to the polymorphism of the HLA system, many patients have to be transplanted with a HLA mismatched donor. However, the immunogenicity of an HLA mismatch is not the same for every individual. Structural comparison of the mismatched HLA antigen with the patient's own HLA antigens is helpful for the definition of the optimal HLA mismatch for a particular patient. The requirement of an optimal mismatch seems to be different for the T cell and B cell repertoire. HLA antibody formation is most likely to occur if the mismatched HLA antigen has many foreign epitopes whereas a T cell response needs a certain degree of similarity between the mismatched HLA antigen and the patients own HLA antigens. Therefore, selection of the optimally mismatched donor may differ dependent on the main effector cell in the clinical situation which one would like to avoid.

REFERENCES

1. Doxiadis II, Smits JM, Schreuder GM, Persijn GG, van Houwelingen HC, van Rood JJ, Claas FH. Association between specific HLA combinations and probability of kidney allograft loss: The taboo concept. Lancet 1996;348: 850-53.
2. Duquesnoy RJ. Clinical usefulness of HLAMatchmaker in HLA epitope matching for organ transplantation. Cur Opin Immunol 2008;20:594.
3. Dankers MK, Witvliet MD, Roelen DL, et al. The number of amino acid triplet differences between patient and donor is predictive for the antibody reactivity against mismatched human leukocyte antigens. Transplantation 2004;77:1236.
4. Goodman RS, Taylor CJ, O'Rourke CM, et al. Utility of HLAMatchmaker and single antigen HLA-antibody detection beads for identification of acceptable mismatches in highly sensitized patients awaiting kidney transplantation. Transplantation 2006;81:1331.

5. Heemskerk MB, Cornelissen JJ, Roelen DL, van Rood JJ, Claas FH, Doxiadis II, Oudshoorn M. Highly diverged MHC class I mismatches are acceptable for haematopoietic stem cell transplantation. Bone Marrow Transplant 2007; 40:193-200.
6. Claas FH, Roelen DL, Mulder A, Doxiadis II, Oudshoorn M, Heemskerk M. Differential immunogenicity of HLA class I alloantigens for the humoral versus the cellular immune response: "towards tailor-made HLA mismatching". Hum Immunol 2006;67(6):424-29.
7. Gökmen MR, Lombardi G, Lechler RI. The importance of the indirect pathway of allorecognition in clinical transplantation Curr Opin Immunol 2008;20(5):568-74
8. Velardi A. Role of KIRs and KIR ligands in hematopoietic transplantation. Curr Opin Immunol. 2008;20(5):581-87.

Chapter 28

The Role of HLA Typing in Hematopoietic Stem Cell Transplantation

Frank T Christiansen

INTRODUCTION

It is now over 40 years since the first successful transplant of hematopoietic stem cells (HSC) in bone marrow was successfully undertaken for the treatment of a case of severe combined immunodeficiency.[1] This pioneering work followed extensive earlier studies in experimental animals where the feasibility of this approach was demonstrated and the importance of matching for genes in the major histocompatibility complex (MHC) was shown—reviewed in.[2] Having shown that sustained engraftment of donor hematopoietic stem cells could be achieved and that they can develop into mature hematopoietic cells, this technique was adapted to treat hematological malignancies by using the allograft to rescue patients following extensive myeloablative therapy.[3] For a review of the early history of the bone marrow transplant see Dupont, et al.[4] Subsequently this life-saving treatment has been applied to an increasing number of conditions including a range of congenital immunodeficiencies, aplastic anemias, hematological malignancies including lymphomas and myeloablative syndromes and a range of inherited disorders including various disorders of red cell function such as thalassemias and hemoglobinopathies and various metabolic disorders including a range of lipid storage diseases. Now more than 20,000 new transplants are reported every year to international transplant registries such as the Center for International Blood and Bone Marrow Transplant Research (i.e. CIBMTR) and the European Group for Blood and Bone Marrow Transplantation (i.e. EGBBMT). In addition, from the initial use of MHC genotypical matched siblings, the source of stem cell donors now includes partially matched related donors, including those with a complete haplotype mismatch, unrelated donors selected based on HLA matching, and cord blood units collected at the time of delivery, whilst more recently donor stem cells have been obtained from peripheral blood following various protocols which mobilize peripheral blood stem cells (PBSC).

The main barriers to successful allogeneic hematopoietic stem cell transplantation (HSCT) are immunological complications due to the immune response to histocompatibility antigens – the process of allorecognition. Because the transfer of bone marrow or mobilized PBSC results in the transfer of immunocompetent cells from the donor, these allogeneic reactions can occur in two directions, namely graft-versus-host disease (GVHD), a potentially fatal reaction, and host-versus-graft (HVG) response which can lead to failure of engraftment or rejection of transiently engrafted stem cells. Much of the progress achieved in HSCT over the years can be attributed to improvements in HLA typing techniques which identify the HLA class I and class II molecules within the human MHC and which has allowed better matching unrelated donors for patients requiring HSCT. This chapter describes the importance of HLA antigens as targets for the alloresponse and their influence on outcome in HSCT, and how information on HLA matching is used for both related and unrelated donor selection for treatment of hematological and other disorders.

SELECTION OF FAMILY DONORS

Prior to the development of extensive panels of HLA-typed unrelated donor, the only suitable donor was an HLA identical sibling. HLA alleles are inherited in a Mendelian fashion with inheritance of one allele from each parent, and the HLA alleles at each of the loci from each parent are inherited *en bloc* as a single haplotype. Recombination between the loci occurs relatively infrequently; occurring approximately 0.8 percent of all meiotic division between HLA-A and –B and a similar frequency between HLA-B and –DRB1. As a result there is a 1 in 4 chance that any one sibling will share the same maternal and paternal haplotypes with each sibling. Unless recombination has occurred, such matched siblings will share identical HLA alleles at all loci, and in addition they will share identitiy at all intervening gene loci between the extremes of the defined haplotypes – usually between HLA-A and –DRB1. They do not necessarily share identity at all other minor histocompatibility antigens encoded on other chromosomes and, on average, will only share 50 percent of all such genes. These so-called minor histocompatibility antigens can also be the target for allorecognition leading to GVH and graft versus leukemia (GVL) responses. Nonetheless HLA identical siblings remain the ideal allogeneic donor and serve as a reference point in any studies examining the impact of matching HLA in mismatched non-identical related donor or unrelated donor transplants.

Identification of HLA Identical Sibling Donor

In family, studies HLA typing is used to determine whether two siblings share the same maternal and paternal HLA haplotypes. This therefore requires identification of the two maternal and two paternal haplotypes. It is not sufficient to simply demonstrate that the two siblings share the same HLA antigen at HLA-A, -B and –DRB1. There are a number of situations where such apparent identity may occur in the absence of sharing both haplotypes;

i. One (or indeed both) parent(s) is homozygous for an HLA antigen inherited by the patient. For example, the parent is homozygous at HLA-A, -B and –DR. In this case, the parent's two haplotypes appear to be identical based on the HLA typing information available but they may have differences at other HLA loci which have not been typed, for example HLA-C, -DQ or –DP. Also, when only low or intermediate level HLA typing has been performed, it is possible high resolution typing would show heterozygosity.

ii. The possibility of unidentified recombination in one of the siblings. If one parent is apparently homogenous at one locus, e.g. HLA-DR, it is possible that recombination may have occurred between the two haplotypes without this being recognized. If typing additional loci e.g. HLA-DQ or -DP is informative, it may be possible to exclude recombination.

iii. Case of alternative parentage (usually paternity) where the two alternative parents share by chance the same HLA antigens at the loci typed. It is possible, however, they are different at other loci not typed.

Given these caveats it is important that the HLA typing undertaken in a family study unequivocally identifies all four haplotypes at least HLA-A, -B and –DRB. Usually this requires typing of as many members of the family as possible, including both parents whenever possible, and all available siblings. In many cases, it is possible to identify all four haplotypes with only intermediate level HLA typing and in such circumstances high resolution typing or typing of additional loci will not be necessary as the donor and recipient will be identical at the allele level at these loci and at all other HLA loci, at least those within the extremes of the identified haplotype. When it is not possible to identify all four haplotypes, then it is necessary to confirm identity between the donor and recipient by high resolution typing and typing the other HLA loci (e.g. HLA-C, -DQB1, -DPB1). Whilst this will not prove the sharing of haplotypes identical by decent, it will increase the likelihood that this is the case, and in any event, confirm identity at all HLA loci. By such criteria such a donor would be as well-matched at the HLA loci as any unrelated donor.

Search for a Related Donor in the Extended Family

In most Western countries, with the small family sizes, only some 30 percent of patients will find a suitable family donor. In such circumstances an alternative is required. With the development of extensive donor registries, a suitable well-matched, unrelated donor can be found for some 70-80 percent of all patients. However, there remains a number of cases where a suitable donor cannot be found. This often occurs in patients from ethnic minority groups or those of mixed ethnic background who have HLA types which are poorly represented in current donor registries. In such circumstances, it is possible to search for a donor in the extended family who shares with the patient one haplotype which is identical by decent and who fortuitously may also be matched with the patient for at least some of the HLA- antigens encoded on the non-shared haplotypes. In general, the haplotype with the uncommon set of alleles is tracked through the family searching for relatives who share the more common antigens present on the other haplotype.

This approach, pioneered by the Seattle group, has been applied more widely resulting in transplants with acceptable graft outcome.[5-7]

Use of One Haplotype Matched (Haploidentical) Family Donors

Although the number of patients transplanted through searches in the extended family has been relatively small and has less application now given the availability of donor registries, in some cases, it still provides the only opportunity to provide a suitable matched donor. This approach should be considered where it seems unlikely that a well-matched unrelated donor will be found in registries. Transplants using partially-matched family donors have been very informative in defining the levels of HLA matching required for successful outcome, and provided some of the first clear evidence for the importance of HLA matching.[8,9] From these studies several points became clear. Firstly, the risk of graft failure and the incidence and severity of acute GVHD increased with increasing mismatches at HLA-A, -B, and –DR.[10-12] Secondly, the direction (or vector) of the HLA mismatching was important – the risk of graft failure correlated with mismatches in the HVG direction, whilst the risk of acute GVHD correlated with mismatches in the GVH direction. Thirdly, the data showed different effects of HLA class I and class II mismatches – class II mismatches (HLA-DR and –DQ) were associated with increased risk of acute GVHD, while class I mismatches, particularly multiple mismatches, were associated with graft failure.[13] A number of studies have shown that the outcome of transplants from related donors with a limited number of HLA mismatches can approach the results obtained with HLA-identical siblings.[14-17] In all these studies, it has been shown that a number of patients, who would otherwise not had a donor, were able to achieve a satisfactory outcome. The data also indicated that when unrelated donors are being used, good HLA matching would be required.

TRANSPLANTATION USING UNRELATED DONORS

Factors Allowing the Development of Unrelated Transplantation

Given that for some two thirds of patients, a suitably matched related donor cannot be identified, in the early 1970s investigators turned to using unrelated donors but with only limited ability to achieve good HLA matching due to limitations of available HLA typing methods. The initial results were at best problematic with failure of engraftment and acute GVHD being major problems limiting its application.[18-20] In 1980, the Seattle group described the successful treatment of a ten-year-old girl with acute lymphoid leukemia (ALL).[21] In this case the donor and recipient were matched for two very common caucasoid HLA haplotypes, and as a consequence, the donor was probably very well-matched. The patient had an uncomplicated course with no evidence of GVHD. This case, and others that followed, clearly showed the feasibility of using unrelated donors providing good HLA matching could be achieved.

Over the past two decades, two major developments have facilitated the widespread application of HSCT using an unrelated donor viz: (i) the development of improved methods of HLA typing resulted in better definition of HLA polymorphism and (ii) the development of international registries of HLA typed volunteer donors. Initially HLA typing was defined by serological methods but with the development of molecular techniques and the specific cloning and subsequent sequencing of HLA genes it is now possible to precisely define each allele at the DNA sequence level. Details of HLA polymorphism and methods for HLA typing are covered elsewhere in this book. Currently HLA allele identity between donor and recipient is defined based on matching within the antigen recognition site (ARS) domains which are responsible for peptide binding and HLA interactions with antigen receptors on T cells and B cells and with receptors on NK cells (KIR) which regulate NK cell activation. For HLA class I genes these ARS domains correspond to exons 2 and 3 and for class II genes exon. Generally it is thought that differences in the ARS are responsible for allorecognition and the generation of alloimmune responses. More recently, additional polymorphisms have been identified in the other regions of the HLA genes which include the additional extracellular Ig-like domain, transmembrane and intracytoplasmic regions of the molecules. Little is known of the functional relevance of these polymorphisms and to date there have been no studies reported on their relevance in HSC transplantation.

The HLA system is extremely polymorphic and despite some alleles being relatively common, the presence of linkage disequilibrium between HLA alleles at different loci and the presence of a relatively limited number of founder or conserved ancestral haplotypes,[22] there is extensive diversity of HLA phenotypes present in the human population.[23,24] The ability to find a well-matched donor therefore depends upon the availability of large international panels of volunteer donors who have been HLA typed and their development over the last two decades have facilitated unrelated donor HSCT. Following the initial pioneering work of the Anthony Nolan appeal in establishing the first volunteer donor panel, other registries were established including the establishment of the National Marrow Donor Program in the United States in 1986 and the establishment of the Australian Bone Marrow Registry in 1990. Bone Marrow Donors Worldwide (BMDW), sponsored by the Europdonor Foundation in Leiden, The Netherlands, lists the HLA typings reported by most of the national registries and is available through the internet (www.bmdw.org).[25] Currently over 12 million donors, including umbilical cord blood (CB) units, are listed by BMDW which has been of enormous value in facilitating international donor searches and planning therapeutic strategies for individual patients.

Role of HLA Matching in Unrelated HSCT

With the widespread use of unrelated donors numerous studies have examined the effects of HLA matching on various outcomes following transplantation. Over the years, these studies have examined HLA matching defined at various HLA loci or combinations of loci and at different degrees of HLA resolution which has been largely influenced by the available technology. In addition, a wide range of outcome parameters have been measured including graft rejection usually defined in terms of failure to engraft, acute GVHD variously graded according to clinical scoring parameters and with their varying cut-offs for severity, chronic GVHD, incidence of transplant related mortality (TRM), overall survival (OS), disease free survival, and relapse. The effects of HLA matching have been examined in many ways. Often only a mismatched donor is available and under these circumstances, selection of the preferred donor will require knowledge of which mismatches are preferable. The impact on outcome of mismatches at individual HLA loci or the qualitative effects of increasing numbers of HLA-mismatches have been studied. Whether certain mismatches at a particular locus or whether certain donor-recipient mismatch combinations are less likely to invoke an alloresponse – so-called "permissible" mismatches, has been examined. The effects of mismatches of particular combinations of alleles and more recently the matching effects of MHC haplotypes rather than individual HLA loci, have also been examined. With the recognition of other polymorphic genes within the MHC, including a number which are important in the immune response, the possibility that mismatches at these loci are important has also more recently been reviewed. In the subsequent sections each of these will be considered. Only more recent studies utilizing high resolution molecular techniques have been considered. The extensive literature on HLA matching and its impact on graft failure, GVHD and mortality up until 2001 has been excellently described in an extensive review by Petersdorf et al, 2002.[26] The reader is referred to this review for details of the early literature. More recent reviews have been provided by Bray et al 2008[27] and Petersdorf et al, 2008.[28]

Effect of Mismatches at Individual HLA Loci

It has been well recognized for some time that the ideal HSC donor should be matched at all HLA loci especially HLA-A, -B, -C, -DRB1, and –DQB1 (i.e. so-called 10/10 match) using molecular techniques. A number of studies have shown that matching at all 5 loci (the impact of HLA-DP will be considered separately) lowers the risk of acute GVHD and improves overall survival.[29-34]

In many cases, a 10/10 fully matched donor cannot be identified but a number of donors mismatched for a single allele at a single locus are available. Thus knowledge of the risks associated with mismatches at each locus would assist in donor selection. To obtain such data requires studies of large patient numbers and most studies have not had the power to address this question adequately. Four recent studies of large patient cohorts have provided some important data addressing this key question.[31,35-37] Three are large multicenter studies and the other a large single center study. All have used molecular, high resolution typing usually at the four digit allele level, and all have studied patient cohorts whose donors were selected based on initial low level (or at best intermediate level) class I typing but at least intermediate level class II typing. All, with the exception of the Japanese study, included only leukemia patients. All studies reported the effects of mismatching on survival or mortality whilst only two reported the results on acute GVHD, rejection and disease relapse.

The major findings of these studies are summarized in Table 28.1 which shows for each HLA locus the hazard or odds ratio (HR or OR) and associated P value for a mismatch at that locus. In terms of patient survival, which is clinically the most important outcome parameter to measure, several points are evident. Overall a detrimental effect of mismatches at HLA-A, -B, and –C was observed,

Table 28.1: Effects of single locus HLA mismatches on outcome in unrelated HSCT- shown are the HLA loci, hazard ratio/odds ratio and p values for those loci showing a significant association

Centre	n	Diseases	Ethnic group	Survival/Mortality Locus–HR/OR	P	Acute GVHD Locus–HR/OR	P
NMDP[35]	3857	ALL AML	Cauc	A - 1.50 B - 1.25 C[#] - 1.22 DRB1 - 1.42	<0.001 .09 .004 .003	A - 1.62 B - 1.63 C[#] - 1.60 DRB1 - 1.20	.007 .002 <.001 ns
FHCRC[31]	948	Leukemia MDS	Cauc	(A - 1.64)* (B - 2.55)* C - 3.18* (DRB1 - 3.21)* (DQB1 - 1.81)*		NR	
IHWC[36]	4796	CML AML ALL MDS	Jap/Cauc	A - 1.37$ B - 1.98$ C - 1.65$ DRB1 - 1.32$ DQB1 - 1.17$	.02 .0001 .0001 ns ns	NR	
JMDP[37]	1790	AML ALL CML	Jap	A - 1.36 B - 1.40 C - 1.17 DRB1 - 0.92 DQB1 - 1.28 DPB1 - 1.06	<.001 .002 .067 ns ns ns	A - 1.22 B - 1.43 C - 1.29 DRB1 - 1.15 DQB1 - 1.02 DPB1 - 1.39	.03 .003 .006 ns ns <.001

NMDP = National Marrow Donor Program, USA
FHCRC = Fred Hutchinson Cancer Research Centre, USA
IHWC = International Histocompatibility Workshop Conference
JMDP = Japan Marrow Donor Program
HR = Hazard ratio
OR = Odds ratio
NR = Not reported
[#]Broad antigen mismatch only
*p values not given, brackets indicate non significant
$Low risk patient data shown
&especially ALL

though the effects did vary between the studies. For example, in all three studies in Caucasians, mismatches at HLA-C (specifically mismatches at the serological level rather than the four digit allele level) had a profound effect but this was not observed in the Japanese cohort. A strong effect of HLA-C mismatches on survival has also been observed in an additional single center study using a non-myeloablative conditioning protocol.[38] The effects of mismatches at HLA-A was evident in both racial groups whereas HLA-B had a somewhat variable effect though was generally associated with poorer outcome. Interestingly a separate analysis of a National Marrow Donor Program (NMDP) cohort by Wade et al showed mismatches at HLA-A or –B within serological cross-reactive groups (CREG) were as detrimental on acute GVHD and survival as those outside these CREGS.[39] The effect of HLA-class II mismatches was also variable. Whilst the NMDP study showed a strong effect on survival, a significant effect could not be found in the other caucasoid studies, though in all cases the hazards ratios (HR) were all greater than 1.0. No effect of class II mismatch was evident in the Japanese study. It does seem, in caucasoids at least, that HLA-DQB1 mismatches carry the lowest risk. However, in the NMDP study, a mismatch at HLA-DQB1, when present in addition to mismatches at other loci, was associated with a worse outcome. It is perhaps important to note that all cohorts included only small numbers of transplants in which the donor was mismatched only at HLA-DQB1, especially at the broad serological level. Hence, it may be premature to make definitive statements about the importance of HLA-DQB1 matching. In terms of the likelihood of acute

GVHD, in the two studies in which this parameter was reported, in both Caucasoids and Japanese, mismatches at HLA-A, -B, and -C were associated with increased risk, whereas in both studies mismatches at HLA -DRB1 or – DQB1 were not associated with acute GVHD. Interestingly in those studies where the data was reported, the effects of HLA mismatching on outcome measures were most evident in those patients considered clinically at low risk whereas in high-risk patients, the increase in overall mortality may obscure the impact of HLA matching.

Effect of the Total Number of HLA Mismatches

The early studies of outcome in one haplotype mismatched (i.e. haploidentical) related donor transplants first showed the cumulative effects of multiple HLA mismatches on graft outcome (see section 2.2). This observation has now been confirmed in matched unrelated donor studies.[34,35,40] In the NMDP study reported by Lee, increasing the number of HLA mismatches was associated with clinically important and statistically worse outcomes, particularly overall survival (Table 28.2). Each additional HLA mismatch was associated with absolute unadjusted survival differences of 9 to 10 percent and the differences in survival for 7/8 vs 8/8 and for 6/8 vs 7/8 were significant (both $p < 0.001$). The results of a multivariable model showed the relative risk for a single HLA mismatch was 1.25 ($p < 0.001$), and 1.65 ($p < 0.001$) for two HLA mismatch. These effects were shown to be independent of other patient characteristics known to influence outcome such as patient age, race, diagnosis, CMV status, and disease status. Whilst the impact of disease risk state on survival was greater than HLA mismatch, the impact of HLA mismatch on survival was evident in all disease risk categories and was greatest in those with early disease. It was also evident that multiple class I mismatches and class I plus class II mismatches were associated with poorer outcome than single mismatches.

Similar findings were reported by Loiseau et al in a study of French patients.[34] They reported that increasing numbers of mismatches at HLA-A, -B, -C, -DRB1, or DQB1 were associated with an increased risk of acute GVHD and overall survival. In univariate analysis the cumulative survival at three years was 45 percent for donor recipient pairs with zero mismatches compared to 31 percent for pairs with one mismatch ($p = 0.03$) and 23 percent for pairs with >1 mismatch ($p = 0.002$).

Importance of HLA-DP Mismatches

Historically matching HLA-DP has lagged behind matching for other HLA-loci. This has been largely due to the previous lack of adequate typing methods and it is only with the development of molecular typing for this locus that the influence of HLA-DP matching has been studied. HLA-DP shares structural similarity with the other class II molecules. It can present peptides, is highly polymorphic and is expressed on antigen presenting cells so it is likely that it will serve as a histocompatibility antigen. The strong linkage disequilibrium associated between HLA-DRB1 and –DQB1 is not evident for HLA-DP and therefore many transplant donor-recipient pairs matched on the basis of HLA-DRB1 will not be matched at HLA-DP. Indeed in a study of 423 donor-recipient pairs transplanted through the Anthony Nolan Trust, only 17 percent were HLA-DPB1 identical whilst 51 percent had one mismatch and 33 percent two mismatches. Even amongst the pairs who were completely matched at the other five HLA loci (-A, -B, -C, -DRB1, -DQB1) only 29 percent were completely matched at HLA-DPB1.[41] Therefore in historical transplants, HLA-DP mismatching will be very common and could be contributing to allorecognition and the clinical outcome of transplantation.

Table 28.2: Effect of increasing HLA mismatching on survival					
Degree of match	No	Relative risk	P	Survival [#] 1 yr[¥]	5 yr
Fully Matched (8/8)[φ]	1840	1.00		52%	37%
Single Match (7/8/)	985	1.26	<0.001	43%	29%
Double Mismatch (6/8)	633	1.66	<0.001	33%	22%
Triple Mismatch (5/8)	275	1.64	<0.001	NR	NR
Quadruple Mismatch (4/8)	91	2.05	<0.001	NR	NR

Modified from Lee et al 2007[35]
φ   Matched at HLA-A, -B, -C, -DRB1
\#   Unadjusted survival outcome
¥   7/8 vs 8/8 RR 1.25 p <0.001: 6/8 vs 7/8 RR 1.31 p <0.001

A number of studies have addressed the role of HLA-DP matching in HSCT.[35,41-44] The first suggestion that HLA-DP matching may be important was provided by Varney, et al[42] who showed a significant improvement in patient survival in HLA-DP matched compared to mismatched cases. Even when mismatches at the other HLA loci were excluded, an increased frequency of severe acute GVHD was noted. Similarly a study by Loiseau showed incompatibility at both HLA-DPB1 loci was associated with an increased risk of severe acute GVHD and a poorer survival.[43] In the large NMDP study previously described, although an association of HLA-DPB1 mismatching with acute GVHD and a trend towards a decreased risk of relapse were observed, there was no effect on survival.[35]

Two recent studies in large independent cohorts both provide similar findings and give insights into the seemingly unique contribution of HLA-DP to disease relapse.[41,44] Shaw et al undertook an analysis of 5929 patients who received a myeloablative conditioning regimen and either T replete or T-depleted marrow for a range of hematological disorders studied as part of the International Histocompatibility Working Group (IHWG).[44] After adjusting for the effects of other factors known to influence outcome including matching at other HLA loci, they showed that compared to the matched group, HLA-DPB1 mismatching was associated with an increased risk of severe acute GVHD (HR 1.22, p = 0.005) and reduced risk of relapse (HR 0.78, p = 0.002) and in both instances this effect was evident for those with one or two HLA-DPB1 mismatches. However, they were unable to show an overall effect on survival. These results were essentially similar to those found by Shaw et al in a smaller cohort of T-cell depleted donor marrow from the Anthony Nolan Trust.[41] Taken together these results suggest HLA-DPB1 matching should be considered in donor selection, particularly when selecting from a number of 10/10 matched donors, though other factors described below should also be taken into account.

Identification of Permissible Epitope Mismatches

The studies described in the preceding sections suggest that not all HLA mismatches at all HLA loci are equally immunogenic. Differences in amino acid polymorphisms at specific sites within the HLA molecule, particularly those involved in T-cell receptor recognition, may identify particularly harmful mismatches at a particular locus by virtue of their impact on T-cell responses and T-cell effects on graft rejection, GVHD or graft-versus leukemia (GVL). Differences in *in vitro* allorecognition of class I molecules by T-cells due to differences in amino acids at specific sites have already been described. Using a series of T-cell clones recognizing a HLA-B8 restricted CMV a viral peptide, McDonald et al showed such clones from HLA-B8 positive individuals were also capable of specific allorecognition of HLA-B*4402 alloantigens. However, these clones only poorly recognized HLA-B*4403.[45] The loss of allorecognition was shown to be due to the substitution of a Leu amino acid HLA-B*4403 for an Asp at position 156 in HLA-B*4402 and the structural basis for these differences in interaction of the T-cell receptor has been described. In this context, a mismatch for the amino acid Leu at position 156 could be considered a permissible epitope mismatch for such HLA-B8 individuals. A number of studies have now been undertaken examining the impact of amino acid differences at specific positions on HLA molecules between donor and recipient on transplant outcome in an attempt to define "permissible" and "non-permissible" epitope mismatches.

Permissible HLA-DP Mismatches

The existence of permissible mismatches at HLA-DP has now been demonstrated. Using the ability of CD4 positive T-cell clones isolated from a patient who rejected a HSCT allograft from a donor only mismatched at HLA-DPB*0901,[46] to lyse a series of allogeneic HLA-DP mismatched targets, Zino et al observed a series of T-cell reactivity patterns. They suggested these patterns could be explained by the expression of an epitope shared by a defined subset of HLA-DPB1 alleles that determined these HLA-DP specific alloresponses.[47] Three immunogenic groups of alleles were proposed-immunogenic group 1 alleles; intermediate group 2 alleles and; poorly immunogenic group 3 alleles which lacked this specific T-cell epitope. The structural basis for these groupings was determined by the various combinations of amino acids present on the six hypervariable regions of the HLA DPβ chain. On this basis each of the common HLA-DP alleles was assigned to one of these three groups. Based on these groupings a matching algorithm was developed which would allow prediction of HLA-DP alloreactivity in a GVH or host, versus donor (HVD) direction; combinations of donor-recipient matching for these –DP immunogenic groups would be either "permissive" or "non-permissive".

In an initial retrospective analysis of 118 unrelated grafts who were completely matched at all other HLA loci, Zino et al showed that those cases whose donor had non-permissive mismatches at HLA-DP in the GVH direction had a significantly higher probability of developing acute GVHD and transplant related mortality but not of relapse. A non-significant trend for increased survival was also observed.[48] In a second study of a small cohort of thalassemia patients, this group also showed that those transplants with non-permissive mismatches in the HVG direction had a statistically significant increased risk of graft rejection and reduced thalassemia free survival.[49]

More recently the same group has modified their original algorithm by incorporating additional functional data to now include four T-cell epitope groups of HLA-DP molecules and thus a reclassification of the permissive and non-permissive grouping of HLA-DP mismatches.[50] They have evaluated the effect of this new algorithm in a cohort of 621 adult oncohematologic patients receiving myeloablative or reduced conditioning regimens. They showed that, in line with other studies (see section 3.5), there was no effect of HLA-DP mismatching on survival without taking into account their immunogenicity. However, when the patients with a HLA-DP mismatched transplant were classified as receiving an HLA non-permissive or permissive HLA-DP mismatch, those with permissive mismatches had a significantly greater two years survival (55% vs 33%, p = 0.005) which was due to a reduced risk of non relapse mortality. Importantly the effect of non-permissive mismatches on overall mortality was similar in the 10/10 and 9/10 mismatch pairs and in both those with early and advanced disease.[50] Using an approach analyzing the effects of mismatches at each of six hypervariable regions within exon 2 of the HLA-DPB1 molecule, Shaw showed that one of these regions, hypervariable region D (amino acids 65-69) had significant impact on outcome.[51] Those with no epitope mismatch had a significantly better survival when compared to those with either one of two mismatches (51% versus 46% respectively, P = 0.013). Of the two polymorphic amino acid positions within this epitope, only a mismatch at position 65 influenced overall survival (49% in compatible versus 35% in incompatible, P = 0.039). If the findings of these studies can be confirmed in other retrospective studies and it should be relatively easy to undertake these studies on some of the already existing large cohorts, then this algorithm could be used in donor selection, certainly in distinguishing between similarly 10/10 or 9/10 matched donors.

Permissible Mismatches at Other HLA Loci

The first systematic attempt to identify the impact on transplant outcome of different amino acid substitutions in HLA molecules was undertaken by Ferrara et al.[52] In a series of 100 HSC transplants completely matched for HLA-DR and -DQ, 40 were completely matched for HLA-A, -B, and -C and 60 had one or more mismatches at class I. For each class I mismatch the positions of amino acid discrepancies between the donor and recipient were identified. The impact of such differences at each amino acid site on transplant outcome parameters was then determined. Numerous polymorphic positions were identified. Disparity at position 116 was shown to correlate with an increased risk of transplant related mortality (HR2.36, p = 0.01) and acute GVHD (HR2.47, p = 0.03). When the mismatch pairs were compared to all other pairs, the actuarial risk estimate for overall three years survival was 62 percent for those without the disparity compared to 36 percent for those with the disparity (p = 0.004). These data suggested that donor-recipient amino acid mismatches at position 116 may be particularly detrimental to transplant outcome and should therefore be avoided. Interestingly amino acid 116 is on the floor of the peptide binding groove and would therefore influence peptide binding but not make direct contact with the T cell receptor. Within the scope of this study, discrepancies at other positions, at least those ten or so for which there was sufficient statistical power to detect an effect, may be less immunogenic and donors with such mismatches could preferentially be selected from amongst potential single class I mismatched donors.

These initial findings have now been extended by Kawase et al.[53] In a series of elegant analyses of 5210 Japanese Marrow Donor Program transplants, they systematically identified all specific donor-recipient allele mismatch combinations at each HLA locus including HLA-DRB1 and –DQB1 and, for those which occurred more than ten times, the effects of each of these allele mismatch combinations on outcome was compared to the matched group. Amongst all combinations tested, 16 "non-permissive" mismatch combinations were identified. Those pairs who had one or two or more non-permissive mismatches had a progressively higher incidence of acute GVHD and a poorer overall survival than those with non-permissive mismatches (but HLA allele mismatches) and the fully matched group (Table 28.3). Strikingly outcome in those with no non-permissive mismatches was not different to the fully

Table 28.3: Impact of number of non-permissive mismatches on acute a GVHD and overall survival

Match category	N	No of events[b]	Severe a GVHD HR[a]	P	Survival	P
Full Match	972	129	1.0	NA	1.0	NA
Zero non-permissive	2446	411	1.0	0.996	1.06	0.315
One non-permissive MM	571	211	2.22	<0.001	1.51	<0.001
>One non-permissive MM	61	36	3.68	<0.001	2.25	<0.001

[a]by a multivariable analysis – see ref for details
[b]Event = No of occurrences
MM = Mismatch
Modified from Kawase et al Blood 2007[53]

matched group suggesting these donors truly did have permissive HLA mismatches.

By a similar series of analyses the effects of specific donor-recipient amino acid mismatch combinations were evaluated. Donor-recipient disparity for Tyr9A-Phe9A at HLA-A and Tyr9C-Ser9C, Asn77C-Ser77C, Lys80C-Asn80C, Tyr99C-Phe99C, Leu116C-Ser116C, Arg156C-Leu156C at HLA-C were each associated with significantly increased risks of acute GVHD and, in most cases with poorer survival. Interestingly, of these six amino acid positions, 2 of these, positions 77 and 80 in HLA-C, are associated with KIR2DL ligand binding, whilst the remaining four are all important positions for peptide binding and T-cell recognition. Position 116 was the position identified as important in the study of Ferrara.[53] Many of the other "permissible" amino acid mismatch combinations at positions in the residues are not accessible to the T-cell receptor nor influence the specificity of the peptide binding groove. Taken together, the data from the studies of HLA-DP and of class I mismatches suggest all HLA mismatches are not equally immunogenic. The approaches outlined have identified important amino acid mismatches which probably should be avoided in the clinical setting and perhaps also allow the identification of "permissible" epitopes. If this data can be replicated and shown to be valid in other populations then it offers a practical basis for the selection of mismatched unrelated donors.

Haplotype Matching

Within a family, siblings who share two haplotypes are the ideal HSCT donor. Because the two haplotypes within the family are identical by descent, the donor-recipient pairs will necessarily be identical at all HLA loci and will also be identical for all other genes and intervening sequences within the defined MHC haplotype. On the other hand, unrelated individuals matched simply on the basis of their HLA type do not necessarily share the same degree of match. Firstly, they may not be completely matched within the HLA genes unless complete sequencing of all the HLA genes is undertaken. Secondly, they may not be matched for the polymorphic blocks which are present throughout the MHC.[54,55] Whilst it has been shown that many combinations of HLA alleles and multiple HLA loci predict the presence of highly conserved ancestral haplotypes comprising a series of highly conserved DNA segments or blocks, historical recombination has occurred between such haplotypes.[22] It is thus possible that even when common combinations of HLA alleles are present, they may not be in cis position on the same haplotype or share the same surrounding block structure. Thus given the generally better outcome observed in matched sibling transplants, it has been suggested that donor-recipient matching at the level of haplotype blocks or the entire haplotype will provide better outcomes than simply matching the individual HLA-loci.

Several approaches to haplotype matching have been described. For a number of years the Perth group has used a "block matching" technique to compare donor recipient matching for blocks of polymorphic DNA around HLA-B (beta-block) and around HLA-DRB1 (delta-block).[54,55] In a series of studies they showed that transplants occurring between "block matched" donor recipient pairs had superior outcome compared to those using mismatched pairs,[56,57] even amongst those who were matched at the allele level for the associated HLA locus.[58]

A second approach has used microsatellites within the MHC. These polymorphic markers scattered throughout the MHC may mark or tag identical genomic segments or blocks of DNA[59] and thus donors matched for these markers might also be matched for these segments. As part of the IHWG, among 900 donor recipient pairs completely matched at HLA-A, -B, -C, -DRB1 and DQB1, the effects of matching at each of 14 MHC microsatellite markers on mortality was determined.[59] Mismatching for two of these markers, at BATC2A in the central MHC region and D62105 in the class I region telemeric of HLA-A, were each associated with a significant risk of death whilst four others showed a suggestive association.[60] This data, together with the block-matching data, suggest non-HLA polymorphisms within segments of the MHC haplotype, contribute to graft outcome.

Another approach to haplotype matching has been described by the Seattle group. They have developed a novel DNA microarray method by which the cis/trans relationship of alleles at HLA-A, -B, and –DRB1 can be determined.[61] By comparing these relationships in donors and recipients who were completely matched at HLA-A, -B, and -DRB1 (but heterozygous at HLA-B and HLA-A and/or HLA-DRB1) they were able to classify these patients as either MHC haplotype matched or haplotype mismatched. Some 20 percent of cases were indeed haplotype mismatched. MHC haplotype mismatching was associated with a statistically significant increased risk of severe acute GVHD (OR 4.51, p<0.0001) and a lower risk of disease recurrence (HR 0.45, p = 0.03) though, perhaps reflecting opposing effects of these two outcomes, there was no effect on survival.[62] These data provide further evidence that additional polymorphisms within the MHC may be important in determining transplant outcome. Candidate sites would include any gene encoding polymorphic determinants that could function as histocompatibility antigens or that could be presented as peptides and there are potentially many in the MHC. They also suggest that where there is the potential to select amongst a number of fully HLA matched donors there may be an advantage in selecting those in whom the HLA alleles are in the same cis relationship to those identified in the patient. Indeed in most cases, because of prior family studies, this arrangement will be known in the patient, though it is not known usually known for unrelated donors from international volunteer donor registries.

Importance of HLA Antibodies

It has been known for some 40 years that donor specific sensitization is an important factor in allogeneic transplantation. Sensitization to HLA antigens resulting in the production of HLA, antibodies can occur following exposure to nonself HLA antigens through blood transfusion, pregnancy with exposure of the mother to fetal cells bearing paternal antigens, and prior transplantation. The first two of these mechanisms are applicable to many patients requiring HSCT and HLA, antibodies can be detected in a proportion of such patients. Such donor specific HLA, antibodies have traditionally been detected by a complement dependant cytotoxicity (CDC) assay. Whilst the role of HLA-antibodies and a positive crossmatch in predicting graft outcome has been extensively studied in solid organ transplantation,[63] there has been relatively little literature on the relevance of a positive crossmatch and of donor specific HLA antibodies in HSCT.

In transplants involving HLA identical sibling donors, the donor will necessarily be completely matched at all HLA loci. Therefore, even in sensitized recipients with HLA antibodies, these will not be directed against the donor. This will also be true in fully matched unrelated donors. However, in transplants involving mismatched donors, there is the possibility that the recipient may have HLA antibodies directed against the mismatched HLA antigens on the donor cells. Early data from the Seattle group clearly showed that the presence of donor specific antibodies as detected by the CDC crossmatch assay were associated with graft failure.[64] In a review by Hansen et al, they reported that amongst HLA identical siblings, graft failure (i.e. failure of donor cells to become established in the recipient) occurred in only 2 percent of transplants using HLA identical sibling donors compared to 9 percent in transplants using donors mismatched for one haplotype. Importantly amongst the latter group, graft failure occurred in 13 of 21 (62%) of cases with a positive CDC or flow cytometry crossmatch against donor lymphocytes compared to only 35 of 501 (7%) of cases with a negative crossmatch.[64] Similar findings have been reported more recently by Ottinger et al [65] in a retrospective, single center, matched pair study. They showed that the risk of graft failure was greater in the 30 cases with a positive crossmatch than the matched controls (p< 0.04).[65] The data from these studies clearly show the importance of donor-specific HLA-antibodies. In many centers crossmatching is routinely performed against all mismatched donors and a positive crossmatch is generally considered a contraindication to transplantation. Presumably as a result of such practice, very little additional data on the relevance of a positive crossmatch has been published.

The performance of a crossmatch has however often proven problematic. Obtaining suitable cell preparations and adequate viable cell numbers from international donors can be difficult. However, the availability of new solid phase, single antigen bead assays has meant that it is now possible to detect DSAs previously not recognized[66] and it is now possible to perform a "virtual" crossmatch based on the donor's HLA and the specificities of the HLA-antibodies detected in the recipient.[67]

Two recent preliminary studies suggest that HLA DSAs detected by solid phase assays are important in HSCT. In a study facilitated through the NMDP, Bray et al identified 37 cases in whom there was a failure of sustained donor cell engraftment, and 78 controls with successful engraftment who were matched for disease, disease status, graft type, patient age and year of transplant.[68] Pretransplant sera from both patients and controls were then assayed for HLA antibodies by a solid phase, Luminex based, single bead assay. Among the 37 failed patients, 11 (30%) had HLA antibodies against donor class I and/or class II antigens compared to only 3 (4%) of the controls. All donor specific class II antibodies were against HLA-DP antigens, perhaps reflecting the greater degree of mismatching which occurs at this locus. The effect of HLA class I or class II directed antibodies was similar and was also shown to be independent of cell dose or patient CMV status, two factors also found to be predictive of graft outcome. Similar findings have also been reported by Takanashi et al in a Japanese cohort of 374 unrelated cord blood transplants.[69] All recipients were tested for HLA antibodies including the use of single antigen beads to characterize the HLA specificity of the antibodies. HLA antibodies were detected in 43(15%) and in eight these were shown to be donor specific. The Kaplan-Meier estimate of engraftment for recipients with DSAs was only 58 percent compared to 93 percent for those without DSA ($p=0.02$). A more recent retrospective single center study has suggested a positive cytotoxic crossmatch was a poor predictor of rejection.[70] However, the majority of cases were completely HLA matched and none had a major HLA-mismatch and the authors did not test for autoantibodies against lymphocytes. Nonetheless they showed one out the four with a positive T cell crossmatch failed to engraft and multivariate analysis showed a positive B cell crossmatch was associated with a significantly higher risk of graft rejection.

The results from these studies indicate that the presence of donor specific HLA antibodies is an important predictor of graft failure. Additional evidence of the importance of preformed antibody to HSC engraftment has also been provided in two studies in mice. Both studies using mouse models of allogeneic bone marrow engraftment, showed that preformed alloantibody, and not T cells, was the initial and major barrier to successful engraftment.[71,72] As suggested by Bray et al, current "Standard of Practice" should include testing all recipients for HLA antibodies (both class I and class II and donors excluded, if they carry mismatched antigens against which the patient has specific HLA antibodies.[68] Such a procedure can probably replace the traditional CDC crossmatch assay and greatly facilitate selection of the most appropriate HLA-mismatched donor.

USE OF UNRELATED DONOR UMBILICAL CORD BLOOD TRANSPLANTATION

Use of Cord Blood Units

The first successful umbilical cord blood (CB) transplant from an HLA identical sibling in a child with severe Fanconi anemia was reported by Guckman et al in 1989,[73] and the first use of CB from an unrelated, only partially HLA matched donor was reported by Kurtzberg in 1996.[74] Subsequently a number of studies have now shown that the results of HSC transplants, using unrelated CB (UCB) donors, can be comparable to those using unrelated bone marrow or mobilized peripheral blood stem cell (PBSC) donors. Whilst, these studies have been predominantly in pediatric cases, with the use of multiple UCB donors, better risk patients and submyeloblative preparative regimens, UCB transplants are being increasingly applied to adult patients. As of 2008 there are some 50 public CB banks around the world with over 260,000 CB units stored and CB from unrelated donors are being increasingly utilized clinically. As the HLA matching requirements seem less stringent than those for bone marrow or mobilized PBSC, UCB transplantation is providing access to HSC therapy for many patients in whom a well-matched unrelated adult donor is not available.

In comparison with transplants using adult bone marrow or PBSC, a unit of cord blood has approximately a log fewer hematopoietic progenitor cells[75] and are also functionally partially T-cell depleted. For grafts using adult donors, cell numbers are well above transplant threshold and with the exception of T-depleted grafts and those occurring in the presence of donor specific alloantibodies, graft failure is uncommon. This is not true for UCB transplants. Many studies have shown that UCB transplantation is associated with a higher incidence of graft failure and delay in hematopoietic engraftment with its associated clinical risks. The cell dose, usually measured in terms of total nucleated count (TNC), CD34 positive cell count or colony forming units (CFU) per kilogram body weight of the recipient, has been shown to be a major factor determining success. Limited cell numbers has been a major limitation to the widespread application of UCB to adult patients. Detailed discussion of the cell dose requirement for successful engraftment is beyond the scope of this article and has been reviewed elsewhere.[76] However, it seems more is better. In general a TNC dose of greater than 3.7×10^7/kg is required for consistent engraftment. Most centers target a TNC dose of at least 5×10^7/kg and generally a minimum of 2×10^7/kg is required, a level which is rarely achieved with a single cord blood unit for an adult patient.

Despite the limitation of cell dose, UCB offers a number of advantages over other sources of allogeneic unrelated HSC. Firstly, cord blood units are already banked and processed and therefore, more readily available for use. There is a lower risk of transmitting infections by latent viruses such as a CMV and EBV and there is an ability to undertake careful screening of the mother at the time of collection and subsequently on further clinical follow-up, prior to use of the CB unit. There is no risk to the donor and a product which would otherwise be discarded is used. There is lack of donor attrition due to age, unavailability or the development of an intervening illness whilst, it seems that CB can be stored for at least ten years without loss of potency. Cord blood banks in general provide a greater access to some ethnic and cultural groups who have not been major volunteers through adult donor registries. Transplants using CBs have been associated with lower risk and less severe acute and chronic GVHD, despite major HLA disparity. This seems to be due to the lower number of mature T-cells in the CB graft and to the relative unresponsiveness of these T-cells to alloantigens. Because of the ability to use CBs with greater degrees of HLA disparity, they are being increasingly used in those patients who cannot find a well-matched donor in the adult donor registries. Nonetheless as described below, HLA matching is an important factor in determining outcome and needs to be considered in donor selection. In general selection of the most suitable UCB donor involves a balance between, on the one hand the need for adequate cell dose, and on the other, generally getting the best HLA matched unit.

Importance of HLA Matching in UCB Transplantation

A detailed consideration of the importance of HLA matching in UCB transplants is beyond the scope of this article and only the findings of the major studies will be reviewed. The reader is also referred to two excellent recent reviews.[76,77] The impact of HLA mismatching following transplantation using UCB units has been studied in a number of studies which are summarized in Table 28.4.[78-85] Each study will not be reviewed in detail but several general points are worth highlighting. It is important to note that in all studies, at least one outcome measure was shown to be adversely affected by increased HLA mismatches. An effect on engraftment has been shown in almost all studies reflecting the critical requirement for adequate cell dose, which seems to be particularly the case in HLA mismatched transplants. The effects on acute GVHD seem least striking, again perhaps reflecting the overall low prevalence of acute GVHD following UCB transplants. In general most studies have

Table 28.4: Summary of studies examining the effects of HLA-mismatches on various clinical outcome parameters following transplantation using UCB

Study	N	Mismatch Comparisons	Outcome parameters				
			Engraftment	GVHD	Relapse	TRM	Survival
Rubinstein[78]	861	0 vs ≥1	↓[b]	↑	N/A	↑	↓
Wagner[79]	102	0-1 vs 2	0	0	N/A	0	↓
Gibbons[81]	755	0 vs 1 vs 2	↓	N/A	N/A	N/A	↓
Gluckman[80]	550	0 vs 1 vs 2 vs 3/4	(↓)	↑[a]	↓	N/A	0
Eapen[83]	503	0 vs 1 vs 2	↓	0	↓	↑	↓
Barker[82]	608	0 vs 1 vs 2 vs 3	N/A	N/A	N/A	↑	N/A
Kurtzberg[84]	191	0-1 vs ≥2	↓[b]	↑[a]	0	N/A	(↓)
Matsuno[85]	152	0=1 vs 2	↓	(↑)	N/A	N/A	0

↑ = Mismatch associate with increased risk   ↓ = Mismatch associated with decreased risk
0 = no effect   N/A = Not examined   ( ) = trend only
[a] = severe (Grade III-IV)   [b] = Neutrophils

shown increased HLA mismatches are associated with increased transplant related mortality (TRM) and poorer survival. Clearly then, despite less stringent HLA matching requirements, HLA matching is important.

In reviewing these studies, several other points need to be considered. Generally in these studies HLA matching has only been considered at the HLA-A, -B and -DRB1 loci with class I typing usually being defined at the broad serological level and HLA-DR at a molecular level but only at an intermediate level of resolution. Very few studies have examined the impact of high resolution typing. This was considered in a study reported by Kurtzberg, where retrospective high resolution typing was undertaken and the effects of both the initial and final level of typing were considered. The higher definition of HLA mismatch generally resulted in a greater impact on outcome, though these effects were small.[84] One other study from a single center has shown that higher resolution typing, including typing of additional loci, did not show a dramatic effect on outcome, though the power of this study was limited.[86]

Secondly, perhaps reflecting the use of CB transplants for those for whom a well-matched adult donor is not available, transplants using CB generally have considerable degrees of mismatch, even when defined only at a broad level, at HLA-A, -B, and -DRB1. Very few have ideal matching with over 90 percent of transplants being performed with at least one major mismatch. Thus, most studies have compared various degrees of mismatch often with limited power within each of the mismatch categories. At this stage there is no consensus as to which mismatches (class I or II) or which loci (HLA-A, -B or -C or HLA-DR, -DQ) are preferable. Gluckman et al suggested the presence of both class I and or class II mismatches was associated with a higher incidence of severe acute GVHD and delayed engraftment,[80] whilst another study showed some evidence that HLA-DR mismatches are less well tolerated.[87] The effects of mismatches at other loci, e.g. HLA-C and HLA-DQB1 have not been adequately studied. Few studies have examined the quantitative effect of increasing numbers of mismatches and in those in which an effect has been observed, these have generally been small but the power of such studies has been limited.

Thirdly, the majority of these studies have been undertaken in children, predominantly with hematological malignancy. The effects of mismatches on overall survival in such cases is likely to be affected by the counter balancing benefit of reduced acute GVHD observed in CB transplants and the potential for decreased graft versus leukemia effects.

Fourthly, there have been suggestions that the effects of HLA mismatch are most apparent when cell dose is low and that increasing cell dose can at least partially reduce the impact of HLA disparity on survival.[79] Eapen et al showed that recipients of CB with low cell dose and one or two HLA mismatches had worse outcomes.[83] In Eurocord data the negative effects of 2-4 HLA mismatches on engraftment could be overcome by higher cell dose.[88] Given these apparent interactive effects, studies examining the effects of HLA matching should take account of cell dose in multivariate analysis. This has been done in very few studies and may account for a possible masking of the effects of HLA matching.

Finally, to overcome the limitations of cell dose in adults, transplantation using two cord blood units has been recently introduced and is now being more widely used.[89-91] Whilst, this has resulted in better engraftment and outcome, particularly in adult patients, usually by one month only one cord contributes to the hemopoiesis in the recipient. HLA matching does not seem to be a factor in determining which CB unit engrafts and the importance of HLA matching in the units has not been established. At this stage no definitive statements can be made about the role of HLA matching in selecting CB units for double unit transplants. However, it would seem reasonable that at least one cord unit should have a higher cell dose and at least some degree of matching between the cord units and recipient should be sought.

Selection of Donor CB Unit

Despite the evidence that transplants using CB donors do not have the strict requirements for HLA matching as those using HSC, nonetheless HLA matching, together with cell dose, is an important factor influencing outcome. Most centers primarily select a cord blood on the basis of cell dose requiring at least a TNC dose of 3.7×10^7/kg and preferably at least 5×10^7/kg. If multiple units with good cell dose are available then the unit with the best match is used. In the event that only units with a marginal cell dose are being available, then the CB unit should be well-matched (6/6) or a double unit transplant should be considered. The Texas Transplant Institute has suggested an algorithm for cord blood unit selection with a target cell dose of TNC $>5 \times 10^7$/kg, taking account of HLA match,[76] which gives a guide to the approach adopted by transplant centers in selecting the most appropriate CB unit.

FINDING A SUITABLE HSC DONOR

It is now well established that HSCT is the best treatment for a large range of clinical conditions. Such therapy requires the identification of the most suitable allogeneic HSC donor. Several basic principals are important to consider in any search and the selection of the best donor. Firstly, it is important that the various therapeutic options are considered and the decision to undertake HSCT, if a suitable donor can be identified is fully discussed with the patient. A search for a donor should not be initiated unless there is at least a prospect of proceeding to transplantation. Secondly, the disease risk category and clinical urgency, particularly in relation to patients with leukemia, needs to be determined. Generally three levels of risk: low, intermediate and high, have been used. Such categorization is important in that it provides a good indication of the likelihood of successful transplant outcome, the relative importance of HLA-matching of the donor and the urgency in finding a suitable donor. Transplantation outcome is less favorable with increasing risk category and the best outcome can be achieved with low risk patients transplanted with a well-matched donor. Donor searching is often a critical balance between the benefits of using a well-matched donor versus the risks of a lengthy search delaying transplantation. Thirdly, the likelihood of finding a suitable donor requires an up front evaluation of the patient's HLA genotype and haplotypes which allows an estimation of the likelihood of finding a suitably matched donor. Such estimates are best based on high resolution, preferably allele level typing, of the patient at HLA-A, -B, -C, and –DRB1. A search on bone marrow donors worldwide (www.bmdw.org), which can be undertaken online by the HLA laboratory or transplant center, is particularly helpful and provides a list of potential donors of both adult and cord blood units with various degrees of HLA match and the donor registry in which they are located. Finally, close collaboration between the clinician caring for the patient and the donor search coordinator and the HLA laboratory, is particularly helpful.

On the basis of the data reviewed in this chapter, it is clear that from the histocompatibility point of view, the best donor is the donor with best HLA match and that any HLA mismatch should be considered a bad mismatch. However, it is often not possible to identify a completely matched donor, in which case donors with some degree of mismatch may need to be considered. The following section describes a possible hierarchical approach to donor selection and provides some guidelines on donor selection within each of the possible match levels. The National Marrow Donor program has also recently provided guidelines for HLA matching requirements for unrelated hematopoietic cell transplants.[27]

HLA Identical Sibling Donors

Despite the recent evidence that transplant outcome using a matched unrelated donor can approach that using a HLA identical sibling, the latter remains the allogeneic HSC donor of choice. If HSCT is being considered, family studies should be initiated as soon as possible. It is important that, whenever possible, the paternal and maternal haplotypes in the patient and siblings are unequivocally identified and the potential donor is shown to share two haplotypes with the patient. This requires the typing of as many family members as possible including both parents if available. In the first pass, it is often sufficient to undertake intermediate level typing at HLA-A, -B, and –DRB1 and if the haplotypes can be assigned unequivocally, higher resolution typing or typing of additional loci is not required. However, it is important that identity of the donor and recipient is confirmed by HLA typing on repeat separate samples. This avoids any potential mislabeling or handling errors at the time of collection or by the HLA laboratory.

In the event that more than one HLA identical sibling is identified, HLA-DPB1 typing should be considered to ensure a recombination between HLA-DRB1 and –DPB1 has not occurred. If this has been excluded, other non-HLA factors such as gender, CMV status, or age maybe considered in selecting between HLA identical sibling donors.

It is not always possible to unequivocally identify the HLA haplotypes in the family and in such circumstance additional high resolution typing at all HLA loci including HLA-DPB1 should be undertaken on the patient and the potential donor. If identity at these loci is confirmed, this will increase the likelihood that the patient and donor share the same maternal and paternal haplotypes but in any event would mean such a donor would be at least as well-matched as any unrelated donor.

In the event that a suitable donor is not identified in the family, high resolution, preferably allele level, typing at HLA-A, -B, -C, and –DRB1 at a minimum should be undertaken on the patient and a donor search initiated. The search strategy should take account of the patient's HLA genotype and risk category and clinical urgency.

Potential Donors Matched at HLA-A, -B, -C and -DRB1

The data reviewed previously indicate that ideally an unrelated donor should be matched at the allele level at HLA-A, -B, -C and -DRB1 and probably –DQB1. Most donors in registries have not been typed at this level, often lacking allele level typing, particularly at the class I loci, or often without any typing information at HLA-C and -DQB1. A search for the most suitable donor should focus on those listed potential donors with the highest probability of being matched at the allele level at all loci. Knowledge of the patient's alleles and haplotypes and their frequencies within different populations (i.e. common or rare) can guide in the selection of those donors on whom additional HLA typing should be performed. Programs such as HapLogic provided through NMDP can provide estimates of the likelihood that a donor will be matched at the allele level and be matched at the non typed HLA-loci. High resolution typing of a number of such potential donors should be undertaken. The numbers on whom this should be undertaken will depend upon the clinical urgency and patient's HLA genotype. For those with common alleles or haplotypes, high resolution typing of 3- 5 donors will usually be sufficient. For patients with rarer alleles or uncommon haplotype combinations, where the probability of matching is low, many more may need to be typed and even then a suitable donor may not be identified. Donors matched at the allele level at HLA-A, -B, -C, -DRB1 and –DQB1 (i.e. 10/10) can be considered suitable. In the event that more than one such donor is identified then HLA-DPB1 typing could be considered. In many cases, the donors will be mismatched at least one HLA-DPB1, locus. Depending on urgency and available funding, typing of additional donors seeking complete HLA-DP match donor could be undertaken. Alternatively donors with "permissible matches" (see section 3.4.1) could be selected. Selection might also be based on the presence of a donor-recipient haplotype match where the HLA alleles are known to be in the same cis relationship. However, haplotype assignment on the donor is almost never known and the techniques for haplotype assignment are not widely available and such an approach must be considered experimental at this stage. Other donor factors such as gender, age, CMV status may also be considered.

Single HLA Antigen Mismatched Donors

In the event that a fully matched (i.e. 10/10) donor is not available, a single HLA-mismatched donor can be considered. Transplants using such donors generally have a higher incidence of adverse outcome events but satisfactory long-term survival can be achieved. In patients with high and intermediate risk disease, the benefits of HLA mismatching are less evident and for such patients, it may be preferable to proceed with a single antigen mismatched donor than delay transplantation whilst seeking a 10/10 matched donor.

When selecting a mismatched donor it seems that all mismatches should be considered bad. One should select the donor with as few mismatches as possible and those with multiple mismatches (with a possible exception of the additional mismatch being at HLA-DP) should be avoided. At this stage, it is not possible to state whether a mismatch at any one locus is preferable to any other, though it does seem that a single mismatch at HLA-DQB1 might have the lowest risk. When considering selection from amongst donors with a single allele mismatch at a particular locus, it is not possible to make any specific recommendations. Whilst, it is possible that not all mismatches are equally bad and that there may be some "permissible mismatches", with the possible exception of HLA-DP, there is insufficient data to make recommendations at this stage on the most appropriate specific allele mismatches at individual HLA loci.

If an HLA mismatched donor is being considered, the patient should be tested for HLA antibodies, using modern solid phase assays and the specificity of any HLA antibodies present should be determined. This is particularly important for those patients who may have been sensitized through pregnancy or blood transfusion. If HLA antibodies are present, then donors mismatched for these antigens, including HLA-DPB1, should be excluded. Given the lack of evidence to guide donor selection from amongst those with a single HLA mismatch, other non-HLA donor factors such as gender, age, CMV status or time in procuring the donor may be taken into account.

Alternative Allogeneic Donors

If no completely matched or suitable single HLA antigen mismatched donor can be identified, several alternatives can be considered. A CB unit may be suitable, particularly for pediatric cases. In general, the TNC is the critical requirement in CB unit selection with a TNC of at least 3.7×10^7/kg being required, though in general the greater the cell number the better. If CB units with a high cell count are available then such units with only an HLA 4 out of 6 match (at HLA-A, -B, and –DRB1) can be considered suitable. Often such units can be identified, at least for children. For cords with a better HLA match, a somewhat lower TNC may be acceptable. The patient disease may also be a factor and in diseases where a graft-versus leukemia effect is not required, CB units may be particularly indicated. In adult patients, where it is usually not possible to identify a single cord with a suitable cell count, double CB units may be an option. Whilst the initial data is encouraging, there is still relatively limited experience with this approach and it should only be undertaken where the various therapeutic options are carefully considered. When selecting multiple CB units, it is probably reasonable to select units with as high a cell count as possible and to try and ensure that they have at least 4 at out of 6 HLA-match.

Other possible donors that may be considered are mismatched haploidentical family donors. In some cases, through an extended family search, donors sharing one haplotype with the patient and with some degree of matching on the non-shared haplotype might be identified. Such donors may be suitable though these are probably high risk. Alternatively complete haplotype mismatched family donors may also be used using various T cell depletion protocols or with a non-myeloablative preparative regimen. Such treatments should only be considered using standardized protocols and for patients in whom no other donor is available.

SUMMARY

Much progress has been made in HSCT and this therapy is now a well established treatment, offering the prospect for long-term cure for a number of malignant and non-malignant diseases. There has been a steady improvement in the outcome and the availability of better HLA typing techniques has meant that outcome using unrelated donors is now approaching those found in sibling transplants. The indications and criteria for using allogeneic HSCT have evolved. Finding suitable donors for all patients who would benefit from such therapy remains a major challenge and is one of the significant barriers to its increasing use. Understanding the mechanisms and basis for allorecognition and the immunogenicity of particular mismatch combinations with the hope of identifying permissible mismatches remains a challenge. A successful HSC program requires the support of a histocompatibility laboratory and an effective interaction between the clinician, histocompatibility, scientists, donor search coordinators and the donor registries and transplant centers.

REFERENCES

1. Gatti RA, HJ Meuwissen, HD Allen, R Hong, RA Good. Immunological reconstitution of sex-linked lymphopenic immunological deficiency. Lancet 1968;2:1366-69.
2. Thomas ED, R Storb. The development of the scientific foundation of haematopoietic cell transplantation based on animal and human studies. In Haematopoietic Cell Transplantation 1999;Vol. 2, SJ Forman, KG Blume, ED Thomas (Eds). Wiley-Blackwell, pp. 1-11.
3. Thomas ER, Storb RA, Clift A, Fefer FL, Johnson PE, Neiman KG, Lerner H. Glucksberg CD Buckner. Bone-marrow transplantation (first of two parts). N Engl J Med 1975;292:832-43.
4. Dupont B. Immunology of hematopoietic stem cell transplantation: A brief review of its history. Immunol Rev 1997;157:5-12.
5. Anasetti C, JA Hansen. Bone marrow transplantation from HLA partially matched related donors and unrelated volunteer donors. In Bone Marrow Transplantation SJ, Forman KG, Blume, ED Thomas (Eds): Wiley, John & Sons, Incorporated 1994;665-69.
6. Ottinger H, M Grosse-Wilde, A Schmitz, H Grosse-Wilde. Immunogenetic marrow donor search for 1012 patients: A retrospective analysis of strategies, outcome and costs. Bone Marrow Transplant 1994;14 (Suppl 4):S34-S38.
7. Schipper RF, JD'Amaro, M Oudshoorn. The probability of finding a suitable related donor for bone marrow transplantation in extended families. Blood 1996;87: 800-04.
8. Beatty PG, RA Clift, EM Mickelson, B B Nisperos, N Flournoy, PJ Martin, J E Sanders, P Stewart, CD Buckner, R Storb, ED Thomas, JA Hansen. Marrow transplantation from related donors other than HLA-identical siblings. N Engl J Med 1985;313:765-71.
9. Powles RL, GR Morgenstern, HE Kay, TJ McElwain, HM Clink, PJ Dady, A Barrett, B Jameson, MH Depledge, JG Watson, J Sloane, M Leigh, H Lumley, D Hedley, SD Lawler, J Filshie, B Robinson. Mismatched family donors for bone-marrow transplantation as treatment for acute leukaemia. Lancet 1983;1:612-15.
10. Anasetti C, D Amos, PG Beatty, F R Appelbaum, W Bensinger, CD Buckner, R Clift, K Doney, PJ Martin, E Mickelson, B Nisperos, J O'Quigley, R Ramberg, JE Sanders, P Stewart, R Storb, KM Sullivan, RP Witherspoon, ED Thomas, JA Hansen. Effect of HLA compatibility on engraftment of bone marrow transplants in patients with leukemia or lymphoma. N Engl J Med 1989;320:197-202.
11. Beelen DW, HD Ottinger, A Elmaagacli, B Scheulen, O Basu, B Kremens, W Havers, H Grosse-Wilde, UW Schaefer. Transplantation of filgrastim-mobilized peripheral blood stem cells from HLA-identical sibling or alternative family donors in patients with hematologic malignancies: A prospective comparison on clinical outcome, immune reconstitution, and hematopoietic chimerism. Blood 1997;90:4725-35.

12. Anasetti C, PG Beatty, R Storb, PJ Martin, M Mori, JE Sanders, ED Thomas, JA Hansen. Effect of HLA incompatibility on graft-versus-host disease, relapse, and survival after marrow transplantation for patients with leukemia or lymphoma. Hum Immunol 1990;29:79-91.
13. Ottinger HD, S Ferencik, DW Beelen, M Lindemann, R Peceny, AH Elmaagacli, J Husing, H Grosse-Wilde. Hematopoietic stem cell transplantation: Contrasting the outcome of transplantations from HLA-identical siblings, partially HLA-mismatched related donors, and HLA-matched unrelated donors. Blood 2003;102:1131-37.
14. Gaziev D, M Galimberti, G Lucarelli, P Polchi, C Giardini, E Angelucci, D Baronciani, P Sodani, B Erer, M D. Biagi, M Andreani, F Agostinelli, M Donati, S Nesci, N Talevi. Bone marrow transplantation from alternative donors for thalassemia: HLA-phenotypically identical relative and HLA-nonidentical sibling or parent transplants. Bone Marrow Transplant 2000;25:815-21.
15. Drobyski WR, J Klein, N Flomenberg, D Pietryga, DH Vesole, DA Margolis, CA Keever-Taylor. Superior survival associated with transplantation of matched unrelated versus one-antigen-mismatched unrelated or highly human leukocyte antigen-disparate haploidentical family donor marrow grafts for the treatment of hematologic malignancies: Establishing a treatment algorithm for recipients of alternative donor grafts. Blood 2002;99:806-14.
16. Caillat-Zucman S, F Le Deist, E Haddad M Gannage, L Dal Cortivo, N Jabado, S Hacein-Bey-Abina, S Blanche, JL Casanova, A Fischer, M Cavazzana-Calvo. Impact of HLA matching on outcome of hematopoietic stem cell transplantation in children with inherited diseases: A single-center comparative analysis of genoidentical, haploidentical or unrelated donors. Bone Marrow Transplant. 2004;33:1089-95.
17. Bunin N, R Aplenc, A Leahey, E Magira, S Grupp, G Pierson, D Monos. Outcomes of transplantation with partial T-cell depletion of matched or mismatched unrelated or partially matched related donor bone marrow in children and adolescents with leukemias. Bone Marrow Transplant 2005;35:151-58.
18. Speck B, FE Zwaan, JJ van Rood, JG Eernisse. Allogeneic bone marrow transplantation in a patient with aplastic anemia using a phenotypically HL-A-identifcal unrelated donor. Transplantation 1973;16:24-28.
19. Horowitz SD, FH Bach, T Groshong, R Hong, EJ Yunis. Treatment of severe combined immunodeficiency with bone-marrow from an unrelated, mixed-leucocyte-culture-non-reactive donor. Lancet 1975;2:431-33.
20. O'Reilly RJ, B Dupont, S Pahwa, E Grimes, EM Smithwick, R Pahwa, S Schwartz, JA Hansen, FP Siegal, M Sorell, A Svejgaard, C Jersild, M Thomsen, P Platz, PL'Esperance, RA Good. Reconstitution in severe combined immunodeficiency by transplantation of marrow from an unrelated donor. N.Engl.J Med 1977;297:1311-18.
21. Hansen JA, RA Clift, ED Thomas, CD Buckner, R Storb, ER Giblett. Transplantation of marrow from an unrelated donor to a patient with acute leukemia. N Engl J Med 1980;303:565-67.
22. Degli-Esposti MA, AL Leaver, FT Christiansen, CS Witt, LJ Abraham, RL Dawkins. Ancestral haplotypes: Conserved population MHC haplotypes. Hum Immunol 1992;34:242-52.
23. Muller CR, G Ehninger, SF Goldmann. Gene and haplotype frequencies for the loci HLA-A, HLA-B, and HLA-DR based on over 13,000 German blood donors. Hum.Immunol 2003;64:137-51.
24. Hurley CK, M Fernandez-Vina, WH Hildebrand, HJ Noreen, E Trachtenberg, TM Williams, LA Baxter-Lowe, AB Begovich, E Petersdorf, A Selvakumar, P Stastny, J Hegland, RJ Hartzman, M Carston, S Gandham, C Kollman, G Nelson, S Spellman, M Setterholm. A high degree of HLA disparity arises from limited allelic diversity: Analysis of 1775 unrelated bone marrow transplant donor-recipient pairs. Hum Immunol 2007; 68:30-40.
25. Oudshoorn M, A van Leeuwen, H G vd Zanden, JJ van Rood. Bone Marrow Donors Worldwide: A successful exercise in international cooperation. Bone Marrow Transplant 1994;14:3-8.
26. Petersdorf EW, C Anasetti, PJ Martin, JA Hansen. Tissue typing in support of unrelated hematopoietic cell transplantation. Tissue Antigens 2003;61:1-11.
27. Bray RA, CK Hurley, NR Kamani, A Woolfrey, C Muller, S Spellman, M Setterholm, DL Confer. National marrow donor program HLA matching guidelines for unrelated adult donor hematopoietic cell transplants. Biol Blood Marrow Transplant 2008;14:45-53.
28. Petersdorf EW. Immunogenomics of unrelated hematopoietic cell transplantation. Curr Opin Immunol 2006;18:559-64.
29. Morishima Y, T Sasazuki, H Inoko, T Juji, T Akaza, K Yamamoto, Y Ishikawa, S Kato, H Sao, H Sakamaki, K Kawa, N Hamajima, S Asano, Y Kodera. The clinical significance of human leukocyte antigen (HLA) allele compatibility in patients receiving a marrow transplant from serologically HLA-A, HLA-B, and HLA-DR matched unrelated donors. Blood 2002;99:4200-06.
30. Flomenberg N, LA Baxter-Lowe, D Confer, M Fernandez-Vina, A Filipovich, M Horowitz, C Hurley, C Kollman, C Anasetti, H Noreen, A Begovich, W Hildebrand, E Petersdorf, B Schmeckpeper, M Setterholm, E Trachtenberg, T Williams, E Yunis, D Weisdorf. Impact of HLA class I and class II high-resolution matching on outcomes of unrelated donor bone marrow transplantation: HLA-C mismatching is associated with a strong adverse effect on transplantation outcome. Blood 2004;104:1923-30.
31. Petersdorf EW, C Anasetti, PJ Martin, T Gooley, J Radich, M Malkki, A Woolfrey, A Smith, E Mickelson, JA Hansen. Limits of HLA mismatching in unrelated hematopoietic cell transplantation. Blood 2004;104:2976-80.
32. Greinix, HT, I Fae, B Schneider, A Rosenmayr, A Mitterschiffthaler, B Pelzmann, P Kalhs, K Lechner, WR

Mayr, GF Fischer. Impact of HLA class I high-resolution mismatches on chronic graft-versus-host disease and survival of patients given hematopoietic stem cell grafts from unrelated donors. Bone Marrow Transplant 2005;35:57-62.

33. Chalandon Y, JM Tiercy, U Schanz, T Gungor, R Seger, J Halter, C Helg, B Chapuis, A Gratwohl, A Tichelli, DF Nicoloso, E Roosnek, JR Passweg. Impact of high-resolution matching in allogeneic unrelated donor stem cell transplantation in Switzerland. Bone Marrow Transplant 2006;37:909-16.

34. Loiseau P, M Busson, ML Balere, A Dormoy, JD Bignon, K Gagne, L Gebuhrer, V Dubois, I Jollet, M Bois, P Perrier, D Masson, A Moine, L Absi, D Reviron, V LePage, R Tamouza, A Toubert, E Marry, Z Chir, JP Jouet, D Blaise, D Charron, C Raffoux. HLA association with hematopoietic stem cell transplantation outcome: The number of mismatches at HLA-A, -B, -C, -DRB1, or -DQB1 is strongly associated with overall survival. Biol Blood Marrow Transplant. 2007;13:965-74.

35. Lee SJ, J Klein, M Haagenson, LA Baxter-Lowe, DL Confer, M Eapen, M Fernandez-Vina, N Flomenberg, M Horowitz, C K Hurley, H Noreen, M Oudshoorn, E Petersdorf, M Setterholm, S Spellman, D Weisdorf, TM Williams, C Anasetti. High-resolution donor-recipient HLA matching contributes to the success of unrelated donor marrow transplantation. Blood 2007;110:4576-83.

36. Petersdorf EW, T Gooley, M Malkki, M Horowitz. Clinical significance of donor-recipient HLA matching on survival after myeloablative hematopoietic cell transplantation from unrelated donors. Tissue Antigens 2007;(69 Suppl) 1:25-30.

37. Morishima Y, T Yabe, K Matsuo, K Kashiwase, H Inoko, H Saji, K Yamamoto, E Maruya, Y Akatsuka, M Onizuka, H Sakamaki, H Sao, S Ogawa, S Kato, T Juji, T Sasazuki, Y Kodera. Effects of HLA allele and killer immunoglobulin-like receptor ligand matching on clinical outcome in leukemia patients undergoing transplantation with T-cell-replete marrow from an unrelated donor. Biol Blood Marrow Transplant 2007;13:315-28.

38. Ho VT, HT Kim, D Liney, E Milford, J Gribben, C Cutler, SJ Lee, J H Antin, RJ Soiffer, E P Alyea. HLA-C mismatch is associated with inferior survival after unrelated donor non-myeloablative hematopoietic stem cell transplantation. Bone Marrow Transplant 2006;37:845-50.

39. Wade JA, CK Hurley, SK Takemoto, J Thompson, SM Davies, TC Fuller, G Rodey, DL Confer, H Noreen, M Haagenson, F Kan, J Klein, M Eapen, S Spellman, C Kollman. HLA mismatching within or outside of cross-reactive groups (CREGs) is associated with similar outcomes after unrelated hematopoietic stem cell transplantation. Blood 2007;109:4064-70.

40. Arora M, DJ Weisdorf, SR Spellman, M D Haagenson, JP Klein, CK Hurley, GB Selby, JH Antin, NA Kernan, C Kollman, A Nademanee, P McGlave, MM Horowitz, EW Petersdorf. HLA-identical sibling compared with 8/8 matched and mismatched unrelated donor bone marrow transplant for chronic phase chronic myeloid leukemia. J Clin Oncol 2009;27:1644-52.

41. Shaw BE, SG Marsh, NP Mayor, NH Russell, JA Madrigal. HLA-DPB1 matching status has significant implications for recipients of unrelated donor stem cell transplants. Blood 2006;107:1220-26.

42. Varney MD, S Lester, J McCluskey, X Gao, BD Tait. Matching for HLA DPA1 and DPB1 alleles in unrelated bone marrow transplantation. Hum Immunol 1999;60: 532-38.

43. Loiseau P, H Esperou, M Busson, R Sghiri, R Tamouza, M Hilarius, C Raffoux, A Devergie, P Ribaud, G Socie, E Gluckman, D Charron DPB1 disparities contribute to severe GVHD and reduced patient survival after unrelated donor bone marrow transplantation. Bone Marrow Transplant. 2002;30:497-502.

44. Shaw BE, TA Gooley, M Malkki, JA Madrigal, AB Begovich, MM Horowitz, A Gratwohl, O Ringden, SG Marsh, EW Petersdorf. The importance of HLA-DPB1 in unrelated donor hematopoietic cell transplantation. Blood 2007;110:4560-66.

45. Macdonald WA, AW Purcell, NA Mifsud, LK Ely, DS Williams, L Chang, JJ Gorman, CS Clements, L Kjer-Nielsen, DM Koelle, SR Burrows, BD Tait, R Holdsworth, AG Brooks, GO Lovrecz, L Lu, J Rossjohn, J McCluskey. A naturally selected dimorphism within the HLA-B44 supertype alters class I structure, peptide repertoire, and T cell recognition. J Exp Med 2003;198:679-91.

46. Fleischhauer K, E Zino, B Mazzi, E Sironi, P Servida, E Zappone, E Benazzi, C Bordignon. Peripheral blood stem cell allograft rejection mediated by CD4(+) T lymphocytes recognizing a single mismatch at HLA-DP beta 1*0901. Blood 2001;98:1122-26.

47. Zino E, G Frumento, S Marktel, MP Sormani, F Ficara, S Di Terlizzi, AM Parodi, R Sergeant, M Martinetti, A Bontadini, F Bonifazi, D Lisini, B Mazzi, S Rossini, P Servida, F Ciceri, C Bonini, E Lanino, G Bandini, F Locatelli, J Apperley, A Bacigalupo, GB Ferrara, C Bordignon, K Fleischhauer. A T-cell epitope encoded by a subset of HLA-DPB1 alleles determines non-permissive mismatches for hematologic stem cell transplantation. Blood 2004;103:1417-24.

48. Zino E, L Vago, S Di Terlizzi, B Mazzi, L Zito, E Sironi, S Rossini, C Bonini, F Ciceri, MG Roncarolo, C Bordignon, K Fleischhauer. Frequency and targeted detection of HLA-DPB1 T cell epitope disparities relevant in unrelated hematopoietic stem cell transplantation. Biol Blood Marrow Transplant 2007;13:1031-40.

49. Fleischhauer K, F Locatelli, M Zecca, MG Orofino, C Giardini, P De Stefano, A Pession, AM Iannone, C Carcassi, E Zino, G La Nasa. Graft rejection after unrelated donor hematopoietic stem cell transplantation for thalassemia is associated with nonpermissive HLA-DPB1 disparity in host-versus-graft direction. Blood 2006; 107:2984-92.

50. Crocchiolo R, E Zino, L Vago, R Oneto, B Bruno, S Pollichieni, N Sacchi, MP Sormani, J Marcon, T Lamparelli, R Fanin, L Garbarino, V Miotti, G Bandini, A Bosi, F Ciceri, A Bacigalupo, K Fleischhauer. Non-permissive HLA-DPB1 disparity is a significant independent risk factor for mortality after unrelated hematopoietic stem cell transplantation. Blood, 2009;114:1437-44.

51. Shaw BE. The clinical implications of HLA mismatches in unrelated donor haematopoietic cell transplantation. Int J Immunogenet 2008;35:367-74.

52. Ferrara GB, A Bacigalupo, T Lamparelli, E Lanino, L Delfino, A Morabito, A M Parodi, C Pera, S Pozzi, MP Sormani, P Bruzzi, D Bordo, M Bolognesi, G Bandini, A Bontadini, M Barbanti, G Frumento. Bone marrow transplantation from unrelated donors: The impact of mismatches with substitutions at position 116 of the human leukocyte antigen class I heavy chain. Blood 2001;98:3150-55.

53. Kawase T, Y Morishima, K Matsuo, K Kashiwase, H Inoko, H Saji, S Kato, T Juji, Y Kodera, T Sasazuki. High-risk HLA allele mismatch combinations responsible for severe acute graft-versus-host disease and implication for its molecular mechanism. Blood 2007;110:2235-41.

54. Abraham LJ, C Leelayuwat, G Grimsley, MA Degli-Esposti, A Mann, WJ Zhang, FT Christiansen, RL Dawkins. Sequence differences between HLA-B and TNF distinguish different MHC ancestral haplotypes. Tissue Antigens 1992;39:117-21.

55. Ketheesan N, S Gaudieri, CS Witt, GK Tay, DC Townend, FT Christiansen, R L Dawkins. Reconstruction of the block matching profiles. Hum Immunol 1999;60:171-76.

56. Tay GK, CS Witt, FT Christiansen, D Charron, D Baker, R Herrmann, LK Smith, D Diepeveen, S Mallal, J McCluskey, S Lester, P Loiseau, H Teisserenc, J Chapman, B Tait, RL Dawkins. Matching for MHC haplotypes results in improved survival following unrelated bone marrow transplantation. Bone Marrow Transplant 1995;15:381-85.

57. Witt C, D Sayer, F Trimboli, M Saw, R Herrmann, P Cannell, D Baker, FT Christiansen. Unrelated donors selected prospectively by block-matching have superior bone marrow transplant outcome. Hum Immunol 1999;61:85-91.

58. Kitcharoen K, CS Witt, AV Romphruk, FT Christiansen, C Leelayuwat. MICA, MICB, and MHC Beta Block Matching in Bone Marrow Transplantation: Relevance to Transplantation Outcome. Hum Immunol 2006;67:238-46.

59. Foissac A, M Salhi, A Cambon-Thomsen. Microsatellites in the HLA region: 1999 update. Tissue Antigens 2000;55:477-509.

60. Malkki M, T Gooley, M Horowitz, E W Petersdorf. MHC class I, II, and III microsatellite marker matching and survival in unrelated donor hematopoietic cell transplantation. Tissue Antigens 2007;69 (Suppl 1):46-49.

61. Guo Z, L Hood, M Malkki, EW Petersdorf. Long-range multilocus haplotype phasing of the MHC. Proc. Natl. Acad. Sci USA 2006;103:6964-69.

62. Petersdorf EW, M Malkki, TA Gooley, PJ Martin, Z Guo. MHC haplotype matching for unrelated hematopoietic cell transplantation. PLoS Med 2007;4:e8.

63. Gebel HM, RA Bray, P Nickerson. Pretransplant assessment of donor-reactive, HLA-specific antibodies in renal transplantation: Contraindication vs risk Am J Transplant 2003;3:1488-1500.

64. Hansen JA, E Petersdorf, PJ Martin, C Anasetti. Hematopoietic stem cell transplants from unrelated donors. Immunol Rev 1997;157:141-51.

65. Ottinger HD, V Rebmann, KA Pfeiffer, DW Beelen, B Kremens, V Runde, UW Schaefer, H Grosse-Wilde. Positive serum crossmatch as predictor for graft failure in HLA-mismatched allogeneic blood stem cell transplantation. Transplantation 2002;73:1280-85.

66. Tait B. Solid phase assays for HLA antibody detection in clinical transplantation. Current Opinion in Immunology. Ref Type: In Press, 2009.

67. Bingaman AW, CL Murphey, J Palma-Vargas, F Wright. A virtual crossmatch protocol significantly increases access of highly sensitized patients to deceased donor kidney transplantation. Transplantation 2008;86:1864-68.

68. Bray R, Rosen-Bronson S, Haagenson M, Klein J, Flesch S, Vierra-Green C, Spellman S, Anasetti C. The detection of donor-directed, HLA-specific alloantibodies in recipients of unrelated hematopoietic cell transplantation is predictive of graft failure. Blood. 110,2009. Ref Type: Abstract.

69. Takanashi M, K Fujiwara, H. Tanaka, M. Satake, K Nakajima. The impact of HLA antibodies on engraftment of unrelated cord blood transplants. Transfusion 2008;48:791-93.

70. Mattsson J, A Nordlander, M Remberger, M Uhlin, J Holgersson, O Ringden, D Hauzenberger. Cytotoxic crossmatch analysis before allo-SCT is a poor diagnostic tool for prediction of rejection. Bone Marrow Transplant, 2009 (in press).

71. Taylor PA, MJ Ehrhardt, MM Roforth, JM Swedin, A Panoskaltsis-Mortari, JS Serody, BR Blazar. Preformed antibody, not primed T cells, is the initial and major barrier to bone marrow engraftment in allosensitized recipients. Blood 2007;109:1307-15.

72. Xu H, PM Chilton, MK Tanner, Y Huang, C L Schanie, M Dy-Liacco, J Yan, ST Ildstad. Humoral immunity is the dominant barrier for allogeneic bone marrow engraftment in sensitized recipients. Blood 2006;108:3611-19.

73. Gluckman E, HA Broxmeyer, AD Auerbach, HS Friedman, GW Douglas, A Devergie, H Esperou, D Thierry, G Socie, P Lehn, Hematopoietic reconstitution in a patient with Fanconi's anemia by means of umbilical-cord blood from an HLA-identical sibling. N Engl J Med 1989;321:1174-78.

74. Kurtzberg J, M Laughlin, ML Graham, C Smith, JF Olson, EC Halperin, G Ciocci, C Carrier, C E Stevens, P Rubinstein. Placental blood as a source of hematopoietic stem cells for transplantation into unrelated recipients. N Engl J Med 1996;335:157-66.

75. Grewal SS, J N Barker, SM Davies, JE Wagner. Unrelated donor hematopoietic cell transplantation: Marrow or umbilical cord blood? Blood 2003;101:4233-44.
76. Wall DA, KW Chan. Selection of cord blood unit(s) for transplantation. Bone Marrow Transplant 2008;42:1-7.
77. Kamani N, S Spellman, CK Hurley, JN Barker, FO Smith, M Oudshoorn, R Bray, A Smith, TM Williams, B Logan, M Eapen, C Anasetti, M Setterholm, DL Confer. State of the art review: HLA matching and outcome of unrelated donor umbilical cord blood transplants. Biol Blood Marrow Transplant 2008;14:1-6.
78. Rubinstein P, CE Stevens. Placental blood for bone marrow replacement: The New York Blood Center's program and clinical results. Baillieres Best Pract Res Clin Haematol 2000;13:565-84.
79. Wagner JE, JN Barker, TE Defor, KS Baker, BR Blazar, C Eide, A Goldman, J Kersey, W Krivit, ML MacMillan, PJ Orchard, C Peters, DJ Weisdorf, NK Ramsay, SM Davies. Transplantation of unrelated donor umbilical cord blood in 102 patients with malignant and nonmalignant diseases: Influence of CD34 cell dose and HLA disparity on treatment-related mortality and survival. Blood 2002;100:1611-18.
80. Gluckman E, V Rocha, W Arcese, G Michel, G Sanz, KW Chan, TA Takahashi, J Ortega, A Filipovich, F Locatelli, S Asano, F Fagioli, M Vowels, A Sirvent, JP Laporte, K Tiedemann, S Amadori, M Abecassis, P Bordigoni, B Diez, PJ Shaw, A Vora, M Caniglia, F Garnier, I Ionescu, J Garcia, G Koegler, P Rebulla, S Chevret. Factors associated with outcomes of unrelated cord blood transplant: Guidelines for donor choice. Exp Hematol 2004;32:397-407.
81. Gibbons R. Statistical Report: Analysis of the NYBC, NMDP and NHLBI cord blood data. In Cord Blood: Establishing a National Haematopoietic Stem Cell Bank Program. EA Meyer, K Hanna, K Gebbie, eds. National Academies Press 2005;273-82.
82. Chaubey SK, AK Sinha, E Phillips, DB Russell, H Falhammar. Transient cardiac arrhythmias related to lopinavir/ritonavir in two patients with HIV infection. Sex Health 2009;6:254-57.
83. Eapen, M, P Rubinstein, MJ Zhang, C Stevens, J Kurtzberg, A Scaradavou, FR Loberiza, RE Champlin, JP Klein, MM Horowitz, JE Wagner. Outcomes of transplantation of unrelated donor umbilical cord blood and bone marrow in children with acute leukaemia: A comparison study. Lancet 2007;369:1947-54.
84. Kurtzberg J, VK Prasad, SL Carter, JE Wagner, LA Baxter-Lowe, D Wall, N Kapoor, EC Guinan, SA Feig, EL Wagner, NA Kernan. Results of the Cord Blood Transplantation Study (COBLT): Clinical outcomes of unrelated donor umbilical cord blood transplantation in pediatric patients with hematologic malignancies. Blood 2008;112:4318-27.
85. Matsuno N, A Wake, N Uchida, K. Ishiwata, H Araoka, S. Takagi, M Tsuji, H Yamamoto, D Kato, Y Matsuhashi, S Seo, K Masuoka, S Miyakoshi, S Makino, A Yoneyama, Y Kanda, S Taniguchi. Impact of HLA disparity in the graft-versus-host direction on engraftment in adult patients receiving reduced-intensity cord blood transplantation. Blood, 2009;114:1689-95.
86. Kogler G, J Enczmann, V Rocha, E Gluckman, P Wernet. High-resolution HLA typing by sequencing for HLA-A, -B, -C, -DR, -DQ in 122 unrelated cord blood/patient pair transplants hardly improves long-term clinical outcome. Bone Marrow Transplant 2005;36:1033-41.
87. van Heeckeren, WJ, LR Fanning, HJ Meyerson, P Fu, HM Lazarus, BW Cooper, WW Tse, T L Kindwall-Keller, J Jaroscak, MR Finney, RM Fox, L Solchaga, M Forster, RJ Creger, MJ Laughlin. Influence of human leucocyte antigen disparity and graft lymphocytes on allogeneic engraftment and survival after umbilical cord blood transplant in adults. Br J Haematol 2007;139:464-74.
88. Gluckman E. V Rocha. Donor selection for unrelated cord blood transplants. Curr Opin Immunol 2006;18:565-70.
89. Barker JN, DJ Weisdorf, TE Defor, BR Blazar, PB McGlave, JS Miller, CM Verfaillie, JE Wagner. Transplantation of 2 partially HLA-matched umbilical cord blood units to enhance engraftment in adults with hematologic malignancy. Blood 2005;105:1343-47.
90. Majhail NS, CG Brunstein, JE Wagner. Double umbilical cord blood transplantation. Curr Opin Immunol 2006;18:571-75.
91. Ballen KK, TR Spitzer, BY Yeap, S McAfee, BR Dey, E Attar, R Haspel, G Kao, D Liney, E Alyea, S Lee, C Cutler, V Ho, R Soiffer, JH Antin. Double unrelated reduced-intensity umbilical cord blood transplantation in adults. Biol Blood Marrow Transplant 2007;13:82-89.

Chapter 29

The Role of HLA Matching and Recipient Sensitization in Organ Allograft Outcome

Brian D Tait

INTRODUCTION

There are two aspects to consider when assessing the role of HLA in clinical transplantation. Firstly HLA molecules expressed on donor cells are recognized as nonself by the recipient, the resultant immune response being expressed clinically in the form of organ rejection. The rejection response can involve both antibody (humoral) and cell mediated mechanisms. Minimizing the HLA differences therefore between donor and recipient can reduce the likelihood of rejection occurring. The HLA matching effect on solid organ transplantation will be a major theme of this chapter.

The second aspect is the role that antibodies to both HLA class 1 and class 2 molecules play in the rejection process and strategies to both prevent rejection in patients who are previously sensitized to HLA antigens, or who develop antibodies post-transplant. The techniques for detection of HLA antibodies will also be discussed in this chapter.

Early studies on HLA matching in renal transplantation established the principle and importance of HLA matching in improving graft outcome.[1,2] Given our current understanding of the extensive polymorphism of the HLA genes it is somewhat surprising when viewed in retrospect that associations with matching were observed with the limited appreciation of HLA polymorphism at the time. Even more convincing were the studies which established that the presence of HLA antibodies as detected by the microlymphocytotoxicity assay[3] (commonly referred to as the complement dependent cytotoxicity assay or CDC) were associated with early rejection in kidney transplantation.[4,5] This discovery led to the establishment of the pretransplant crossmatch which involved testing the patients' serum against donor cells by CDC, which is also discussed in this chapter. Subsequently the crossmatch became a mandatory requirement for all forms of solid organ transplantation.

ORGAN DONORS

When discussing the role of HLA matching in organ transplantation it is important to specify the type of donor used in the transplant procedure. For example in renal transplantation living related, living unrelated and deceased donor organs can be used. Obviously only deceased donors can be used for heart transplantation but recent developments have permitted both lung and liver transplants to be used from living related donors. The obvious advantages of living donation are firstly that in the case of related donors the level of recipient/donor matching in many cases is superior to that obtained with deceased donors, and secondly for both related and unrelated living donation the cold ischemia time, the prolongation of which can negatively influence both short and long-term graft function, is greatly reduced from that obtained with deceased donors.

An additional variable with respect to deceased organ donors is that while most donations over recent years have been on the basis of brain death criteria, in response to insufficient donors being available for the increasing numbers of patients on the transplant waiting lists, there has been a resurgence in the use of organs from non-heart beating donors.

From a matching and crossmatching perspective living donation provides additional time to determine compatibility between recipient and donor. It allows repeated crossmatching in the case of doubtful results and also permits the use of antibody ablation techniques to be administered in the case of living renal donation where donor specific antibodies are present. This aspect will be discussed in detail under the section *Crossmatch conversion—The role of antibody ablation technology.*

Living unrelated renal donation has taken on a new perspective with the introduction of paired kidney exchange (PKE) schemes. The basis behind the PKE concept is that potential recipient/donor pairs who are prevented from proceeding to transplantation due to blood group or HLA antibody incompatibility may obtain suitably matched organs by simply exchanging donors. Obviously where many patients are involved in a PKE scheme the possibilities of exchange are increased and may involve a 3 way or 4 way exchange. Such schemes require good software support in order to maximize the exchange possibilities and strict uniform criteria across transplant centers relating to the definition of a match.

HLA Matching and Organ Transplantation

Introduction

The definition of the HLA system and its polymorphism in the early 1960s, relied solely on the recognition of serological epitopes. Sera obtained from both multiparous females who formed HLA antibodies as a result of exposure to paternally inherited HLA antigens expressed by fetal tissue, and from patients who had experienced reactions in response to blood transfusions served as the source of HLA antibodies. These antibodies were used in a microlymphocytotoxicity assay utilizing lymphocytes as the target cells for HLA typing.[3] The degree of polymorphism identified in these early days of transplantation was limited and only the class 1 loci HLA-A and HLA-B were recognized, yet surprisingly a beneficial effect on graft survival of matching donors and renal transplant recipients for these two loci was demonstrated.[2] With the discovery and nomenclature standardization of the DR antigens at the 7th International Workshop the effect of matching for DR antigens could also be studied. Numerous studies followed showing a beneficial effect on renal graft survival of matching at HLA- A, B and DR.[6-11] Debate followed on the relative importance of the 3 loci in transplant matching and whether more emphasis should be placed on matching at HLA-A and B or HLA-DR.[12-16] The general consensus emerging was that HLA-B matching appeared more important than HLA-A matching while HLA-B and DR were of equal importance. The difference seen between HLA-A and HLA-B was borne out by subsequent studies which showed that in assays of T cell function there are numerically more precursor T cells capable of recognizing HLA-B differences than HLA-A differences.[17,18]

These findings resulted in various methods of matching patients on a renal transplant waiting list with deceased donors. Many of these algorithms involve a points system where points are lost as a result of a donor incompatibility with the patient. In some algorithms more points are allotted to an HLA-B or DR mismatch than an HLA-A mismatch.

The methods derived for matching therefore, were based on serologically derived epitopes rather than sequenced alleles. The introduction of molecular techniques for HLA genotyping allowed some of these techniques to be used in the renal transplant matching procedure but essentially the level of matching remains at the serological epitope level. There are several reasons for this. Firstly, when a deceased donor becomes available for renal donation there is a limited time in which to retrieve the kidney and perform the transplant, since prolonged cold ischemia time can have a negative impact on the function of the transplanted organ. This time constraint therefore does not permit the use of more sophisticated methods for HLA genotyping such as sequencing in order to assign sequenced alleles. Secondly, the renal transplant waiting lists are not sufficiently large to allow matching of recipients and donors at the allele level. Thirdly, the graft survival results obtained with matching at the epitope level are excellent and the capacity for improvement is limited. The current immunosuppressive drugs available for use in transplantation have narrowed the gap between the graft survival curves for well matched and the poorly matched grafts. The other point to be appreciated is that the discovery of the HLA-C, –DRB3, –DRB4,-DRB5,-DQA1,-DQB1,-DPA1 and DPB1 genes has had little impact on the way kidneys are matched for transplantation. The principle reasons for this is the strong linkage disequilibrium (LD) observed between alleles at HLA-B and HLA-C and between HLA-DRB1 and either DRB3, 4 or 5. Matching for antigens at both HLA-B and –DRB1 results in a degree of matching at the other loci by virtue of this LD. It must be noted however, that the indirect effect of matching by LD is somewhat weakened by matching for antigens rather than alleles. Matching for DPA1 and DPB1 has never been performed prospectively because these antigens cannot be satisfactorily detected by serological means due to their low level of expression on the cell surface.

Finally, there is a scientific as well as practical reason for matching at the serological level. Antibody based rejection poses a more serious risk to graft loss than cellular immunity which is well controlled by current immunosuppressive protocols. Matching for epitopes recognized by B cells therefore appears a rational approach. However, this is tempered by the fact that historically serologically defined epitopes shared between HLA molecules have not been taken into account when matching for transplantation. This aspect is discussed further in the section *Matching in the 21st Century*.

The impact of HLA matching and factors which influence its effect on graft survival are discussed below.

Data Source

The collaborative transplant (CTS) database was established by Gerhard Opelz in Heidelberg, Germany in 1982. As of 2009 data has been freely submitted from over 400 transplant centers in 43 countries worldwide on all forms of solid organ transplantation. There are data on over 300,000 renal transplants in the database. Because the data has been collected over a 10 years span it is possible to analyze both short-term and long-term effects of variables on graft outcome.

One of the criticisms leveled at the CTS database is that the data is derived from so many transplant centers of varying expertise that misleading conclusions may be made which are not applicable to transplant centers worldwide. The opposing argument however is that given the large numbers used in the analyses any heterogeneity effects will become minimal and that statistically significant associations represent findings of true biological significance. No one transplant center would be able to perform all the analyses reported in the CTS and obtain statistical significance due to lack of patient numbers. The CTS database therefore has made an extraordinary contribution to our understanding of factors which impact on all facets of transplant outcome and the reader is encouraged to visit the CTS database at http://www.ctstransplant.org/

Most of the analyses reported in the following have been obtained from the CTS database. Where papers from individual transplant centers are quoted the appropriate reference are used.

HLA Matching for Renal Transplantation

When analyzing the effect of matching, it is conventional to describe differences between donor and recipient as mismatches. A mismatch (MM) is described as an HLA antigen present in the donor which is absent in the recipient. That is a mismatch represents an HLA antigen which the patient is able to recognize as foreign and mount an immune response against it in the form of either cytotoxic T cells or antibodies, which are able to attack the graft. This process is expressed clinically as a rejection episode and can result in loss of the graft.

As shown in Figure 29.1 the data from the CTS study clearly demonstrates that there is a direct association between the number of donor/recipient HLA-A,-B, and -DR mismatches (shown as 0-6 MM) and graft survival in patients receiving their first renal transplant. The data shown is for deceased donor transplants and includes over 136,000 recipients transplanted between 1985 and 2007. The approximate graft survival frequencies for 0 and 6 MM groups at various time points are as follows: 1 year; 91 percent, 81 percent 2 years; 87 percent, 75 percent 10 years; 57 percent, 40 percent respectively. There are several important points which can be made about these data. Firstly the majority of the difference in the time/survival curves between the best matched and worst matched grafts has appeared by 1 year post-transplant. From this point onwards the lines run almost

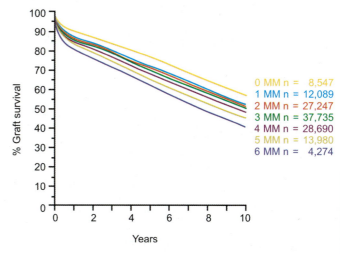

Fig. 29.1: Shows the effect of recipient donor HLA mismatching on primary renal graft survival in a cohort of 132,562 patients. Data is analyzed according to mismatches where each A, B or DR antigen present on the donor but not recipient is counted as one mismatch. The data includes patients transplanted between 1985 and 2007. The effect of mismatching can be seen in the first year post-transplant. Beyond that time point the graphs for each mismatching group are parallel, with each group losing approximately 5% of grafts per year (CTS K-21101-0209)

parallel although the worst matched 6 MM grafts tend towards a steeper decline in graft survival. Secondly although the effect of HLA matching is evident at an early post-transplant period there is a continuing loss of kidneys over time in all matching level groups. The conclusions that can be drawn from this type of analysis is that there is an acute rejection period where kidneys are lost early in the post-transplant period which is highly correlated with the degree of HLA matching. Secondly after patients have overcome this early acute period there is an ongoing chronic loss phase where patients lose kidneys due partly to ongoing antibody mediated rejection, so called chronic rejection. The ongoing loss rate appears fairly constant across all matching grades and is approximately 4 percent per year.

The efficacy of immunosuppressive therapy has improved dramatically over the last 20 years. However, when the matching analysis is restricted to those patients transplanted between 2002 and 2007, graft survival is improved in all groups compared with the earlier data regardless of matching, but the difference between the well matched and the worst matched groups remains.

Figure 29.2 shows an identical analysis for patients receiving a second or subsequent transplant. As with the first graft analysis over 31,000 patients included in the analysis were transplanted between 1985 and 2007. The graft survival figures for the 0 and 6 MM groups at various time points are as follows: 1 year; 85 percent, 74 percent 2 years; 82 percent, 67 percent 5 years; 69 percent, 53 percent respectively. As with the first transplant analysis the major impact of the HLA matching effect is evident at 1 year and from that point onwards the survival curves are parallel. The major differences between the first transplant and retransplant graft survival rates are firstly at each point in time the survival rates are inferior in the second transplant group. For example, the 0MM group in the first transplant analysis had approximate graft survival rates of 91 percent and 87 percent at 1 and 2 years compared with 85 percent and 82 percent in the re-transplant patients. The difference in graft survival between the best and worst matched groups in the retransplants also appears to be greater than in the primary grafts. The differences observed between the primary and subsequent graft cohorts is most likely accounted for by the fact that many patients are sensitized to HLA antigens by their first grafts and hence represent a higher risk group.

HLA Sensitization and the Matching Effect

Sensitization refers to the state of immunization to HLA antigens as detected by the presence of HLA antibodies. When testing pretransplant patients for the presence of HLA antibodies a large panel of HLA typed cells is used for screening in the microlymphocytotoxicity test. The percentage of cells in the panel to which the recipient is sensitized is referred to as the panel reactive antibody percentage or PRA. A PRA of 50 percent therefore, indicates the patients serum is reactive with 50 percent of the panel cells. Antibody screening is discussed further in the section on *HLA antibodies and their impact on renal allograft survival*.

The dramatic impact of HLA sensitization on the matching effect in both primary and secondary and subsequent transplants is shown in Figures 29.3 and 29.4. Again the data are for patients transplanted between 1985 and 2007. The difference between the best HLA matched group (0MM) and the worst matched group (6MM) with respect to graft survival in primary transplant patients is approximately 19 percent, 20 percent and 22 percent at 1, 2 and 5 years respectively, greater differences than that seen in the total first transplant cohort. The difference in graft survival between the best and worst HLA matched groups in the second transplant patients is approximately 21 percent, 22 percent and 23 percent at 1, 2 and 5 years respectively. However, the graft survival figures at each point in time for each matching group are inferior to that seen in the total second transplant groups.

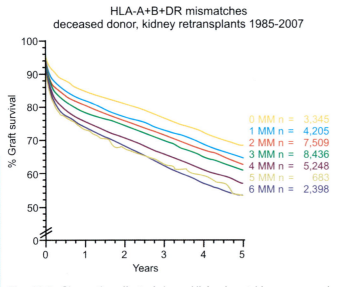

Fig. 29.2: Shows the effect of donor HLA mismatching on second transplant graft survival in a cohort of 31,824 patients. The data includes transplants performed between 1985 and 2007. At every time point the survival for each matching group is inferior to that seen in the comparable matching group for primary transplants (CTS K-21501-0209)

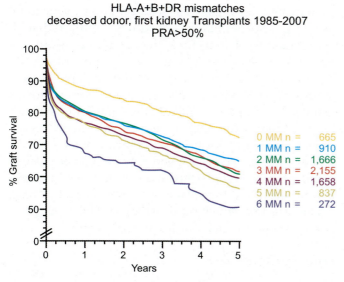

Fig. 29.3: Shows the effect of donor HLA mismatching on primary renal graft survival in patients sensitized with a PRA>50%. The data includes 8,163 patients transplanted between 1985 and 2007. All mismatching groups have inferior graft survival at each time point compared with the comparable matching group in the total primary transplant group (CTS K-21141-0209)

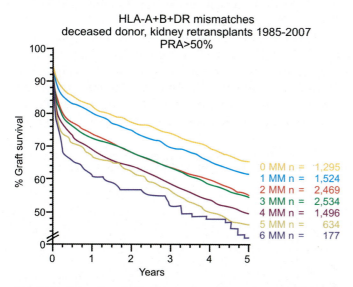

Fig. 29.4: Shows the effect of donor mismatching on second transplant survival in patients sensitized with a PRA>50%. The data includes over 10,129 patients transplanted between 1985 and 2007. The effect of mismatching has the greatest effect in this group with all mismatching groups having inferior graft survival at each time point compared with the comparable matching group in the total second transplant group (CTS K-21511-0209)

The dramatic impact sensitization has on the HLA matching effect probably reflects the presence of undetected HLA sensitization to donor specific antigens given that the specificity of HLA sensitization in the majority of these patients was defined by the CDC techniques. This is supported by the observation that most of the difference seen in graft survival rates between the total group and the sensitized group is evident at 6 months post-transplant suggestive of more rapid acute rejection, perhaps suggestive of donor specific pre-sensitization in a proportion of patients. The effect of sensitization on HLA matching and graft survival appears to be diminished by the use of sensitive solid phase assays for detection of HLA sensitization. Using these techniques and avoiding HLA antigens to which the patient is sensitized results in graft survival that is comparable to that seen in non-sensitized renal transplant patients.[19]

Recipient Race

The American dataset included within the CTS data clearly shows a dramatic effect of recipient race on the association of HLA matching with graft survival rates. While there is a clear effect of improved graft survival with HLA matching in African Americans the graft loss for each matching group is approximately 15-20 percent greater than that seen in the Caucasian group of patients. For example, at 5 years the graft survival rate in Caucasian patients is approximately 64 percent for the 6MM group and 72 percent for the 0MM group. In contrast the comparable figures in the African American dataset is 45 percent for the 6MM group and 59 percent for the 0 and 1MM groups combined (combined due to relatively low numbers). Given the recipients and donors are matched at the generic antigen level there may be a greater number of undetected allele mismatches in the African American patients than the Caucasian patients given that a large proportion of African American patients will have received kidneys from Caucasian donors. It is beyond the scope of this chapter to explore other reasons hypothesized to explain this phenomenon but nevertheless the results highlight the possibility that there may be other racial factors which play a role in determining transplant outcome.

Relevance of HLA Matching in Other Forms of Solid Organ Transplantation

Historically the early results demonstrating the important role of HLA matching and pre-sensitization centered on renal transplantation and established the crossmatch and HLA matching as mandatory criteria for a successful renal transplant program. However, the introduction of other forms of solid organ transplantation were not accompanied initially by the same mandatory requirements for crossmatching. More recent results have shown however that crossmatching is a prerequisite for successful transplantation of heart, lung and liver. While matching also seems to be a variable associated with improved graft survival in heart and lung transplantation there are problems in introducing HLA matching as part of the clinical decision-making for reasons outlined below.

Heart Transplantation

Figure 29.5 is from the CTS dataset and shows the HLA matching effect in a cohort of over 25,000 orthotopic heart transplants. The matching effect is similar to that seen in renal transplants but of a smaller magnitude. The separation of the graphs showing graft survival based on matching grades (0-2, 3, 4, 5, 6 MM based on A,B and DR) are clearly present at 1 year and the difference between the best and worst matched groups at this time point is approximately 4 percent. From that point on the graphs run almost parallel with a graft survival difference between the 0-2MM and the 6MM groups of approximately 6 percent at 5 years post-transplant.

Although there is a significant effect of HLA matching in heart transplantation it has been difficult to apply this information in the clinical setting for several reasons. Firstly, patient waiting lists for heart transplants are not sufficiently large to apply an effective HLA matching strategy. Secondly, the cold ischemia times tolerated by hearts is approximately 6-7 hours, compared with approximately 24 hours for kidneys, which is insufficient time for extensive exchange between geographically separate transplant units in order to give a donor heart to the best matched patient. Thirdly, there are size constraints in transplanting hearts. Unlike kidneys the size of the heart has to be matched to that of the recipient. Finally clinical urgency is a high priority in heart transplantation. Unlike kidney patients who can spend long periods on dialysis waiting for the best matched kidney some heart patients require lifesaving transplants in a short period of time. All these factors mitigate against the use of HLA matching as a selection criteria in cardiac transplantation.

Liver Transplantation

Figure 29.6 shows the CTS data on HLA matching in over 17,000 worldwide liver transplants performed between 1988 and 2007. There is no apparent advantage shown for any of the matching groups. The one year graft survival for liver transplantation is approximately 77 percent at 1 year which decreases to 64 percent at 5 years and 53 percent at 10 years.

The lack of the matching effect in liver transplantation is a topic which has created a great deal of interest with respect to the mechanisms involved and the differences between liver and other forms of solid organ transplants. One of the key differences is that the liver contains large numbers of hematopoietic cells which are released from

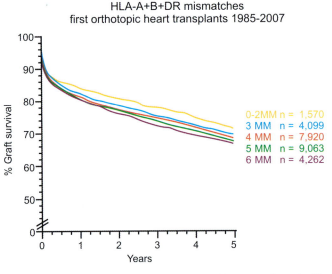

Fig. 29.5: Shows the effect of donor mismatching on graft survival in 26,914 first orthotopic heart transplants performed between 1985 and 2007. Although there is significant effect of HLA mismatching on transplant survival the effect is not as marked as that observed in renal transplantation (CTS H-21101-0809)

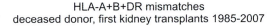
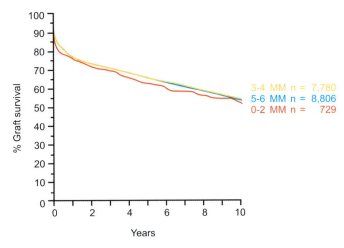

Fig. 29.6: Shows the effect of donor HLA mismatching on graft survival in 17,513 first liver transplants performed between 1985 and 2007. No significant effect of mismatching is observed (CTS L-21101-0209)

the graft and circulate in the recipient circulation. Many of these cells circulate for a prolonged period of time and develop a state of microchimerism in the recipient which may lead to a state of tolerance. Microchimerism is more commonly observed in liver transplantation than other forms of transplantation and may explain the absence of rejection on the withdrawal of immunosuppressive drugs in some patients which has been reported in the literature over the past 20 years. The influx of donor cells into the recipient circulation in liver transplant patients can also lead to graft-versus-host disease which again is more common in liver transplants.

Matching in the 21st Century

Two developments over recent years have challenged the notion of matching based on generic serologically defined antigens particularly in highly sensitized patients. The first was the introduction of molecular typing in defining the degree of HLA polymorphism. It soon became evident that included within serologically defined groups there were many sequence variants or alleles and in many cases these differences were capable of recognition by T cells. The serological definition of HLA antigens is therefore based on epitopes which in the majority of cases are shared between alleles within a serological group and also in some cases shared between alleles of different serological groups. The second development was the introduction of the solid phase assays and in particular the Luminex system for the detection of HLA antibodies in patients awaiting a transplant. The fine definition provided by the single antigen beads has revealed antibodies to allele specific epitopes not previously recognized by CDC techniques. For example, an A*2403 patient who developed an antibody to A*2402 carried by her renal donor, which was associated with rejection.[20]

When highly sensitized patients' antibody profiles are analyzed by Luminex it is possible to demonstrate in many cases that the antibody reactivity can be explained by immunization to a limited number of shared epitopes rather than a large number of antibodies directed at many generic level antigens. With the information provided by molecular typing methods and the precise definition of antibody epitopes it would seem more rational to be applying matching based on epitope sequences. An algorithm has been devised by Duquesnoy et al[21] which assigns amino acid triplets located in polymorphic sites to describe the minimal requirements for a serologically recognized epitope. Using this approach Duquesnoy's group have defined most of the class 1 and class 2 epitopes recognized by both allosera and monoclonal reagents.[22,23] El Awar et al using mouse monoclonal antibodies and eluted or absorbed allosera to define epitopes have described a similar list of sequences which explains most anti-HLA antibody reactivity.[24,25] It has been further shown in renal transplantation that the more triplet mismatches that occur between donor and recipient the higher the frequency of post-transplant immunization and consequently a higher rate of graft rejection.[26] The triplet approach can also be used to define acceptable mismatches in highly sensitized patients. By identifying triplets to which the patient is not immunized combinations of acceptable donor HLA mismatches have been identified which permits transplantation to proceed with a high rate of success.[27]

The definition of acceptable and unacceptable HLA mismatches in organ allocation in order to firstly reduce the number of potential immunizing epitopes and secondly to provide a rational matching approach for highly sensitized patients would seem to be an approach which should be adopted worldwide and would no doubt result in improvement of graft survival particularly for HLA sensitized patients.

HLA ANTIBODIES AND THEIR IMPACT ON RENAL ALLOGRAFT SURVIVAL

Antibodies directed at non-self-HLA determinants expressed on donor cells can result in antibody mediated rejection of the transplanted organ. HLA antibodies produced in the recipient can be either pre-existing in which case the patient is said to be presensitized, or can form post-transplant in response to exposure to foreign HLA antigen on the graft. There are different forms of rejection caused by either antibody (both HLA and non-HLA) or reactive T cells. The reader is referred to a description of the Banff criteria for classifying renal rejection.[28]

When the recipient blood vessels are anastomosed to the vessels on the donor graft the recipient blood flows into the graft and is exposed to endothelial cells lining the donor vessels. Since, these cells express both class 1 and class 2 antigens any pre-existing HLA antibodies in the recipient can attack the cells via fixation of complement and activation of the complement attack complex. This rapid process is termed hyperacute rejection and has become rare in recent years due to the introduction of more sensitive methods of antibody detection. When it occurs it is manifest often in the first few hours but certainly in the first few days post-transplant. HLA antibodies formed *de novo* can be responsible for early and late acute rejection which occurs in the first post-transplant year.[29] Chronic allograft nephropathy which includes chronic rejection is also associated with the presence of both class 1 and class 2 HLA antibodies.[30] The detection of these antibodies post-transplant can be a good predictor of the eventual fate of the graft. HLA antibodies precede the rise in creatinine levels indicating failing renal function. The detection of antibodies in some cases has predicted graft loss several years later.[31] The association of HLA antibodies with chronic rejection has also been observed in heart and lung transplantation.[32]

Despite the association of HLA antibodies with hyperacute, acute and chronic rejection it became evident with the use of the sensitive solid phase assays for detecting HLA antibodies there are some patients with low titre antibodies who have uneventful post-transplant courses. This phenomenon was observed when ABO incompatible renal transplants were first performed and referred to as *antibody accommodation*.[33] Accommodation also occurs with HLA antibodies and is said to exist when donor specific antibodies can be detected in the patient in the absence of any discernible immunological damage to the transplanted organ. There are several possible explanations for the mechanism underlying antibody accommodation which include interference in the complement cascade by CD59,[34] the presence of non-complement fixing antibodies which may block the activity of complement fixing antibodies[35] and the activation of non-apoptopic genes which activate the endothelial cell survival pathway and protect the cell from complement mediated damage.[36]

The presence of potentially damaging HLA antibody can be detected in the graft by performing biopsies of the transplanted organ. Using a monoclonal antibody directed at human C4d, a product of the classical complement cascade, and detection of binding by either immunofluorescence or histochemistry on frozen or paraffin embedded tissue, deposits of C4d can be detected on the endothelial cells lining the capillaries of the transplanted organ. This has become one of the routine tests for diagnosing antibody mediated rejection.

Methods for HLA Antibody Screening

Historically HLA antibody testing of potential transplant recipients was performed using the CDC assay. The process involved testing the patients' sera against a large panel of cells either un-fractionated or enriched for T cells, in order to test for the presence of HLA class 1 antibodies. The cells were obtained from normal individuals designed to represent the majority of known HLA class 1 antigens. Very few laboratories screened all patients routinely for the presence of class 2 antibodies as there was little evidence until the 1990s, that the presence of donor specific HLA class 2 antibodies was a contraindication to transplantation. Prior to the introduction of erythropoietin blood transfusions were given regularly to potential transplant patients on the waiting list. As a result it was imperative to screen patients regularly for the presence of HLA antibodies, usually on a monthly basis to detect any potentially new sensitization. In addition, antibody levels obtained by CDC tend to fluctuate over time in renal dialysis patients largely due to the changing composition of panels used for testing and also the lack of reproducibility of the CDC assay. Regular testing therefore generates cumulative data on the pre-sensitization status of patients and this information can be used to make decisions on the suitability of prospective donors. The introduction of erythropoietin into clinical practice and the use of solid phase assays has resulted in less frequent testing but more accurate assessment of a patient's antibody profile.

The introduction of solid phase assays for the detection of HLA antibodies over the past 10 years has revolutionized the practice of pre- transplant testing and to a large extent replaced the CDC method as the method of choice for antibody screening. The introduction of these techniques into clinical testing laboratories has allowed the detection of sensitization in patients not possible with the less sensitive CDC assay and has permitted an evaluation of the importance of class 2 donor specific antibodies in organ transplantation.

Solid Phase HLA Antibody Detection Methods

The solid phase assays consists of three main types. First introduced into the routine laboratory was the enzyme linked immunosorbent assay (ELISA) specifically modified for the detection of HLA antibodies.[37-39] Purified HLA molecules derived from cell lines are adhered to the bottom of wells in multi-well testing trays. The test serum is added and if an HLA antibody is present it binds to the appropriate HLA molecule. A second enzyme linked anti-human IgG antibody is then added followed by a substrate which changes color in the presence of the enzyme. The extent of color change can be measured on a colorimeter. The specificity of the HLA antibody can be deduced from the pattern of reaction with the array of HLA molecules used.

The second generation of solid phase assays consists of dye impregnated beads bound with recombinant HLA molecules or molecules extracted from cell lines. Two fluorescent dyes are present in differing ratios which gives each type of bead a unique fluorescent signal. One hundred beads are used whose specific signal indicates the HLA molecule or molecules bound. Test serum is added to the beads and the HLA antibody present binds to the appropriate bead or beads which are then detected using a second fluorescent labeled anti- human IgG antibody. There are two methods for the detection of the bound antibody. The first method involves analysis in a flow cytometer, a channel shift indicating the binding of HLA antibody to the beads.[40] The second method[41] which has become the preferred technique in many routine laboratories involves the use of a Luminex (Luminex Corporation, Texas, USA) fluorocytometer containing two lasers. One laser excites the dye in the bead while the other excites the fluorophore bound to the second antibody. The combination of the two signals indicates the presence and the specificity of the bound HLA antibody.

There are three levels of specificity testing using the bead technology. The first involves beads that contain a multitude of either class 1 or class 2 molecules which are used to determine if there are HLA antibodies present in a serum sample. The second level utilizes beads with molecules from one cell line attached which are useful for estimating the panel reactive antibody (PRA) percentage. The third level uses beads with one recombinant HLA molecule attached, the so called single antigen beads (SAG). The use of SAG has enabled sera with complex mixtures of antibodies to be accurately dissected and has enabled the identification of antibodies directed at loci such as HLA-DRB3,-DRB4,-DRB5, -DQA1, -DQB1,-DPA1 and DPB1 which was not possible using the CDC technique.

All three solid phase assay approaches have proved to be more sensitive than CDC in detecting HLA antibodies. The bead assay is the most sensitive with ELISA being of intermediate sensitivity. The use of these assays has revealed HLA antibodies in many potential transplant patients which test negative when tested by CDC. The important question is how clinically relevant are these low level antibodies in the transplant setting.

Antibodies Detected by Solid Phase Assays but not CDC and their Role in Graft Rejection

When comparing antibody screening results obtained by CDC with solid phase assays several factors have to be considered. Firstly CDC detects both complement fixing HLA IgG and IgM antibodies while the solid phase assays only detect IgG unless the tests are run in parallel using both IgG and IgM second antibodies. Antibodies detected by CDC can be identified as IgM by the use of dithiothreitol (DTT) in the antibody antigen reaction which reduces the IgM antibody by destroying the disulphide bonds and hence rendering the reaction negative. The role of HLA IgM antibodies in renal transplant rejection however is somewhat controversial with some reports claiming they are not graft damaging[42-44] while a recent report[45] demonstrated an association of IgM HLA antibodies with renal graft rejection incidence and loss.

The second issue to be considered is the fact that the CDC assay will detect any antibody that reacts with a lymphocyte. In some cases therefore reactivity in the CDC can be due to non-HLA antibodies. In contrast because the solid phase assays employ isolated HLA molecules as the target any reactivity by definition is directed at HLA epitopes.

The third and most critical issue is the fact that while the solid phase assays are a great deal more sensitive than CDC they do not discriminate between complement binding (CB) and non-complement binding (NCB) antibodies. The role of NCB antibodies in graft rejection has not been elucidated although there is evidence that they are present in approximately a quarter of eluates from explanted renal grafts.[46] Modification of the Flow Cytometry technique to measure complement C4 production as a result of complement binding to HLA antibodies has revealed that a percentage of patients have mixtures of both CB and NCB HLA antibodies.[47,48] This emphasizes the importance of defining the complement binding status of antibodies prior to deciding whether or not to proceed with a transplant. One study in heart transplant patients[49] using a modification of the Luminex assay to define the complement binding status of HLA antibodies reported that while patients with CB donor specific (DSA) HLA antibodies detectable by Luminex had inferior graft survival, patients with donor specific NCB HLA antibodies had a graft survival intermediate between those patients with CB DSA and those patients negative for DSA.

Keeping in mind the above points there is now an emerging literature which suggests that the presence of solid phase detectable donor directed HLA antibodies and in particular those detected by the Luminex technique are associated with rejection in several cohorts of patients.[49-53] However, it is also clear that a proportion of patients transplanted with DSA detected only by solid phase techniques have uneventful post-transplant outcomes. Since the solid phase assays are more sensitive than CDC, antibodies that are detected only by the solid phase assays by definition will fall into the low titer range. This can be measured by converting the mean fluorescence index (MFI) obtained using the Luminex technique into molecules of equivalent soluble fluorochrome (MESF).[54] The threshold for CDC positivity is approximately 250,000 while Flow Cytometry which has a similar sensitivity to the Luminex assay detects HLA antibodies with a MESF as low as 18,000-25,000.[55]

Detection of Class 2 Antibodies

One of the most important advantages of the solid phase assays and in particular the single antigen (SAG) bead assay has been the ability to define accurately HLA class 2 antibodies and their role in graft rejection. In addition to antibodies to DRB1 coded antigens antibodies to products of the DRB3, DRB4, DRB5, DQA1, DQB1, DPA1 and DPB1 loci have also been described.[56] The accuracy in definition provided by the SAG assay has also allowed the definition of antibodies to class 2 epitopes shared by several molecules.

MICA and MICB Antigens

The MICA and MICB are highly polymorphic genes which are located in the MHC class 3 region. The structure of the MIC molecules has some homology with the classical HLA-A, B, C molecules with the exception that there is no binding to beta -2 microglobulin and no functional peptide binding groove. The MIC molecules function as stress molecules with limited cell distribution and are upregulated under certain conditions. They are expressed on monocytes, fibroblasts, epithelial cells including gastric epithelium and endothelial cells. Their expression on endothelial cells means that they are targets for antibodies capable of causing humoral rejection. Their upregulation during stress can potentiate their role as targets during organ rejection. There have been several reports in the literature during the last several years which have highlighted the direct role played by antibodies to the MIC molecules in antibody mediated renal rejection.[57-59]

RECIPIENT/DONOR CROSSMATCHING

Pretransplant crossmatching is an essential component of the matching process in solid organ transplantation. The principle underlying crossmatching is the detection of HLA and other antibodies which are specific to the donor (so called donor specific antibodies or DSA). This has been achieved by using a number of technological approaches but the common theme between them is the testing of patients' serum samples for reactivity against patient's cells. The early discovery in the 1960s, that HLA antigens were expressed on lymphocytes circulating in the blood led to early use of isolated donor lymphocytes as the target cell in the crossmatch assay. This has essentially remained the general approach to the present day.

The importance of pretransplant crossmatching was first established in renal transplantation but more recently other forms of solid organ transplantation and in hematopoietic stem cell transplantation (HSCT).

This review will focus on the various technological approaches to crossmatching and the interpretation of positive results in a clinical setting.

Historical Perspective

The earliest method used for detecting HLA antibodies was leukoagglutination which proved to lack reproducibility and viability of granulocytes *in vitro* presented a problem. Paul Terasaki at UCLA overcame these problems by introducing the use of isolated lymphocytes as the target cell and developing a test which could be performed in a microwell using small volumes of sera and became known as the microlymphocytotoxicity or complement dependent cytotoxicity test (CDC).[3]

Principles of the CDC Crossmatch

The basic principle of the crossmatch test is to test the patient's serum for donor specific HLA antibodies by reacting with donor lymphocytes.

One or two microliters of a patient's serum is aliquoted into the wells of a plastic Terasaki typing tray. Two microliters of donor lymphocytes at a concentration of 1×10^6 cells/ml (2,000 cells) are added to the cells. If antibody is present in the serum it binds to the appropriate HLA molecule on the cell membrane. Rabbit serum is then added as a source of complement which mediates lysis of the cells in the presence of specific antibody. Vital dyes are added which can be used to assess the degree of cell lysis. By comparing degrees of cell lysis in the test well with control wells containing normal human serum the presence of donor specific antibody in the patient serum can be ascertained.

Separation of Lymphocytes

Until the mid 1990's lymphocytes were isolated by a density gradient technique. This method uses isopaqueficoll as the separating medium and mononuclear cells harvested at the interface after centrifugation at a specified gravity force. This method provided mononuclear cells of varying purity and the cells obtained consisted of monocytes, and B and T lymphocytes. Since T cells express only HLA class 1 but B cells both HLA class 1 and class 2 molecules further separation was required if information on the class of antibody was required.

This method was superseded by the introduction of magnetic bead technology. Magnetic beads with specific monoclonal antibodies directed at either T cell or B cell specific antigenic epitopes are bound to the appropriate cell type and separated from buffy coat samples by adherence to a magnet. This method provides B and T cells of very high purity for use in the CDC test.

Dyes to Assess Degree of Cytotoxicity

The dye initially used in the CDC test was Eosin. Eosin is a red dye of high molecular weight which can only gain access to the interior of a cell if the membrane has been damaged. Cells whose membranes have been damaged by complement dependent antibody activity therefore permit the passage of Eosin across the membrane staining the cell red. Examining the contents of the wells under a phase contrast microscope allows the visual identification of cells which have undergone lysis due to antibody activity. Adding formaldehyde after Eosin preserved the integrity of the reaction and extends the time over which the result can be read.

Eosin was eventually replaced by Acridine orange and Ethidium Bromide. The advantage of this method is that both lysed and non-lysed cells are stained with the appropriate microscope filters. Lysed cells are stained red with Ethidium Bromide and non-lysed cells green with Acridine orange.

Variations on the CDC Test

Several variations have been added to the CDC test over the years in an effort to increase the sensitivity of the test. These variations include increasing the length of the incubation periods and adding a second antibody in the form of an anti-human IgG antibody.

In order to make the test specific for IgG antibody serum treatment with dithiothreital (DTT) which reduces the pentameric IgM structure was also introduced.

Application of the CDC Crossmatch to Compatibility Testing in Transplantation

Renal Transplantation

It became evident early in renal transplantation that transplanting across a positive crossmatch was associated with hyperacute rejection.[4,5] However, not all transplants suffered this fate and there are several explanations for this observation. Firstly, the early transplants were performed using lymphocytes from either whole blood or spleen with any degree of specific cell death being considered a contraindication. In the absence of lymphocyte fractionation approximately 10 percent of mononuclear cells in peripheral blood and 40 percent in spleen are B lymphocytes. Since, B cells express both HLA class 1 and class 2 molecules some patients were transplanted with a positive B cell crossmatch which may have been due to donor specific HLA class 2 antibodies or to low level class 1 antibodies which are more reactive with B cells than T cells due to their increased expression of class 1 molecules. An additional factor was the presence of antibodies specific for monocytes. Secondly, some patients have auto antibodies reactive with autologous and allogeneic lymphocytes and give the appearance of a positive crossmatch. Thirdly, the date of the serum used in the crossmatch and its proximity to the date of the transplant can be a critical factor in determining the result of the crossmatch and the ultimate fate of the graft. It is imperative therefore to determine the reason for a positive crossmatch before exclusion of a potential donor. Some of the factors requiring consideration are discussed below.

IgM Antibodies—Auto and Alloreactive

When assessing antibodies in potential renal transplant recipients, it is important to include an auto-crossmatch as part of the workup. This involves testing the patient's serum against autologous lymphocytes a positive result being indicative of the presence of autoantibody. Most autoantibodies which react with autologous lymphocytes are of the IgM class. Treatment of the patient's serum with dithiothreitol (DTT) destroys the structure of the pentameric IgM molecule and renders the autologous crossmatch negative. One important issue with this approach however is that in patients who have a mixture of autoantibodies and IgM HLA alloantibodies, the latter is also reduced and is no longer detectable. An alternative approach to inactivating IgM autoantibodies involves heating the serum sample to 63°C. But as with DTT treatment the loss of detection of IgM alloantibodies is still an issue.

Interpreting a positive crossmatch that reduces with DTT should be done in combination with antibody screening results. If a solid phase antibody screening test is performed using an IgM second antibody it is possible to determine if the antibody has HLA specificity and is donor specific. Failing access to this technology screening of the serum can be performed by CDC with and without DTT and an assessment made of the IgM antibody specificity.

Monocyte Specific Antibodies

Antibodies specific for monocytes but non-reactive with lymphocytes are known to be associated with renal graft rejection. Some of these antibodies are clearly not directed at MHC coded antigens as they have been linked to rejection in donor/recipient HLA identical transplants.[60] When crossmatching was first introduced in the 1960s, these antibodies would have been detected in a proportion of patients due to the fact that unfractionated mononuclear cells were used as targets. With the introduction of magnetic bead technology and the use of purified cell populations these antibodies are no longer detected routinely.

Some of the antigens to which monocyte antibodies are directed are also shared with endothelial cells.[61] Since the, endothelial cells lining the donor vasculature are the first cells the recipient circulation comes in contact with it appears the monocyte/endothelial cell shared antigens are the ones involved in graft rejection. Recently a crossmatching kit has been produced which uses endothelial precursor cells as the target cell and renal graft rejection has been shown to be associated with the presence of antibodies specific to these cells.[62]

The targets of endothelial antibodies can be endothelial specific or antigens shared between monocytes and endothelial cells such as MICA and MICB.[63]

HLA Class 2 Antibodies

HLA class 2 antibodies are detected by their reactivity with B lymphocytes and non-reactivity with T lymphocytes. However, reactivity with B lymphocytes can be due to reasons other than the presence of class 2 antibodies. Interpreting positive B cells crossmatches therefore requires information on the HLA antibody specificities detected by previous screening of the patient's serum. Confirmation that the antibody concerned is class 1 in most cases would exclude proceeding with the transplant other than in the living related situation where time would permit antibody ablation processes to be carried out. The situation with respect to donor specific class 2 antibodies is less clear cut.

The advent of solid phase antibody detection methods has permitted a more accurate assessment of the role of class 2 antibodies in renal transplant rejection. There is a paucity of publications linking positive B cell crossmatches due to class 2 antibodies with renal rejection.[64] However, since, the introduction of solid phase assays and particularly the Luminex assay for identifying class 2 antibodies there has been a clear link established between donor specific class 2 antibodies and renal transplant glomerulopathy and rejection.[65-67] It would seem therefore that a positive crossmatch due to class 2 antibodies increases the risk of rejection.

THE RELEVANCE OF CDC CROSSMATCHES IN OTHER SOLID ORGAN TRANSPLANTS

Surprisingly when cardiac, lung and liver transplantation were introduced there was little attention paid to the CDC crossmatch assay as a means of predicting likely rejection. In fact many of these forms of transplantation proceeded in the face of a positive CDC crossmatch. However, mounting evidence supported by solid phase assay screening for HLA antibodies has confirmed that the presence of donor specific antibodies either presenting as a positive crossmatch or in some cases below the threshold of CDC detection can be associated with both acute and chronic rejection.

Heart

In a retrospective study of crossmatching in pediatric cardiac transplantation Wright et al[68] demonstrated that patients with a positive crossmatch and/or a positive panel reactive antibody (PRA) had a significantly raised risk of graft failure. The negative consequences of a positive crossmatch is supported by additional data examining the effects of both class 1 and class 2 antibodies detected by solid phase assays. Donor specific HLA antibodies are associated with transplant vasculopathy[69] and an increased rate of rejection and decreased patient survival.[49] As with renal transplantation immunization to MICA is also associated with acute rejection and its associated vasculopathy.[70] A recent report has linked non-HLA IgM lymphocytotoxic antibodies detected by CDC with ischemic damage and primary allograft failure leading to decreased survival.[71] If independently confirmed this finding will lead to a re-interpretation of the importance of non-HLA antibodies detected in the crossmatch procedure.

Lung

As with heart transplantation the importance of crossmatching prior to lung transplantation is borne out by studies which have shown detrimental effects of both HLA class 1 and class 2 antibodies on transplant outcome.[72-74] The presence of either donor specific class 1 or class 2 HLA antibodies is associated with allograft dysfunction which may result in broncholitis obliterans syndrome (BOS).[74] Hyperacute rejection of lung transplants rarely occurs although when it does appears quite severe and has been shown to be associated with the presence of HLA DSA.[75,76] In one case the antibody was only detected by a solid phase assay being undetectable by CDC.[76] The rejection episode proved fatal which underlines the need for sensitive methods of pretransplant HLA antibody detection to complement the crossmatch results when deciding whether or not to proceed with a transplant.

The long-term presence of both class 1 and class 2 HLA antibodies post-transplant either formed *de novo* or pre-existing is associated with chronic rejection in many forms of solid organ transplantation including lung.[77]

Liver

The general consensus is that antibody mediated rejection occurs to a lesser extent in liver transplant than in other forms of solid organ transplantation. However, several studies have shown poorer outcome in crossmatch positive compared to crossmatch negative transplants in both deceased donor and living donor situations.[78-81] In a large study of living related liver transplants in Japan positive crossmatches were associated with lower survival particularly in older and female recipients. A recent study compared positive and negative crossmatch groups in association with HLA antibody detection by Flow bead technology with clinical outcome.[82] Although acute rejection was not different between the groups there was an increased graft loss in the antibody positive patients, most of the losses occurring in the first post-transplant year.

Additional Crossmatch Techniques

Flow Cytometry

Besides CDC the most commonly used crossmatch technique utilizes Flow Cytometry. Basically the Flow cytometer (fluorescent activated cell sorter FACS) consists of a light beam which is focused at right angles on a cell chamber though which cells pass in a fluid stream. The light is reflected from cells in a manner dependent on their physical properties. The deflected light is captured by photodectors which detect forward and side light scatter as well as signals emitted by specific fluorochromes. In the crossmatch application specific fluorescein labeled monoclonal antibodies are used to identify the cell population under study, in this case B and T lymphocytes. The patient's serum is incubated with the donor cells and then washed to remove unbound antibody. A second fluorescein labeled anti-human IgG (or IgM) antibody is then used which binds to the patient's primary antibody. Passing the cells through the Flow Cytometer will then identify the type of cell and whether or not the patient's antibody has bound.[83]

Flow cytometry crossmatching (FCXM) sometimes referred to as FACS crossmatching has proved to be more sensitive than the CDC technique and there are numerous papers describing the association of a positive FACS result with increased incidence of rejection in renal transplantation including cases where the CDC crossmatch was negative. The effect appears more marked when the positive crossmatch is due to HLA class 1 antibodies.[84-93]

As with CDC both rejection incidence and reduced survival have been demonstrated with positive FACS crossmatches in heart and liver transplantation.[94-97]

Although more sensitive than CDC the Flow crossmatch does not differentiate between complement and non-complement fixing antibodies. However, a recent paper by Saw et al[98] describes a method enabling the Flow crossmatch to simultaneously measure the presence of HLA antibody and complement binding.

ELISA-based Crossmatching

An ELISA crossmatch technique has been developed (GTI, Wisconsin USA) called the antibody monitoring system (AMS) which involves the detergent solubilization of donor lymphocytes. The membrane glycoproteins are added to wells of a microtiter tray containing a bound monoclonal antibody to either HLA class 1 or class 2 molecules. After washing to remove the unbound glycoproteins the recipient's serum is added. Donor specific antibody present in the patients'serum bind to the HLA molecule. Goat anti-human IgG antibody conjugated to alkaline phosphatase is then added which when bound is detected with a p-nitrophenyl phosphate substrate, the readout being a color change. Being an ELISA based method the sensitivity is greater than that obtained with CDC and can be applied as a pre-transplant crossmatch procedure or alternatively as a post-transplant monitoring assay. The use of this method post-transplant avoids the necessity of storing viable donor lymphocytes. Aliquots of the solubilized material can be stored and used when required.

Luminex Crossmatch

As with the ELISA technique a Luminex crossmatch is essentially the same method that is used for antibody screening with the exception that in the crossmatch situation donor MHC molecules are attached to the beads. This is achieved by using beads coated with monoclonal antibodies to either class 1 or class 2 molecules. Cell lysates of donor lymphocytes are prepared by treatment with nonionic lysis buffer. The lysate is incubated with the beads which enables binding of the donor HLA molecules. After washing to remove excess lysate the recipient serum sample is added followed after an incubation period by anti-human IgG conjugated with phycoerythrin. Fluorescent intensity is then measured on the Luminex cytometer as previously described for antibody screening. Being a Luminex based technology this method of crossmatching like the ELISA crossmatch is more sensitive than CDC. In a recent retrospective study of the importance of the Luminex crossmatch in renal transplantation Billen et al[99] demonstrated that approximately 20 percent of patients with a negative CDC crossmatch had a positive Luminex crossmatch due either to donor specific class 1 or class 2 antibodies. While there was no observed short-term effect in the Luminex crossmatch positive group long-term graft survival was significantly lower in those patients with class 1 antibodies directed at the donor, while donor specific class 2 antibodies appeared to have no long-term deleterious effects.

The Luminex crossmatch would appear to have a role in future matching for renal transplantation and like the ELISA method is amenable to post-transplant crossmatch monitoring.

The Virtual Crossmatch

With the excellent definition of HLA antibodies now possible with the solid phase techniques some transplant centers are placing more emphasis on the antibody screening results rather than the actual crossmatch, particularly if CDC crossmatching is the only technique available. Some centers therefore have abandoned the crossmatch procedure and rely solely on HLA antibody screening results to determine if a donor is acceptable to a particular recipient. In the absence of any detectable class 1 or class 2 HLA donor specific antibodies it is deemed safe to proceed with the transplant. While logically this approach seems acceptable most centers however, still include the crossmatch within the matching algorithm as added proof of recipient/donor compatibility.

Crossmatch Conversion—The Role of Antibody Ablation Technology

As stated earlier a positive crossmatch particularly due to HLA class 1 antibodies is considered a contraindication in solid organ transplantation. However, new approaches taken in the last 8-10 years has made it possible to convert a positive living related or unrelated donor crossmatch to negative.[100-102] This is achieved by a process called antibody ablation. The aim of antibody ablation is to remove or greatly reduce antibody in the circulation of the recipient hence rendering the crossmatch negative. This process however does not remove circulating plasma cells and therefore the antibody often re-appears after transplantation. It does avoid hyperacute rejection however and in the majority of cases the subsequent re-appearance of antibody can be countered post-transplant by further antibody ablation procedures and careful immunological monitoring of the patient.

Although there are several variations on the antibody ablation technique the essential elements are firstly the use of plasma exchange (PE) to physically reduce the amount of circulating antibody and secondly the administration of pooled intravenous immunoglobulin (IVIG). Rituximab (an anti-CD20 monoclonal) is also now used as an adjunct therapy. CD20 is expressed on B cells but not mature plasma cells so while there is no removal of antibody secreting cells some centers have reported positive benefits of using this drug in combination with IVIG and/or PE.[103,104]

IVIG is prepared from the plasma fractionation of 3000-6000 blood donors and consists of Cohn fraction 2 which is >95 percent IgG. Originally used for passive transfer of anti-pathogen antibodies in immunodeficiency cases, renewed interest in the mode of action was stimulated by the observation that IVIG has a suppressive effect on HLA antibody production in renal patients awaiting a transplant.[105] It has also been used effectively to reduce autoantibodies in autoimmune disease patients.[106] There have been many proposed mechanisms suggested for the mode of action of IVIG including Fc receptor mediated effects, interference in the complement cascade, and effects on T cells and cytokines.[107] However, the most intriguing proposed mode of action is the passive transfer of anti-idiotypic antibodies with HLA specificity.[108] Such antibodies could conceivably reduce the amount of circulating antibody by forming complexes with the primary anti-HLA antibody and also either block or eradicate B cells with the appropriate B cell receptor. *In vitro* evidence for such a mechanism includes the observation that the current serum of some patients who have falling HLA antibody levels is able to abrogate the activity of the peak antibody serum in a lymphocytotoxicity assay.[109]

REFERENCES

1. Lee HM, Hume DM, Vredevoe DL, Mickey MR, Terasaki PI. Serotyping for homotransplantation. IX Evaluation of leukocyte antigen matching with clinical course and rejection types. Transplantation 1967;5(4):1040-45.
2. Ogden DA, Porter KA, Terasaki PI, Marchioro TL, Holmes JH, Starzl TE. Chronic renal homograft function. Correlation with histology and lymphocyte antigen matching. American Journal of Medicine 1967;43(6):837-45.
3. Terasaki PI, McClelland JD. Microdroplet assay of human cytotoxins Nature 1964; 204:998-1000.
4. Morris PJ, Williams GM, Hume DM, Mickey MR, Terasaki PI. Serotyping for homotransplantation XII Occurrence of cytotoxic antibodies following kidney transplantation in man. Transplantation 1968;6(3):392-99.
5. Patel R, Terasaki PI. Significance of the positive crossmatch test in kidney transplantation. New Eng J Med 1969;280(14):735-39.
6. Persijn GG, Gabb BW, Van Leeuwen A. Matching for HLA antigens of A, B and DR loci in renal transplantation by Eurotransplant. Lancet 1968; 1(8077):1278-81.
7. Persijn GG, Cohen B, Van Rood JJ. Eurotransplant: Improved graft survival through HLA-A,-B and DR-matching and prospective blood transfusion policy. Dialysis and Transplantation 1979;8(5):493-97.
8. Festenstein H, Pachoula-Papasteriadis C, Sachs JA. Collaborative scheme for tissue typing and matching in renal transplantation X. Effect of HLA-A, B, D, and DR matching and pretransplant blood transfusions on 769 cadaver renal grafts. Transplantation Proceedings 1979;11(1):752-55.
9. Van Hooff JP, Van Hooff-Eijkenboom YEA, Kalff MW. Kidney graft survival, clinical course, and HLA-A, B, and D matching in 208 patients transplanted in one centre. Transplantation Proceedings 1979;11(2):1291-92.
10. Albrechtsen D, Bratlie A, Kiss E. Significance of HLA matching in renal transplantation. A prospective one centre study of 485 transplants matched or mismatched for HLA-A, B, C, D, and DR antigens. Transplantation 1979; 28(4):280-84.
11. Lenhard V, Dreikorn K, Rohl L. Results of kidney transplantation in relation to HLA-A, B, DR matching and quality of donor organ. Proceedings of the European Dialysis and Transplant Association 1980;17:450-56.
12. Albrechtsen D, Flatmark A, Jervell J. Significance of HLA-D/DR matching in renal transplantation. Lancet 1978;2(8100):1126-27.
13. Ting A, Morris PJ. Powerful effect of HLA-DR matching on survival of cadaveric renal grafts Lancet 1980;2(8189):282-85.
14. Moen T, Albrechtsen D, Flatmark A. Importance of HLA-DR matching in cadaveric renal renal transplantation. A prospective one centre study of 170 transplants. New Eng.J. Medicine 1980;303(15):850-54.
15. D'Apice AJF, Sheil AGR, Tait BD, Bashir HV. Controlled trial of of HLA-A, B versus DR matching in cadaveric renal transplantation. Transplant Proceedings 1981;13(1):938-41.
16. MacLeod AM, Mason RJ, Catto GRD. HLA and renal transplantation: Yet another approach. Journal of Medical Genetics 1981;18(6):461-63.
17. Zhang L, Van Bree S, Van Rood JJ, Claas FHJ. The effect of individual HLA-A and –B mismatches on the generation of cytotoxic T lymphocyte precursors. Transplantation 1990;50(6):1008-10.
18. Roelen DL, Van Bree SPMJ, Van Beelen E, Schanz U, Van Rood JJ, Claas FHJ. Cytotoxic T lymphocytes against HLA-B antigens are less naive than cytotoxic T lymphocytes against HLA-A antigens. Transplantation 1994;57(3):446-50.
19. Bray RA, Nolen JDL, Larsen L, Pearson T, Newell KA, Kokko K, Guasch A, Tso P, Mendel JB, Gebel HM. Transplanting the highly sensitized patient: The Emory algorithm. American J Transplantation 2006;6(10):2307-15.
20. Pancoska C, Breed R, Harris P, Sonuga B, Venzon I. Emergent PRA technologies may detect unexpected antibodies in the sera of solid organ transplant recipients. One Lambda Advanced LABMAS Workshop, Los Angeles, August 14-17th, 2007.
21. Duquesnoy RJ. HLAMatchmaker. A molecularly based algorithm for histocompatibility determination. Description of the algorithm. Human Immunology 2002;63(5):339-52.
22. Duquesnoy RJ, Marrari M. Correlation between Terasaki's HLA class 1 epitopes and HLAMatchmaker defined eplets on HLA-A,-B and C antigens. Tissue Antigens 2009;74(2):117-33.

23. Mararri M, Duquesnoy RJ. Correlation between Terasaki's HLA class 2 epitopes and HLAMatchmaker defined eplets on HLA-DR and –DQ antigens. Tissue Antigens 2009; 74(2):134-46.
24. El-Awar N, Lee J-H, Tarsitani C, Terasaki PI. HLA class 1 epitopes: Recognition of binding sites by mAbs or eluted alloantibody confirmed with single recombinant antigens. Human Immunology 2007;68(3):17-180.
25. El-Awar N, Terasaki PI, Cai J, Deng CT, Ozawa M, Nguyen A. Epitopes of the HLA-A, B, C, DR, DQ and MICA antigens. Clinical Transplants 2007;175-94.
26. Claas FHJ, Roeln DL, Dankers MKA, Persijn GG, Doxiadis IIN. A critical appraisal of HLA matching in today's renal transplantation. Transplantation Reviews 2004;18(2):96-102.
27. Duquesnoy RJ, Takemoto S, De Lange P, Doxiadis IIN, Schreuder GMTh, Persijn GG, Claas FHJ. HLA Matchmaker: A molecularly based algorithm for histocompatibility determination. III. Effect of matching at the HLA-A, B amino acid triplet level on kidney transplant survival. Transplantation 2003; 75(6):884-89.
28. Solez K, Colvin RD, Racusen LC, Haas M, Sis B, Mengel M, Halloran PF, et al. Banff 07 classification of renal allograft pathology. Updates and future directions. American J. Transplantation 2008;8(4):753-60.
29. Girnita AL, Girnita DM, Zeevi A. Role of anti-HLA antibodies in allograft rejection. Current Opinion in Organ Transplantation 2007;12(4):420-25.
30. Ozawa M, Terasaki PI, Lee JH, Castro R, Alberu J, Alonso C, Alvarez I, Toledo R, Alvez H, et al. 14th International HLA and Immunogenetics Workshop: Report on the prospective chronic rejection project. Tissue Antigens 2007; 69(Supp1):174-79.
31. Worthington JE, Martin S, Al-Husseini DM, Dyer PA, Johnson RWG. Post-transplantation production of donor HLA specific antibodies as a predictor of renal transplant outcome. Transplantation 2003;75(7):1034-40.
32. Terasaki PI. Humoral theory of transplantation. American J Transplantation 2003;3(6):665-73.
33. Chopek MW, Simmons RL, Platt JL. ABO- incompatible kidney transplantation: Initial immunopathologic evaluation. Transplant Proceedings 1987; 19:4533-57.
34. Hung Y, Qiao F, Abagyan R, Hazard S, Tomlinson S. Defining the CD59-C9 binding interaction. Journal of Biological Chemistry 2006; 281(37) 27398-404.
35. Koch CA, Khalpey ZI, Platt JL. Accommodation: Preventing injury in transplantation and disease. Journal of Immunology 2004;172:5143-48.
36. Hanto DW. ABO-incompatible transplantation: Accommodation by upregulation of protective genes-A hypothesis. International Congress Series 2006; 1292: 53-60.
37. Kao KJ, Scornik JC, Small JC. Enzyme linked immunoassay for anti-HLA antibodies-an alternative to panel studies by lymphocytotoxicity. Transplantation 1993;55(1):192-96.
38. Worthington JE, Robson AJ, Sheldon S, Langton A, Martin S. A Comparison of enzyme- linked immunoabsorbent assays and flow cytometry techniques for the detection of HLA specific antibodies. Hum. Immunol 2001;62(10): 1178-84.
39. Monien S, Salama A, Schonemann C. ELISA methods detect HLA antibodies with variable sensitivity. Int J Immungenet. 2006;33(3):163-66.
40. Rebibou JM, Chabod J, Bittencourt MC, Thevenin C, Chalopin JM, Herve P, Tiberghien P. Flow PRA evaluation for antibody screening in patients awaiting kidney transplantation. Transpl. Immunol 2000;8(2):125-28.
41. Colombo MB, Haworth SE, Poli F, Nocco A, Puglisi G, Innocente A, Serafini M, Messa P, Scalamogne M. Luminex technology for anti-HLA antibody screening: Evaluation of performance and of impact on laboratory routine. Cytometry B Clin.Cytom. 2007;72(6):4645-71.
42. Smith JD, Danskine AJ, Rose ML, Yacoub MH. Successful renal transplantation in the presence of donor specific HLA IgM antibodies. Trans Proc 1992;27:664.
43. Tardif GN, McCalmon RT. Successful renal transplantation in the presence of donor specific HLA IgM antibodies. Trans.Proc 1995;27 (1):664-65.
44. Suzuki M, Ishida H, Komatsu T, Kennoki T, Tshizuka T, Tanabe K. Kidney transplantation in a recipient with anti-HLA antibody IgM positive. Transplant Immunology 2009;21(3):150-54.
45. Stastny P, Ring S, Lu C, Arenas J, Han M, Lavingia B. Role of immunoglobulin (Ig) –G and IgM antibodies against donor human leukocyte antigens in organ transplant recipients. Human Immunology 2009;70(8): 600-604.
46. Heinemann FM, Roth I, Rebmann V, Arnold ML, Witzke O, Wilde B, Spriewald BM, Grosse-Wilde H. Immunoglobulin isotype-specific characterization of anti-human leukocyte antigen antibodies eluted from explanted renal allografts. Hum.Immunol 2007;68 (6):500-06.
47. Wahrmann M, Exner M, Regele H, Derfler K, Kormoczi GF, Lhotta K, Zlabinger GJ, Bohmig JA. Flow cytometry based detection of HLA alloantibody mediated classical complement activation. J Immunological Methods 2003;275:149-60.
48. Wahrmann M, Exner M, Schillinger M, Haidbauer B, Regele H, Kormoczi GF, Horl WH, Bohmig GA. Pivotal role of complement fixing HLA antibodies in pre-sensitized kidney allogaft recipients. American. J Transplantation 2006;6(5 Pt1) 1033-41.
49. Smith JD, Hamour IM, Banner NR, Rose M. C4d fixing Luminex antibodies – A new tool for prediction of graft failure after heart transplantation. American Journal of Transplantation. 2007;7:2809-15.
50. Gibney EM, Cagle LR, Freed B, Warnell SE, Chan L, Wiseman AC. Detection of donor specific antibodies using HLA coated microspheres. Another tool for kidney transplant risk stratification. Nephrology Dialysis and Transplantation 2006;21:2625-29.

51. Gupta A, iveson V, Varagunam M, Bodger S, Sinnott P, Thuraisingham RC. Pretransplant donor specific antibodies in cytotoxic negative crosmatch kidney transplants: Are they relevant? Transplantation 2008; 85(8):1200-04.
52. van den Berg-Loonen EM, Billen EVA, Voorter CVM, van Heurn LWE, Claas FHJ, van Hooff JP, Christiaans MHL. Clincal relevance of pre-transplant donor-directed antibodies detected by single antigen beads in highly sensitized renal transplant patients. Transplantation. 2008, 85(8):1086-90.
53. Castillo-Rama M, Castro MJ, Bernardo I, Meneu-Diaz JC, Elola-Olaso AM, Calleja-Antolin SM, Romo E, Morales P, Moreno E, Paz-Artal E. Preformed antibodies detected by cytotoxic assay or multibead array decrease liver allograft survival: Role of human leukocyte antigen compatibility. Liver Transplantation 2008;14(4):554-62.
54. Vaidya S. Clinical importance of anti-human leukocyte antigen–specific antibody concentration in performing calculated panel reactive antibody and virtual crossmatches. Transplantation 2008;85(7):1046-50.
55. Vaidya S, Partlow DA, Suskind b, Gugliuzzi K. Prediction of crossmatch outcome of highly sensitized patients by single and/or multiple antigen bead Luminex assay. Abstract 870.The First Joint International Transplant Meeting, Boston Massachussetts July 2006.
56. Duquesnoy R, Awadalla Y, Lomago J, Jelinek L, Howe J, Zern D, Hunter B, Martell J, Girnita A, Zeevi A. Retransplant candidates have donor specific antibodies that react with structurally defined HLA-DR,DQ,DP epitopes. Transplant Immunology 2008;18(4):352-60.
57. Terasaki PI, Ozawa M, Castro R. Four years follow-up of a prospective trial of HLA and MICA antibodies on kidney graft survival. Am J Transplant 2007;7(2):408-15.
58. Panigrahi A, Gupta N, Siddiqui JA, Margoob A, Bhowmik D, Guleria S, Mehra NK. Post-transplant development of MICA and anti-HLA antibodies is associated with acute rejection episodes and renal allograft loss. Hum.Immunol 2007;68(5):362-67.
59. Alvarez-Marquez A, Aquilera I, Gentil MA, Caro JL, Bernal G, Alonso JF, Acevedo MJ, Cabello V, Wichmann I ,Gonzales-Escribano MF, Nunez-Roldan A. Donor-specific antibodies against HLA,MICA, and GSTT1 in patients with allograft rejection and C4d depostion in renal biopsies. Transplantation 2009; 1:94-99.
60. Cerilli J, Bay W, Brasile L. The significance of the monocyte crossmatch in recipients of living related HLA identical kidney grafts. Human Immunology. 1983;7(1):45-50.
61. Stastny P. Endothelial monocyte antigens in man. Transplantation Proceedings 1978;10(4):875-77.
62. Breimer ME, Rydberg L, Jackson AM, Lucas DP, Zachary AA, Melancon JK, Visger JD, Pelletier R, Saidman SL, Williams WW, Holgersson J, Tyden G, Klintmalm GK, Coultrup S, Sumitran-Holgersson S, Grufman P. Multicenter evaluation of a novel endothelial cell crossmatch test in kidney transplantation. Transplantation 2009;87(4):549-56.
63. Zwimmer NW, Dole K, Stastny P. Differential surface expression of MICA by endothelial cells, fibroblasts, keratinocytes and monocytes. Human Immunology 1999;60( ):323-30.
64. Le Bas-Bernardet S, Hourmant M, Velentin M, Paitier C, Gral-Classe M, Curry S, Follea G, Soulillou J-P, Bignon JD. Identification of the antibodies involved in B-cell crossmatch positivity in renal transplantation. Transplantation 2003;75(4):477-82.
65. Lee PC, Ozawa M. Reappraisal of HLA antibody analysis and crossmatching in kidney transplantation. Clinical Transplants 2007;219-226.
66. Issa N, Cosio FG, Gloor JM, Sethi S, Dean PG, Moore SB, Degoey S, Stegall MD. Transplant glomerulopathy: Risk and prognosis related to anti-human leukocyte antigen clas 2 antibody levels. Transplantation 2008;86(5):681-85.
67. Duquesnoy RJ. Human leukocyte antigen class 2 antibodies and transplant outcome. Transplantation 2008;86(5):638-40.
68. Wright EJ, Fiser WP, Edens RE, Frazier EA, Morrow WR, Imamura M, Jaquiss RDB. Cardiac transplant outcomes in pediatric patients with pre-formed anti-human leukocyte antigen antibodies and/or positive retrospective crossmatch. Journal of Heart and Lung Transplantation 2007;26(11):1163-69.
69. Kaczmarek I, Deutch MA, Kauke T, Beiras-Frnanadez A, Schmoeckel M, Vicol C, Sodian R, Reichart B, Spannagl M, Ueberfuhr P. Donor –specific HLA antibodies: Long-term impact on cardiac allograft vasculopathy and mortality after heart transplantation. Experimental and clinical transplantation: Official Journal of the Middle East Society for Organ Transplantation 2008;6(3):229-35.
70. Kauke T, Kaczmarek I, Dick A, Schmoeckel M, Deutch M-A, Beiras-Frnandez A, Reichart B, Spannagl M. Anti-MICA antibodies are related to adverse outcome in heart transplant recipients. Journal of Heart and Lung Transplantation 2009;28(4):305-11.
71. Smith JD, Hamour IM, Burke MM, Mahesh B, Stanford RE, Haj-Yahia S, Robinson DR, Kaul P, Yacoub MH, Banner NR, Rose ML. A re-evaluation of the role of IgM non-HLA antibodies in cardiac transplantation. Transplantation 2009;87(6):864-71.
72. Morrell MR, Patterson GA, Trulock EP, Hachem RR. Acute antibody-mediated rejection after lung transplantation. Journal of Heart and Lung Transplantation 2009;28(1):96-100.
73. Girnita AL, Lee TM, McCurry KR, Baldwin WM, Yousem SA, Detrick B, Pilewski J, Toyoda Y, Jelinek L, Lomago J, Zaldonis D, Spichty KJ, Zeevi A. Anti-human leukocyte antigen antibodies, vascular C4d deposition and increased soluble C4d in bronchoalveolar lavage of lung allografts. Transplantation 2008;86(2):342-47.
74. Bharat A, Kuo E, Steward N, Aloush A, Hachem R, Trulock EP, Patterson GA, Meyers BF, Mohanakumar T. Immunological link between primary graft dysfunction and chronic allograft rejection. Annals of Thoracic Surgery 2008; 86(1):189-97.

75. de Jesus Peixoto Comargo J, Marcantonio Camargo S, Marcelo Schio S, Noguchi Machuca T, Adelia Perin F. Hyperacute rejection after single lung transplantation: A case report. Transplantation Proceedings 2008;40(3): 867-69.
76. Masson E, Stern M, Chabod J, Thevenin C, Gonin F, Rebibou J-M, Tiberghein P. Hyperacute rejection after lung transplantation caused by undetected low-titer anti-HLA antibodies. Journal of Heart and Lung Transplantation. 2007; 26(6):642-45.
77. Ozawa M, Terasaki PI, Catro R, Alberu J, Morales-Buenrostro L, Alvarez, L, et al. 14th International HLA and Immunogenetics Workshop prospective chronic rejection project: A three years follow-up analysis. Clinical Transplants 2007:255-60.
78. Nikaein A, Backman I, Jennings L, Levy MF, Goldstein R, Gonwa T, Stome MJ, Klintmalm G. HLA compatibility and liver transplant outcome. Improved patient survival by HLA and crossmatching. Transplantation 1994;58 (7):786- 92.
79. Muro M, Sanchez-Bueno F, Moya-Quiles MR, Martin L, Torio A, Minguela A, Sanchis MJ, Garcia-Alonso AM, Parrilla P, Alvarez-Lopez MR. Liver allograft survival in specifically presensitized recipients with a positive T lymphocyte crossmatch. European Journal of Immunogenetics 2001;28(2):265.
80. Suehiro T, Shimada M, Kishikawa K, Shimura T, Soejima Y, Yoshizumi T, Hashimoto K, Mochida Y, Maehara Y, Kuwano H. Influence of HLA compatibility and lymphocyte crossmatch-matching on acute cellular rejection following living donor adult liver transplantation. Liver International 2005; 25(6):1182-88.
81. Kasahara M, Kiuchi T, Takakura K, Uryuhara K, Egawa H, Asonuma K, Uemoto S, Inomata Y, Ohwada S, Morishita Y, Tanaka K. Post-operative flow cytometry crossmatch in living donor liver transplantation: Clinical significance of humoral immunity in acute rejection. Transplantation.199, 67(4):568-75.
82. Muro M, Marin L, Miras M, Moya-Quiles R, Minguela A, Sanchez–Bueno F, Bermejo J, Robles R, Ramirez P, Garcia-Alonso A, Parrilla P, Alvarez-lopez MR. Liver recipients harbouring anti-donor preformed lymphocytotoxic antibodies exhibit a poor allograft survival at the first year after transplantation: Experience of one centre. Transplant Immunology 2005;14(2):91-107.
83. Horsburgh T, Martin S, Robson AJ. The application of flow cytometry to histocompatibility testing. Transplant Immunology 2000;8(1):3-15.
84. Ogura k, Terasaki PI, Johnson C, Mendez R, Rosentahl JT, Ettenger R, Martin DC, Dainko F, Cohen L, Mackett T, Berne T, Barba L, Leiberman E. The significance of a positive flow cytometry crossmatch test in primary kidney transplantation. Transplantation 1993;56(2):294-98.
85. Talbot D. Flow cytometric crossmatching in human organ transplantation. Transplant Immunology 1994;2(2):138-39.
86. Talbot D, White M, Shenton BK, Bell A Forsythe JLR, Proud G, Taylor RMR. Flow cytometric crossmatching in renal transplantation—The Long term outcome. Transplant Immunology 1995;3(4):352-55.
87. Nelson PW, Eschliman P, Shield CF, Aeder MI, Luger AM, Pierce GE, Bryan CF. Improved graft survival in cadaveric renal transplantation by flow crossmatching. Archives of Surgery 1996;131(6):599-603.
88. Cassens U, Garritsen H, Kelsch R, Sibrowski W. Flow cytometric crossmatch in solid organ transplantation. Infusiontherapie und Transfusionmedizin 1998; 25(1): 8-14.
89. Bryan CF, Baier KA, Nelson PW, Luger AM, Martinez J, Pierce GE, Ross G, Shield CF, Warady BA, Aeder MI, Helling TS, Muruve N. Long-term graft survival is improved in cadaveric renal transplantation by flow cytometric crossmatching. Transplantation 1998;66(12): 1827-32.
90. O' Rourke RW, Osorio RW, Friese CE, Lou CD, Garavoy MR, Bachetti P, Ascher NL, Melzer JS, Roberts JP, Stock PG. Flow cytometry crossmatching as a predictor of acute rejection in sensitized recipients of cadaveric renal transplants. Clinical Transplantation 2000;14(2):167-73.
91. Kaprinski M, Rush D, Jeffery J, Exner M, Regele H, Dancea S, Pochinco D, Birk P, Nickerson P. Flow cytometric crossmatching in primary renal transplant recipients with a negative anti-human globulin enhanced cytotoxicity crossmatch. Journal of the American Society of Nephrology 2001; 12(12):2807-14.
92. Abdel Rahman AS, Fahim NM, El Sayed AA, El Hady SA, Ahmad YS. Comparative study between cytotoxicity and flow cytometry crossmatches before and after renal transplantation. The Egyptian Journal of Immunology/Egyptian Association of Immunologists 2005;12(2):77-89.
93. Ilham MA, Winkler S, Coates E, Rizzello A, Rees TJ, Asderakis A. Clinical significance of a positive flow crossmatch on the outcomes of cadaveric renal transplants. Transplant Proceedings 2008;40(6):1839-43.
94. Ogura K, Terasaki PI, Koyama H, Chia J, Imagawa DK, Busuttil RW. High one month liver graft failure rates in flow cytometry crossmatch-positive recipients. Clinical Transplantation 1994;8(21):111-15.
95. Aziz S, Ahmad Hassantash S, Nelson K, Levy W, Kruse A, Reichenbach D, Himes V, Fishbein D, Allen MD. The clinical significance of flow cytometry crossmatchng in heart transplantation. Journal of Heart and Lung Transplantation 1998;17(7):686-92.
96. Kasahara M, Kiuchi T, Takakura K, Uryuhara K, Egawa H, Asonuma K, Uemoto S, Inomata Y, Ohwada S, Morishita Y, Tanaka K. Postoperative flow cytometry crossmatch in living donor liver transplantation: Clinical significance of humoral immunity in acute rejection. Transplantation 1999; 67(4):568-75.
97. Bishay ES, Cook DJ, Starling RC, Ratliff NB, White J, Blackstone EH, Smedira NG, McCarthy PM. The clinical significance of flow cytometry crossmatching in heart transplantation. European Journal of Cardio-Thoracic Surgery 2000;17(4):362-69.

98. Saw CL, Bray RA, Gebel HM. Cytotoxicity and antibody binding by flow cytometry: A single assay to simultaneously assess two parameters. Cytometry Part B-Clinical Cytometry 2008;74(5):287-94.
99. Billen EVA, Christiaans MHL, van den Berg-Loonen EM. Clinical relevance of Luminex donor-specific crossmatches: Data from 165 renal transplants. Tissue Antigens 2009;74:205-12.
100. Zachary AA, Montgomery RA, Ratner LE, Samaniego-Picota M, Haas M, Kopchaliiska D, Leffell MS. Specific and durable elimination of antibody to donor HLA antigens in renal transplant patients. Transplantation 2003; 76(10):1519-25.
101. Montgomery RA, Zachary AA. Transplanting patients with a positive donor-specific crossmatch: A single centre's perspective. Paediatric Transplantation 2004;8(6): 535-42.
102. Jordan SC, Locke JE, Montgomery RA. Desensitization protocols for crossing leukocyte antigen and ABO-incompatible barriers. Current Opinion in Organ Transplantation 2007;12(4):371-78.
103. Lefaucheur C, Nochy D, Andrade J, Verine J, Gautreau C, Charron D, Hill GS, Glotz D, Suberbielle-Boissel C. Comparison of combination plasmapheresis /IVIG /Anti-CD20 versus high-dose IVIG in the treatment of antibody-mediated rejection. American Journal of Transplantation 2009;9(5):1099-1107.
104. Jordan SC, Peng A, Vo AA. Therapeutic strategies in management of the highly HLA-sensitized and ABO-incompatible transplant recipients. Contributions to Nephrology 2009;162:13-26.
105. Jordan SC, Tyan D, Stablein D, McIntosh M, Rose S, Vo A, Tyoda M, Davis C, Shapiro r, Adey D, Milliner D, Graff R, Steiner R, Ciancio G, Sahney S, Light J. Evaluation of intravenous immunoglobulin as an agent to lower allosensitization and improve transplantation in highly sensitized adult patients with end stage renal disease: Report of the NIH IG02 trial. Journal of the American Society of Nephrology 2004;15(12):3256-62.
106. Negi V-S, Elluru S, Siberil S, Graff-Dubois S, Mouthon L, Kazatchkine MD, Lacroix-Desmazes S, Bayry J, Kaveri SV. Intravenous immunoglobulin: An update on the clinical use and mechanisms of action. Journal of Clinical Immunology 2007;27(3):233-45.
107. Negi VS, Murmu V, Kaveri SV, Swaminathen RP, Das AK. Intravenous immunoglobulin: Mechanism of action and clinical uses. Biomedicine 2008; 28(1):3-8.
108. Seite J-F, Shoenfeld Y, Youinou P, Hillion S. What are the contents of the magic draft IVIg? Autoimmunity Reviews 2008;7(6):435-39.
109. Paterson GE, Walker RG, Tait BD. A screening assay to simultaneously determine the presence and specificity of HLA anti-idiotypic antibodies. Transplant Immunology 1993;3:192-97.

Chapter 30

Organ Transplantation: Post-transplant Antibody Monitoring and Associated Mechanisms

Mary E Atz, Elaine F Reed

INTRODUCTION

In the past, T-cells were implicated as the central regulatory and effector cells involved in graft rejection. Most of the current therapies to prevent or treat rejection target T-cell function. For renal and cardiac transplants these treatments have improved short-term graft survival to 88-95 percent in the first year. In spite of this success, acute rejection episodes still occur and long-term allografts often end up with chronic rejection. Recent evidence suggests that a majority of these rejection episodes occur because of antibody involvement. Antibodies specific for HLA molecules on the donor endothelium are now indicated to play a major role in antibody mediated rejection (AMR). In fact, the prognosis of AMR is generally worse and requires a different type of therapy than T-cell mediated acute rejection.[1] Some time ago, AMR often went undiagnosed and unclassified because reliable morphological and immunohistochemical markers were not available. This all changed with the introduction of complement component 4d (C4d) immunostaining which proved to be a promising marker of AMR.[2] Interestingly, data on the sensitivity of a C4d as a marker for AMR was shown to be controversial. As the investigation continued subsequent studies found associations between C4d and the development of post-transplant anti-HLA antibodies. A majority (78-95%) of C4d positive patients also were positive for circulating donor specific antibodies (DSA). These results have led to the recommendation that the diagnosis of AMR should include both DSA testing and C4d staining.[3,4]

There is evidence to suggest that the development of post-transplant anti-HLA antibody production plays a role in long-term graft survival. Circulating anti-HLA antibodies are associated with a risk for later heart and renal graft loss. There is growing support for a role of anti-HLA antibodies in both acute and chronic rejection.[5] This suggests that monitoring for the production of anti-HLA antibodies post-transplant can be a useful test for diagnosing and classifying AMR patients who are at risk for early graft dysfunction.

The presence of anti-HLA antibodies following transplantation can be detrimental to the graft. The mechanisms for understanding the role of anti-HLA antibodies in rejection are best studied using endothelial cells (ECs), which are the main targets of the antibodies. The ligation of HLA molecules on ECs has been shown to induce both the proliferation and survival pathways. The mechanisms underlying these pathways and the role of anti-HLA antibody at the donor endothelium will be discussed in detail. In addition, other mechanisms of AMR will be discussed including the effect of anti-HLA antibodies on airway epithelial cells in terms of lung transplantation and anti-HLA antibody induced exocytosis and cytokine production.

ACUTE ANTIBODY MEDIATED REJECTION

The diagnostic criteria defining acute AMR (AAMR) include clinical indication of acute graft dysfunction, histological evidence of tissue injury, C4d deposition and the presence of circulating HLA-specific antibodies or other DSA. AAMR is evident in renal transplantation when serum creatinine levels rise quickly. It is often severe and resistant to high doses of steroids and anti-lymphocyte antibody treatments. AAMR can occur at anytime after transplantation (within days to years). A timely diagnosis and an optimal treatment are crucial for graft survival when AAMR occurs.

Halloran et al were the first to identify that acute rejection in renal allografts could be associated with post-transplant anti-HLA DSA production and described this as a unique phenomenon carrying a poor prognosis. This study postulated that the 'complement-neutrophil pathway' was likely the main pathophysiological mechanism of AAMR.[6] Feucht et al showed the deposition of C4d in the peritubular capillaries (PTC) of renal allografts is strongly associated with poor prognosis and raised the possibility that antibodies were involved.[2] These observations were further extended in a study showing that most patients (95%) with DSA at the time of rejection had extensive C4d deposition, signifying that the presence of circulating alloantibody may have a pathogenic role. Additionally this brought forth the notion that the combination of DSA monitoring and C4d staining may be a useful technique for the early diagnosis of AMR.[4,7-9]

CHRONIC ANTIBODY MEDIATED REJECTION

Chronic rejection is a leading cause of late heart, lung and kidney graft loss; affecting more than 40 percent of recipients within the first 5 years after transplantation. Transplant arteriosclerosis (TA) is a hallmark of chronic rejection and is described by diffuse, concentric intimal thickening resulting in vessel occlusion within the transplanted organ. The presence of circulating HLA-specific antibodies is common in patients with long-term allografts. Post-transplant production of anti-donor HLA class I and class II molecules are risk factors for early graft loss and the development of TA. Evidence of these circulating antibodies can be detected months to years before any sign of graft dysfunction, suggesting the progression of antibody-mediated injury might be slow.[10]

Patients with chronic antibody mediated rejection (CAMR) can be characterized by C4d deposition in biopsies and most of these patients have circulating DSA specific for HLA molecules. C4d appears to be a predictor of the development of chronic allograft dysfunction. However, in recent studies in ABO incompatible transplants, C4d deposition has been found in the absence of the histological changes associated with AMR. In human allografts, complement regulation and how it is affected by antibody binding against blood group and HLA antigens continue to be vital areas of future investigation.

Along with the evidence of donor specific anti-HLA antibodies and C4d deposition, CAMR is also characterized by intimal proliferation of the arteries and mononuclear cell infiltration. To elucidate the association between development of anti-donor HLA antibodies and chronic rejection it has been postulated that anti-donor HLA antibodies contribute to the development of chronic rejection by ligating to class I molecules on the endothelium and smooth muscle of the graft causing both survival and proliferation signal transduction. Data supporting this hypothesis are discussed later in this chapter under "Mechanisms of AMR".

DSA MONITORING

The mounting evidence that anti-HLA antibodies play a role in acute and chronic allograft rejection presented a need to detect these antibodies in a clinically relevant manner. Thus, post-transplant monitoring of anti-HLA antibodies may be useful in identifying patients at risk for acute and/or chronic rejection in heart, lung and renal transplantation.

The success of antibody monitoring has been aided by technological advances in the purification of the HLA antigens as well as the generation of recombinant HLA molecules. Purified antigens permit the HLA molecules to be coupled to a solid matrix. These assays are known as "membrane-independent" because they essentially lack the interference of proteins found on intact cell membranes. The use of enzyme-linked immunosorbent assay (ELISA) was the first solid phase method used for assessing HLA-specific antibodies. Additionally, multiplexed bead arrays have been developed for analysis of anti-HLA antibodies bound to antigen coated microspheres by flow cytometry or Luminex®. These assays have helped to further define HLA specificity.[11]

The development of anti-HLA antibodies following transplantation is positively associated with chronic rejection of heart and renal allografts. Additionally in heart allografts, the frequency of rejection episodes, production of anti-donor HLA antibodies, and persistence of donor HLA alloantigens were all found to be associated with an increased risk of developing TA which is a major indicator of chronic rejection.[12] When renal transplant patients were examined prospectively for the development of anti-HLA antibodies there was a strong association between the production of DSA, AMR and early graft dysfunction. Additionally, in a multicenter large-scale prospective study the presence of HLA antibodies was confirmed in patients with well-functioning grafts and this detection predicted later graft failure.[13] These studies demonstrate that monitoring DSA production after transplantation may aid in the ability to identify patients at risk for AMR, early graft dysfunction and/or the development of chronic rejection.

The utilization of post-transplant antibody monitoring is made possible because of advancements in techniques which are sensitive for the detection of the antibodies and the determination of donor specificity. Antibody testing is additionally beneficial because it provides a means to monitor the patient in a less invasive manner than protocol biopsy; it is less expensive and can be repeated often. Post-transplant antibody monitoring is essential to graft survival because the development of anti-donor antibodies is the initial response against the allograft while complement activation (as shown by C4d deposition) is a secondary event as are other non-complement mediated mechanisms of AMR. The details of these mechanisms will be discussed later in the next section of this chapter.

As the above studies have described, the detection of post-transplant DSA poses danger for patients with well-functioning grafts; the next question faced is what action should be taken once a patient tests positive for antibodies in their peripheral blood. It has been recommended that to treat and prevent AMR, first antibody producing cells should be inhibited or depleted, secondly, the antibodies should be removed or blocked and lastly, the antibody mediated tissue injury should be impeded or held off for as long as possible via anticoagulation or glucosteroid therapies.[14] These approaches were shown to be effective for different patients under different circumstances, but much is still unknown about how these therapies or others could be used to prevent and/or treat AMR.

MECHANISMS OF AMR

Complement Activation

The primary effects of antibody binding to HLA molecules on the allograft endothelium cause damage via several distinct pathways which are all complement dependent. These pathways include formation of membrane attack complex (MAC), soluble complement factors that recruit inflammatory cells and phagocytosis mediated by complement receptors recognizing complement fragments. Antibody mediated complement activation appears to have a role in AAMR. A complete description of complement activation is reviewed elsewhere.[15] Simply stated (Fig. 30.1), the process begins

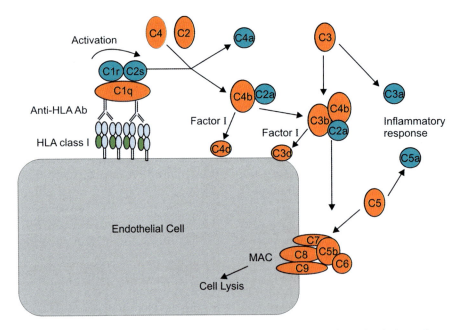

Fig. 30.1: Antibody binding to HLA molecules on the allograft endothelium leads to activation of the classical complement pathway. Complement activation begins when anti-HLA antibodies interact with complement component 1q (C1q). C1q cleaves C1r allowing activated C1r to activate C1s. C1s is the enzyme that activates C2 and C4. C4 is cleaved by C1s into a small C4a fragment and large C4b fragment. C4b can be inactivated by factor I which produces C4d which then covalently binds to the endothelium. C3 is cleaved into a small C3a and a large C3b fragment. The C3b fragment can be inactivated by factor I and produces C3d which can bind to the endothelium. Additionally C5 is cleaved into C5a and C5b framents. C3a and C5a are chemoattractants involved in mediating the inflammatory response. The process ends with the formation of terminal complement components. These components form the MAC which leads to cell lysis or leakage

when antibody interacts with complement component 1q (C1q). The next steps involve soluble peptide and bound molecule generation and ends with the formation of terminal complement components. These components form the MAC which leads to cell lysis or leakage. The part of this pathway which generates C4d begins when C1q cleaves C1r subsequently permitting activated C1r to activate C1s. C1s is the enzyme that activates C2 and C4. C4 is cleaved by C1s into a small C4a fragment and large C4b fragment. C4b becomes inactivated by factor I resulting in C4d which remains covalently bound to the tissue thereby making it a robust *in situ* marker of complement activation. No functional activity of C4d has been reported; therefore C4d is only useful as a marker of antibody deposition and complement activation. C4d is eventually cleared from the tissue and in response to treatment it can be cleared within 8 days.

The fundamental step in regulation and activation of the complement cascade occurs after C4 activation. The pathophysiological effect of complement requires activation of a final common pathway and if activation is prevented at C4, so that C3 is not activated, then it is possible that graft injury may be prevented or limited. In addition to C4d production, factor I cleaves C3b and produces C3d which is also a stable marker of complement activation. C4d occurs less frequently in normal tissue then C3d deposition so it has been the favored marker for AMR. Although, there is evidence to suggest that C3d may be a useful marker in cases of severe rejection because the split products of C3 have more pro-inflammatory functions than C4 split products.[16]

Another effect of complement is that it can activate ECs. Upon EC activation there is increased production of pro-inflammatory cytokines. Thus, complement activation is thought to mediate AAMR because it recruits inflammatory cells to the chemoattractants C3a and C5a. The receptors for these chemoattractants are found on neutrophils and macrophages. C3a and C5a receptors are also found on the surface of ECs. When these receptors bind C3a and C5a produced after complement activation the ECs undergo cytoskeleton changes, cytokine release and increase the expression of adhesion molecules, cytokines and chemokines.[17] Evidence thus far indicates that complement activation contributes to graft dysfunction and that complement fixation is a mechanism underlying AAMR.

HLA Antibody Induced Cytokine Production

As discussed above, complement is a mediator of AMR which has been shown to promote inflammation by inducing both cytokine release and production. Interestingly, when non-complement activating antibodies cross-link HLA molecules they can also activate ECs and promote inflammation. HLA antibody activation of ECs induces the production of IL-1α, IL-8 and monocyte chemotactic protein 1 (MCP-1) which then results in the recruitment of neutrophils and monocytes to the endothelium. HLA antibodies are also involved in stimulating NK cells, macrophages and neutrophils through their Fc receptors. The activated macrophages can produce TNF-α and IL-1α which also contribute to EC activation.

Immunoglobulin knockout (IgKO) mice which have impaired B-cell development are unable to produce antibodies. In a cardiac transplant model, when IgKO mice are passively transferred with proinflammatory IgG2b monoclonal antibodies against donor MHC, AAMR occurred and was dose-dependent. While AAMR does not occur in the mice passively transferred with IgG1 alloantibodies that do not activate complement. However, when IgG1 alloantibodies are combined with a subthreshold dose of IgG2b alloantibodies rejection does occur suggesting that IgG1 alloantibodies contribute to the EC injury caused by IgG2b alloantibodies. Furthermore, *in vitro*, IgG1 is shown to stimulate MCP-1 in mouse ECs in the absence of complement.[18] These data indicate that the non-complement activating antibodies enhance the injury induced by complement-activating alloantibodies. The mechanism of how non-complement activating antibodies contribute to the rejection process appears to be via the stimulation of chemokine production from ECs.

To extend on this idea, a recent experiment showed that when monoclonal alloantibodies to donor MHC antigens were passively transferred into an IgKO heart recipient mouse, acute rejection occurred and the expression of MCP-1, IL-6 and IL-1α were increased compared to non-rejecting transplanted mice. Additionally, *in vitro* results showed that sensitized ECs produced high levels of MCP-1 and KC and when macrophages are added to these ECs, increased levels of IL-6, MCP-1, KC, Rantes and TIMP-1 were observed. When ECs were sensitized with IgG1 monoclonal alloantibodies and grown with mononuclear cells from Fcγ-Receptor II KO graft recipients the levels of MCP-1 and IL-6 were lower compared to co-cultures with wild-type mononuclear cells. Furthermore, the levels of these cytokines were also lower when ECs were stimulated with F(ab')2 fragments of antibody.[19] These data suggest that IgG1 monoclonal antibodies to MHC class I antigens augment graft injury by stimulating ECs to produce MCP-1 and through their Fc receptors activate mononuclear cells. These results indicated that more understanding of MHC antibody induced cytokine production is essential in understanding macrophage and neutrophil recruitment during AMR.

HLA Antibody Induced Endothelial Cell Exocytosis

HLA antibody ligation of HLA molecules on ECs contributes to the pathogenesis of AMR. HLA ligation is linked to EC swelling, platelet aggregation and macrophage accumulation. The mechanisms underlying this type of EC injury are not well understood, but EC exocytosis is thought to have a role.[20] EC exocytosis is calcium mediated and proceeds when Weibel-Palade bodies within ECs fuse to the plasma membrane consequently releasing von Willebrand factor (VWF) and externalizing P-selectin. Released VWF mediates platelet aggregation and P-selectin externalization triggers leukocyte rolling. *In vitro*, when ECs are stimulated with HLA class I antibody, EC exocytosis occurs in a dose-dependent manner (Fig. 30.2). The cross-linking of HLA molecules appears to be necessary to stimulate exocytosis. This is shown by results suggesting that the bivalent F(ab')2 fragment of the HLA class I antibody W6/32 is effective at eliciting exocytosis, while the monovalent Fab fragment is not. *In vivo*, these effects have been investigated using a mouse model of transplantation. Two human skin grafts were transplanted onto SCID mice. These grafts maintain superficial dermal human microvessels and when the mice are injected with an MHC class I antibody and the graft is harvested there is evidence of EC exocytosis.

To expand upon these results another *in vivo* model of transplantation has been established. In this model skin from a B10. A mouse is transplanted onto a Balb/c nude mouse. Because the nude mice have no T-cells the development of cellular rejection is prevented and the production of IgG antibodies is inhibited. The mice are MHC incompatible so in order to induce an antibody mediated reaction, alloantibody to B10. A MHC is injected into the nude mice. The endothelium is ligated by the anti-donor MHC antibody and leukocyte rolling and activation is induced. The platelet activation also mediates leukocyte localization at the transplant endothelium. These experiments imply that MHC class I antibody ligation to ECs can cause vascular inflammation via EC exocytosis. If this plays a role in the

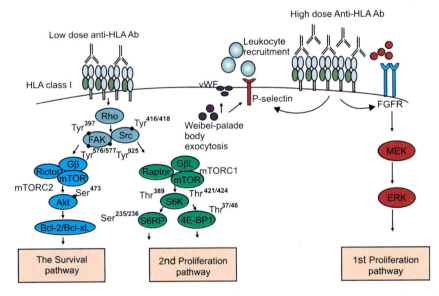

Fig. 30.2: The capacity of HLA class I molecules to transduce signals depends on the antibody concentration and the degree of molecular aggregation. High doses of anti-HLA class I antibody bind to class I molecules on the surface of EC and result in a proliferative response. Two signaling pathways have been described that regulate class I mediated cell proliferation. The first pathway involves the initiation of intracellular signals that synergize with the FGFR to stimulate cell proliferation via the MAPK signaling pathway. The second proliferation pathway is mediated through the activation of mTORC1, S6K and S6RP. The ligation of class I molecules with low doses of anti-HLA class I antibodies stimulates the survival pathway through the phosphorylation of Src, FAK and paxillin followed by downstream activation of the PI3K/Akt/mTORC2 pathway and increased expression of cell survival proteins. In addition, when ECs are stimulated with HLA class I antibody, EC exocytosis occurs in a dose-dependent manner. Exocytosis occurs when Weibel-Polade bodies within ECs fuse to the plasma membrane and release von Willebrand factor (VWF) and externalize P-selectin. Released VWF mediates platelet aggregation and P-selectin externalization triggers leukocyte rolling

pathogenesis of AMR then it may be important to elucidate means which would limit this early inflammatory response. In doing so this may contribute to promoting graft survival. As an example, the therapeutic target P-selectin glycoprotein ligand-1 (PSGL-1) is shown to play a role in organ targeting during inflammation in animal models, and its inhibition provides an attractive anti-inflammatory strategy.

The Effects of HLA Antibody Ligation on Airway Epithelial Cells

In another process, which is less well-understood, the development of DSA against HLA class I molecules has also been associated with bronchiolitis obliterans syndrome (BOS) after lung transplantation. BOS is a hallmark of chronic lung allograft rejection. The etiology and pathogenesis of BOS is not well characterized, but airway epithelial cells (AEC) are thought to be involved. *In vitro* studies show that when AECs are stimulated with a HLA class I monoclonal antibody they undergo cell proliferation, induce growth factor production and apoptosis; all of which may be contributing to BOS.[21] Additionally, in an animal model of chronic lung allograft rejection in which murine heterotopic tracheal allografts develop obliterative airway disease (OAD) it has been shown that the airway epithelium plays an essential role in the development of OAD. The murine model also established that anti-HLA antibodies play an important role in the development of OAD. The findings from this model suggest that DSA to HLA class I molecules may contribute to the pathogenesis of BOS in patients by inducing cellular activation, proliferation and apoptosis. The activation of AECs may also hasten local inflammation resulting in macrophage and granulocyte infiltration. Thus, during the process of antibody mediated lung allograft rejection AECs appear to be the major immunological targets.

HLA Antibody Induced Endothelial Cell Proliferation

EC activation by antibody is also seen in the absence of complement or inflammatory cells and these processes might contribute to the pathogenesis of AMR. It is hypothesized that complement fixation may be required for AAMR and that complement-independent mechanisms may be involved in CAMR.[1] Evidence for this is found when HLA class I molecules are ligated by class I antibodies *in vitro* and EC proliferation is observed. For example, the ligation of HLA class I molecules results in increased tyrosine phosphorylation, NF-κB levels and induces cell proliferation in both human umbilical vein and heart microvascular ECs. Additionally, non-complement fixing HLA antibodies activated mouse ECs *in vitro* to produce CCL2 and CXCL1 and this response is increased in the presence of TNF. This transcriptional activation is thought to be relevant to the arterial proliferation characteristic of CAMR which results in vessel occlusion and fibrosis of the graft.

The capacity of HLA molecules to transduce proliferative signals is directly related to the density of HLA antigen on the EC surface. This implies that the mechanism for EC proliferation involves the capacity at which the antibody is able to crosslink the HLA class I molecule. INF-γ treatment increases the expression of both class I and class II antigens on ECs and is accompanied by a proliferation response. Nevertheless, this does not entirely explain the mechanism of proliferation. HLA class I molecules do not have intrinsic kinase activity so in order to stimulate cell proliferation it is likely that they must associate with other molecules in order to transduce signals.

Anti-HLA class I antibody binding to class I molecules on the surface of ECs results in a proliferative response thus implicating HLA class I antibodies in chronic rejection and the development of TA. Consequently, it is imperative that the signaling events which occur after class I ligation be characterized. To understand more about this mechanism, two signaling pathways have been described that regulate class I mediated cell proliferation (Fig. 30.2). One pathway involves the initiation of intracellular signals that synergize with the fibroblast growth factor receptor (FGFR) to stimulate cell proliferation.[22] The second proliferation pathway is mediated through the activation of the mammalian target of rapamycin (mTOR) complex 1, S6 kinase (S6K) and S6 ribosomal protein (S6RP).[23]

The primary mechanism of EC proliferation is thought to occur via the first pathway (Fig. 30.2); where the engagement of HLA class I molecules by anti-HLA antibodies leads to tyrosine phosphorylation of intracellular proteins, increased FGFR cell surface expression and increased proliferative responses to basic FGF (bFGF).[24] HLA class I ligation on ECs causes FGFR in intracellular stores to be redistributed to the plasma membrane in a dose-dependent manner. In addition, when ECs are stimulated with the highest doses of anti-HLA antibody the maximum degree of HLA class I mediated FGFR expression and EC proliferation is observed.

The intracellular signals transduced by antibody ligation of HLA class I molecules on EC utilize tyrosine kinases to transduce intracellular signals. HLA class I ligation stimulates Src phosphorylation and mediates FGFR translocation to the nucleus, but Src kinase activity is not necessary for class I mediated redistribution of FGFR to the plasma membrane. Src is also involved in class I mediated phosphorylation of FAK and paxillin.[22] The FAK autophosphorylation site Tyr[397] binds Src and PI3 Kinase (PI3K), and Src binding at this site promotes maximal FAK catalytic activity. Interestingly, an intact cytoskeleton is required for HLA class I induced tyrosine phosphorylation of FAK and paxillin. Further exploration of cytoskeleton changes induced by HLA class I ligation on ECs has revealed that Rho GTPase and Rho-kinase (ROK), which are involved in promoting stress fiber formation and focal adhesions, are implicated in the class I signaling pathway. HLA class I ligation induces Rho activation and increases stress fiber formation. When Rho GTPase and ROK are blocked the HLA class I phosphorylation of paxillin and FAK are inhibited.[25] These data suggest that the cytoskeleton is involved in the signaling process, possibly because actin-dependent clustering of molecules might be necessary to elicit the class I signaling events.

To learn more about the specific role that FAK plays in the class I signaling pathway, FAK has been knocked down using small interfering RNA (siRNA) technology.[26] These data showed definitively that siRNA depletion of FAK protein does not inhibit class I mediated upregulation of FGFR. Presently, the signaling pathway responsible for HLA class I induced FGFR translocation is unknown and requires further investigation. Interestingly, the inhibition of FAK protein expression by siRNA does not reduce FGFR expression. On the other hand, FAK knockdown does block HLA class I stimulated cell cycle proliferation in the presence and absence of bFGF. This implies that the involvement of FAK is essential to class I-mediated EC proliferation downstream of bFGF ligand binding to FGFR. It remains to be determined whether there is a direct association between FGFR and FAK, but several studies have described cross-talk between FGFR and focal adhesion complexes. Overall these studies implicate FAK and the adaptor protein paxillin as important targets of class I induced tyrosine phosphorylation as well as the cytoskeleton.

The second pathway involved in the regulation of HLA class I induced proliferation is mediated via the activation of mTOR complex 1 (mTORC1), S6K and S6RP (Fig. 30.2).[23] The FAK autophosphorylation site Tyr[397] promotes the assembly of a signaling complex with PI3 kinase (PI3K). *In vitro* studies show that when ECs are treated with HLA class I antibodies PI3K and Akt Ser[473] are phosphorylated. It is well established that Akt downstream signaling regulates both cell survival and cell proliferation through the activation of S6K and S6RP.[27] *In vitro* studies using human aortic ECs demonstrate that after HLA class I antibody ligation S6RP undergoes rapid phosphorylation. This phosphorylation event is dependent on Src, which is displayed when ECs are pre-treated with the Src inhibitor PP2 and S6RP phosphorylation is abolished. Additionally, it has been shown HLA class I mediated S6RP phosphorylation requires an intact cytoskeleton. In an attempt to further characterize S6RP's role in this pathway it has been shown that two pharmacological inhibitors of PI3K (wortmanin and LY294002) inhibit HLA class I induced S6RP phosphorylation. These results offer substantiation that HLA class I mediated phosphorylation of S6RP is mediated by the PI3K/Akt pathway and this activation is vital for eliciting EC proliferation. Treatment of ECs with anti-HLA class II antibodies also increases S6RP protein phosphorylation.[28]

The *in vitro* evidence showing HLA class I and II mediated phosphorylation of S6RP leads to EC proliferation prompted an exploration of the significance of anti-HLA antibody mediated proliferation pathway in the setting of AMR *in vivo*. Cardiac allograft biopsies from patients with and without evidence of AMR were examined by immunohistochemistry for increased phosphorylation of S6RP in capillary ECs. Increased S6RP phosphorylation within the biopsy samples was found to be significantly associated with the diagnosis of AMR, circulating anti-HLA class I and class II antibodies and with the deposition of C4d on the endothelium. Therefore, in the *in vivo* setting, S6RP appears to serve as an indicator of anti-HLA antibody mediated cell proliferation and may prove to be a useful biomarker for the diagnosis of AMR in cardiac allografts.

Additional evidence contributing to the second proliferation pathway involves mTORC1 which is upstream of S6RP. mTOR is a functionally diverse serine/threonine kinase which forms two discrete complexes, mTORC1 and mTOR complex 2 (mTORC2). mTORC1 contains mTOR, regulatory associated protein of TOR (raptor) and GβL. mTORC1 activates p70 ribosomal S6K and eukaryotic initiation factor 4E-binding protein 1 (4E-BP1) which results in cell proliferation and increased protein synthesis. mTORC2 contains mTOR, rapamycin-insensitive companion of TOR (rictor) and GβL. Its role is to modulate the phosphorylation of PKCα and via Rho GTPase activation is involved in actin cytoskeleton regulation. mTORC2 can also phosphorylate Akt at Ser^{473} and plays a role in the phosphorylation of the Thr^{308} site of Akt via phosphoinositide-dependent kinase 1 (PDK1). mTORC2 interacts with stress-activated protein kinase-interacting protein 1 (Sin1), an adaptor protein which acts to preserve mTORC2 integrity and facilitate Akt phosphorylation at Ser.^{473}

There is still much work required to fully understand mTOR signaling complex formation and the activation of downstream signaling pathways following HLA class I ligation. The work that has been done thus far shows that when HLA class I molecules are ligated by anti-HLA antibodies the mTOR pathway is activated and cell proliferation is induced. When mTOR protein expression is depleted using siRNA, HLA class I-mediated phosphorylation of proteins downstream of mTORC1 and mTORC2 are inhibited. In fact, if either total mTOR or raptor is knocked down, HLA class I-induced endothelial cell proliferation is completely blocked; while the knockdown of rictor inhibits class I mediated EC proliferation to a lesser extent. In addition, HLA class I mediated activation of Akt at Ser^{473} is regulated by mTORC2, but not mTORC1. These results show that mTORC1 and mTORC2 have distinct mechanisms involved in signal transduction which leads to the activation of cell proliferation, but it appears that they function cooperatively.

The significance and mechanism of mTORC1 and its role in cell proliferation has been studied and defined.[29] On the other hand, mTORC2 and its participation in cell proliferation are less understood. Recently, a novel role for mTORC2 in HLA class I and integrin mediated activation has been characterized.[30] These data show that HLA class I or integrin stimulation of ECs, but not growth factor, induces the phosphorylation of ERK. ERK 1/2 are members of a serine/threonine family of kinases which are activated by various growth factors, cell surface receptors, integrins and HLA class I. This activation is critical for cell proliferation, differentiation, survival and actin cytoskeleton remodeling. The knockdown of mTOR or rictor by siRNA inhibits HLA class I mediated-induced phosphorylation of ERK at Thr^{202}/Try^{204}, but with growth factor stimulation there is no phosphorylation inhibition. Interestingly, raptor knockdown does not affect ERK activation. This suggests that the ligation of HLA class I molecules by class I antibodies on the surface of ECs mediates ERK 1/2 activation via an mTORC2 dependent pathway. Moreover, these data contribute to the notion that mTORC1 and mTORC2 have distinctive roles in cell signaling.

Based on the *in vitro* and *in vivo* evidence of HLA class I mediated proliferation signaling events described above a heterotopic heart transplant mouse model was developed in order to characterize the underlying mechanisms of AMR.[31] To examine the specific effects of anti-MHC antibody on signal transduction in endothelial cells this model requires a mouse in which alloreactive T and B cells are absent. Therefore, a B6.RAG1 KO was selected as the recipient. The donor is a fully MHC-incompatible BALB/c heart. In order to imitate the characteristics of human AMR the recipients are passively transfused with anti-donor MHC class I antibodies. Histological examination of the hearts revealed evidence of microvascular changes and complement deposition in capillaries. Stimulation with the MHC class I antibody showed increased phosphorylation of ERK, mTOR, S6K and S6RP at day 30 specifically localized at the endothelium. This suggests that the presence of post-transplant anti-HLA antibodies *in vivo* contributes to the activation of signaling cascades within the endothelium which elicit the proliferation pathway. These markers therefore, could provide a useful signature to understand the mechanism of AMR in human transplant patients.

In an attempt to further characterize the mechanism of HLA induced phorphorylation of ERK at Thr^{202}/Tyr^{204}, ECs were treated with the drug rapamycin. Rapamycin targets mTOR and is used as an immunosuppressive drug; in organ transplantation it is used to prevent rejection. Rapamycin dissuades the development of cardiac allograft vasculopathy because it functions to inhibit proliferation. The end result is a decrease in intimal thickening.[32] Rapamycin inhibits the kinase activity of mTORC1 by forming a complex with FKBP12. It was originally thought that mTORC2 was insensitive to rapamycin, but this perception has been arguable. The consequence of varying treatment time periods of rapamycin on mTORC2 has been investigated. In context of HLA class I induced activation of mTORC2; data revealed that long-term exposure to rapamycin inhibits the phosphorylation of ERK at Thr^{202}/Tyr.^{204} The effect of rapamycin on HLA class I induced signaling requires further exploration.

Another aspect of HLA class I induced EC proliferation involves the mechanism of how HLA molecules elicit an intracellular signaling cascade despite having no signaling motif within their cytoplasmic domain. It has been postulated that HLA class I molecules must interact with an accessory protein in order to transduce downstream signaling cascades. A current hypothesis suggests that members of the integrin family may be involved in this process. Evidence for this is based on data which shows that integrin ligation leads to the phosphorylation of ERK in many cell types. When ECs are ligated with fibronectin an mTORC2 dependent phosphorylation of ERK is induced which is similar to HLA class I molecules.

In summary, these studies identified several key molecules involved in HLA class I induced cell proliferation signaling in ECs (Fig. 30.2). Specifically two signaling pathways have been described, but the upstream mechanisms whereby HLA class I molecules elicit the signals which explain the above phosphorylation events are unknown. Given the likeness between the HLA class I and integrin signaling pathways, it is imperative to determine whether HLA class I molecules and integrins work together to transmit signals in ECs.

THE ROLE OF HLA ANTIBODIES IN ACCOMMODATION

Accommodation vs AMR

The capacity of a graft to acquire resistance to immune mediated injury is the basis of accommodation. In general, accommodation occurs when an organ allograft functions normally despite the presence of anti-donor antibodies.[33] Sensitized patients with high levels of circulating anti-HLA antibodies usually experience hyperacute rejection following transplantation. Currently hyperacute rejection is an uncommon occurrence because it is evaded by screening recipients using a pretransplant cross-match to identify patients with circulating donor specific HLA antibodies. Delayed AMR still can occur and it has been shown to be prevented by anti-donor antibody depletion using plasmapheresis or immnoabsorption prior to transplantation. The return of donor HLA class I antibodies often results in rejection, but in some cases accommodation occurs.

In the clinical setting when DSA to HLA molecules are found in the absence of graft dysfunction accommodation is said to occur. However, when patients have circulating HLA donor specific antibodies there is a greater chance of graft loss at a later time. Therefore accommodation is either fleeting or insufficient to avert chronic rejection from occurring at a later time point. Indeed, long-term and absolute accommodation has not been documented for HLA molecules. Nevertheless, the fact that the allograft can continue to function in spite of the return of donor specific anti-HLA class I antibodies suggests that when the HLA class I molecule becomes ligated by antibody this may actually promote the survival signaling cascade and this may mediate resistance to graft injury. If this is true, then it implies that HLA class I ligation must initially induce accommodation and then over time the signal induces rejection. The mechanism of the EC response to antibody ligation in which there is a shift between accommodation and rejection remains to be investigated. Perhaps, this shift could be explored by investigating the HLA class I induced EC survival and proliferation pathway balance. The details of proliferation pathway were discussed above and in the next section the survival pathway will be detailed.

HLA Antibody Induced Endothelial Cell Survival

FAK has been established as a critical mediator regulating growth factor and integrin signaling, cell survival, cell proliferation and cell migration. The findings discussed above show that FAK phosphorylation is central to the regulation of the HLA class I signaling pathway. Based on the multifunctional role of FAK it was hypothesized that HLA class I ligation could also be facilitating cell survival. To test this hypothesis, FAK was knocked down in ECs using siRNA and it was found that the phosphorylation of PI3K and Akt induced by class I antibody ligation was reduced.[26] These data demonstrated that FAK was central to HLA class I induced EC survival (Fig. 30.2).

Activation of the survival pathway after HLA class I ligation on ECs is evident by the increased phosphorylation of PI3K and Akt along with the upregulation of antiapoptotic proteins Bcl-2 and Bcl-X_L.[34] Additionally, ligation of class I molecules by anti-HLA antibody resulted in phosphorylation of the apoptosis-inducing protein Bad at Ser[136] and Ser[112] and sequestration of Bad with 14-3-3. HLA class I induced ECs treated with wortmannin (PI3K inhibitor) show reduced expression of Bcl-2, demonstrating a PI3K/Akt dependent pathway in the up-regulation of these cell survival proteins.

As mentioned above, the greatest level of cell proliferation was observed at the highest dose of anti-HLA class I treatment. Interestingly, the ability of HLA class I antibody ligation to induce the survival pathway is also dependent on antibody concentration where the maximum expression of Bcl-2 and Bcl-X_L is observed when ECs are stimulated with a low dose of class I antibody. Additionally, Akt phosphorylation levels peak when ECs are treated with the lowest class I antibody dose. Activation of the EC survival pathway and induction of antiapoptotic proteins in the presence of anti-HLA class I antibodies is consistent with the concept of allograft accommodation.

It is unclear how accommodation is induced in transplanted allografts and it is also unknown how ECs respond to physiological stimuli which result in accommodation. Activation of the survival pathway has the potential to provide clues for these mechanisms. In order to elucidate the role of HLA class I EC signal transduction which leads to phenotypic changes consistent with accommodation, *in vitro* and *in vivo* models have been developed. Salama et al were the first to present experiments which led to the development of these models of accommodation.[35] In this study, highly sensitized renal transplant patients were cleared of anti-HLA antibodies by immunoabsorption and this was shown to promote accommodation *in vivo*. Anti-donor antibodies returned in 4/7 patients yet they did not show any indication of AMR and instead, there was an up-regulation of Bcl-X_L which is EC specific. These findings were further substantiated *in vitro*, when human umbilical vein ECs were exposed to low concentrations of anti-HLA antibodies and subsequently expressed high levels of Bcl-X_L, and were resistant to complement-mediated lysis, while exposure to high levels of anti-HLA antibodies caused EC activation and low Bcl-X_L expression. These data strengthen the *in vitro* experiments discussed above which suggest that activation of the survival pathway following HLA class I ligation is dependent on antibody concentration.

Additional experiments for understanding HLA class I induced accommodation were provided by Narayanan et al. Employing an *in vitro* model it was shown that at sub-saturating HLA class I antibody concentrations, human aortic ECs are resistant to antibody and complement mediated cell lysis.[36] Consequently, these ECs were said to have induced accommodation. Gene expression studies demonstrated that accommodated ECs expressed high levels of *Bcl-X_L*, *Bcl-2* and *HO-1*. Moreover, the accommodated phenotype was shown to be regulated by the PI3K/Akt pathway.

Bcl-X_L expression in EC has been suggested to be a marker which could be used to define the accommodation process in human renal allografts. This suggestion, along with the *in vitro* findings which also implicate the stimulation of pro-survival genes, point to the fact that it is necessary to determine whether these findings can be validated *in vivo*. Therefore, cardiac biopsies with evidence of AMR were examined by immunohistochemistry for Bcl-2 protein expression. Increased Bcl-2 expression was found within the graft endothelium which correlated with the presence of circulating anti-HLA class I antibodies, but not circulating class II antibodies. Patients without AMR and without circulating antibodies showed no indication of Bcl-2 expression. The outcome of these results demonstrates that the survival pathway is activated, but only when circulating anti-HLA class I antibodies are present. It will be essential to observe Bcl-2 expression in accommodated cardiac biopsies as well as Bcl-X_L, which may be activated independently from Bcl-2. Evidence for this hypothesis comes from data which shows that when the PI3K/Akt pathway is blocked with the pharmacological inhibitor wortmannin HLA class I induced expression of Bcl-2 is inhibited. But, after ECs are treated with wortmannin the expression Bcl-X_L is unaffected; suggesting that Bcl-X_L may be activated independent of PI3K/Akt.

Further investigation into the survival pathway revealed that the adaptor protein rictor complexes with mTOR and functions as an upstream kinase of Akt at Ser^{473} to regulate cell survival machinery. The ligation of HLA class I molecules by anti-class I antibodies stimulates mTOR rictor complex formation in ECs.[23] To explore the role of mTORC2 in class I mediated survival signaling rictor was knocked down. ECs transfected with rictor siRNA and stimulated with HLA class I antibodies showed decreased Akt phosphorylation at Ser.^{473} These results implicate mTORC2 as a regulator of HLA class I induced cell survival signaling. Interestingly, the knockdown of rictor does not affect class I-mediated activation of S6K at Thr,^{389} the downstream target of mTORC1. Together these experiments reinforce the notion that mTORC1 and mTORC2 play distinct roles in HLA class I mediated signaling in ECs.

Akt activation can promote cell survival via the upregulation of the anti-apoptotic protein Bcl-2 or by sustaining nutrient transporters and receptors via an mTOR dependent mechanism. As discussed above, the effect of long-term exposure to rapamycin may result in inhibition of mTORC2 function by preventing complex assembly. After HLA class I ligation, if ECs are exposed to rapamycin for a brief time period there is no effect on mTORC2 or its capacity to phosphorylate Akt at Ser.^{473} Conversely, ECs with long-term (>2 hours) exposure to rapamycin display mTORC2 formation disruption and the phosphorylation of Akt at Ser^{473} is blocked. In addition, prolonged exposure to rapamycin reduces HLA class I-induced Bcl-2 expression, which is consistent with the study showing rapamycin treatment long-term inhibits Akt survival signals. Further evidence for the effect of drugs is shown when after rapamycin treatment a large number of ECs are found to be going through apoptosis following serum starvation and after vascular endothelial growth factor stimulation. These results suggest that while rapamycin is valuable for abrogating EC proliferation and initmal thickening, long-term exposure may hinder the activation and up-regulation of HLA class I mediated survival proteins. Further investigation of these data is required as the effects of this drug are important in transplantation.

In summary, the data discussed in Sections HLA Antibody Induced Endothelial Cell Proliferation and HLA Antibody Induced Endothelial Cell Servival indicate that the ligation of HLA class I molecules on the surface of ECs results in two different but related outcomes: cell survival and cell proliferation (Fig. 30.2). The capacity of ECs to transduce survival or proliferative signals depends on the degree of HLA antibody induced molecular aggregation which is based on the concentration of the antibody, the affinity and the level of antigen expression. The proliferation pathway is activated by high concentrations of anti-HLA antibodies and can promote cell proliferation via two pathways; one that involves synergy with FGFR signaling and another which activates mTORC1, S6K and S6RP. The survival pathway is triggered by low concentrations of anti-HLA class I antibodies and involves activation of the PI3K/mTORC2/Akt pathway. HLA class I antibodies have the ability to activate these pathways in ECs. For the survival pathway the activation of mTORC2 and phosphorylation of Akt Ser,^{473} which results in upregulation of "protective proteins" such as Bcl-2 on EC, appears to be consistent with an acquired state of accommodation. Although, it remains to be seen whether class I mediated signaling by low concentrations of anti-HLA antibodies can provide long-term graft accommodation. The class I activation of ECs is complicated by the fact that the proliferation pathway is also activated. mTORC1 phosphorylates S6K at sites Thr^{389} and Thr^{421}/Ser^{424} and 4E-BP1 at Thr.$^{37/46}$ Together this leads to increased protein translation and cell proliferation. The mTOR inhibitor rapamycin is effective at inhibiting HLA class I mediated proliferation and thus appears to represent a targeted therapy for treatment and prevention of chronic rejection. However, the actions of this drug require more investigation given that exposure to rapamycin inhibits class I mediated Bcl-2 expression suggesting it may impede accommodation induction and compromise graft outcome.

THE PRODUCTION OF NON-HLA ANTIBODIES

Allograft survival and function is complicated by the presence of antibodies which mediate the process of rejection. As described above, the ability to monitor DSA production of HLA antibodies after transplantation has proved to be important for both AAMR and CAMR. An immune response against non-HLA antigens has also been noted to affect allograft function and survival. Evidence for this is shown when AMR occurs in HLA-identical sibling transplants. This book is intended to focus on HLA, but for the topic of this chapter it is essential to mention that non-HLA antibodies are also relevant during post-transplant monitoring.

The relevance of non-HLA antibodies was confirmed in a large-scale collaborative study in which recipients from HLA-identical sibling transplants were examined for lymphocytotoxic panel-reactive antibodies (PRA).[37] Patients with no PRA have significantly higher 10-year graft survival compared to patients with 1-50 percent PRA or patients with >50 percent PRA. These findings suggested that PRA reactivity was highly associated with long-term graft loss in kidney transplantation in HLA-identical sibling donors. This study implicated the relevance of non-HLA immunity in the development of chronic rejection.

While the implication of non-HLA antibodies in humoral immunity is apparent, the characterization of non-HLA antibodies remains a difficult task. Most non-HLA antigens are directed against autoantigens and seldom appear to recognize alloantigens. Thus, the presence of non-HLA antibodies may be diagnostically useful even though an effector mechanism may not exist. In general, these antibodies can be termed anti-endothelial cell antibodies (AECA). Antibodies directed against the endothelium are implicated in tissue injury for both renal and cardiac transplants. The non-HLA AECA recognize EC antigens and activate ECs for pathogenicity. Consequently, it is essential that these antibodies be identified and their role in rejection explored.

Antibodies directed against the angiotension type 1 (AT$_1$) receptor have been implicated in rejection of renal allografts via the activation of intracellular signaling cascades. The endogenous ligand of the AT$_1$ receptor is angiotension II and its binding activates multiple signal transduction cascades that regulate several processes, including cellular proliferation, fibrosis, smooth muscle cell hyperplasia, extracellular matrix accumulation, pro-inflammatory responses and immune modulation. In renal allograft recipients agonistic antibodies against the AT_1 receptor have been shown to be associated with severe vascular rejection. In addition this group of patients experienced malignant hypertension. Therefore, the role of antibodies against the AT_1 receptor in the pathogenesis of renal rejection has been investigated.[38] In contrast to HLA-antibodies, the actions of anti-AT_1 receptor antibodies appear to be solely complement-independent. On the other hand, the activation of intracellular signaling is comparable to the results with anti-HLA antibodies. For instance, it was shown that the antibodies targeting the AT_1 receptor stimulated phosphorylation of ERK in ECs and smooth muscle cells. Moreover, in smooth muscle cells, anti-AT_1 receptor antibodies were shown to increase the DNA binding activity of the transcription factors activator protein 1 (AP-1) and nuclear factor-kB (NF-κB), which are known to be downstream of ERK. The transcription factors AP-1 and NF-κB regulate the expression of genes involved in inflammatory responses and coagulation. The role of anti-AT_1 receptor antibodies in allograft rejection has also been explored *in vivo* using an animal model. When antibodies against the AT_1 receptor are passively transferred to recipients in a rat-kidney transplantation model evidence of both vasculopathy and hypertension were observed. Currently, there is not an explanation for the mechanism of the extreme vascular pathology observed in renal allografts with circulating anti-AT_1 receptor antibodies. One question yet to be answered includes whether or not the phenomenon observed via anti- AT_1 receptor antibodies truly represents rejection or if it is an auto-immune response triggered by the post-transplantation environment.

Another non-HLA target implicated in the pathogenesis of allograft rejection is vimentin. Vimentin is an intermediate filament protein primarily expressed in the intima and media of both normal and diseased coronary arteries. The production of antivimentin antibodies in cardiac transplant patients is associated with development of transplant vasculopathy.[39] In renal transplantation, an autoimmune response to vimentin is shown to be frequently associated with graft loss. Using a mouse model of cardiac transplantation, the production of anti-vimentin antibody was also found to be associated with accelerated rejection. In this model, it was demonstrated that anti-vimentin antibodies activate ECs by inducing the expression of P-selectin on the microvessels of hearts. Another mechanism of EC activation by anti-vimentin antibodies is shown when the antibodies stimulate leukocytes to release platelet-activating factor, thereby inducing platelet activation followed by adherence to the endothelium. The role of antivimentin antibodies in rejection remains unclear. Further complications are shown in non-human primate studies in which antivimentin antibodies appear to play a contributing role in chronic cardiac vasculopathy and rejection, but not in renal allograft rejection. The production of antivimentin antibodies clearly has consequences for the allograft, but to fully understand this mechanism more studies must be carried out.

A third non-HLA antibody that has been described to play a role in rejection targets the major histocompatibility complex class I chain-related genes A and B (MICA and MICB) loci. The MICA and MICB genes encode cell surface glycoproteins which share homology with HLA class I molecules, but do not associate with β2-microglobulin. MICA is expressed on ECs and is therefore considered to be a possible target of allograft response.[40] The presence of MICA antibodies which are reactive to microvascular ECs have been shown is several cases of hyperacute rejection and primary allograft thrombosis. In patients positive for MICA antibodies the MICA antigen is found to be upregulated in endomycardial biopsies and is associated with cardiac allograft rejection. In renal allograft biopsies there is an up-regulation of MICB expression post-transplant and this increase in associated with MHC class II antigen induction and leukocyte infiltration. There have been several lines of evidence demonstrating a correlation between the presence of anti-MICA/MICB antibodies and different states of allograft failure, but the actual mechanism of these antibodies actions has yet to be determined.[41, 42]

It is clear that post-transplant antibody screening is important for not only HLA-antibody production, but for non-HLA antibodies. The antibodies described above contribute to the complexity of antibody monitoring and enhance the importance of studies which aim to determine to role of these antibodies in rejection and general immune response.

CONCLUSION

The development of post-transplant anti-HLA antibody production contributes to long-term graft survival. Monitoring for the production of such antibodies can be useful for diagnosing and classifying AMR patients. In fact there is growing evidence that anti-HLA antibodies play a role in both acute and chronic AMR. The advancements in post-transplant antibody monitoring have aided the diagnosis, treatment and prevention of AMR. While much has been learned from patient monitoring the mechanisms of how antibodies affect the graft are still not fully understood.

Several mechanisms of how HLA antibodies contribute to AMR have been described. The utility of C4d as a marker of graft dysfunction underscores the importance of complement-dependent mediated mechanisms. Complement activates ECs and increases the production of pro-inflammatory cytokines and contributes to graft dysfunction which leads to AAMR (Fig. 30.1). Another mechanism of AMR involves cytokine production. ECs can be activated by non-complement activating antibodies which ligate HLA molecules. This activation yields an increase in the production of IL-1α, IL-8 and MCP-1and neutrophil and monocyte recruitment to the endothelium. Ligation of class I molecules by antibodies also results in EC exocytosis which contributes to the pathogenesis of AMR by inducing platelet aggregation and neutrophil and macrophage accumulation. Finally, a major area of study concerning HLA class I induced EC activation involves the ability of HLA antibodies to contribute to EC proliferation. Two distinct yet contributory pathways result following HLA class I ligation by anti-HLA class I antibodies (Fig. 30.2). These pathways both induce EC proliferation and this has been described to be a mechanism for the development of CAMR.

The ligation of HLA class I molecules by anti-HLA class I antibodies can activate EC survival (Fig. 30.2). It is not understood if class I mediated survival signaling results in the allograft and it is also unclear how ECs respond to physical stimuli which result in accommodation. The activation of survival signals in ECs following class I ligation by anti-HLA antibodies may offer clues to the mechanisms of this phenomenon.

In addition to HLA antibody monitoring it is important to note that non-HLA antibodies such as anti-vimentin, anti-AT_1 receptor and anti-MICA/MICB antibodies may also be advantageous to monitor as they have been shown to contribute to various stages of rejection process. The identification of these antibodies and others contributes to the complexity surrounding post-transplant antibody production monitoring. Additionally, the mechanisms involving antibodies and their role in AMR contribute to the complexity of understanding the rejection process.

KEY ISSUES

This chapter details the background and current knowledge surrounding post transplant antibody monitoring and the associated mechanisms. Certain aspects of each of these topics are still under investigation and should provide insight into future directions that surround AMR studies. As discussed above, the evidence that HLA antibodies are likely to be the main cause of chronic graft rejection supports post-transplant monitoring of antibodies to identify patients at risk. One of the benefits of antibody testing is that if offers a less invasive way to monitor the patient compared to biopsy and it can be repeated often. In the case of renal transplantation the antibody appears much earlier than the increase in serum creatinine and therefore may permit therapies to begin sooner. Future studies which improve the identification of the HLA epitopes should be useful in differentiating DSA from natural antibodies, which appear to be produced in response to non-HLA environmental stimuli.

The mechanisms of HLA antibody induced EC activation which contributes to AMR are still being uncovered. There is a complex interaction of intracellular signaling pathways activated within the ECs following antibody ligation of HLA, which either contribute to rejection or induce accommodation. By focusing on the pathways involved in these processes and how they are either working independently from each other or cross-talking will offer an enhanced perspective as to what causes a cell to proliferate or to permit the induction of the survival pathway. Knowledge about the survival pathway along with proliferation pathway activation can help to elucidate the molecular mechanisms of accommodation and chronic rejection. Revelation of these pathways indicates that in the future, drugs could be developed which are targeted to prevent proliferation and promote accommodation thereby improving the success of transplantation.

Finally, the results discussed in this chapter also have the potential to be clinically applicable. The levels of circulating antibody can be critical in determining whether either the survival or the proliferation pathway is activated. High antibody titers increase EC proliferation, while low titers augment expression of anti-apoptotic proteins. This suggests that patients who develop high levels of antibodies to more than one of the donor's mismatched HLA antigens may be at increased risk for developing chronic rejection. Furthermore, this information emphasizes the notion that depletion of DSA prior to transplantation may provide the allograft with an increased likelihood of survival. Lastly, there is evidence to suggest that there may be a common pathway between accommodation and other forms of acquired resistance to injury; conceivably elucidation of mechanism of HLA antibody induced accommodation and rejection may provide further insight into the mechanisms surrounding other disease states.

ACKNOWLEDGMENTS

This work was supported by the National Institute of Allergy and Infectious Diseases Grant RO1 AI 42819, the National Heart, Lung and Blood Institute Grant RO1 HL 090995 and the Novartis Grant 20072118 to EFR and the National Science Foundation Graduate Research Fellowship Award to MEA.

REFERENCES

1. Colvin RB, Smith RN. Antibody-mediated organ-allograft rejection. Nat Rev Immunol 2005;5:807-17.
2. Feucht HE, Schneeberger H, Hillebrand G, Burkhardt K, Weiss M, Riethmuller G, et al. Capillary deposition of C4d complement fragment and early renal graft loss. Kidney Int 1993;43:1333-8.
3. Takemoto SK, Zeevi A, Feng S, Colvin RB, Jordan S, Kobashigawa J, et al. National conference to assess antibody-mediated rejection in solid organ transplantation. Am J Transplant 2004;4:1033-41.
4. Reed EF, Demetris AJ, Hammond E, Itescu S, Kobashigawa JA, Reinsmoen NL, et al. Acute antibody-mediated rejection of cardiac transplants. J Heart Lung Transplant 2006;25:153-9.
5. Turgeon NA, Kirk AD, Iwakoshi NN. Differential effects of donor-specific alloantibody. Transplant Rev (Orlando) 2009;23:25-33.
6. Halloran PF, Schlaut J, Solez K, Srinivasa NS. The significance of the anti-class I response. II. Clinical and pathologic features of renal transplants with anti-class I-like antibody. Transplantation 1992;53:550-5.
7. Crespo M, Pascual M, Tolkoff-Rubin N, Mauiyyedi S, Collins AB, Fitzpatrick D, et al. Acute humoral rejection in renal allograft recipients: I. Incidence, serology and clinical characteristics. Transplantation 2001;71:652-8.
8. Lones MA, Czer LS, Trento A, Harasty D, Miller JM, Fishbein MC. Clinical-pathologic features of humoral rejection in cardiac allografts: A study in 81 consecutive patients. J Heart Lung Transplant 1995;14:151-62.
9. Girnita AL, McCurry KR, Yousem SA, Pilewski J, Zeevi A. Antibody-mediated rejection in lung transplantation: Case reports. Clin Transpl 2006;508-10.
10. Cai J, Terasaki PI. Post-transplantation antibody monitoring and HLA antibody epitope identification. Curr Opin Immunol 2008;20:602-6.
11. Zachary AA, Leffell MS. Detecting and monitoring human leukocyte antigen-specific antibodies. Hum Immunol 2008;69:591-604.
12. Reed EF, Hong B, Ho E, Harris PE, Weinberger J, Suciu-Foca N. Monitoring of soluble HLA alloantigens and anti-HLA antibodies identifies heart allograft recipients at risk of transplant-associated coronary artery disease. Transplantation 1996;61:566-72.
13. Terasaki PI, Ozawa M, Castro R. Four-year follow-up of a prospective trial of HLA and MICA antibodies on kidney graft survival. Am J Transplant 2007;7:408-15.
14. Cai J, Terasaki PI. Humoral theory of transplantation: Mechanism, prevention, and treatment. Hum Immunol 2005;66:334-42.
15. Oksjoki R, Kovanen PT, Meri S, Pentikainen MO. Function and regulation of the complement system in cardiovascular diseases. Front Biosci 2007;12:4696-708.
16. Baldwin WM, 3rd, Kasper EK, Zachary AA, Wasowska BA, Rodriguez ER. Beyond C4d: Other complement-related diagnostic approaches to antibody-mediated rejection. Am J Transplant 2004;4:311-8.
17. Albrecht EA, Chinnaiyan AM, Varambally S, Kumar-Sinha C, Barrette TR, Sarma JV, et al. C5a-induced gene expression in human umbilical vein endothelial cells. Am J Pathol 2004;164:849-59.
18. Rahimi S, Qian Z, Layton J, Fox-Talbot K, Baldwin WM, 3rd, Wasowska BA. Non-complement- and complement-activating antibodies synergize to cause rejection of cardiac allografts. Am J Transplant 2004;4:326-34.
19. Lee CY, Lotfi-Emran S, Erdinc M, Murata K, Velidedeoglu E, Fox-Talbot K, et al. The involvement of FcR mechanisms in antibody-mediated rejection. Transplantation 2007;84:1324-34.
20. Yamakuchi M, Kirkiles-Smith NC, Ferlito M, Cameron SJ, Bao C, Fox-Talbot K, et al. Antibody to human leukocyte antigen triggers endothelial exocytosis. Proc Natl Acad Sci USA 2007;104:1301-6.
21. Jaramillo A, Smith CR, Maruyama T, Zhang L, Patterson GA, Mohanakumar T. Anti-HLA class I antibody binding to airway epithelial cells induces production of fibrogenic growth factors and apoptotic cell death: A possible mechanism for bronchiolitis obliterans syndrome. Hum Immunol 2003;64:521-9.
22. Jin YP, Singh RP, Du ZY, Rajasekaran AK, Rozengurt E, Reed EF. Ligation of HLA class I molecules on endothelial cells induces phosphorylation of Src, paxillin, and focal adhesion kinase in an actin-dependent manner. J Immunol 2002;168:5415-23.
23. Jindra PT, Jin YP, Rozengurt E, Reed EF. HLA class I antibody-mediated endothelial cell proliferation via the mTOR pathway. J Immunol 2008;180:2357-66.
24. Bian H, Harris PE, Reed EF. Ligation of HLA class I molecules on smooth muscle cells with anti-HLA antibodies induces tyrosine phosphorylation, fibroblast growth factor receptor expression and cell proliferation. Int Immunol 1998:10:1315-23.
25. Lepin EJ, Jin YP, Barwe SP, Rozengurt E, Reed EF. HLA class I signal transduction is dependent on Rho GTPase and ROK. Biochem Biophys Res Commun 2004;323: 213-7.
26. Jin YP, Korin Y, Zhang X, Jindra PT, Rozengurt E, Reed EF. RNA interference elucidates the role of focal adhesion kinase in HLA class I-mediated focal adhesion complex

formation and proliferation in human endothelial cells. J Immunol 2007;178:7911-22.
27. Hay N, Sonenberg N. Upstream and downstream of mTOR. Genes Dev 2004;18:1926-45.
28. Lepin EJ, Zhang Q, Zhang X, Jindra PT, Hong LS, Ayele P, et al. Phosphorylated S6 ribosomal protein: A novel biomarker of antibody-mediated rejection in heart allografts. Am J Transplant 2006;6:1560-71.
29. Kim DH, Sarbassov DD, Ali SM, King JE, Latek RR, Erdjument-Bromage H, et al. mTOR interacts with raptor to form a nutrient-sensitive complex that signals to the cell growth machinery. Cell 2002;110:163-75.
30. Jindra PT, Jin YP, Jacamo R, Rozengurt E, Reed EF. MHC class I and integrin ligation induce ERK activation via an mTORC2-dependent pathway. Biochem Biophys Res Commun 2008;369:781-7.
31. Jindra PT, Hsueh A, Hong L, Gjertson D, Shen XD, Gao F, et al. Anti-MHC class I antibody activation of proliferation and survival signaling in murine cardiac allografts. J Immunol 2008;180:2214-24.
32. Mancini D, Pinney S, Burkhoff D, LaManca J, Itescu S, Burke E, et al. Use of rapamycin slows progression of cardiac transplantation vasculopathy. Circulation 2003;108:48-53.
33. Tang AH, Platt JL. Accommodation of grafts: Implications for health and disease. Hum Immunol 2007;68:645-51.
34. Jin YP, Fishbein MC, Said JW, Jindra PT, Rajalingam R, Rozengurt E, et al. Anti-HLA class I antibody-mediated activation of the PI3K/Akt signaling pathway and induction of Bcl-2 and Bcl-xL expression in endothelial cells. Hum Immunol 2004;65:291-302.
35. Salama AD, Delikouras A, Pusey CD, Cook HT, Bhangal G, Lechler RI, et al. Transplant accommodation in highly sensitized patients: A potential role for Bcl-xL and alloantibody. Am J Transplant 2001;1:260-9.
36. Narayanan K, Jaramillo A, Phelan DL, Mohanakumar T. Pre-exposure to sub-saturating concentrations of HLA class I antibodies confers resistance to endothelial cells against antibody complement-mediated lysis by regulating Bad through the phosphatidylinositol 3-kinase/Akt pathway. Eur J Immunol 2004;34:2303-12.
37. Opelz G. Non-HLA transplantation immunity revealed by lymphocytotoxic antibodies. Lancet 2005;365:1570-6.
38. Dragun D. Agonistic antibody-triggered stimulation of Angiotensin II type 1 receptor and renal allograft vascular pathology. Nephrol Dial Transplant 2007;22:1819-22.
39. Jurcevic S, Ainsworth ME, Pomerance A, Smith JD, Robinson DR, Dunn MJ, et al. Antivimentin antibodies are an independent predictor of transplant-associated coronary artery disease after cardiac transplantation. Transplantation 2001;71:886-92.
40. Sumitran-Holgersson S, Wilczek HE, Holgersson J, Soderstrom K. Identification of the nonclassical HLA molecules, mica, as targets for humoral immunity associated with irreversible rejection of kidney allografts. Transplantation 2002;74:268-77.
41. Quiroga I, Salio M, Koo DD, Cerundolo L, Shepherd D, Cerundolo V, et al. Expression of MHC class I-related Chain B (MICB) molecules on renal transplant biopsies. Transplantation 2006;81:1196-203.
42. Zou Y, Stastny P, Susal C, Dohler B, Opelz G. Antibodies against MICA antigens and kidney-transplant rejection. N Engl J Med 2007;357:1293-300.

Chapter 31

The Influence of NK Cell Alloreactivity on Hematopoietic Stem Cell Transplantation

Campbell Stewart Witt

INTRODUCTION

Since the report in 2002 by Ruggeri et al[1] demonstrating the effectiveness of NK cell alloreactivity in haploidentical stem cell transplants, many contradictory reports have appeared concerning the role of NK alloreactivity in haploidentical, matched unrelated donor (MUD) and HLA identical sibling transplants. To those outside the field, it must be bewildering to try and identify any consistency in the reported effects of NK alloreactivity. Indeed, it has been bewildering to those of us in the field. However, some recent studies have provided clues as to why such contradictory findings have emerged and suggest that we may yet learn to reliably exploit NK alloreactivity. There is increasing evidence that the beneficial effects of donor NK alloreactivity are dependent on the transplant protocol. The aim of this review is to organize the various findings and attempt to account for the apparently conflicting literature.

KIR RECEPTORS AND NK ALLOREACTIVITY

Until the early 1990s, it was generally believed that human alloreactivity was the preserve of T cells. In 1988 and the early 1990s, several papers from the Moretta laboratories demonstrated that a small percentage of NK clones were able to lyse allogeneic PHA blasts.[2,3] Different NK clones lysed different targets thereby defining several distinct allo-specificities.[4] Further experiments established that these target cell specificities are encoded by the HLA-C and HLA-B genes.[5-8] Curiously however, target cells were lysed by alloreactive NK cells if they lacked the HLA gene product ("missing self"), thereby establishing that NK cell alloreactivity was very different to T cell alloreactivity ("altered-self"). Experiments by Colonna[7,9,10] revealed that all HLA-C alleles can be divided into two groups defined by an asparagine or lysine at amino acid 80 of the alpha-2 domain and that the specificity of some alloreactive NK clones was determined by the absence of one or other of these dimorphic epitopes on target cells. Absence of an allele with the relevant amino acid at residue 80 resulted in lysis of the target. Additional NK clones showed specificity for a similar epitope on HLA-B alleles.[11,12] Two HLA-B allele groups could be identified corresponding to the well-known serological specificities Bw4 and Bw6, determined by amino acids in the vicinity of residues 77-80. However, in the case of Bw4 and Bw6, only NK clones capable of lysing targets lacking the Bw4 epitope have been identified. NK clones lysing targets lacking the Bw6 specificity have not been identified. The precise amino acids conferring the Bw4 epitope as determined by NK cell lysis have only recently been determined.[13,14] Although the mechanism by which this phenomenon occurred was not known at the time, it was referred to as the "missing self" model of NK cell lysis[15] because alloreactive NK clones that lysed targets lacking a particular HLA epitope could only be found in individuals whose HLA type included that epitope. The mechanism by which the absence of a ligand could trigger NK mediated lysis was revealed with the discovery of the killer cell immunoglobulin-like receptor (KIR) family of receptors.[9,12,16,17] Many of the KIR family members encoded inhibitory receptors that prevent NK cell activation when they engaged their ligand on a potential target cell. The involvement of inhibitory receptors also implies the existence of activation receptors that allow an NK cell to recognise when a potential target cell has been encountered. Thus the two receptor model of NK cell mediated alloreactivity invokes activating receptors that engage relatively ubiquitous ligands on potential target cells and inhibitory receptors that prevent target cell lysis if their HLA ligand is engaged on the target cell. Different members of the inhibitory KIR receptor family recognize the C1, C2 and Bw4 epitopes (reviewed in Rajalingham, this issue). In an individual whose HLA type does not include a particular epitope, NK cells with the inhibitory KIR for that epitope are reduced in number and functionally silenced ("disarmed") to prevent autoreactivity (See Rajalingham et al in this volume for a detailed review).

NK ALLOREACTIVITY SHOWN TO BE CLINICALLY RELEVANT

Although it had been known for many years that F1 murine NK cells were capable of rejecting parental strain bone marrow grafts (consistent with a reaction to missing-self) (reviewed in[18]), it was not until 2002 that Velardi's group demonstrated the relevance of NK alloreactivity to human bone marrow transplantation.[1] Acute myeloid leukaemia (AML) patients receiving a transplant from a haploidentical donor with potential NK alloreactivity had a 60 percent 5-year survival, whereas those receiving a transplant from a donor without potential NK alloreactivity had only a 5 percent survival. These impressive survival figures were achieved through significantly lower incidences of relapse, rejection and GHVD when donors had potential NK alloreactivity towards their recipient. In this study, potential NK alloreactivity was said to be present when the patient lacked one of the three KIR inhibitory ligands (C1, C2, Bw4) that was present in the donor. Murine models[1] were used to demonstrate that rejection was prevented by alloreactive donor NK cells eliminating recipient T cells. Similarly, acute GVHD was prevented by alloreactive donor NK cells eliminating recipient APC and relapse was prevented by donor alloreactive NK cells eliminating residual leukaemia cells. Interestingly, the reduced relapse rate and improved survival was not observed in acute lymphocytic leukaemia (ALL) patients. The failure to prevent relapse in ALL patients was suggested to be due to the inability of NK cells to lyse ALL cells which lack accessory NK ligands such as ICAM-1.[19] These remarkable results stimulated many groups to retrospectively analyze their own transplant cohorts to determine whether the same effects could be shown in their own haploidentical transplants and matched unrelated donor (MUD) transplants in which HLA-C was mismatched.

MODELS OF ALLOREACTIVITY

Three approaches have been applied to analyzing the influence of NK cells and their ligands on graft outcome. The "ligand incompatibility" model is strongly grounded in NK cell biology and assumes that if the recipient's HLA type lacks one or more KIR ligands (C1, C2 or Bw4) that are present in the donor, then the donor NK cells will be alloreactive towards the patient (potential NK alloreactivity in the GVH direction). This is the model behind the Perugia data and supporting murine experiments. In this model, ligand incompatibility is necessary but not sufficient to generate NK cell alloreactivity. In order for the potential NK alloreactivity to be realized, the donor must also have the gene encoding the inhibitory KIR receptor for the mismatched ligand. Not all donors have the relevant KIR gene. However, as each of the genes for the inhibitory KIR receptors is present in ~95 percent of the population,[20,21] the assumption that a KIR gene is present in the donor will be correct 95 percent of the time even if the KIR gene repertoire has not been formally demonstrated. Thus, in some studies the donor KIR gene repertoire is formally determined to enable a more accurate analysis of the ligand incompatibility model whereas in other studies it is not. The simpler model is illustrated in Figure 31.1. As KIR ligands will always be matched in HLA identical siblings, the ligand incompatibility model is not relevant to these transplants. The ligand incompatibility model is also not relevant to MUD transplants in which the donor and recipient are matched at all loci. However, many MUD transplants have been performed with donors who were mismatched at HLA-C and therefore ligand incompatibility may well be relevant in such transplants.

In contrast to the ligand incompatibility model, the "missing ligand" model takes no account of the donor's HLA type (Fig. 31.1). The missing ligand model posits that in the early post-transplant period, newly developing NK cells expressing inhibitory KIR temporarily fail to achieve tolerance towards cells lacking ligands. For example, NK cells expressing KIR2DL1 developing in a patient whose HLA type does not include the C2 epitope would normally fail to become "armed" or "licensed" to recognize targets lacking C2. In the missing ligand model, it is suggested that such cells are temporarily, and inappropriately, aggressive towards cells that lack C2, the inhibitory ligand for KIR2DL1. During this period such alloreactive NK cells might exert the same beneficial effects observed in the ligand incompatibility model. Subsequently, when a normal bone marrow environment is re-established, such developing NK cells would not

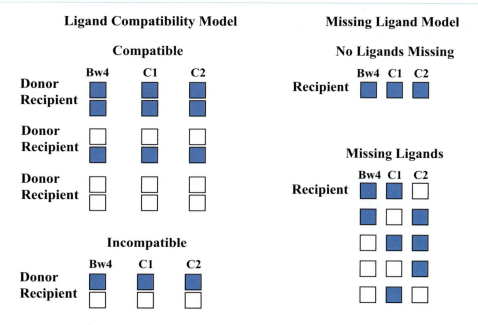

Fig. 31.1: The "ligand compatibility model" (left) considers both the donor and recipient HLA types. Each of the Bw4, C1 and C2 epitopes can be considered separately. If the donor's HLA type includes the epitope and the recipient's HLA type does not, then they are incompatible. The "missing ligand model" (right) only considers the recipient's HLA type. If any of the three epitopes is missing from the recipient's HLA type, the recipient is said to be missing a ligand

be armed for killing and would be tolerant to cells lacking C2 in the usual way. As the missing ligand model is not dependent on the donor's HLA type, it is applicable to all forms of stem cell transplantation, though it has not been studied after autologous transplants.

A third approach that has been applied to analyzing the influence of NK alloreactivity on transplant outcome is to relate outcome to the presence of particular KIR genes, or the total number of KIR genes in the donor, usually without reference to the HLA type of the patient or donor. There is no clear biological basis to this approach though it might be envisaged that the greater the number of KIR receptors, the more likely it is that a difference in KIR ligands between the donor and recipient will be detected by donor NK cells. In more elaborate versions of this approach (with even less biological basis), the difference between donor and recipient KIR repertoire is related to outcome.

PUZZLING ASPECTS OF NK ALLOREACTIVITY IN STEM CELL TRANSPLANTATION

The Effect of Donor-recipient Ligand Incompatibility on Outcome is Rarely Neutral

Numerous retrospective studies have examined the influence of ligand incompatibility on outcome. These studies rarely fail to show an effect but surprisingly, they often show opposite effects. A minority of reports find significantly beneficial effects while the majority find significantly deleterious effects. It is possible that this simply represents reporting bias, i.e. analyses that fail to find an effect are not submitted for publication and those that are submitted, simply represent type I errors. Alternatively, donor NK cells may have beneficial or deleterious effects depending on the transplant protocol. The possibility that NK cells might have potential for both beneficial and deleterious effects is suggested by results of murine experiments. While murine experiments[1] demonstrate that NK cells can prevent GVHD by eliminating recipient APC and thereby preventing their interaction with donor T cells, there is also evidence that NK cells can participate as effector cells in GVHD lesions[22,23] and are even *essential* for the development of GVHD in murine models.[24] If T cells are allowed to initiate GVHD, it is possible that NK cells are recruited to participate as effector cells. Variation in the relative number of donor T cells and NK cells in the graft might determine whether recipient APC have the opportunity to interact with donor T cells. A low T: NK cell ratio would favor NK mediated elimination of APC thereby preventing interaction with donor T cells whereas a high T: NK cell ratio would favor T cell interaction with APC and thus GVHD.

Evidence that the presence of donor T cells in the graft influences the outcome of NK alloreactivity has received support from two human studies. Yabe et al[25] compared the influence of potential NK alloreactivity in 1395 MUD transplants in which patients were not given ATG and 91 transplants in which ATG was administered as part of the transplant protocol. In transplants without ATG, ligand incompatibility was strongly associated with increased GVHD which translated into an adverse effect on overall survival (OS). In contrast, in transplants that included ATG, ligand incompatibility was associated with a significantly reduced incidence of GVHD. This study strongly supports the notion that potential NK alloreactivity can have opposite effects depending on the number of donor T cells. However, it is certainly not the case that all studies employing ATG report beneficial effects of ligand incompatibility and other protocol differences are also likely to be important. In addition to possible effects of the T: NK cell ratio on T-cell interaction with APC, Cooley et al[26] have provided evidence that donor T cells may also influence the development of NK alloreactivity in newly forming NK cells in the post graft period. They specifically set out to determine the influence of T cells in the graft on NK cell reconstitution and function by comparing data from 37 T-depleted unrelated donor grafts and 40 T-replete grafts. Their data showed that T cells in the graft, while not influencing NK cell recovery in terms of absolute numbers of NK cells, did delay the acquisition of KIR receptors on newly developing NK cells in the recipient. Thus, 100 days after transplant, 50.6 percent of NK cells expressed KIR receptors in T-depleted transplants compared with 35.2 percent in T-replete transplants. As inhibitory KIR mediate NK alloreactivity, a delay in acquisition of KIR receptors may impede the development of NK alloreactivity sufficiently to prevent its benefits from being realized. As might be predicted by this model, patient survival was poorer in those transplants in which KIR acquisition was delayed.

Origin and Longevity of NK Alloreactivity in the Recipient

Another puzzle that remains to be explained is the origin and longevity of alloreactive donor NK cells in T-depleted transplants. Modern T cell depletion methods, as used in the current Perugia protocol, consist of CD34 cell selection which effectively depletes NK cells as well as T cells. Could the small number of residual NK cells in the graft be sufficient to mediate lysis of the host's residual leukaemia cells, T cells and APC? Alternatively, could the beneficial effects of alloreactive NK cells be mediated by NK cells newly derived from donor stem cells in the patient? The two possibilities are not mutually exclusive. As acute GVHD often develops within 30 days of the transplant, if alloreactive NK cells were to prevent GVHD by eliminating recipient APCs before they interact with donor T cells, this would need to occur almost as soon as the transplant takes place and it seems unlikely that newly developing NK cells reach significant numbers in time to achieve this. The elimination of residual leukaemia cells might take place over a longer period and could therefore be a function of newly developing NK cells. This would require that newly developing NK cells are alloreactive towards the patient, i.e. armed to recognize missing donor antigens as if they had developed in the donor's body. Such arming would require interaction with ligands of the donor's HLA type during development. The nature of the cells whose HLA type influences NK cell arming during development is as yet unknown. If the relevant cell type were not of hematopoietic origin, then NK cells developing in the recipient milieu would be tolerant of the recipient's HLA type and therefore, not alloreactive. If the relevant cell type were of donor hematopoietic origin, then developing NK cells would continue to be alloreactive, presumably for the life of the patient. This would appear to constitute a very effective, life-long anti-leukemic mechanism but begs the question: why do such NK cells not attack recipient nonhematopoietic tissues which lack the relevant inhibitory ligand, particularly as there is evidence that NK cells can be effector cells in GVHD?[22,23] Post-transplant monitoring of NK cells for alloreactivity ought to help clarify these questions, but the data appears contradictory at this point. Several groups have monitored post graft NK cells for KIR expression or alloreactivity. In both the HLA identical[27] and allogeneic settings,[26,28] NK cells in the immediate post-transplant period have been reported to have a relatively immature phenotype with a large proportion expressing NKG2A and a small proportion expressing KIR receptors, suggesting low potential for alloreactivity. In another phenotypic study, Vago et al[29] enumerated the number of "single KIR positive" NK cells, a phenotype associated with alloreactivity, in the post-transplant period of T-depleted, haploidentical grafts. At 30 and 60 days post-transplant, NK cells were invariably NKG2A+, a phenotype inconsistent with alloreactivity. Single KIR positive NK cells did not reappear in appreciable numbers until 75 days post-transplant. It is possible that the transplant protocol, which included donor T cell add back at day 30, may have impeded the reappearance of alloreactive NK cells. In contrast to Vago et al,[29] Ruggeri et al[30] monitored functional anti-recipient NK alloreactivity in 24 recipients of haploidentical transplants and found alloreactive NK cells were present early in the post graft period. Anti-recipient alloreactive NK clones, demonstrated in functional assays, were detectable in most patients 1-3 months post-transplant with frequencies similar to those in the donor prior to transplantation. Subsequently the frequency of such alloreactive cells declined, being lower at 4-7 months, detectable at low frequencies in only 2 of 9 patients at 12 months, and not detectable subsequently. This suggests that developing NK cells develop according to donor HLA type in the first few months post-transplant but eventually adopt a functional phenotype consistent with their maturation having been influenced by the patient's HLA type. Pende et al[28] also found NK clones that were functionally alloreactive towards the recipient in the early post-transplant period but in contrast to Ruggeri et al[30] such cells were still present several years after transplantation in numbers similar to those that existed in the donor prior to transplantation. Locatelli et al[31] also found donor-derived NK cells with alloreactivity towards the patient in two childhood ALL patients (6% of NK cells at 3 months and 5 years in one patient; 5% and 2.5% at 6 months and 2 years after transplant in the second patient). Triplett, et al [32] also detected NK cells capable of lysing recipient leukemia cells 3 months post-transplant in one patient. Therefore these important questions of how soon after transplant donor-derived NK cells can be detected and for how long they remain detectable, require further clarification.

OTHER STUDIES HIGHLIGHTING THE TRANSPLANT PROTOCOL-DEPENDENT NATURE OF THE INFLUENCE OF NK ALLOREACTIVITY ON OUTCOME

Brunstein et al[33] compared the influence of ligand incompatibility in 102 cord blood transplants performed with reduced intensity conditioning (RIC) and 155 cord blood transplants performed with myeloablative conditioning (MAC). In RIC transplants, ligand incompatibility was associated with a significant increase in the incidence of grade III-IV GVHD and this translated into a significantly worse OS. Neither effect was observed in the MAC transplants. Why the deleterious effects of NK alloreactivity should be apparent in the RIC cohort and not the MAC is not clear. It is possible that more intense conditioning regimen reduced the number of residual recipient antigen presenting cells, which are critical in initiating GVHD by interaction with donor T cells. Total body irradiation (TBI) may also increase the effectiveness of NK alloreactivity as radiation has been shown to up-regulate stress related molecules such as MIC and ULPB that are ligands for the NK cell activating receptor NKG2D[34] thereby making recipient hematopoietic cells more susceptible to lysis by donor NK cells.

DATA FROM HAPLOIDENTICAL TRANSPLANTS

The beneficial effect in haploidentical transplants of NK alloreactivity first published by the Perugia group in 2002 and again confirmed in an update of their findings[30] still has not been reproduced by any other group (Table 31.1). The table shows that no other group has found benefit. Two small under-powered studies showed no effect and three other studies showed poorer outcome. Of the three studies showing poorer outcome, two analyzed T-replete transplants and the single study utilizing T-depletion used a T-depletion method that was less thorough than the Perugia protocol. The inability of other groups using different protocols to reproduce the success of the Perugia group reinforces the idea that successful exploitation of NK alloreactivity may be critically dependent on the protocol. Protocols that fail to efficiently deplete donor T cells *in vitro*[36,37] result in an increased frequency of acute GVHD when potential donor alloreactivity is present and this may prevent other benefits of NK alloreactivity from being realised. Under these protocols, HLA-C mismatches consistent with ligand incompatibility appear to increase rather than decrease the risk of acute GVHD and fail to produce a GVL effect. The studies in Table 31.1 are discussed briefly below highlighting the aspects of the transplant protocol that differed from the Perugia protocol.

Leung et al[35] studied 17 childhood cases of myeloid and 19 childhood cases of lymphoid leukemia. They failed to find a beneficial effect of NK alloreactivity based on the ligand incompatibility model but did find a beneficial effect based on the missing ligand model. However, although the missing ligand model produced a significant survival advantage and the ligand incompatibility model did not, the small number of transplants did not have the power to demonstrate a significant difference *between* the two models. This publication prompted the Perugia group to reanalyze their own data comparing the two models of alloreactivity.[30] Their reanalysis reaffirmed the ligand

Table 31.1: Studies investigating whether ligand mismatching benefits or disadvantages outcomes of haploidentical stem cell transplants

Reference	PRO (%)[a]	TBI (%)[b]	BM (%)[c]	M:L:O[d]	T-DEP (%)[e]	ATG (%)[f]	CD3[g]	CD34[h]	ALLO (n)[i]	REJ[j]	GVHD[k]	Relapse[l]	Surv[m]
Ruggeri 2002[1]	0	100	0	34:0:0	100	100	3.7	>13	34	√***	√***	√***	√***
Leung 2004[35]	0	100	0	17:19:0	100	100	<3.0	?	8	-		-	
Vago 2008[29]	0	30	0	44:3:9	100	100	1.0	11.3	27	-	-	-	-
Bishara 2003[36]	0	100	0	28:24:10	100	100	11.0	8.6	14	-	X**	-	X**
Huang 2007[37]	100	0	B+P[n]	71:40:0	0	100	15000	?	18	-	X***	X**	X***
Zhao 2007[38]	100	0	100	47:17:0	0	100	17500	2.6	15	-	X***	-	X*

Studies are arranged to group together those finding similar associations with outcome.
[a] % of patients who received GVHD prophylaxis.
[b] % patients receiving TBI.
[c] percentage of bone marrow grafts as opposed to PBSC.
[d] proportion of myeloid:lymphoid:other patients.
[e] % patients receiving T-depleted grafts.
[f] % patients receiving ATG.
[g] CD3 x 10^4/kg.
[h] CD34 x 10^6/kg.
[i] Number of transplants with ligand incompatibility model.
[j] effect of ligand mismatching on rejection/graft failure.
[k] effect of ligand mismatching on acute GVHD.
[l] effect of ligand mismatching on relapse rate.
[m] effect of ligand mismatching on survival.
[n] all patients received bone marrow + peripheral blood stem cells.
? = data not provided.
X: deleterious effect found.
√: beneficial effect found.
-: no effect found at p< 0.10.
*=p< 0.1, **=p< 0.05,
***=p< 0.01.
Blank cells for rejection, GVHD, relapse and survival indicate that these outcomes were not reported on.

incompatibility model as the best predictor of outcome in the Perugia data. There was no benefit associated with the missing ligand model.

Vago et al[29] analyzed 44 transplants in mostly myeloid patients using a protocol very similar to that used in Perugia but failed to show any clinical benefit of ligand incompatibility. The protocol differed from the Perugia protocol in that TBI was not used in 70 percent of the transplants and, in an attempt to protect recipients from infections in the early post-transplant period, donor T cells were added back to the recipient at day 30 in most cases. It is possible that these two deviations from the Perugia protocol, particularly the addition of donor T cells, may have prevented the beneficial effects expected.

Bishara et al[36] studied 62 mostly adult patients including 28 with myeloid malignancies but failed to show any benefit of donors with potential NK alloreactivity. In fact, in that study, such donors resulted in a significantly higher incidence of acute GVHD and significantly poorer survival. Although the protocol was similar to the Perugia protocol, the method of T-depletion resulted in three times more T cells contaminating the stem cells and this may have been a sufficient number of T cells to interfere with the beneficial effects of NK alloreactivity. A three-fold increase in T cells may seem a relatively small increase but it was apparently sufficient to result in a considerably increased incidence of acute GVHD (50% grade II-IV compared to 9% in Perugia).

Huang et al[37] studied 111 patients, including 71 with myeloid malignancies, receiving T-replete grafts. In addition to using T-replete grafts, patients were given both G-CSF mobilized peripheral stem cells as well as bone marrow resulting in high T cell numbers accompanying the graft. Additional departures from the Perugia protocol included the use of chemotherapy-based myeloablation rather than TBI and GVHD prophylaxis. The authors failed to find a beneficial effect of potential NK alloreactivity. To the contrary, potential NK alloreactivity was associated with increased frequencies of relapse, GVHD and poorer survival.

Interestingly, the association between ligand incompatibility and increased GVHD was only present in those patients receiving higher T cell doses. This interaction between T cell dose and ligand incompatibility was highly significant (p< 0.00001) and supports the notion that ligand incompatibility exacerbates GVHD in the presence of donor T cells.

Zhao et al [38] studied 64 patients including 47 with myeloid malignancies receiving T-replete grafts. Transplants in which donors had ligand incompatibility experienced a significantly increased incidence of GVHD and poorer survival. In addition to using T-replete grafts, the transplant protocol did not include TBI and included GVHD prophylaxis.

Triplett et al [32] described a case report illustrating the applicability of the haploidentical approach to childhood ALL. An ALL patient who had received a conventional allograft from an HLA identical sibling subsequently developed multiple complications including grade III GVHD and leukemia relapse. A subsequent T-cell depleted graft from the haploidentical, ligand incompatible father had an uncomplicated course with neutrophil engraftment on day 10 and molecular remission on day 16 which persisted to the time of reporting (16 months post transplant). NK cells taken from the patient 3 weeks after transplant had assumed the donor's KIR expression pattern and were capable of killing the patient's leukemic blasts. This successful outcome occurred despite the omission of TBI from the transplant protocol.

Stern et al [39] studied 118 patients (67 with AML and 51 with ALL) patients transplanted in Perugia (n=90) and Pavia (n=28) who had been transplanted according to the Perugia protocol. The beneficial effect of potential NK alloreactivity was evident but as most of the patients from Perugia had been reported in previous publications, it would not be appropriate to consider this an independent confirmation of the earlier results from Perugia. The main purpose of this study was to report on the better survival of patients receiving a graft from their mother as opposed to fathers or haploidentical siblings. Despite the overall advantage of mothers over fathers, haploidentical fathers with ligand incompatibility also gave better outcomes than fathers without ligand incompatibility. Why mothers were advantageous is not clear but as haploidentical sisters did not give the same benefits as mothers, this argues against donor sex being the critical factor and suggests a role for *in utero* exposure of the mother to the child's paternal HLA antigens. The authors suggested that maternal exposure to the father's haplotype *in utero* may have resulted in a small number of alloreactive maternal anti-father T cells being transferred in the graft and subsequently proliferating to produce a GVL effect in addition to any NK cell mediated GVL effect.

STUDIES ANALYSING THE LIGAND INCOMPATIBILITY MODEL IN UNRELATED DONOR AND CORD BLOOD TRANSPLANTATION

In addition to the studies in haploidentical transplants, numerous groups have examined the effects of ligand incompatibility on the outcome of unrelated donor and cord blood transplants. Most of the studies reviewed below address the question of whether ligand incompatibility provides any clinical benefit. Therefore, the transplants with ligand incompatibility (i.e. HLA mismatched donors) are compared with transplants in which the donor was ligand compatible. The ligand compatible group includes HLA-C *allele* matched transplants and HLA-C allele mismatched (but ligand compatible) transplants. As the ligand incompatible group has more HLA mismatching on average, we should not be surprised if outcomes are worse in this group but the hypothesis predicts better outcomes. The p-values in table 2 relate to this question. The studies in Table 31.2 have been arranged so as to group together those that find similar effects on outcome. Only a few of the larger studies attempt to determine whether, among HLA-C mismatched transplants, ligand incompatibility or compatibility provides better outcome. Some of the larger studies that address this question are discussed in more detail below.

Studies Finding Evidence for a Deleterious Effect, or No Effect of Ligand Incompatibility

Morishima et al[40] studied 1790 patients, including 577 AML, 596 CML and 617 ALL patients all treated with T-replete grafts and relatively uniform transplant protocols in terms of GVHD prophylaxis. None received ATG. Most (82%) received TBI. In AML and CML, KIR ligand incompatibility significantly increased the incidence of grade III-IV GHD (p< 0.005 and p< 0.001, respectively) and although the trend was similar in ALL, it was not significant (p = 0.11). KIR ligand incompatibility was a significant risk for mortality, particularly in AML (p< 0.005) and CML (p< 0.001), but less of a risk in ALL (p=0.09). This study enabled a comparison of the effect of KIR ligand incompatibility (in the GVH direction) to be compared with KIR ligand compatibility among HLA-C mismatched transplants thereby allowing the effect of the amino acids at residue 80 to be compared with mismatching at other residues. KIR ligand incompatibility among HLA-C mismatched patients resulted in lower survival in ALL (p=0.04), AML (p=0.01) and CML (p< 0.001) than for those HLA-C mismatched but ligand compatible. Thus, KIR ligand incompatibility was disadvantageous relative to HLA matched transplants and also a particularly deleterious kind of HLA-C mismatch among HLA-C mismatched transplants. Although this is consistent with the deleterious effect being NK cell mediated, it does not formally exclude the possibility that mismatching at residue 80 engenders particularly strong T cell allo-responses.

While ligand incompatibility had no significant effect on relapse in myeloid leukemias, it significantly *increased* the incidence of relapse in ALL. This result is particularly surprising and informative. Despite the fact that NK alloreactivity can provide a GVL effect in the T-depleted setting, there are several reports of significantly increased relapse rates (Table 31.2) in the T-replete setting. In the report by Morishima et al,[40] HLA-C allele mismatching, without reference to KIR ligand incompatibility, was associated with a significantly reduced incidence of relapse in ALL; presumably a T cell mediated GVL effect. However, if the HLA-C allele mismatch constituted KIR ligand incompatibility, this effect was completely reversed such that relapse was significantly *more* frequent. This suggests that NK alloroeactivity in T-replete grafts can nullify a T cell mediated GVL effect. It is difficult to conceive an explanation for this effect. One possibility might be that NK-mediated elimination of recipient APC prevents priming of donor T cells that would otherwise mediate a GVL effect. This would be a particular problem in ALL where there is less likelihood of an NK-mediated GVL effect.[1]

In this study the authors were also able to show that mismatching for KIR ligands in the HVG direction also predicted rejection in patients who had initially engrafted supporting the same finding in DeSantis et al.[41]

Farag et al[42] studied 1397 patients with myeloid leukemia receiving T-replete transplants. The majority of patients received TBI but did not receive ATG. Comparison of transplants from KIR ligand incompatible donors with HLA matched donors enabled the question of whether there is an advantage in deliberate KIR ligand incompatibility over HLA matched transplants to be addressed. KIR ligand incompatibility resulted in significantly more grade III-IV GVHD, TRM, relapse and mortality. Among HLA mismatched transplants (any locus), KIR ligand incompatibility resulted in significantly lower survival rates compared to KIR ligand compatible transplants. Non-significant trends for worse outcome with ligand incompatibility were also observed for TRM and relapse. These data are largely consistent with the findings of Morishima et al.[40]

HSU et al[43] studied 1770 patients, including 1022 myeloid malignancies, receiving T-replete grafts. In the 428 transplants in which there was HLA mismatching at the either the HLA-B or HLA-C locus, they asked whether KIR ligand incompatible pairs resulted in better outcome than KIR ligand compatible pairs. This analysis differs from that in most other studies in which HLA-B and HLA-C matched transplants are included among the ligand matched group. They were unable to show any advantage in relation to relapse or survival of ligand incompatibility. The transplants were performed in multiple centres employing different transplant protocols. If there are protocol-dependent effects of ligand mismatching, it may be difficult to detect them in this type of study.

Brunstein et al[33] studied 257 patients with a mixture of hematological malignancies, including 122 myeloid cases, receiving cord blood transplants. The patients tended to be young with a mean age of 15 years. They were analyzed as subgroups receiving myeloablative (n=155) or reduced intensity conditioning (n=102). Both groups received TBI but a lower dose in the reduced intensity group. Approximately 35 percent received ATG. In the myeloablative group, KIR ligand incompatibility had no significant effect on acute GVHD, relapse or survival. However, in the reduced intensity group, KIR ligand incompatibility resulted in significantly more grade III-IV acute GVHD (p< 0.01), increased TRM (p=0.03) and this translated into poorer survival (p=0.03). Why the deleterious effects of KIR ligand mismatching should be evident only in the reduced intensity group is not clear but a greater number of residual APC after RIC compared to MAC may be relevant.

Studies Finding Evidence for a Beneficial Effect of Ligand Incompatibility

Giebel et al[44] studied 130 transplants performed in three European centres, including 87 myeloid malignancies receiving T-replete grafts. The transplant protocol included ATG and 48 percent of patients received TBI. This is the only study of MUD transplants in which a beneficial effect of ligand mismatching on patient survival has been observed. The survival benefit appeared to be due primarily to a significantly reduced relapse rate in transplants with potential NK alloreactivity, although a trend (p= 0.08) towards less severe acute GHVD was also observed. Although this report is the only one to report a survival advantage with ligand mismatching in MUD transplants, two other reports[45-47] have observed a lower incidence of relapse in ligand mismatched transplants. Most reports of MUD transplants have failed show a benefit of ligand mismatching. It is therefore of interest to try and identify those aspects of the transplant protocol that may have resulted in the unique findings of this group. The almost exclusive use of bone marrow cells in this study, as opposed to PBSC which would contain a greater number of T cells, combined with the use of ATG may have resulted in sufficiently high NK:T cell ratio that NK cell recovery was not impeded. The only other study that also used exclusively bone marrow as the stem cell source and that included ATG was that by Lowe et al.[48] While most other single centre studies tend to find adverse effects of ligand mismatching on outcome, the study by Lowe et al found the effect of ligand mismatching to be essentially neutral with respect to GVHD and relapse and just a trend (p< 0.1) towards poorer survival. Thus, while not resulting in a beneficial effect, the combined use of bone marrow and ATG may have been sufficient to prevent the deleterious effects found in most other studies from being realized.

Yabe et al[25] reanalysed the transplants from Morishima et al[40] but included transplants in which ATG had been used in order to determine whether T-depletion influenced the effects of KIR ligand incompatibility. As previously reported,[40] there was a significantly increased incidence of grade III-IV GVHD in KIR ligand incompatible transplants in which ATG was not used (p=0.001). Remarkably, in the ATG group, KIR ligand incompatibility protected against GVHD (p = 0.04). Although only small numbers of ATG transplants with KIR ligand mismatch were available for analysis, this appears to give strong support to the notion that ligand incompatiblity can result in completely opposite effects depending on number of T cells present in the graft.

Willemze et al[49] studied 218 patients with AML (n=94) or ALL (n=124) in complete remission receiving a single-unit unrelated cord blood transplant from a KIR ligand compatible or incompatible cord unit. As the patients were mostly childhood cases with an average age of 13 years, most ALL cells would be expected to be susceptible to NK-mediated lysis and therefore susceptible to NK cell alloreactivity. 56 percent of the cohort received TBI and 81 percent received ATG. The analysis performed by these authors was slightly unconventional in that it included HLA-A3 and HLA-A11 (purported to be ligands for the NK receptor KIR3DL2) as KIR ligands. Inclusion of HLA-A3 and HLA-A11 was necessary for some findings to reach statistical significance but similar trends were observed when HLA-A3 and A11 were excluded. In AML, the 2-year relapse rate was reduced if the cord unit included KIR ligand incompatibility (5 ± 4 versus 36 ± 7%, p = 0.005). The benefit in relation to relapse also translated into and improved 2-year LFS (73% v 38%, p=0.012). Although similar trends were present in the ALL cases, they were not significant (p=0.1 for improved survival). KIR ligand compatibility had no significant effect on the incidence of GVHD. The results of Brunstein et al[33] who found deleterious effects of ligand incompatibility are in stark contrast to those of Willemze et al.[49] Therefore the differences between the two studies are of particular interest. One difference is the more frequent use of ATG in Willemze's study (81% v 35% in Brunstein's study) which may tend to favor beneficial NK alloreactivity. The effect of combining two cords (Brunstein), which could have been mismatched with each other at HLA-C or HLA-B, is difficult to predict. The other factor that differed substantially between the studies was the CD34 dose. Brunstein's patients received approximately four fold more CD34+ cells, but Brunstein's patients and Willemze's patients received similar TNC doses (3.5 and 3.0 x 10^7/kg, respectively). It is unclear whether the difference in CD34 numbers results from technical differences between USA and European cord banks in the way CD34 cells are enumerated or whether this difference reflects real differences in the composition of the grafts which influence clinical outcome.

Kroger et al[47] studied 142 patients with multiple myeloma receiving ATG followed by T-replete grafts. Donors with ligand incompatibility resulted in less relapse (p< 0.0001) but this did not translate into an improved OS. The reduced relapse rate is consistent with evidence that NK cells are capable of lysing myeloma cells[50] and may therefore be a useful tool in the treatment of myeloma.

Although some studies of MUD transplants have employed *in vitro* T-depletion, those studies used older methods for T-depletion resulting in 2-logs more T cells than is achieved for haploidentical transplants using modern methods. Table 31.2 shows that the majority of studies find that KIR ligand incompatibility in T-replete MUD transplants results in significantly poorer clinical outcomes than for KIR ligand compatible transplants. This strongly argues that there is no benefit in deliberately selecting donors with an HLA-B or -C mismatch in order to generate ligand incompatibility in standard T-replete transplant protocols. In most of the studies in Table 31.2, the KIR ligand incompatible group has been compared to all other transplants, which will include HLA-C matched and HLA-C mismatched but KIR ligand compatible transplants. Clearly this finding can be partly explained by T cell alloreactivity towards the ligand incompatible transplants. The question of whether KIR ligand incompatible donors result in poorer outcomes than HLA-C mismatched but KIR ligand compatible donors has only been addressed by the larger studies. The studies of Farag et al[42] and Morishima et al[40] suggest that HLA-C mismatches producing ligand incompatibility tend to do worse than other HLA mismatches and should be avoided. Although this implicates NK alloreactivity as the cause of the poorer outcomes, the possibility that mismatches at residue 80 generates particularly vigorous T cell allo-reactions cannot be ruled out. The study by Yabe et al[25] strongly suggests that the potentially beneficial effects of NK alloreactivity may be nullified by using T-replete transplant protocols. This finding appears to explain, why so many studies find an adverse effect of ligand incompatibility on relapse when the opposite would be expected based on the Perugia data. Nevertheless, it also appear that the use of ATG in T-replete transplants protocols can sometimes result in sufficient T cell depletion that the benefits of NK alloreactivity can be achieved[44] but this is not a universal finding and other factors must be involved.

STUDIES ANALYZING THE MISSING LIGAND MODEL

The missing ligand model, in its most commonly applied form, is a function of only the patient's HLA type. In this respect, it might be used to predict outcome for particular patients but does not provide any scope for selecting more advantageous donors. In more sophisticated analyses, the donor's inhibitory KIR gene repertoire is also considered but as most donors have genes for all inhibitory KIR, there is still little scope for applying this information to donor selection. There is relatively little evidence from NK cell biology that this model should be considered. Nevertheless, some studies have found that transplant outcomes are consistent with the missing ligand model (Table 31.3). The effects are often only present in certain subsets of transplants. On the other hand, when an effect of the missing ligand model is found, it is generally restricted to reduced relapse in the myeloid subset of patients, consistent with the greater ability of NK cells to lyse myeloid leukemia cells than lymphoid leukemia cells.

Studies Finding Evidence Supporting the Missing Ligand Model

Miller et al[51] studied 2062 patients with myeloid leukemia receiving MUD transplants facilitated through the NMDP. Transplants were not selected by transplant protocol and therefore presumably included a mixture of T-depleted and non-T-depleted transplants and protocols that may have included ATG and TBI, or not. In the total study cohort, recipients missing KIR ligands showed no significant differences to those with a full complement of ligands (C1, C2, Bw4). After stratifying patients according to disease status, recipients missing KIR ligands were found to have less relapse in AML and CML patients in first chronic phase within one year from diagnosis (RR = 0.54, p=0.03). This effect was independent of T-depletion and independent of donor HLA type (i.e. the effect was not explained by the ligand incompatibility model). In the subset of CML patients in chronic phase and at least one year since diagnosis, missing KIR ligands was associated with an increased incidence of grade II-IV GVHD (RR=1.58, p=0.008).

Hsu et al[43] studied relapse rates and survival in 1770 patients with hematological malignancies, including 1022 myeloid patients, receiving T-replete grafts from MUD donors. There was no selection on transplant protocols that included ATG or TBI. Consistent with the study of Miller et al,[51] no effect of missing ligands was observed in the total cohort. In the subset of transplants in which the donor was HLA mismatched (at any locus), the relapse rate was lower among those with a missing ligand (p=0.004). This effect was independent of disease type (AML, CML, ALL), but did not translate into a significantly improved survival. The reduced relapse rate was not seen in the HLA matched cohort. Patients transplanted at different stages of disease were not analyzed separately to enable comparison with Miller et al.[51]

Table 31.2: Studies investigating whether ligand mismatching benefits or disadvantages outcomes in unrelated donor transplants

Reference	Donor	Subgroup	PRO[a]	TBI (%)[b]	BM (%)[c]	M:L:O[d]	T-DEP (%)[e]	ATG (%)[f]	CD3[g]	CD34[h]	ALLO (n)[i]	REJ[j]	GVHD[k]	Relapse[l]	Surv[m]
Brunstein 2009[33]	CORD	RIC[q]	100	98	cord	43:50:9	0	29	1300	4.5	33		X***	-	X**
Brunstein 2009[33]	CORD	MAC[q]	100	94	cord	79:67:9	0	39	1300	4.3	41		-	-	-
Davies 2002[68]	MUD		100	+/-	100	71:35:59	34P	?	~100	?	62	-	X*	-	X***
Yabe 2008[25]	MUD		100	81	100	1173:617:0	0	6	~1000t	?	81	X***		-	X***
Morishima 2007[69]	MUD		100	82	100	577 AML	0	0	~1000	?	31	X**	X***	-	X***
Morishima 2007[69]	MUD		100	82	100	596 CML	0	0	~1000	?	36	X**	X***	-	X***
Morishima 2007[69]	MUD		100	82	100	617 ALL	0	0	~1000	?	30	X**	-	X**	X*
Farag 2006[42]	MUD		100	92	?	1397:0:0:	22P	14	~1000	?	137		X***	X**	X***
De santis 2005[41]	MUD		100	+/-	63	42:17:45	9P	?	370	35	16	-	X**	X**	X**
Bornhauser 2004[70]	MUD			100	47	118:0:0	19	100	?	45	15	-	-	X**	-
Schaffer 2004[71]	MUD			+/-n	62	132:54:0	7	100	?	?	18	-	-	-	X***
Kroger 2006a[57]	MUD		100	40	47	90:52:0	0	100	?	62	22	-	-	X**	X**
Lowe 2003[48]	MUD		100	100	100	69:33:3	100P	100	~100	?r	?	-	-	-	X*
Miller 2007[51]	MUD	EM[s]	?	?	?	534:0:0	+/-	+/-	?	?	44		-		
Miller 2007[51]	MUD	EC1[s]	?	?	?	479:0:0	+/-	+/-	?	?	60		-		
Miller 2007[51]	MUD	IM[s]	?	?	?	702:0:0	+/-	+/-	?	?	71		-		
Hsu 2006[43]	MUD		100	?	?	?	0	?	?	?	189		-		-
Sun 2005[61]	MUD		100	41	50	65:0:0	0	0	?	?	5		-	-	-
Elmaagalci 2005[45]	MUD		100	100	61:39	236:0:0	0	?	?	?	29	-	-	√**	-
Giebel 2003[44]	MUD		100	48	96:4	87:38:5	0	100	?	4.3	20	-	√*	√*	√***
Beelen 2005[46]	MUD		100	100	+/-	137:0:0	0	0	?	?	48	X**	-	√**	-
Kroeger 2006b[47]	MUD		100	0	37:63	0:0:73	0	100	?	?	8	-		√***	-
Willemze 2009[49]	CORD		100	56	cord	94:124:0	0	81	?	1.3	50		-	√**	√**
Willemze 2009[49]	CORD	Myeloid	100	56	cord	94:0:0	0	81	?	1.3	50				√**
Willemze 2009[49]	CORD	Lymphoid	100	56	cord	0:124:0	0	81	?	1.3	50				√*
Yabe 2008[25]	MUD	ATG	100	?	100	?	0	100	~1000	?			√**	-	-

Studies are arranged to group together those finding similar associations with outcome.
[a]% of patients who received GVHD prophylaxis.
[b]% patients receiving TBI.
[c]percentage of bone marrow grafts as opposed to PBSC.
[d]proportion of myeloid:lymphoid:other patients.
[e]% patients receiving T-depleted grafts.
[f]% patients receiving ATG.
[g]CD3 x 10^4/kg.
[h]CD34 x 10^6/kg.
[i]Number of transplants with ligand incompatibility model.
[j]effect of ligand mismatching on rejection/graft failure.
[k]effect of ligand mismatching on acute GVHD.
[l]effect of ligand mismatching on relapse rate.
[m]effect of ligand mismatching on survival.
[n]includes patients with either treatment but proportions not stated.
[p]T-depeletion by older, less efficient methods.
[q]RIC=reduced intenstity conditiong, MAC = myeloablative conditioning.
[r]not stated.
[s]EM = Early myeloid leukaemia, EC1 = early CML > 1 year from diagnosis, IM = intermediate myeloid disease.
[T]estimated based on usual values for T-repleate transplants.
? = data not provided. X:deleterious effect found.
√:beneficial effect found.
-:no effect found at $p<0.10$.
*=$p< 0.1$,
**=$p< 0.05$,
***=$p< 0.01$. p-values are for comparisons of transplants with ligand mismatch v all other transplants. Blank cells for rejection, GVHD, relapse and survival indicate that these outcomes were not reported on.

Table 31.3: Studies investigating whether missing ligands benefits or disadvantages outcomes

Reference	Donor	Subgroup	PRO^a (%)^b	TBI	BM (%)^c	M:L:O^d	T-DEP (%)^e	ATG (%)^f	CD3^g	CD34^h	REJ^j	GVHD^k	Relapse^l	Surv^m
Cook 2004[55]	SIB		100	56	?	0:108:0	?	?	?	?			-	
Cook 2004[55]	SIB		100	90	?	112:0:0	?	?	?	?				X***
Hsu 2005[52]	SIB		100	100	100	ALL:45	100	?	85	?	-	-	-	
Hsu 2005[52]	SIB		100	100	100	AML:72	100	?	85	?		-	√**	√**
Hsu 2005[52]	SIB		100	100	100	CML:61	100	?	85	?		-	-	-
Sun 2005[61]	MUD		100	41	50	65:0:0	0	0	?	?		-	-	-
Hsu 2006[43]	MUD	HLA matched (n=581)	?^{m}	?	+/-^{n}	1022:180:0	0	?	?	?		-	-	
Hsu 2006[43]	MUD	Mismatched (n=622)	?	?	+/-	1022:180:0	0	?	?	?		√***	-	
Miller 2007[51]	MUD	Early myeloid	?	?	?	536:0:0	+/-	?	?	?	-	√**		
Miller 2007[51]	MUD	Late myeloid	?	?	?	1526:0:0	+/-	?	?	?	X***	-		
Kroger 2006[57]	MUD		Y	40	47	90:52:0	0	100	?	62	-	-	-	
Sobecks 2007[54]	SIB		100	0	100	AML:60	0	0	?	19.4	-		√**	√**
La nasa 2007[53]	SIB		100	0	100	THAL:45	0	0	?	?		√***		

^{a}% of patients who received GVHD prophylaxis.
^{b}% patients receiving TBI.
^{c}percentage of bone marrow grafts as opposed to PBSC.
^{d}proportion of myeloid:lymphoid:other patients.
^{e}% patients receiving T-depleted grafts.
^{f}% patients receiving ATG.
^{g}CD3 x 10^4/kg.
^{h}CD34 x 10^6/kg.
^{i}effect of ligand mismatching on rejection/graft failure.
^{j}effect of ligand mismatching on acute GVHD.
^{k}effect of ligand mismatching on relapse rate.
^{l}effect of ligand mismatching on survival.
^{m}data not provided.
^{n}includes patients with either treatment but proportions not stated.
X:deleterious effect found.
√:beneficial effect found.
-:no effct found at p< 0.10.
*=p< 0.1,
**=p< 0.05,
***=p< 0.01.
Blank cells for rejection, GVHD, relapse and survival indicate that these outcomes were not reported on.

Hsu et al[52] studied 178 patients with various hematological malignancies, including 148 myeloid cases, receiving T-depleted grafts from HLA matched siblings. T -depletion was achieved using older methods so that the mean T cell dose was nearly 2 logs higher (8-9 × 10^5/ kg) than would be achieved by modern methods. In order to evaluate more accurately the missing ligand model, the donor KIR gene repertoire was determined. No effect of missing ligands on acute GVHD could be shown. No effect of missing ligand on relapse rate could be shown in ALL or CML patients but in the combined AML, MDS group, the incidence of relapse was lower in patients missing at least one ligand (p = .04). This translated into a significantly improved disease free survival (DFS) (p = 0.014) and OS (p =0.03). Furthermore, AML and MDS patients missing two HLA ligands had a higher DFS and OS than patients lacking a missing a single ligand. These findings are in contrast to Hsu et al[43] in MUD transplants where a beneficial effect of missing ligands was only observed in HLA mismatched patients. The missing ligand effect is hypothesised to be mediated by a period of "aberrant" NK cell development during which NK cells are not entirely tolerant to self-ligands. To date, there has not been any studies examining the influence of T- depletion on the period of aberrant NK cell development. As the beneficial effect was observed in relatively T-depleted transplants, it will be of interest to determine whether T cells affect this aspect of NK cell development.

La Nasa et al[53] studied 45 thalassemia patients receiving T-replete grafts from MUD donors. With one exception, all donors were matched at HLA-C. All donors were also matched at all other HLA loci with the exception of DPB1. In thalassemia, leukemia relapse is not an issue but the incidence of grade II-IV acute GVHD was analyzed. If a beneficial effect of NK alloreactivity on GVHD were anticipated, one might expect it to work in the same way as in haploidentical transplants wherein recipient antigen presenting cells are eliminated by alloreactive NK cells thereby preventing their initiation of GVHD. One would therefore expect recipients missing ligands to experience less GVHD. Indeed, HLA-C ligand homozygous patients (ligand missing) had a lower risk of developing grade II-IV acute GVHD (HR=8.7, p=0.007) compared to C1/C2 heterozygous patients. This finding contrasts with that of Miller et al[51] in which patients missing ligands experienced more GVHD. Patients who were homozygous at HLA-C (missing ligand) had a higher risk of graft rejection (HR = 20.5, p=0.009). This finding is not consistent with a missing ligand model in which alloreactive donor NK cells might eliminate residual recipient T cells, which would otherwise reject the graft.

Sobecks et al[54] studied 60 AML patients receiving T-replete grafts from HLA identical siblings. The transplant protocol included neither TBI nor ATG. In contrast to the findings of Cook et al[55] HLA-C homozygous patients (i.e. those missing a ligand) had a significantly lower relapse rate than C1/C2 heterozygous patients ($p<0.05$) and this translated into improved survival ($p=0.02$). These findings are consistent with the missing ligand model and with the findings of Hsu et al.[52]

Studies Finding no Evidence in Support of the Missing Ligand Model

Cook et al[55] studied 220 patients, including 112 myeloid and 108 lymphoid leukaemias, receiving grafts from HLA identical siblings. Details of the transplant protocol were not provided. Only patient survival was analyzed with respect to the ligand status of the patient. No effect was observed in lymphoid leukemia patients. In myeloid leukemia patients, those who were homozygous for the C2 ligand (missing C1) had inferior survival ($p<0.005$). Furthermore, the effect of C2 homozygosity was restricted to those transplants in which the donor's KIR repertoire included KIR2DS2, an activating KIR postulated to be a receptor for the C1 ligand. These observations are not consistent with the missing ligand model in which C2 homozygosity (missing the C1 ligand) would be expected to confer a survival advantage. As T-depletion is not often used in sibling transplants, it is possible that the apparently opposite effects of missing ligand found in this study and that of Hsu et al[52] is due to the use of T-depletion in Hsu et al.

The number of studies in which the effect of missing ligands has been analyzed is probably too small at this point to enable any clear conclusions to be drawn. As the effects of ligand incompatibility appear to be so protocol-dependent, the same may be true in relation to the missing ligand model. Additional studies should aim to select patients with uniform transplant protocols or select a sufficient number of transplants to enable comparisons of transplant protocols

STUDIES ANALYZING THE INFLUENCE OF DONOR KIR RECEPTOR GENE REPERTOIRE

As is the case for the ligand incompatibility model, it is surprising how few studies fail to find any association between the donor's KIR genotype and outcome. However, as with the ligand incompatibility model, both favourable and adverse effects are reported to be associated with the KIR genotype of the donor. Some reports have analyzed outcomes in terms of donors who have a KIR B haplotype or not. As most donors are either homozygous or heterozygous for the KIR A haplotype, the KIR A haplotype is a constant. As the KIR B haplotype has inhibitory and activating KIR genes that are not present on the KIR A haplotpye, the presence of the KIR B haplotype is highly correlated with an increased number of activating KIR genes and a higher total number of KIR genes.

Studies Finding Evidence that More KIR Genes is Favorable

Cooley et al[56] studied 448 AML patients receiving transplants from T-replete, MUD donors. The three-year OS was significantly higher after transplantation from a donor with at least one KIR B haplotype (KIR B/x donors) ($p=0.007$). Multivariate analysis demonstrated a 30 percent improvement in the relative risk of relapse-free survival with KIR B/x donors compared to donors who were homozygous for the KIR A haplotype ($p=0.002$). B/x donors were associated with a higher incidence of chronic GVHD ($p=0.03$), but not of acute GVHD, relapse, or TRM.

Kim et al[34] studied 44 leukemia patients of various types receiving grafts from MUD donors most of whom were matched with their donors at the class I HLA loci. No convincing associations with the number of activating or inhibitory KIR was demonstrated though donors with more than 12 KIR genes (including the framework genes KIR2DL4, KIR3DL2, KIR3DL3) showed significantly decreased frequencies of severe acute GVHD compared with donors with less than 11 KIR genes ($P<0.05$).

Kroger et al[57] studied 142 patients with various types of leukemia receiving grafts from MUD donors. The transplant protocol included ATG. Transplants from donors with only the group A haplotype ($p=0.003$) or with low number of activating KIR genes ($p=0.005$) resulted in reduced relapse rate with improved disease-free survival ($p=0.04$). This effect was seen only in acute myeloid leukemia/myelodysplastic syndrome and to a less extent in chronic myeloid leukemia. No effect was seen for acute lymphoblastic leukemia.

Mancusi et al[58] studied 74 AML patients receiving haploidentical, T-depleted transplants. A trend for improved event-free survival was observed in transplants from donors with B haplotype genes (48% vs 23%, p=0.066). The improved survival was not related to a difference in relapse rate. Rather transplants from donors with the KIR B haplotype had a markedly reduced TRM (59% vs 30%, p=0.03).

Savani et al[59] studied 54 patients with various leukemias receiving T-depleted grafts from HLA identical siblings. A higher total number of KIR genes (total, activating only or inhibitory only) was associated with protection against relapse (total KIR, p=0.002, activating KIR, p=0.006, inhibitory KIR, p=0.01).

Verheyden et al[60] studied 65 patients with a variety of malignancies receiving HLA identical sibling transplants 52 percent of which were T-depleted. The presence of two activating KIRs, KIR2DS1 and KIR2DS2, in the donor was associated significantly reduced risk of relapse (17% versus 63%, p=0.018).

De Santis et al[41] studied 104 transplants for haematological malignancies and other disorders receiving grafts from MUD donors. Donors with a high number of KIR genes were associated with less GVHD ($p < 0.00005$) and improved survival ($p < 0.02$). As the number of inhibitory and activating genes was highly correlated, the protective effect could not be attributed to one or the other.

Studies Finding Evidence that More KIR Genes is Neutral or Unfavorable (Table 31.4)

Sun et al[61] studied 65 AML patients receiving T-replete grafts from MUD donors. They derived a complicated algorithm of KIR compatibility, which best explained outcomes in their study. They did not observe any association between the number of donor activating KIR and GVHD nor between donors having a KIR B haplotype and GVHD.

Hsu et al[62] studied relapse rates and survival in 1770 patients with hematological malignancies, including 1022 myeloid patients, receiving T-replete grafts from MUD donors. No effect of activating KIR2DS1 or KIR2DS2 or the total number of activating KIR genes was observed. Transplants were performed in many different transplant centres with varying transplant protocols.

Table 31.4: Studies investigating whether a greater number of donor KIR genes benefits or disadvantages outcomes													
Reference	Donor	PRO[a]	TBI (%)[b]	BM (%)[c]	M:L:O[d]	T-DEP (%)[e]	ATG (%)[f]	CD3[g]	CD34[h]	REJ[i]	GVHD[j]	Relapse[k]	Surv[m]
De Santis 2005[41]	MUD	100	+/-	63	42:17:45	9	?	370	35	-	√***	-	√***
Cook 2004[55]	SIB	100	90		112:0:0	?[m]	?	?	?				√***
Cooley 2009[56]	MUD	?	?	88	448:0:0	0	?	?	?			-	√***
Savani 2007[59]	SIBS	100	100	33	39:15:0	100	?	2	54		√**	√***	√***
Verheyden 2005[60]	SIBS	47	97	73	49:16:0	52	0	>45	?		-	√**	-
Kim 2007[34]	MUD	?	?	?	30:7:7	?	?	?	?		√*		
Kroger 2006[47]	MUD	100	40	47	90:52:0	0	100	?	62			X***	X***
Mcqueen 2007[72]	SIBS	?	?	11	113:61:0	?	?	?	?		X**		X**
Triplett 2009[73]	MUD	+/-[n]	100	?	59:0:0	13+27	100	494	51				X**
Giebel 2009[64]	MUD/SIB	100	20	54	78:22:0	0	68	4900			-	X**	X**
Clausen 2007[63]	SIB	100	27	0	?	0	0	28700	74				X**
Yabe 2008[25]	MUD	100	81	100	n=187	0	6	?	?		X**	-	-
Sun 2005[61]	MUD	100	41	50	65:0:0	0	0	?	?		-	-	-
Hsu 2007[62]	MUD/SIB	100	?	?	?	0	?	?	?			-	-

Studies are arranged to group together those finding similar associations with outcome.
[a]% of patients who received GVHD prophylaxis.
[b]% patients receiving TBI.
[c]percentage of bone marrow grafts as opposed to PBSC.
[d]proportion of myeloid:lymphoid:other patients.
[e]% patients receiving T-depleted grafts.
[f]% patients receiving ATG.
[g]CD3 x 10^4/kg.
[h]CD34 x 10^6/kg.
[i]effect of ligand mismatching on rejection/graft failure.
[j]effect of ligand mismatching on acute GVHD.
[k]effect of ligand mismatching on relapse rate.
[l]effect of ligand mismatching on survival.
[m]not stated in publication.
[n]includes patients with either treatment but proportions not stated.
X:deleterious effect found.
√:beneficial effect found.
-:no effect found at p< 0.10.
*=p< 0.1,
**=p< 0.05,
***=p< 0.01.
Blank cells for rejection, GVHD, relapse and survival indicate that these outcomes were not reported on.

Clausen[63] studied 43 patients with various hematological malignancies including 18 with AML or MDS receiving T-replete grafts from HLA identical siblings. Donors with three or more activating KIRs resulted in a significantly higher incidence of non-relapse mortality compared to donors with only one or two activating KIRs (40% versus 0%, p = 0·01).

Giebel[64] studied 100 patients with various hematological malignancies receiving T-replete grafts of either bone marrow or PBSC from either HLA identical siblings or MUDs. Despite being a study of mixed patient types and transplants, the comprehensive analyses of the role of activating KIR genes using different models was extremely informative. Given the bewildering array of findings in relation to NK alloreactivity and often the necessity to break patient cohorts into sub-cohorts in order to find a significant effect, readers of the field may wonder whether the associations reported are mostly type I errors caused by analyzing the data in so many different ways. By presenting all the data generated by different models, it was clear in this study that some models produced multiple significant p-values whereas others produced none. The presence of KIR2DS1, KIR2DS2, or KIR2DS5 in the donor, the presence of the KIR B haplotype in the donor and the total number of activating KIR in the donor were all associated with higher relapse and mortality. As these genes are all found on the KIR B haplotype it is not surprising that these different ways of analyzing activating KIR all showed the same associations. In contrast, all methods of analyzing *patient* activating KIR failed to show any associations with relapse or mortality. This is consistent with donor lymphocytes being more likely to mediate post graft effects. Further analysis of donor activating KIR taking into account whether the same KIR gene was present in the recipient or not, did not reveal any new associations with relapse or mortality that were not already significant or nearly significant in the simpler analysis just considering the donor KIR gene. Surprisingly, the presence in the donor of KIR2DS1, KIR3DS1, and the number of activating KIR was associated with an increased risk of acute GVHD but only if these genes were absent in the recipient. Why the absence of the KIR gene in the recipient should be important is difficult to envisage.

Most studies have reported some kind of effect of a greater number of KIR genes on various aspects of outcome. However, reports of adverse effects on outcome are just as common as reports of beneficial effects on outcome. Some authors analyzed this in terms of donors having a KIR B haplotype while others analyzed the total number of KIR genes or activating KIR genes. All of these measures of KIR gene number are highly correlated. It is noteworthy that one of the largest studies[62] did not detect any effect of KIR number on outcome. It is possible that this simply means that the other studies with such disparate results all represent type I errors. Alternatively, the effect of increasing numbers of KIR genes is just as sensitive to transplant protocol as appears to be the case for the ligand incompatibility model. If this is the case, then the failure of Hsu et al to detect any effect may be the result of including transplants from a large number of transplant centres with diverse transplant protocols. Additional studies would help clarify this issue.

CONCLUSION

It is clear from the number of studies of potential NK alloreactivity by whatever model that completely opposite effects on outcome can be observed. While we still do not completely understand the variables affecting outcome, it is becoming clearer that donor T cells prevent the beneficial effects of donor NK alloreactivity from being realized. Whether this is solely due to the disruptive effects of acute GVHD on the reconstituting immune system is unclear. Nevertheless it appears that potential NK alloreactivity can result in more severe GVHD and greater likelihood of relapse in the context of some transplant protocols and attempts to harness NK alloreactivity by deliberately mismatching donor and recipient must await better understanding of the variables. Factors that are likely to decrease donor T cell numbers include the use of bone marrow as opposed to PBSC, *in vitro* T-depletion and ATG. Other factors that have a theoretical basis for influencing the activity of NK cells include TBI, and GVHD prophylaxis. The up-regulation of ligands for NKG2D on leukemia cells has already been discussed. GHVD prophylaxis may tend to reduce any graft versus leukemia effect of potential alloreactivity due to the immunosuppressive effect of corticosteroids and cyclosporine on NK cell activity[65,66] and KIR expression.[67] Until the variables that determine whether NK alloreactivity results in beneficial or deleterious effects are known, it would seem prudent to adhere closely to the Perugia protocol.

REFERENCES

1. Ruggeri L, M Capanni, E Urbani, K Perruccio, WD Shlomchik, A. Tosti, S Posati, D Rogaia, F Frassoni, F Aversa, MF Martelli, A Velardi. Effectiveness of donor natural killer cell alloreactivity in mismatched hematopoietic transplants. Science 2002;295:2097-2100.

2. Ciccone E, O Viale, D Pende, M Malnati, R Biassoni, G Melioli, A Moretta, EO Long, L Moretta. Specific lysis of allogeneic cells after activation of CD3- lymphocytes in mixed lymphocyte culture. J Exp Med 1988;168:2403-08.
3. Moretta A, C Bottino, D Pende, G Tripodi, G Tambussi, O Viale, A Orengo, M Barbaresi, A Merli, E Ciccone, L Moretta. Identification of four subsets of human CD3-CD16+ natural killer (NK) cells by the expression of clonally distributed functional surface molecules: Correlation between subset assignment of NK clones and ability to mediate specific alloantigen recognition. J Exp Med 1990;172:1589-98.
4. Ciccone E, D Pende, O Viale, C Di Donato, G Tripodi, AM Orengo, J Guardiola, A Moretta, L Moretta. Evidence of a natural killer (NK) cell repertoire for (Allo) antigen recognition: Definition of five distinct NK-determined allospecificities in humans. J Exp Med 1992;175:709-18.
5. Ciccone E, M Colonna, O Viale, D Pende, C Di Donato, D Reinharz, A Amoroso, M Jeannet, J Guardiola, A Moretta, T Spies, J Strominger, L Moretta. Susceptibility or resistance to lysis by alloreactive natural killer cells is governed by a gene in the human major histocompatibility complex between BF and HLA-B. Proc Natl Acad Sci USA 1990;87:9794-97.
6. Ciccone E, D Pende, O Viale, C Di Donato, AM Orengo, R Biassoni, S Verdiani, A Amoroso, A Moretta, L Moretta. Involvement of HLA Class I alleles in natural killer (NK) cell-specific functions: Expression of HLA-Cw3 confers selective protection from lysis by alloreactive NK clones displaying a defined specificity (specificity 2). J Exp Med 1992;176:963-71.
7. Colonna M, T Spies, JL Strominger, E Ciccone, A Moretta, L Moretta, D Pende, O Viale. Alloantigen recognition by two human natural killer cell clones is associated with HLA-C or a closely linked gene. Proc Natl Acad Sci USA 1992;89:7983-85.
8. Colonna M, EG Brooks, M Falco, GB Ferrara, JL Strominger. Generation of allospecific natural killer cells by stimulation across a polymorphism of HLA-C. Science 1993;260:1121-24.
9. Cella M, A Longo, GB Ferrara, JL Strominger, M Colonna. NK3-specific natural killer cells are selectively inhibited by Bw4-positive HLA alleles with isoleucine 80. J Exp Med 1994;180:1235-42.
10. Colonna M, G Borsellino, M Falco, GB Ferrara, JL Strominger. HLA-C is the inhibitory ligand that determines dominant resistance to lysis by NK1- and NK2-specific natural killer cells. Proc Natl Acad Sci USA 1993;90:12000-12004.
11. Gumperz JE, V Litwin, JH Phillips, LL Lanier, P Parham. The Bw4 public epitope of HLA-B molecules confers reactivity with natural killer cell clones that express NKB1, a putative HLA receptor. J Exp Med 1995;181:1133-44.
12. Colonna M, J Samaridis. Cloning of immunoglobulin-superfamily members associated with HLA-C and HLA-B recognition by human natural killer cells. Science 1995;268:405-08.
13. Foley BA, D De Santis, E Van Beelen, L J Lathbury, FT Christiansen, CS Witt. The reactivity of Bw4+ HLA-B and HLA-A alleles with KIR3DL1: Implications for patient and donor suitability for haploidentical stem cell transplantations. Blood 2008;112:435-43.
14. Sanjanwala B, M Draghi, PJ Norman, LA Guethlein, P Parham. Polymorphic sites away from the Bw4 epitope that affect interaction of Bw4+ HLA-B with KIR3DL1. J Immunol 2008;181:6293-6300.
15. Ljunggren HG, K Karre. In search of the "missing self": MHC molecules and NK recognition. Immunol Today 1990;11:237-44.
16. Litwin V, JE Gumperz, P Parham, JH Phillips, LL Lanier. NKB1: A natural killer cell receptor involved in the recognition of polymorphic HLA-B molecules. J Exp Med 1994;180:537-43.
17. Colonna M, H Nakajima, F Navarro, M Lopez-Botet. A novel family of Ig-like receptors for HLA class I molecules that modulate function of lymphoid and myeloid cells. J Leukoc Biol 1999;66:375-81.
18. Bennett M. Biology and genetics of hybrid resistance. Adv Immunol 1987;41:333-445.
19. Ruggeri L, M Capanni, M Casucci, I Volpi, A Tosti, K Perruccio, E Urbani, RS Negrin, MF Martelli, A Velardi. Role of natural killer cell alloreactivity in HLA-mismatched hematopoietic stem cell transplantation. Blood 1999;94:333-39.
20. Uhrberg M, NM Valiante, BP Shum, HG Shilling, K Lienert-Weidenbach, B Corliss, D Tyan, LL Lanier, P Parham. Human diversity in killer cell inhibitory receptor genes. Immunity 1997;7:753-63.
21. Witt CS, C Dewing, DC Sayer, M Uhrberg, P Parham, FT Christiansen. Population frequencies and putative haplotypes of the killer cell immunoglobulin-like receptor sequences and evidence for recombination. Transplantation 1999;68:1784-89.
22. Ferrara JL, FJ Guillen, PJ van Dijken, A Marion, GF Murphy, SJ Burakoff. Evidence that large granular lymphocytes of donor origin mediate acute graft-versus-host disease. Transplantation 1989;47:50-54.
23. Rhoades JL, ML Cibull, JS Thompson, PJ Henslee-Downey, CD Jennings, HP Sinn, SA Brown, TR Eichhorn, ML Cave, DA Jezek. Role of natural killer cells in the pathogenesis of human acute graft-versus-host disease. Transplantation 1993;56:113-20.
24. Ghayur T, TA Seemayer, PA Kongshavn, JG Gartner, WS Lapp. Graft-versus-host reactions in the beige mouse. An investigation of the role of host and donor natural killer cells in the pathogenesis of graft-versus-host disease. Transplantation 1987;44:261-67.
25. Yabe T, K Matsuo, K Hirayasu, K Kashiwase, S Kawamura-Ishii, H Tanaka, A Ogawa, M Takanashi, M Satake, K Nakajima, K Tokunaga, H Inoko, H Saji, S Ogawa, T Juji, T Sasazuki, Y Kodera, Y Morishima. Donor killer immunoglobulin-like receptor (KIR) genotype-patient cognate KIR ligand combination and antithymocyte globulin preadministration are critical

factors in outcome of HLA-C-KIR ligand-mismatched T cell-replete unrelated bone marrow transplantation. Biol Blood Marrow Transplant 2008;14:75-87.

26. Cooley S, V McCullar, R Wangen, T L Bergemann, S Spellman, DJ Weisdorf, JS Miller. KIR reconstitution is altered by T cells in the graft and correlates with clinical outcomes after unrelated donor transplantation. Blood 2005; 106:4370-76.

27. Shilling HG, KL McQueen, NW Cheng, JA Shizuru, RS Negrin, P Parham. Reconstitution of NK cell receptor repertoire following HLA-matched hematopoietic cell transplantation. Blood 2003;101:3730-40.

28. Pende D, S Marcenaro, M Falco, S Martini, ME Bernardo, D Montagna, E Romeo, C Cognet, M Martinetti, R Maccario, MC Mingari, E Vivier, L Moretta, F Locatelli, A Moretta. Anti-leukemia activity of alloreactive NK cells in KIR ligand-mismatched haploidentical HSCT for pediatric patients: Evaluation of the functional role of activating KIR and re-definition of inhibitory KIR specificity. Blood 2008;113:3119-29.

29. Vago L, B Forno, MP Sormani, R Crocchiolo, E Zino, S Di Terlizzi, MT Lupo Stanghellini, B Mazzi, SK Perna, A Bondanza, D Middleton, A Palini, M Bernardi, R Bacchetta, J Peccatori, S Rossini, MG Roncarolo, C Bordignon, C Bonini, F Ciceri, K Fleischhauer. Temporal, quantitative, and functional characteristics of single-KIR-positive alloreactive natural killer cell recovery account for impaired graft-versus-leukemia activity after haploidentical hematopoietic stem cell transplantation. Blood 2008;112:3488-99.

30. Ruggeri L, A Mancusi, M Capanni, E Urbani, A Carotti, T Aloisi, M Stern, D Pende, K Perruccio, E Burchielli, F Topini, E Bianchi, F Aversa, MF Martelli, A Velardi. Donor natural killer cell allorecognition of missing self in haploidentical hematopoietic transplantation for acute myeloid leukemia: Challenging its predictive value. Blood 2007; 110:433-40.

31. Locatelli F, D Pende, R Maccario, MC Mingari, A Moretta, L Moretta. Haploidentical hemopoietic stem cell transplantation for the treatment of high-risk leukemias: How NK cells make the difference. Clin Immunol 2009.

32. Triplett B, R Handgretinger, CH Pui, W Leung. KIR-incompatible hematopoietic-cell transplantation for poor prognosis infant acute lymphoblastic leukemia. Blood 2006;107:1238-39.

33. Brunstein CG, JE Wagner, DJ Weisdorf, S Cooley, H Noreen, JN Barker, T DeFor, MR Verneris, BR Blazar, JS Miller. Negative effect of KIR alloreactivity in recipients of umbilical cord blood transplant depends on transplantation conditioning intensity. Blood 2009;113:5628-34.

34. Kim, SY, HB Choi, HY Yoon, EJ Choi, B Cho, HK Kim, YJ Kim, HJ Kim, CK Min, DW Kim, JW Lee, WS Min, CC Kim, TG Kim. Influence of killer cell immunoglobulin-like receptor genotypes on acute graft-vs-host disease after unrelated hematopoietic stem cell transplantation in Koreans. Tissue Antigens (69 Suppl) 2007;1:114-17.

35. Leung W, R Iyengar, V Turner, P Lang, P Bader, P Conn, D Niethammer, R. Handgretinger. Determinants of antileukemia effects of allogeneic NK cells. J Immunol 2004;172:644-50.

36. Bishara A., D De Santis, CC Witt, C Brautbar, FT Christiansen, R Or, A Nagler, S Slavin. The beneficial role of inhibitory KIR genes of HLA class I NK epitopes in haploidentically mismatched stem cell allografts may be masked by residual donor-alloreactive T cells causing GVHD. Tissue Antigens 2004;63:204-11.

37. Huang XJ, XY Zhao, DH Liu, KY Liu, LP Xu. Deleterious effects of KIR ligand incompatibility on clinical outcomes in haploidentical hematopoietic stem cell transplantation without in vitro T-cell depletion. leukemi 2007;21:848-51.

38. Zhao XY, XJ Huang, KY Liu, LP Xu, DH Liu. Prognosis after unmanipulated HLA-haploidentical blood and marrow transplantation is correlated to the numbers of KIR ligands in recipients. Eur J Haematol 2007;78:338-46.

39. Stern M, L Ruggeri, A Mancusi, ME Bernardo, C de Angelis, C Bucher, F Locatelli, F Aversa, A Velardi. Survival after T cell-depleted haploidentical stem cell transplantation is improved using the mother as donor. Blood 2008;112:2990-95.

40. Nguyen S, M Kuentz, JP Vernant, N Dhedin, D Bories, P Debre, V Vieillard. Involvement of mature donor T cells in the NK cell reconstitution after haploidentical hematopoietic stem-cell transplantation. Leukemi 2008; 22:344-52.

41. De Santis D, A Bishara, CS Witt, A Nagler, C Brautbar, S Slavin, and FT Christiansen. HLA natural killer cell HLA-C epitopes and killer cell immunoglobulin-like receptors both influence outcome of mismatched unrelated donor bone marrow transplants. Tissue Antigens 2005;65: 519-28.

42. Farag SS, A Bacigalupo, M Eapen, C Hurley, B Dupont, MA Caligiuri, C Boudreau, G Nelson, M Oudshoorn, J van Rood, A Velardi, M Maiers, M Setterholm, D Confer, PE Posch, C Anasetti, N Kamani, JS Miller, D Weisdorf, SM Davies. The effect of KIR ligand incompatibility on the outcome of unrelated donor transplantation: A report from the center for international blood and marrow transplant research, the European blood and marrow transplant registry, and the Dutch registry. Biol Blood Marrow Transplant 2006;12:876-84.

43. Hsu KC, T Gooley, M Malkki, C Pinto-Agnello, B Dupont, JD Bignon, M Bornhauser, F Christiansen, A Gratwohl, Y Morishima, M Oudshoorn, O Ringden, JJ van Rood, E Petersdorf. KIR ligands and prediction of relapse after unrelated donor hematopoietic cell transplantation for hematologic malignancy. Biol Blood Marrow Transplant 2006;12:828-36.

44. Giebel S, F Locatelli, T. Lamparelli, A Velardi, S. Davies, G Frumento, R Maccario, F Bonetti, J Wojnar, M Martinetti, F Frassoni, G Giorgiani, A Bacigalupo, J Holowiecki. Survival advantage with KIR ligand incompatibility in hematopoietic stem cell transplantation from unrelated donors. Blood 2003;102:814-19.

45. Elmaagacli AH, H Ottinger, M Koldehoff, R Peceny, NK Steckel, R Trenschel, H Biersack, H Grosse-Wilde, DW Beelen. Reduced risk for molecular disease in patients with chronic myeloid leukemia after transplantation from a KIR-mismatched donor. Transplantation 2005;79: 1741-47.

46. Beelen DW, HD Ottinger, S Ferencik, AH Elmaagacli, R Peceny, R Trenschel, H Grosse-Wilde. Genotypic inhibitory killer immunoglobulin-like receptor ligand incompatibility enhances the long-term antileukemic effect of unmodified allogeneic hematopoietic stem cell transplantation in patients with myeloid leukemias. Blood 105:2594-2600.

47. Kroger N, B Shaw, S Iacobelli, T Zabelina, K Peggs, A Shimoni, A. Nagler, T Binder, T Eiermann, A Madrigal, R Schwerdtfeger, M Kiehl, HG Sayer, J Beyer, M Bornhauser, F Ayuk, AR Zander, DI Marks. Comparison between antithymocyte globulin and alemtuzumab and the possible impact of KIR-ligand mismatch after dose-reduced conditioning and unrelated stem cell transplantation in patients with multiple myeloma. Br J Haematol 2005;129:631-43.

48. Lowe EJ, V Turner, R Handgretinger, EM Horwitz, E Benaim, GA Hale, P Woodard, W Leung. T-cell alloreactivity dominates natural killer cell alloreactivity in minimally T-cell-depleted HLA-non-identical paediatric bone marrow transplantation. Br J Haematol 2003;123:323-26.

49. Willemze R, CA Rodrigues, M Labopin, G Sanz, G Michel, G Socie, B Rio, A Sirvent, M Renaud, L Madero, M Mohty, C Ferra, F Garnier, P Loiseau, J Garcia, L Lecchi, G Kogler, Y. Beguin, C Navarrete, T Devos, I Ionescu, K Boudjedir, AL Herr, E Gluckman, V Rocha. KIR-ligand incompatibility in the graft-versus-host direction improves outcomes after umbilical cord blood transplantation for acute leukemia. leukemi 2009;23:492-500.

50. Frohn C, M Hoppner, P Schlenke, H Kirchner, P Koritke, J Luhm. Anti-myeloma activity of natural killer lymphocytes. Br J Haematol 2002;119:660-64.

51. Miller JS, S Cooley, P Parham, SS Farag, MR Verneris, KL McQueen, LA Guethlein, EA Trachtenberg, M Haagenson, MM. Horowitz, JP Klein, DJ Weisdorf. Missing KIR ligands are associated with less relapse and increased graft-versus-host disease (GVHD) following unrelated donor allogeneic HCT. Blood 2007;109:5058-61.

52. Hsu KC, CA Keever-Taylor, A Wilton, C Pinto, G Heller, K Arkun, RJ O'Reilly, MM. Horowitz, B Dupont. Improved outcome in HLA-identical sibling hematopoietic stem cell transplantation for acute myelogenous leukemia (AML) predicted by KIR and HLA genotypes. Blood 2005.

53. La Nasa G, R Littera, F Locatelli, C Giardini, A Ventrella, M Mulargia, A Vacca, N Orru, S Orru, E Piras, G Giustolisi, D Lisini, S Nesci, G Caocci, C Carcassi. Status of donor-recipient HLA class I ligands and not the KIR genotype is predictive for the outcome of unrelated hematopoietic stem cell transplantation in beta-thalassemia patients. Biol Blood Marrow Transplant 2007;13:1358-68.

54. Sobecks RM, EJ Ball, JP Maciejewski, LA Rybicki, S Brown, M Kalaycio, B Pohlman, S Andresen, KS Theil, R Dean, BJ Bolwell. Survival of AML patients receiving HLA-matched sibling donor allogeneic bone marrow transplantation correlates with HLA-Cw ligand groups for killer immunoglobulin-like receptors. Bone Marrow Transplant 2007;39:417-24.

55. Cook MA, DW Milligan, CD Fegan, PJ Darbyshire, P Mahendra, CF Craddock, PA Moss, DC Briggs. The impact of donor KIR and patient HLA-C genotypes on outcome following HLA-identical sibling hematopoietic stem cell transplantation for myeloid leukemia. Blood 2004; 103:1521-26.

56. Cooley S, E Trachtenberg, TL Bergemann, K Saeteurn, J Klein, CT Le, SG Marsh, LA Guethlein, P Parham, JS Miller, DJ Weisdorf. Donors with group B KIR haplotypes improve relapse-free survival after unrelated hematopoietic cell transplantation for acute myelogenous leukemia. Blood 2009;113:726-32.

57. Kroger N, T Binder, T Zabelina, C Wolschke, H Schieder, H Renges, F Ayuk, J Dahlke, T Eiermann, A Zander. Low number of donor activating killer immunoglobulin-like receptors (KIR) genes but not KIR-ligand mismatch prevents relapse and improves disease-free survival in leukemia patients after in vivo T-cell depleted unrelated stem cell transplantation. Transplantation 2006;82: 1024-30.

58. Antonella Mancusi, Loredana Ruggeri, Karina McQueen, Katia Perruccio, Franco Aversa, Massimo F.Martelli, Peter Parham, Andrea Velardi. Donor Activating Kir Genes and Survival after Haplo-Identical Hematopoietic Transplantation. Blood. Nov 2004(104), 2219. 2009. Ref Type: Generic

59. Savani BN, S Mielke, S Adams, M Uribe, K Rezvani, AS Yong, J Zeilah, R Kurlander, R Srinivasan, R Childs, N Hensel, AJ Barrett. Rapid natural killer cell recovery determines outcome after T-cell-depleted HLA-identical stem cell transplantation in patients with myeloid leukemias but not with acute lymphoblastic leukemia. leukemi 2007;21:2145-52.

60. Verheyden S, R Schots, W Duquet, C Demanet. A defined donor activating natural killer cell receptor genotype protects against leukemic relapse after related HLA-identical hematopoietic stem cell transplantation. Leukemi 2005;19:1446-51.

61. Sun JY, L Gaidulis, A Dagis, J. Palmer, R Rodriguez, MM Miller, SJ Forman, D Senitzer. Killer Ig-like receptor (KIR) compatibility plays a role in the prevalence of acute GVHD in unrelated hematopoietic cell transplants for AML. Bone Marrow Transplant 2005;36:525-30.

62. Hsu KC, C Pinto-Agnello, T Gooley, M Malkki, B Dupont, EW. Petersdorf. Hematopoietic stem cell transplantation: Killer immunoglobulin-like receptor component. Tissue Antigens 2007;69 Suppl 1:42-45.

63. Clausen J, D Wolf, AL Petzer, E Gunsilius, P Schumacher, B Kircher, G Gastl, D Nachbaur. Impact of natural killer cell dose and donor killer-cell immunoglobulin-like receptor (KIR) genotype on outcome following human leucocyte antigen-identical haematopoietic stem cell transplantation. Clin Exp Immunol 2007;148:520-28.
64. Giebel S, I Nowak, J Dziaczkowska, T Czerw, J Wojnar, M Krawczyk-Kulis, J Holowiecki, A Holowiecka-Goral, M Markiewicz, M Kopera, A Karolczyk, S Kyrcz Krzemien, P Kusnierczyk. Activating killer immunoglobulin-like receptor incompatibilities enhance graft-versus host disease and affect survival after allogeneic hematopoietic stem cell transplantation. Eur J Haematol, 2009.
65. Giebel S, J Dziaczkowska, J Wojnar, M Krawczyk-Kulis, M Markiewicz, T Kruzel, I Wylezol, K Nowak, K Jagoda, J Holowiecki. The impact of immunosuppressive therapy on an early quantitative NK cell reconstitution after allogeneic haematopoietic cell transplantation. Ann Transplant 2005; 10:29-33.
66. Muller C, G Schernthaner, J Kovarik, W Kalinowska, CC Zielinski. Natural killer cell activity and antibody-dependent cellular cytotoxicity in patients under various immunosuppressive regimens. Clin Immunol Immunopathol 1987;44:12-19.
67. Wang H, B Grzywacz, D Sukovich, V McCullar, Q Cao, AB Lee, BR Blazar, DN Cornfield, JS Miller, MR Verneris. The unexpected effect of cyclosporin A on CD56+. Blood 2007;110:1530-39.
68. Davies SM, L Ruggieri, T DeFor, JE Wagner, DJ Weisdorf, JS Miller, A Velardi, BR Blazar. Evaluation of KIR ligand incompatibility in mismatched unrelated donor hematopoietic transplants. Killer immunoglobulin-like receptor. Blood 2002;100:3825-27.
69. Morishima Y, T Yabe, K Matsuo, K Kashiwase, H Inoko, H Saji, K Yamamoto, E Maruya, Y Akatsuka, M Onizuka, H Sakamaki, H Sao, S Ogawa, S Kato, T Juji, T Sasazuki, Y Kodera. Effects of HLA allele and killer immunoglobulin-like receptor ligand matching on clinical outcome in leukemia patients undergoing transplantation with T-cell-replete marrow from an unrelated donor. Biol Blood Marrow Transplant 2007;13:315-28.
70. Bornhauser M, R Schwerdtfeger, H Martin, KH Frank, C Theuser, G Ehninger, F Locatelli, A Velardi, S Giebel. Role of KIR ligand incompatibility in hematopoietic stem cell transplantation using unrelated donors. Blood 2004;103: 2860-61.
71. Schaffer M, K J Malmberg, O Ringden, HG Ljunggren, M Remberger. Increased infection-related mortality in KIR-ligand-mismatched unrelated allogeneic hematopoietic stem-cell transplantation. Transplantation 2004;78: 1081-85.
72. McQueen, KL, KM Dorighi, LA Guethlein, R Wong, B Sanjanwala, P Parham. Donor-recipient combinations of group A and B KIR haplotypes and HLA class I ligand affect the outcome of HLA-matched, sibling donor hematopoietic cell transplantation. Hum Immunol 2007;68:309-23.
73. Triplett BM, EM Horwitz, R Iyengar, V Turner, MS Holladay, K Gan, FG Behm, W Leung. Effects of activating NK cell receptor expression and NK cell reconstitution on the outcomes of unrelated donor hematopoietic cell transplantation for hematologic malignancies. leukemi 2009;23:1278-87.

Chapter 32

Minor Histocompatibility Antigens in Biology and Medicine

Eric Spierings, Els Goulmy

INTRODUCTION

Minor histocompatibility (H) antigens are peptides derived from polymorphic self proteins that can differ between individuals. Minor H peptides are presented by the various MHC class I and class II molecules (Fig. 32.1). The MHC/minor H peptide complexes can function as transplantation barriers in allogeneic HLA-matched hematopoietic stem cell (SC) and in solid organ transplantation and induce immune responses in pregnancy.[1-4] Early murine studies demonstrated skin graft rejection by non-H2-encoded transplantation antigens in H2-identical mouse strains.[5,6] In humans, the impact of the minor H antigenic systems became apparent in 1976, through a serious clinical problems following HLA-identical sibling SC transplantation (SCT).[1] Although *in vitro* techniques unequivocally showed cellular activities between the HLA-identical donor and the SC recipient,[7,8] it was not until 1995 that the molecular characteristics of human minor H antigens were, clarified.[9-11] The chemical identification was instrumental for novel research aiming at understanding the immunobiology of minor H antigenic systems and at exploring the possibilities of their clinical usefulness in SCT and solid organ transplantation.

Here, we review our current knowledge on the immunobiology of human minor H antigens and discuss their relevance in transplantation.

THE IMMUNOBIOLOGY OF HUMAN MINOR H ANTIGENS

The Genetic Basis for Minor H Antigen Polymorphisms

Polymorphisms of genes between related and unrelated individuals form the genetic basis for minor H immunogenic T-cell epitopes. The most frequently observed form of polymorphism leading to minor H antigens is the non-synonymous single nucleotide polymorphism (SNP). Here, a single nucleotide difference in the genome results in a different amino acid in the peptide. Examples thereof have been described for the autosomally encoded minor H antigens HA-2,[11] HA-1,[12] HB-1,[13] HA-8,[14] HA-3,[15] ACC-1 and ACC-2,[16] SP110,[17] CTSH,[18] LB-ECGF,[19] LB-ADIR-1,[20] ACC-6,[21] CD19,[22] LB-PI4K2B-1,[23] and C19 orf 48.[24] Also all Y-gene encoded minor H antigens identified so far display non-synonymous SNP-like alterations, although most HY antigens display more than one SNP compared to their X-gene counterpart. Occasionally, a SNP leads to a stop codon instead of an altered amino acid, as observed for PANE1.[25] Here, the 3' RNA is not translated and a truncated protein is produced. Alternatively, SNPs can lead to changes in intron splicing, resulting in loss of a complete exon.[21]

Minor H antigen polymorphisms can also arise from so called deletion-insertion polymorphisms (DIPs). In these cases, one allele of the minor H gene has one or more extra nucleotide(s) when, compared to the other allele. If the DIP comprises a full triplet of nucleotides, the resulting protein will contain an extra-amino acid. Minor H antigens with a full triplet DIP have, however, not yet been described. The only DIP-based minor H antigen identified to date is LRH-1, consisting of a single nucleotide DIP leading to a shift in the open reading frame of the protein.[26]

Minor H antigen polymorphisms may also result from copy number variation (CNV). In humans, CNVs encompass more DNA than SNPs and DIPs. CNVs can result in either too many or too few of the dosage sensitive genes. The, as yet, one example with CNV is UGT2B17.[27] Its immunogenic allele is encoded on chromosome 4. A

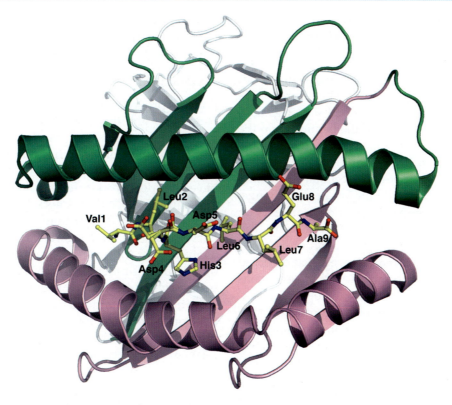

Fig. 32.1: Crystal structure of the minor H antigen HA-1 in the peptide binding groove of HLA-A*0201 (Protein Data Bank no. 3FT3). In green the alpha-1 domain and in pink the alpha-2 domain. Residues of the minor H antigen HA-1 are listed by the amino acid name and their position in the HA-1 peptide. Image kindly provided by Dr D Housset, Grenoble, France

non-immunogenic allele is non-existing, since its chromosomal counterpart has been deleted.

Mechanisms of Minor H Antigenic T-Cell Epitope Generation

As outlined above, the polymorphisms leading to alloimmune responses, as for example observed after SCT, often comprises a single nucleotide difference between recipient and donor. Various studies have investigated how these small differences can have such a significant immunological impact. Basically, two main mechanisms for the immunogenicity of genomic polymorphisms leading to minor H antigens have been described; the one mechanism occurs at the genomic, transcription or translational level; the other at the antigen processing and presentation level. Both mechanisms will be discussed and exemplified below.

Minor H Antigen Immunogenicity Resulting from Genomic/Transcription/Translation Differences

The immunogenicity of minor H antigens can be due to differences in the genome or in the transcription/translation of the genomic sequences. As already mentioned above, these involve mechanisms as a frameshift due to a DIP for LRH-1.[26] As DIPs result in a codon shift, all amino acids encoded after the DIP differ between the two alleles. This frame shift can be maintained for the remaining of the gene. It should however, be noted that alternative open reading frames have a higher frequency of stop codons leading to abrogation of the protein. This is the case for LRH-1, where, the LRH-1[4C] allele results in a protein of 146 amino acids compared to 422 amino acids for LRH-1[5C]. The sequence following the stop codon will not be translated. As a result thereof, these parts of the gene can theoretically contain additional minor H T-cell epitopes. Other mechanisms are copy number variation for UGT2B17,[27] introduction of a translation termination codon for PANE1,[25] and alternative splicing as observed for ACC-6.[21] All of the latter three mechanisms have in common that a potential allelic counterpart is not produced. The fact that (a part of) a protein is absent, opens the possibility for more minor H antigens encoded by one single genomic locus. Data on UGT2B17 confirm this assumption.[27-29]

Minor H Antigen Immunogenicity Resulting from Minor H Antigen Processing and Presentation Differences

The presentation of minor H antigens by HLA class-I and -II molecules on the cell surface depends on proper intracellular antigen processing. These processes comprise ubiquitinilation, degradation by proteasomes into peptides and translocation of the peptides into the ER, as well as the capacity of the peptides to bind HLA molecules.[30] As shown in previous studies on viral cytotoxic T-cell (CTL) epitopes, intracellular processing can be prohibited by a single amino acid exchange, resulting in absence of the MHC/peptide complexes on the cell surface.[31-33] These rules of processing and presentation also apply for the generation of minor H antigens. Differential proteasomal cleavage was observed for HA-3.[15] The non-immunogenic HA-3^M allele contains a proteasome cleavage site, destroying nonameric HA-3^M peptides and thus preventing cell-surface presentation of them. This cleavage site is absent in the immunogenic HA-3^T allele. Differential TAP translocation between two alleles of autosomally encoded minor H antigens was exemplified by Brickner, et al for HA-8;[14] the immunogenic HA-8^R peptide can efficiently be translocated into the ER via TAP molecules, whereas, its allelic counterpart HA-8^P peptide cannot. HLA-peptide stability and dissociation appeared to be essential for the generation of HA-1.[34] The immunogenic HA-1^H peptide forms a stable complex with the HLA-A2 molecule, with half-life values of more than 9 hr at 37°C. The non-immunogenic HA-1^R peptide, however, dissociates rapidly from the HLA-A2 molecule, displaying half-life values of less than 8 minutes. The HA-1^R peptide most likely already dissociates intracellular and never reaches the cell surface.

Minor H Antigen Immunogenicity Resulting from Differential T-cell Recognition

All above-described mechanisms imply a loss or absence of cell surface expression of one of the minor H antigen alleles. In these situations, the immune recognition pattern is thus unidirectional with regard to its presentation by the same HLA molecule. Yet, there are exceptions to the rule of unidirectionality. To date, bidirectional immune recognition in association with the same HLA allele has been described for the minor H antigens HB-1[13,35] and ACC-1.[16,36] As both minor H alleles can be presented at the cell surface, the T-cell receptor must be able to discriminate between the two alleles. Bidirectional minor H antigens have an advantage over unidirectional minor H antigens since bidirectionality evidently increases the number of patients eligible for minor H antigen-based immunotherapeutic applications.[37]

Genomic Minor H Antigen Typing

Both the progress in the genomic identification of minor H antigens and the growing interest in the application of minor H antigens as therapeutic tools require a simple and uniform allele-specific minor H antigen-typing protocol. Various methods for minor H antigen typing have been described including allele-specific PCR based on sequence-specific primers (SSP-PCR), PCR-RFLP, gene-specific PCR, real-time PCR, PCR with melting curve analyses, and reference strand conformation analysis (RSCA) (reviewed in).[38] We recently, reported on the development of a uniform methodology for genotyping of molecularly identified minor H antigens.[39] Additionally, a minor H antigen database has been developed providing information on the potential clinical relevance of the minor H antigen-typing results for the relevant donor/recipient pair (www.lumc.nl/dbminor).

Minor H Antigen Population Diversity

Logically, once new genetic systems are defined, population genetics are the fundamental analyses to be carried out. Moreover, the entrance of the minor H antigens as immunotherapeutic tools in the clinic (see below) demands estimation of their potential applicability in the different ethnic groups. A multi-center study comprising a worldwide analysis on the phenotype frequencies of minor H antigens provided for the first time the global phenotype frequencies of the 10 autosomally encoded minor H antigens identified at the initiation of the study.[37]

The results of this study can be summarized as follows; small and for some minor H antigens significant differences in the genotype and phenotype frequencies in the various ethnic populations were observed for all autosomally encoded minor H antigens. The highest variation among the ethnic populations was observed for UGT2B17. The phenotype frequency of UGT2B17 appeared to be geographically correlated on the Eurasian continents (Fig. 32.2), with the lowest frequency of the gene deletion in Western Europe (5%) and the highest in Eastern Asia (70% in Japan). For the other minor H antigens, the differences between populations were less pronounced. For example for the HA-1 immunogenic phenotype, the frequencies ranged from 60 to 75 percent. No geographical correlation could be observed for this minor H antigen.

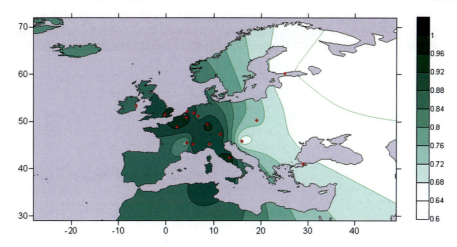

Fig. 32.2: Geospatial analyses of the phenotype frequencies of UGT2B17 in the European White Populations. Red dots represent the centers from which the frequency data were obtained. Numbers in the scaling indicate the proportion of individuals with the immunogenic phenotype. Numbers on the axis indicate the geographical coordinates in grades

Minor H Antigens in Biology—Key Points

- Minor H antigens result from genomic differences including SNPs, DIPs, and CNVs
- The immunogenicity of minor H antigens can be explained by:
  - Differential transcription/translation:
    - CNVs
    - Translation termination codons
    - DIPs
    - Alternative splicing
  - Differential antigen processing:
    - Proteasome-mediated cleavage
    - TAP translocation
    - HLA/peptide binding
- Minor H antigen phenotype frequencies can differ between ethnic populations
- These frequencies are relevant in the various clinical settings.

MINOR H ANTIGENS IN MEDICINE

The immune recognition of minor H antigens is a typical example of HLA-restricted recognition by T-cells in man.[1] Consequently, minor H antigen-specific cellular immune responses are readily generated in the HLA-matched transplantation settings. Interestingly, minor H antigenic immune responses are now known to occur in the physiological situation of HLA haplo-mismatched pregnancy as well.[3] Studying these naturally-occurring minor H antigen-specific immune reactions is crucial for understanding the minor H antigen immunobiology and provides the necessary information for the relevance of these histocompatibility systems for transplantation.

Below, the current knowledge on the minor H antigen-related responses both in the clinical settings and in pregnancy is summarized.

Minor H Antigens in Stem Cell Transplantation

In HLA-identical SCT, minor H antigens are key molecules driving allo-immune responses both in Graft-versus-Host-Disease (GvHD) and in Graft-versus-Tumor (GvT) reactivity.[40] Dissection of this apparent dual function of minor H antigens became evident through the observation of their different modes of tissue and cell expression, i.e. hematopoietic system restricted or broad.[41] Evidently, broadly expressed minor H antigens cause immune responses in both arms (GvHD and GvT) of Graft versus Host (GvH) responses. Indeed, the Y-chromosome encoded HY antigens, most of which are broadly expressed (Table 32.1), have been reported to clinically contribute to Graft versus Leukemia (GvL) activity.[42] CTLs specific for the broadly expressed HY antigen can be detected in association with leukemia remission.[43]

The involvement of broadly expressed minor H antigens, such as HY, in the GvHD arm of SCT was first shown by functional *in vitro* assays; CTLs directed to broadly expressed minor H antigens lyse, amongst others, cell types affected during GvHD, such as fibroblasts, melanocytes, and keratinocytes.[41] To further address this issue, skin sections were incubated with CTLs specific for the broadly expressed minor H antigen, A2/HY, or for the hematopoietic system-restricted minor H antigens HA-1 and HA-2. CTLs specific for the A2/HY minor H antigen induced severe GvH reactions of grades III–IV, while CTLs specific for HA-1 and HA-2

Table 32.1: The currently molecularly identified minor H antigens encoded by genes on the Y-chromosome. The mechanism explaining their immunogenicity has not yet been identified for any of these minor H antigens

Minor H antigen	HUGO Gene names		Tissue distribution
A1/HY	USP9Y	Ubiquitin specific peptidase 9, Y-linked	Broad
A2/HY	KDM5D	Lysine (K)-specific demethylase 5D	Broad
A33/HY	TMSB4Y	Thymosin, beta 4, Y-linked	Unknown
B27/HY	DDX3Y	DEAD (Asp-Glu-Ala-Asp) box polypeptide 3, Y-linked	Restricted
B52/HY	RPS4Y1	Ribosomal protein S4, Y-linked 1	Restricted
B60/HY	UTY	Ubiquitously transcribed tetratricopeptide repeat gene, Y-linked	Broad
B7/HY	KDM5D	Lysine (K)-specific demethylase 5D	Broad
B8/HY	UTY	Ubiquitously transcribed tetratricopeptide repeat gene, Y-linked	Restricted
DQ5/HY	DDX3Y	DEAD (Asp-Glu-Ala-Asp) box polypeptide 3, Y-linked	Broad
DR15/HY	DDX3Y	DEAD (Asp-Glu-Ala-Asp) box polypeptide 3, Y-linked	Broad
DRB3*0301/HY	RPS4Y1	Ribosomal protein S4, Y-linked 1	Broad

induced no or weak GvH reactions.[44] Since T-cells directed to hematopoiesis-restricted minor H antigens do not target the non-hematopoietic skin components, they may not be involved in local GvHD. This skin explant assay, however, does not provide a complete picture of GvHD, because antigen presenting cells (APCs) easily migrate out of the skin samples during its *in vitro* processing. Therefore, we recently developed specific T-cell staining reagents to directly study the specificity of T-cells infiltrated in the skin of sex-mismatched SCT recipients. Indeed, these *in situ* results fortify the presence of HY-specific T-cells in skin samples taking from male patients suffering from acute GvHD after sex-mismatched SCT (Kim et al manuscript in preparation).

As opposed to the combined GvHD and GvL activity of the broadly expressed minor H antigens, the activity of the hematopoietic system-specific minor H antigens is directed towards the GvL arm of SCT. So far, most autosomally encoded minor H antigens demonstrate expression limited to, but expressed on all cells of the hematopoietic system, including leukemic cells and leukemic progenitor cells (Table 32.2). *In vitro* experiments demonstrated that CTLs specific for HA-1 and HA-2 are capable of lysing leukemic cells.[45] Clinically, CTLs specific for the hematopoiesis-restricted minor H antigens HA-1 and HA-2 coincide with remission of hematological malignancies after donor lymphocyte infusion (DLI).[46]

Strikingly, some of the hematopoietic system-restricted minor H antigens show additional expression on a variety of solid tumor cells and are especially relevant for the GvT activity.[47-49] Whereas, the former group of minor H antigens is crucial in the GvL responses, the latter group of minor H antigens with additional expression on solid tumor cells can be exploited as curative tools for SC-based immunotherapy of both hematological malignancies and solid tumors. A recent clinical-related study wherein HA-1, HA-3 and HA-8 CTLs lysing carcinoma cells were, isolated from renal cell cancer patients with clinical responses after allogeneic SCT, further underlined the participation of minor H antigens in the GvT response.[50]

CLINICAL APPLICATION OF MINOR HISTOCOMPATIBILITY ANTIGENS

For clinical application, HLA-matched minor H antigen-mismatched recipient/donor combinations are selected based on their incompatibility of the relevant minor H antigen. Minor H antigens differ in their phenotype frequencies in the various ethnic populations, therewith determining the number of patients eligible for minor H antigen based immunotherapy.[37] The high phenotype frequency of HLA-A2 in combination with a relatively high disparity rate for HA-1 in all ethnic populations studied, currently mark HA-1 as the most favorable minor H antigen for clinical application in all ethnic populations. Similar results, however limited to only one or two ethnic groups, were obtained for the minor H antigens ACC-1, ACC-2, and HB-1^Y. The ACC-1 minor H antigen is restricted to the Asian/Pacific population,

Chapter 32 ■ Minor Histocompatibility Antigens in Biology and Medicine

Table 32.2: The currently molecularly identified minor H antigens encoded on autosomal genes ordered by chromosome. N.A. = not available

Chrom	Minor H antigen	HLA restriction	HUGO Gene name		Tissue distribution	dbSNP	Mechanism for immunogenicity
1	LB-ADIR-1	HLA-A2	TOR3A	Torsin family 3, member A	Restricted	rs2296377	Unknown
2	SP110	HLA-A3	SP110	SP110 nuclear body protein	Restricted	rs1365776	Unknown
4	LB-PI4K2B-1	HLA-DQ6	PI4K2B	Phosphatidylinositol 4-kinase type 2 beta	Broad	rs313549	Unknown
4	UGT2B17	HLA-A29	UGT2B17	UDP glucuronosyltransferase 2 family, polypeptide B17	Restricted	N.A.	Copy number variation
4	UGT2B17	HLA-B44	UGT2B17	UDP glucuronosyltransferase 2 family, polypeptide B17	Restricted	N.A.	Copy number variation
4	UGT2B17	HLA-A2	UGT2B17	UDP glucuronosyltransferase 2 family, polypeptide B17	Restricted	N.A.	Copy number variation
5	HB-1	HLA-B44	HMHB1	Histocompatibility (minor) HB-1	Restricted	rs161557	TCR (bidirectional)
7	HA-2	HLA-A2	MYO1G	Myosin IG	Restricted	rs61739531	Unknown
9	HA-8	HLA-A2	KIAA0020	KIAA0020	Broad	rs2173904	TAP translocation
15	ACC-1	HLA-A24	BCL2A1	B-cell leukemia/lymphoma 2 related protein A1	Restricted	rs1138357	TCR (bidirectional)
15	ACC-2	HLA-B44	BCL2A1	B-cell leukemia/lymphoma 2 related protein A1	Restricted	rs3826007	Unknown
15	CTSH/A31	HLA-A31	CTSH	Cathepsin H	Restricted	rs2289702	Unknown
15	CTSH/A33	HLA-A33	CTSH	Cathepsin H	Restricted	rs2289702	Unknown
15	HA-3	HLA-A1	AKAP13	A kinase (PRKA) anchor protein 13	Broad	rs7162168	Proteasome mediated digestion
16	CD19	HLA-A2	CD19	CD19 molecule	Restricted	rs2173904	Unknown
17	LRH-1	HLA-B7	P2RX5	Purinergic receptor P2X, ligand-gated ion channel, 5	Restricted	rs5818907	Frame shift
18	ACC-6	HLA-B44	HMSD	Histocompatibility (minor) serpin domain containing	Restricted	rs9945924	Alternative splicing
19	HA-1/A2	HLA-A2	HMHA1	Histocompatibility (minor) HA-1	Restricted	rs1801284	HLA binding stability
19	HA-1/B60	HLA-B60	HMHA1	Histocompatibility (minor) HA-1	Restricted	rs1801284	Unknown
19	C19orf48	HLA-B7	C19orf48	Chromosome 19 open reading frame 48	Restricted	rs5818907	Unknown
19	SLC1A5	HLA-B61	SLC1A5	Solute carrier family 1 (neutral amino acid transporter), member 5	Unknown	rs3027956	Unknown
22	LB-ECGF-1	HLA-B7	TYMP	Thymidine phosphorylase	Broad	N.A.	Unknown
22	PANE1	HLA-A3	CENPM	Centromere protein M	Restricted	N.A.	Stop codon

with 6.5 percent disparity in sibling pairs and 12.1 percent in MUD pairs. Similarly, ACC-2 can only be applied in a significant proportion of the pairs in the Caucasian and Mulatto population, as counts for HB-1^Y. Finally, estimating the chance of having at least one mismatch for a hematopoietic system-restricted minor H antigen out of the eight hematopoietic system-restricted minor H antigens included in this study, revealed 21.2 percent and 33.6 percent for Caucasian sibling and MUD pairs respectively, and 7.4 percent and 11.9 percent for the Black population, respectively. In all these estimations, the HLA allele phenotype frequencies of the respective populations were, taken into account. Since the report of this study on 10 minor H antigens, 13 novel minor H antigens have been identified. It is estimated that the current set of 23 minor H antigens leads to at least one disparity in more than 50 percent of the SCT MUD pairs in the Caucasian population.

Two modalities currently apply minor H antigens for anti-tumor therapy in the HLA-matched but minor H antigen-mismatched SCT setting. The one modality is the adoptive transfer of *in vitro* generated SC donor-derived minor H antigen-specific CTLs. The other, a more practical and far less laborious strategy, is post-SCT 'vaccination'. Both strategies, which are shortly discussed below, are currently ongoing in clinical phase I/II studies.[40]

Cellular Adoptive Immunotherapy

Disparity between HLA-matched donor and recipient for hematopoietic system restricted or solid tumor-specific minor H antigens can be applied as immunogens for cellular adoptive immunotherapy of hematological malignancies and solid tumors after allogeneic SCT and DLI respectively. Transfer of human minor H antigen-specific CTLs is successful in the treatment of human leukemia and solid tumors in an experimental non-obese diabetic/severe combined immunodeficiency mouse model.[51,52] This approach is possible in humans because minor H antigen-specific CTLs can be generated in large numbers in vitro by co-culturing of donor lymphocytes with donor-derived dendritic cells (DCs) which are minor H peptide-loaded or retrovirally transduced with the minor H gene.[53,54] Artificial APCs coated with HLA-A2/minor H antigen complexes, CD80 and CD54 might help to selectively enrich minor H antigen-specific CTLs for adoptive immunotherapy.[55]

Alternatively, transfer of minor H antigen-specific T-cell receptor (TCR) genes into peripheral blood mononuclear cells of the SCT donor can be explored. In vitro, successful transfer of TCR specific for the minor H antigens HA-2[56] or HA-1[57] has been demonstrated. Implementation of the TCR gene transduced cells into clinical trials is currently not opportune. Two crucial barriers still have to be overcome. Firstly, the relatively low avidity of the transferred TCRs is associated with (in vitro) low lysis capacity. Secondly, autoreactivities caused by TCR rearrangements cannot be excluded.

Interestingly, minor H antigens could potentially be applied in a partly HLA-mismatched setting of SCT. This supposition is based on in vitro results demonstrating the generation of CTLs specific for the self-antigens HLA-A2/cyclin-D1,[58] and the minor H antigen HA-1[59] in an HLA-mismatched setting, the so-called allo-restricted peptide-specific T-cells. Although really challenging and with a potential broad applicability, undesired alloreactivity is a major problem of this approach. As to the best of our knowledge, so far no protocols exist with which non-self HLA/minor H antigen specific CTLs can reliably be generated at clinical grade.

Vaccination

In the concept of minor H antigen vaccination, the relevant recipient-specific minor H peptides are administered to the SC recipient after SCT and/or after DLI. The goal is to further enhance the donor-derived minor H antigen-specific immune response via T-cells that have already been primed in vivo by minor H antigen-expressing host APCs.[47] The observation that HA-1- and HA-2-specific CTLs emerge after DLI following allogeneic SCT, underscores the feasibility of this approach.[60,61] Minor H antigen vaccination will boost minor H antigen-specific CTLs in patients with partial or full donor chimerism—i.e. when host APCs are progressively being replaced by minor H antigen-negative donor APCs. The protocol for optimally boosting minor H antigen-specific CTLs by vaccination is still unknown. Variables such as the choice of delivery system (naked DNA, recombinant vectors, short peptides, long peptides, recombinant protein or peptide-loaded DCs), dose, route of administration, frequency of vaccination and immunological adjuvants still need to be determined.[62,63]

A potential danger for life-long anti-tumor reactivity is the development of peripheral or central tolerance against tumor minor H antigens. Allogeneic SCT, however, provides the unique option of partially overcoming tolerance by repetitive deliveries of non-tolerant mature CTLs via DLI. Phase I and II minor H peptide vaccination studies have been started recently in non-myeloablative SCT for hematological malignancies promoting minor H antigen specific CTL responses in combination with DLI.[40]

Minor H Antigens in Solid Organ Transplantation

Several studies have reported a detrimental role for minor H antigen-specific T-cells in solid organ graft survival.[64] Noteworthy, a beneficial role, i.e. a tolerogenic effect of minor H antigen mismatches in renal transplantation – exists as well. This effect has been described in a report on a female recipient transplanted with a kidney from her HLA-identical sister.[65] Five years after transplantation, the recipient explicitly requested to discontinue treatment with immunosuppressive drugs permanently. Thirty years later, the transplanted kidney was still tolerated and well-functioning. Donor and recipient minor H antigen typing revealed that the donor was homozygous for the immunogenic HA-1^H allele, while the recipient was homozygous for the non-immunogenic HA-1^R allele. Interestingly, minor H antigen HA-1-specific CTLs were, identified in the tolerant patient's peripheral blood. Yet, minor HA-1-specific T-regulator cells were, also isolated from the same recipient, as was demonstrated in trans-vivo delayed type hypersensitivity (tvDTH) tests. The regulatory activity of these T-cells in the latter assays was dependent on three factors; the immunogenic HA-1^H minor H peptide, TGF-β, and, to a lesser extent, IL-10. Since HA-1 is only expressed by hematopoietic cells and thus absent on the non-hematopoietic kidney parenchymal cells, the regulation of host-versus-graft responses via HA-1 is supposed to act via the mechanism of linked suppression.

As mentioned above, the peripheral blood of the recipient also contained HA-1-specific effector T-cells. The regulatory and effector T-cell populations could be separated by FACS based on their differential staining intensity after incubation with HLA-A2/HA-1^H tetrameric complexes. The tetramer-bright staining T-cells were effector T-cells, while tetramer-dim staining T cells displayed a regulatory phenotype. Further *in vitro* studies on these T-cell populations showed an additional role of CTLA-4, indicating that cell-cell contact is involved in the regulation of these HA-1-specific immune responses. The maintenance of the HA-1-specific regulatory and effector T-cell populations in the recipient suggests the presence of a continuous source of HA-1 antigen *in vivo*. Due to the absence of HA-1 on the non-hematopoietic kidney parenchymal cells, these sources should be searched for in hematopoietic (stem) cells co-transplanted with the kidney or could be due to exchange of such cells during pregnancy. Cai, *et al* indeed detected HA-1^H-positive T-cell- and DC-microchimerism.[65] Since, the kidney recipient not only gave birth to an HA-1^H-positive daughter prior to transplantation, but was herself delivered by an HA-1^H positive mother, the origin of this microchimeric cells (i.e. from mother, daughter, or kidney donor) remains to be elucidated.

Minor H Antigens in Pregnancy

Minor H antigen immunization also occurs over HLA barriers as exemplified by minor H antigen-specific responses observed in pregnancy; namely, examination of multiparous women demonstrated that pregnancy can lead to allo-immune responses against the infant's paternal minor H antigens.[3] Similarly, minor H antigen-specific CTLs directed at the non-inherited maternal minor H antigens could be demonstrated in cord blood.[4] Interestingly, both minor H antigen sensitization and tolerization occur in mothers and in their adult offspring.[66] It is clear that this natural occurring allogeneic situation is a most interesting source for studying minor H antigen immunization patterns in all its aspects providing the basic information for transplantation-related reactions and development of minor H antigen-based immunotherapeutic strategies.

Minor H Antigens in Medicine—Key Points

- Immune responses to minor H antigens have been observed in relation to:
  - Stem cell transplantation
  - Organ transplantation
  - Pregnancy
- Tissue and cell expression of minor H antigens are either ubiquitous or restricted.
- Immune responses to minor H antigens are involved in:
  - Graft versus host disease
  - Graft versus leukemia/Graft versus tumor responses
  - Graft rejection
  - Graft tolerance
- Minor H antigens are currently used as immunogens to boost GvL/GvT after SCT responses with:
  - Cellular adoptive transfer of minor H antigen specific T-cells
  - Vaccination of the recipient after transplantation

KEY ISSUES

Genomic typing for minor H antigens has been implemented in many HLA typing laboratories. Information on the minor H phenotype is needed to identify patient/donor pairs eligible for minor H antigen-based immunotherapy in the setting of allogeneic SCT. HLA-matched patients/donors should be incompatible for the patient-specific tumor minor H antigen. The availability of matched unrelated SCT donors may facilitate the selection of donors mismatched for minor H antigens expressed on the malignancy of the patient. Additional information on the minor H antigen immunization status of SCT donors is useful as well. Namely, pregnancy induces immunization against minor H antigens, resulting in either sensitization or tolerization for minor antigens; either status can be expected in female and male SC donors.[67] Similarly, cord blood samples contain antigen-experienced CTLs recognizing maternal minor H antigens.[4] Currently, we analyze the impact of this naturally acquired minor H antigen immunization for subsequent minor H antigen immunotherapy.

Overall, the current number of molecularly identified minor H antigens still limits the actual clinical potential. A significant number of minor H antigens were, reported to display a restricted tissue expression pattern, potentially allowing the use of these antigens in enhancing graft-versus-leukemia effects. However, only three hematopoietic system-restricted minor H antigens have so far been demonstrated to be additionally expressed on solid tumors. The immunotherapeutic potential of minor H antigens demands serious searches for new minor H antigens and analyses of their phenotype frequency, tissue distribution, and functional membrane expression. Newly identified minor H antigens that meet the prerequisites for specific immunotherapy for malignancies, such as membrane expression by malignant cells, offer additional curative tools for SC-based immunotherapy for various hematological malignancies and solid tumors. A serious search for tumor cell-specific minor H antigens expressed by common HLA alleles is urgently needed.

As for solid organ transplantation, successful induction of life-long immunological tolerance to allogeneic minor H antigens has key priority, considering the high risk to develop malignancies caused by continuous use of immunosuppressive drugs. Pregnancy leads to minor H antigen-specific CTLs but also to the induction of minor H antigen-specific regulatory T-cells in mutual mother/child direction.[66] This information needs further exploration; for example, by identifying renal transplant recipients for pre-existing minor H antigen-specific regulatory T-cells. Similarly, monitoring of recipients after HLA-matched minor H antigen-mismatched renal transplantation may be used to guide in tapering of immunosuppressive agents.

ACKNOWLEDGMENTS

We are grateful to Dr Dominique Housset for providing the image of the crystal structure of HA-1 in HLA-A*0201. The work has been funded in part by the Netherlands Organization for Scientific Research (NWO), the Dutch Cancer Foundation, the Macropa Foundation, National Institutes of Health (NIH) under contract 1R01CA118880-01A1, and the Leiden University Foundation (pilot grant).

REFERENCES

1. Goulmy E, Termijtelen, A, Bradley, BA, van Rood, JJ. Alloimmunity to human H-Y. Lancet 1976;2:1206.
2. Goulmy E, Bradley, BA, Lansbergen, Q, van Rood, JJ. The importance of H-Y incompatibility in human organ transplantation. Transplantation 1978;25:315-19.
3. Verdijk RM, Kloosterman A, Pool J, et al. Pregnancy induces minor histocompatibility antigen-specific cytotoxic T-cells: Implications for stem cell transplantation and immunotherapy. Blood 2004;103:1961-64.
4. Mommaas B, Stegehuis-Kamp, JA, Van Halteren, AG, et al. Cord blood comprises antigen-experienced T cells specific for maternal minor histocompatibility antigen HA-1. Blood 2004;105:1823-27.
5. Graff RJ, Bailey DW. The non-H-2 histocompatibility loci and their antigens. Transplant Rev 1973;15:26-49.
6. Schultz, JS, Beals, TF, Petraitis, FP. Contributions of H-2 and non H-2 genetic barriers. Immunogenetics 1976;3:85-96.
7. Goulmy, E, Gratama, JW, Blokland, E, Zwaan, FE, van Rood, JJ. A minor transplantation antigen detected by MHC-restricted cytotoxic T lymphocytes during graft-versus-host disease. Nature 1983;302:159-61.
8. van Els, CA, D'Amaro, J, Pool, J et al. Immunogenetics of human minor histocompatibility antigens: their polymorphism and immunodominance. Immunogenetics 1992;35:161-65.
9. Wang W, Meadows LR, den Haan JM, et al. Human H-Y: A male-specific histocompatibility antigen derived from the SMCY protein. Science 1995;269:1588-90.
10. Goulmy E, Pool J, van den Elsen PJ. Interindividual conservation of T-cell receptor beta chain variable regions by minor histocompatibility antigen-specific HLA-A*0201- restricted cytotoxic T-cell clones. Blood 1995;85:2478-81.
11. den Haan JM, Sherman NE, Blokland E, et al. Identification of a graft versus host disease-associated human minor histocompatibility antigen. Science 1995; 268:1476-80.
12. den Haan JM, Meadows LM, Wang W, et al. The minor histocompatibility antigen HA-1: A diallelic gene with a single amino acid polymorphism. Science 1998;279:1054-57.
13. Dolstra H, Fredrix H, Maas F, et al. A human minor histocompatibility antigen specific for B cell acute lymphoblastic leukemia. J Exp Med 1999;189:301-08.
14. Brickner AG, Warren EH, Caldwell JA, et al. The immunogenicity of a new human minor histocompatibility antigen results from differential antigen processing. J Exp Med 2001;193:195-206.
15. Spierings E, Brickner AG, Caldwell JA, et al. The minor histocompatibility antigen HA-3 arises from differential proteasome-mediated cleavage of the lymphoid blast crisis (Lbc) oncoprotein. Blood 2003;102:621-29.
16. Akatsuka Y, Nishida T, Kondo E, et al. Identification of a Polymorphic Gene, BCL2A1, Encoding Two Novel Hematopoietic Lineage-specific Minor Histocompatibility Antigens. J Exp Med 2003;197:1489-500.
17. Warren EH, Vigneron NJ, Gavin MA, et al. An antigen produced by splicing of noncontiguous peptides in the reverse order. Science 2006;313:1444-47.
18. Torikai H, Akatsuka Y, Miyazaki M, et al. The human cathepsin H gene encodes two novel minor histocompatibility antigen epitopes restricted by HLA-A*3101 and -A*3303. Br J Haematol 2006;134:406-10.
19. Slager EH, Honders MW, van der Meijden ED, et al. Identification of the angiogenic endothelial cell growth factor-1/thymidine phosphorylase as a potential target for immunotherapy of cancer. Blood 2006;107:4954-60.
20. van Bergen CA, Kester MG, Jedema I, et al. Multiple myeloma-reactive T cells recognize an activation-induced minor histocompatibility antigen encoded by the ATP-dependent interferon-responsive (ADIR) gene. Blood 2007; 109:4089-96.

21. Kawase T, Akatsuka Y, Torikai H, et al. Alternative splicing due to an intronic SNP in HMSD generates a novel minor histocompatibility antigen. Blood 2007; 110:1055-63.
22. Spaapen RM, Lokhorst HM, van den OK, et al. Toward targeting B cell cancers with CD4+ CTLs: Identification of a CD19-encoded minor histocompatibility antigen using a novel genome-wide analysis. J Exp Med 2008; 205:2863-72.
23. Griffioen M, van der Meijden ED, Slager EH, et al. Identification of phosphatidylinositol 4-kinase type II beta as HLA class II-restricted target in graft versus leukemia reactivity. Proc Natl Acad Sci USA 2008;105:3837-42.
24. Tykodi SS, Fujii N, Vigneron N, et al. C19orf48 encodes a minor histocompatibility antigen recognized by CD8+ cytotoxic T cells from renal cell carcinoma patients. Clin Cancer Res 2008;14:5260-69.
25. Brickner AG, Evans AM, Mito JK, et al. The PANE1 gene encodes a novel human minor histocompatibility antigen that is selectively expressed in B-lymphoid cells and B-CLL. Blood 2006;107:3779-86.
26. de Rijke B, van Horssens-Zoetbrood A, Beekman JM, et al. A frame-shift polymorphism in P2X5 elicits an allogeneic cytotoxic T lymphocyte response associated with remission of chronic myeloid leukemia. J Clin Invest 2005;115:3506-16.
27. Murata M, Warren EH, Riddell SR. A Human Minor Histocompatibility Antigen Resulting from Differential Expression due to a Gene Deletion. J Exp Med 2003;197: 1279-89.
28. Terakura S, Murata M, Warren EH, et al. A single minor histocompatibility antigen encoded by UGT2B17 and presented by human leukocyte antigen-A*2902 and -B*4403. Transplantation 2007;83:1242-48.
29. Kamei M, Nannya Y, Torikai H, et al. HapMap scanning of novel human minor histocompatibility antigens. Blood 2009;113:5041-48.
30. Pamer E, Cresswell P. Mechanisms of MHC class I—restricted antigen processing. Ann Rev Immunol 1998;16: 323-58.
31. Beekman NJ, van Veelen PA, van Hall T, et al. Abrogation of CTL epitope processing by single amino acid substitution flanking the C-terminal proteasome cleavage site. J Immunol 2000;164:1898-905.
32. Ossendorp F, Eggers M, Neisig A, et al. A single residue exchange within a viral CTL epitope alters proteasome-mediated degradation resulting in lack of antigen presentation. Immunity 1996;5:115-24.
33. Theobald M, Ruppert T, Kuckelkorn U, et al. The sequence alteration associated with a mutational hotspot in p53 protects cells from lysis by cytotoxic T lymphocytes specific for a flanking peptide epitope. J Exp Med 1998;188: 1017-28.
34. Spierings E, Gras S, Reiser JB, et al. Steric hindrance and fast dissociation explain the lack of immunogenicity of the minor histocompatibility HA-1Arg Null allele. J Immunol 2009;182:4809-16.
35. Dolstra H, de Rijke B, Fredrix H, et al. Bi-directional allelic recognition of the human minor histocompatibility antigen HB-1 by cytotoxic T lymphocytes. Eur J Immunol 2002;32:2748-58.
36. Kawase T, Nannya Y, Torikai H, et al. Identification of human minor histocompatibility antigens based on genetic association with highly parallel genotyping of pooled DNA. Blood 2008;111:3286-94.
37. Spierings E, Hendriks M, Absi L, et al. Phenotype Frequencies of Autosomal Minor Histocompatibility Antigens Display Significant Differences among Populations. PLoS Genet 2007;3:e103.
38. Spierings E, Goulmy E. Molecular typing methods for minor histocompatibility antigens. Methods Mol Med 2007;134:81-96.
39. Spierings E, Drabbels J, Hendriks M, et al. A uniform genomic minor histocompatibility antigen typing methodology and database designed to facilitate clinical applications. PLoS ONE 2006;1:e42.
40. Hambach L, Goulmy E. Immunotherapy of cancer through targeting of minor histocompatibility antigens. Curr Opin Immunol 2005;17:202-10.
41. de Bueger MM, Bakker A, van Rood, JJ, van der Woude F, Goulmy E. Tissue distribution of human minor histocompatibility antigens. Ubiquitous versus restricted tissue distribution indicates heterogeneity among human cytotoxic T lymphocyte-defined non-MHC antigens. J Immunol 1992;149:1788-94.
42. Gratwohl A, Hermans J, Niederwieser D, van Biezen A, van Houwelingen HC, Apperley J. Female donors influence transplant-related mortality and relapse incidence in male recipients of sibling blood and marrow transplants. Hematol J 2001;2:363-70.
43. Takami A, Sugimori C, Feng X, et al. Expansion and activation of minor histocompatibility antigen HY-specific T cells associated with graft-versus-leukemia response. Bone Marrow Transplant 2004;34:703-09.
44. Dickinson AM, Wang XN, Sviland L, et al. In situ dissection of the graft-versus-host activities of cytotoxic T cells specific for minor histocompatibility antigens. Nat Med 2002;8:410-14.
45. van der Harst D, Goulmy E, Falkenburg J, et al. Recognition of minor histocompatibility antigens on lymphocytic and myeloid leukemic cells by cytotoxic T-cell clones. Blood 1994;83:1060-66.
46. Marijt W, Heemskerk M, Kloosterboer F, et al. Hematopoiesis-restricted minor histocompatibilty antigens HA-1- or HA-2-specific T cells can induce complete remissions of relapsed leukemia. Proc Natl Acad Sci 2003;100:2742-47.
47. Mutis T, Goulmy E. Hematopoietic system-specific antigens as targets for cellular immunotherapy of hematological malignancies. Semin Hematol 2002;39: 23-31.
48. Klein CA, Wilke M, Pool J, et al. The Hematopoietic System-specific Minor Histocompatibility Antigen HA-1 Shows Aberrant Expression in Epithelial Cancer Cells. J Exp Med 2002;196:359-68.

49. Fujii N, Hiraki A, Ikeda K, et al. Expression of minor histocompatibility antigen, HA-1, in solid tumor cells. Transplantation 2002;73:1137-41.
50. Tykodi S, Warren E, Thompson J, et al. Allogeneic hematopoietic cell transplantation for metastatic renal cell carcinoma after nonmyeloablative conditioning: toxicity, clinical response, and immunological response to minor histocompatibility antigens. Cinical Cancer research 2004;10:7799-811.
51. Hambach L, Nijmeijer BA, Aghai Z, et al. Human cytotoxic T lymphocytes specific for a single minor histocompatibility antigen HA-1 are effective against human lymphoblastic leukaemia in NOD/scid mice. Leukemia 2006;20:371-74.
52. Hambach L, Vermeij M, Buser A, Aghai Z, van der KT, Goulmy E. Targeting a single mismatched minor histocompatibility antigen with tumor-restricted expression eradicates human solid tumors. Blood 2008;112: 1844-52.
53. Mutis T, Verdijk R, Schrama E, Esendam B, Brand A, Goulmy E. Feasibility of immunotherapy of relapsed leukemia with ex vivo- generated cytotoxic T lymphocytes specific for hematopoietic system- restricted minor histocompatibility antigens. Blood 1999;93:2336-41.
54. Mutis T, Ghoreschi K, Schrama E, et al. Efficient induction of minor histocompatibility antigen HA-1-specific cytotoxic T-cells using dendritic cells retrovirally transduced with HA- 1-coding cDNA. Biol Blood Marrow Transplant 2002;8:412-19.
55. Oosten LE, Blokland E, Van Halteren AG, et al. Artificial antigen-presenting constructs efficiently stimulate minor histocompatibility antigen-specific cytotoxic T lymphocytes. Blood 2004;104:224-26.
56. Heemskerk MH, Hoogeboom M, de Paus RA, et al. Redirection of antileukemic reactivity of peripheral T lymphocytes using gene transfer of minor histocompatibility antigen HA-2-specific T-cell receptor complexes expressing a conserved alpha joining region. Blood 2003;102:3530-40.
57. Mommaas B, Van Halteren AG, Pool J, et al. Adult and cord blood T cells can acquire HA-1 specificity through HA-1 T-cell receptor gene transfer. Haematologica 2005; 90:1415-21.
58. Sadovnikova E, Jopling LA, Soo KS, Stauss HJ. Generation of human tumor-reactive cytotoxic T cells against peptides presented by non-self HLA class I molecules. Eur J Immunol 1998;28:193-200.
59. Mutis T, Blokland E, Kester M, Schrama E, Goulmy E. Generation of minor histocompatibility antigen HA-1-specific cytotoxic T cells restricted by nonself HLA molecules; a potential strategy to treat relapsed leukemia after HLA-mismatched stem cell transplantation. Blood 2002;100:547-52.
60. Marijt WA, Heemskerk MH, Kloosterboer FM, et al. Hematopoiesis-restricted minor histocompatibility antigens HA-1- or HA-2-specific T cells can induce complete remissions of relapsed leukemia. Proc Natl Acad Sci USA 2003; 100:2742-47.
61. Kircher B, Stevanovic S, Urbanek M, et al. Induction of HA-1-specific cytotoxic T-cell clones parallels the therapeutic effect of donor lymphocyte infusion. Br J Haematol 2002;117:935-39.
62. Scheibenbogen C, Letsch A, Schmittel A, Asemissen AM, Thiel E, Keilholz U. Rational peptide-based tumour vaccine development and T cell monitoring. Semin Cancer Biol 2003;13:423-29.
63. Figdor CG, de VI, Lesterhuis WJ, Melief CJ. Dendritic cell immunotherapy: Mapping the way. Nat Med 2004;10: 475-80.
64. Dierselhuis M, Goulmy E. The relevance of minor histocompatibility antigens in solid organ transplantation. Curr Opin Organ Transplant 2009.
65. Cai J, Lee J, Jankowska-Gan, E, et al. Minor H Antigen HA-1-specific Regulator and Effector CD8+ T Cells, and HA-1 Microchimerism, in Allograft Tolerance. J Exp Med 2004;199:1017-23.
66. van Halteren AG, Jankowska-Gan E, Joosten A, et al. Naturally acquired tolerance and sensitization to minor histocompatibility antigens in healthy family members. Blood 2009;114:2263-72.

Chapter 33

Unrelated Marrow Donor Registries

S Tulpule, JA Madrigal

INTRODUCTION AND BACKGROUND

Transplantation of hematopoietic stem cells derived from the bone marrow or peripheral blood of matched related or unrelated donors, or the umbilical cord, has become the standard of care for patients with hematological malignancies. Its clinical application also include treatment of immune deficiency disorders, metabolic disorders and bone marrow failure syndromes.

One of the limitations to the application of the procedure has been the lack of HLA matched donors. In most situations, the donor of first choice is a HLA-matched sibling. It is estimated that, in European Caucasoid patients requiring a hematopoietic stem cell transplant only 30 percent would have a HLA matched sibling. In patients without a related donor, a Volunteer Unrelated Donor (VUD) search is initiated. Many studies now show the outcome of VUD transplants to be similar to that of HLA-matched sibling transplants.

Currently there are more than 13 million unrelated stem cell donor worldwide. They are made up from 60 stem cell donor registries from 44 countries, and 42 cord blood banks from 26 countries.[1] Bone Marrow Donors Worldwide (BMDW) is an organization that works towards collecting the HLA phenotypes of volunteer stem cell donors and cord blood units. It is also responsible for the co-ordination of their worldwide distribution. However, approximately only 30 percent of VUD searches result in identification and availability of a suitably matched bone marrow donor. In order to increase the probability of a match, registries in countries all over the world in Europe, North America, Australia, Asia, Africa and South America have increased their efforts to improve the number of donors on their register.

Data from the National Marrow Donor Program (NMDP) indicate that it takes a median of 4 months to complete searches that result in a transplantation. A proportion of patients succumb to their disease while awaiting a suitable HLA matched VUD. Donor searches in patients of non European Caucasoids, result in an even lower success because of less chance of finding a suitable donor. These results have stimulated the search for other potential sources of hematopoietic stem cells one of them being cord stem cells.

Worldwide, registries have their own organisational set up and pattern, to find a suitable match for a patient. Within each registry, the co-ordinating centre works with the donor recruitment centres and transplant centres to identify hematopoietic stem cells which are a potential match. In the UK, the Anthony Nolan Trust runs and maintains it's registry including donor recruitment. It also has its in-house laboratory where all the donors are tissue typed and therefore has centralisation of all the services. In Bone Marrow Donors World Wide, the HLA phenotypes of more than 13 million unrelated stem cell donors including cord stem cells are collected and combined in matching programmes.

TRANSPLANT ACTIVITY

Given below is a snap shot of donor numbers in the major registries worldwide.

The large bone marrow donor registries

Name	Total Donors	%ABDR typed
NMDP (US)	5,375,853	87.4
ZKDR (Germany)	3,645,872	66.3
Ezer Mizion (Israel)	487,470	75.9
Anthony Nolan (UK)	402,373	82.1
Japan	344,121	100
IBMDR (Italy)	327,610	68.4
BBMR (UK)	310,806	94.2
Buddhist Tzu Chi Stem Cells Center (Taiwan)	291,168	87.7

Unrelated Donor Registries in the UK

At the time of writing there were a total of 759,974 UK donors. The split between the 3 UK registries is as under. The year the registry was established is shown in brackets.

ANT (1974) - Anthony Nolan Trust — 395,135
BBMR (1987) - British Bone Marrow
    Registry — 310,541
WBMDR (1989) - Welsh Bone Marrow
    Donor Registry — 54,298

International v/s UK Activity (WMDA 2007 Statistics)

A survey of 69 participating registries (inc Brazil and China) revealed that 0.2 percent of the worldwide population is a registered potential HPC donor compared to 1.2 percent of UK population. Similarly 0.07 percent of all the listed worldwide donors actually donated in 2007. This is comparable to 0.07 percent of all UK donors and 0.09 percent of ANT donors.

There were 32,387 new patients worldwide referred for unrelated donor searches of which 1260 were new UK patients. 48,005 donors world-wide provided CT samples, of which 3205 were for the UK, with 2004 from the ANT. There were 9,484 adult donations were recorded world-wide with 67 percent being PBSC donations. There were 550 adult donations for the UK out of which 368 were from the ANT. Out of the total UK adult donations 67 percent were PBSC of which 73 percent were from the ANT).

Looking at the International Activity

- 42 percent of transplants (from adult donors) were performed using donors from another country
- 3,029 patients received HPC-M (BM)
- 5,974 patients received HPC-A (PBSC)
- 1,350 patients received HPC-C (cord blood).

Looking at UK Activity in 2007

- 1260 new patients referred for searches
- 704 had their search extended internationally by end of 2007
- 221 transplants from ANT donors to patients referred from UK centres
- 75 transplants from BBMR (British Bone Marrow Registry) donors and 22 from WBMDR (Welsh Bone Marrow Donor Registry) donors to patients referred from UK centers
- 318 transplants from an international donor/cord unit to UK patients (241 adult 77 CB)
- 32 UK transplant centers performed at least one unrelated donor transplant (range 1-40).

Looking at UK activity in 2008, it showed an increasing trend of activity in keeping with data from other larger registries worldwide.

- 1414 new patients were referred for searches
- 857 had their search extended internationally by end of 2007
- There were 212 transplants from ANT donors to patients referred from UK centers
- There were 171 transplants from ANT donors to patients overseas
- There were 359 transplants from an international donor/cord unit to UK patients (265 adult 91 CB)
- A total of 33 UK transplant centers performed at least one unrelated donor transplant (range 1-19).

STRUCTURE OF REGISTRIES

The World Marrow Donor Association (WMDA) is an international collaboration of organisations and individuals involved in hematopoietic stem cell donation and transplantation. It has developed guidelines to facilitate the international exchange of hemopoietic stem cells through working groups in the area of donor registries, clinical issues, ethics, quality assurance and information technology. In 2003, the WMDA began an accreditation program for national donor registries to ensure uniform standards for international donor exchange.

The collaboration between international donor and cord blood registries is essential in ensuring an optimal supply and efficiency in exchanging stem cell donors worldwide for patients in need of a HCT.

Registries worldwide differ in their structure and operations. This is largely dependent upon the set up of the local health services, funding and allied organisations. The 3 main aspects important to the development of a registry are recruitment of donors, HLA typing of the donors and provision of a matched donor. Registries world wide have 1 or all 3 under one organisation like the Anthony Nolan Trust, or most which type the HLA from third party labs which have undergone the required accreditation and quality assessments. The structure of the Anthony Nolan Registry is briefly outlined below.

Prototype ANT

The Anthony Nolan Trust was established in 1974, by Shirley Nolan, as the world's first volunteer unrelated bone marrow donor register. The trust is one of the largest unrelated donors registries in the world.

The 3 main sections of the Trust are:
- Operations and Donor Recruitment
- Research
- Laboratory services.

The Operations division is a very busy section. Responsibilities include:
- Maintaining an active volunteer register, through donor recruitment, retention and tracing strategies.
- Processing the search request and reporting results to the requesting center, including a report of international panels for UK centers.
- Co-ordinating blood samples from both the Anthony Nolan Trust donors and international donors required for further match testing at the Anthony Nolan Histocompatibilty laboratories or other laboratories both in the UK and overseas.
- Co-ordinate the testing and procurement of cord bloods from international cord blood banks.
- Co-ordinating the donation procedure in the event of a donor/patient match, both nationally and internationally.
- Monitoring the Anthony Nolan Trust donor's physical, emotional and psychological well being during and post donation.

Operations Department

The organizational set up for an unrelated donor marrow registry is summarized in Figure 33.1.

Donor Recruitment Manager

- Updates and manages donor database.
- Promotes and secures active recruitment of bone marrow donors, working predominantly with organisations and groups from within the corporate, private and public sectors as well as individuals, community groups and social organisations in a designated region.

Search Manager

- Includes the complex procedure related to HLA identification and matching of donors and patients involved in the bone marrow transplant.
- Procures samples for confirmatory typing from international donors at the request of UK transplant centers.

Preharvest Manager

- Locates and contacts Anthony Nolan Donors and procures samples for confirmatory typing as requested by the transplant centers for further testing prior to final identification as donor of choice.

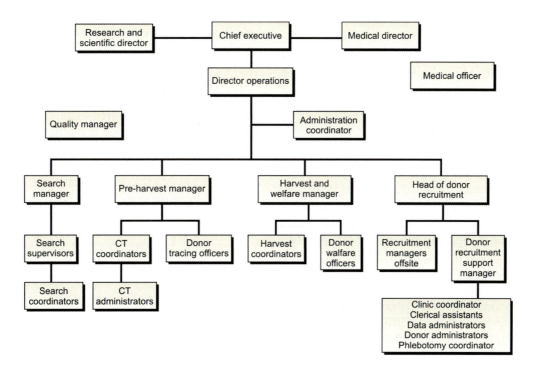

Fig. 33.1: Operational set up at the Anthony Nolan Trust

Harvest and Welfare Manager
- Co-ordinates procurement of donations and follows up on donor welfare post donation.
- Maintains volunteer courier database.

Laboratory Services

The Histocompatibility laboratory services are divided into teams, which work in close co-ordination with each other. They are:
- New Donor Typing.
- Confirmatory Typing.
- Clinical Services.
- High Resolution Typing.
- Solid Organ Team.
- Support Staff.

New Donor Typing

This team is responsible for work as per ANT protocols. This includes:
- Luminex SSOP – Intermediate resolution typing
- HLA-A, -B, -C, –DRB1 and –DQB1 on all samples
- CMV status

HLA TYPING WITHIN REGISTRIES

One of the important aspects of a registry is the resolution of HLA typing for it's first time donors. It is debatable whether increasing the typing resolution to allelic level for all 5 loci- HLA-A, B, C, DRB1 and DQB1 results in an increased frequency of a fast and successful 10/10 match. With technological advances and the need to find a match in the shortest possible time within financial boundaries, registries are constantly reviewing their policies towards achieving this goal.

In 2003, under the auspices of the WMDA, a survey was conducted looking at new donor typing in registries.[2] There were over 1 million HLA typing requests including over 918,000 requests for typing of new volunteers for entry into their databases from registries worldwide. The registries used up to 28 HLA laboratories to perform the typing. The registries using more than one typing laboratory differed in their requirements for HLA testing with one third having no requirements for resolution, loci required, or testing methods. HLA-A, -B, -DRB1 was routinely done for new donors by almost half of the registries. However, a quarter typed only HLA-A, -B. Additional loci tested included, DRB3/4/5, DQB1, and HLA-C. HLA class I was typed by both DNA-based methods and serology with half of the registries collecting only low resolution typing. 77 percent of registries typed more than 50 percent of their new volunteers by oligonucleotide probe-based testing, although other methods like sequence-specific priming and sequence-based typing were used. It was clear, however, that other methods, were used for some samples to reach the resolution required for the typing. DNA-based methods were used by most registries to type DRB1.

Impact on Informatics

Given the varying resolution of HLA typing and changes in typing methods, registries need to be prepared to meet this bioinformatics challenge. A method to collect HLA data by the registry from most HLA typing methods would be quite useful. This could then be incorporated in software programmes allowing exchange of information between the laboratories and the registry. The WMDA Information Technology Working Group has proposed a set of guidelines for use of HLA nomenclature for international exchange.[3]

Transplant centers typically search for allele-level HLA matches for their patients. Similarly registries are continually finding ways to maximize the chances of a 'match' with one of their donors. To do this, given the varying resolutions for HLA typing, registries would need to find ways to predict the potential of allele matches among volunteer donors typed at low to intermediate resolution. Although population genetics can be helpful, applying it to large registries to assist with donor selection would need established systems and pathways in place making this a challenging task. The National Marrow Donor Program has defined allele-level haplotypes for HLA-A, B, DRB1 and has incorporated this information into their search and matching algorithm. At the Anthony Nolan Trust (ANT) registry, a software package Cactus, being developed at the ANT, is able to assess HLA diversity patterns in the UK. This is based on a population genetics analysis using data derived from 268,000 individuals of a north European Caucasoid population. The analysis is performed using using allele, haplotype, and phenotype frequencies. The differences observed between regions of the UK could provide useful information to the registry to focus their recruitment strategies.

Strategies for New Donor Typing

Unrelated donor registries must make decisions on the methods used to HLA type new donors based on various factors including available finances and donor diversity. The approaches change over time with respect to the level of resolution and loci tested based on costs, advances in technologies and emerging clinical outcome data from matching studies.

A comparison of new donor typing strategies for three European registries was undertaken.[4] These were the France Greffe de Moelle (FGM), France; The Czech National Marrow Donors Registry (CNMDR), Czech Republic; and The Anthony Nolan Trust (ANT), UK. They looked at HLA and donor factors.

The age and sex of donors did not influence the HLA typing strategy of the FGM Register; however, both the ANT and CNMDR had additional testing of some of the new donors. The ANT had undertaken additional HLA-C and DQB1 testing on all male donors aged 30 years or younger. The CNMDR also performed additional testing on males under 35 years of age (HLA-C, two-digit testing; B*35, *44 and DRB1*04, *11, *13 sub typing). Of interest, the two larger and older registries (ANT and FGM) have more female than male donors; however, within the fully typed portion of these registries, male donors make up the largest percentage.

To improve the quality of the data on the register, all the three registries felt the need to have a system that would select donors for additional HLA typing. All the three registries had specific 'projects' in place. The ANT performed additional sub typing on particular HLA types, e.g. DRB1*04 sub typing. The CNMDR undertook additional HLA-C typing of donors possessing 'promiscuous' HLA-B types, e.g. HLA-B*51 is associated with several HLA-C alleles. The FGM were introducing a new policy for new donor testing whereby all new donors would be HLA-A and B tested only and, similar to the CNMDR, only those donors who did not possess common HLA-A and B haplotypes were further tested for HLA-DR and DQ. The FGM has also undertaken additional projects, e.g. HLA-C testing, where the HLA-C type is used to predict the HLA-B allele type.

None of the registries reported any logistical problems in selecting donors for additional testing.

In another survey[5] of 4 registries which included the NMDP-USA, Welsh Registry-UK, DKMS-Germany and the Japanese Registry, strategies for new donor testing were looked at.

The 3 main factors that determined the methodology for HLA typing for new volunteer donors were 1) funding, 2) the potential for the donor to contribute desirable characteristics such as racial or ethnic diversity, younger age, or male sex and 3) meeting the needs of the patients. Of these three factors, funding was most important factor that determined the methodology and loci typed in the registries Luminex methodology (Japan) or in-house preparation of sequence specific primer reagents (Wales, UK) were quite cost effective methods, yet retaining quite a high level of resolution. The highest level of resolution attained by sequence based typing was used only when sufficient funding was available.

In the German register, all newly recruited donors were only HLA-A and -B typed. Which donors go on to have HLA-DRB1 typing depended upon factors like phenotype, age, and sex, accounting for approximately 50 percent of their new donors. Focused recruitment efforts increased the diversity by contributing new phenotypes at a rate of nearly 47 percent for the Welsh Register and 30 percent for the NMDP. For the Welsh register, these are prioritized for complete HLA-A, B, C, DRB1, DQB1 typing. In the United States, typing for intermediate resolution HLA-A, B, DRB1 is fully funded by the government.

Most registries attempt to recruit donors from diverse ethnic backgrounds. However, this information may not be available for selecting donors depending upon the laws in different countries.

The issue of whether to type donors already on the registry at higher resolution or to recruit more donors is a topic of debate. This implies spending financial resources on increasing the level of resolution and number of loci of existing donors, or by prospectively typing new donors in this way. An effective prospective typing program should consider the phenotypes of the donors, non-HLA factors (age or sex), and the needs of transplant physicians in determining the final loci and level of resolution. The NMDP conducted a study of 2217 Black donors. The typing of the HLA-A, -B, -C loci was upgraded to intermediate resolution and the HLA-DRB1 to high resolution. The request rate of these 'highly' typed donors was compared with a control pool without additional typing. There was results showed a 50 percent reduction in requests for the higher matched donors. This showed that when allele data are known, the mismatched donors are clearly distinguished and avoided. However, similar studies in Germany showed increased utilization of donors with higher resolution typing.

TYPING OF POTENTIAL AND SELECTED DONORS[6]

Method

Complete sequence of exons 2 and 3 for class I and exon 2 for class II molecules by sequencing-based typing is thought to be the best technique for typing potential and selected typing. It has fewer problems with ambiguities and null alleles and the possibility to establish a completely automated system.

Increasingly labs are switching from serology to molecular typing methods. Various studies have shown a high frequency of typing errors using serological methods. Although some consider HLA class I serology as useful to detect null alleles, after sequencing of exons 2 and 3 for class I, only a minority remain undetected.

Resolution

Four-digit typing (allele level) of human leukocyte antigen (HLA)-A, -B, -C, -DRB1, and –DQB1 is required to assess the suitability of a stem cell donor. The complete sequence of exon 2 for class II and exons 2 and 3 for class I molecules needs to be determined to resolve all ambiguities that contribute to the amino acid changes in those regions of the HLA molecule that are relevant to histocompatibility.

Sequence Specific Priming (SSP) or probing (such as sequence-specific oligonucleotide) may not detect novel alleles or null alleles that differ only by single nucleotide differences and frequently do not resolve all ambiguities. Sequencing-based typing (SBT) uncovers these variations, especially when allele-separating techniques are applied. Sequencing exons 2 and 3 can detect over 50 percent of currently known null alleles.

High level resolution typing is becoming the standard in Germany and USA. Potential donors typed to high resolution level are selected in preference to intermediate typed donors.

Systems are now available to make high resolution typing cost-effective and achievable. This translates into a reduction in length of donor search time leading to improved outcome. Figure 33.2 is a graph for new alleles found worldwide.

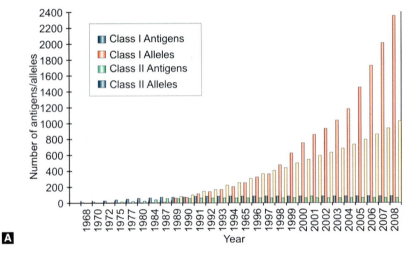

HLA Antigens and Alleles 1968–2008					
HLA-A	HLA-B	HLA-C			
733(24)	1115(49)	392(9)			
HLA-E	HLA-F	HLA-G			
9	21	42			
HLA-DRA	HLA-DRB	HLA-DQA 1	HLA-DQB1	HLA-DPA1	HLA-DPB1
3	697(20)	34	95 (7)	27	132
HLA-DMA	HLA-DMB	HLA-DOA	HLA-DOB		
4	7	12	9		
MICA	MICB	TAP1	TAP2		
65	30	7	4		

Figs 33.2A and B: (A) Increasing number of HLA class I and class II antigens and alleles defined by serology and molecular methods respectively over 40 year period. (B) A summary of the total number of alleles known at various loci in the HLA region. Figures in parenthesis indicate serologically identified specificities

Options for High Resolution Typing

Sequencing Based Typing

- Can be a cost-effective option but currently requires high degree of analysis skills
- Automation of set-up processes required for high throughput
- Bespoke system developed in-house not standardised across all loci
- Should be possible to achieve a 4 to 5 day turnaround time

Luminex High Definition Beads

- Comparatively easy to convert current system
- High throughput/three day turnaround time can be achieved
- Can be made a very cost-effective
- Protocols require no additional equipment.

Emulsion PCR Technology

Race

Information about racial background is helpful in certain situations where one encounters rare alleles and nonfrequent genotypes. This information could be potentially useful in searches in population- specific registries.

The NMDP suggest that it is advisable to match at the allele level for HLA-A, B, C and DRB1.[7] If a donor is required urgently,[6] the patient's HLA-A, -B, -DRB high-resolution typing data should be submitted to the registry for a donor search. If there is low resolution typing information available from family analysis, it might help identify possible haplotypes and point towards the presence of a rare allele. The haplotype and linkage disequilibrium can predict allelic variants of HLA-C and -DQB1 that are associated with the patient's HLA-B and -DRB typing results. In such situations it is advisable to do high resolution typing for HLA-C and -DQB1 before starting the search. Ambiguous typing results should be resolved while the search for a donor is conducted. Racial background might be helpful in such situations.

In less urgent donor search requests, searches should be based on high-resolution typing of the patient's HLA-A, -B, -C, -DRB, and -DQB alleles. When donors are identified, their high-resolution typing for HLA-A, -B, and -DRB is required. All potential donors may be typed simultaneously and use a strategy for resolving the expected ambiguities based on the patient's HLA typing results. HLA-C and -DQB1 might be included if multiple allelic variants are predicted based on linkage disequilibrium with HLA-B and DRB, respectively. No further testing is carried out for multiple HLA-A, -B, or -DRB mismatches. HLA-C and -DQB1 typing should be continued for matched donor samples. For a single mismatched donor, the donor's HLA-C and -DQB1 high-resolution typing should be included to evaluate overall matching. Again here, haplotype and race information may be useful.

Urgency of Requests

Most labs use typing methods that can provide results within a matter of hours. Although it is not necessary to have multiple typing strategies for urgent versuss non urgent requests[6], urgent samples need to be prioritized for typing and non included in the batch setup for nonurgent samples. It is useful to have a strategy to address typing drop outs (i.e. missed alleles), discrepancies due to potential new alleles, and to confirm sample identity.

Non-HLA Loci

Increasingly, non-HLA loci are being shown to be important in transplant outcome. It is possible that, in the future, registries may be asked to provide information on these non-HLA loci as part of donor testing. Some transplant centers already use information on compatibility of minor antigens [especially minor Histocompatibility Antigen number one (HA-1)] for donor selection to increase the graft vs leukemia effect by mismatching for these antigens in the graft vs host direction.

Typing Ambiguities

Unlike the Anthony Nolan Trust, where all the HLA typing is done in-house, a lot of registries get their HLA typing done from 1 or more laboratories outside of their organization. There may be occasions relating to HLA typings that do not resolve to one or two broad allele groups making it difficult to enter the typing into the registry database. Protocols vary from lab to lab, and the registry should request that the typing laboratory resolve such ambiguous typing results. As a result registries need to make policies that include criteria for HLA typing laboratories.

Typing ambiguities should be resolved, although this is dependent on the situation and cost, and some times can be impractical. The patient and finally selected donor should be typed at the highest resolution and ambiguities thus should be resolved. For other potential donors, resolving ambiguities is not required and can be omitted or postponed. Different laboratories use different methods to resolve ambiguities. Methods include locus-specific single amplification, covering all exons needed to resolve ambiguities, for sequencing; selective amplification and subsequent sequencing of specific alleles [group-specific allele primer (SAP)]. In some cases SSP and sequence-specific oligonucleotide probe (SSOP) approaches resolve ambiguities. Ambiguities that are difficult or near to impossible to resolve should be considered for relevance based upon, for example allele frequency in the population. Race and haplotype information might be informative. It would be efficient if protocols to resolve those are generally available and reference DNA accessible.

DONOR HEALTH

One of the objectives of a donor registry is to create a pool of healthy, well-selected and well-informed donors who would have the highest likelihood of getting selected for a specific patient. If a donor is deferred for any reason especially medical reasons, there is a considerable loss of time, effort and resources, not to mention the potential impact on the treatment of a patient awaiting a transplant. It is therefore of paramount importance to have policies in place to evaluate the donor's health before being recruited onto the register and then finally selected for donation. The WMDA[8] has made specific recommendations in this regard to provide donor centres with the general principles and minimum requirements for donor registration and further evaluation for specific conditions. The 2 main aspects of such an approach are one to safeguard the donor's own health, and secondly to protect the recipient from transmissible diseases. At recruitment, donor centres commonly use questionnaires which give an indication of donor health and these can be explored further if need be. Few questions are directed at self-exclusion. Once on the register, it can be several years before the donor comes up as a potential match, at which point a follow up questionnaire is sent through. Similarly, a transmissible infectious disease profile is conducted on the blood tests collected at registration at some registries and again once a name comes up as a potential match. Once a final selection is made, the donor then undergoes a thorough medical including physical examination and an expanded transmissible disease profile. As standards and regulatory procedures vary from country to country, donor centres must consider their local requirements while designing screening strategies.

The clinical working group at the WMDA[9] maintain an anonymous register of serious events in the donor after donation as well as the product at collection.

The SEAR (Serious Events Adverse Effects Registry) reporting system started in 2001. Over 80 percent of the donor registries worldwide participate in the SEAR project. The SEAR database gives a good insight in the occurrence of serious events and adverse effects in relation to stem cell donation by unrelated donors.

The SPEAR (Serious Product Events and Adverse Effects Registry) reporting system started in 2007. The SPEAR database gives a good insight in the serious events and adverse effects in relation to URD-SC harvest and processing. The system has been set up in accordance with the WMDA standards, JACIE-FACT standards and EU Directive on Tissues and Cells.

STEM CELL MOBILIZATIONS AND DONOR SAFETY

GCSF

Traditionally, stem cells have been collected after bone marrow harvests. However, this approach does mean that the donor needs to spend at least 1 night in the hospital. In addition there is the morbidity related to anaesthesia, pain from the procedure post harvest, time off from work and need to check the blood count post harvest and action if required. From the donor's perspective, all these add to the cost and time. For a few years now, stem cells have been mobilised using growth factors. These have an excellent safety profile and are generally well tolerated by the donors. It is usually done as a day procedure and the donor can go back to their usual routine within a day or two. There are no concerns regarding anaesthetic risks, although the donors do need to take the GCSF injections for 4 days. Currently, two forms of recombinant human G-CSF are available for mobilization of haemopoietic stem cells. Both of these are licensed in the UK for use in healthy donors. Lenograstim is a Chinese hamster ovary-derived G-CSF consisting of 174 amino acids with 4 percent carbohydrate, indistinguishable from native G-CSF. Filgrastim is an *Escherichia coli*-derived G-CSF, differing from lenograstim in being non-glycosylated and in having an extra methionine group at the N-terminal end of the peptide chain.

As per The Anthony Nolan Trust policy, the G-CSF injections were coordinated by a fully qualified nurse from Healthcare at Home. This is an independent healthcare company which provides healthcare services to individuals within their own homes in the UK. Under normal circumstances, the nurse remains with the donor for 1 hour after each injection to ensure that no adverse events have occurred. This is done for a total of 3 days. The fourth injection is given at the peripheral blood stem cell collection centre. The Healthcare at Home nurse is fully trained to manage adverse reactions, should they occur and carries the appropriate emergency kit to deal with an allergic response to the drug.

The NMDP conducted a study,[10] looking at donation and recovery experiences of rst-time BM and PBSC donors. The donations were from November 2001 through March 2006. From the donor's perspective these stem cell sources carry different recovery and safety proles. Most of BM and PBSC donors experienced some symptoms during the course of their donation. Pain was the number 1 symptom for both groups of donors. BM donors most often reported pain at the collection site (82% back or hip pain), whereas PBSC donors most often reported bone pain (97%) at various sites during filgrastim administration. Fatigue was the second most reported symptom by both BM and PBSC donors (59% and 70%, respectively). PBSC donors reported a median time to recovery of 1 week compared to a median time to recovery of 3 weeks for BM donors. Both BM and PBSC donors experienced transient changes in their WBC, platelet, and hemoglobin counts during the donation process, with most counts returning to baseline values by 1 month post-donation and beyond. Serious adverse events were uncommon, but these events occurred more often in BM donors than PBSC donors.

Peripheral Blood Progenitor Cells (PBPC) are increasingly being used as a source of hematopoetic stem cells for allogeneic transplantation because of technical ease of collection and shorter time required for engraftment. Traditionally, granulocyte-colony stimulating factor (G-CSF) has been used to obtain the peripheral blood stem cell graft. Although regimens using G-CSF usually succeed in collecting adequate numbers of PBPC from healthy donors, a small number will mobilize stem cells poorly and may require multiple large volume aphaeresis or bone marrow harvesting. Although G-CSF is generally well tolerated in healthy donors, it may be associated with bone pain, headache, myalgia and rarely life threatening side effects like stroke, myocardial infarction and splenic rupture.

Although, Granulocyte-colony stimulating factor (G-CSF) is widely administered to donors who provide peripheral blood stem cells (PBSC) for individuals who undergo hematopoietic stem cell transplants, questions have been raised about the safety of G-CSF in this setting. The Research on Adverse Drug Events and Reports (RADAR)[11] project investigators reviewed the literature on G-CSF-associated adverse events in healthy individuals or persons with chronic neutropenia or cancer. Toxicities identiûed included bone pain and rare instances of splenic rupture, allergic reactions, ares of underlying autoimmune disorders, lung injury and vascular events. Among healthy individuals, four patients developed splenic rupture shortly after G-CSF administration and three patients developed acute myeloid leukemia 1 to 5 years after G-CSF administration. Registry studies identied no increased risks of malignancy among healthy individuals who received G-CSF before PBSC harvesting.

In a study done at Tel Aviv University, Nagler et al[12] (2004), reported finding specific abnormalities in lymphocytes from healthy donors who had received G-CSF. These were very similar to the changes seen in lymphocytes from people with malignant diseases. The abnormalities included loss of synchrony in allelic replication timing (epigenetic) and aneuploidy (genetic). The loss of synchrony in allelic replication timing was a transient phenomenon consistent with the view that changes in the blood due to G-CSF are transient and do not last very long. However, the aneuploidy persisted during the study period even after the asynchrony in replication timing corrected. This appeared to contradict the view that G-CSF induced changes were transient.

Following this in December 2006, Bennett et al[13] reported five cases of hematological malignancy occurring in normal individuals following exposure to hematopoietic growth factors. Three cases described lymphoid malignancies (non-Hodgkin lymphoma and chronic lymphocytic leukaemia) occurring months to years after receipt of an investigational agent (pegylated, recombinant megakaryocyte growth and development factor). The two additional cases, however, were identified among 200 healthy donors who had received filgastrim (recombinant human granulocyte colony-stimulating factor; rhG-CSF, Neupogen) as a mobilising agent for collection of peripheral blood stem cells (PBSC) for allogeneic transplantation. The transplant recipients for these latter two donors were their own siblings, each with acute myelogenous leukaemia (AML). The donors themselves also developed AML 4–5 years following filgrastim exposure.

Based on these reports, the Immunobiology Working Party (IWP) of the EBMT, took action to clarify the potential risk of using G-CSF in unrelated bone marrow donors (UBMD). A Working Group Committee in collaboration with the World Marrow Donor Association (WMDA) and the National Marrow Donor Program (NMDP) was held and undertook an evaluation of the existing data from all worldwide Registers. This gave confidence to believe that apparently there is no increase in malignancy in voluntary UBMD who receive G-CSF for mobilization.

The IWP of the EBMT are currently performing a joint study to perform cytogenetic analysis on UBMD both retrospectively and prospectively. It will include in this group, bone marrow donors and patients with malignancies as control.

This study is being performed under the umbrella of EMBT and in collaboration with members of The Anthony Nolan Research Institute, Royal Free and University College Medical School, British Bone Marrow Registry, NMDP and Chugai Pharma UK.

Newer Agents

New agents are being developed as an alternative to GCSF. The pegylated form of filgrastim *(pegfilgrastim)* has a longer elimination half-life because of decreased serum clearance and might be a convenient alternative for stem cell mobilization. There are a few case reports of the use of pegfilgratim for stem cell mobilizations in healthy family and unrelated donors with good effect.[14] However, large studies are required to validate their effectiveness and safety profile.

AMD3100 (Plerixafor) is one such compound. It is a bicyclam compound that inhibits the binding of stromal cell derived factor-1 (SDF-1) to its cognate receptor CXCR4. CXCR4 is present on CD34+ hematopoetic progenitor cells and its interaction with SDF-1 plays an important role in the homing of CD34+ cells in the bone marrow. Inhibition of the CXCR4-SDF1 axis by AMD3100 releases CD34+ cells into the circulation, which can then be collected easily by apheresis.

A recently published report[15] demonstrated that large numbers of CD34+ cells were rapidly mobilized in healthy volunteers following a single subcutaneous injection of AMD3100. This was comparable to the number of CD34+ cells collected from historical controls receiving 5 days of G-CSF prior to stem cell mobilization. Side-effects to this agent were mild and transient with no serious complications reported. The ability to collect a large quantity of PBPC with a single injection of this drug makes this an attractive agent for mobilizing donors of allogeneic PBSC.

Another study looked at AMD3100 induced PBSC's from sibling donors. The results of this trial support the hypothesis that directly targeting the interaction between CXCR4 and SDF-1/CXCL12 is an effective strategy to reduce the length of time required to procure a functional HLA matched sibling donor hematopoietic allograft. In two-thirds of the donors, a single injection of AMD3100 just 4 hours after its administration induced the mobilization of sufcient numbers of HSPCs to reconstitute durable trilineage hematopoiesis. This was in contrast to the 4 to 5 days of G-CSF administration typically required to procure an adequate number of HSPCs for transplantation. AMD3100 appeared to be at least as safe as G-CSF in the short term. Donors experienced no long-term consequences with at least a median follow-up of 9 months after donation. Longer follow-up and greater numbers of donors would be needed to assess the overall safety of AMD3100.

However, the immune reconstitution profiles of AMD3100 mobilized cells, in terms of lymphocyte content (T cell, B cell, NK cell, immuno-regulatory T cell), T cell polarization status (TH1 versus TH2), status of antigen presenting cells (DC1 versus DC2), alloreactive potential, and preservation of reactivity to infectious agents (e.g. EBV, CMV) are unknown. Consequently, whether AMD3100 mobilized PBPC would be suitable for use as an allograft is uncertain.

The US FDA has approved the use of Plerixafor for mobilization of hematopoietic stem cells in conjunction with GCSF.

RESEARCH

Depending on the set up and available resources, registries may have an associated research programme. This is an important aspect into developing new insights into the application of stem cell transplants and cellular therapy. Almost all registries collect data on clinical outcomes and activities that are published annually either internally or externally in peer reviewed journals. Linking clinical data with immunological and genetic data would give insights into transplant biology. Research at the NMDP is co-ordinated through its affiliate the Center for International Blood and Marrow Transplant Research (CIBMTR).[16] Similarly research at the Anthony Nolan Trust is facilitated via the Anthony Nolan Research Institute. The main groups are the HLA- informatics group, the Immunotherapy group and the Clinical Research Group. Prof. J Alejandro Madrigal who is also the current president of the EBMT currently heads it.

QUALITY

Quality Control (QC) is a system of routine technical activities, to measure and control the quality of the inventory as it is being developed. The QC system is designed to:

 i. Provide routine and consistent checks to ensure data integrity, correctness, and completeness;
 ii. Identify and address errors and omissions;
 iii. Document and archive inventory material and record all QC activities.

Quality Assurance (QA) activities include a planned system of review procedures conducted by personnel not directly involved in the inventory compilation/development process.

The NMDP[17] has published a report of BM donations from 1987 to 2007 and PBSC donations from 1994 to 2007. It looked at multiple parameters – single and multiple collections, product collected but not infused, GCSF administered but product not collected, central line placement, Peripheral blood CD34+ cell mobilisation and PBSC yield, positive microbiological cultures in BM and PBSC grafts, non standard transport, compromised bags and product clotting.

It is good practice to implement quality control and quality assurance (QA/QC) procedures in place. Depending upon local guidelines and regulations, joining local or national QA/QC schemes is an independent verification of the procedures and SOP's in place (e.g. NEQUAS in the UK). This especially important for histocompatibility labs and donor centres. The outcome of the QA/QC process help in identifying errors if any and a re-think or modification of SOP's, eventually helping to improve the performance.

ACKNOWLEDGMENTS

BE Shaw[1,3], P Makoni[1], SGE Marsh[1], JM Goldman.[1,2]
[1]The Anthony Nolan Trust, The Royal Free Hospital, London, UK.
[2]Department of Hematology, Imperial College, London, UK.
[3]Section of Hemato-oncology, The Royal Marsden Hospital, London, UK.

REFERENCES

1. Bone Marrow Donors Worldwide. www.bmdw.org
2. Hurley CK, Maiers M, Marsh SGE et al. Overview of registries, HLA typing and diversity, and search algorithms. Tissue Antigens. 2007: 69; suppl 1: 3–5.
3. Bochtler W, Maiers M, Oudshoorn et al. World Marrow Donor Association Guidelines for use of HLA nomenclature and its validation in the data exchange among hematopoietic stem cell donor registries and cord blood banks. Bone Marrow Transplantation. 2007; 737-41.
4. Little AM, Jindra P, Raffoux C. Strategies for new donor typing based on donor HLA type or donor characteristics. Tissue Antigens. 2007: 69; suppl 1: 8-9.
5. Setterholm M, Morishima Y, Pepperall J et al. Strategies for typing new volunteer donors Tissue Antigens. 2007: 69; suppl 1: 6-7.
6. Oudshoorn M, Horn PA, Tilanus M et al. Typing of potential and selected donors for transplant: Methodology and resolution Tissue Antigens. 2007: 69; suppl 1: 10-12.
7. Hurley C, Lowe L, Logan B et al. National Marrow Donor Program HLA-Matching Guidelines for unrelated marrow transplants. Biol Bld Marrow Transplant. 2003; 9:610-15.
8. Sacchil N, Costeas P, Hartwell L et al. Hematopoietic stem cell donor registries: World Marrow Donor Association recommendations for evaluation of donor health. Bone Marrow Transplantation 2008; 42: 9-14.
9. WMDA- www.worldmarrow.org
10. Miller JP, Perry EH, Price TH et al. Recovery and Safety Proles of Marrow and PBSC Donors: Experience of the National Marrow Donor Program Biology of Blood and Marrow Transplantation. 2008; 14:29-36.
11. Tigue CC, McKoy JM, Evens AM et al. Granulocyte-colony stimulating factor administration to healthy individuals and persons with chronic neutropenia or cancer: An overview of safety considerations from the Research on Adverse Drug Events and Reports project Bone Marrow Transplantation. 2007; 40: 185-92.
12. Nagler A, Korenstein-Ilan A, Amiel A et al. Granulocyte colony-stimulating factor generates epigenetic and genetic alterations in lymphocytes of normal volunteer donors of stem cells. Experimental Hematology. 2004;32:122-30.
13. Bennett CL. Hematological malignancies developing in previously healthy individuals who received haematopoietic growth factors: Report from the Research on Adverse Drug Events and Reports (RADAR) project. British Journal of Hematology. 2006; 135:642-50.
14. Kobbe G, Bruns I, Fenk R, et al. Peglgrastim for PBSC mobilization and autologous haematopoietic SCT Bone Marrow Transplantation 2009;43:669-77.
15. Conrad Liles W, Broxmeyer HE, Rodger E et al. Mobilization of hematopoietic progenitor cells in healthy volunteers by AMD3100, a CXCR4 antagonist. Blood. 2003;102:2728-30.
16. Horowitz MM. The role of registries in facilitating clinical research in BMT: Examples from the Center for International Blood and Marrow Transplant Research Bone Marrow Transplantation. 2008; 42: S1-S2.
17. Bolan C, Hartzman R, Perry E et al. Donation Activities and Product Integrity in Unrelated Donor Allogeneic Hematopoietic Transplantation: Experience of the National Marrow Donor Program. Biol Bld Marrow Transplant. 2008; 14:23-28.

Chapter 34

An Overview of Statistical Methods for Disease Gene Mapping Using Data on Related and Unrelated Individuals

Indranil Mukhopadhyay, Saurabh Ghosh, Partha P Majumder

INTRODUCTION

One of the most important and challenging problems in human genetics is to map genes that are responsible for a disease. This endeavor is important because it allows one to predict, or to estimate the chance, whether an individual will be affected with the disease under consideration. Mapping and identifying genes responsible for a disease is also a pre-requisite for understanding the biology and pathophysiology of the disease. The endeavor is challenging, especially for a disease that is controlled by multiple genes, because environmental factors almost always interact with genetic factors to determine disease outcome. This implies that the outcome of a disease may differ between individuals even if they have the same genotypes at the locus that causes the disease. For a disease that is determined not by a single gene but by multiple genes, the impact of any one of these genes on disease outcome may be low and hence difficult to detect.

Aside from various molecular biological methods, localizing genes responsible for a disease can be done by collecting and analyzing data and DNA samples from members of families or even from sets of unrelated individuals affected (case) and unaffected (control) individuals. The data that are collected from each individual included in the sample (family sample or case-control sample) are: (a) disease phenotype, and (b) genotypes at a number of loci, called marker loci, whose chromosomal locations are known. The analysis of these data involves estimation of the extent of co-segregation of alleles at the marker locus with disease, either within families (family data) or at the population level (case-control data). If the marker locus is in the vicinity of the disease locus, there will be higher co-segregation. If the marker locus is physically far away from the disease locus, then alleles at the two loci will segregate independently. In other words, the strength of co-segregation determines the proximity of the marker locus to the disease locus. If the marker locus is found to be in proximity to the disease locus, then the chromosomal position of the disease locus becomes known since the position of the marker locus is known a priori.

It is of paramount importance to carefully collect information on the disease phenotype. Misdiagnosis of an affected individual as unaffected, or the vice-versa, can completely drown the chance of mapping genes for the disease. This fact is often underappreciated. The clinical phenotype of the disease must be well-defined, clinical evaluations of every individual in the sample must be done very carefully, especially because clinical symptoms or clinical-biochemistry profiles of two different diseases can often overlap.

The choice of markers also has to be judicious. The most important factor to be considered in choosing a marker is to be sure that the proportion of heterozygotes at the locus is reasonably high (as close to 50% as possible if the locus has two segregating alleles, but certainly not close to 10%). Depending on whether the researcher has a set of favorite "candidate" genes, the markers may be chosen from these genes. If the researcher has no favorite genes, then an agnostic approach may be taken and a large set of markers spanning the entire human genome may be selected. Another criterion to bear in mind in selecting marker loci is that adjacent markers should not be "too close" or "too far" from each other. With the completion of the Human Genome Project and the HapMap Project, choice of markers has become easier than before, because the data from these projects have been used to create a public-domain database (www.hapmap.org). This database contains relevant and useful information on millions of markers that is helpful in making a judicious choice of markers for a gene-mapping study.

LINKAGE ANALYSIS

Concept of Co-segregation and Data Requirement for Linkage Analysis

We assume that precise chromosomal locations of markers chosen in a study are known. If a family study design is used, then the statistical method for analyzing these data for detection of co-segregation is called linkage analysis. Co-segregation is a tendency for alleles at two or more loci to be inherited together in families, and so members in families with the same disease phenotype would share same allele, or at least show a significantly enhanced chance of sharing, at the marker locus. This is because when two loci are close to each other, then there is reduced recombination between them. Two genes are said to be completely linked if a doubly heterozygous individual (that is, an individual who is heterozygous at both the loci under consideration) can produce only non-recombinant gametes. On the other hand, such linkage is absent (recombination is free), when the proportions of recombinant and non-recombinant haplotypes produced by the individual are equal.

Since transmission of haplotypes (haploid gametes with a specific combination of alleles at the loci under consideration) from parents to children would help in identifying the recombination events, linkage analysis cannot be carried out using unrelated individuals, but requires observations on relatives. Thus for linkage analysis, data on a group of related individuals or members of family or pedigree are required. A *pedigree* may be defined as a set of relatives with known relationships among individuals. Pedigree members can be of two types: *Founders* and *nonfounders*. Founders are individuals whose parents are not in the pedigree whereas nonfounders have their parents in the pedigree. Usually, founders are assumed to be unrelated individuals and drawn at random from the population under study. For linkage analysis, data on pedigrees is more valuable than data on nuclear families, because in multi-generation pedigrees a large number of meiotic events (each of which can result in recombinant or a non-recombinant haplotype through crossing-over) can be observed.

Sometimes, it may be difficult to distinguish between recombinant and non-recombinant haplotypes produced by a parent. For example, at a pair of loci with alleles (A, a) and (B,b), consider the Ab haplotype produced by a parent with genotype Ab/ab. Since the parent is homozygous at the second locus, Ab can be a recombinant (if there is a crossover) or a non-recombinant (in case of no crossover) haplotype. Therefore, to distinguish between these cases, the parent must be heterozygous at both the loci, i.e., doubly heterozygous. Only then the parent would be *potentially informative* for linkage. Thus a mating is potentially informative for linkage between two specific loci when at least one of the parents is a double-heterozygote.

Thus, for linkage analysis we require data (disease status and marker genotypes) on members of pedigrees or on sets of related individuals (e.g. extended families, nuclear families, sibling-pairs, etc).

In a small 3-generation pedigree as in Figure 34.1, consider two loci jointly, locus 1 with two alleles, A and a, locus 2 with two alleles B and b. Figure 34.1 shows an artificial family in which two grandparents are both doubly homozygous: the grandfather is homozygous for the alleles A (at locus 1) and B (at locus 2), and the grandmother is homozygous for the alleles a (at locus 1) and b (at locus 2). The mother (daughter of two grandparents) must have received alleles A and B from the grandfather and alleles a and b from the grandmother. Thus the mother received the AB haplotype from her father and the ab haplotype from her mother.

In principle, a doubly heterozygous individual, i.e. individual with heterozygous genotypes at both the loci (A/a, B/b) received his or her A allele in coupling with either

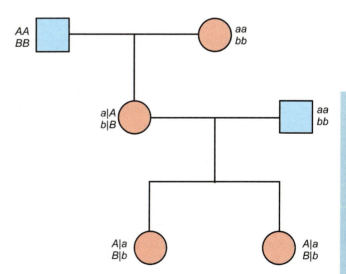

Fig. 34.1: An illustrative example to establish concepts

the B or the b allele from one parent. These two possibilities are distinguished as the two *phases* of a double heterozygote (more than two phases exist in individuals heterozygous at more than two loci). Depending on the alleles of interest, one of the two phases is called *coupling* and the other is called *repulsion*. Suppose that the two loci were on the same chromosome and further suppose that one member of the chromosome pair had alleles AB and the other ab. Thus we write the genotype as ab|AB, the vertical bar indicating which allele were on the same chromosome, i.e. their phase. Thus AB/ab is in coupling; Ab/aB is in repulsion. The phase plays an important role in developing the method for testing the presence or absence of linkage. Ignoring the phase information might induce biases leading to a completely wrong conclusion about the presence of linkage.

Test for Linkage

Although crossover events cannot be directly observed, using the techniques of linkage analysis, the results of recombination are observable by tracing which grandparent the alleles at the two loci originally came from. Two loci, A and B, separated by a single crossover event will thus appear as a recombinant. If the two loci are separated because of two crossover events, they will appear as a non-recombinant since the transmitted alleles will have originated from the same chromosome. Such an event is indistinguishable from zero crossovers unless one observes a third locus, C, between A and B with recombinants both between A and C and between C and B. Thus, in general, we can say that a recombination relates to an odd number of crossovers whereas a non-recombination to an even number. We define recombination fraction (denoted by θ) as the proportion of recombinant gametes transmitted to offspring. If the recombination fraction is small, the probability of two or more recombination events is extremely small indeed; so a recombinant is likely to relate to a single crossover and a non-recombinant to zero crossover. As the crossover rate becomes large, multiple crossovers will become common so that eventually the probability of an even number of events is same as the probability of an odd number of crossovers; hence the limiting value of the recombination fraction becomes ½. Thus, $\theta = 0.5$ would indicate the situation that the odd number of crossovers and the even number of crossovers are equally probable, assuming Mendel's second law of independent segregation. Hence, we can propose the null hypothesis as H_0: $\theta = 0.5$ for testing of linkage between two loci.

When the two loci are very tightly linked (that is, θ is much less than 0.5 or nearly close to zero) almost always the same haplotypes will be transmitted to the offspring. The closer the value of θ to zero, the tighter is the linkage between the two loci. Hence, the alternate hypothesis is H_1: $\theta < 0.5$. Thus $\theta = 0.5$ implies that the two genes segregating independently, or are unlinked, whereas $\theta = 0$ indicates that the genes are very tightly linked or very rarely (theoretically, never) does a recombination occur between them. Hence, to test for linkage we test H_0: $\theta = 0.5$ against H_1: $\theta < 0.5$.

The LOD-score Method

A *direct counting method* was used to estimate the recombination fraction at the initial stages of human linkage analysis. Suppose one could observe recombinations directly. Also suppose that one locus is an unknown disease susceptibility locus with alleles t and T and the other is a known marker locus with alleles m and M. As mentioned earlier, only doubly heterozygous parents (genotypes tm|TM or tM|Tm) are informative for linkage. Depending on the parents' linkage-phase, the probability of each of the four possible haplotypes being transmitted to the offspring is given in Table 34.1 (Thomas, 2004). The entries that involve θ are those for transmission from double heterozygotes.

In principle, we try to determine, for those parent-offspring pairs in which a parent is doubly heterozygous, the number of meiotic events in which the transmitted haplotype is a recombinant or a non-recombinant. Let r and s be the numbers of recombinant and non-recombinant haplotypes, respectively. Also let $n = r+s$ be the total number of informative meioses. An estimate of θ would be given as $\hat{\theta} = r/n$ and one could use this estimate of θ to test for linkage.

Table 34.1: Haplotype transmission through the process of recombination

Parental genotype	Transmitted haplotype			
	t m	t M	T m	T M
t m | t m	1	0	0	0
t m | T M	0.5	0.5	0	0
t M | t M	0	1	0	0
t m | T m	0.5	0	0.5	0
t m | T M	$(1-\theta)/2$	$\theta/2$	$\theta/2$	$(1-\theta)/2$
t M | T m	$\theta/2$	$(1-\theta)/2$	$(1-\theta)/2$	$\theta/2$
t M | T M	0	0.5	0	0.5
T m | T m	0	0	1	0
T m | T M	0	0	0.5	0.5
T M | T M	0	0	0	1

However, when linkage-phase of the double-heterozygote parent is not known, or there is incomplete penetrance at the disease locus, as is usually the case with human data, genotype-phenotype relationship gets blurred; the direct method, therefore, can extract only a limited amount of information from the actual data, sometimes in a biased manner. Thus instead of this direct count method, the human genetic linkage analysis generally uses the relative pair or lod score methods based on likelihood of the observed data.

In 1922, Fisher developed the maximum likelihood method as a general statistical estimation procedure that allows an efficient estimation of recombination fractions. Likelihood is a measure of the plausibility of the observed data. Its value depends on the values of θ and also the assumed probability distribution. If we calculate the likelihood for a number of values of θ, the plausibility of the data will be highest for one specific value of θ, which is then taken to be a good estimate. This is known as *maximum likelihood estimate (MLE)* of θ. Plugging the maximum likelihood estimate (MLE) into the likelihood and considering the ratio of likelihoods under the alternative hypothesis to that under the null hypothesis, Fisher subsequently developed a testing procedure, which could be used to test the presence of linkage. The *odds* in favor of H_1 versus H_0 are expressed in terms of the likelihood ratio, $L(H_1)/L(H_0)$ and common logarithm using base 10 of this ratio is called *lod score* (Morton, 1954).

In linkage analysis involving two loci, the two basic hypotheses of interest are no-linkage (H_0) and linkage (H_1) between the two loci under consideration, defined in terms of recombination fraction as H_0: $\theta=0.5$ and H_1: $\theta<0.5$. Thus the **logarithm of the odds** of linkage vs. no-linkage, is the same as the logarithm of the ratio of the likelihood of observing the data under H_1 to that under H_0, i.e. $Z(\theta) = \log_{10}[L(\theta)/L(0.5)]$. This lod score can be used as a measure of support for the linkage against absence of linkage. For example, if observations consist of r recombinants and $n-r$ non-recombinants, the corresponding lod score is given by

$$Z(\theta) = \begin{cases} n\log_{10}(2) + r\log_{10}(\theta) + (n-r)\log_{10}(1-\theta) & \text{if } \theta > 0 \\ n\log_{10}(2) & \text{if } \theta = 0 \text{ and } r = 0 \\ -\infty & \text{if } \theta = 0 \text{ and } r > 0 \end{cases}$$

where the domain is usually $0 \leq \theta \leq 0.5$. A plot of $Z(\theta)$ over different values of θ would give an idea about the value of θ for which we can get the maximum value of $Z(\theta)$. It is to be noted that the combined lod score for a given number of independent families is just the sum of the lod scores for individual families. However, if there is linkage, the maximum lod score tends to increase with an increasing number of families. Once it reaches or exceeds 3, linkage is generally considered significant (Morton, 1954). We now move towards evaluating likelihood function or lod score for a small pedigree. Figure 34.2 presents a two-generation family with parents and four offspring.

We assume that the father as likely to be $TM|tm$ as $Tm|tM$. If the father has genotype $TM|tm$, the first three offspring are non-recombinants and the last offspring is a recombinant. On the other hand, if the father has genotype $Tm|tM$, the first three offspring are recombinants and the last offspring is a non-recombinant. Hence,

$$\begin{aligned} P(\text{data}|\theta) &= P(\text{parents' data } | \theta) \times P(\text{offspring data } | \text{ parents' data}, \theta) \\ &= P(\text{parents' data}) \times \left\{ \frac{1}{2}\left[((1-\theta)/2)^3 \cdot \theta/2\right] \right. \\ &\quad \left. + \frac{1}{2}\left[(\theta/2)^3 \cdot (1-\theta)/2\right] \right\} \end{aligned}$$

Thus, given the data, this can be treated as the likelihood of the family, $L(\theta)$ which can be maximized to get an estimate of θ. If the phase is known, the likelihood can take a simpler form; but when the phase of the parental haplotype(s) is (are) unknown, the likelihood calculation must take all possible of phases, given the genotypes, into account.

The general formula for determining the likelihood of observed data on any arbitrary multi-generation family is complex because of the complex nature of dependence within the data set. Since most members within a family

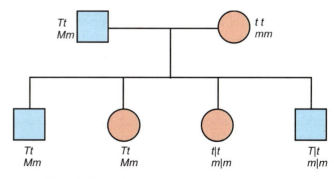

Fig. 34.2: An illustrative example with parents and four children

are genetically related, their observations on disease phenotype and marker genotypes are not independent. A major breakthrough in statistical genetics was obtained by Elston and Stewart (1971), when having noted that genotypes of offspring of a pair of parents are all independent conditional on the genotype data of the parents, they were able to recursively derive the likelihood function of data on members of a family of any arbitrary complexity. The three major components of this general likelihood are: (1) genotype probabilities for the founders, (2) transmission probability of the offspring genotypes given the parental genotypes, and (3) probabilities of an individual being affected for the possible genotypes at the putative disease locus. The general form of the likelihood function is complex, and is, of course, a function of the recombination fraction. Explicit analytical form of the estimator of the recombination fraction is nearly impossible to derive. The likelihood is therefore numerically maximized with respect to θ (and, other parameters, such as allele frequencies, if unknown) using a recursive algorithm. Since this numerical maximization is computationally heavy, an easier way is to calculate the value of the likelihood function for different values of θ (0.001, 0.05, 0.1, 0.2, 0.3 and 0.4, is the standard set of values used) and plot these values against θ. The value of θ for which the likelihood function attains its maximum is the best estimate of θ. At this value of θ, if the value of the lod score exceeds 3, then it is inferred that the marker locus and the putative disease locus are linked. Since the chromosomal location of the marker locus is precisely known, with the estimated value of θ one can make a reasonable guess – with the help of a mapping function (Thomas, 2004) – about the physical location of the disease locus.

SIB-PAIR ANALYSIS

Allele Sharing Methods

In linkage analysis, as described above, one requires data on a set of families, either nuclear or extended (preferred). However, it is possible to draw inferences on linkage even with data on pairs of relatives. In terms of data collection, the simplest form of data are data on pairs of affected siblings. Analyses of such data from the viewpoint of detecting linkage uses allele-sharing statistics and are termed affected sib-pair (ASP) analyses. The basic paradigm is that since both the sibs in an affected sib-pair have the disease allele at the trait locus, they must have inherited the same allele from their parents. Hence, they tend to share more inherited alleles at the trait locus than at random.

Concept of ibd: An Example

The extent of allele sharing is measured by a quantity called identity-by-descent (ibd) score, which is defined as the proportion of ancestral alleles shared by two individuals identical by descent. For pair of siblings, the most common ancestors are the two parents. For example, if the genotypes of the two parents at a locus are AB and CD and those of the two sibs are AC and BD, their ibd score is 0; if the genotypes of the sibs were AC and AD, then it would be ½ and if the genotypes of both the sibs were BC, it would be 1. However, if the genotypes of the two parents were AB and AC, and those of the sibs were AB and AC, it is important to note that although each of the sibs has inherited one A allele, the inheritance is not identical by descent and hence, the ibd score in this case would be 0.

Test for Linkage

In general, the ibd score for a pair of sibs at any locus assumes three values 0, ½ and 1 with probabilities ¼, ½ and ¼, respectively. Thus, the expected (that is, average) ibd score at a locus is ½. However, if both the sibs are affected, they are more likely to share at least one allele identical by descent at the trait locus, and hence their expected ibd score at the trait locus will be greater than ½. This property of excess allele sharing is also exhibited at marker loci that are physically close to the trait locus. Hence, a statistical test for the extent of allele sharing can be used to test for linkage between a marker locus and the trait locus. The test statistic is given by $(p\text{-}0.5)/\sqrt{(1/8n)}$ where p is the mean ibd score of a set of n independent sib-pairs, and is distributed as standard normal (that is, a Gaussian distribution with mean = 0 and variance = 1) in the absence of linkage between the marker and the trait locus (which is the null hypothesis, as mentioned in earlier sections). Thus, we reject the null hypothesis of no-linkage if the observed value of the test statistic exceeds 1.96. We note here that while this statistic can be used when the ibd score can be determined unambiguously, as in the above examples, we need to modify it slightly when the ibd score cannot be determined unambiguously, as in the case of homozygous parents.

Pros and Cons

The major advantage of affected sib-pair analysis is that the data requirement is minimal and hence, compared to pedigree-based linkage analysis, it is relatively much easier to obtain the complete phenotype and genotype information required for the analyses. For example, it does not require phenotype information on parents. Analyses based on only affected sib-pairs circumvent the problem of age-at-onset encountered in analyses involving unaffected individuals. (For most late-onset diseases, at any particular age an individual may be free of the disease under consideration, but may actually carry the disease allele.) Moreover, these analyses are model-free (for example, these analyses do not require information on the mode of inheritance of the disease) and hence, more robust to violations in underlying distributional and genetic assumptions. However, affected sib-pair analyses suffer from some inherent limitations. It is statistically much less powerful than linkage analyses based on large pedigrees, since sib-pair data contain minimal information on recombination, which forms the basis for detecting linkage. This means that if a disease and a marker locus are linked and $\theta = 0.1$, then it may be possible to detect this linkage (using the lod-score method) with data from 10 families each with 10 members (that is, a total of 100 individuals), while it may require several hundred affected sib-pairs to detect this linkage. The test statistic is not very efficient for marker loci that are not sufficiently polymorphic as the sib-pair ibd score cannot be determined unambiguously if parents are homozygous. In summary, while affected sib-pair analyses are robust, they compromise on statistical power for detecting linkage.

ASSOCIATION ANALYSIS

The most popular statistical method for identifying genes for diseases is the population-based case-control approach. Case-control studies test for allelic or genotypic association between a marker locus and the disease locus. Unlike tests for linkage, which require data on families, tests for association can be performed using population-based data, and hence are advantageous from the point of data requirement.

Case-control Design

Genotype data at various marker loci are collected on a set of unrelated affected individuals (called "cases") and an independent set of unrelated unaffected individuals (called "controls"). Since the aim is to test whether there is a significant difference in the genotypic or allelic distribution between cases and controls, the two groups needs to be matched in terms of other confounding variables like age, sex, exposure to environmental hazards known to be associated with the disease, etc. as differences in these variables between the two groups may result in false positive inferences about the genetic association of a locus with the disease.

An Example

Suppose we have collected genotype data at a biallelic locus with alleles A and a on 1200 cases and 1200 controls. The genotypic and allelic distributions are provided in Table 34.2. By considering the 2 x 2 table of allelic distributions, we find that the frequency of the allele A is 0.6 among cases and 0.3 among controls. Thus, a z-test for equality of proportions of the A allele among cases and controls yields a z-score 20.86 with p-value < 0.001 indicating a significant over-representation of the allele A among cases. Similarly, the Odds Ratio based on the above 2 x 2 table [(1440 x 1680)/ (720 x 960)] is 3.5 with p-value < 0.001, indicating a significant risk associated with the A allele. The two tests are equivalent when sample sizes are large, though not exactly identical. However, neither of the two tests is appropriate if any of the cell frequencies is very small. In such a case, Fisher's exact test (which is based on all possible permutations of the cell frequencies) needs to be performed.

Population Stratification

If the sample comprises a mixture of genetically heterogeneous subpopulations (for example, from different ethnic groups) having different allele frequencies at a locus, case-control studies may yield spurious association results. We consider the same example provided in the previous section (Table 34.2). Suppose the sample is in reality a mixture of two subpopulations 1 and 2. In subpopulation 1, the frequencies of the three genotypes AA, Aa and aa among cases are 560, 160 and 80, respectively; while among controls, the corresponding frequencies are 140, 40 and 20. In subpopulation 2, the frequencies of the three genotypes among cases are 40, 80 and 280; while among controls, these frequencies are 100, 200 and 700,

Table 34.2: Genotypic and allelic distributions in cases and controls at a biallelic locus

	Genotypes			Alleles	
	AA	Aa	aa	A	a
Cases	600	240	360	1440	960
Controls	240	240	720	720	1680

respectively. The genotypic and allelic distributions in the two subpopulations are provided in Table 34.3. We emphasize that the genotype frequencies of Table 34.2 are equal to the sum of the genotype frequencies of the two subpopulations provided in Table 34.3. We observe that the frequency of allele A is 0.8 among both cases and controls in subpopulation 1; while the frequency of A is 0.2 among both cases and controls in subpopulation 2. Hence, there is no difference in allele frequencies between cases and controls in either of the two subpopulations, but as shown in the previous section, there is significant evidence of allelic association in the pooled population. Thus, the observed association in the pooled population is in reality a statistical artifact induced by pooling two genetically heterogeneous subpopulations. In other words, if we had analyzed the data given in Table 34.2, without taking into account the fact that the data have arisen from a mixture of two subpopulations, we would falsely infer that there is association between the locus and the trait/disease, when in fact there is no association. Thus, in population association studies, it is of critical importance to draw samples – both cases and controls – from a homogeneous population. Sometimes there is covert population stratification, within an apparently homogeneous population. It is, therefore, best to actually test for population stratification using the genetic data generated in an association study, and take appropriate safeguards against population stratification when analyzing the data.

Methods to Safeguard Against Population Stratification

Statistical methods adjusting for population stratification is currently an active area of research. There are currently three methods which attempt to correct for population stratification: Genomic Control (Devlin et al, 2001), Structure (Pritchard et al, 2000) and Eigenstrat (Price et al, 2002). The "Genomic Control" approach chooses a large set of markers, unlinked to the polymorphism under study and preferably selectively neutral. The association test statistic needs to be adjusted by a factor depending on the median of the values of the chi-square statistic for the case-control data at these markers. The "Structure" approach adjusts for population stratification by estimating allele frequencies of each sub-population within the data and ancestry of the alleles. However, the method requires *a priori* classification of individuals into sub-populations. The "Eigenstrat" approach is based on principal components analysis involving explicit modeling of ancestry differences between cases and controls along continuous axes of variation. The resulting correction is specific to a candidate marker's variation in frequency across ancestral populations.

Circumventing the Problem of Population Stratification

An alternative to population-based case-control studies that circumvents the problem of population stratification is the family-based tests for association. The simplest of these tests is the Transmission Disequilibrium Test or TDT (Spielman et al, 1993) that examines whether there is a preferential transmission of a specific marker allele from a heterozygous parent to an affected offspring. The data required for such analyses are trios comprising a pair of parents of whom at least one is heterozygous at a biallelic marker locus and an affected offspring. The method tests whether the two marker alleles have been transmitted in equal proportions from the heterozygous parents using a chi-squares statistic. In the presence of linkage and association between the marker locus and the disease locus, there will be a preferential transmission of one of the marker alleles from heterozygous parents to affected offspring. For example, suppose we have collected data on 100 trios in which exactly one parent is heterozygous at a marker locus with alleles M and m. Thus, the TDT will compare the frequencies of transmissions of M and m from the 100 heterozygous parents. Suppose the frequencies of transmissions of M and m from these parents are 60 and 40, respectively. Then, the value of the TDT statistic is $(60-40)^2 / (60+40) = 4$, which has a p-value of 0.045 indicating a bias in the transmission pattern of the two alleles from heterozygous parents to affected offspring. Since these tests do not involve estimation of allele frequencies and are conditional on parental genotypes, they are protected

Table 34.3: Genotypic and allelic distributions for two genetically heterogeneous subpopulations within the population presented in Table 34.2

	Subpopulation 1				
	Genotypes			Alleles	
	AA	Aa	aa	A	a
Cases	560	160	80	1280	320
Controls	140	40	20	320	80
	Subpopulation 2				
	Genotypes			Alleles	
	AA	Aa	aa	A	a
Cases	40	80	280	160	640
Controls	100	200	700	400	1600

against population stratification. In other words, when the investigator is unsure whether the case and control samples are derived from a genetically homogeneous population, it is preferable to collect data on trios and carry out a transmission-disequilibrium test, to guard oneself against drawing false inferences.

SAMPLE SIZE AND STATISTICAL POWER

Unless the sample size is adequate, there may not be sufficient statistical power to detect the association of genotypes/alleles/haplotypes on disease (affection) status. Inadequate sample size, with inadequate statistical power to test the null hypothesis of association, can result in a false inference. Therefore, during the design of an association study, it is important to assess what should be the sample size for detecting an association of a given strength for preassigned values of the level of significance and statistical power. This is not an easy task, since it requires considerable prior information. Usually power of the statistical test for association depends on several factors such as the genotype/allele frequencies at the locus under consideration among groups of affected and unaffected individuals, the strength of association (usually expressed as relative risk, RR) that is to be detected and the statistical power that is desired by the investigator for a fixed level of significance (usually held fixed at 0.05). It can be algebraically shown that for any test usually the power increases with the increase in sample size and vice versa.

For purposes of illustration, we consider a simple scenario. Consider a disease that is determined by a single one autosomal locus with two alleles at which genotypes have been determined for a number of affected individuals and an equal number of unaffected individuals. Under this scenario, the sample size (n) for each group is calculated using the following formula:

$$n \text{ (each group)} = \frac{(p_0 q_0 + p_1 q_1)(z_{1-\alpha/2} + z_{1-\beta})^2}{(p_1 - p_0)^2}$$

where,

p_0 = proportion of genotype among unaffected individuals (controls)

p_1 = proportion of genotype among affected individuals (cases) = $p_0 \times RR$, where RR = Relative Risk = p_1/p_0, $q_1 = 1 - p_1$, $q_0 = 1 - p_0$

$z_{1-\alpha/2}$ = value of the standard Normal [N(0,1)] distribution corresponding to the level of significance, α; which equals 1.96 at $\alpha=0.05$ (for a two-sided test)

$z_{1-\beta}$ = value of the standard Normal [N(0,1)] distribution corresponding to the desired value of statistical power; which equals 0.84 for a power of 80%

Consider the following example:

Suppose, $p_0 = 10\%$, RR = 1.8, $p_1 = (p_0)(RR) = (0.10)(1.8) = 0.18$. Hence,

$q_1 = 1 - p_1 = 1 - 0.18 = 0.82$

$q_0 = 1 - p_0 = 1 - 0.10 = 0.90$

$z_{1-\alpha/2} = 1.96$ (corresponding to a two-sided test at level $\alpha = 0.05$)

$z_{1-\beta} = 0.84$ (corresponding to a power of 80%).

Then, the sample size n (for each group, case and control) is calculated as:

$$n = \frac{[(0.1)(0.9) + (0.18)(0.82)][1.96 + 0.84]^2}{(0.18 - 0.10)^2}$$

$$= \frac{(0.2376)(7.84)}{0.0064} = 291.06 = 291 \text{ (approx.)}$$

For the above values of p_0 (=0.10), α (=0.05) and power (=0.80), one can compute sample size requirements for different values of RR, as in Table 34.4.

From the above equation, it is also easy to see that the statistical power can be calculated for a given sample size (n) for plausible values of p_0, α and RR. The above formula will require slight modifications when there are multiple alleles. It is expected that the statistical power of the proposed sample size be calculated for plausible values of the genotype frequency (p_0) among non-responders and for clinically-relevant values of the relative risk (RR). Alternatively, the sample size requirement to attain a reasonable statistical power (say, 80%) may be calculated. Plausible values of genotype frequencies may be obtained from pilot studies or from the literature, if available.

Table 34.4: Sample size requirement for a case-control study for various values of Relative Risk (RR) for genotype frequency of 10% among controls, level of significance of 5% and statistical power of 80%

Postulated RR	Required sample size (n) per group
1.2	3834
1.3	1769
1.5	682
1.8	291
2.0	196
2.5	97
3.0	59

However, in linkage study the mathematical formula for calculating power corresponding to a statistical test for linkage is very complicated and cannot be written in a compact form. Hence, the only way to calculate the power in such cases is to simulate data under the scenario guided by plausible alternative hypotheses. Here the power depends on the family structure, allele frequency, prevalence, and several other parameters. It also depends on the disease models considered if parametric linkage methods are to be used. There are some software packages that can be used to calculate the power using simulation methods (Ott, 1989). Basically the computer programs simulate a large number of possible sets of marker data for each family of the same structure as an observed family, with user-specified values of the number of alleles, their frequencies, and the recombination fraction between the disease and marker loci, and calculate the lod-score. From the set of values of the lod-scores thus obtained from a large number of simulation runs, the empirical probability that lod-score will exceed 3 (or any other specified value) can be obtained and, thus, these simulation results can be used to evaluate the overall power of the study. From this value of the empirical power one can calculate the sample size required to get a high enough value of power. The most popular software packages for this purpose are SIMLINK (Boehnke and Ploughman, 1997) and FastSLINK (Weeks, Ott and Lathrop, 1990) [See section 6.2 for web site addresses of these software packages].

SOME PUBLIC-DOMAIN SOFTWARE RESOURCES

Many of the methods described above cannot be used without the help of computers. Various software packages have been developed for these analyses. We list some of the popular software packages below that are available freely in the public-domain. We also list a package (PLINK) for analyzing from a genome-wide scan, although we have not described specifics of the methodologies for analyzing such data. References can be found in the user manual of this package.

LINKAGE ANALYSIS IN PEDIGREES

Linkage

- *web/ftp*: ftp://linkage.rockefeller.edu/software linkage
- *Operating systems:* MS-DOS, OS2, UNIX, VMS

Merlin

- *web/ftp:* http://www.sph.umich.edu/csg/abecasis/Merlin
  http://www.sph.umich.edu/csg/abecasis/Merlin/download
- *Operating systems:* UNIX. LINUX

Genehunter

- *web/ftp:* http://www.broad.mit.edu/ftp/distribution/software/genehunter/ *Operating systems:* UNIX]

Sample-size Determination for Linkage Analysis Using Simulation

- SIMLINK: http://csg.sph.umich.edu/boehnke/simlink.php
- FastSLINK: http://watson.hgen.pitt.edu/register/soft_doc.html

Test for Association/Linkage between Disease Phenotypes and Haplotypes by Utilizing Family-based Controls

- FBAT
- *web/ftp:* http://www.biostat.harvard.edu/~fbat/fbat.htm
- *Operating systems:* UNIX, Solaris, Linux, MS-Windows, Mac (MacOS X/Darwin)

Population Substructure Analysis

Eigensoft/Eigenstrat

- *web/ftp:* http://genepath.med.harvard.edu/~reich/EIGENSTRAT.htm; *Operating systems:* Linux]

Structure

- *web/ftp*: http://pritch.bsd.uchicago.edu/software.html
- *Operating systems:* MS-DOS, MS-Windows, UNIX(Solaris), Linux]

Transmission Disequilibrium Test and Sib Transmission Disequilibrium Test

- TDT/S-TDT
- *web/ftp:* http://genomics.med.upenn.edu/spielman/TDT.htm
  Operating systems: MS-Windows (95/NT)

Whole-genome Association Analysis Toolset

PLINK [web/ftp: http://pngu.mgh.harvard.edu/purcell/plink/]

BIBLIOGRAPHY

1. Boehnke, M., Ploughman, LM. SIMLINK. A Program for Estimating the Power of a Proposed Linkage Study by Computer Simulation. Version 4.12, 1997.
2. Chotai J. On the lod score method in linkage analysis. Ann Hum Genet 1984;48:359-78.
3. Devlin B, Roeder K, Wasserman L. Genomic control, a new approach to genetic-based association studies. Theor Popul Biol 2001;60:155-66.
4. Elston RC, Stewart J. A general model for the genetic analysis of pedigree data. Hum Hered 1971;21:523-42.
5. Fisher RA. On the mathematical foundations of theoretical statistics. Philos Trans Roy Soc London Ser. A 1922;222:309-68.
6. Morton NE. Sequential tests for the detection of linkage. Am J Hum Genet 1955;7: 277-318.
7. Ott J. Computer-simulation methods in human linkage analysis. Proc. Natl. Acad Sci USA 1989;86:4175-78.
8. Ott J. Analysis of Human Genetic Linkage. The John Hopkins University Press, Baltimore, 1999.
9. Price AL, Patterson NJ, Plenge RM, Weinblatt ME, Shadick NA, Reich D. Principal components analysis corrects for stratification in genome-wide association studies. Nat Genet 2006;38:904-09.
10. Pritchard JK, Stephens M, Rosenberg NA, Donnelly P. Association in structured populations. Am J Hum Genet 2000;67:170-81.
11. Spielman RS, McGinnis RE, Ewens WJ. Transmission test for linkage disequilibrium: the insulin gene region and insulin-dependent diabetes mellitus (IDDM). Am J Hum Genet 1993;52:506-16.
12. Thomas DC. Statistical Methods in Genetic Epidemiology. Oxford University Press, Oxford, 2004.
13. Weeks DE, Ott J, Lathrop GM. SLINK. A general simulation program for linkage analysis. Am J Hum Genet 1990;47:A204.

Index

A

Abacavir 334
Accessing information from external source 131
Acquired immune deficiency syndrome (AIDS) 305
Acridine orange 175
Activation receptors 6
Acute
    anterior uveitis 259
    antibody mediated rejection 510
Adaptive
    immune system 19
    immunity 11
Additional
    crossmatch techniques 503
    disease predisposing genes besides HLA 270
    features of MHC genes and molecules 72
    reading 76
Adiponectin gene 246
Affected sib-pairs 205
AG processing in class I pathway 93
Age-related macular degeneration 150
AIDS-associated HLA alleles target distinct intervals of disease course 297
Air-borne environmental mycobacteria 365
Airway hyper responsiveness 27
Allele
    frequency database 123
    sharing methods 570
Alloantisera 175
Allopurinol 340
Alloreactivity on outcome 529
Allorecognition by
    B lymphocytes 465
    CD4 positive T cells 467
    CD8 positive cells 466
    NK cells 468
Alpha fetoprotein 450
Alternative
    allogeneic donors 485
    pathway of complement activation 10

Alzheimer's disease 10
Amino acid 87
Amplification of
    TH17 cells 29
    TR1 cells 35
Ancestral haplotypes 146, 323
Andrenocorticotrophic hormone 71
Antenatal HLA testing 452
Anthony Nolan
    bone marrow trust 453
    trust 453
Antibodies to other antigens 221
Antibody-dependent cell-mediated cytotoxicity 5, 16
Anticardiolipin antibodies 436
Anti-cyclic citrullinated antibodies 276
Antigen
    presenting cells 17, 75, 86, 425
    processing machinery molecules in human cancers 69
    recognition in T-cell immunity 98
Antinuclear antibody 436
Antiphospholipid antibodies 436
Antiviral factor 315
Arlequin 133
Aromatic amine anticonvulsants 340
Arthritis 282
Asian Indian donor marrow registry 460
Aspirin therapy 440
Assay design 180
Attenuation of TH17 responses 33
Atypical hemolytic uremic syndrome 150
Autoantibodies 220
Autoimmune disease 416, 147

B

B cell
    antigen receptor 15
    development 14
    effector functions 15
    signaling 15, 16
B lymphocytes 14, 18
Bacille Calmette-Buérin (BCG) 365
Beçhet's disease 107

Bone marrow 3
    donors
        program in Singapore 456
        worldwide 133
    transplantation 49
Borderline
    lepromatous 389
    tuberculoid 389
Brain 3

C

C. aethiops 167
C4 genes 78
Caboxypeptidase 221
Campylobacter 271
Candida albicans 32, 313
Candidate gene studies 374
Captain of death 387
Carbamazepine 340
Carboxyfluoroscein diacetate 175
Cardiovascular diseases 148
Catechol-O-methyltransferase 359
Catholic hematopoietic stem cell bank 456
CDNA
    amplification 162
    sequencing 162
Cellular
    adoptive immunotherapy 550
    markers of T1D 221
Center for HIV-AIDS vaccine immunology 326
Cercopithecinae 167, 169
Cercopithecinae subfamily 167
Cervical adenitis 365
Chemiluminescent detection 160
Chemokines 3, 309
Chlamydia 259
Chromosomal region 400
Chronic antibody mediated rejection 511
Circumventing problem of population stratification 572
Classical pathway of complement activation 10

Clinical
　application of minor histocompatibility antigens 548
　description of ankylosing spondylitis 259
　implications of
　　TNF 70
　　variable KIR-HLA interactions 414
Clonal expression of KIR receptors 412
Clustal X 133
Codominant expression and recombination 74
Cohort study 322
Collagen-induced arthritis 30, 280
Colony forming units 481
Color development for alkaline phosphatase 161
Common lymphoid
　precursor 15
　progenitors 11
Comparative genomics 350, 361
Comparative genomics in
　coding regions 354
　non-coding regions 359
Comparative genomics might uncover susceptibility genes for human diseases 360
Complement
　activation 512
　binding 499
　component
　　C2 137
　　C4 142
　dependant
　　cytotoxicity 480
　　lymphomicrocytotoxicity test 175
　factor B 140
　genes in central region of MHC 135
Complementarity determining regions 89, 104
Computer programs for development of SBT for HLA 188
Concept of IBD 570
Conclusions on
　differential immunogenicity of HLA mismatch 468
　HLA-G evolution 169
Congenital adrenal hyperplasia 71
Conserved extended haplotypes 146
Convergence of immunoendocrine pathways 434
Coronavirus 313
C-reactive protein 10
Crohn's disease 259, 271, 372
Crossmatch conversion 504

Cycle sequencing 189
Cynomolgous monkey 167
Cytokines 3, 19
Cytoplasm 82
Cytotoxic T
　cells 93
　lymphocyte 229
　　associated antigen-4 gene 229
Czech national marrow donors registry 559

D

Data from haploidentical transplants 529
DBMHC anthropology 133
Deficiency of complement
　component
　　C2 138
　　C4 144
　factor B 141
Dendritic cells 3, 4, 19, 313, 391
Dengue virus 313
Deoxyribonucleic acid 387
Detection of
　allelism 160
　class 2 antibodies 500
Development of T cells in thymus 11
Dideoxynucleotides 188
Different cytokines 5
Differentiation of
　TH17 cells 28
　TH2 cells 25
　TR1 cells 34
Digestion 161
Direct
　allorecognition 467
　reprogramming of adult cells 450
Discovery of
　first HLA antigens 44
　histocompatibility antigen II and H-2 complex 43
　HLA-B27 259
　TH17 cells 28
Disease
　burden 387
　free survival 455
　heterogeneity 271
　progression 391
Dithiothreitol 501
Diversity region 15
DNA
　based methods 177
　sequencing 189
Donor
　bone marrow 455

　health 562
　recruitment manager 557
　selection strategies 449
DP subregion 67
DQ subregion 67
DR subregion 66
Drug
　hypersensitivity syndromes 332
　induced liver disease 341
DSA monitoring 511
Duffy antigen receptor for chemokines 313
Dyes to assess degree of cytotoxicity 501

E

Early experimental allotransplantations 42
Ebola virus 313
Effect of
　HLA interaction with KIR on AIDS progression 299
　individual HLA alleles on AIDS progression 293
　mismatches 474
　total number of HLA mismatches 476
　HLA antibody ligation on airway epithelial cells 515
Eigensoft 574
Eigenstrat 574
ELISA-based crossmatching 503
Embryonic stem cells 450
Emulsion PCR technology 561
Endoplasmic reticulum 93
Enzyme-linked immunosorbent assay 140
Epitopes 176
European Bioinformatics Institute 81
Evaluation of selective pressure on coding regions 352
Evolution 164
Evolving role of HLA-E and HLA-F 431
Exon-intron organization of KIR genes 410
Experimental
　approaches in genetic studies 367
　model of arthritis 280

F

Fetomaternal interface 434
　immunomodulation 429
Fibroblast growth factor receptor 515
Ficoll gradient centrifugation 176
Finding suitable HSC donor 484

Flow cytometry 503
Flucloxacillin 341

G

Gene of complement
    component C2 and its regulation 138
    factor B and its regulation 141
Genehunter 574
Generation of new alleles 120
Genes 376
    influencing viral entry 309
    involved in anti-HIV immune response 314
Genetic
    architecture of mycobacterial diseases 365
    basis for minor H antigen polymorphisms 544
    contribution to immune response 392
    determinants of type 1 diabetes 219
    module of complement component C4 and its regulation 143
    polymorphisms in pro- and anti-inflammatory cytokines 323
    spectrum of human infectious diseases 369
    structure 61
Genetics of type
    1 diabetes 205
    2 diabetes 241
Genome
    screens 399
    wide association studies 209, 241
Genomic minor H antigen typing 546
Genotype-phenotype association studies 368
Glutamic acid decarboxylase 208, 220
Graft-versus
    host disease 49
    leukemia 477
    tumor effect 415
GWA studies for T2D genes 248

H

H. influenzae 148
Haplotype 47, 73
    data 126
    matching 479
    segregation in families 74
Heart 502
    transplantation 496
Heat shock 398
    proteins 425

Helicobacter pylori 313
Hematopoietic
    cells 5
    growth factors 3
    stem 449
        cell 15, 471
        cell transplantation 49, 415, 449, 500, 525
Hemolytic uremic syndrome 150
Heparin therapy 440
Hepatitis C virus 313
Herpes simplex virus 339
HFE gene 65
Highly exposed persistently seronegative 322
Histocompatibility 43
    locus 2 43
History of HLA 42
HLA and
    disease 121
        associations 104
    drug
        hypersensitivity 318
        reactions 332
    HIV mimicry 319
    spondyloarthropathies 259
    T1D autoantibodies 208
    transplantation 121
    vaccination 122
HLA antibody induced
    cytokine production 513
    endothelial cell
        exocytosis 514
        proliferation 515
        survival 518
HLA
    architecture of HIV disease pathogenesis 292
    association studies in mycobacterial diseases 394
    B27
        disease association 260
        homozygosity and disease association 260
        positive versus negative disease 262
        prevalence 261
    C influences AIDS progression through interaction with KIR 300
    class 1
        associations 319
        peptide-binding motifs 89
        region genes 61
        structure 86

class 2
    antibodies 502
    associations 321
    polymorphism and AIDS progression 297
    region genes 66
    structure and nature of bound peptides 95
class 3 region genes 69
complex 44, 205
E 76, 159, 161, 163, 164
F 64, 159, 162, 163
G 63, 159, 162-164, 168
gene organization and structure 61
heterozygous advantage 315
identical sibling 452
    donors 484
KIR interactions modulate NK cell responses 318
matched stem cell bank 451
matching and organ transplantation 492
maternal
    fetal sharing 427
    paternal/couple sharing 427
molecules 86
nomenclature 79
    committee 46
polymorphism and nomenclature 96
SBT and importance of quality control 194
sensitization and matching effect 494
sharing and virus transmission 315
supertypes 322
system 425
transgenic mice 281
typing technologies 175
Host genetic
    determinants 387
    HIV-1/AIDS infection 305
    underlies disease susceptibility 365
Host immune response to mycobacterial infections 391
Human
    chorionic gonadotrophin 450
    cytotoxic T cells 53
    diseases 365
    diversity in KIR-HLA compound genotypes 413
    dopamine receptor D2 gene 359
    health and disease 350
    immunodeficiency virus 305
    immunology 97
    leukocyte antigen 61, 170, 276, 374, 449

major histocompatibility complex 61
TH17 cells 29
Hybridization 160, 161
Hypotheses to explain pathogenic role of HLA-B27 269

I

Ideal donor 452
Identification of
    chromosomal regions carrying major susceptibility genes 372
    HLA identical sibling donor 472
    permissible epitope mismatches 477
Immune
    epitope database 133
    response 52
        genes 219
    system 3, 163
Immunobiological function of HLA class I and II antigens 52
Immunobiology of human minor H antigens 544
Immunogenetic 97
    databases 119
    mechanisms of celiac disease 254
Immunogenetics of rheumatoid arthritis 276
Immunoreceptor tyrosine-based inhibitory motif 6
Implications of GWA studies 248
Importance of HLA
    antibodies 480
    DP mismatches 476
    matching in UCB transplantation 482
Inadequate donor pool 460
Indeterminate leprosy 389
Indirect allorecognition 467
Infections 148
Inflammatory
    bowl disease 24
    diseases 163
Influence of NK cell alloreactivity 525
Initiation of bone marrow registries 453
Innate
    immune system 19
    immunity 3
Insulin
    autoantibodies 220
    receptor substrate-2 gene 246
Insulinoma-associated protein 2 220
Interaction codons 101
Interaction of class II molecules in arthritis 286
Interferon-gamma 398
Interleukin
    1RA 398
    2 receptor 210
International histocompatibility workshops (IHWSs) 45, 50, 477
Intravenous immunoglobulin infusion therapy 439
Introduction to immune system 1
Isotypes of complement component C4 142

J

Joint United Nations Program 305

K

Killer
    activating receptor associated protein 6
    cell immunoglobulin receptors 6
    inhibitory receptors 375
KIR
    genomic organization 408
    HLA in infection 415
    receptors 122, 525
Klebsiella pneumoniae 271, 313
Korean marrow donor program 456

L

Laboratory services 558
Lectin pathway 10, 136
Leishmania 23, 24
Ligand for KIR receptors 412
Listeria monocytogens 21
Liver 3, 503
    transplantation 496
LOD-score method 568
Logarithm of odds 209
Luminex
    crossmatch 504
    high definition beads 561
Lung 3, 503
Lupus anticoagulant 436
Lymph nodes 3
Lymphocyte choriomeningitis virus 53
Lymphoid tissues 3

M

M. avium 365
M. chelonae 365
M. fascicularis 167
M. flavescens 365
M. fortuitum 371
M. intracellulare 365
M. malmoense 365
M. marinum 365
M. mulatta 167
M. paratuberculosis 372
M. smegmatis 365
M. ulcerans 365
Macrophages 3
Magnetic beads 177
Major
    histocompatibility complex 43, 48, 52, 56, 61, 136, 119, 223, 315, 376, 425, 449
    immune response complex 56
    system of leukocyte antigens 79
Management of RSA 437
Mannan binding lectin 437
Map of MHC and genomic structure 76
Matched unrelated donor 455
Maturity-onset diabetes of young 241, 242
Maxam-Gilbert method 188
Measles 313
Mechanisms of minor H antigenic T-cell epitope generation 545
Membrane
    attack complex 10, 11, 136
    proteins 5
Mendelian susceptibility to mycobacterial diseases 370
Method for
    HLA antibody screening 498
    HLA typing 189
    isolating lymphocytes 176
Methods to
    safeguard against population stratification 572
    study influence of genes on human disease 393
MHC and
    non-MHC genes in tuberculosis and leprosy 386
    rheumatoid arthritis 276
MHC class 1
    chain related gene 226
    peptides 90
MHC
    class 2 molecules 94
    haplotypes 323
Minor H antigen population diversity 546
Minor H antigens in
    biology 547
    medicine 547, 551
    pregnancy 551

solid organ transplantation 550
    stem cell transplantation 547
Minor histocompatibility antigens in biology and medicine 544
Miscarriage 424
Mixed lymphocyte culture 46, 80
Model of
    alloreactivity 526
    NK cell development 5
    rheumatoid arthritis 280
    study genetic aspects of T1D 221
Molecules 96
Monocyte specific antibodies 502
Monogenic diabetes 242
Multiple genes control HIV-1/AIDS 308
Murine leukemia virus 315
Mycobacteria 23, 24
Mycobacterial
    infections 400
    pathogens 365
Mycobacterium
    africanum 365
    bovis 365
    leprae 392
    tuberculosis 313, 365

N

N. brasiliensis 26, 27
N. meningitidis 148
National Marrow Donor Program 131, 555
Natural
    killer cells 3, 18, 53, 406, 407
    resistance 307, 374
Neonatal diabetes 243
Neuraminidase treated sheep erythrocytes 176
Nevirapine 338
Next generation sequencing 184
    technologies 188
Nippostrongylus brasiliensis 27
NK
    alloreactivity 525, 528
    cell licensing 412
    receptors 6
NKG2
    family receptors 6
    ligand 7
NKT cells 7
Nomenclature 72
Non-classical
    class 1 genes 62
    HLA 319
Non-complement binding 499
Non-genetic triggers 271

Non-HLA
    genes in mycobacterial infections 396
    genetic associations 280
    loci 561
    T1D susceptibility genes 209
Non-MHC
    genetic contribution 270
    mediators of RSA 436
Nonrandom codon usage 358
Non-syncitium inducing 309
Normal pregnancy 424
Nucleotide
    polymorphism of KIR genes 411
    substitution rate 357, 358
Nylon wool columns 176

O

Old world primates 167
Oligonucleotide labelling 160
Options for high resolution typing 561
Organ
    donors 491
    transplantation 510
Overview of genotype-phenotype association studies 368

P

Paired kidney exchange 492
Partially matched donor 452
Paternal lymphocyte alloimmunization therapy 437
Pathogenesis of mycobacterial infections 387
PCR
    based methods 177
    single strand conformation polymorphism 179
Peptide
    hypothesis 269
    presenting molecule 168
Peripheral blood transplantation 455
Peritoneum 3
Permissible HLA-DP mismatches 477
Peyers' patches 3
Physiological functions of activating receptors 7
Planned immunization 259
Plasma cell glycoprotein PC-1 gene 245
Plasmodium
    falciparum 351
    vivax 309
Pneumocystis carinii 32
Polygenic type 2 diabetes 244
Polymerase chain reaction 73, 160, 175, 177

Polymorphism 72, 162
Polymorphism in
    humans 168
    pongidae 168
Polymorphism of HLA-B27 264
Population
    demographic data 124
    stratification 571
    studies 120
    substructure analysis 574
Post-transplant antibody monitoring and associated mechanisms 510
Pregnancy 164
Prehybridization 161
Principles of
    CDC crossmatch 500
    dye terminator cycle sequencing 180
Production of non-HLA antibodies 520
Proteasomes 77
Protects against AIDS progression 299
Protein tyrosine kinase 6
Pseudogenes 64
Pulmonary
    surfactant proteins 398
    tuberculosis 399
Purified protein derivative 374

R

Race 561
Rare alleles 129
Recipient race 495
Recombinase activation gene 15
Recurrent spontaneous abortions 424
Reference strand conformational analysis 177
Regional differences in transplantation activity 455
Relevance of
    HLA matching 495
    polymorphism in TNF gene 70
Renal transplantation 501
Restriction fragment length polymorphism 175, 177
Reverse transcription 162
Rheumatoid
    arthritis 276, 277
    factor 276
RNA extraction 162
Role of
    antibody ablation technology 504
    autoantibodies 436
    dendritic cells 5
    HLA
        antibodies in accommodation 518
        in normal pregnancy 426

matching in unrelated HSCT 474
typing in hematopoietic stem cell transplantation 471
International Histocompatibility Workshops 50
non-classical HLA antigens in pregnancy 424
rare HLA alleles 317
shared epitope in arthritis 284
toll-like receptors 401

S

S. pneumoniae 148
Salmonella 271
Sample size and statistical power 573
Schistosoma mansoni 27
Selected non-HLA candidate gene studies 377
Selection of
   donor CB unit 483
   family donors 471
   HLA alleles 120
Separation of lymphocytes 500
Sequence
   analysis software requirements for HLA SB 190
   based typing 175, 187
Sequence specific
   hybridization technique 73
   oligohybridization 175, 178
   primer amplification 175
Sequencing based typing 180, 561
Serology 175
Several loci in HLA chromosomal region 46
Shared epitope and autoantibodies 279
Shigella 271
Shistosoma mansoni 313
Sib transmission disequilibrium test 574
Single
   HLA antigen mismatched donors 485
   nucleotide polymorphisms 244
   specific oligonucleotide typing 160
   strand conformation polymorphism 175
Slot blotting 160
Solid
   organ transplantation 415, 495
   phase HLA antibody detection methods 498
Sources of hematopoietic stem cells 450
Spleen 3
Spondylitis 259
Spondyloarthropathies 259
Spontaneous
   abortion 424
   controllers 307
Stain dead cells 175
Staphylococcus aureus 341
Stem cell transplantation in Asian region 456
Step. pneumonia 10
Stevens-Johnson syndrome 339
Stromal cell derived factor 312
Structure of
   HLA 53
   registries 556
Studies analyzing
   ligand incompatibility model 531
   missing ligand model 534
Studies finding evidence supporting missing ligand model 534
Syndromes of drug toxicity and HLA 332
Systemic
   disease 365
   lupus erythematosus 24, 72

T

T cell
   development 11
   effector functions 12
   receptor 53, 406
   signaling 11
   subsets 19
T gondii 24, 33
T lymphocytes 11, 18
Tapasin 68, 77
Test for linkage 568, 570
T_H1 cells and
   autoimmunity 24
   immune responses 20
   infection 23
T_H1 specific transcription factors 23
T_H17 cells and
   autoimmunity 31
   immune responses 28
T_H17 responses and
   infection 32
   transcription factors 31
T_H2 cells and
   immune responses 25
   infections 27
   transcription factors 26
Thai Red Cross Society 457
Third party donor cell immunization 440
Thrifty genotype 352
Thymus 3
Tissue antigens 48, 97
Toll-like receptor 19, 354, 391, 401
Total nucleated count 481
Toxic epidermal necrolysis 339
Toxoplasma 23, 24
Transmission disequilibrium test 574
Transplant activity 555
Trichinella spiralis 27
Trophoblast membrane infusion 439
Tryptophan 141
Tuberculosis 387
Tumor 163
   immunotherapy 416
   necrosis factor 69, 70, 122, 226, 397
   rejection antigen 450
Type 1 diabetes 219
Type 2 diabetes 241

U

Ulcerative colitis 259
Uniparental disomy 450
Unique diversity of HLA in Indian population 458
Unrelated
   donor searches 454
   marrow donor registries 555
Urgency of requests 561
Use of
   cord blood units 481
   one haplotype matched family donors 473
   unrelated donor umbilical cord blood transplantation 481

V

Vaccination 550
Variable number of tandem repeats 139, 227
Variations of complement
   component C2 139
   factor B 141
Variations on CDC test 501
Viral infections 163
Virtual crossmatch 504

W

Washing 160, 161
Whole-genome association analysis toolset 575
World marrow donor association 454-456

X

Ximelagatran 341

Y

Yersinia 271